Ben Cao Gang Mu Dictionary

Volume One

The publisher gratefully acknowledges the generous support of the
Joan Palevsky Literature in Translation Endowment Fund
of the University of California Press Foundation.

Ben Cao Gang Mu Dictionary

Volume One

Chinese Historical Illness Terminology

Zhang Zhibin and Paul U. Unschuld

A Volume of the
Ben Cao Gang Mu Dictionary Project

Paul U. Unschuld, General Editor

University of California Press

University of California Press, one of the most distinguished university presses in the United States, enriches lives around the world by advancing scholarship in the humanities, social sciences, and natural sciences. Its activities are supported by the UC Press Foundation and by philanthropic contributions from individuals and institutions.
For more information, visit: www.ucpress.edu.

University of California Press
Oakland, California

Library of Congress Cataloging-in-Publication Data

Ben cao gang mu dictionary / edited by Zhang Zhibin, Paul U. Unschuld.
volumes cm
Includes bibliographical references.
Contents: volume 1. Chinese historical illness terminology
ISBN 978-0-520-28395-4 (cloth : alk. paper) -- ISBN 0-520-28395-3 (cloth : alk. paper)
1. Li, Shizhen, 1518-1593. Ben cao gang mu. 2. Medicine, Chinese--History--16th century. 3. Medicine, Chinese--Dictionaries. 4. Materia medica, Vegetable--China. I. Zhang, Zhibin, 1953- editor. II. Unschuld, Paul U. (Paul Ulrich), 1943- editor. III. Title: Dictionary of the Ben cao gang mu.

RS180.C5B45 2015
615.3'210951--dc23

2014018742

Manufactured in the United States

19 18 17 16 15 14 13 12 11 10

10 9 8 7 6 5 4 3 2 1

The paper used in this publication meets the minimum requirements of ANSI/NISO Z39.48-1992 (R 1997) (Permanence of Paper).

CONTENTS

Acknowledgments

The research leading to the preparation of this volume of the *Ben cao gang mu Dictionary* was financed by Stiftung Volkswagenwerk. The institutional framework enabling us to pursue this project was the Horst-Goertz-Stiftungsinstitut, Charité-Universitätsmedizin Berlin, funded by the Horst-Goertz-Foundation from 2006 through 2013. Martin Huber, Klaus Neugebauer and David Dornier generously provided us with additional support to continue our work into 2014 and complete the compilation of this volume. Prof. Zhang Zhibin of the Research Institute for the History of Medicine and Medical Literature of the China Academy of Chinese Medical Sciences in Beijing laid the foundations to the present volume by researching and documenting all Chinese data required. The authors of and contributors to the other volumes of this project, Zheng Jinsheng, Paul D. Buell, Nalini Kirk, and Ulrike Unschuld all participated in countless sessions to jointly discuss and possibly solve difficult issues. Siglinde Mooney assisted in technical matters. Christine Hu gave the manuscript its final layout. We are most grateful to all these individuals and institutions for their belief in this project and their conceptual as well as financial support.

I. INTRODUCTION

1. The Ben cao gang mu Project

This is the first volume of a project aimed at providing better access to the *Ben cao gang mu* (*BCGM*) 本草綱目, China's great encyclopedia of pharmaceutical lore, first published in 1598 and designated a world cultural heritage in 2012. In addition to the current volume, which focuses on identification and explanation of the occurrence and meaning of approximately 4,500 illness terms in the *BCGM*, three additional volumes will complete the *Ben cao gang mu Dictionary*. They include a second volume dedicated to verifying and localizing geographical designations and a third identifying all book titles and authors named in the *BCGM*. A fourth volume will offer a historical survey of the identifications of all pharmaceutical substances mentioned in the *BCGM*.

The illness terminology encountered in the *BCGM* reflects Chinese observations and theorization of more than 1,500 years. The terms employed often fail to overlap with modern biomedical terminology. Their correct translation and interpretation, based on an application of historical and philological principles, are preconditions for a meaningful reading of the pharmaceutical and therapeutic data gathered not only in the *BCGM* but also in countless other premodern works using the same terminology. While the *BCGM* is a huge repository of Chinese historical illness terminology, it cannot be said to reflect the entirety of premodern illness terms. The *BCGM* is first of all a pharmaceutical encyclopedia. The illness terms encountered in the text are those used in pharmaceutical treatments. Also, for the most part the *BCGM* quotes from earlier printed sources. That is, it documents local folk-medical usages less often. The same applies to illness terms restricted to acupuncture. Since Chinese pharmaceutical treatment has played a significant role in apotropaic therapies cherished by large parts of the Chinese population of all social strata up to the present day, illness terms associated with demon possession and requests for exorcistic treatments are well represented in the *BCGM*.

Of similar importance to users of the *Ben cao gang mu Dictionary* is a correct reading of the geographical designations that the *BCGM* provides in the context of pharmaceutical drug descriptions. As is well known, the history of geographical designations over the two millennia of the Chinese Empire is rather complex. Administrative structures and regions changed again and again. A geographical designation may have been valid for centuries or for a few decades only. For the unprepared reader of the *BCGM* it is often impossible to locate a historical place name, quoted from a source written centuries earlier, and find its current equivalent. The therapeutic value of herbal substances strongly depends on the composition of the soil the herb emerges from, the climate accompanying its growth, and further environmental factors. Hence volume 2 of the *Ben cao gang mu Dictionary* examines all geographical designations found in the *BCGM* and identifies them in today's terms. Again, such information on the *BCGM* has not been available; it will be invaluable for correctly appreciating the drug lore in that encyclopedia.

Volume 3 of the *Ben cao gang mu Dictionary* is devoted to identifying all book titles and their authors in the *BCGM*. The creation of the *BCGM* was directed by Li Shizhen 李時珍 (1518–93), a physician who continued a family tradition of healers after failing to leave the lowly regarded realm of professional medicine and enter the esteemed class of civil servants. Li Shizhen wrote in his retrospective introductory remarks that he had engaged various family members to support him; the true size of his team remains unknown. It is obvious that collaboration between the members of his team lacked strict standardization in citing earlier authors and their texts. Names of authors can have several variants that do not always clearly point to one specific person. Even more confusing are book titles: one book title may appear in four or five different versions, some of which are also used for other books with similar titles. We have traced each quote in the *BCGM* to its source to provide potential users of the encyclopedia with reliable information on titles and authors.

The fourth and final volume of the *Ben cao gang mu Dictionary* offers data on the scientific identification of the approximately two thousand pharmaceutical substances listed in the *BCGM*. The *BCGM* quotes texts from one and a half millennia earlier, and one cannot be sure that an item sold under a specific name in our own time or in the sixteenth century is identical with the one designated by the same name in antiquity, during the Tang or the Song era. However, beginning in the nineteenth century scientists set out to identify and catalogue Chinese herbal substances in terms of modern botanical nomenclature. An examination of animal and mineral substances followed soon afterwards. That is, at least in view of the actual market situation during the past two centuries, a reliable identification is available for most of the pharmaceutical substances recorded in the *BCGM*. More than a few users of the *BCGM* will approach the encyclopedia with an interest in clinical application of its pharmaceutical lore. For them, as well as for historians of medicine and pharmacy, such information is crucial.

The *Ben cao gang mu Dictionary* project owes its conception and realization to an earlier plan to prepare a first annotated English translation of the *BCGM*. The *BCGM* is more than an outstanding example in a long series of materia medica literature written in China over a period of two thousand years. It may be justly called the single most impressive work on medical-pharmaceutical natural history of China's imperial age. Chinese scholars have written and published innumerable medical and pharmaceutical books since the beginnings of a distinct Chinese medicine in the second and first centuries BCE. By preparing translations of the *Huang di nei jing su wen* 黃帝內經素問 (short: *Su wen*) and of the *BCGM* based, for the first time, on a strict application of European philological standards, we meant to provide reliable access to two of the most remarkable literary compendia signaling the beginning and the final culminating period in the development of Chinese medicine as an independent tradition of health care ideas and their clinical application.

The *Su wen* is a compilation of dozens of short texts written during the earlier and later Han dynasties by unknown authors. These persons were influenced by a completely new mode of understanding human life and its integration in the larger dynamics of a natural universe. The contents of the *Su wen* challenged established worldviews accepting the power of gods, ancestors, and demons over the length and quality of human life. The authors of the *Su wen* were the first in China to claim that human life depended on natural laws independent of time, place, and human or numinous beings. In their own time they appear to have occupied a rather marginal position in society. Their names have not been recorded. Their texts survived in a feeble tradition of transmissions. It was only in the twelfth century that they began receiving broader attention among the formally educated elite. Even in the subsequent centuries of the second millennium CE the basic notions of systematic correspondences in nature, idealized in the doctrines of yin-yang and the Five Phases, never penetrated beyond a small upper crust of people in Chinese society.

The *Su wen* is witness to the earliest consolidation of Chinese medical theory in textual form. When during the Tang dynasty the physician Wang Bing 王冰 created the body of text known today as the *Su wen* by adding to a text of approximately sixty thousand characters another large text of approximately thirty thousand characters on the theory of the Five Periods and the Six Qi (*wu yun liu qi* 五運六氣), the latter section too had been transmitted since the Han dynasty. The fact that it was not mentioned in a single bibliographical work further attests to a long-term marginality of the contents of the *Su wen*. Only if we reconstruct the Han era pronunciation of the Wang Bing addenda does it become obvious that these chapters cannot have been written in post-Han times. The mnemonic rhymes make sense only in their Han-era pronunciation. Whether for lack of interest or for other reasons unknown today, the basic tenets of Chinese medical theory as formed in the *Su wen* were neither questioned nor substantially further developed in subsequent centuries. They became the canonized theoretical foundations of acupuncture and thus remained "as is" until the Song-Jin-Yuan period of the thirteenth through the fifteenth centuries, when a short-lived attempt is documented in Chinese pharmaceutical literature to establish a pharmacology of systematic correspondences, that is, an explanatory model of drug effects on the human organism based on the yin-yang and Five Phases doctrines.

The *BCGM* signifies an opposite pole to the *Su wen* and its contribution to a tradition of a secular science of systematic correspondences. The *BCGM* is the apex of what has been the basis of Chinese disease treatment since time immemorial, that is, materia medica and associated pharmaceutical lore. The earliest documentation of a diverse materia medica in China prepared from natural and manmade substances may be found in the so-called Mawangdui manuscripts unearthed from a tomb near Changsha in the province of Hunan in the early 1970s.[1] Throughout the imperial era and up to the sixteenth century, Chinese pharmaceutical knowledge developed continuously and most impressively. The number of natural and manmade substances recognized as therapeutically valuable increased from a few hundred listed in the Mawangdui manuscripts to almost two thousand in the *BCGM*. Authors of recipe literature gathered tens of thousands of formulas—the mainstay of historical Chinese medicine. Pharmaceutical treatment of disease remained free, as indicated above, of Chinese medical theory of systematic correspondences until the emergence of Song Neo-Confucianism generated an intellectual climate stimulating a merger of theory and pharmaceutical clinical practice. However, the inroads of theory into pharmaceutical treatments remained superficial. All available evidence suggests that the use of yin-yang and Five Phases theory in pharmaceutical therapy remained limited to a small number of healers.

When Li Shizhen and his team of unknown size sat down to compile the *BCGM*, they strove to gather information as comprehensive as possible on herbal, animal/human, mineral, and manmade substances used in China for therapeutic purposes. With this goal in mind, the *BCGM* was intended as a receptacle to be filled with data from literature of various genres often written many centuries ago, as well as from numerous contemporary sources found in different geographical regions of the Chinese Empire and beyond. Inevitably, the wide net that was cast to catch all available knowledge brought together a rather heterogeneous array of data expressed in terms that originated in different times and diverse cultural environments. The diversity of origins of the information collected is particularly evident in the naming of illnesses that readers encounter in the almost 1,900 entries devoted in the *BCGM* to pharmaceutical items.

2. The Heterogeneity of Early Illness Terminology

The geographical dimensions of the Chinese Empire were too vast, and its internal cultural diversity was too pronounced, for all those engaged in therapeutic activities to ever agree on one binding homogeneous terminological system that might be called a nomenclature. This is why the terminology of traditional Chinese healing, especially in materia medica and recipe literature, comprises a much larger number of terms denoting disease, malady, and illness than does any national European language.

The naming of illnesses has a long history in Chinese literature. The earliest extensive texts listing numerous therapeutic indications in a medical context are the Mawangdui medical manuscripts from around 200 BCE and the biography of

---

1 D. Harper, *Early Chinese Medical Literature: The Mawangdui Medical Manuscripts* (London: Routledge, 1998).

Chunyu Yi 淳于意 in Sima Qian's 司馬遷 *Shi ji* 史記 a hundred years later.[2] These texts, as well as various nonmedical ones such as the etymological dictionary *Shuo wen jie zi* 說文解字 of 121 CE and the first known materia medica text, the *Shen nong ben cao jing* 神農本草經 of possibly the first century CE, already offer examples of a wide range of types of disease terms. They include historical labels such as *wen nüe* 溫瘧, "warmth *nüe*"—presumably referring to malaria—the meaning of which can be known only from an added listing of illness signs covered by these terms. Then there are descriptive labels such as *han re* 寒熱, "[alternating sensations of] cold and heat," as well as descriptive labels with early pathological theorization, such as *da fu shui zhong* 大腹水腫, "enlarged abdomen, a swelling with water." Some terms are entirely based on etiological theory, such as *zhong feng* 中風, "struck by wind," and *shang han* 傷寒, "harm caused by cold." Others indicate subtle understandings of internal tubular structures and the pathological consequences resulting from their clogging, such as *ju* 疽 and *yong* 癰. Both refer to "impediments" or "obstructions" leading to abscesses, boils, and further ailments. Still others evidence their origin in premedical belief systems such as demonology, as in the case of *zhong'e* 中惡, "struck by the malign." Finally, a term like *huo luan* 霍亂 may simply be the Chinese pronunciation of a term known along the entire Silk Road from Southeast Europe to the Far East to communicate a health problem that may have been encountered all the way along, namely cholera. We find terms similarly suggesting a foreign source in the *Su wen*, whose core contents originate from a period between the second century BCE and the second century CE and from additions later on. Two millennia ago, a term like *fei xiao* 肺消, "lung consumption," was phonetically as close to the ancient Greek term *phthisis* as *huo luan* was to cholera. Tuberculosis may have been equally prevalent along the road as disorders of merchants' and other travelers' digestive tracts.

Ever since, Chinese observers and authors have greatly expanded their vocabulary to describe human illness and ailments. The heterogeneity of this vocabulary has likewise increased over time.

One difficulty in appropriately interpreting and translating ancient Chinese illness terminology has to do with a change in linguistic aesthetics. Whereas the oldest examples of illness terms suggest that one single character was used in literary documents to signify an illness or a disease, at some time compounds of two or more characters appear to have appealed to their users. This means that often enough two different characters with similar meanings were combined. One example is *ji ju* 積聚, "accumulation and collection." No conceptual difference exists between the two elements of this compound. More problematic are compounds ending with the character *feng* 風, "wind," or *qi* 氣, "qi." A compound including the term for "wind" may signify two meanings. First, the illness in question was caused by an intrusion into the organism by wind. This may result in blockages, concretions, pain, and other pathological conditions. However, often enough the character for "wind" is added to signify a changing location of the ailment's manifestation, such as pain or

2 E. Hsu, *Pulse Diagnosis in Early Chinese Medicine: The Telling Touch* (Cambridge: Cambridge University Press, 2010.

concretions, in the human body. Here the concept of "wind"—as something that exists because it moves—is transferred to the movement of an ailment in the body. It is not always easy to immediately distinguish between the two different usages of "wind" in illness terminology.

The problem is even harder to solve when the character *qi* is added to an illness designation. Again, the term may signify some pathological or pathogenic dynamics associated with qi. However, the character *qi* may have been added simply for stylistic reasons to generate a compound rather than use a single-character term. The translation of such terms in this dictionary seeks to recreate in the target language English as close an approximation as possible to the original linguistic style and contents of ancient Chinese illness terminology. Hence, whether *qi* is added for conceptual or simply for stylistic reasons is a matter not to be decided by the translator. The term is added in the English word just as it was added to a core concept in the Chinese original.

3. The Concept of Disease and Symptoms

When, with the appearance of Sima Qian's *Shi ji* around the year 90 BCE or shortly thereafter, intellectuals whose names failed to enter historical records created the medicine of systematic correspondences, this entirely novel understanding of human physiology and pathology rested on conceptual foundations supplied by the yin-yang and Five Phases doctrines. The new approach to coping with physical and mental illness in what was perceived as a social and natural environment of permanent violence was introduced to explain illness in purely theoretical terms and to leave only the description of symptoms to everyday language. Bleeding, sores, cough, loss of hair, infertility, menstrual cramps, vomiting, fever, and countless other ailments were supposed to be associated with irregularities in the flow of qi and blood in the human organism. These irregularities in turn were supposed to be linked to irregularities in the constant dynamics of domination and revenge in the coexistence of yin and yang factors, or a failing adaptation of the human organism to the natural course of the Five Phases, equally understood to be constantly engaged in mutual overcoming and generation.

That is, during the closing centuries of the first millennium BCE, Chinese medical intellectuals undertook a most decisive conceptual step in their understanding of bodily and mental suffering that eventually led to a distinction between what in modern terminology might be called a disease and its symptoms. Disease is a theoretical construct. Symptoms are its manifestations. The new medicine went beyond the approach of merely providing illness with a label and seeking means to cure it. It distinguished between external signs and the internal pathological conditions responsible for these signs.

The earliest evidence of this development is documented in the *Su wen*. An example is a passage in its treatise 38. It shows the separation between an underlying pathological condition, sometimes called *ben* 本, "root" or "basis," that is purely theoretical, here "heart cough," and the various signs resulting from this "root," understood as *biao* 表, "outer garments" or "external signs":

心咳之狀，咳則心痛，喉仲介介如梗狀，甚則咽腫喉痺
The appearance of heart cough. When [patients] cough then their heart aches. They have an obstructing sensation in the throat, as if there were a stick. In severe cases, the gullet is swollen and the throat is thick.

Several terminological constructs were introduced to convey the relationship between "root" and "external signs." Disease and suffering were named variously *bing* 病, *ji* 疾, and *huan* 患. These characters have remained in use ever since and are indiscriminately applied to what might be called, from a Western perspective, ailments, illness, or disease in the sense of symptoms and underlying disease. However, in the *Su wen* these terms were often understood as conditions giving rise to external evidence signaling an internal pathological state. These signs were termed *zhuang* 狀, literally "physical appearance," as in the example of signs of heart cough given above; *hou* 候, literally "to inquire," "to observe," or "signs to be observed"; and *zheng* 徵, literally "evidence."

Applying Western terminological categories of "disease" and "symptom" to explain the relationship between a theoretical disease entity, such as *fei yong* 肺癰, "lung obstruction-illness," and its consequences, such as chest pain, vomiting of blood, and fever, may be justified in many cases. In a narrow sense, a disease is a pathological condition deep inside the human organism, perceptible to medical experts only by means of their diagnostic competence and theoretical training. A symptom of such a "hidden" disease is a sign that is perceptible/visible to both patients-laypersons and experts-healers. However, neither in Western nor in Chinese medicine does a clear conceptual line separate "disease" from "symptoms." For example, the compound *lou xue* 漏血, "leaking blood," is used to signify both an "illness sign" and a "pathological condition." That is, in one context "leaking blood" is identified as a consequence of a certain pathological condition; in another context it is a pathological condition itself with no further underlying pathological condition. Such dual usage of a single term or one identical compound is a common phenomenon in Chinese medical disease terminology. The compound *qi ji* 氣急, "qi urgency," is one of countless further examples. It was used to denote an "illness sign" associated with the "pathological condition" of *chuan* 喘, "panting," and it appeared also as a "pathological condition" itself, identical with *chuan* 喘, "panting."

4. Technical Terminology

In acupuncture the identification of an underlying disease condition in terms of the doctrines of systematic correspondences became a nationwide acknowledged standard. This was not at all the case in Chinese pharmaceutical treatment until the twelfth century, and it remained a superficial and short-lived attempt associated with Song-Jin-Yuan pharmacological ideology thereafter. Illness terminology in the context of Chinese materia medica remained tied to a wording largely free of hints at the doctrines of yin-yang and the Five Phases. This is not to say that there was no specific technical language (*Fachsprache*) in Chinese vernacular disease terminology. From early on illnesses were labeled with terms that may not have been easily or immediately comprehended by all strata of even the literate population. Many such labels were deliberately constructed to consist of a radical *ni* 疒 signifying "illness" (originally "bedridden") and an additional element. The latter may have simply hinted at the complete character's pronunciation, which in turn reflected a historical naming of an illness. The character *zhen* 疹, "rash" or "papule," is an example. It also appears written 軫 in medical texts. *Zhen* 軫 is the "cross-board at the rear end of an ancient carriage." An association of this meaning with skin problems such as rashes or papules is difficult to imagine. Hence, one may assume that the word *zhen* was historically used to signify certain pathological changes of the skin. The term 軫 may have been used simply for its pronunciation; the term 疹 may have been constructed to integrate this pronunciation into medical terminology.

In quite a few instances the element combined with the radical *ni* 疒 was associated with the nature of the illness it was supposed to signify. Examples include the following:

> 疔 *ding*, "pin-illness"; 痃 *xian*, "string-illness"; 疽 *ju*, "impediment-illness"; 癩 *lai*, "repudiation-illness"; 癧 *li*, "pervasion-illness"; 㿉 *tui*, "prominence-illness"; 癰 *yong*, "obstruction-illness"; 癃 *long*, "protuberance-illness"; 瘜 *xi*, "tumor-illness"; 疝 *shan*, "elevation-illness"; 瘭 *biao*, "flaming-heat-illness"; 瘕 *jia*, "conglomeration-illness"; 痞 *pi*, "obstacle-illness"; 痢 *li*, "free-flux illness"; 疵 *ci*, "blemish-illness"; 癲 *dian*, "peak-illness"; 瘑 *guo*, "lair-illness"; 瘋 *feng*, "wind-illness"; 瘟 *wen*, "warmth-illness"; 疰 *zhu*, "attachment-illness"; 癖 *pi*, "aggregation-illness"; 癥 *zheng*, "concretion-illness"; 癆 *lao*, "exhaustion-illness"; 瘢 *ban*, "macule-illness."

The addition, for example, of the radical *ni* 疒 to *lao* 勞, "exhaustion," makes clear that *lao* 癆 is a pathological state of exhaustion. The addition of the radical *ni* 疒 to *ban* 斑 ("speck, spot, macule") makes clear that *ban* 瘢 are pathological conditions of the skin. In all instances, the English translation aims at offering an immediate understanding of what the Chinese term appears to have referred to. The inclusion of "-illness" in each of the English versions may at times read somewhat awkwardly but appears necessary to signify the intentional pathological nature of the conditions described.

Some of these terms could also be rendered with vernacular illness terms familiarly used in Western languages. Thus 痢 *li*, "free-flux illness," appears to have covered diarrhea and dysentery. 癲 *dian*, "peak-illness," signifies illnesses associated with the "peak" of the human body, namely the head. That is, a "peak-illness" is a mental illness. 癩 *lai*, "repudiation-illness," is a term paralleling the German term *Aussatz* for leprosy. Lepers were "repudiated" from society, in German *ausgesetzt*, not only because of the contagiousness of their disease but also because of the possibly repulsive appearance of their physical body. Interestingly, all special terms known to signify leprosy in ancient Europe and China appear to have begun with the phoneme **le*: *(e)le-phantiasis* (not to be confused with the modern pathology of "elephantiasis"), *leu-ke*, *le-prosy*, in ancient Europe, and *lei/lai* in China. Like *huo* *luan*/cholera and *fei xiao*/phthisis, the **le*-illness may have been common knowledge along the Silk Road from the eastern Mediterranean all the way to China.

No principle is without exceptions. Numerous ancient Chinese terms signified by their radical *ni* 疒 as illness terminology will appear in this dictionary with English terms that are commonly used in the target language too. Here no attempt has been made to arrive at a translation reflecting possible images conveyed by the Chinese term. For example, 癘 wan, "epidemic," is of course a character consisting of *ni* 疒, "illness," and *wan*, the character meaning "ten thousand." Hence the term could be translated as "disease affecting a myriad of people." Similarly, the term *jie* 痎 links the radical *ni* 疒, "illness," and *jie* 皆, "all." Maybe this was meant to signify "an illness affecting all." In both cases a simple rendering as "epidemic" appeared preferable. The character 痎 is used often in conjunction with *nüe* 瘧, "malaria." *Jie nüe* 痎 瘧 may therefore be translated as "epidemic malaria." Whether the compound *jie nüe* 痎瘧, which was already used in the *Su wen*, is an older writing of the same term or whether it signifies two different diseases, *jie* 痎, "*jie*-illness," and *nüe* 瘧, "malaria," is not clear. After all, the pronunciations of 痎 and 痎 may have differed significantly in the distant past.

The term 痘 *dou* could be rendered as "bean-illness" to convey to English readers the image implied by the Chinese character. However, the term is used for smallpox to this day, and we must avoid unnecessary confusion. Keep in mind that the labeling of conditions with these terms in ancient China (as in premodern Europe) lacked the far-reaching diagnostic differentiation that is required to consider a one-to-one association between what these terms were meant to describe centuries—if not millennia—ago and what today's readers have in mind when they encounter these terms in the twenty-first century. More or less, these labels come close to their modern diagnostic categorization. However, their ancient meaning was not necessarily identical with today's understanding. Further examples of Chinese terms signified by the radical *ni* 疒 as belonging to illness terminology and translated with familiar English terms include the following:

> 瘍 *yang*, "ulcer"; 痔 *zhi*, "piles"; 痛 *tong*, "pain"; 癇 *xian*, "epilepsy"; 痙 *jing*, "spasms"; 痹 *bi*, "blockage"; 皰 *bao*, "blister"; 瘡 *chuang*, "sores"; 瘰 *lou*, "scrofula"; 瘢 *ban*, "wound"; 痕 *hen*, "scar"; 痰 *tan*, "phlegm"; 疹 *zhen*, "papules"; 疫 *yi*, "epidemics."

It is worthwhile to take a closer look at some of these examples.

The two terms *ju* 疽 and *yong* 癰 referred to above are represented by characters resulting from a deliberate combination of the radical *ni* 疒 with one additional element, in this case *ju* 沮 (lit. "impediment" and "corruption"), omitting the radical "water," and *yong* 雝 (used in antiquity with the same meaning as *yong* 壅, lit. "to stop up," "obstruction"), modified to 用 in the modern abbreviated character. In the medicine of systematic correspondences these two terms were used to form a yin-yang pairing signifying internal cloggings resulting in dermal or subdermal tissue destruction, such as festering abscesses. However, they may have been in use before the emergence of such a theoretical framework to signify ailments seen with the naked eye or perceived through the touch of one's fingers and hence may have been construed to convey meanings such as "corruption-illness" for a decaying skin surface in the case of *ju* 疽 and "walled-up location where pus collects"[3] in the case of *yong* 癰.

An example of a character that may have been constructed to convey an image that is also known in Western medical terminology is the character *long* 癃, a combination of the radical *ni* 疒 and *long* 隆, "a high mountain with steep slopes on its four sides." That is, a suitable literal translation of the term *long* 癃 might be "bedridden/ill with a protuberance." The description of the signs associated with this disease suggests that the character *long* 癃 was chosen here to denote a state one might identify in hindsight as a prostate disease. To avoid an implication of a one-to-one overlap of *long* 癃 with the Western medical concept of prostate disease and to reflect the image conveyed by the original character, the translation chosen for this dictionary is "protuberance-illness."

The term *ding* 疔 is another example. Here, too, the radical *ni* 疒 signifying "illness" is combined with a meaningful second character indicative of the nature of the illness concerned. *Ding* 丁 is a "nail" or "pin." The appearance of the illness *ding* 疔, literally "bedridden/ill with a pin," is that of an acute festering developing between skin and subdermal tissue, with a small size, deep-reaching root and hardness. Chao Yuanfang 巢元方, the author of the seventh-century *Zhu bing yuan hou lun* 諸病源候論, the earliest Chinese text on the origins and signs of disease, wrote: "When it first becomes active it rises like a pinhead. Hence one speaks of 'pin sores.'" In contrast to *long* 癃, "protuberance-illness," the illness *ding* 疔 has no corresponding pathological concept or designation in modern medicine. The translation chosen is "pin-illness," to remain as close as possible to the original Chinese meaning.

Examples of terms in which the element added to the radical *ni* 疒 for a pathological condition or sign offers no clear-cut hint at the reason underlying its selection are the following:

疸, "*dan*-illness"; 癬, "*xuan*-illness"; 疥, "*jie*-illness"; 疳, "*gan*-illness."

They are given in the present dictionary as semitranslated/semitransliterated terms. In the English compounds, the radical *ni* 疒 is reflected by the word "-illness," the added element is simply given in pinyin, transliterating the pronunciation of either the entire character or only that added element.

These disease labels remain inaccessible in their pictographic meaning. An example is *dan* 疸. Neither the symptoms associated with this illness nor an explicit attempt at an explanation by an ancient author, as was provided by Chao Yuanfang for *ding* 疔, suggests a reason for combining the character *ni* 疒, signifying "illness," with *dan* 旦, the latter signifying the sun rising above the horizon, or "dawn." The character *dan* 疸 may have been designed to convey an ancient term pronounced *dan* for an illness so well known to everyone in the field that it required no further identification, or it may simply be a modification—that was easier to write—of

---

3 D. Harper, 1998, 290. E. Hsu, 2010, 123 ff.

the character combining *ni* 疒 with *dan* 單, literally "solitary," referring to what is described in the *Su wen* as an illness resulting from a "solitary" presence of heat qi. In this case, I have chosen to render 癉 in the present dictionary as "solitary [heat] illness." In combination with the character *huang* 黃, "yellow," and given descriptions of a patient's condition to this effect, an identification of a "yellow *dan*-illness 黃疸" as jaundice appears justified.

The term *gan* 疳 poses a different difficulty in finding a suitable English equivalent. A combination of the character *ni* 疒 signifying "illness" with the character *gan* 甘, "sweet," *gan* 疳 is used to label diseases affecting spleen and stomach, organs associated in the Five-Phases worldview with the flavor "sweet." In some cases *gan* 疳 is used to denote ailments resulting from a one-sided consumption of sweet items. Hence a translation of *gan* 疳 as "sweets-illness" appears to make sense. However, the term is also used to denote illnesses that cannot easily be associated with either the spleen and stomach or the consumption of sweet food, as when *gan* 疳, "*gan*-illness," is said to be caused by worms in the patient's intestinal tract. Hence, the present dictionary has provided the entry with the heading "*gan* 疳, *gan*-illness; sweets-illness" to permit a flexible adaptation to the various usages of the term in Chinese medical and pharmaceutical literature. A singular usage of the compound *ya gan* 牙疳, "dental *gan*-illness," combined with the term *qing tui* 青腿, "black legs," in the medical text *Yi zong jin jian* 醫宗金鑒 of 1742, to signify the disease scurvy, may be seen as a further hint at the association of *gan*-illness with malnutrition.

5. Vernacular-Descriptive Terms

Given the lack of a "dead" metalanguage such as the combination of ancient Greek and Latin available to European medicine in the centuries following the Renaissance, Chinese writers resorted to several strategies to build up their specific disease terminology. A first approach may be called vernacular-descriptive. The combination of *bei* 背, "back of the human body," and *jiang* 強, "stiff," to form the compound *bei jiang* 背強 may have been understood by virtually everyone, literate or not. It signifies a "stiff back" with difficulties in bending and stretching. The compound *ao tong* 懊痛, "annoyance with pain," similarly describes a feeling a patient may have experienced after excessive consumption of alcoholic beverages. The compound *ji man* 急滿, "tightness and fullness," likewise describes an ailment from the perspective of a patient's sensations. In his *Zhu bing yuan hou lun* of the early seventh century, Chao Yuanfang described the illness as follows: "The disease develops into failure to defecate and urinate. [It is associated with] a feeling of fullness and pain in the head and neck, of tightness and fullness in the lower abdomen. Patients are not in peace, neither when they are up nor when they sit down."

Such vernacular-descriptive illness terms are not restricted to single characters or binomials. *Bian nong xue* 便膿血 is easily understandable as a reference to "relief (i.e., defecation) with pus and blood." *Bao zhu xia po* 暴注下迫 is an example of a four-character wording. The appearance of this term in the *BCGM* can be traced for about one and a half millennia to the earliest text of the medicine of systematic correspondences, the *Su wen*, where an author chose to describe a violent diarrhea as "sudden outpour with downward pressing." Even compounds of six and seven characters are seen occasionally when the description of a specific condition necessitates a lengthy wording such as *chan hou bai xue chong xin* 產後敗血沖心, "rotten blood surging to the heart following delivery." *Chan hou xue ben ru si zhi* 產後血奔入四肢 describes a situation conceptualized as "blood hastening to enter the four limbs following delivery." Vernacular-descriptive illness terms of this type have remained in constant use in materia medica literature and recipe texts into the present. They are an unavoidable consequence of the absence of a technical nomenclature developed by experts for experts.

In some instances modern translations found in Chinese-English dictionaries of traditional medical terminology prefer not to elucidate the images inherent in an illness term introduced as a meaningful vernacular-descriptive term long ago. The terms signifying numbness provide an example. Beginning with the Tang era, traceable to the *Qian jin yao fang* 千金要方 of Sun Simiao 孫思邈 (581-682?), the two characters *ma* 麻, "hemp," and *mu* 木, "log," were combined to *ma mu* 麻木 to signify a loss of sensitivity. Hence, *ma mu* 麻木 may justly be translated as "numbness." Still, this dictionary translates the term differently. A literal translation as "hemp and logs" would be as irritating as misleading; a patient can hardly be said to suffer from "hemp and logs" in his legs. In this case, a compromise appears to be meaningful: "[numbness of] hemp and logs." Though we have avoided such explanatory brackets in parentheses as much as possible, this case is an exception.

6. Terms Reflecting the Mechanics of the Human Organism

A different approach to the naming of illness resorted to a physiological and pathological understanding based on everyday know-how that also entered the medicine of systematic correspondences. Here the human organism was seen as a system of long-term storage facilities, *zang* 藏, and short-term storage facilities, *fu* 府, interconnected by ducts or conduits, *jing* 經, literally "warp thread." Blood and qi were considered the normal contents transported through this system. Rheum, pus, snot, bad odors, and various intruders such as moisture, wind, and heat were identified as pathological and had to be removed from the organism. Associated with this understanding of the organism were illness concepts such as "blockage," "aggregation," "abiding [item]," and many other terms transferred from a knowledge of simple mechanics in daily life to a conceptualization of human pathology.

An example is *bi* 痺, "blockage" or "numbness." The sensation of numbness was associated with a notion of the flow of qi and blood being blocked by pathogenic intruders such as wind and cold. *Bi* 痺 is homophone with *bi* 閉, a character used in daily life to describe "closure." Both characters appear as illness terms; the former is the result of a modification of a vernacular term to a technical illness term. Such terms lend themselves to countless combinations with more specific terms. An example is *bi long* 閉癃, "closure with protuberance-illness." Given the observation that the flow of urine is restrained by a protuberance-illness, this compound links the vernacular term for "closure" with the technical term *long* 癃.

Some terms link such a simple mechanical understanding of the human organism's "storage facilities" and the network of conduits with more sophisticated concepts found in the medicine of systematic correspondence. An example is the term *pi wei xu* 脾胃虛, "spleen and stomach depletion," an abbreviation of "spleen depletion" and "stomach depletion." At least the stomach must have been known as an anatomical entity to virtually every adult from time immemorial. "Depletion," though, has two levels of meaning. An empty or "depleted stomach" is first of all a colloquial expression requiring no expert explanation in most cultures. Given the functional proximity in Chinese culture of spleen and stomach, "spleen and stomach depletion" may simply be a reference to an insufficient supply of food with the result of a weakened organism, or to a loss, primarily through diarrhea, of food contents before they can be digested. Chao Yuanfang offered a definition to this effect when he stated: "This is a free-flux illness [i.e., diarrhea] that has lasted for an extended period of time and may change into [abdominal] distension and fullness; it may also . . . cause vomiting." However, as a technical term used by medical experts, *xu* 虛, "depletion," conveys an additional notion when combined with the word for one of the long-term storage facilities, *zang* 藏, such as the lungs, heart, spleen, liver, or kidneys. In this conceptual context, a spleen depletion refers to a significant loss of qi in the long-term storage facility "spleen." Such a "depletion" is harmful because it generates free space to be entered by intruders from outside the human organism or from a neighboring storage facility within the organism. Terms like *pi wei xu* 脾胃虛 are not defined in materia medica and recipe literature. Their meaning was evident both to laypersons and, as technical terms, to medical experts.

Although referring equally to simple mechanics assumed to work in the human organism, a term like *pi yu* 脾鬱, "pent-up spleen [qi]," may have been more meaningful to experts than to laypersons. Understanding its significance required at least a superficial acquaintance with the basic physiological concepts of the medicine of systematic correspondences. In this context, the spleen is supposed to receive qi from the stomach, process it, and supply it to the remaining long-term storage facilities. If the functions of the spleen are restrained, it will be unable to feed the lungs, heart, liver, and kidneys, with all kinds of unfortunate consequences. In such a case, the qi may be "pent up" in the spleen, a disease with signs described in the *San yin ji yi bing zheng fang lun* 三因極一病證方論, published by Chen Yan 陳言 in 1174, as follows: "When the liver qi is not balanced and manages to overcome the spleen, [this brings forth] pent-up spleen [qi] and [this qi] fails to move. This results in nodular amassments with saliva turning into foam. The qi of the depots [i.e. long-term storage facilities] is locked in, and the qi of the palaces [i.e. short-term storage facilities] cannot move freely. As a result, the stomach is distended with a feeling of fullness, and the [movement in the] vessels is string-like and retarded." Evidently, this is a definition written by an expert for experts. The level of theorization required to comprehend this explanation may have been beyond the reach of the general public.

7. Locally Specific Terms

Unrelated to the conceptual realm of the medicine of systematic correspondences and possibly enigmatic to the general public are terms that nevertheless appear to have originated from a local or an otherwise specific popular culture. An example is the term *bie jia* 鱉瘕, "turtle[-shaped] conglomeration-illness," cited in the *BCGM* twenty-three times. It is conceptually related to the term *bie zheng* 鱉癥, "turtle[-shaped] concretion-illness," cited five times, and to the term *qi bie* 氣鱉, "qi turtle," which appears six times. These terms reflect an assumption to the effect that certain pathogenic conditions may result in the growth of a turtle in the human organism. The reference to a "turtle" was more than simply a metaphor. Chao Yuanfang in his *Zhu bing yuan hou lun* suggested this when he wrote: 鱉瘕者，謂腹中瘕結如鱉狀是也, "'Turtle[-shaped] conglomeration-illness' is to say: these are conglomeration-illness nodes in the abdomen that have the shape of a turtle." Yang Shiying 楊士瀛 in his *Ren zhai zhi zhi fang lun* 仁齋直指方論 of 1264 differentiated between "turtles" formed by an interaction of blood with wine and those resulting from blood congealing with qi when he wrote: 腹中鱉瘕：平時嗜酒，血入於酒則為酒鱉；平時多氣，血凝於氣則為氣鱉, "Abdominal turtle conglomeration-illness: When someone regularly indulges in drinking wine, when his blood enters the wine, this will result in 'wine turtle.' When someone regularly has much qi, the blood congeals with the qi, and this will result in 'qi turtle.'" Presumably, Yang Shiying's was an attempt to give some scholarly credence to an ancient folk term by associating it with regular medical concepts such as blood, qi, and the consumption of an alcoholic beverage. Chao Yuanfang's more realistic idea appears to have survived until recent times. Drawings in nineteenth- and early twentieth-century folk-medical manuscripts show the location and concrete appearance of a "turtle" growth in the human body.

8. Demon Belief Terms

The cultural or regional context that gave rise to the idea of a "turtle" growing in the human abdomen may be difficult to trace. In contrast, a large number of "irregular" illness terms in the *BCGM* signify the widespread and millennia-long transmission, even in a work compiled by a representative of regular Chinese medicine such as Li Shizhen, of terms originating in a belief system acknowledging the existence of demons and their ability to harm human health. Some of these terms were given definitions in earlier medical and nonmedical texts suggesting an English translation that would be impossible if one were to start from the Chinese characters forming the term.

An example is the term *ba bing* 魃病. The etymological dictionary *Shuo wen jie zi* 說文解字 of 100 CE identified the demon *ba* 魃 as *han gui* 旱鬼, or "drought demon." This dictionary therefore translates *Ba bing* 魃病 as "drought demon disease." Another example is the term *xiao er qi bing* 小兒魃病. The author of the recipe collection *Tai ping sheng hui fang* 太平聖惠方 of 978–92 must have felt a need to explain this term to his readers. He wrote:

> 小兒所有此魃病，由婦人懷妊之時，有惡神導其腹中胎妒嫉而制服他小兒令病也。…治小兒生十餘月後，母又有娠，令兒精神不爽，身體萎瘁，名為魃病
> Children have this *qi* 魃 disease when their mother is pregnant [again] and a malign demon causes jealousy against the fetus in the abdomen and then takes control over the other children and makes them have a disease.

The explicit reference to jealousy hints at a notion of what is called sibling rivalry today and suggests a translation of *qi bing* 魃病 as "jealousy demon disease."

An imagined negative relationship between a suckling and a mother's unborn child may also have been the rationale underlying the term *ji bing* 繼病, literally "transmission disease." This is a disease first afflicting a suckling and then the fetus in the once-again pregnant mother's womb. The *BCGM* quoting the *Jia you ben cao* 嘉祐本草 of 1061 explained the term as follows:

> 繼病者，母有娠乳兒，兒病如瘧痢，他日相繼腹大，或瘥或發。他人有娠，相近亦能相繼也。北人未識此病，
> Transmission disease: A mother is pregnant and has a suckling. The suckling has a disease resembling malaria free-flux illness. The next day it is transmitted [to the fetus] and causes the [mother's] abdomen to increase in size. This may go into remission and then break out again. When another person is pregnant and comes close, a transmission is possible too. The people in the North do not know this disease.

To this quote Li Shizhen added a commentary:

> 繼病亦作魃病，魃乃小鬼之名，謂兒羸瘦如魃鬼也，
> Transmission disease is also named drought demon disease. Drought demon is the name of a small demon. That is to say, the child is as emaciated as a drought demon.

However, elsewhere in the *BCGM*, the author quoted from the *Tang ben cao*'s 唐本草 entry on "a white horse's eyes," *bai ma yan* 白馬眼, which in the *Tang ben cao* were recommended to treat *xiao er qi* 小兒魃, "children's jealousy demon." In the *BCGM*, this was modified to *xiao er ba bing* 小兒魃病, "drought demon disease in children."

That is, while the conceptual foundation of some terms resulting from a belief in the illness-causing potential of demons is obvious, in the *BCGM* these terms are met outside their original conceptual context. Medical authors from those of the Tang era *ben cao* 本草 works to Li Shizhen in the sixteenth century may or may not have shared the belief in the potential of demons to cause illness. Sufficient textual evidence exists, however, for the assumption that at least in the *BCGM* the ancient demon terms may have simply been labels of diseases that had lost their original significance. This is comparable to the use of the term *stroke* in English today. It is no longer associated with its connotation of a demon striking a person and causing loss of consciousness, sudden immobility, and further unexpected conditions.

The move away from a term meaningful in the demon belief system to labels surviving in a different conceptual context is apparent from the modification over time of terms originally meant to convey a notion of demon possession, such as *gui zhu* 鬼注. The character *zhu* 注 was used in the *Shi jing* 詩經 of the late Zhou era in the sense of "water flowing into," and it appeared in the dictionary *Er ya* 爾雅 of about the 2nd century BCE in the sense of "to attach to." That is, the notion of demon possession is expressed in the Chinese term *gui zhu* 鬼注 as "demon influx" or "demon attachment." Apparently, in a regular medical context the term *zhu* 注 was an alien import from its very beginning and required explanation and modification.

An early explanation was provided by Chao Yuanfang when he wrote:

> 注之言住也，言其連滯停住也。人有先無他病，忽被鬼排擊，當時或心腹刺痛，或悶倒地，如中惡之類，其得瘥之後，餘氣不歇，停住積久，有時發動，連滯停住，乃至於死。死後注易傍人，故謂之鬼注
>
> *Zhu* 注, "influx," stands for *zhu* 住, "to stay with; to be attached to." That is to say, the [disease] stays with/is attached to [a patient] for an extended period of time. When someone originally had no other disease and then was suddenly attacked by a demon, his heart and abdomen may experience a piercing pain. Or he experiences heart-pressure and falls to the ground, as if struck by the malign. After this has been cured, there may be additional qi that have not left. They stay for long, and at times they break out. This continues for an extended period of time until [the patient] dies. After he has died, [these qi] flow over into a bystander. Hence one speaks of "demon influx."

While the existence of demons is not explicitly denied here, a medical notion of qi is introduced to explain the pathological dynamics. At some time, the character *zhu* 注 appears to have been replaced by its homophone *zhu* 疰. *Zhu* 疰 is a deliberate combination of the character *ni* 疒 signifying "illness" with the character *zhu* 主. The latter is that segment of *zhu* 注/住 that indicates its pronunciation. This way the new character *zhu* 疰 retained the pronunciation of *zhu* 注/住 while at the same time it alienated the term from its original demon belief context and integrated the concept of "influx" and "attachment" into a more regular medical terminology. The term *zhu* 疰 is translated in this dictionary as "attachment-illness."

Henceforth, even the concept of "demon possession" appears to have been mostly written, at least in printed medical literature, with the characters *gui zhu* 鬼疰. An example is the compound *gui zhu xi tong* 鬼疰心痛, "heart-ache because of a demon attachment-illness." However, the label *zhu* 疰 was removed even further from its original context when it was also used to form compounds such as *lao zhu* 勞疰, "overexertion attachment-illness," *chong zhu* 蟲疰, "bug attachment-illness," *du zhu* 毒疰, "poison attachment-illness," *re zhu* 熱疰, "heat attachment-illness," *leng zhu* 冷疰, "cold attachment-illness," and *shi zhu* 食疰, "food attachment-illness."

As late as in the twelfth century, Chen Yan 陳言 in his *San yin ji yi bing zheng fang lun* 三因極一病證方論 explained to his readers why all these illnesses included the label *zhu* 疰:

> 以疰者、注也，病自上注下，與前人相似，故曰疰
> This is because *zhu* 疰 is *zhu* 注, "to flow into." The disease flows from above to below, and appears similar to [its appearance in] previously [affected] persons. Hence it is called *zhu* 疰.

The communicable nature of *zhu* diseases alluded to here was emphasized by other authors too. In English, a term like *zhu* 注 permitting a reading of "to flow into" and "to attach to" is not available. With *zhu* 疰 occurring mostly in compounds retaining a demonological flavor, this dictionary has chosen to remain with the definition of "attachment-illness" suggested by Chao Yuanfang.

9. This Dictionary's Underlying Principles

The limited number of examples of Chinese illness terms discussed above may suffice to leave users of the *Ben cao gang mu Dictionary* of illness terms and of premodern Chinese materia medica and recipe literature with at least a rough idea of the heterogeneity of Chinese traditional illness terminology. The extreme difficulty of grouping and categorizing these terms on the basis of their conceptual systems is further aggravated by terminologically unclear boundaries between terms signifying causes, pathological mechanisms, diseases, symptoms, and occasionally even therapies. A brief remark is also needed on the anatomical-morphological specificity of ancient Chinese organ terms. There can be no doubt that as early (or as late) as during the Han dynasty all major anatomical components of the human organism were known to Chinese medical experts and, given the absence of a terminology exclusively used by these experts, to educated laypersons too. Hesitation voiced by Western authors in the late twentieth century to translate *fei* 肺 as "lung," *gan* 肝 as "liver," et cetera, has been overcome as knowledge of the contents of ancient texts has improved. Questioning a translation of *gan* 肝 as "liver" or *xue* 血 as "blood" today would be the same as questioning the translation of *bi* 鼻 as "nose" and *er* 耳 as "ears." The anatomical and material entity is the same in the ancient and modern understanding—only the functions assigned differ. The one exception is the term and concept of *xin* 心, usually translated as "heart." Like the respective hieroglyph in ancient Egyptian papyri and *kard-* in ancient Greek medical texts, *xin* 心 covers both heart and stomach. Apparently, *xin* 心 was meant to signify a "center," and this center was varyingly identified as heart and as stomach. When the *BCGM* refers to 心氣痛, "heart qi pain," it mostly means pain in the stomach duct. Interestingly, in the *Su wen* 素問 at least one quote suggests a link of both meanings: In *Su wen* treatise 10, the term *xin bi* 心痹, "heart blockage," is defined as follows:

> 積氣在中，時害於食，名曰心痹。得之外疾，思慮而心虛
> Accumulated qi in the center. Occasionally this is harm caused by food. It is called heart blockage. If one gets it as an external disease, [the reason is that] one thinks and ponders [about something] and the heart is depleted.

Readers of premodern Chinese medical texts need to be aware of this dichotomy. It is not always clear which anatomicial entity is meant in a statement.

This dictionary offers definitions and historical data on illness terms encountered in the *BCGM*. Reliance on a list included in the *BCGM* section *Bai bing zhu zhi yao* 百病主治藥, "Pharmaceutical Substances to Treat the Hundreds of Diseases," would lead one to assume that Li Shizhen acknowledged only about two hundred diseases. This small number may indeed have composed the entire range of disease names Li Shizhen regarded as sufficient to cover the horizon of human suffering. However, the number of disease terms scattered throughout the *BCGM* text, with its innumerable quotations from earlier sources, exceeds this number by far.

A complete list of therapeutic indications encountered in the *BCGM* comprises approximately eighteen thousand illness states. Examples are *er san shi nian tou feng bu yu* 二三十年頭風不愈, "head wind that has not been cured for twenty to thirty years"; *er yin bu tong* 二陰不通, "the two yin[-orifices] are not passable"; *er bian bu li* 二便不利, "the two reliefs [of stools and urine] are not free"; *er bian bu tong chang ji* 二便不通脹急, "the two reliefs [of stools and urine] do not pass, the intestines are tight"; *er bian bu tong* 二便不通, "the two reliefs [of stools and urine] do not pass"; *er bian bu jin* 二便不禁, "the two reliefs [of stools and urine] cannot be restrained"; *er bian bi* 二便閉, "the two reliefs [of stools and urine] are blocked"; *er bian guan ge* 二便關格, "the two reliefs [of stools and urine] are locked up." This dictionary has not given all of these phrases separate entries.

To arrive at a manageable and meaningful selection of entries, we have identified basic terms, such as *chuang* 瘡, "sores," and composite terms combining basic terms with a modifying term. Such a combination must result in a changed meaning not immediately understood, as in the case of *yin chuang* 陰瘡, "yin sores," or sores affecting a person's private parts. We have not taken into account composites of basic terms with simple additions that do not have a new meaning resulting out of this composition. Examples are combinations of the basic term *chuang* 瘡 with a body part, such as *jiao chuang* 腳瘡, "leg sores"; *zu chuang* 足瘡, "foot sores"; *mian chuang* 面瘡, "facial sores"; *shou chuang* 手瘡, "hand sores"; and *ti chuang* 體瘡, "body sores." These compounds have not been given an entry of their own.

9.1. Pseudocomposites

In listings of illness terms one often encounters composites of two terms that are, in fact, pseudocomposite terms. They are not standard, and their terms are grouped together simply as items in a list failing to generate a new meaning. The text passage 古方治風毒痹厥諸酒, "all types of wines from ancient recipes to treat wind poison, blockage, and recession" offers an example. The first compound, *feng du* 風毒, "wind poison," is a standard composite term. It receives an entry of its own because it refers to a pathogenic evil qi including the characteristics of both *feng* 風, "wind," and *du* 毒, "poison." In contrast, the following two characters *bi jue* 痹厥 represent simply the listed items of "blockage" and "recession," both of which are treated in separate entries. Some compounds, though, are neither pseudo- nor true composites. They signify often-seen combinations of two illnesses closely associated with each other. Examples are *wan die* 踠跌, "[injury from] fracturing and falling," and *tu nü* 吐衄, "spitting [blood] and spontaneous external bleeding." Such compounds have also been given entries.

The application of this principle has resulted in a selection of approximately 4,500 term entries.

9.2. Two Terms—One Meaning

Numerous therapeutic indications are phrased with different characters expressing, as composites, identical meanings. Examples are the two terms *fu zhang* 腹脹 and *du zhang* 肚脹. Both are used to signify "abdominal distension." The first appears in the *BCGM* 126 times, the second only 9 times. In such instances, on the basis of their frequency of appearance we have identified one term, here *fu zhang* 腹脹, as the standard term, and the second, here *du zhang* 肚脹, as an alternative designation. A standard term is given a more detailed entry than an alternative designation.

Fu zhang **腹脹, abdominal distension** [126]

① AN *du zhang* 肚脹; *lu zhang* 胪脹, the abdominal wall is distended. IS of a) an uncomfortable feeling of fullness and pressure in the abdominal region. *SW* 19: 脈盛，皮熱，**腹脹**，前後不通，悶瞀，此謂五實, "An abounding [movement in the] vessels, a hot skin, an **abdominal distension**, [defecation and urination] in front and in back are not passable; mental and physical pressure, these are called the five repletions." b) A concrete distension and massive swelling of the abdominal region. *TPSHF* 19: 治乾霍亂，不吐不瀉，**腹脹**如鼓，心胸痰壅，宜服此方, "To cure dry cholera, when one neither vomits nor has diarrhea, and if there is drum-like **abdominal distension**, with the heart and chest congested by phlegm, it is advisable to ingest this recipe."

② PC with abdominal distension. *ZBYHL* 15: 脾氣盛，為形有餘，則病**腹脹**, "When spleen qi abounds, one's physical appearance has an excess. This leads to the disease of **abdominal swelling**."

Du zhang **肚脹, abdominal distension** [9]

IS identical with → *fu zhang* 腹脹①. *RHZ* SE *ma bian cao* 馬鞭草：通月經，治婦人血氣**肚脹**，月候不勻, "It makes the monthly period pass and cures women with **abdominal distension** resulting from blood and qi, with menstrual irregularity."

Another example is the therapeutic indication "difficult birth." In the *BCGM* it is expressed with two terms of identical characters in opposite sequence signifying an identical meaning: *nan chan* 難產 and *chan nan* 產難. The former appears in the *BCGM* ninety-one times and is therefore regarded as standard term; the latter appears only fifty-three times and is listed as an alternative designation.

The two terms for "pin sores," *ding chuang* 丁瘡 [27] and *ding chuang* 疔瘡 [58], may be used here as an example of departing from the principle of identifying a standard term that is used more often than others of identical meaning. In ancient medical texts of Tang and Song times, the character 疔 was not used at all. Books like *Zhou hou fang* 肘後方, *Zhu bing yuan hou lun* 諸病源候論, *Qian jin yao fang* 千金要方 and *Qian jin yi fang* 千金翼方, *Wai tai mi yao* 外臺秘要, *Tai ping sheng hui fang* 太平聖惠方, and *Sheng ji zong lu* 聖濟總錄 always refer to *ding chuang* 丁瘡. The term *ding chuang* 疔瘡 appears for the first time in a *Si ku quan shu* 四庫全書 edition of the *Pu ji fang* 普濟方, possibly as a modification introduced by a Qing era editor. Hence we have identified *ding chuang* 丁瘡 as a standard term, although it is encountered in the *BCGM* only twenty-seven times, and have made *ding chuang* 疔瘡, with fifty-eight occurrences, an alternative designation, despite the latter's more numerous appearances in the *BCGM*.

9.3. One Term—Different Meanings

The same term may appear in different contexts with different meanings. An example is *xia xie* 下泄; it appears in the *BCGM* thirteen times, to designate (1) an illness sign, *zheng zhuang* 症狀; (2) a pathological condition, *bing zheng* 病證; (3) a pathological mechanism, *bing ji* 病機; and (4) a therapeutic approach, *zhi fa* 治法. For example, in the section *Huang lian* fu fang 黃連附方, "[Pharmaceutical Substance] *huang lian*, Attached Recipes," the term *xia xie* 下泄 appears in the passage 氣痢後重：裡急或下泄, "Qi free-flux illness with a feeling of heaviness in one's behind, internal tension, and occasionally a discharge with outflow." Here it is used to designate an illness sign (IS) to be translated as "discharge with outflow." In the section *Ji luan bai* zhu zhi, 雞卵白 主治, "Egg White, Main Indications," it appears in the passage 止煩滿咳逆，小兒下泄，婦人產難, "It stops irritation and fullness with cough and [qi] countermovement, discharge with outflow in children, and difficult birth in women." Here, *xia xie* 下泄 is used to designate a pathological condition (PC). In the section Bai bing yin chui 百病陰吹, "The Hundred Diseases—Vaginal Flatulence," it appears in the passage 婦人胃氣下泄，陰吹甚喧, "Women with discharge and outflow of stomach qi experience extremely noisy vaginal flatulence." Here *xia xie* 下泄, "discharge and outflow," is used to designate a pathological mechanism (PM). Finally, in the section *Pu xiao,* fa ming 朴消 發明, "*pu xiao*, Explanatory Notes," it appears in the passage 內經云：鹹味下泄為陰, "The Inner Classic states: salty flavor causing draining is yin." Here *xia xie* 下泄 is used to designate a therapeutic approach (TA) of "draining."

Hence in the present dictionary the term *xia xie* 下泄 has received the following entry:

***Xia xie* 下泄, discharge with outflow; to drain** [13]
① IS identical with → *xie xie* 泄瀉, outflow ①. *SW* 45: 少陰厥逆，虛滿嘔變，下泄清，治主病者, "Recession with counterflow in the minor yin [conduit results in the following]: depletion with a change to fullness, vomiting, and a **discharge with clear outflow**. Treat the [conduit] ruling the disease."

② PC identical with → *xie xie* 泄瀉, outflow②, *YD* SE hou po 厚朴：大溫。主下泄，腹痛, "Very warm. Controls **discharge with outflow** with abdominal pain."
③ PM of a disease-caused downward movement of qi that normally moves upward. *LS* 22: 氣下泄，不治, "**Discharge with outflow** of qi. Do not treat."
④ TA CD of numerous different therapies aiming at stimulating excretion, draining liquids, facilitating intestinal passage, causing qi to move down, and removing extravascular blood. *SWBJQYBMJ* Fj 上涌下泄，奪其病之大勢, "Causing upward gushing and **discharge with outflow** will take its major strength away from any disease."

9.4. Meanings Selected by Li Shizhen

As this is a dictionary of the *BCGM*, it should reflect the meanings assigned to terms by Li Shizhen. Such an approach confronts three possibilities. First, authors in former times may have assigned a different meaning to a term than Li Shizhen did. Second, different authors in former times may have associated different meanings with one single term, and Li Shizhen may have agreed with one of them. Third, all former authors may have used a specific term with a certain meaning, and Li Shizhen may have added yet another meaning.

An example is the term *xue xia* 血下. It is used as a distinct term in the *BCGM* thirteen times. In former times it was associated with the general meaning of "bleeding," "blood loss," or "hemorrhage," identical with today's *chu xue* 出血. Hence the following passage from the *Wai tai mi yao* 外臺秘要, chapter 3:

> 療天行毒病，鼻衄是熱毒，血下數升者方
> All types of recipes to cure diseases resulting from epidemic poison, nosebleed because of heat poison, and bleeding with a loss of several *sheng*.

In contrast, in the *BCGM*, all thirteen occurrences associate the term 血下 with vaginal bleeding. Hence, the entry devoted to *xue xia* 血下 begins as follows:

> ***Xue xia* 血下, blood discharge** [13]
> IS of bleeding in women through their yin orifice, i.e., vagina.

Another example is *zang nüe* 臟瘧. In the *BCGM*, under the substance entry *fu zi* 附子, *pi han nue ji* 脾寒瘧疾, "malaria illness associated with spleen cold," Li Shizhen quotes a passage from the book *Ji sheng fang* 濟生方:

> 五臟氣虛，陰陽相勝，發為臟瘧，寒多熱少，或但寒不熱，宜七棗湯主之
> When the qi in the five depots is depleted, and yin and yang [qi] dominate alternatingly, this effuses as depot-specific malaria. There is more often a feeling of cold than of heat, or there is only a feeling of cold and not heat. The decoction with seven pieces of *zao* is appropriate to control this.

However, the original text of the *Ji sheng fang* 濟生方 was worded differently:

> 七棗湯，治五臟氣虛，陰陽相勝，作為痎瘧，不問寒熱先後，與夫獨作、疊作、間日，悉主之
> Decoction with seven pieces of *zao* serves to treat qi depletion of the five depots, with yin and yang [qi] dominating alternatingly, resulting in *jie* and malaria. Regardless of whether a feeling of cold or heat sets in first or second, or whether one [such cold or hot feeling] appears alone, whether [these feelings] appear accumulated or every second day, [this medication] will master them all.

In the *BCGM* the term *jie nüe* 痎瘧 appears eight times. At least three possibilities can be imagined for interpreting this compound. It may be read as a genuine composite, in the sense of "*jie*-malaria," that is, "the *jie* variant of malaria." It may also be simply a combination of two characters used to signify, in two different regions or traditions, the same illness. Or it may be an enumeration of two distinct illnesses, "*jie* and *nüe*," with the symptoms of *nüe* in all instances described in terms reminiscent of malaria. In such cases, a more cautious approach has been chosen. The heading of the entry in the dictionary translates *jie nüe* 痎瘧 as "*jie* and malaria."

In contrast, the term *zang nüe* 臟瘧, literally "depot[-specific] malaria," appears in the *BCGM* only once and is attested nowhere in earlier medical-pharmaceutical literature. It may have been a writing error or a new creation by Li Shizhen or someone else of his team, perhaps as an abbreviated version of the term *wu zang nüe* 五臟瘧, "five types of depot[-specific] malaria." This term is already attested in the Tang era *Wai tai mi yao* 外臺秘要 and appears in the *BCGM* twice. It may have originated in the context of *Su wen* treatise 36 attributing a characteristic *nüe*-disease to the "depots and palaces" in the human organism. Despite its unclear origin, the term *zang nüe* 臟瘧 has been given an entry in this dictionary.

The term *gui tai* 鬼胎 is an example of designations that appear in pre-*BCGM* texts with several different meanings, whereas the *BCGM* conveys only one of these meanings. Prior to the publication of the *BCGM* it was used to express three meanings. A first meaning is found in chapter 42 of Chao Yuanfang's *Zhu bing yuan hou lun* 諸病源候論:

> 若榮衛虛損，則精神衰弱，妖魅鬼精，得入於藏，狀如懷娠，故曰鬼胎也
> If camp and guard [qi] are depleted and harmed, the essence spirit is weakened. All types of specters and demon-spirits will be able to enter the depots, and the resulting condition resembles a pregnancy. Hence it is called "demon fetus."

This is a description of a pseudopregnancy assumed to have been caused by the presence of demons in any of the depots. A second meaning of the compound is conveyed in chapter 77 of the *Tai ping sheng hui fang* 太平聖惠方:

治婦人經脈不通，癥塊脹滿，腹有鬼胎方
Recipe to cure women with a blockage of conduit vessels, concretions with distension and a feeling of fullness, and a demon fetus in the abdomen.

Here the term refers to a "demon fetus" that is in fact a "concretion" generated by blocked flow of qi and blood through the conduit vessels. A third meaning is given in the final chapter of the *Nü ke bai wen* 女科百問:

雄黃丸，治妊娠是鬼胎，致腹中黑血數下，腹痛。…服後…初下清水，次下蟲如馬尾狀無數，病極者下蛇蟲，或如蝦卵雞子，或如白膏，或如豆汁
Pills with *xiong huang* serve to treat a pregnancy that is in fact a demon fetus. It causes frequent downward passage of black blood from within the abdomen, accompanied by abdominal pain. . . . After having ingested this . . . [the patient] will pass clear water first. Then innumerable bugs will be discharged resembling hair from a horse tail. When the disease has reached an extreme, [patients] will discharge snake bugs. Sometimes they resemble shrimp eggs or chicken eggs, sometimes a white paste, or bean juice.

Here the term may refer to a molar pregnancy. An examination of the ten occurrences of *gui tai* in the *BCGM* shows that it is used throughout to signify only the notion conveyed by the quote from the *Tai ping sheng hui fang*, a concretion-illness. Hence this is the definition given in the dictionary entry first. It is followed by a quote from a very early, if not the earliest known, literary source, conveying the meaning found in the *BCGM*. The complete entry reads as follows:

Gui tai **鬼胎, demon fetus** [10]
PC of → *zheng jia* 癥瘕, concretion-illness and conglomeration-illness, assuming an appearance of pregnancy, with blocked menses and abdominal distension. *TPSHF* 77: 治婦人經脈不通，癥塊脹滿，腹有**鬼胎**方, "Recipe to cure women with a blockage of conduit vessels, concretions with distension and a feeling of fullness, and a **demon fetus** in the abdomen."

The term *mu nüe* 牡瘧, "male malaria," is known from three earlier appearances in medical literature. In the *Jin gui yao lüe* 金匱要略, chapter 1, one finds the following wording:

牡蠣湯，治牡瘧
Decoction with *mu li* serves to treat *mu*-malaria.

The term *mu* in *mu li* 牡蠣, literally "male oysters," and *mu nüe* 牡瘧, literally "male malaria," is identical. One might speculate that "male malaria" is a disease associated with heat, and since oysters originate from the sea they are classified as yin and are considered, because of the terminological link by means of *mu*, to be able to counter a yang disease. However, the text itself says nothing on a hot or cold nature of the disease. In Sun Simiao's *Qian jin yao fang* 千金要方, chapter 10, the following statement appears:

> 蜀漆散，多寒者牡瘧也
> Powder with *shu qi*. Those [cases of malaria] with a dominating feeling of cold, they are called *mu nüe*, "male malaria."

In Wang Tao's *Wai tai mi yao* 外臺秘要, chapter 5, the information given in the *Jin gui yao lüe* and in the *Qian jin yao fang* is combined, but instead of *mu nüe* the text speaks of *pin nüe*, literally "female malaria":

> 多寒者名牝瘧，牡蠣湯主之方
> Those with a dominating feeling of cold are called *pin nüe*. The decoction with *mu li* is a recipe to control it.

Centuries later, the *Pu ji fang* 普濟方, chapter 197, repeats the former version:

> 病者寒多不熱 名曰牡瘧
> Those with a dominant feeling of cold and no feeling of heat, they are called *mu nüe*, "male malaria."

The *BCGM*, in the entry of *chang shan shu qi* 常山蜀漆, "*Shu qi* from Chang shan," writes:

> 牡瘧，獨熱不冷者
> *Mu nüe* are those with a feeling of heat only, and the absence of a feeling of cold.

Hence, the entry in this dictionary shows the change of meanings conveyed by *mu nüe* 牡瘧 over time and reads as follows.

> ***Mu nüe* 牡瘧, male malaria** [3]
> PC of → *nüe ji* 瘧疾, malaria ailment, with a predominance of heat over cold sensations. *BCGM* SE *chang shan shu qi* 常山蜀漆, quoting *WTMY*: 牝瘧多寒者, "Cases of female malaria are those with much cold sensation," writes: **牡瘧**，獨熱不冷者, "Cases of **male malaria** are those with only heat sensation and no cold."

9.5. Meanings Introduced by Li Shizhen

An example of an entry pointing out a peculiar position held by Li Shizhen, while also drawing attention to older views, is *wu dan* 五疸, "five types of *dan*-illness." The *Jin gui yao lüe* 金匱要略, chapter 2, lists

> *huang dan* 黄疸, "yellow *dan*-illness"; *jiu dan* 酒疸, "wine *dan*-illness"; *gu dan* 穀疸, "grain *dan*-illness"; *nü lao dan* 女勞疸, "*dan*-illness resulting from exhaustion with women"; *hei dan* 黑疸, "black *dan*-illness,"

as the "five types of *dan*-illness."

The *Zhou hou fang* 肘後方, chapter 4, has omitted "black *dan*-illness" and has split *nü lao dan* into *nü dan*, or *dan*-illness resulting from intercourse with women, and *lao dan*, or *dan*-illness resulting from exhaustion.

> 疸病有五種，謂黃疸，穀疸，酒疸，女疸，勞疸也
> There are five types of *dan*-illness: *huang dan*, *gu dan*, *jiu dan*, *nü dan*, and *lao dan*.

The *BCGM*, section *Bai bing zhu zhi yao* 百病主治藥, "Pharmaceutical Substances to Treat the Hundreds of Diseases," offers yet another, hitherto unrecorded, definition of only *huang dan*, "yellow *dan*-illness":

> 黃疸：有五，皆屬熱濕。有瘀熱，脾虛，食積，瘀血，陰黃
> There are five types of *huang dan*; all are associated with heat and moisture. They include *yü re* [*huang dan*] 瘀熱[黃疸], "stagnant heat" [yellow *dan*-illness]; *pi xu* [*huang dan*] 脾虛[黃疸], "spleen depletion" [yellow *dan*-illness]; *shi ji* [*huang dan*] 食積[黃疸], "food accumulation" [yellow *dan*-illness]; *yü xue* [*huang dan*] 瘀血[黃疸], "stagnant blood" [yellow *dan*-illness], and *yin huang* 陰黃, "yin jaundice."

However, in the entry for *zhu* 豕, "swine," *zhi gao* fu fang 脂膏附方, "Attached Recipes with Lard," the *BCGM* quotes the *Zhou hou fang* offering a list reminiscent of the phrasing in the *Jin gui yao lüe*:

> 五種疸疾：黃疸、穀疸、酒疸、黑疸、女勞疸
> Five types of *dan*-illness: *huang dan*, "yellow *dan*-illness"; *gu dan*, "grain *dan*-illness"; *jiu dan*, "wine *dan*-illness"; *hei dan*, "black *dan*-illness"; *nü lao dan*, "*dan*-illness resulting from exhaustion with women."

Hence the complete entry in the present dictionary reads as follows:

> ***Wu dan* 五疸, five types of *dan*-illness** [4]
> PC referring to five different types of → *huang dan* 黃疸, yellow *dan*-illness. *BJ* SE *zi cao* 紫草: 主心腹邪氣, **五疸**, "It controls evil qi in the heart and abdomen, and the **five types of *dan*-illness**."

The "five types of *dan*-illness" have been defined differently by medical authorities. The most widely accepted definition originates from the *Jin gui yao lüe*: *gu dan* 穀疸, "grain *dan*-illness"; *jiu dan* 酒疸, "wine *dan*-illness"; *hei dan* 黑疸, "dark *dan*-illness"; *nü lao dan* 女勞疸, "*dan*-illness resulting from exhaustion with women"; *huang dan* 黃疸, "yellow *dan*-illness." This definition is repeated in the *BCGM*, substance entry *zhu* 豕, "swine," *Zhi gao* fu fang 脂膏附方, "Attached Recipes with Lard," with only a modification from *nü lao dan* 女勞疸 to *nü dan* 女疸, "female *dan*-illness." In contrast, the *BCGM*'s section Bai bing zhu zhi yao 百病主治藥, "-Pharmaceutical Substances to Treat the Hundreds of Diseases," lists *yü re huang dan* 瘀熱黃疸, "stagnant heat yellow *dan*-illness"; *pi xu huang dan* 脾虛黃疸, "spleen depletion yellow *dan*-illness"; *shi ji huang dan* 食積黃疸, "food accumulation yellow *dan*-illness"; *yü xue huang dan* 瘀血黃疸, "stagnant blood yellow *dan*-illness," and *yin huang* 陰黃, "yin jaundice."

9.6 Error and Intention: The Divergence of the BCGM from Its Sources

To provide comprehensive data on individual natural and manmade pharmaceutical drugs, the *BCGM* is known to have relied on numerous earlier texts. Some such sources were compiled more than a millennium ago, others possibly only a few years or decades before Li Shizhen made use of them. The older a primary source, however, the more likely it is that Li Shizhen had access to them only through later secondary sources, such as Song dynasty encyclopedias. A comparison of the wording of quotes from earlier texts frequently shows more or less significant deviations from the original texts. The question here is whether such divergences were intentional or simply the result of careless copying or erroneous reading. A clear distinction between these two possibilities is not always possible. If divergences were intentional, they may have resulted from an advanced nosological or therapeutic understanding or simply from a change in terminological aesthetics. A few examples may illustrate various forms the divergences in the *BCGM* have taken from its sources.

9.6.1. Intentional Divergence—in Style

In its description of the therapeutic effects of *wu jing* 蕪菁, the *BCGM* based its text on the Song dynasty recipe work *Tai ping sheng hui fang* 太平聖惠方. There the description of the illness to be cured is as follows:

> 身體腫強，舌乾燥硬
> The body is swollen and stiff. The tongue is dry and hard.

The *BCGM* shortened this to

> 身體強，舌乾硬
> The body is stiff. The tongue is desiccated and hard.

That is, a two-times-four-characters wording was changed to a two-times-three-characters phrase.

The Tang era recipe book *Zhen yuan ji yao guang li fang* 貞元集要廣利方 describes the therapeutic effects of *bi jie* 萆薢 as follows:

> 療丈夫腰脚痹，緩急，行履不穩者
> It heals males experiencing blockages affecting the lumbar region and legs, with alternating episodes of slackening and tension, so that they are unable to walk steadily.

In the *BCGM*, this information is repeated as follows:

> 腰脚痹軟，行履不穩者
> The lumbar region and legs experience blockage with slackening, with patients being unable to walk steadily.

Here the *BCGM* has moved from a two-times-six-characters wording to a two-times-four-characters statement. Similarly, the following deviation from the original wording may also be attributed to an intention to shorten a statement and make it appear more precise:

The following statement on the therapeutic potential of *wo niu* 蝸牛 in the *Zi mu mi lu* 子母秘錄, a gynecological and pediatric text also of the Tang dynasty, is quoted in the *BCGM*:

> 小兒鼻下兩道赤者名曰䘌，亦名赤鼻疳
> When the two paths below the noses of children are red, this is called "hidden worms." Another name is "red nose *gan*-illness."

The *BCGM* rewords this as

> 小兒鼻䘌：鼻下兩道赤色，有疳
> Nose with hidden worms in children: the two paths below the nose assume a red color. They have a *gan*-illness.

Even more with an eye to offering short, precise data on illness in its therapeutic advice, the *BCGM* quotes the following effects of *xiong* 熊 from the Song dynasty recipe work *Tai ping sheng hui fang* 太平聖惠方:

> 治小兒疳瘡蟲蝕鼻
> It cures children with *gan*-illness sores, and bugs/worms eroding their nose.

In the *BCGM* this therapeutic indication is narrowed down to

> 小兒鼻蝕
> Nasal erosion in children

While a comparison of *BCGM* quotes with its source texts suggests a general tendency to shorten original wordings, a comparison of the following two versions shows a difference in style but no difference in their lengths.

The Song dynasty recipe work *Sheng ji zong lu* 聖濟總錄 of the twelfth century contains the following description:

> 咽喉如有物噎塞，飲食不下
> The throat has a feeling as if there were a gullet occlusion with a blockage; beverages and food do not descend.

The *BCGM* changes this statement to

> 咽喉妨礙，如有物吞吐不利
> Throat blockage as if there were an item that fails to move regardless of whether one intends to swallow it or spit it out.

9.6.2. Intentional Divergence—in Technical Terms

Possibly as a consequence of a change in describing a loss of consciousness in technical terms including the cause of unconsciousness, a statement on the effects of *fu long gan* 伏龍肝 in the seventh-century Tang recipe book *Qian jin bei ji fang* 千金備急方 was reworded in the *BCGM*. The original statement reads:

> 鬼魘不悟
> Demonic nightmares and unconsciousness

The *BCGM* wrote:

> 魘寐暴絕
> Nightmare with sudden cut-off [of qi]

The term *bu wu* 不悟, "not awake," is a vernacular description of unconsciousness. It was replaced by a technical term possibly unfamiliar to medical laypersons but known to experts in the theory of qi flow in the human organism, and the consequences of an interruption, or "cut-off," of this flow.

Similarly, a quote in simple vernacular from the *Qian jin yi fang* 千金翼方, also from the seventh century, reads more "professionally" in the *BCGM*. Again, a common-language description is replaced by a term emphasizing a hidden cause. The original listing of conditions to be treated with *tan huo* 炭火 includes

> 卒噦
> Sudden retching

The *BCGM* writes:

> 卒然咽噎
> Sudden gullet occlusion

One may wonder whether the following change of wording has followed the same rationale. The *Shi zhai bai yi xuan fang* 是齋百一選方, a recipe work from the southern Song era of the twelfth century, refers to

> 心神不安
> restless spirit of the heart

The *BCGM*, once again changing perspective from a description to an underlying cause, writes:

> 心神不足 "heart spirit [qi] insufficiency"

9.6.3. Erroneous Divergence

The *Ben cao shi yi* 本草拾遺, a Tang dynasty book on the pharmaceutical use of victuals, says of garlic/chives, *jiu* 韭,

> 止泄白膿
> It ends outflow of white pus.

The *BCGM* writes:

> 止泄血膿
> It ends outflow of blood and pus.

Given the close resemblance of the two characters *bai* 白, "white," and *xue* 血, "blood," in—perhaps—a handwritten or erroneously wood-carved source text, the change from "white pus" to "blood and pus" may not have been intentional.

Not infrequently, the *BCGM* has illness terms that are not found in earlier texts. The origin of such innovations is often beyond our reach. In some cases, however, it is virtually certain that Li Shizhen or one of his team members simply introduced a writing error. The term *da bai yi* 大白蟻, "big termite," may serve as an example. It appears in the *BCGM* only once. The *BCGM* entry for *ming* 茗, "tea," in the section *cha zi* fu fang 茶子附方, "Attached Recipes with *cha zi*," has

> 頭腦鳴響：狀如蟲蛀，名大白蟻。以茶子為末，吹入鼻中，取效。楊拱，醫方摘要
> A ringing sound in the brain, as if there were insects boring, is called "big termite." Grind *cha zi* to a powder and blow into the nose. This is effective. Yang Gong. [Quoted from] *Yi fang zhai yao.*

The original text, in *Yi fang zhai yao* 醫方摘要, a recipe book published in 1572, that is, while the *BCGM* was being compiled, has

> 頭內有蟲蛀響聲，名天白蟻。用茶子細末，吹入鼻中，效
> If in the head there is a ringing sound of insects boring, this is called "heaven's termite." Prepare a fine powder from *cha zi* and blow this into the nose. Effective.

This suggests that *da bai yi* 大白蟻 may simply be an erroneous writing of *tian bai yi* 天白蟻. A comparison with further texts supports this. In the *Yi xue gang mu* 醫學綱目, a book on clinical medicine of 1389, the text states:

> 頭內如蟲蛀響，名天白蟻。用茶子細末，吹鼻中
> If in the head there is a ringing [sound] as if there were insects boring, this is called "heaven's termite." Prepare a fine powder from *cha zi* and blow into the nose.

Similarly, a hundred years after the *BCGM*, the *Zhang shi yi tong* 張氏醫通 of 1695, in chapter 5, wrote:

> 頭內如蟲蛀響者，名天白蟻…丹方：用茶子為細末，吹鼻中
> If in the head there is a ringing [sound] as if there were insects boring, this is called "heaven's termite." . . . Recipe for an elixir: prepare a fine powder from *cha zi* and blow into the nose.

That is, the new term "big termite," *da bai yi* 大白蟻, resulting most likely from an erroneous writing of the character *tian* 天, "heaven," as *da* 大, "big," was not continued by authors in subsequent times.

9.6.4. Divergence—Reasons Unclear

Numerous quotes in the *BCGM* show substantial changes in the documentation of therapeutic indications for pharmaceutical drugs. It is unclear what caused these modifications. They are too fundamental to suggest an unintentional divergence, and they often lack a medical-theoretical or clinical rationale. For those interested in tracing the therapeutic effects of historically transmitted Chinese recipes and single pharmaceutical drugs, such discrepances between source text and *BCGM* quote suggest to never rely on the *BCGM* only but also to take the source text into account. A few examples serve to illustrate this. The *Yao xing lun* 藥性論, a materia medica book possibly of the Song era, writes on the effects of *ma bo* 麻勃:

> 一百二十種惡風，黑色遍身苦癢
> [It cures] 120 types of malign wind, the entire body assumes a dark complexion and suffers from itching.

The *BCGM* has

> 一百二十種惡風，黑色遍身苦痹攣
> [It cures] 120 types of malign wind, the entire body assumes a dark complexion with blockage cramps.

The *Ying tong bai wen* 嬰童百問, a pediatric book of the fifteenth century, writes in its description of the therapeutic effects of *zi bei* 紫貝:

> 瘡痘入眼
> Sores of smallpox enter the eyes.

The *BCGM* writes

> 瘢疹入目
> Macule-illness and papules enter the eyes.

The *Xiao er yao zheng zhi jue* 小兒藥證直訣, a pediatric book of the twelfth century, in its description of the therapeutic effects of *hou po* 厚朴, writes:

小兒吐瀉或誤服冷藥，脾虛生風，因成慢驚
When children vomit and have outflow, or if they mistakenly ingest medication with a cold nature, their spleen will be depleted and generate wind. Hence this generates slow fright.

The *BCGM* changes this to

小兒吐瀉，胃虛及有痰驚
When children vomit and have ouflow, their stomach is depleted and they have phlegm fright.

10. The Structure of the Entries of this Dictionary

Each dictionary entry begins with the pinyin transcription and the Chinese characters of the term to be introduced. This is followed by an English translation and, in brackets, a number referring to the number of occurrences of that term in the *BCGM*. If this occurrence is frequent, this is indicated by [p], or *passim*. The heading of an entry may also include references to alternative names (AN), alternative writings (AW), and abbreviated designations (AD) of the term in question.

The entry itself begins with a categorization of the term based on a classical Chinese understanding distinguishing between pathological condition (PC) and illness sign (IS). The former is the condition thought to exist in the organism. The latter is a condition resulting from a pathological condition. One identical illness term may be used in historical writings to signify both a pathological condition and an illness sign. A third most frequently encountered categorization is that of etiological agent (EA), reflecting a notion underlying much of illness conceptualization in Chinese as well as European traditional medicine: that is, illness must have a cause, and for an effective treatment the cause should be identified. For all abbreviations used in the entries, see the Abbreviations List at the front of this book. Entries of terms that we have identified as secondary to a standard term of equal meaning refer readers to the entry of the standard term itself. Different classifications of one single term, such as pathological condition (PC), illness sign (IS), therapeutic approach (TA), and etiological agent (EA), are indicated by numbers ①, ②, ③, and so on. Different meanings within these classifications are indicated by a), b), c), and so on. Following its classification, each term is defined on the basis of its usage in the *BCGM*. This is followed by a quote from an earlier, if not the earliest known, medical text elucidating the meaning conveyed by the term in this source. In very few instances, a term found in the *BCGM* was identified only in a text published after the appearance of the *BCGM*. All terms have been translated into English. Where a subsequent term requires a translation identical with the preceding, the translation is not repeated.

If a term is used in the *BCGM* in a form different from an obvious source, both the original source and the modified wording in the *BCGM* are quoted. Titles of texts quoted are given as abbreviations. A complete list of all these titles is provided in a first appendix following this dictionary. Abbreviated titles of source texts are followed by numbers indicating a chapter (e.g., *QJYF* 4 for *Qian jin yao fang, juan* 4), a treatise (e.g., *SW* 44 for *Su wen*, treatise 44), or other types of numbered sections (e.g., *SHL* 229 for *Shang han lun*, paragraph 229; *NJ* 56, for *Nan jing*, difficult issue number 56) where a text passage quoted may be found. Quotes from materia medica books are referred to by the title of the book followed by a reference to the respective substance entry [SE] in that book (e.g., *BJ* SE *wan jiao* 蔓椒 for *Ben jing*, substance entry *wan jiao* 蔓椒). Quotes from the *BCGM* that can be traced to an earlier source text are indicated accordingly (e.g., *BCGM* SE *ren ru* 人乳 quotes *HSYT*: 治风火证，养老尤宜, "It cures wind and fire condition, and is particularly well-suited for nourishing old people"). Often a quote from an earlier source text appears in a modified wording in the *BCGM*. This is indicated by the following structure: *BCGM* SE [substance name] quoting [source text] writes: [BCGM text] (e.g., *BCGM* SE *bie* 鳖 quoting *SHZBL* 4: 斑豆烦喘, "Macule smallpox with vexation and panting," writes: 瘢痘烦喘, "Macule-illness with smallpox, with vexation and panting"). When quotes from the *BCGM* or from earlier texts include references to pharmaceutically used herbal, mineral, and animal substances, their names are provided in the entries with their pinyin transliteration. An identification of these transliterations in terms of the botanical, mineralogical, and zoological definitions is provided in a second appendix to this dictionary.

Berlin, 2014

II. BEN CAO GANG MU DICTIONARY

1. Abbreviations

AD	Abbreviated Designation
AN	Alternative Names
AW	Alternative Writing
CC	Climatic Condition
CD	Combined Designation
DC	Disease Classification
EA	Etiological Agent.
Fj	First juan
IS	Illness Sign
Lj	Last juan
Mj	Middle juan
N	Note
PC	Pathological Condition
PE	Pharmacological Effect
PI	Pathological Item
PM	Pathological Mechanism
PN	Physiological Notion
PP	Pathological Product
PTP	Pharmaceutical-technological Procedure
PQ	Pharmacological Quality
PS	Pharmaceutical Substance
PuQ	Pulse Quality
RE	Recipe Entry
SE	Substance Entry
SEC	Secondary Etiological Condition
TA	Therapeutic Approach
TE	Therapeutic Effect
VPC	Veterinary Pathological Condition
WBC	Wang Bing commentary

2. Dictionary

- A -

***Ai chuang* 癌瘡, tumor sores** [2]
PC of → *chuang* 瘡, sores, conditions that form peaks and reach deep into the tissue, with separate entities next to each other, and a poisonous root kept deep inside and boring through the interior. *PJF* 288: 黃芩散，**癌瘡**爛腫化惡膿，止痛活血，以洗之, "The powder with *huang qin* is used for washing **tumor sores** with festering and swelling, and transforming to a malign putrescence. It ends the pain and quickens the blood".

***An ding* 暗疔, pin-illness with dim vision** [4]
PC of red → *ding chuang* 丁瘡, pin sores, with a protrusion on top that is often accompanied by loss of consciousness and/or restlessness. *PJF* 274: 亦治**暗疔**，瘡頭凸紅色，使人昏懵狂惶者, "It also cures **pin-illness with dim vision** where the top of the sores protrudes and assumes a red color while causing that person to become unconscious or turn wild".

***An feng* 暗風, dim-vision wind** [16]
PC of sudden dizziness or transient unconsciousness. *WTMY* 13: 廣濟療痃氣，心忪，骨蒸熱，**暗風**，鱉甲丸方, "Recipe for pills with *bie jia*: widely helpful in the treatment of string-illness qi, heart agitation, bone steaming with heat, and **dim-vision wind**".

***An mu* 暗目, dimmed eyes** [2]
PC identical with → *mu an* 目暗, dim vision. *BCGM* SE *qing yu* 青魚 quoting *KBBC*: 主目暗, "It controls dim vision", writes: 點**暗目**, "Drip into **dimmed eyes**".

***Ao nao* 懊憹, anguish** [7]
IS of dryness and heat in the heart and chest, with vexation and heart-pressure accompanied by an inability to calm down. *SHL* 76: 反覆顛倒，心中**懊憹**，梔子豉湯主之, "Repeated peak inversion with **anguish** in the heart; the decoction with *zhi zi* and *chi* will master this".

***Ao tong* 懊痛, annoyance with pain** [2]
IS identical with → *fan teng* 煩疼, vexing pain. *ZHF* 4: 酒疸者，心**懊痛**，足脛滿，小便黃, "In the case of wine *dan* illness, one experiences **annoyance with pain** in the heart and a feeling of fullness in legs and shins. The urine is yellow".

- B -

***Ba ban tou feng* 八般頭風, the eight types of head wind** [3] AN *ba zhong tou feng* 八種頭風, the eight types of head wind.

PC DC of eight types of → *tou feng* 頭風, head wind. *FKJYMF* 21: 治**八般頭風**：草烏尖、細辛去苗，各等分,黃丹少許, "To cure **the eight types of head wind**: *cao wu*, top quality, *xi xin*, remove the sprouts, equal amounts. Add a little *huang dan*".

***Ba bing* 魃病, drought-demon disease** [6]

PC identical with → *xiao er qi bing* 小兒魃病, jealousy-demon disease in children. *BCGM* Bai bing zhu zhi yao 百病主治藥 quoting *TBC* SE *bai ma yan* 白馬眼：小兒魃, "children's jealousy-demon", writes: 小兒**魃病**, "**drought-demon disease** in children".

***Ba dan* 八疸, the eight types of *dan*-illness** [4]

A definition of ***ba dan* 八疸** is found nowhere in medical literature. *BJ* SE *bai ying* 白英：主寒熱，**八疸**，消渴，補中益氣, "It controls alternating sensations of cold and heat, **the eight types of *dan*-illness**, as well as melting with thirst, and supplements the center and increases qi".

***Ba li* 八痢, the eight types of free-flux illness** [4]

PC CD of eight types of → *li ji* 痢疾, free-flux illness ailment. *SJZL* 172: 治小兒天瘹客忤，五疳**八痢**，十二驚癇，青黛丸方, "To cure children dangling [like a fish] from a hook from heaven and suffering from a visitor's hostility, the five types of *gan* illness and **the eight types of free-flux illness**, as well as the twelve types of fright epilepsy: [ingest] the recipe for the pills with *qing dai*".

***Ba xian* 八癇, the eight types of epilepsy** [1]

PC CD of → *xian ji* 癇疾, epilepsy ailment, classified into eight categories. They include → *feng xian* 風癇, wind epilepsy; → *jing xian* 驚癇, fright epilepsy; and → *shi xian* 食癇, food epilepsy; as well as the five types of epilepsy associated with the five depots: heart, liver, spleen, lung, and kidneys. *HYBC* SE *ran she dan* 蚺蛇膽：主小兒**八癇**, "It controls the **eight types of epilepsy** in children".

***Ba zhong tou feng* 八種頭風, the eight types of head wind** [1]

PC DC identical with → *ba ban tou feng* 八般頭風, the eight types of head wind. *BCGM* SE *bi ma* 蓖麻 quotes *XZF*: **八種頭風**，蓖麻子、剛子各四十九粒去殼，雀腦芎一大塊，搗如泥，糊丸彈子大，綫穿掛風處陰乾。用時先將好末茶調成膏子塗盞內，後將炭火燒前藥烟起，以盞覆之。待烟盡，以百沸葱湯點盞內茶藥服之。後以綿被裹頭臥，汗出避風, "For **the eight types of head wind** take 49 *bi ma* seeds and *gang* seeds and remove the hard shell, as well as 1 large lump of *que nao xiong*. Pound these until they become a pulp, and prepare pills of the size of bullets. Pierce them with a cotton thread and hang them in a windy place in the shade. When they are to be applied, first prepare a paste from the powder of good tea and smear the inside of a cup with it. Then burn the medication mentioned above until smoke rises, and cover it with the cup. Wait until no more smoke develops and then pour a decoction with *cong* that has boiled a hundred times on the tea and have [the patient] ingest this medication. Next cover his head with a cotton quilt and have him lie down. Once he sweats the wind will be dispersed".

Bai beng **白崩, white collapse** [7]

PC of a) large quantities of sticky, white liquid emitted through the vaginal tract. *MJ* 9: **白崩**者，形如涕, "The physical appearance of **white collapse** is that of snivel". b) → *beng zhong* 崩中②, collapsing center, with the blood leaving the vaginal tract being accompanied by large quantities of a white, sticky liquid. *ZBYHL* 38: 崩中之病，是傷損衝任之脈，衝任之脈皆起於胞內，為經脈之海。勞傷過度，衝任氣虛，不能統制經血，故忽然崩下，謂之崩中。五臟皆稟血氣，五臟之色，隨臟不同；傷損之人，五臟皆虛者，五色隨崩俱下，其狀**白崩**形如涕, "The disease of 'collapsing center' is associated with damage to the throughway and controller vessels. Both the throughway and the controller vessel emerge from the uterus; they constitute the sea for all conduit vessels. In the case of excessive exhaustion, the qi of the throughway and controller [vessels] is depleted, and they are no longer capable of controlling the menstrual blood. Hence there is a sudden collapse downward, called 'collapsing center'. All the five depots rely on blood and qi, and the colors of the five depots differ depending on each depot. Persons who have been subjected to damage to the extent that all their five depots are depleted, they will experience a collapse of all five colors. The form this assumes is that of **white collapse**, with the physical appearance of snivel".

Bai bing **百病, the one hundred diseases; all diseases** [117] AN *wan bing* 萬病, the ten thousand diseases.

CD of all types of PC. These may be all diseases, or a large group of diseases classified by a specific prefix as, for example, 丈夫莖中百病, "All diseases of the male stalk", 婦人百病, "All diseases of women", 小兒百病, "All diseases of children". *SW* 62: **百病**之生，皆有虛實, "When the **one hundred diseases** develop, there is always a depletion or a repletion [involved]".

Bai bo **白駁, white variegation** [13]

PC identical with → *bai dian feng* 白癜風, white patches wind. *QJYF* 23 SE *man li yü zhi* 鰻鱺魚脂：治凡身諸處**白駁**漸漸長似癬, "Cures all cases of slowly growing **white variegation** similar to *xuan*-illness at any location on the body".

Bai bo feng **白駁風, white variegation wind** [5]

PC identical with → *bai dian feng* 白癜風, white patches wind. *TPSHF* 24: 治**白駁風**諸方, "All recipes to treat **white variegation wind**".

Bai chong **白蟲, white worm** [20]

EA, PC; AD of → *cun bai chong* 寸白蟲, inch-long white worm. *BJ* SE *ya zi* 牙子：去**白蟲**，一名狼牙, "It removes **white worm**; another name is *lang ya*".

Bai chuang **敗瘡, decay sores** [9]

PC CD of → *chuang* 瘡, sores, conditions that have not been cured for an extended period of time, and where local tissue has decayed assuming a dark color and dries, without new tissue being generated. *BJ* SE *lü ru* 藺茹：主蝕惡肉，**敗瘡**死肌, "It controls the erosion of bad flesh, **decay sores**, and dead muscles".

Bai dai **白帶, white [discharge from below the] belt** [28] AN *bai wo* 白沃.
PC of → *dai xia bing* 帶下病, diseases of discharge from below the belt, with a discharge of white matter from the vagina. *QJYF* 4: 龍骨散，治腹下十二病絕產，一曰**白帶**，二曰赤帶, "Powder with *long gu* cures the twelve diseases of the lower abdomen that result in childlessness. The first is named '**white [discharge from below the] belt**'. The second is called 'red [discharge from below the] belt'".

Bai dan **白丹, white cinnabar** [1]
PC of → *dan du* 丹毒, cinnabar poison, with rashes of unclear red color brought forth by a combination of heat poison and wind cold. *ZBYHL* 31: **白丹**者，初發癢痛，微虛腫，如吹，疹起不痛不赤面白色。由挾風冷，故使色白也, "As for **white cinnabar**, in its early stages there is itching and pain, and a slight empty swelling, as if inflated. When papules rise there is no pain, and no redness, but the face assumes a white complexion. This is because wind cold is involved. This lets the color turn into white".

Bai dian **白癜, white patches** [12]
PC identical with → *bai dian feng* 白癜風, white patches wind. *ZBYHL* 31: 皮肉色變白，與肉色不同，亦不癢痛，謂之**白癜**, "When skin and flesh change color, and no longer resemble the color of flesh, and if there is neither itching nor pain, this is called '**white patches**'".

Bai dian feng **白癜風, white patches wind** [30] AD *bai dian* 白癜, white patches. AN *bai bo* 白駁, white variegation; *bai bo feng* 白駁風, white variegation wind.
PC of white skin patches without pain and itching. *QJYF* 23: 九江散，治**白癜風**, "The Nine Rivers Powder cures **white patches wind**".

Bai han **白汗, white sweat** [3]
IS. Possibly a writing error of either → *zi han* 自汗, spontaneous sweating, or *po han* 魄汗, sweat associated with the body soul. *SW* 21: 真虛痟心，厥氣留薄，發為**白汗**, "The true [qi] is depleted and makes the heart feel pain. The receding qi remains [at one place] and beats. It develops into **white sweat**".

Bai he **百合, a hundred convergences** [5]
PC AD of → *bai he bing* 百合病, disease of a hundred convergences. *QJYF* 10: 傷寒方下，**百合**第十二, "Recipes for harm caused by cold, final section, **a hundred convergences**, number twelve".

Bai he bing **百合病, disease of a hundred convergences** [12] AD *bai he* 百合, a hundred convergences.
PC of a mental disease that may appear in many different combinations of symptoms but includes absent-minded expression, depressed mood, and general dissatisfaction with movement, lying down, drinking and eating. Possibly because the name of this disease was identical with the name of the lily flower, *bai he* 百合, this herb was used for treatment. Hence the name of the disease is usually translated as "lily disease" in English. *JGYL* Fj: **百合病**者，百脈一宗，

悉致其病也, "As for the **disease of a hundred convergences**, all possible (lit.: a hundred) vessels may contribute to this disease".

Bai hu bing 白虎病, **white tiger disease** [1]

PC identical with → *li jie feng* 歷節風, pervading joints wind. *BCSY* SE *bai shi zi* 白師子：主**白虎病**，向東人呼為歷節風, "It controls the **white tiger disease**. The people towards the East call it 'pervading joints wind'". *WTMY* 13: 其疾晝靜而夜發，發即徹髓，酸疼乍歇，其病如虎之嚙，故名**白虎之病**也, "This disease is dormant during daytime and breaks out during the night. When it breaks out it cuts through to the marrow. The pain stops at times. This disease feels like being bitten by a tiger. Hence it is called '**white tiger disease**'".

Bai hu feng 白虎風, **white tiger wind** [11]

PC of → *tong feng* 痛風, pain wind, characterized by aching bone joints with the pain increasing during the night and reaching into the bone marrow. *TPSHF* 22: 治**白虎風**，痛徹骨髓，晝靜夜發，宜服酸棗仁散方, "To treat **white tiger wind** with pain penetrating into the bones and their marrow, that is calm during daytime and breaks out during the night, the recipe to ingest the 'powder with *suan zao* kernels' is advisable".

Bai hu zheng 白虎證, **white tiger condition** [2]

PC in the course of harm caused by cold disease where evil heat abounds and floods the yang brilliance conduit, and then spreads through the entire body, but not forming dry nodes of the feces yet, with high fever, profuse sweating, much thirst, and a vast and massive movement in the vessels as regularly seen signs. *PJF* 142: 遍身出汗，此為熱越，**白虎證**也, "When one sweats all over his body, this is exuberant heat. It is the **white tiger condition**".

Bai jing lao wu 百精老物, **all types of ancient spirit beings** [2]

EA identical with → *e gui* 惡鬼, malign demon. *MYBL* SE *sheng ma* 升麻：主解百毒，殺**百精老物**殃鬼，辟温疫，瘴氣，邪氣，蠱毒, "It controls the dissolution of all types of poison. It kills **all types of ancient spirit beings** and calamitous demons, and eliminates warmth epidemics, miasmatic qi, evil qi, and *gu* poison".

Bai ju 敗疽, **decay impediment-illness** [1]

PC CD of → *ju* 疽, impediment-illnesses, developing in a body in a rather deficient condition that has not been healed for an extended period of time, with locally rotten tissue that turns black and is desiccated and where there is no sign of new tissue growth. *BJ* SE *bai ji* 白及：主癰腫惡瘡**敗疽**, "It controls obstruction-illnesses, swelling, malign sores, and **decay impediment-illnesses**".

Bai lai 白癩, **white repudiation-illness** [10]

PC of → *lai* 癩, repudiation-illness, with the patient's voice turning hoarse, the eyeballs becoming white with unclear vision, numbness of the four limbs, the joints in the limbs feeling hot and painful, hands and feet being slack and weak, and the body covered with white papules. *ZBYHL* 2: 身體手足隱疹起，往往正白在肉里，鼻有瘜肉，目生白珠當瞳子，視無所見，此名**白癩**, "Dormant papules emerge all over the body, the hands and the feet. Often genuine whiteness appears in the flesh. The nose develops tumorous flesh-growths. The eyes develop white pearls at the location of the pupil. [Patients] do not see anything. This is called '**white repudiation-illness**'".

Bai lai feng chuang **白癩風瘡, white repudiation-illness wind sores** [2]
PC of → massive wind disease with white papules on the skin. *BCGM* SE *ai* 艾 quotes *ZHF*: **白癩風瘡**，干艾隨多少，以浸曲釀酒如常法，日飲之，覺痹即瘥, "[To treat] **white repudiation-illness wind sores**, take an appropriate amount of dried *ai*, soak [in water], add yeast and prepare a wine the usual way. [Have the patient] drink this everyday until a feeling of numbness sets in. This is the cure".

Bai li **白痢, white free-flux illness** [28]
PC of thin stool interspersed with white mucus, or of → *li ji* 痢疾, free-flux illness ailment, with stool consisting of white mucus only. *QJYF* 15: 凡**白痢**屬冷，赤痢屬熱, "All cases of **white free-flux illness** are associated with cold; red free-flux illness is associated with heat".

Bai mo **白膜, white membrane** [6]
PC identical with → *bai yi* 白翳, white shade. *BJ* SE *qin pi* 秦皮：除熱，目中青翳**白膜**, "It eliminates heat and removes greenish shades and **white membranes** from the eyes".

Bai tu **白秃, white baldness** [73] AN *tu chuang* 秃瘡, baldness sores; *la li* 蠟梨, polished pear; *la li* 臘梨, preserved pear.
PC of → *tou chuang* 頭瘡, head sores, with grey-white crumbs and specks emerging from one's hair base and itching, slowly growing into countless larger flakes of white crust and loss of hair as major sign. In former times it was believed that this type of sore is caused by pinworms, hence it mostly affects people in their early years and cannot be cured for a long time. *BJ* SE *song zhi* 松脂：主疽，惡瘡，頭瘍，**白秃**, "It controls impediment-illnesses, malign sores, head ulcers, and **white baldness**".

Bai wo **白沃, white downpour** [5]
PC identical with → *bai dai* 白帶, white [discharge from below the] belt. *BJ* SE *fan shi* 礬石：主寒熱，泄痢，**白沃**，陰蝕, "It controls alternating sensations of cold and heat, diarrhea/free-flux illness, **white downpour**, and erosion in the genital region".

Bai xie **白屑, white scaling** [20]
PP CD of fine, small scaling or secretions shed by the skin at locations affected by pathological change. *ZBYHL* 35: 乾癬，但有匡郭，皮枯索，癢，搔之**白屑**出是也, "Dry *xuan*-illness: when it has just one outer wall, the skin is dried up, it itches, and when scratched it sheds a **white scaling**".

Bai xie **百邪, the one hundred evils** [24]
① EA CD of all evil qi evoked by curses released by ghosts and demon spirits. *MYBL* SE *jiu* 酒：主行藥勢，殺**百邪**惡毒氣, "It is capable of transporting the effects of pharmaceutical substances, and it kills the qi of **one hundred evils** and malign poison".

② CD of all PC resulting from curses released by ghosts and demon spirits. *YXL* SE *shi chang sheng* 石長生：治疥瘙，逐諸風，治**百邪**鬼魅, "It cures *jie*-illness and *xuan*-illness, removes all types of wind, and cures **the one hundred evils** and demonic seduction-specters".

Bai xie mei **百邪魅, the one hundred evil seduction-specters** [1]
PC identical with *gui mei* 鬼魅②, demonic seduction-specters. *BCGM* SE *shi chang sheng* 石長生 quoting *YXL*: 百邪鬼魅, "The one hundred evil demonic seduction-specters", writes: **百邪魅, "The one hundred evil seduction-specters"**.

Bai xuan **白癬, white *xuan*-illness** [5]
PC of → *xuan* 癬, *xuan*-illness a), with a white lesion. The skin is dried up and thick, and itches. *MYBL* SE *bai ji* 白及：除**白癬**疥蟲, "It removes **white *xuan*-illness** and *jie*-illness bugs".

Bai xue **敗血, rotten blood** [39]
① PI identical with → *e xue* 惡血①, malign blood. *HJJF* 8: 婦人產後**敗血**不盡，血迷、血運, "[For] women who experience following delivery an incomplete discharge of **rotten blood**, blood[-induced] mental confusion, blood[-induced brain] movements".
② PC identical with → *e xue* 惡血②, malign blood. *BCTJ* SE *lan shi* 藍實：治婦人**敗血**甚佳, "It is very good for curing women with **rotten blood**".

Bai yi **白翳, white shade** [5] AN *bai mo* 白膜.
PC of → *mu yi* 目翳, eye shade, with a white, speckled membrane. *MYBL* SE *xian shi* 莧實：主**白翳**，殺蛔蟲, "It controls **white shade** and kills roundworms".

Bai yin **白淫, white overflow** [11]
PC of white mucus excreted from one's urinary tract/genital region as a result of excessive sexual intercourse or unfulfilled desires. *SW* 44: 思想無窮，所願不得，意淫於外，入房太甚，宗筋弛縱，發為筋痿，及為**白淫**, "When pondering is without limits, when one does not get what he had longed for, when [lewd] sentiments flow unrestrained to the outside and when one enters the [women's] chambers excessively, [then] the basic sinew slackens. This develops into sinew dysfunction. It also causes **white overflow**".

Bai you feng **白游風, white roaming wind** [1]
PC. The white variant of → *chi bai you feng* 赤白游風, red-white roaming wind. *BCGM* SE *wo luo* 蝸螺, recipe attached to sub-entry *rou* 肉：**白游風**腫，螺螄肉入鹽少許，搗泥貼之，神效, "For **white roaming wind** with swelling add a small amount of salt to *luo si* meat, pound to pulp, and apply externally. Wondrously effective".

Bai you zhen **白游疹, white roaming papules** [1]
PC identical with → *bai zhen* 白疹, white papules. *BCGM* SE *wu lan si can* 烏爛死蠶 quoting *BCSY*: 白死蠶主白游，赤死蠶主赤游，並塗之。游，一名疹也, "White dead silkworms control white roaming, red dead silkworms control red roaming. For both they are to be applied externally. Another designation of

you is *zhen*, papules", writes: 白死者主**白游疹**, 赤死者主赤游疹, "White dead ones control **white roaming papules**; red dead ones master red roaming papules".

Bai zhang **白障, white screen** [1]
PC quotation error. *BCGM* SE *ying yu* 蘡薁 quoting *BCSY*: 滴目中，去熱翳赤障, "Dripped into the eyes it will remove heat shade and red screen", writes: 滴入目中，去熱翳，赤**白障**, "Dripped into the eyes it will remove heat shade and red and **white screen**". Further, in Bai bing zhu zhi yao 百病主治藥 *BCGM* quotes the same passage as 點熱翳，去**白障**, "Dripped onto a heat shade it will remove a **white screen**".

Bai zhen **白疹, white papules** [1] AN *bai you zhen* 白游疹, white roaming papules. PC, white variant of → *feng zhen* 風疹, wind papules. *ZBYHL* 2: **白疹**得天陰雨冷則劇，出風中亦劇, "**White papules** turn to the worse if one encounters heaven's yin as rain and cold. If outdoors one is struck by wind they turn for the worse too".

Bai zhuo **白濁, white turbidity** [102]
① IS of turbid, white urine. In serious cases it assumes a pasty, fatty condition. In former times it was assumed that this results from a mixture of urine with sperm. *QJYF* 19: 治虛損，小便**白濁**，夢泄方, "Recipe for dream ejaculation: It cures depletion injury and **white turbidity** of the urine". *BCGM* commonly refers to this as a male condition, with only one exception where a case of white turbidity, resulting from a mixture of urine with minute particles, was observed in a woman.
② PC with turbid, white urine as major sign. In former times it was believed that such a condition results from excesive lust and deliberation. *ZBYHL* 4 lists 虛勞小便**白濁**候, "Signs of depletion exhaustion and **white turbidity** of urine".

Ban **斑, macule** [p] AW 瘢, macule-illness.
① IS of red, purple or in severe cases even black macules developing on the skin. When the dots are large they may develop flakes. In general, though, when stroking the afflicted dermal region one does not feel an elevation. *ZBYHL* 8: 體如被打，發**斑**，此皆其候, "The body looks as if beaten and develops **macules**. All these [conditions] are its signs".
② PC a) of the development of macules. *ZBYHL* 9: 凡發**斑**不可用發表藥，令瘡開泄，更增斑爛，表虛故也, "Whenever **macules** appear one must not use pharmaceutical substances to open up the exterior. They would cause the sores to open and discharge liquid, and the festering of the macules would be further increased because of a depletion in the exterior". b) identical with → *dou chuang* 痘瘡, smallpox sores. *TPSHF* 18: 治熱病**斑**發，須臾遍身，皆戴白漿, "To cure heat disease with the appearance of **macules**. After a short while they cover the entire body, with all of them containing a thick, white liquid.".

Ban **瘢, macule-illness** [p]
PC identical with → *ban* 斑, macule. *TYBC* Xu 序：醫壘元戎、陰證略例、**瘢**論萃英、錢氏補遺等書，安樂之法，湯液本草統之, "The approaches to peace and happiness documented in books such as *Yi lei yuan rong*, *Yin zheng lue*

li, *Ban lun cui ying*, ("A Collection of the Best Writings on **Macule-Ilnness**"), and *Qian shi bu yi* are all gathered in the *Tang ye ben cao*".

***Ban* 瘢, scar** [p]
PC of a scar or mark on the skin. *ZHF* 5: 甘家松脂膏，療熱瘡，尤嗍膿，不痂無**瘢**方, "Mr. Gan's ointment with *song zhi* is a recipe to cure heat sores, and in particular to suck pus, without leaving a crust or **scar**".

***Ban chan* 半產, miscarriage** [5] AN *xiao chan* 小產.
PC of spontaneous miscarriage at a stage of pregnancy when the fetus has assumed a child's physical appearance. *JGYL* Lj: 婦人有漏下者，有**半產**後因續下血都不絕者, "It may be that a woman experiences dribbling discharge because after a **miscarriage** blood continues to be discharged without coming to an end".

***Ban chuang* 瘢瘡, macule-illness sores** [6] AW *ban chuang* 斑瘡.
PC identical with → *ban chuang* 斑瘡, macule sores. *BCGM* SE *shui ping* 水萍 quoting *SYDXF* 11: 豌豆瘡入目, "Pea[-like] bean sores enter the eyes", writes: **瘢瘡**入目, "**Macule-illness sores** enter the eyes".

***Ban chuang* 斑瘡, macule sores** [10] AW 瘢瘡, macule-illness sores.
PC identical with → *dou chuang* 痘瘡, smallpox sores. *WTMY* 3 quotes *ZHF*: 比歲有病天行發**斑瘡**，頭面及身須臾周匝，狀如火瘡，皆戴白漿，隨決隨生，不即療，劇者數日必死, "Near the age of 1 year, [the child] suffered from heaven-sent **macule sores**. Head, face and the entire body were all covered in no time. It looked like fire sores. They all contained thick white fluid. Where [a sore] burst open, another one grew. There was no way to cure this. In severe cases death is inevitable within a few days".

***Ban dou* 瘢痘, macule-illness with smallpox** [10] AW 斑痘；斑豆.
PC identical with → *dou chuang* 痘瘡, smallpox sores. *BCGM* SE *bie* 鱉 quoting *SHZBL* 4: 斑豆煩喘, "Macule smallpox with vexation and panting", writes: **瘢痘**煩喘, "**Macule-illness with smallpox**, with vexation and panting".

***Ban dou* 斑痘, macules with smallpox** [3]
PC identical with → *ban dou* 瘢痘, macule-illness with smallpox. *PJF* 403: 葛根麥門冬散，治小兒熱毒**斑痘**，頭痛壯熱，心神煩悶, "Powder with *ge gen* and *mai men dong* cures heat poison [generating] **macules with smallpox** in children. Their head aches and they have a high fever. Heart and spirit experience vexation and heart-pressure".

***Ban dou* 斑豆, macules with beans** [4]
PC identical with → *ban dou* 瘢痘, macule-illness with smallpox. *SJZL* 169: 治小兒**斑豆**瘡退熱躁，沖和散方, "Recipe for a 'powder that is both vigorous and gentle' to cure **macules with bean** sores in children; it removes the heat and the restlessness".

***Ban hen* 瘢痕, wound scar** [41]
PC of a scar remaining after a wound or sores have healed, leaving the texture of the skin permanently altered. *QJYF* 6: 治**瘢痕**凸出方, "Recipe to cure **wound scar** protrusion".

Ban sheng ku si **半身枯死, unilateral withering and necrosis** [1]

IS identical with → *pian ku* 偏枯, unilateral withering. *BCSY* SE *fu she* 腹蛇: 有患大風及諸惡風，惡瘡瘰癧，皮膚頑痹，**半身枯死**，皮膚手足臟腑間重疾，並主之, "If someone suffers from massive wind and all types of malign wind, malign sores and scrofula with pervasion-illness, stubborn skin blockage, **unilateral withering and necrosis,** [that is,] any serious disease in the region of skin, hands and feet, and depots and palaces, it will master these all alike".

Ban zhen **瘢疹, macule-illness and papules** [4]

PC identical with → *dou chuang* 痘瘡, smallpox sores. *BCGM* SE *zi bei* 紫貝 quoting *YTBW*, Ying tong bai wen 嬰童百問: 瘡痘入眼, "Sores of smallpox enter the eyes", writes **瘢疹**入目, "**Macule-illness and papules** enter the eyes".

Ban zhen **斑疹, macules and papules** [7]

PC CD of → *ban* 斑, macule, and → *zhen* 疹, papules. *SJZL* 27: 毒氣內盛，因表虛，熱毒乘虛出於皮膚，發為**斑疹**, "When poison qi abounds internally, following a depletion in the exterior, heat poison will avail itself of this depletion and appear in the skin where it effuses as **macules and papules**".

Ban zhen du **斑疹毒, poison of macules and papules** [2]

PC identical with → *ban zhen* 斑疹, macules and papules. *BCGM* SE *e shi* 惡實: 消**斑疹毒**, "It dissolves the **poison of macules and papules**".

Bao bing **暴病, sudden and violent disease** [2] AN *bao ji* 暴疾, sudden and violent ailment.

CD of all PC with a sudden and violent onset, and taking a rather dramatic course. *QJYiF* 20: 主心腹**暴病**,若中惡客忤，心腹脹滿刺痛，口噤氣急，停屍卒死者, "It controls **sudden and violent diseases** affecting heart and abdomen, as if being struck by the malign, or experiencing a visitor's hostility. Heart and abdomen extend and have fullness associated with a piercing pain. The jaws are clenched, and the qi [moves] urgently. [Patients] assume the appearance of a corpse that has succumbed to a sudden death".

Bao bu chu **胞不出, the placenta fails to appear** [1]

PC identical with → *bao yi bu xia* 胞衣不下, the placenta fails to descend. *YD* SE *ma you* 麻油: 治產難，**胞不出**, "To cure difficult birth, with **the placenta failing to appear**".

Bao bu luo **胞不落, the placenta fails to descend** [1]

PC identical with → *bao yi bu xia* 胞衣不下. *MYBL* SE *zao jia* 皂莢: 除咳嗽，囊結，婦人**胞不落**, "It removes cough, pouch nodes, and [helps] women when **the placenta fails to descend**".

Bao chi mu **暴赤目, severely red eye** [3]

PC identical with → *bao chi yan* 暴赤眼. *BCYY* SE *gu wen qian* 古文錢: 少時常自患**暴赤目**，腫痛，數日不能開, "In my youth I often suffered from **severely red eyes**, with swelling and pain. I could not open them for several days".

Bao chi yan **暴赤眼, severely red eye** [7] AN *bao chi mu* 暴赤目.

PC of → *chi yan* 赤眼, red eyes, with a violent, abrupt and serious appearance. *TPSHF* 32: 治**暴赤眼**，腫澀疼痛，宜服犀角散方, "For treating **severely red**

eyes, with swelling, roughness, and pain, the recipe to ingest the powder with *xi jiao* is advisable".

Bao feng **暴風, violent wind** [16]

① A baneful climatic phenomenon, able to turn into → *feng xie* 風邪, wind evil. *ZBYHL* 10: 節氣不和，寒暑乖候，或有**暴風**疾雨, "If the seasonal qi fails to agree with [what should be the proper qi], and if cold and summer heat run counter [to normal], or if there happen to be **violent winds** and severe rain".

② PC. A sudden occurrence of → *zhong feng* 中風, being struck by wind. *WTMY* 14: **暴風**手足癱廢，言語謇澀, "In the case of violent wind hands and feet are paralyzed, one's speech is stuttering and rough". *BCGM* refers to various related pathological conditions including *bao feng tong* 暴風痛, violent wind with pain, *bao feng kou jin* **暴風**口噤, violent wind with clenched jaw, bao feng sao yang 暴風瘙癢, violent wind with itching.

Bao ji **暴疾, sudden and violent ailment** [2]

PC identical with → *bao bing* 暴病， sudden and violent disease. *BJ* SE *ji tou shi* 雞頭實：補中除**暴疾**，益精氣, "It supplements the center and eliminates **sudden and violent ailments**. It fills the essence qi".

Bao leng **暴冷, violent cold** [7]

① EA of a sudden and violent cold evil. *QJYF* 5: 小兒嫩弱，其外則易傷，**暴冷**折其陽, "Weak and tender children: their outer sections are easily harmed. **Violent cold** cuts their yang".

② PC brought forth by a violent cold. *MYBL* SE *gao liang jiang* 高良薑：主**暴冷**，胃中冷逆，霍亂腹痛, "It controls **violent cold**, cold counterflow in the stomach, and cholera with abdominal pain".

Bao li **暴痢, violent free-flux illness** [14]

PC of → *li ji* 痢疾, free-flux illness, with a sudden onset and a violent course of the disease. *QJYF* 15: 如陟厘丸、烏梅丸、松皮散等，**暴痢**服之，何有不瘥, "If patients suffering from **violent free-flux illness** ingest the pills with *zhi li*, the pills with *wu mei*, and the powder with *song pi*, how could it be that they are not cured?!"

Bao lin **暴淋, violent dripping** [1]

PC of → *lin bing* 淋病, dripping disease, with a sudden onset and a violent course. *BCYY* SE *xiao mai* 小麥：小麥，**暴淋**煎湯飲, "For **violent dripping**, prepare a decoction of *xiao mai* for ingestion".

Bao lou **胞漏, uterine leaking** [2]

PC identical with → *lou tai* 漏胎, dribbling fetus. *QJYF* 4: 女人**胞漏**，下血不可禁止, "Females with **uterine leaking**, [that is,] a discharge of blood that cannot be stopped".

Bao man **飽滿, satiation and fullness** [2]

① IS of an uncomfortable feeling of having eaten beyond repletion. *PJF* 172: 青空湯，治傷酒食**飽滿**, "Blue sky decoction cures harm caused by [consumption of] wine and food to **satiation and fullness**".

② Refers to the condition of satiation experienced by a person after having dined. *BCJJZ* preface: 病在骨髓者，宜**飽滿**而在夜, "When the disease is in the bone marrow, it is advisable [to take medication] after one has eaten to **satiation and fullness** at night".

***Bao qi* 暴氣, violent qi** [3]
PC of a sudden, violent outbreak of disease. *LS* 1: 員利針者，大如氂，且員且銳，中身微大，以取**暴氣**, "The round-sharp needle has the size of a hair. It is both round and pointed. In its middle it is a little more massive. It serves to eliminate **violent qi**".

***Bao qiang* 抱槍, spear holder** [2]
EA identical with → *she gong* 射工①, archer. *BCGM* SE *xi gui chong* 溪鬼蟲：酉陽雜俎謂之**抱槍**, "The *YYZZ* calls it **spear holder**".

***Bao re* 暴熱, fulminant heat** [27]
PC of rather severe → *re bing* 熱病, heat disease, characterized by a sudden outbreak. *BJ* SE *bai jiang* 敗醬：主**暴熱**，火瘡赤氣, "It controls **fulminant heat**, fire sores, red qi". *BCGM* speaks of numerous types of fulminant heat, such as *bao re chuan xi* 暴熱喘息, fulminant heat with pant-breathing; *bao re re li* 暴熱熱痢, fulminant heat with heat free-flux illness; *bao re xia xue* 暴熱下血, fulminant heat with a discharge of blood.

***Bao shui* 暴水, sudden water** [4]
PC of a very acute and dramatic → *shui zhong* 水腫, edema, affecting primarily the abdomen with distension and a feeling of fullness. *ZBYHL* 21: **暴水**者，先腹滿, "In the case of **sudden water**, the abdomen has a feeling of fullness first".

***Bao si* 暴死, sudden [appearance of] death** [5]
PC identical with → *cu si* 卒死. *SW* 62: 血之與氣並走於上，則為大厥，厥則**暴死**，氣復反則生，不反則死, "When the blood and the qi both move upwards, this is a massive recession. [Massive] recession causes **sudden [appearance of] death**. If the qi turns back again, [the patient] will live; if it does not turn back, [he] will die".

***Bao tai se* 胞胎澀, rough [passage of] placenta and fetus** [1]
PC of → *nan chan* 難產, difficult birth, because of blood depletion and insufficient body liquids. *BCGM* hua ji 滑劑, lubrication remedies: **胞胎澀**者，黃葵子、王不留行之屬, "In the case of a **rough [passage of] placenta and fetus**: *huang kui zi* and *wang bu liu xing* belong to this group [of lubricating medications]".

***Bao tui* 暴㿗, sudden prominence-illness** [1]
PC of sudden emergence of → *yin tui* 陰㿗, yin (i.e. scrotal) prominence-illness. *MYBL* SE *hai zao* 海藻：療皮間積聚，**暴㿗**, "It cures accumulations and collections in the skin, and **sudden prominence-illness**".

***Bao wang* 暴亡, sudden [appearance of] death** [8]
PC identical with → *cu si* 卒死. *SW* 74 *WBC*: 絕粒服餌，則不**暴亡**, "If one stops eating grain, and consumes substitutes instead, one will not have a **sudden [appearance of] death**".

***Bao xie* 暴泄, violent outflow** [12] AW *bao xie* 暴瀉.

PC of a rather sudden onset of a violent form of → *xie xie* 泄瀉②, outflow. *QJYF* 30: 大都、太白，主**暴泄**，心痛腹脹, "[Needling the insertion holes] *da du* and *tai bai* controls **violent outflow**, heartache and abdominal distension".

***Bao xie* 暴瀉, violent outflow** [3]

PC identical with → *bao xie* 暴泄. *SJZL* 40 lists li lu wan 藜蘆丸, pills with li lu: 治霍亂，赤白冷熱等利，及**暴瀉**, "They cure free flow of the types of cholera, red and white [discharge], cold and heat [free-flux illness], and also **violent outflow**".

***Bao xie* 暴下, violent downpour** [4]

PC a) identical with → *bao xie* 暴泄, violent outflow. *QJYF* 15: 附子湯，治**暴下**積日不住及久痢方, "Decoction with *fu zi* is a recipe for treating **violent downpour** that lasts for days without ending, as well as prolonged free-flux illness". b) of blood discharged abruptly and in large quantities from a female's genital organ. *BCGM* often uses it together with the term *beng zhong* 崩中, collapsing center, and speaks of *beng zhong bao xia* 崩中**暴下**, "collapsing center with **violent downpour**", which is profuse uterine bleeding. *SJZL* 152: 衝任氣虛，則經血不能制約，故令**暴下**, "When the qi is depleted in the throughway and contoller [vessels], the menstrual blood can no longer be restrained. Hence this leads to **violent downpour**".

***Bao xin tong* 暴心痛, violent heartache** [5]

PC of → *xin tong* 心痛, heartache, with a most violent onset. *QJYF* 17: 治**暴心痛**，面無顏色慾死者方, "Recipe to cure **violent heartache**, with the patient having no complexion and being about to die". Note: usages of *xin* 心, heart, may refer to the anatomical heart or to the stomach.

***Bao yao* 暴夭, sudden [appearance of] death** [5]

PC identical with → *cu si* 卒死. *SW* 49 *WBC*: 臟有偏絕，則有**暴夭**, "Once [the qi of] a depot has been cut off unilaterally, **sudden [appearance of] death** results".

***Bao yi bu chu* 胞衣不出, the placenta fails to appear** [13]

PC identical with → *bao yi bu xia* 胞衣不下, the placenta fails to descend. *MYBL* SE *ou shi* 藕實：帶下百病，產難，**胞衣不出**, "[It cures] all diseases of discharge from below the belt, difficult birth, and **failure of the placenta to appear**".

***Bao yi bu luo* 胞衣不落, the placenta fails to descend** [1]

PC identical with → *bao yi bu xia* 胞衣不下. *MYBL* SE *hu ma* 胡麻：以作油，微寒，利大腸，**胞衣不落**, "The oil prepared from it is slightly cold. It stimulates passage in the large intestine, and [helps when] **the placenta fails to descend**".

Bao yi bu xia **胞衣不下, the placenta fails to descend** [25] AN *tai yi bu xia* 胎衣不下; *bao yi bu chu* 胞衣不出; *yi bu xia* 衣不下; *bao yi bu xia* 包衣不下; *bao bu chu* 胞不出, the placenta fails to appear; *bao yi bu luo* 胞衣不落; *bao bu luo* 胞不落.

PC following the birth of a fetus with the placenta failing to be expelled for an extended period of time. *QJYF* 12 RE qi po wan bing wan 耆婆萬病丸, "granny's pills for a myriad of of diseases": 婦人諸疾，**胞衣不下**，服二丸如小豆，取吐利即出, "For all types of ailments of women, and when **the placenta fails to descend**, ingest two pills of the size of small beans. This is to take advantage of [this recipe's] effects to cause vomiting and free-flux illness, stimulating [the placenta] to appear".

Bao yin **暴喑, sudden muteness** [2]

PC with a sudden loss of voice as major sign. *SJZL* 191: 治**暴喑**氣哽，喉痹咽腫，不得息, "To treat **sudden muteness** and qi occlusion, with throat blockage and gullet swelling, and an inability to find rest".

Bao yi bu xia **包衣不下, the placenta fails to descend** [1]

PC identical with → *bao yi bu xia* 胞衣不下. *BCGM* SE *ji li* 蒺藜 quotes *HSF*: 催生下衣難產，胎在腹中，並**包衣不下**, "It hastens delivery and makes the placenta come down in the case of difficult birth, when the fetus remains in the abdomen, and **the placenta fails to descend**".

Bao zhang **飽脹, satiation and distension** [3]

IS of having eaten to more than one's fill with a feeling of distension. *BCJJZ* SE *xiao shi* 消石：主療熱，腹中**飽脹**，養胃消谷，去邪氣, "It controls the cure of heat, and in the abdomen a feeling of **satiation and distension**. It nourishes the stomach and digests solid food. It eliminates evil qi".

Bao zheng **暴癥, sudden concretion-illness** [8]

PC of → *zheng* 癥, concretions that appear suddenly and grow very fast. *MYBL* SE wei xian 薇銜：主**暴癥**，逐水，療痿蹶, "It controls **sudden concretion-illness**, eliminates water, and cures dysfunction with [a tendency to] fall".

Bao zhong **暴腫, sudden and violent swelling** [8]

IS of a sudden, violent appearance of a swelling, either topical or affecting the entire body. *ZHF* 5: 身體頭面，忽有**暴腫**處如吹方, "Recipe for body, head, and face showing places of a **sudden and violent swelling** as if inflated".

Bao zhong feng **暴中風, violent wind stroke** [9]

PC of sudden onset of a hot body and mental confusion brought about by taking in wind heat. *BJ* SE *bai wei* 白薇：主**暴中風**，身熱肢滿，忽忽不知人, "It controls **violent wind stroke**, with a hot body, a feeling of fullness in the limbs, and mental confusion including an inability to recognize people".

Bao zhu xia po **暴注下迫, sudden outpour with downward pressing** [1]

PC of sudden, violent watery diarrhea. *SW* 74: 諸嘔吐酸，**暴注下迫**，皆屬於熱, "All [cases of] vomiting sour [matter], **sudden outpour with downward pressing**, without exception they are associated with heat".

***Bei fa* 背發, effusion of the back** [1]
PC identical with → *fa bei* 發背. *BCGM* Bai bing zhu zhi yao 百病主治藥 quoting *ZHF*: 發背欲死 writes **背發**欲死, "**Effusion of the back** [so serious] that one wishes to die".

***Bei han* 背寒, the back is cold** [2]
IS of a feeling of cold in the back. *ZBYHL* 5: 其人必眩，**背寒**而嘔, "This person will be dizzy. His **back is cold**, and he vomits".

***Bei jiang* 背強, stiff back** [4]
IS of stiff back with difficulties to move. *BJ* SE *sang shang ji sheng* 桑上寄生：主腰痛，小兒**背強**，癰腫, "It controls lower back pain, **stiff back** in children, and obstruction-illnesses with swelling".

***Bei yang chuang* 悲羊瘡, sad sheep sores** [1]
PC identical with → *zou pi qu chuang* 走皮趨瘡, sores running through the skin. *BCGM* SE *zi wei* 紫葳quotes *RZZZF*: 走皮趨瘡：滿頰滿頂，浸淫濕爛，延及兩耳，癢而出水，發歇不定。田野名**悲羊瘡**, "Sores running through the skin: they cover cheeks and the entire top of the head with soaking moisture and a festering extending to the two ears. They itch and release liquid, with irregular periods of activity and dormancy. In the countryside this is named **sad sheep sores**".

***Ben tun* 奔豚, running piglet** [51] AW 賁豚. AN *shen ji* 腎積, kidney accumulation
PC of a → *ji* 積, accumulation, associated with the kidneys. It assumes the shape of a piglet and affects the lower abdomen. It may ascend to below the heart, and it moves upward and downward at irregular intervals. It is accompanied by panting with counterflow, a feeling of fullness and pain, and cannot be cured for an extended period of time. *BJ* Xu li shang 序例上：夫大病之主，有…**奔豚**上氣，咳逆嘔吐, "Now, among the major illnesses are…**running piglet** with rising qi, cough and vomiting".

***Ben tun* 賁豚, running piglet** [7]
PC identical with → *ben tun* 奔豚. *NJ* 56: 腎之積，名曰**賁豚**，發於少腹，上至心下，若豚狀，或上或下無時。久不已，令人喘逆，骨痿，少氣, "Accumulations related to the kidneys are called '**running piglets**'. They develop in the lower abdomen and extend upward to below the heart. Like a piglet, they move up or down unexpectedly. They last a long time without ending. They make the [afflicted] person pant with [qi] counterflow, and they cause bone dysfunction and shortness of qi".

***Beng* 崩, collapse** [p]
PC identical with → *beng zhong* 崩中, collapsing center. *SW* 7: 陰虛陽搏謂之**崩**, "When the yin is depleted and the yang beats, this is called '**collapse**'".

***Beng chi* 崩赤, collapsing red** [1]
PC identical with → *chi beng* 赤崩, red collapse. *PJF* 330: 治傷中**崩赤**，用醍醐杵汁拌酒，煎沸，空心服一盞, "To treat harm to the center with **collapsing red**, take milk fat and pound until it becomes a liquid. Mix with wine and heat until boiling. Ingest 1 small cup on an empty stomach".

Beng dai **崩帶, collapsing belt** [8]

PC CD of → *beng zhong* 崩中②, collapsing center, and → *dai xia* 帶下②, discharge from below the belt. *HJJF* 5: **崩帶**虛損，臍腹撮痛，艾醋湯下, "[For treating] **collapsing belt** with depletion harm, and pinching pain in the navel and abdominal region, ingest a decoction with *ai* and vinegar".

Beng lou **崩漏, collapse and leaking** [14]

PC CD of → *beng zhong* 崩中②, collapsing center, and → *lou xia* 漏下, leaking discharge. Collapsing center is often followed by leaking downflow. In some cases they appear alternatingly. *JSF* Fu ren men 婦人門：**崩漏**之疾，本乎一證。輕者謂之漏下，甚者謂之崩中, "The ailments of '**collapse' and 'leaking'** are basically one single condition. Light cases are called 'leaking discharge'; severe cases are called 'collapsing center'".

Beng sha **崩砂, collapsing sand** [1]

PC of the first stage of → *zou ma ya gan* 走馬牙疳, running horse dental *gan*-disease, with bad mouth odor and teeth turning black. *HYKY* 18: 次第齒黑，名曰**崩砂**, "At first in a series [of four stages] the teeth turn black. This is called '**collapsing sand**'".

Beng xue **崩血, collapsing blood** [2]

PC identical with → *xue beng* 血崩, blood collapse. *YXL* SE ai ye 艾葉：能止**崩血**，安胎，止腹痛, "It is able to stop **collapsing blood**, it calms the fetus, and it ends abdominal pain".

Beng zhong **崩中, collapsing center** [171] AN *xue beng* 血崩, blood collapse; AD *beng* 崩, collapse.

PC of excessive vaginal bleeding outside of a menstruation period. *JGYL* Lj: 兼取**崩中**去血，或月水來過多, "[This recipe] is also able to eliminate [conditions such as] **collapsing center** and blood loss, as well as excessive menstruation".

Bi **痹, blockage; numbness** [p]

① PC of a) wind, cold, moisture evil entering the conduits and generating barriers to the flow of qi and blood, which in turn leads to pain, cramps, and stiffness of joints and muscles, in some cases including morphological changes such as swelling and distension, or impediment of one's movement . *SW* 43: 風寒濕三氣雜至, 合而為**痹**也, "When the three qi wind, cold, and moisture arrive together, they merge and cause a **blockage**". b) Wind evil closing the skin, with a thickening and numbness of the skin, and pain or itching. *ZBYHL* 2: 凡**痹**之類, 逢熱則癢, 逢寒則痛, "All cases of **blockage** type [disease], if [patients] happen to encounter heat, this will result in itching. If they encounter cold, this will cause pain". c) Being struck by wind evil, resulting in either one half of the body or hands and arms being paralyzed as major sign. *JGYL* Fj: 風之為病, 當半身不遂；或但臂不遂者, 此為**痹**, "When wind causes a disease, if either one half of the body or only his arms do no longer follow his will, this is '**blockage**'". d) Conditions resulting from a blocked passage of qi and blood. *SW* 10: 血凝於膚者為**痹**, "When the blood congeals in the skin, this is **blockage**". *LS* 10 氣往來行, 則為癢；留而不去, 則**痹**, "When qi moves in and out, this causes itching.

When it stays and fails to leave, this causes **blockage**". e) Identical with → *nao bi* 腦痹, brain blockage. *BCGM* SE *fu shi* 浮石 quotes *RZZZF*: 頭核腦痹：頭枕後生痰核，正者為腦，側者為**痹**, "head kernel, brain blockage: When a phlegm kernel develops behind the head, those in the center are 'brain', those developing at the side are '**blockage**'".

② IS of a) pain, cramps and tightness of joints and muscles, in severe cases including morphological changes such as swelling and distension. *ZBYHL* 6: 若產婦中風寒, 身體強痛, 不得動搖者, 便溫服一劑, 因以寒水浴即瘥。以浴後, 身有**痹**處者, 便以寒水洗, 使周遍, "If a woman in the course of delivery is struck by wind cold, with her body being stiff and painful, and if she is unable to move or sway, she should consume one dosage warmed up. If she is then washed with cold water, this will bring the cure. If following the washing the body has regions that have a **blockage**, she is to be washed with cold water all over". b) Identical with → *ma bi* 麻痹②, hemp[-like numbness] blockage. *ZHF* 3: 服從一合始, 以微**痹**為度, "Consume beginning with a dosage of 1 *he*, and end when a weak feeling of **numbness** sets in". c) All types of phenomena including a blocked passage, mostly exchangeable with *bi* 閉 and *bi* 秘. *YXL* SE *gui* 桂：除咳逆, 結氣擁**痹**, "It eliminates cough with [qi rising] contrary to its normal direction, bound qi, and **blockages**".

***Bi* 躄, inability to walk** [5]

PC identical with → *wei bi* 痿躄, dysfunction with an inability to walk. *BJ* SE *wu jia pi* 五加皮：益氣療**躄**，小兒不能行, "It increases qi and cures **inability to walk**, when children cannot walk".

***Bi bing* 鼻病, nasal diseases** [2]

All types of PC affecting the nose. *ZHF* 8: 耳、**鼻病**，可以綿裹莽草膏塞之, "For ear and **nasal diseases** wrap the ointment with *mang cao* in silk and stuff into the [afflicted ear or nose]". *ZBYHL* 29 has a section on **鼻病**諸候, "All signs of **nasal diseases**".

***Bi gan* 鼻干, desiccated nose** [5]

IS of either a feeling of having a dry nose or of an appearance of the nose as if it contained no liquid. *SW* 31: 二日陽明受之，陽明主肉，其脈挾鼻絡於目，故身熱目疼而**鼻干**，不得臥也, "On the second day, the yang brilliance [conduits] receive it. The yang brilliance rules the flesh; its vessels line the nose on both sides and enclose the eyes. Hence, the body is hot, the eyes are painful, and the **nose is desiccated**. One cannot lie down".

***Bi gan* 鼻疳, nasal *gan*-illness** [7]

PC of → *gan chuang* 疳瘡, *gan*-illness sores, with redness and itching in the nose, and affecting the region between nose and lips. In severe cases mouth and teeth turn red and fester. *TPSHF* 87: 鼻中赤癢，壯熱多啼，皮毛干焦，肌膚消瘦，咳嗽上氣，下痢無恆，鼻下連唇生於赤爛，故名**鼻疳**也, "Nasal redness and itching. Strong heat and much weeping. Skin and hair are scorched. Muscles and skin wane and are emaciated. Cough with rising qi. Irregular discharge with free-flux illness. The region from the nose to the lips turns red and festers. Hence this is called '**nasal *gan*-illness**'".

Bi han **痹寒, blocking cold** [1]
PC identical with → *han bi* 寒痹, cold blockage. *MYBL* SE *shu er* 鼠耳：主**痹寒**，寒熱，止咳, "It controls **blocking cold** and alternating sensations of cold and heat, and stops cough".

Bi hong **鼻洪, nose flood** [13]
PC of profuse → *bi nü* 鼻衄②, nosebleed. *SLBC* SE *chuan di tai* 船底苔：治**鼻洪**吐血，淋疾, "It cures **nose flood**, blood spitting, and drippling ailments".

Bi huan **痹緩, blockage with slackening** [1]
IS identical with → *bi ruan* 痹軟. *PJF* 155: 萆薢丸，治丈夫腰脚**痹緩**，急行不穩, "Pills with *bi jie* cure males experiencing **blockage with slackening** affecting lumbar region and legs. When they walk fast, they are unable to walk steadily".

Bi ji **痹疾, blockage ailment** [2]
PC identical with → *bi* 痹, blockage. *SYDXF* 13: 兼治**痹疾**，半身麻木, "It also cures **blockage ailments**, with one half of the body turned [numb like] hemp and logs".

Bi jie **閉結, closed and bound** [7]
IS, PC identical with → *bian bi* 便閉, constipation. *SJZL* 47: "腹中痛楚，時復冷滑，或即**閉結**, "There is a feeling of pain in the abdomen. There may be a repeated feeling of cold, with smooth [diarrhea]. In some cases [stool] may be **closed and bound**".

Bi liang beng dao **鼻梁崩倒, nose beam collapse** [1]
IS of an inversion of the nose beam resulting from a fracture of the nasal bone. *SYDXF* 13: 大風惡疾，雙眼昏，咫尺不辨人物，髮眉自落，**鼻梁崩倒**，肌膚瘡如苔蘚，勢若不救, "In the case of the malign ailment of massive wind, vision of both eyes is dimmed. One cannot recognize others even at a very close distance. The hair and the eyebrows fall off by themselves. The **nose beam collapses**. The skin develops sores as if this were moss. It appears as if no intervention could bring relief".

Bi long **閉癃, closure with protuberance-illness** [1]
PC identical with → *long* 癃 a), protuberance-illness. *LS* 2: 實則**閉癃**，虛則遺溺, "Repletion leads to **closure with protuberance-illness**; depletion brings forth [involuntary] loss of urine".

Bi luan **痹攣, blockage cramps** [1]
IS of numbness together with cramps. *QJYF* 7: 石斛酒，治風虛氣滿，脚痛**痹攣**，弱不能行方, "Wine with *shi hu*, a recipe to cure wind [intruding into a state of] depletion and qi fullness, with pain and **blockage cramps** affecting one's legs, and resulting in weakness and an inability to move". However, in the *BCGM* this term is documented only as a result of what may be a copying error: *BCGM* 百病主治藥 quoting *YXL* Ma bo zhu zhi 麻勃主治：一百二十種惡風，黑色遍身苦癢, "120 types of malign wind, the entire body assumes a dark complexion and suffers from itching", writes: 麻勃，一百二十種惡風，

黑色遍身苦**痹攣**, “*Ma bo*, [It cures] 120 types of malign wind, the entire body assumes a dark complexion with **blockage cramps**”.

***Bi mian zi feng* 鼻面紫風, purple-nose-and-face wind** [1]

PC identical with → *jiu zha* 酒齇, wine sediments. *BCGM* SE *shi liu huang* 石硫黃quoting *XMLF* 3: 面鼻生紫赤風刺癮疹, 俗呼為肺風者, “Face and nose grow purple-red wind thorns and hidden papules. A colloquial term is 'lung wind'”, speaks of **鼻面紫風, purple-nose-and-face wind**”. and defines it as resulting from 風熱上攻陽明經絡, “Wind heat rising and attacking yang brilliance conduits and network conduits”.

***Bi mu* 痹木, blockage [with numbness like a] log** [4] AN *mu bi* 木痹, log[-like numbness with] blockage.

IS identical with → *ma mu* 麻木, [numbness of] hemp and logs. *BCGM* SE *ji* 雞 quoting *QJYF* 13: 治頭風方, “Recipe to cure head wind”, writes: 頭風**痹木**, “Head wind and **blockage [with numbness like a] log**”.

***Bi ni* 鼻䘌, nose with hidden-worms** [2] AN *bi xia chi ni* 鼻下赤䘌, hidden worms with redness below the nose.

PC of → *ni* 䘌, hidden-worms, disease with redness and festering below both nostrils in children. *BCGM* SE *wo niu* 蝸牛 quoting *ZMML*: 小兒鼻下兩道赤者名曰䘌，亦名赤鼻疳, “When the two paths below the nose of children are red, this is called 'hidden worms'. Another name is 'red nose *gan*-illness'”. writes: 小兒**鼻䘌**：鼻下兩道赤色，有疳, “**Nose with hidden worms** in children: the two paths below the nose assume a red color. They have a *gan*-illness”.

***Bi nü* 鼻衄, nosebleed** [91]

① IS of nosebleed. *QJYF* 5: 小兒未滿百日傷寒，**鼻衄**，身熱，嘔逆, “When children are harmed by cold during the first one hundred days of their life, they [will suffer from] **nosebleed**, a hot body, and vomiting with counterflow”.

② PC of nosebleed. *ZBYHL* 29: 血氣俱熱，血隨氣發出於鼻，為**鼻衄**, “If both blood and qi are hot, the blood will follow the qi and leave through the nose. This is **nosebleed**”.

***Bi qi* 痹氣, blocked qi** [6]

PC a) identical with → *bi* 痹①, blockage. *LS* 7: 病**痹氣**，痛而不去者，取以毫針, “If someone suffers from **blocked qi** with pain that fails to go away, remove it with the fine needle”. b) DC of conditions brought forth by sluggish qi and blood stasis, with a cold body as characteristic sign. *SW* 34: 是人多**痹氣**也，陽氣少，陰氣多，故身寒如從水中出, “This person has much **blocked qi**. [His] yang qi is diminished; [his] yin qi is present in large quantities. Hence, the body is as cold as if it had just come out of water”.

***Bi qiu* 鼻鼽, nasal congestion** [3]

PC with profuse snivel flow accompanied by nasal congestion. *QJYF* 30: 至陰、通谷，主**鼻鼽**清涕出, “[Piercing the holes] *zhi yin* and *tong gu* controls **nasal congestion** with clear snivel flow”.

Bi re **痹熱, blockage with heat** [1]

PC identical with → *re bi* 熱痹, heat blockage. *MYBL* SE *wu yu* 烏芋：主消渴，**痹熱**，温中益氣, "It controls melting with thirst and **blockage with heat**, warms the center and increases qi".

Bi ruan **痹軟, blockage with slackening** [3]

IS of slackening and loss of strength resulting from a → *bi bing*, 痹病, blockage disease. *BCGM* SE bi jie 萆薢 quoting *ZYGLF*: 療丈夫腰脚痹，緩急，行履不穩者, "It heals males experiencing blockages affecting the lumbar region and legs, with alternating episodes of slackening and tension, so that they are unable to walk steadily", writes: 腰脚**痹軟**，行履不穩者, "Lumbar region and legs experience **blockage with slackening**; patients are unable to walk steadily".

Bi ruo **痹弱, blockage with weakness** [7]

IS of pain, numbness, and slackening. *MYBL* SE shi hu 石斛：逐皮膚邪熱痱氣，脚膝疼冷**痹弱**, "It eliminates from the skin evil heat and prickly heat qi, and it relieves legs and knees from pain, cold, and **blockage with weakness**".

Bi sai **鼻塞, nasal congestion** [33] AN *bi zhi* 鼻窒.

① IS of blocked nasal ducts impairing the passage of air. *LS* 8: 肺氣虚則**鼻塞**不利，少氣, "Lung qi depletion causes **nasal congestion**. [The nose is] not open and [patients are] short of qi".

② PC with nasal congestion. *ZBYHL* 48: 氣不宣和，結聚不通，故**鼻塞**也, "When the qi is not spread harmoniously, it will form nodular collections and blockage the passage. Hence there is **nasal congestion**".

Bi se **閉塞, closure** [19]

① IS a) identical with → *da bian mi* 大便秘, constipation. *ZBYHL* 14: 龜行氣，伏衣被中，覆口鼻頭面，正臥，不息九通，微鼻出氣，治**閉塞**不通, "The turtle passes the qi: one lies down burying the face in one's clothes or bedding. Mouth, nose, head, and face are to be covered. One lies straight as if sleeping, and holds the breath nine times. Only very tiny quantities of qi are allowed to leave the nose. This cures [intestinal] **closure** with a failure [of stools] to pass". b) Identical with → *xiao bian bu tong* 小便不通, blocked urination. *YXFM* 2: 大渴引飲，小便淋瀝或**閉塞**不通，脛酸脚熱，此通草主之, "If one is very thirsty and drinks large quantities of liquid, and experiences urinary dripping or **closure** with a complete failure to pass, aching shins and hot legs, this can be controlled by *tong cao*". c) Swelling of the throat inhibiting a patient's ability to breathe or swallow. *WTMY* 2: 集驗療傷寒熱病，喉中痛，**閉塞**不通，烏扇膏方, "The *JiY(F)* cures febrile diseases such as harm caused by cold, pain in the throat, with **closure** and no passage possible, with the recipe for an ointment with *wu fan*".

② PM including all types of pathological processes of closure and blockage of passages. *ZBYHL* 14: 陽盛而外熱者，上焦不通利，皮膚緻密，腠理**閉塞**不通，衛氣不得泄越，故外熱也, "When yang [qi] abounds and there is external heat, the upper burner is not passable, the skin is very tight, with **closure** of the interstice structures and no passage possible, and the guardian qi is unable to flow off. Hence this results in external heat".

***Bi shang zha bao* 鼻上皻皰, sediment blisters on the nose** [1]
PC identical with → *jiu zha* 酒皻, wine sediments. *BCGM* SE *hu shi* 槲實 quotes *TPSHF*: 鼻上皻皰，出膿血者，以泔水煮槲葉，取汁洗之，拭乾，納槲葉灰少許於中，良, "For **sediment blisters on the nose** releasing pus and blood boil the leaves of *hu* with water from washing rice, use the liquid to wash [the blisters], rub them dry, and insert a small amount of a *hu*-leaves ashes into them. Good".

***Bi shi* 鼻蝕, nasal erosion** [1]
PC with a festering nose as major sign. *BCGM* SE *xiong* 熊 quoting *TPSHF* 87: 治小兒疳瘡蟲蝕鼻, "It cures children with *gan*-illness sores and bugs/worms eroding their nose", writes: 小兒**鼻蝕**, "**Nasal erosion** in children".

***Bi shi* 痹濕, blockage with moisture** [2]
PC identical with → *shi bi* 濕痹. *YXL* SE *wu jia pi* 五加皮：治**痹濕**，內不足, "It cures **blockage with moisture**, with an insufficiency of internal [qi]".

***Bi tong* 痹痛, blockage with pain** [37]
IS of a feeling of pain associated with some kind of an obstruction, or pain together with numbness. *BJ* SE *yin yu* 茵芋：諸關節風濕**痹痛**, "[It controls] all types of wind and moisture [causing] a **blockage with pain** in one's joints".

***Bi wai zha liu* 鼻外皻瘤, sediment tumor outside the nose** [1]
PC identical with → *jiu zha* 酒皻, wine sediments. *BCGM* SE *lu feng fang* 露蜂房 quotes *ZHF*: **鼻外皻瘤**，膿水血出。蜂房炙研，酒服方寸匕，日三服, "For **sediment tumors outside the nose**: Roast and grind the beehive and ingest the amount on a square inch spoon. Ingest three times a day".

***Bi weng* 鼻齆, nasal congestion** [6]
PC identical with → *weng bi* 齆鼻, stuffed nose. *MYBL* SE *gui* 桂：止煩止唾，咳嗽**鼻齆**, "It stops vexation and saliva, cough and **nasal congestion**".

***Bi xi* 鼻瘜, nasal tumor-illness** [1]
PC of → *xi rou* 息肉, tumorous fleshgrowths, inside the nostrils. *BCGM* 百病主治藥 quoting *QJYF*: 鼻中息肉, "Tumorous flesh-growth in the nose", writes: **鼻瘜**, "**Nasal tumor-illness**".

***Bi xi* 鼻息, nasal tumorous [flesh-growth]** [3]
PC identical with → *bi xi* 鼻瘜. *BCGM* SE *shi hu sui* 石胡荽：塞**鼻息**，自落，又散瘡腫, "It is to be stuck [into the nose to cause] **tumorous [flesh-growth]** to fall off by themselves, and in addition it disperses sores with swelling".

***Bi xia chi ni* 鼻下赤䘌, hidden-worms with redness below the nose** [1]
PC identical with → *bi ni* 鼻䘌, nose with hidden-worms. *BCGM* Bai bing zhu zhi yao 百病主治藥：黃連同大黃、麝香搽鼻中。末，傅**鼻下赤䘌**, "Apply *huang lian* together with *da huang* and *she xiang* to the inside of the nose. The pulver is applied to **hidden-worms with redness below the nose**".

***Bi xue* 鼻血, nosebleed** [19]
① IS identical with *bi nü* 鼻衄①. *BCTJ* SE *guan zhong* 貫眾：取根為末，水調服一錢匕，止**鼻血**有效, "Prepare a powder from its root and ingest, mixed

with water, a spoonful in the quantity of 1 *qian*. It is effective for stopping **nosebleed**".

② PC identical with → *bi nü* 鼻衄②. *SYDXF* 7: 蘇子降氣湯，治虛壅**鼻血**, "The decoction with *su zi* to bring the qi down cures depletion and obstruction accompanied by **nosebleed**".

***Bi xue* 閉血, blocked [menstrual] blood** [2]

PC identical with → *xue bi* 血閉, [menstrual] blood blockage. *BJ* SE *qu mai* 瞿麥：破胎墮子，下**閉血**, "It breaks a fetus and causes abortion. It brings down **blocked [menstrual] blood**".

***Bi yang* 痹癢, blockage with itching** [2]

IS of a feeling of numbness together with itching. *BCGM* Bai bing zhu zhi yao 百病主治藥 quoting *SLBC* SE *wu zhu yu* 吳茱萸：風瘙癢痛, "Wind causing itching and pain", writes: 頑風**痹癢**, "Stubborn wind causing **blockage with itching**".

***Bi yuan* 鼻淵, nasal deep-source [outflow]** [16] AN *nao xie* 腦瀉, brain efflux; *nao xie* 腦泄; *nao beng* 腦崩, brain collapse; *nao lou* 腦漏, brain leakage; *kong nao sha* 控腦砂, grit impacting the brain; *nao xuan* 腦宣, brain spread.

PC with much snivel that is malodorous, dirty and turbid, or resembles yellow liquid. SW 37: **鼻淵**者，濁涕下不止也, "As for '**nasal deep-source [outflow]**', that is turbid snivel flowing down without end".

***Bi zha* 鼻齇, nose sediments** [1]

PC identical with → *jiu zha* 酒齇, wine sediments. *BCGM* SE li shi 蠡實 quoting *ZHF*: 治面及鼻病酒皶, 以馬藺子花杵傅之，佳, "To treat facial and nasal disease and wine sediments, externally applying *ma li* seeds and flowers is excellent", writes: 面皰**鼻齇**，馬藺子花杵傅之佳, "For facial blister illness and **nose sediments**, pound *ma li* seeds and flowers and apply externally. Excellent".

***Bi zhang* 鼻張, flaring nostrils** [2]

IS of the alar wings of the nose widening towards outside, often associated with panting. *QJYF* 17: 麻黄引氣湯，治肺勞實，氣喘**鼻張**，面目苦腫方, "The 'decoction with *ma huang* to guide the qi' cures lung exhaustion-repletion, with qi panting and **flaring nostrils**, as well as face and eyes suffering from swelling".

***Bi zhi* 鼻窒, nasal congestion** [9]

IS, PC identical with → *bi sai* 鼻塞. *MYBL* SE *yi weng* 蠮螉：療**鼻窒**, "It cures **nasal congestion**".

***Bi zhong* 痹腫, blockage with swelling** [2]

PC identical with → *zhong bi* 腫痹②, swelling with blockage. *ZHF* 8: 並癱瘓不隨，風濕痹不仁，偏枯拘屈口喎，耳聾，齒痛，頭風，**痹腫**，腦中風動, "Simultaneous paralysis on the left and right, wind and moisture blockage with numbness, hemilateral cramps with wry mouth, deafness, toothache, head wind, **blockage with swelling**: wind moving in the brain".

***Bian bi* 便閉, relief closed, constipation** [13]

① IS a) mostly identical with → *da bian mi* 大便秘①, constipation. *QXLF* 54: 瘡科通治方，治諸熱腫，一切風熱瘡證，發熱多汗，大渴**便閉**，"Cure-all recipe in the discipline of sores [therapy]. It cures all types of heat with swelling, all sores as signs of wind heat, with an effusion of heat and copious sweating, massive thirst, and **constipation**". b) Occasionally the *BCGM* refers to 便閉, constipation, as blockage of both stools and urine. *BCGM* Bai bing zhu zhi yao 百病主治藥, Xiao er chu sheng zhu bing 小兒初生諸病, "Diseases of newborn children": **便閉**：胡麻油，初生大小便不通，入芒消少許，煎沸，徐灌即通, "**Constipation**: *hu ma* oil for newborn children with a failure to pass stools and urine. Add a little *mang xiao* and boil until it bubbles. Gently force into the [child's] mouth. This will open the passage".

② PC identical with → *da bian mi* 大便秘②, constipation. *PJF* 138: **便閉**者，大承氣湯下之, "In the case of **constipation**, the 'decoction to massively uphold qi' will bring it down".

***Bian du* 便毒, poison [in the region] of relief** [33] AN *bian yong* 便癰, obstruction-illness in the [region of urination and defecation] relief.

PC of swelling with poison developing in the body region associated with functions of 'minor relief', i.e. urination, and 'major relief', i.e. defecation. *SYDXF* 9: 治**便毒**腫結，因敗精搏血留聚而成, "It cures **poison [in the region] of relief** with swelling and nodes that have developed because of collections resulting from a clash of decayed essence/semen with blood".

***Bian mi* 便秘, relief closed; constipation** [2]

IS identical with → *da bian mi* 大便秘①, constipation. *QJYF* 13: 小兒則**便秘**、口重舌鵝口、聲嘶, "In children it manifests itself as **constipation**, a heavy tongue and goose-mouth, as well as a hoarse voice".

***Bian nan* 便難, relief with difficulty; difficult defecation** [3] AW *da bian nan* 大便難, *da bian se* 大便澀, *da bian nan se* 大便難澀, *da bian jian nan* 大便艱難，*bian se* 便澀.

IS of an urge to defecate that goes along with great difficulties in relieving oneself. *NWSBHL* Mj: 脈弦，四肢滿，**便難**而心下痞, "The [movement in the] vessels is string-like. The four extremities have a feeling of fullness. **Defecation is difficult**, with an obstacle-illness located below the heart".

***Bian ni yi shi* 便溺遺失, uncontrolled [major] relief and loss of urine; incontinence** [1]

IS of uncontrollable discharge of stool and/or urine. *SWBJQYBMJ* Fj: 開腸洞泄，**便溺遺失**，必澀劑以收之, "It opens the intestines and causes outflow, resulting in **stool and urine incontinence**. This requires the intake of astringent remedies to hold [the outflow]".

***Bian nong xue* 便膿血, relief with pus and blood; defecation with pus and blood** [5] AN *xia nong xue* 下膿血, discharge of pus and blood; *xie xue nong* 泄血膿, outflow with pus and blood.

IS of feces carrying pus and blood. *JGYL* Mj 下利，**便膿血**者，桃花湯主之, "In the case of free-flux illness, when **defecation** occurs **with pus and blood**, a decoction with *tao hua* will master this".

Bian se **便澀, relief with roughness; rough defecation** [1]

IS identical with → *bian nan* 便難, difficult defecation. *BCGM* SE *xi xin* 細辛：通少陰及耳竅，**便澀**者宜用之, "It penetrates the minor yin [conduits] and the ear-orifices. It is suitable for [treating] **rough defecation**".

Bian shu **便數, frequent relief; frequent urination** [2]

IS identical with → *xiao bian shuo* 小便數. *BCGM* Bai bing zhu zhi yao 百病主治藥：溲數遺尿, *sou shuo yi niao*: 茴香，止**便數**, "*Hui xiang* ends **frequent urination**".

Bian tang **便溏, relief of viscous liquid; viscous defecation** [3]

IS identical with → *tang xie* 溏泄①, semiliquid outflow. *SHL* 229: 陽明病，發潮熱、大**便溏**、小便自可、胸脅滿不去者，與小柴胡湯, "For diseases of the yang brilliance [conduit], with tidal fever, **viscous defecation**, normal urination, and a feeling of fullness in the chest and flanks that does not subside, give the 'minor decoction with *chai hu*'".

Bian xue **便血, relief with blood; stools with blood** [27]

① IS identical with → *xie xue* 瀉血, blood outflow. *SW* 7: 結陰者，**便血**一升, "In the case of bound yin [qi], **the stools have** one pint of **blood**".

② PC with bloody stools. *SYJY BZFL* 9: 病者大便下血，或清或濁，或鮮或黑，或在便前，或在便後，或與泄物並下，此由內外有所感傷，凝停在胃，隨氣下通，亦妄行之類，故曰**便血**, "The patients' stool has blood. It may be clear or turbid, it may be fresh or dark. It may leave prior to or following defecation, or it may pass down together with other outflow. The reason is always an internal harm. As a result [blood] coagulates and stays in the stomach from where it is passed downward together with the qi. It belongs to the group of disorderly movements. Hence one speaks of '**stools with blood**'".

Bian yong **便癰, obstruction-illness [in the region] of [urination and defecation] relief** [6] AN *xue shan* 血疝, blood elevation-illness.

PC identical with → *bian du* 便毒, poison [in the region] of relief. *RMSQ* 4: 言於大便處害一癰，故名**便癰**也, "That is to say: a harmful obstruction-illness at the location where major relief takes place (i.e. defecation). Hence it is called '**obstruction-illness [in the region] of relief**'".

Biao chuang **熛瘡, flaming-heat sores** [4] AW → *biao chuang* 瘭瘡, flaming-heat-illness sores. AN → *chi biao* 赤熛, red flaming heat.

PC identical with → *re chuang* 熱瘡, heat sores. *ZBYHL* 50: 為風熱毒氣所傷，客於皮膚，生熛漿，而潰成瘡，名為**熛瘡**也, "If one is harmed by the poison qi of wind and heat, it will settle in the skin and generate thick flame liquid which then festers and generates sores. They are called **flaming-heat sores**".

Biao chuang **瘭瘡, flaming-heat-illness sores** [3]

PC identical with → *biao chuang* 熛瘡, flaming-heat sores. *BCGM* SE *wu zhu yu* 吳茱萸 quoting *BBSJ*: 小兒**瘭瘡**：一名火灼瘡，一名火爛瘡。茱萸煎酒，拭之良, "**Flaming-heat-illness sores** in children: another name is 'sores following scorching by fire'. Another name is 'festering fire sores'. Prepare a wine decoction with *zhu yu* and rub the [afflicted regions with it]. Good".

Biao ju **瘭疽, flaming-heat-illness with impediment-illness** [23]
PC CD of → *ju* 疽, impediment-illnesses, initially emerging like a bean kernel from which a root reaches into the depth of the tissue. This is associated with extreme pain. It slowly increases in size and generates several tips filled with pus that look like clusters of rice grains. The surface of the sores is purple-black, and the pus does not come out unimpeded. They often develop on the back of hands and feet. *ZHF* 5: 忽得**瘭疽**著手足肩，累累如米豆，刮汁出，急療之, "If suddenly one develops **flaming-heat-illness with impediment-illness** on the back of his hands and/or feet, clustered like grains of rice or beans, it must be opened to let the sap come out. One must act quickly to cure this". *BCGM* Bai bing zhu zhi yao 百病主治藥：皂莢灰、田螺、鯽魚同亂髮、豬脂熬膏，並傅**瘭疽**, "Mix *zao jia* ashes, *tian luo*, and *ji yu*, and boil with dishevelled hair and lard to prepare a paste. This is to be externally applied to **flaming-heat-illness with impediment-illness**".

Biao xu **表虛, exterior depletion** [7]
PC of an insufficiency of yang qi guarding the body's external sections, with the interstitial structures being loose and relaxed, leading to sweating or to festering papules. *SHL* 218: 沉為在里，而反發其汗，津液越出，大便為難，**表虛**里實, "A deep [movement in the vessels means the disease is in the] interior. If nevertheless sweating is induced body liquids will stray outward and major relief (defecation) becomes difficult. This is, therefore, a situation of **exterior depletion** and interior repletion".

Bie jia **鱉瘕, turtle[-shaped] conglomeration-illness** [23]
PC of → *jia* 瘕, conglomeration-illness, in the abdomen that is shaped like a turtle and moves if squeezed. It was believed that such a condition could result from eating turtles. *ZBYHL* 19: **鱉瘕**者，謂腹中瘕結如鱉狀是也, " '**Turtle[-shaped] conglomeration-illness**'; that is to say: these are conglomeration-illness nodes in the abdomen that have the shape of a turtle".

Bie zheng **鱉癥, turtle[-shaped] concretion-illness** [5]
PC of *zheng* → 癥, concretions that are shaped like a turtle. It was believed that the formation of such concretions resulted from eating turtles. *ZBYHL* 19: **鱉癥**者，謂腹內癥結如鱉之形狀, " '**Turtle[-shaped] concretion-illness**' is to say: concretion-illness nodes in the abdomen with the shape of a turtle".

Bing mu **病目, diseased eye** [6]
PC identical with → *mu ji* 目疾, ailments of the eyes. *RMSQ* 1: **病目**百餘日，羞明隱澀，腫痛不已, "Suffered from a **diseased eye** for more than one hundred days, with photophobia and hidden roughness, swelling and pain that would not end".

Bing wen **病温, warmth disease** [1]
PC identical with → *wen bing*, 温病, warmth disease. *SW* 4: 藏於精者，春不病温, "If essence is stored, there will be no **warmth disease** in spring".

Bo niu ji **伯牛疾, Bo Niu's ailment** [1]
PC referring to the lethal ailment of Confucius' disciple Bo Niu as mentioned in Confucius' *Analects*, Bk. VI, ch. 8. Later commentators have identified it as either *e ji* 惡疾, malign ailment, or → *lai* 癩, repudiation-illness, both terms presumably used for leprosy. *BCJJZ* SE *ran she dan* 蚺蛇膽：真膏多所入藥用，亦云能療**伯牛疾**, "Its genuine paste is often used in medications. It is also said to be able to cure **Bo Niu's ailment**".

Bu de da bian **不得大便, inability to achieve major relief; constipation** [1]
PC of → *da bian mi* 大便秘①, constipation. *WTMY* 27: 備急**不得大便**，或十日一月方, "Recipe from the *Bei ji* for **constipation** lasting from ten days to one month".

Bu de mian **不得眠, inability to sleep** [20]
IS, PC identical with → *bu mian* 不眠. *SHL* 71: 胃中干，煩躁**不得眠**, "Dryness in the stomach with vexation and **inability to sleep**".

Bu de wo **不得臥, inability to sleep; inability to lie down** [16]
IS a) identical with → *bu mian* 不眠①, inability to sleep. *SHL* 303: 心中煩，**不得臥**，黃連阿膠湯主之, "If one experiences vexation in the heart and is **unable to sleep**, a decoction with *huang lian* and *a jiao* will master this". b) A condition of panting with an inability to lie flat. *SW* 34: 夫**不得臥**，臥則喘者，是水氣之客也, "Now, when someone is **unable to lie down** and when, if he lies down, he pants, this is a case of water qi settling as a visitor".

Bu li **不利, not freely passable; impeded** [42]
IS of diminished or blocked functions of the organism. *SW* 5: 年六十，陰痿，氣大衰，九竅**不利**，下虛上實，涕泣俱出矣, "At the age of sixty, the yin (i.e. the sexual organ) [reaches a state of] dysfunction. The qi is severely weakened and the nine orifices are **no** [longer] **freely passable**. Below is depletion; above is repletion. Both snivel and tears are released".

Bu liao liao **不了了, not entirely finished yet** [2]
IS of all types of feeling not well. *SHL* 10: 風家，表解而**不了了**者，十二日愈, "Wind patients: if the exterior has been resolved but [the patient's feeling sick] is **not entirely finished yet**, this will be healed within twelve days".

Bu lu **哺露, breastfeeding-period emaciation** [2]
PC of → *gan* 疳, *gan*-illness, with emaciation, desiccation, abdominal fullness, vexation, and heat . *ZBYHL* 74: 血氣減損，不榮肌肉，而柴辟羸露，其腑臟之不宣，則嗡嗡苦熱，謂之**哺露**也, "When blood and qi are diminished and harmed, and cannot nourish muscles and flesh any longer, with emaciation to the bones and the depots and palaces fail to transmit, and eventually one has a slight feeling of heat, this is called '**breastfeeding-period emaciation**'".

Bu mian **不眠, inability to sleep; insomnia** [28] AN *bu de mian* 不得眠.
① IS of a difficulty to find sleep when it is sleeping time, or waking up again shortly after having fallen asleep. In extreme cases, lying awake all night. *QJYF* 5: 哺食減少，氣息不快，夜啼**不眠**, "It eats less, and breathing is uncomfortable. It cries at night and **cannot sleep**".

② PC of a disease with insomnia. *SJZL* 42, section Dan men 膽門, lists the condition 膽虛**不眠**, gallbladder depletion with **insomnia**.

Bu neng ru **不能乳, inability to take breast-milk** [4]
IS of children who cannot be breast-fed because of a disease or pain. *TPSHF* 82: 小兒鵝口，**不能乳**方, "Recipe for children with goose-mouth and an **inability to take breast-milk**".

Bu neng yan **不能言, inability to speak** [15]
IS identical with → *bu yu* 不語①, speechlessness. *ZHF* 1: 卒忤停屍，**不能言**者，桔梗燒二枚，末之，服, "If suddenly one encounters something hostile and turns into an immobile corpse, and **cannot speak**, [take] two pieces of roasted *jie geng*, grind to a powder and ingest".

Bu neng yu **不能語, inability to speak** [6]
IS identical with → *bu yu* 不語①, speechlessness. *ZBYHL* 48: **不能語**者，語聲不出，非牙關噤也, "If someone is **unable to speak**, [that is,] he fails to produce speech sounds, this is not a case of clenched teeth".

Bu neng yuan shi **不能遠視, inability to see into the distance; shortsightedness** [3]
PC with distant objects appearing unclear as major sign. *ZBYHL* 28: 精華之氣衰弱，故**不能遠視**, "The essence qi is weak. Hence one **cannot see into the distance**".

Bu ren **不仁, insensitivity; numbness** [44]
IS of a diminuition or complete loss of the skin's and tissue's sensitivity, so that one is unable to feel cold or heat, pain or itching. *SW* 34: 榮氣虛則**不仁**，衛氣虛則不用, "Depletion of camp qi results in **insensitivity**. Depletion of guardian qi results in loss of function".

Bu ru **不乳, failure to accept breast-milk** [16]
① AN *bu xia ru* 不下乳, failure to ingest breast-milk. IS of children who do not drink breast-milk. *QJYF* 卷 15: 治少小下痢，苦熱不食，傷飽**不乳**方, "Recipe to cure discharge with free-flux illness of very young children, when they suffer from heat and fail to eat, with harm from satiation and **failure to accept breast-milk**".
② PC CD of conditions among children who do not take breast-milk. *BCGM* Bai bing zhu zhi yao 百病主治藥：小兒初生諸病：沐浴、解毒、便閉、無皮、不啼、**不乳**、吐乳，目閉，血眼, "All diseases of newborns: [they are to be] washed and poison is to be dissolved; [they may suffer from] constipation, absence of skin, failure to cry, **failure to accept breast milk**, spitting of breast milk, closed eyes, blood eyes, [etc.]".

Bu shi ren **不識人, failure to recognize persons; unconsciousness** [20]
IS identical with → *bu sheng ren shi* 不省人事, failure to recognize persons or items. *ZHF* 8: 口不能言，冒昧**不識人**, "[Patients] cannot speak. They are benighted and **fail to recognize persons**".

Bu shou **不收, inability to contract; failure to receive** [45]
IS of a) limbs and trunk, joints and sinews that are slack and have no strength so that they cannot be moved. 肢體、關節、筋脈緩弱無力，不任動作。*SW* 69:

甚則肌肉萎，足痿**不收**, “If [the excess of the qi of soil] is severe, the muscles and the flesh decay. The legs become dysfunctional and **cannot be contracted**”. b) Body organs that irrevocably descend from their regular position. *TPSHF* 86: 瀉痢頻並，下部開張，肛門**不收**, “Diarrhea and free-flux illness frequently occur together. The [body's] lower parts open and distend. The anus [prolapse] **cannot be contracted**”. c) Inability to control the “essence spirit”, i.e. mental disorder. *ZZJ* Fj: 精神**不收**，此五臟之虛也, “When the essence spirit **cannot be held together**, this is because of a depletion of the five depots”. d) An inability of the eyes to collect light and to see things clearly. *YJQW* Fj: 久則光**不收**，遂為廢疾, “After an extended period of time [the eyes] **do not receive** light. This results in a disability ailment”. e) Wounds unable to close and heal properly by themselves. *WKLL* 3: 兩月餘氣血復而瘡亦愈，但一口**不收**, “Over a period of more than two months qi and blood recovered and the wounds healed too. Only one opening **failed to contract”.**

Bu shui **不睡, inability to sleep** [19]

① IS, PC identical with → *bu mian* 不眠, insomnia. *BCSY* SE *ku zhu sun* 苦竹筍：主**不睡**，去面目並舌上熱黃, “It controls **inability to sleep** and removes heat yellowness from face, eyes and tongue”.

② TE of preventing a person from falling asleep. *MYBL* SE *ma* 馬：頭骨，主喜眠，令人**不睡**, “Its skull bones master an inclination to sleep; they make people **unable to sleep**”.

Bu sui **不隨, paralyzed; [body parts] do not follow [one's will]** [20]

IS identical with → *bu sui* 不遂. *ZBYHL* 1: 其狀半身**不隨**，肌肉偏枯, “Its appearance is such that one half of the body **does not follow [one's will].** Muscles and flesh wither on their own”.

Bu sui **不遂, paralyzed; [body parts] do not follow [one's will]** [60]

AW 不隨. IS of an inability of any body part to move according to one's will. *JGYL* Fj 夫風之為病，當半身**不遂**。或但臂**不遂**者，此為痹, “In the case of diseases caused by wind, if one half of the body **does not follow [one's will]**, with sometimes only an arm **not following [one's will]**, this is blockage”.

Bu ti **不啼, failure to cry** [4]

PC with the inability of a newborn to immediately cry. *YYXS* 4: 若**不啼**，灸至五七壯，灸了以封臍散封之, “When it **fails to cry** cauterize five to seven times. Once cauterized cover it with the ‘powder to cover the umbilicus’”.

Bu wu **不寤, failure to awake** [5]

IS of a difficulty to awake from sleep. *ZHF* 1: 臥忽**不寤**，勿以火照, “If unexpectedly someone **fails to awake** from sleep, do not shine light at him”.

Bu xia ru **不下乳, failure to ingest breast-milk** [1]

IS identical with → *bu ru* 不乳①, failure to take breast-milk. *YXL* SE *rou dou kou* 肉豆蔻：能主小兒吐逆，**不下乳**, “It can master vomiting with counterflow, and **failure to ingest breast-milk**, among children”.

Bu xing ren 不省人, failure to recognize persons; unconsciousness [3]

IS identical with → *bu xing ren shi* 不省人事, failure to recognize persons or items. *BCYY* preface, final section: 此胃中有結熱，故昏瞀**不省人**, "In this case there is bound heat in the stomach. Hence [patients] experience a clouding with dim vision and a **failure to recognize people**".

Bu xing ren shi 不省人事, failure to recognize persons or items; unconsciousness [26] AN *bu zhi ren shi* 不知人事, not to recognize persons or items; *bu zhi ren* 不知人, not to recognize persons; *bu shi ren* 不識人; *bu sheng ren* 不省人.

IS of derangement with a failure to recognize even persons that are close to oneself, or to identify simple items. *TPSHF* 22: 治急風，**不省人事**，宜服雄黃散方, "To cure acute wind with a **failure to recognize people or items**, the recipe to ingest the powder with *xiong huang* is advisable".

_Bu yu_ 不語, speechlessness [90]

① AN *bu neng yan* 不能言; *bu neng yu* 不能語; *yu yan nan chu* 語言難出, impeded speech. PC of an inability to speak brought forth by either mental blockage, diseases affecting the throat, or any other cause. *QJYF* 8: 卒半身不遂，手足拘急不得屈伸，身體冷，或智或痴，或身強直**不語**, "Suddenly one half of the body no longer follows [one's will]. Hands and feet cramp and are tense, and cannot be stretched or bent. In some cases [patients] are conscious, in others not. Sometimes the body is stiff and straight and [patients] **do not speak**".

② PC of children who after completing their third year are still unable to open their mouth and learn how to speak. *QJYF* 5: 治小兒四五歲**不語**方, "Recipe to cure children who at the age of four, five years **do not speak**".

Bu yun 不孕, failure to become pregnant; infertility [3]

① PC identical with → *jue yun* 絕孕①, barred from pregnancy. *SW* 60: 其女子**不孕**，癃痔遺溺, "In females [this disease] **prevents them from becoming pregnant**. [Also, it leads to] protuberance-illness, piles, and [involuntary] loss of urine".

② Identical with → *jue yun* 絕孕②. *BCGM* SE *ma bing lang* 馬檳榔 quotes Wang Ji 汪機：欲斷產者，常嚼二枚，水下。久則子宮冷，自**不孕**矣, "Those who wish to be sterilized should constantly chew two pieces and ingest them with water. After some time, their uterus will be cold. This results in a **failure to become pregnant**".

Bu zhi ren 不知人, failure to recognize persons; unconsciousness [20]

IS identical with → *bu xing ren shi* 不省人事, failure to recognize persons or objects. *BJ* SE *bai wei* 白微：主暴中風，身熱肢滿，忽忽**不知人**, "It controls violent wind stroke, with the body being hot and the limbs giving a feeling of fullness, as well as sudden **failure to recognize persons**".

Bu zhi ren shi 不知人事, failure to recognize persons or items; unconsciousness [7]

IS identical with → *bu xing ren shi* 不省人事. *WTMY* 33 lists 產難，母如死，**不知人事**方, "Recipes for difficult births, when the mother seems to be dead and **fails to recognize persons or objects**".

- C -

***Cao za* 嘈雜, noises** [12]

IS of an uncomfortable vacuity in the stomach, with a feeling of hunger although one is not hungry, and a sensation of pain although there is no pain. *PJBSF* 7: 每覺心中多**嘈雜**，意謂飲作，又疑是蟲, "Whenever one has a feeling of multiple **noises** in the heart (i.e. stomach), one may think this is caused by [the movement of] beverages, one may also hypothesize that bugs/worms are the cause".

***Cha ji* 茶積, tea accumulation** [2]

PC of → *shi ji* 食積②, food accumulation, brought forth by excessive consumption of tea or a chewing of tea leaves that harm spleen and stomach. *SYDXF* 3: 磨積丸，治**茶積**，飲食減少，面黄腹痛, "The 'pills that grind an accumulation' cure **tea accumulation**, with diminished ingestion of beverages and food, a yellow facial complexion, and abdominal pain".

***Chan chang bu shang* 產腸不上, failure of the birth intestine to ascend** [1]

PC identical with → *yin tuo* 陰脫, yin prolapse. *BCGM* SE *zhu tie qi* 諸鐵器：磨刀水，服，利小便，塗脫肛痔核，**產腸不上**, "The water used when grinding knives: ingested it stimulates urination. Apply to prolapse of the rectum, piles, and **birth intestine that fails to ascend**".

***Chan chang bu shou* 產腸不收, failure of the birth intestine to contract** [1]

PC identical with → *yin tuo* 陰脫, yin prolapse. *BCGM* SE *du huo* 獨活 quotes *DMF*: **產腸不收**：用油五斤，煉熟，盆盛。令婦坐盆中，飯久, "For **failure of the birth intestine to contract**: Take 5 *jin* oil, boil thoroughly on fire. Fill a basin with it and let the women sit in the basin for the length of a meal".

***Chan chang tuo chu* 產腸脫出, prolapse of the birth intestine (uterus)** [1]

PC identical with → *yin tuo* 陰脫, yin prolapse. *BCGM* SE *du huo* 獨活 quotes *ZMML*: **產腸脫出**：方同上, "**Prolapse of the birth intestine**: the same recipe as above".

***Chan chang tuo xia* 產腸脫下, prolapse of the birth intestine (uterus)** [1]

PC identical with → *yin tuo* 陰脫, yin prolapse. *BCGM* SE *shi suan* 石蒜 quotes *SYDXF*: **產腸脫下**：老鴉蒜即酸頭草一把，以水三碗，煎一碗半，去滓熏洗，神效, "For **prolapse of the birth intestine**: [take] 1 bundle of *lao ya suan*, i.e. *suan tou cao*, and boil in the amount of water filling 3 bowls down to 1.5 bowls. Discard the dregs and [use the liquid] for fumigation and rinsing. Wondrously effective".

***Chan chuang* 饞瘡, gluttony sores** [3]

PC of → *chuang* 瘡, sores, conditions that emerge on the lips or to the side of the mouth. *BCSY* SE *jia jian* 甲煎：三年者治蟲雜瘡及口旁**饞瘡**、甲疽等瘡, "With those [*jia jian*] that are three years old one may treat sores such as various bug-related sores and **gluttony sores** to the side of the mouth, as well as nails with impediment-illnesses".

Chan diao **顫掉, tremor; trembling** [7]

IS of uncontrolled trembling of hands and feet. *WTMY* 37: 四肢**顫掉**，若有失而悸, "The four limbs **tremble** as if one were greatly agitated because of a loss".

Chan fu pao sun **產婦脬損, damage to a delivering woman's bladder** [2] AN *chan shi shang pao* 產時傷脬, bladder damage at the time of birth; *sheng chan sun pao* 生產損脬, bladder damaged during delivery.

PC with a woman in the course of giving birth having her urinary tract or bladder injured with the result of dribbling urine. *BCGM* SE *juan* 絹 quotes *FRDQLF*: 婦人臨產時傷手胞破，小便不禁, "When a woman has the bladder broken by a [midwife's] hand at the time of delivery, her urine will flow unimpeded", writes: **產婦脬損**：小便淋瀝不斷, "A **delivering woman's bladder damage**: urine drips ceaselessly".

Chan hou bai xue chong xin **產後敗血衝心, rotten blood surging to the heart following delivery** [1]

PC identical with → *chan hou bai xue gong xin* 產後敗血攻心, rotten blood attacking the heart following delivery. *BCGM* SE *yu jin* 鬱金：治血氣心腹痛，**產後敗血衝心**欲死, "It cures pain in heart and abdomen because of blood and qi [stagnation], as well as **rotten blood surging to the heart following delivery** [causing pain so severe that patients] wish to die".

Chan hou bai xue gong xin **產後敗血攻心, rotten blood attacking the heart following delivery** [2] AN *chan hou bai xue ru xin* 產後敗血入心, rotten blood enters the heart following delivery; *chan hou bai chong xin* 產後敗血沖心, rotten [blood] surging to the heart following delivery; *yu xue qiang xin* 余血搶心, residual blood knocks the heart.

PC CD of all types of diseases with vexation and restlessness, distension and heart-pressure, or in severe cases even mental clouding and mad language as their major signs. *BCTJ* SE *jiang huang* 薑黃：蜀人以治氣脹及**產後敗血攻心**，甚驗, "The Shu people use it for treating qi distension and **rotten blood attacking the heart following delivery**. It is very effective".

Chan hou bai xue ru xin **產後敗血入心, rotten blood entering the heart following delivery** [1]

PC identical with → *chan hou bai xue gong xin* 產後敗血攻心, rotten blood attacking the heart following delivery. *BCGM* Bai bing zhu zhi yao 百病主治藥, *kuang huo* 狂惑, madness and delusion: **產後敗血入心**，狂顛見祟，為末，地龍滾過，酒服, "(For treating) **rotten blood attacking the heart following delivery**, with [the woman] being crazy and seeing demons, prepare a powder to be mixed with boiled earthworms, and ingest with wine".

Chan hou ben xue bu ding **產後奔血不定, blood hastening and remaining restless following delivery** [1]

PC identical with → *chan hou yu xue* 產後余血, residual blood following delivery. *YXL* SE *zi wei* 紫葳：止**產後奔血不定**，淋瀝，安胎, "It stops **blood hastening and remaining restless following delivery** and dripping [of urine], and calms the fetus".

Chan hou bi **產後閉, closure following delivery** [2]
PC with constipation because of insufficiencies of qi and blood following delivery. *BCGM* Bai bing zhu zhi yao 百病主治藥 quoting *JSF*: 產後秘塞, "Tight blockage following delivery", writes: **產後閉**, "**Closure following delivery**".

Chan hou chang chu **產後腸出, intestinal prolapse following delivery** [3]
PC identical with → *yin tuo* 陰脫, yin prolapse. *PJF* 357: 治**產後腸出**不收。用枳殼煎湯，溫浸良久，即入, "For **intestinal prolapse following delivery** that fails to contract use a decoction with *zhi ke*. Have [the patient] sit in the warm liquid for an extended period of time, and [the uterus] will recede".

Chan hou chang tuo **產後腸脫, intestinal prolapse following delivery** [3]
PC identical with → *yin tuo* 陰脫, yin prolapse. *BCGM* SE *chun chu* 椿樗 quoting *FRDQLF* 23: 產後子腸下出，不能收拾 writes: **產後腸脫**，不能收拾者, "**Intestinal prolapse following delivery** that cannot be mended".

Chan hou chu nuo **產後搐搦, convulsions following delivery** [3]
PC identical with → *chan hou zhong feng* 產後中風, wind stroke following delivery. *BCGM* SE *biao* 鰾 quotes *JXCB*: **產後搐搦**強直者，不可便作風中，乃風入子臟，與破傷風同。用鰾膠一兩，以螺粉炒焦，去粉為末。分三服，煎蟬蛻湯下, "In the case of **convulsions** and stiffness **following delivery**, one must not act as if this were a wind stroke. Now, when wind enters the child depot, this is identical with wound wind. Take 1 *liang* of *biao jiao*, and burn together with *luo fen*. Discard the powder and grind it to powder. Divide into three portions. Ingest with a *chan tuo* decoction".

Chan hou feng **產後風, wind following delivery** [2]
PC identical with → *chan hou zhong feng* 產後中風, wind stroke following delivery. *JGYL* Lj: **產後風**續續數十日不解，頭微痛，惡寒，時時有熱，心下悶，乾嘔，汗出，雖久，陽旦證續在耳，可與陽旦湯, "If **wind following delivery** continues for tens of days without being resolved, with a slight headache, an aversion to cold and repeated heat spells, heart pressure below the heart, dry vomiting, and sweating, then even though this has existed for some time already, it is still a 'sunrise' condition. [Patients] are to be given a 'sunrise decoction'". [Note: 'Sunrise decoction', *yang dan tang* 陽旦湯, is another name of *gui zhi tang* 桂枝湯, decoction with *gui zhi* 桂枝.]

Chan hou feng **纏喉風, throat-constricting wind** [12]
PC of → *hou bi* 喉痹, throat blockage, with a rapid onset, a swelling of throat and cheeks, and a closure of the throat that makes it impossible to ingest even a liquid. *SJZL* 122: 治**纏喉風**，卒然喉痹，急如奔馬，喉頰俱腫, "To cure **throat-constricting wind** with sudden throat blockage as fast as a galloping horse, and throat and cheeks all swollen".

Chan hou feng bi **纏喉風痹, throat-constricting wind blockage** [3]
PC identical with → *chan hou feng* 纏喉風, throat-constricting wind. *BCGM* SE *xiong huang* 雄黃 quotes *DMF*: **纏喉風痹**：不通欲死者, "**Throat-constricting wind blockage**: This is when [the throat] is impassable and [patients] are about to die".

Chan hou feng chu **產後風搐, wind with tic following delivery** [1]
PC identical with → *chan hou zhong feng* 產後中風, wind stroke following delivery. *BCGM* SE *biao jiao* 鰾膠：燒存性，治婦人產難，**產後風搐**，破傷風痙，止嘔血，散瘀血，消腫毒，伏硇砂, "Burned by maintaining its nature it cures women with difficult delivery, **wind with tic following delivery**, and wind spasms in wounds. It stops vomiting of blood, disperses stagnant blood, dissolves the poison of swellings, and presses down *nao sha*".

Chan hou feng jing **產後風痙, wind spasms following delivery** [3]
PC identical with → *chan hou zhong feng* 產後中風, wind stroke following delivery. *BCGM* Bai bing zhu zhi yao 百病主治藥，Zhu feng 諸風：地黃**產後風痙**，取汁同薑汁交浸焙研，酒服, "For **wind spasms following delivery** Mix *jiang* juice with *di huang* juice, roast over a slow fire, and pulverize to be ingested with wine".

Chan hou ji fu **產後肌浮, muscle surface [swelling] following delivery** [3]
PC of women following delivery with external muscle swelling. *LGPZL* preface: **產後肌浮**，甘皮酒服, "For **muscle surface [swelling] following delivery** ingest *gan pi* with wine".

Chan hou li **產後痢, free-flux illness following delivery** [12]
PC of → *li ji* 痢疾, free-flux illness, affecting women after having given birth. *ZBYHL* 44: **產後痢**若變為血痢，則難治, "If **free-flux illness following delivery** changes to bloody free-flux illness, this is difficult to cure".

Chan hou rou xian **產後肉綫, flesh threads following delivery** [1]
PC with flesh threads that are painful when touched, protruding externally from the birth canal after delivery. *BCGM* SE *sheng jiang* 生薑"：**產後肉綫**，一婦產後用力，垂出肉綫長三四尺，觸之痛引心腹欲絕, "**Flesh threads following delivery**: When a woman presses with force after delivery, she will cause flesh threads of a length of 3 to 4 *chi* to hang down [from her vagina]. When touched there will be pain pulling on the heart and abdomen so severe that she wishes to die".

Chan hou xue ben ru si zhi **產後血奔入四肢, blood hastening to enter the four limbs following delivery** [1]
PC with pain in the four limbs following delivery. *BCGM* Bai bing zhu zhi yao 百病主治藥：狗頭，**產後血奔入四肢**，煮食, "Eat cooked dog's head for [treating] **blood hastening to enter the four limbs following delivery**".

Chan hou xue bi **產後血閉, closure of blood [flow] following delivery** [4] AN *chan xue bu xia* 產血不下， failure to discharge blood following delivery.
PC of a failure of → *e lu* 惡露, malign dew, to be properly discharged following delivery. *BCSY* SE *ji zi* 雞子：主**產後血閉**不下, "It controls **closure of blood [flow] following delivery**, with a failure [of the blood] to be discharged".

Chan hou xue chong **產後血沖, blood surge following delivery** [1]
PC identical with → *chan hou yu xue* 產後余血, residual blood following delivery. *BCGM* SE *qi lin jie* 騏麟竭 quotes *YLJY*: **產後血沖**：心胸滿喘，命在須

臾, "**Blood surge following delivery** [causes] a feeling of fullness in the heart and chest and makes one pant. Life may end any moment".

***Chan hou xue gong* 產後血攻, blood attack following delivery** [4]
PC identical with → *chan hou yu xue* 產後余血, residual blood following delivery. *BCSY* SE *liao qiao* 蓼蕎：**產後血攻**，胸脅刺痛, "**Blood attack following delivery**, with piercing pain in the chest and flanks".

***Chan hou xue luan* 產後血亂, blood unrest following delivery** [1]
PC identical with → *chan hou yu xue* 產後余血, residual blood following delivery. *BCGM* SE *gou* 狗 quotes *JYF*: **產後血亂**：奔入四肢, "**Blood unrest following delivery**: it rushes into the four limbs".

***Chan hou xue shen* 產後血滲, blood seepage following delivery** [1]
PC following delivery with blood discharged together with urine. *FRDQLF* 23: 療**產後血滲**入大小腸, "To cure **blood seepage** into the large and small intestines **following delivery**".

***Chan hou xue xie* 產後血邪, blood evil following delivery** [1]
PC identical with → *chan hou yu xue* 產後余血, residual blood following delivery. *RHZ* SE *zi ran tong* 自然銅：治**產後血邪**, "It cures **blood evil following delivery**".

***Chan hou xue yao fu tong* 產後血咬腹痛, abdominal pain as if bitten caused by blood following delivery** [1]
PC with pain in the lower abdomen resulting from stagnant blood following delivery. *BCGM* SE *wei mao* 衛矛 quoting *RHZ*: 產後血咬肚痛 writes **產後血咬腹痛**, "**Abdominal pain as if bitten caused by blood following delivery**".

***Chan hou yin bu neng he* 產後陰不能合, the yin [gate] is unable to close following delivery** [1]
PC identical with → *chan men bu he* 產門不合, failure of the birth gate to close. *RHZ* SE *shi hui* 石灰：又治**產後陰不能合**，濃煎汁熏洗, "It also cures [women whose] **yin [gate] is unable to close following delivery**. [For this purpose] boil a decoction down to a thick juice and use it for a steaming and bathing [the yin gate]".

***Chan hou yin fan* 產後陰翻, turning inside out of the yin [gate] following delivery** [1]
PC with a woman's birth canal everted to the outside following delivery. *BCGM* SE *ze lan* 澤蘭 quotes *BHJJF*: **產後陰翻**，產後陰戶燥熱，遂成翻花, "**Turning inside out of the yin [gate] following delivery**: When the yin opening is dry and hot following delivery this will result in it turning inside out, resembling the opening of a blossom".

***Chan hou yu ji* 產後余疾, ailments following delivery** [7] AN *chan ru yu ji* 產乳余疾, *zi ru yu ji* 字乳余疾.
PC CD of all types of diseases related to post-partum blood stagnation, qi and blood depletion weakness, as well as breast-feeding. *MYBL* SE *sang shang ji sheng* 桑上寄生：內傷不足，**產後余疾**，下乳汁, "[It cures] internal harm

and insufficiency, as well as **ailments following delivery**. It stimulates breast milk discharge".

***Chan hou yu tong* 產後余痛, pain following delivery** [3]
PC with pain in the lower abdomen. *MYBL* SE *bai jiang can* 白僵蠶：女子崩中赤白，**產後余痛**, "[It cures] collapsing center with red and white [discharge] in women, as well as **pain following delivery**".

***Chan hou yu xue* 產後余血, residual blood following delivery** [3] AN *chan hou xue xie* 產後血邪, blood evil following delivery; *chan hou xue gong* 產後血攻, blood attack following delivery; *chan hou xue chong* 產後血沖, blood surge following delivery; *chan hou xue luan* 產後血亂, blood unrest following delivery; *chan hou ben xue bu ding* 產後奔血不定, blood hastening and remaining restless following delivery.
PC CD of all types of diseases caused by stagnant blood following delivery. *RHZ* SE *wu zhu yu* 吳茱萸：下**產後余血**, "It stimulates the discharge of **residual blood following delivery**".

***Chan hou zhong feng* 產後中風, wind stroke following delivery** [27] AN: *chan hou feng* **產後風**, wind following delivery; *chan hou feng jing* 產後風痙, wind with spasms following delivery; *chan hou feng chu* 產後風搐, wind with tic following delivery; *chan hou chu nuo* 產後搐搦, convulsions following delivery.
PC of → *po shang feng* 破傷風, wound wind, brought about in women after parturition because of an intrusion of wind evil via the puerperal sores. *QJYF* RE *du huo tang* 獨活湯, decoction with *du huo*: 治**產後中風**，口噤不能言, "It cures **wind stroke following delivery** with clenched jaw and an inability to speak".

***Chan lao* 產勞**, childbirth exhaustion [2]
PC identical with → *ru lao* 蓐勞, childbed exhaustion. *BCTJ* SE *ta* 獺：主傳屍勞極，四肢寒瘧，虛汗客熱，亦主**產勞**, "It controls corpse [evil] transmission with extreme exhaustion, cold malaria affecting the four limbs, depletion sweating with visitor heat. It also controls **childbirth exhaustion**".

***Chan li* 產痢, childbirth free-flux illness** [5]
PC identical with → *chan hou li* 產後痢, free-flux illness following delivery. *BCGM* Bai bing zhu zhi yao 百病主治藥 quoting *BCSY ji zi* 雞子：主產後痢, "It controls free-flux illness following delivery", writes: **產痢, "Childbirth free-flux illness"**.

***Chan men bu bi* 產門不閉, failure of the birth gate to close** [1]
PC identical with → *chan men bu he* 產門不合. *BCGM* SE *shi hui* 石灰：產門不閉：產後陰道不閉, "**Failure of the birth gate to close** is a failure of the yin path to close following delivery".

***Chan men bu he* 產門不合, failure of the birth gate to close** [2] AN *chan men bu bi* 產門不閉; *chan hou yin bu neng he* 產後陰不能合, the yin [gate] is unable to close following delivery; *chan hou yin fan* 產後陰翻, yin [gate] turning inside out following delivery.
PC with the birth canal remaining wide open after delivery. *BCGM* Bai bing zhu zhi yao 百病主治藥 (Yin bing 陰病): **產門不合**，石灰，炒熱，淬水洗，

"If the **birth gate fails to close**, roast *shi hui* until it is hot, put it into water and use this to rinse [the yin gate]".

Chan men sheng he **產門生合, congenital birthgate closure** [3]

PC with a congenital closure of the vagina as its sign. *BCGM* SE *shi hui* 石灰 quotes *TBYF*: **產門生合**：不開，用銅錢磨利割開，以陳石灰傅之，即愈, "**Congenital birthgate closure**: When it fails to open use a copper coin and rub to create a sharp cut that opens it. Then apply old *shi hui* to it and it will be cured".

Chan nan **產難, difficult birth** [53]

PC identical with → *nan chan* 難產. BJ SE lou gu 螻蛄：主**產難**，出肉中刺, "It controls **difficult birth**, and serves to remove thorns stuck in one's flesh".

Chan ru yu ji **產乳余疾, additional ailments following delivery** [3]

PC identical with → *chan hou yu ji* 產後余疾. *BJ* SE *xuan shen* 玄參：主腹中寒熱積聚，女子**產乳余疾**, "It controls alternating sensations of cold and heat and accumulations and collections in the abdomen, as well as a female's **additional ailments following delivery**".

Chan she dan du **纏蛇丹毒, twining-snake cinnabar poison** [2]

PC of → *dan du* 丹毒, cinnabar poison, growing like a snake around one's waist. *BCGM* quotes *JJF*: **纏蛇丹毒**：馬蘭、甘草擂醋搽之, "**Twining-snake cinnabar poison**: apply *ma lan* and *gan cao* pounded with vinegar to it".

Chan shi shang pao **產時傷脬, bladder damage at the time of birth** [1]

PC identical with → *chan fu pao sun* 產婦脬損, a delivering woman's bladder damage. *BCGM* SE *juan* 絹：**產時傷脬**，終日不小便，只淋濕不斷, "**Bladder damage at the time of birth** [causes that woman] to be unable to pass urine all day long, with only an unceasing trickling of moisture instead".

Chan xue bu xia **產血不下, failure of blood to be discharged [following] delivery** [1]

PC identical with → *chan hou xue bi* 產後血閉, closure of blood [flow] following delivery. *BCGM* SE *fu qi mo* 釜臍墨 quotes *SSB*: **產血不下**，鍋底墨烟，熱酒服二錢, "[To treat] **failure of blood to be discharged [following] delivery**, ingest 2 *qian* of the black soot from the bottom of a pan, mixed with hot wine".

Chan yun **產運, [brain] movements following delivery; vertigo** [1]

PC identical with → *xue yun* 血運, blood[-induced brain] movements. *BCGM* SE *hong lan hua* 紅藍花 quotes *YEMB*: 新昌徐氏婦，病**產運**已死, "Mr. Xu Xinchang's wife suffered from **[brain] movements following delivery** and died".

Chang chong **長蟲, longworm** [11]

PC identical with → *hui chong* 蛔蟲①, roundworm. *BJ* SE *bai qiu yin* 白蚯蚓：殺**長蟲**，仍自化作水, "It kills **longworms**. They eventually transform themselves into water".

Chang chu **腸出, emergence of intestines** [22]

IS of intestines appearing through an open wound in the abdominal wall. *ZBYHL* 50: 為金刃所傷…自余腹破**腸出**，頭碎腦露，並亦難治, "Following an injury by metal objects, including a sword, … with an **emergence of intestines** from the open abdomen, the head broken to pieces and the brain lying free, this too is difficult to cure".

Chang du **腸毒, intestinal poisoning** [3]
PC identical with → *zang du* 臟毒, depot poisoning. *BCGM* SE *hu* 葫 quoting *JSF*: 蒜連丸治臟毒下血, "Pills with *suan* and *lian* cure depot poisoning with a discharge of blood", writes: **腸毒**下血, "**Intestinal poisoning** with a discharge of blood".

Chang feng **腸風, intestinal wind** [198]
PC of bloody stools with the blood being fresh and red. *SW* 42: 久風入中，則為**腸風**、飧泄, "When wind enters the center over a long period of time, this causes **intestinal wind**, with outflow of [undigested] food". LSZ: 下血，血清者為**腸風**，虛熱生風，或兼濕氣, "If blood is passed down, when the blood is clear, this is **intestinal wind**. In such cases depletion heat has generated wind, sometimes in conjunction with moisture qi".

Chang gu **腸蠱, intestinal *gu*** [2]
PC of a → *li ji* 痢疾, free-flux illness ailment, which is first red and then white and lasts without healing for many years. *WTMY* 25 quoting *ZHF*: 凡病下，應先下白後下赤，若先下赤後下白，為**腸蠱**, "Whenever one suffers from discharge, the normal course is that the discharge is white first and red afterwards. If the discharge is red first and white afterwards, then this is **intestinal *gu***".

Chang hua **腸滑, intestinal smoothness** [10]
① PC identical with → *hua xie* 滑泄, smooth outflow. *TBC* SE *wu shi zi* 無食子：主赤白痢，**腸滑**，生肌肉, "It controls red and white free-flux illness with **intestinal smoothness**, and generates muscles and flesh".
② IS of thin, uncontrollable stool. *QJYF* 43: 治小腸虛寒痛，下赤白，**腸滑**，胸中懊憹，補之方, "To cure depletion in the small intestine with cold pain, red and white discharge, **intestinal smoothness**, and a feeling of vexation in the chest, [use] a recipe for supplementation".

Chang mi **腸秘, intestinal closure** [3]
IS identical with → *da bian mi* 大便秘①, constipation. *BCGM* SE gua lou 栝樓 quoting *BCYY*: 肺燥，熱渴，大腸秘, "Lung dryness; heat with thirst, and large intestine closure", writes: 燥渴**腸秘**, "Dryness, thirst, and **intestinal closure**".

Chang ming **腸鳴, intestinal sounds** [30]
① AN *fu ming* 腹鳴, abdominal sounds; *lei ming* 雷鳴, thunderous sounds. IS of seeping sounds resulting from intestinal peristaltic hyperfunction. *SW* 22: 虛則腹滿**腸鳴**，飧泄食不化, "In the case of depletion, the abdomen is full and there are **sounds in the intestines**. There is outflow of [undigested] food. Food fails to be transformed".
② PC of intestinal sounds. *QJYF* 30: 太白、公孫，主**腸鳴**, "[Needling the holes] *tai bai* and *gong sun* controls **intestinal sounds**".

Chang pi **腸澼, intestinal flush** [40]
PC identical with a) → *li ji* 痢疾, free-flux illness ailment. *SW* 28: **腸澼**下膿血何如, "In the case of **intestinal flush** passing down pus and blood, how does it arise?" b) → *bian xue* 便血, bloody stool. *SW* 28: 腸澼便血何如, "In the case of **intestinal flushing** with bloody stool, how does it arise?"

Chang tan **腸覃, intestinal *tan*** [1]
PC with a swelling and lump present in a woman's lower abdomen despite normal arrival of menstruation. *LS* 57: **腸覃**何如？岐伯曰：寒氣客於腸外, "What about **intestinal *tan***? Qi Bo: Cold qi lodges outside the intestines".

Chang tou ting chu **腸頭挺出, prolapse of the end of the intestine** [2]
PC identical with → *tuo gang* 脫肛, prolapse of the rectum. *ZLBC* SE *xia ma* 蝦蟆 quotes Sun Zhenren 孫真人：**腸頭挺出**，以皮一片，瓶內燒熏挺處, "[To cure] **prolapse of the end of the intestine**, burn a piece of [its] skin in a jar and fumigate the region of the prolapse".

Chang xu **腸虛, intestinal depletion** [9]
PC of a depletion of the large intestine with cold intrusion and diarrhea. *ZBYHL* 4: 夫大腸虛則泄利，胃氣逆則嘔吐。虛勞又**腸虛**胃逆者，故吐利, "Now, when the large intestine has a depletion this results in free outflow. When the stomach qi flows against its proper direction, this brings forth vomiting. If someone has a depletion exhaustion and in addition **intestinal depletion** and stomach [qi] counterflow, he will vomit and have free-flux [illness] as a result".

Chang yong **腸癰, intestinal obstruction-illness** [29] AN *xiao chang yong* 小腸癰, obstruction-illness of the small intestine.
PC of → *yong* 癰, obstruction-illness, developing in the abdominal cavity at the site of the intestines. In general, this is accompanied by fever and spastic pain on the right side of the lower abdomen, where a lump can be felt. *SW* 45: 發**腸癰**不可治, "When this develops into **intestinal obstruction-illnesses**, [the patient] cannot be treated".

Chang yu mian **常欲眠, frequent desire to sleep** [5]
IS identical with → *duo shui* 多睡, profuse sleeping. *MYBL* SE *tong cao* 通草：療脾疸，**常欲眠**，心煩, "It cures spleen *dan*-illness, a **frequent desire to sleep**, and heart vexation".

Chang zhi **腸痔, intestinal piles** [37]
PC of → *zhi chuang* 痔瘡, piles sores, growing to the side of the anus with kernel-like swelling and pain. Patients experience alternating feelings of cold and heat, and bleed. *BJ* SE *bo mu* 蘗木：主五藏腸胃中結熱，黃疸，**腸痔**，止泄痢, "It controls bound heat in the five depots, the intestines, and the stomach, yellow *dan*-illness, as well as **intestinal piles**, and it stops free-flux illness".

Chao re **潮熱, tidal fever** [30]
IS of a fever that sometimes subsides and then develops again, mostly in a daily rhythm. *SHL* 201: 陽明病，脈浮而緊者，必**潮熱**發作有時, "Yang brilliance diseases: if the [movement in the] vessels is at the surface and tight, a **tidal fever** with regular periods will develop".

Che tong **徹痛, penetrating pain** [1] AN *chuan tong* 穿痛.

IS of pain finding its way from one location to another. *QJYF* 27: 上氣短氣咳逆，胸背**徹痛**，灸風門、熱府百壯, "In the case of ascending qi, shortness of qi, and cough resulting from [qi] moving contrary to its normal direction, with **penetrating pain** in chest and back, cauterize the points *feng men* and *re fu* one hundred times".

Che zong **掣瘲, clonic convulsions** [4]

IS identical with → *chi zong* 瘛瘲, clonic spasms. *BCGM* SE *mang cao* 莽草 quotes *WTMY*: 小兒風癇**掣瘲**戴眼，極者日數十發, "Wind epilepsy in children: **clonic convulsions** affect the eyes; in severe cases there are tens of fits each day".

Chen chi **沉滯, deep-seated heaviness** [2]

IS identical with → *chen zhong* 沉重①. *ZHF* 4: 凡男女因積勞虛損，或大病後不復，常若四體**沉滯**，骨肉疼酸, "Whenever males or females have been affected by accumulation exhaustion and depletion injury, or when after a massive disease episode they have not recovered yet, they often experience a feeling as if there were a **deep-seated heaviness** in their four extremities, and bones and flesh have sensations of pain and soreness".

Chen han **沉寒, deep-seated cold; descending cold** [3]

① PC identical with → *gu leng* 痼冷, obstinacy-illness cold. *HJJF* 5 RE *si shen dan* 四神丹, elixir with four wondrous [ingredients]: 治一切**沉寒**痼冷, "It cures all types of **deep-seated cold**, i.e. obstinacy-illness cold".

② PQ of substances with a cold nature and a downward effect. *BCYY* SE *di yu* 地榆：性**沉寒**，入下焦, "Its nature is that of **deep-seated cold**; it enters the lower burner".

Chen shi **沉屍, sunken corpse [qi]** [3]

PC of a twisting pain in the heart and abdomen that recurs repeatedly and cannot be healed for an extended period of time. *ZBYHL* 23: **沉屍**者，發時亦心腹絞痛，脹滿喘急，沖刺心胸，攻擊脅肋, "As for **sunken corpse [qi]**, when it breaks out, one feels a twisting pain in the heart and abdomen, with distension and a feeling of fullness, as well as hectic panting. Heart and chest experience a piercing pain; it also attacks the two flanks".

Chen tong **沉痛, sunken pain** [1]

IS identical with *zhong tong* 重痛, heavy pain. *PJF* 164: 沉香四倍丸，治痰飲，兩臂疼痛，腰腿**沉痛**, "The fourfold pills with *chen xiang* cure phlegm rheum, pain in the two arms, as well as a feeling of **sunken pain** in the lower back and legs".

Chen xue **陳血, aged blood** [2]

① PI of aged extravascular blood. *YXQY* Fj: **陳血**瘀色，熟地黃, "For **aged blood** with [the skin showing] the color of stagnant [blood, use] *shou di huang*".

② EA identical with → *su xue* 宿血①, residual blood. *YXL* SE *fei lian* 飛廉：能破**陳血**，能落胎, "It is capable of breaking through **aged blood** and can bring down a fetus".

Chen zhang **䐜脹, bloating** [1]

IS of a feeling of distension affecting chest and diaphragm. *SW* 5: 濁氣在上，則生**䐜脹**, "When turbid qi is in the upper [regions], this generates **bloating**".

Chen zhong **沉重, deep-seated heaviness; very heavy** [14]

① AN *chen zhi* 沉滯, deep-seated sluggishness. IS of a feeling of unbearable heaviness affecting the entire body or parts of it, together with a sensation of fatigue when one starts moving. *SHL* 316: 腹痛、小便不利，四肢**沉重**疼痛，自下利者，此為有水氣, "Abdominal pain. Anuria. The four limbs are affected by **deep-seated heaviness** and are painful. In the case of spontaneous free-flux illness, this is a situation of a presence of water qi".

② Physical feature of pharmaceutical substances with a heavy mass, identical with → *ti zhong* 體重②, the body feels heavy. *YXQY* Lj: 檳榔性如鐵石之**沉重**，能墜諸藥至於下, "*Bing lang*, by its nature it is **very heavy** like iron or stones. Hence it is able to push all other pharmaceutical substances down into the [body's] lower sections".

Chi bai **齒敗, tooth decay** [1]

PC with rotten teeth as major sign. *WTMY* 22: **齒敗**口臭方，取芎藭，煮一味含之, "Recipe for **tooth decay** and malodorous mouth: Boil a single substance *xiong qiong* in water, and hold the [liquid] in the mouth".

Chi bai dai **赤白帶, red and white [discharge from below the] belt** [59] AN *chi bai wo* 赤白沃, red and white downpour.

PC of → *dai xia bing* 帶下病, disease of discharge from below the belt, with a simultaneous discharge of red and white matter from the vagina. *QJYF* 26: 主女人崩中漏下，**赤白帶**，補虛温中, "It controls women's collapsing center with leaking discharge, **red and white [discharge from below the] belt**, supplements depletions and warms the center".

Chi bai dian feng **赤白癜風, red and white patches wind** [4]

PC identical with → *zi bai dian feng* 紫白癜風, purple and white patches wind. *SJZL* 18: **赤白癜風**，硫黃散塗方, "Recipe for external application of the powder with *liu huang* for [curing] **red and white patches wind**".

Chi bai mo **赤白膜, red and white membrane** [6]

PC identical with → *chi bai yi* 赤白翳, red and white shade. *BJ* SE *jue ming zi* 決明子：主青盲，目淫膚**赤白膜**，眼赤痛，淚出, "It controls green blindness, excess skin and **red and white membranes** in the eyes, red and painful eyes, as well as tearflow".

Chi bai wo **赤白沃, red and white downpour** [4]

PC identical with → *chi bai dai* 赤白帶, red and white [discharge from below the] belt. *BJ* SE *dan xiong ji* 丹雄雞：主女人崩中漏下，**赤白沃**，補虛温中, "It controls women's collapsing center with leaking discharge, **red and white downpour**, supplements depletions and warms the center".

Chi bai yi **赤白翳, red and white shade** [1] AN *chi bai mo* 赤白膜, red and white membrane.

PC CD of → *chi yi* 赤翳, red shade, and → *bai yi* 白翳, white shade. *WTMY* 2 lists 傷寒攻目生瘡兼**赤白翳**方六首, "Six recipes for harm caused by cold affecting the eyes resulting in the growth of sores and at the same time **red and white shades**".

Chi bai you feng **赤白游風, red and white roaming wind** [1]

PC of → *you feng* 游風, roaming wind, characterised by a roaming and erupting nature, sometimes with itching, sometimes with pain, and skin papules and swelling of either red or white color. CD of → *chi you feng* 赤游風, red roaming wind, and *bai you feng* 白游風, white roaming wind. *BYCY* 12: **赤白游風**，屬風熱血熱，蓋血得熱而遊走耳, "**Red and white roaming wind** is associated with wind heat and blood heat. The reason is that the blood moves around because it has been heated".

Chi bai you zhen **赤白游疹, red white roaming papules** [6]

PC CD of → *chi you zhen* 赤游疹, red roaming papules, and → *bai you zhen* 白游疹, white roaming papules. *BCSY* SE *ma zao* 馬藻：搗傅小兒**赤白游疹**, "Pound and apply externally on **red white roaming papules** in children".

Chi bai zhang **赤白障, red and white screen** [1]

PC quotation error. *BCGM* SE *ying yu* 蘡薁 quoting *BCSY*: 滴目中，去熱翳赤障, "Drip into the eyes to remove heat shade and red screen", writes: 滴入目中，去熱翳，**赤白障**, "Drip into the eyes to remove heat shade and **red and white screen**".

Chi bai zhong xia **赤白重下, red and white [free-flux illness] with heaviness [pressuring] downwards** [1]

PC identical with → *chi bai li* 赤白痢, red and white free-flux illness. *BCGM* SE *da dou chi* 大豆豉 quoting *ZHF* 治重下，此即赤白痢也, "To cure heaviness [pressing] downwards, i.e. red and white free-flux illness", writes: **赤白重下**, "**Red and white [free-flux illness] with heaviness [pressing] downwards**".

Chi bai zhuo **赤白濁, red and white turbidity** [11]

PC of urine mixed with a red and white turbid liquid. *SYDXF* 7: 治小便餘瀝，並**赤白濁**, "It cures trickling of residual urine, and also **red and white turbidity**".

Chi ban **赤斑, red macules** [7] AW **赤瘢.**

IS of red → *ban* 斑①, macules, appearing on the skin. *ZHF* 4: 飲酒發**赤斑**黃黑，由大醉當風入水所致，治之方, "Recipe to cure the appearance, following the consumption of wine, of **red macules** – some of which may have turned yellow and black, caused by entering water [possibly: having sexual intercourse] in a state of massive intoxication and an exposure to wind".

Chi ban **赤瘢, red macules** [3]

IS identical with → *chi ban* 赤斑. *BCGM* SE *ling yang* 羚羊 quotes *ZHF*: **赤瘢**如瘡：瘙癢，甚則殺人, "When someone has **red macules** resembling sores, they will itch and in severe cases kill that person".

Chi beng **赤崩, red collapse** [1] AN *hong beng* 紅崩; *beng chi* 崩赤, collapsing red.
PC of red, sticky liquid emitted with the blood of → *beng zhong* 崩中②, collapsing center, through the vaginal tract. *MJ* 9: **赤崩**者形如絳津, "The appearance of **red collapse** is that of deep-red saliva".

Chi bi **赤鼻, red nose** [3]
PC identical with → *jiu zha* 酒齇, wine sediments. *BCGM* SE *shi liu chi* 石硫赤, attached recipes 附方, quotes *SJZL*: **赤鼻**作痛：紫色石亭脂，紅色次之，黃色勿用。研末，冷水調搽，半月絕根, "For a **red nose** that aches: grind purple *shi ting zhi* - red ones are not as good, yellow ones are useless - to a powder and mix with cold water to apply externally. After half a month the root will be severed".

Chi biao **赤熛, red flaming heat** [1]
PC identical with → *biao chuang* 熛瘡, flaming-heat sores. *BC* SE *ji xue cao* 積雪草：主大熱，惡瘡癰疽，浸淫**赤熛**, "It controls massive heat, malign sores, obstruction- and impediment-illnesses, as well as [skin lesions] soaked [with pus and/or liquid] and **red flaming heat**".

Chi bing **瘈病, spasm disease** [1]
PC with → *chi zong* 瘈瘲, clonic convulsions, as its main sign. *BCSY* SE *he ming cao* 合明草：主暴熱淋，小便赤澀，小兒**瘈病**, "It controls violent heat dripping, reddish and rough urination, and in children **spasm disease**".

Chi bing **齒病, tooth disease** [1]
PC identical with → *chi ji* 齒疾, tooth ailment. *BCGM* SE *zao* 棗 quoting *RHZ*: 牙齒有病人切忌啖之, "People with tooth disease must not eat it", writes: 有**齒病**、疳病、蟲䘌人不宜啖棗, "For persons with **tooth disease**, *gan*-disease, and bug-erosion it is not advisable to eat *zao*".

Chi chu **齒齼, dental discomfort** [4] AN *ya chu* 牙齼.
PC with an uncomfortable sensation in one's teeth as major sign. This is often brought about by a consumption of sour items. *RHZ* SE *hu tao* 胡桃：食酸**齒齼**，細嚼解之, "If one experiences **dental discomfort** after having eaten something that is sour, finely chewing [*hu tao*] will bring relief".

Chi ci **赤疵, red blemish-illness** [9]
PC of red speckles of varying size on the skin. They are not elevated and commonly are not associated with any abnormal sensation such as pain and itching. Also, they are not connected to any other physical condition. *ZBYHL* 31: 面及身體皮肉變赤，與肉色不同，或如手大，或如錢大，亦不癢痛，謂之**赤疵**, "If on one's face or body the skin changes to red, and differs from the color of the surrounding flesh, sometimes this being as large as a hand, sometimes as small as a coin, and if there is neither itching nor pain, this is called '**red blemish-illness**'".

Chi dai **赤帶, red [discharge from below the] belt** [9] AN *chi wo* 赤沃, red downpour.
PC of → *dai xia bing* 帶下病, disease of discharge from below the belt, with a discharge of red matter from the vagina. *QJYF* 4: 龍骨散，治腹下十二病絕

產，一曰白帶，二曰**赤帶**, "Powder with *long gu* cures the twelve diseases of the lower abdomen that result in childlessness. The first is named 'white [discharge from below the] belt'. The second is called '**red [discharge from below the] belt**'".

Chi dan **赤丹, red cinnabar** [9] AN *re dan* 熱丹, heat cinnabar; *dan re* 丹熱, cinnabar heat; *re dan du* 熱丹毒, heat cinnabar poison.

PC of → *dan du* 丹毒, cinnabar poison, with massive heat poison and red skin rash. *ZBYHL* 31: **赤丹**者，初發疹起，大者如連錢，小者如麻豆，肉上粟如雞冠肌理, "As for **red cinnabar**, when one first begins to suffer from it, large variants are the size of coins tied together, small ones are the size of sesame kernels. The 'chestnuts' on the flesh resemble the muscle structure of a cockscomb".

Chi ding **赤丁, red pin** [1]

PC identical with → *chi ding chuang* 赤疔瘡, red pin-illness sores. *BCGM* Bai bing zhu zhi yao 百病主治藥：狗寶，同蟾酥諸藥服，治**赤丁**, "*Gou bao* ingested together with *chan su* and the other pharmaceutical substances cures **red pin**".

Chi ding chuang **赤疔瘡, red pin-illness sores** [1] AN *chi ding* 赤丁, red pin.

PC of → *ding chuang* 丁瘡, pin sores, developing on the head and face, or in the region of the joints of hands and feet. When this disease breaks out it quickly leads to a serious condition accompanied by a generation of poison qi that will attack the heart. *BCGM* SE *gou bao* 狗寶 quotes *TXL*: **赤疔瘡**：狗寶丸：用狗寶八分，蟾酥二錢，龍腦二錢，麝香一錢，為末，好酒和丸麻子大，每服三丸, "For **red pin-illness sores**: Pills with *gou bao*: Take *gou bao*, 8 *fen*; *chan su*, 2 *qian*; *long nao*, 2 *qian*; *she xiang*, 1 *qian*. Grind to a powder. Use good wine and prepare pills the size of hemp seeds. Each time ingest 3 pills".

Chi fu yin lan **齒腐齦爛, rotting teeth and gum putrescence** [1]

PC with rotten teeth and festering gums. *BCGM* SE *lu jian* 鹵鹼 quoting *XMLF* 15: 口齒腐蝕出血，斷根宣爛, "The teeth in the mouth have rotted with erosion and are bleeding. This loosens the roots of the teeth, makes them unstable and causes them to fester", writes: **齒腐齦爛**, "**Rotten teeth and gum putrescence**".

Chi gan **齒疳, dental *gan*-illness** [4]

PC identical with → *ya gan* 牙疳. *TPSHF* 34: 又**齒疳**，其齒骨脆爛, "Further there is **dental *gan*-illness**. Here teeth and bones turn brittle and rot".

Chi gen ding chuang **赤根疔瘡, red root pin-illness sores** [1]

PC of → *ding chuang* 丁瘡, pin sores, with an appearance like a red bean and a deep-reaching red color root. *BCGM* SE *ma* 馬 quoting *QJYF* 22: 治赤根丁, "To cure pins with a red root", writes: **赤根疔瘡**, "**Red root pin-illness sores**".

Chi huan **弛緩, relaxed; to slacken** [1]

IS identical with → *huan* 緩①. *SJZL* 162: 產後中風，手足偏枯，筋脈**弛緩**，疼痛無力, "If one has been struck by wind after delivery, hands and feet will show hemilateral withering. The sinew-vessels **slacken**. They ache and have no strength".

***Chi huo dan du* 赤火丹毒, red fire cinnabar poison** [1]

PC identical with → *chi you dan du* 赤游丹毒, red roaming cinnabar poison. *BCGM* SE *yun tai* 芸薹 quotes *SSM*: 貞觀七年三月，予在內江縣飲多，至夜覺四體骨肉疼痛。至曉頭痛，額角有丹如彈丸，腫痛。至午通腫，目不能開。經日幾斃。予思本草芸薹治風游丹腫，遂取葉搗傅，隨手即消，其驗如神也。亦可搗汁服之, "During the *zhen guan* reign period I was in Neijian country where I drank a lot. At night I felt pain in the bones and flesh of all four extremities. At dawn my head ached. On one of my temples I had a cinnabar [poisoning] resembling a bullet. It was swollen and painful. At noon the entire region was swollen, and I could no longer open my eyes. After several days I came close to dying. Then I recalled that the *Ben cao* lists *yun tai* to cure wind roaming cinnabar [poison] swelling. I took its leaves, ground them and smeared [the pulp onto the affected region. The swelling] disappeared immediately. A miraculous effect, indeed. It is also possible to pound it to a juice for internal ingestion". The term → *feng you dan zhong* 風游丹腫, wind roaming cinnabar swelling, appears in the subsequent section Fu fang 附方, Additional Recipes, modified to: *chi you dan du* **赤火丹毒, red fire cinnabar poison**.

***Chi ji* 齒疾, tooth ailment** [3] All PC of the teeth.

BCGM SE *rong yan* 戎鹽 quotes *TBYF*: 牢牙明目：青鹽二兩，白鹽四兩，川椒四兩，煎汁拌鹽炒干。日用揩牙洗目，永無**齒疾**目疾, "To strengthen the teeth and clear the eyes: virid salt, 2 *liang*; white salt, 4 *liang*; *chuan jiao*, 4 *liang*. Boil the latter [in water, remove the dregs, and keep] the liquid to which are added the two types of salt, and heat until dry. Use daily to brush the teeth and wash the eyes, and there will never be **tooth ailments** or eye afflictions".

***Chi lai* 赤癩, red repudiation-illness** [3] AN *xue lai* 血癩, blood repudiation-illness.

PC identical with → *wu lai* 烏癩, black *lai*-illness. *BJ* SE *zhi zi* 梔子：主五內邪氣，胃中熱氣，面赤酒皰皶鼻，白癩**赤癩**，瘡瘍, "It controls the five types of internal evil qi, heat qi in the stomach, red face with wine blisters and a sedimented nose, white repudiation-illness and **red repudiation-illness**, sores and ulcers".

***Chi lan yan* 赤爛眼, red festering eye** [3]

PC identical with → *mu chi lan* 目赤爛, eye redness and festering. *BCGM* Bai bing zhu zhi yao 百病主治藥：青礬，洗**赤爛眼**及倒睫, "*Qing fan* is used to wash **red festering eyes** and inverted eyelashes".

***Chi li* 赤痢, red free-flux illness** [43] AN *hong li* 紅痢.

PC of → *li ji* 痢疾, free-flux illness ailment, with thin stool interspersed with red mucus. *ZBYHL* 17: 血流滲入腸，與痢相雜下，故為**赤痢**, "Blood flows into the intestines where it mixes with free-flux illness and moves downward. Hence one speaks of '**red free-flux illness**'".

***Chi liu* 赤瘤, red tumor** [1]

PC identical with → *dan du* 丹毒, cinnabar poison. *WKJY* Fj: 人身忽然變赤，如塗丹之狀，故謂之丹毒，世俗有云**赤瘤**, "The body of a person suddenly becomes red, as if someone had smeared cinnabar on it. Hence this is called 'cinnabar poison'. The people commonly call this '**red tumor**'".

Chi lou **齒漏, dental leakage** [1]

PC identical with → *chi nü* 齒衄, tooth bleeding. *BCGM* SE *zhu tie qi* 諸鐵器 (*tie ding* 鐵釘): 酒醉**齒漏**，出血不止，燒赤注孔中即止, "For **dental leakage** resulting from intoxification with wine, with incessant bleeding, heat [the iron nails] until they are red and attach them to the opening. This will stop it".

Chi mai guan tong **赤脈貫瞳, red vessels pervading the pupil** [4]

PC of → *mu zhong chi mai* 目中赤脈, red vessels in the eyes, with a network of red threads extending from the white part of the eye to the pupil. *TBC* SE *que shi* 雀屎：雀屎，和男首子乳如薄泥，點目中，弩肉、**赤脈貫瞳**子上者即消, "Sparrow droppings: Mix with the milk for a first male child to prepare a thin paste and swab into the eye. Tumorous flesh growths and **red vessels pervading the pupil** will then dissolve".

Chi mu **赤目, red eye** [92] AN *chi yan* 赤眼.

PC with red eyes, heat and pain, accompanied by swelling, tearflow, and gritty eye secretion. *RHZ* SE ren ru zhi 人乳汁：療**赤目**，使之明潤也, "It cures **red eyes**, and makes them clear and moist".

Chi ni **齒䘌, hidden-worms teeth** [17] AN *ni chi* 䘌齒; *ya ni* 牙䘌; *ya chi xuan ni* 牙齒宣䘌.

PC of → *ni* 䘌, hidden worms, disease with a malodorous liquid excreted. *ZBYHL* 29: 齒䘌者，是蟲食齒至齦，膿爛汁臭，如蝕之狀，故謂之**齒䘌**, "As for **hidden-worms teeth**, this is a condition where worms consume one's teeth down to the gums, with pus, festering, and a malodorous liquid. It appears as if eaten by a bug. Hence the designation 'hidden worms teeth'".

Chi nü **齒衄, spontaneous tooth bleeding** [3] AN *chi xue* 齒血.

PC of a spontaneous tooth bleeding. *JSF* Kou chi men 口齒門：必勝散，治**齒衄**, "The 'powder that will bring victory' cures **spontaneous tooth bleeding**".

Chi pao **赤皰, red blister** [4]

PC identical with → *mian pao* 面皰, facial blister. BJ SE mu lan 木蘭：主身大熱在皮膚中，去面熱**赤皰**酒皶，惡風癲疾，陰下癢濕，明耳目, "It controls massive body heat in the skin and removes facial heat with **red blisters** and wine sediments, malign wind, the ailment of peak-illness, and itching with moisture below one's yin (i.e. intimate) region, and it clears the ears and eyes".

Chi qi **赤氣, red qi** [3]

PC referred to only in the *BJ* and *MYBL*. Its meaning remains unclear. The context suggests an ulcerous condition with red skin, swelling, heat and pain. *BJ* SE *bai jiang* 敗醬：主暴熱，火瘡**赤氣**，疥瘙疽痔, "It controls violent heat, fire sores with **red qi**, *jie*-illness, itching, impediment-illness, and piles".

Chi qu **齒齲, tooth decay** [2]

PC identical with → *qu chi* 齲齒, decayed teeth. *QJYF* 30: 曲鬢、衝陽，主**齒齲**, "[Piercing of the holes] *qu bin* and *chong yang* controls **tooth decay**".

***Chi shu* 齒疏, dental scarcity** [5]
IS with a thinned out row of teeth as major sign. *PJF* 70: 牢牙石燕子散，治牙齒齦肉不固及腎弱**齒疏**, "The 'powder with *shi yan zi* to strengthen the teeth': It cures instability of teeth and gums and kidney weakness with **dental scarcity**".

***Chi teng* 齒疼, toothache** [3]
PC identical with → *ya tong* 牙痛. *QJYiF* 26: **齒疼**，灸外踝上高骨前交脈上七壯, "**Toothache**: Cauterize the vessel crossing in front of the bone elevation above the outer ankle seven times".

***Chi tong* 齒痛, toothache** [49]
PC identical with → *ya tong* 牙痛. *BJ* SE *lang dang zi* 莨菪子：主**齒痛**出蟲，肉痹拘急，使人健行, "It controls **toothache** and eliminates the worms, and flesh blockage with cramps and tension, and enables one to walk strongly again".

***Chi tu* 赤禿, red baldness** [8]
PC of → *tou chuang* 頭瘡, head sores, with red sores, leaking liquid, itching and loss of hair. *ZBYHL* 27: 此由頭瘡，蟲食髮禿落，無白痂，有汁，皮赤而癢，故謂之**赤禿**, "This is because of head sores when bugs/worms eat the hair leading to baldness. There are no white crusts. There is liquid. The skin is red and itches. Hence this is called '**red baldness**'".

***Chi wo* 赤沃, red downpour** [3]
PC identical with → *chi dai* 赤帶, red [discharge from below the] belt. *BJ* SE *shui qin* 水斳：主女子**赤沃**，止血，養精, "It controls women's **red downpour**, stops bleeding, and nourishes the essence".

***Chi xue* 齒血, tooth bleeding** [2]
PC identical with → *chi nü* 齒衄, spontaneous tooth bleeding. *WTMY* 22: 療**齒血**不止方, "Recipe to cure incessant **tooth bleeding**".

***Chi yan* 赤眼, red eye** [54]
PC identical with → *chi mu* 赤目. *ZLBC* SE *huang lian* 黃連 quotes *YXL*: 殺小兒疳蟲。點**赤眼**昏痛，鎮肝去熱毒, "It serves to kill *gan*-illness bugs/worms in children. Dropped into **red eyes** with clouding and pain it will press down liver [qi] and remove heat poison".

***Chi yi* 赤翳, red shade** [6] AN *chi zhang* 赤障, red screen.
PC of → *mu yi* 目翳, eye shade, consisting of a red speckled membrane. *WTMY* 2: 秦皮湯，療毒病沖眼，忽生**赤翳**, "A decoction with *qin pi* cures poison disease rushing against the eyes and causing the sudden growth of a **red shade**".

***Chi yi* 吃噫, hiccough** [2]
PC, IS identical with → *e ni* 呃逆, hiccough with counterflow [of qi]. *RHZ* SE *qu yu rou* 鴝鵒肉：治嗽及**吃噫**，下氣，炙食之, "For treating cough and **hiccough**, in order to make the qi move downwards, consume it roasted".

***Chi you* 赤疣, red wart** [1]
PC of a → *you* 疣, wart, with a pronounced red color. *BCTJ* SE du guan cao 都管草：赤疣，以醋摩其根塗之, "For **red warts**: rub its root with vinegar and apply [the liquid] to the [red wart]".

Chi you dan du **赤游丹毒, red roaming cinnabar poison** [1] AN *re you dan zhong* 熱游丹腫, heat roaming cinnabar-red swelling; *feng you dan zhong* 風游丹腫, wind roaming cinnabar-red swelling; *chi huo dan du* 赤火丹毒, cinnabar poison red-like fire; *chi you huo dan* 赤游火丹, red roaming fire cinnabar.

PC of → *dan du* 丹毒, cinnabar poison, with rashes that seem to be hiding. They move here and there and have no permanent location. *BCGM* quotes *QJYF* with *chi liu zhong dan du* 赤流腫丹毒, red flowing swelling cinnabar poison, and modifies it to *chi you dan du* **赤游丹毒, red roaming cinnabar poison**.

Chi you feng **赤游風, red roaming wind** [6]

PC. The red variant of → *chi bai you feng* 赤白游風, red-white roaming wind. *BCGM* SE *tie xiu* 鐵鏽 quotes *HJJF*: 脚腿紅腫，熱如火炙，俗名**赤游風**。用鐵鏽水塗解之, "When legs and calves are red and swollen, with heat as intensive as if roasted in fire, this is commonly called '**red roaming wind**'. Apply rust water to it to have it resolved".

Chi you feng dan **赤游風丹, red roaming wind cinnabar** [1]

PC identical with → *chi you feng* 赤游風, red roaming wind. *BCGM* SE *wu wei zi* 五味子quotes *XEWSZWLF*: **赤游風丹**，漸漸腫大。五味子焙研，熱酒頓服一錢自消, "[To cure] **red roaming wind cinnabar** associated with a gradual swelling and increase in size, bake *wu wei zi* over a slow fire and grind to a powder. Consume 1 *qian* with hot wine, and it will dissolve".

Chi you feng zheng **赤游風疹, red roaming wind papules** [1]

PC identical with → *chi you feng* 赤游風, red roaming wind. *BCGM* SE *gan jiao* 甘蕉：**赤游風疹**，方同上（芭蕉根搗爛塗之）, "For **red roaming wind papules** the recipe is identical with the preceding one (external application of *ba jiao* root pounded to a pulp)".

Chi you feng zhong **赤游風腫, red roaming wind swelling** [1]

PC identical with → *chi you feng* 赤游風, red roaming wind. *YXGM* 20: 治**赤游風腫**，蕎麥苦酒調敷, "To cure **red roaming wind swelling**: mix *qiao mai* with bitter wine and apply externally".

Chi you huo dan **赤游火丹, red roaming fire cinnabar** [2]

PC identical with → *chi you dan du* 赤游丹毒, red roaming cinnabar poison. *BCGM* SE *he ye* 荷葉, *fu fang* 附方, attached recipes: **赤游火丹**：新生荷葉搗爛，入鹽塗之, "[To cure] **red roaming fire cinnabar**, pound fresh *he ye* to a pulp, add salt, and apply externally".

Chi you zhen **赤游疹, red roaming papules** [1]

PC identical with → *chi zhen* 赤疹, red papules. *BCSY* SE *yun tai* 芸薹：搗葉傅**赤游疹**, "Pound the leaves and paste them on **red roaming papules**".

Chi zha **赤皻, red sediments** [1]

PC identical with → *jiu zha* 酒皻, wine sediments. *BCGM* Zang fu biao ben xu shi yong yao shi 臟腑標本虛實用藥式, *wei* 胃, stomach: 標病：發熱蒸蒸，身前熱，身前寒，發狂譫語，咽痹，上齒痛，口眼喎斜，鼻痛鼽衄**赤皻**, "Its external diseases: effusion of heat with steaming. The body's front is [at times] hot; the body's front is [at times] cold. [Patients] are mad and their speech is incoherent. They have a throat blockage, and the upper teeth ache. Mouth and eyes are slanted. The nose aches, with runny nose, nosebleed and **red sediments**".

Chi zhang **赤障, red screen** [6]

PC identical with → *chi yi* 赤翳, red shade. *YXL* SE *qing yang gan* 青羊肝：主**赤障**，白膜，風淚, "It controls **red screen**, white membrane and wind tearflow".

Chi zhen **赤疹, red papules** [3] AN *you zhen* 游疹, roaming papules; *dan zhen* 丹疹，cinnabar-red papules.

PC of a red variant of → *feng zhen* 風疹, wind papules. *ZBYHL* 2: 熱結成**赤疹**也, "Heat nodes generate **red papules**".

Chi zhong **赤腫, red and swollen** [53] AN *hong zhong* 紅腫; *zhong chi* 腫赤, swollen and red

IS of topical swelling with the skin assuming a red color. *ZBYHL* 31: 發時必在於兩股里，漸引至陰頭而**赤腫**是也, "When it breaks out this will occur inside the two thighs. It gradually extends to the glans penis which will be **red and swollen**".

Chi zhuo **赤濁, red turbidity** [8]

PC of urine mixed with a red, turbid liquid. *QJYF* 30: 腎俞，主小便難，**赤濁**, "[Piercing] the kidney transporter [hole] controls difficult urination, and **red turbidity**".

Chi zi **赤眥, red canthi** [1]

PC with redness of an eye's two canthi as major sign. *BCTJ* SE *rui he* 蕤核：眼風淚癢，或生翳，或**赤眥**，一切皆主之, "It controls all [health problems] such as eyes affected by wind with tearflow and itching, the growth of a shade, and **red canthi**".

Chi zong **瘛瘲, clonic spasms** [14] AW 瘈瘲.

IS of the body sinews alternatingly contracting and relaxing, with uncontrollable spastic movements of hands and feet. *MYBL* SE *sheng xiao* 生消：主風熱癲癇，小兒驚邪**瘛瘲**, "It controls wind heat, peak-illness, and epilepsy, as well as fright evil in children with **clonic spasms**".

Chi zong **瘈瘲, clonic spasms** [26]

IS AW of → *chi zong* 瘛瘲. *BJ* SE *lu feng fang* 露蜂房：主驚癇**瘈瘲**，寒熱邪氣, "It controls fright epilepsy and **clonic spasms**, as well as evil qi of cold and heat".

Chong bing **蟲病, worm diseases** [5]

PC CD of all diseases resulting from the presence of worms. *BCSY* SE *tong tuo mu* 通脫木：藥草，生江南，主**蟲病**，今俗亦名通草, "*Yao cao* grows in the South of the Yangzi. It controls **worm diseases**. Nowadays it is commonly called *tong cao*".

Chong chuang **蟲瘡, bug sores** [24]

PC of → *chuang* 瘡, sores, conditions generated by bugs, insects, worms, etc. *MYBL* SE *fang ji* 防己：散癰腫惡結，諸瘑疥癬**蟲瘡**, "It disperses obstruction-illnesses with swelling, malign nodes, all types of lair-illness, *jie*-illness, *xuan*-illness, and **bug sores**".

Chong die **蟲喋, worm-gnawing** [1]
PC with the growth of parasites in the throat, causing swelling and pain there as a major sign. *SHZBL* 3: 黑龍煎，治咽喉腫痛九種疾…急喉閉、纏喉風、結喉、爛喉、重舌、木舌、遁蟲、**蟲喋**、飛絲入喉, "'Black dragon decoction' cures nine types of ailments of a swollen and aching throat…acute throat closure, throat-constricting wind, bound throat, festering throat, doubled tongue, wooden tongue, run-away bug, **worm-gnawing**, flying silk threads entering the throat".

Chong e **衝惡, surging malignity** [2]
PC of sudden distension and pain affecting the heart and abdomen that cannot be removed by emetics or laxatives. *SYDSF* 8: 卒心腹脹滿，吐利不行，如乾霍亂狀，世所謂**衝惡**是也, "If one suddenly feels distension and fullness in his heart and abdomen, with neither vomiting or purging bringing relief, and if the appearance is that of dry cholera, this is generally called **surging malignity**".

Chong e **重齶, doubled palate** [2] AN *chong e* 重齶.
Pediatric PC with a swelling of the upper palate as if the upper palate consisted of two layers. *SJZL* 167: 小兒初生，上齶有物脹起若懸癰，或如蘆籜盛水之狀者，名曰**重齶**, "When something grows on the upper palate of newborns as if there were an obstruction-illness hanging down, sometimes looking like bamboo sheaths used to scoop up water, this is called '**doubled palate**'".

Chong e **重齶, doubled palate** [1]
PC identical with → *chong e* 重齶. *BCGM* Bai bing zhu zhi yao 百病主治藥：蛇蛻灰，重舌**重齶**，並醋和摻, "*She tui* ashes mixed with vinegar [cure] doubled tongue and **doubled palate**".

Chong ji **蟲積, worm accumulation** [9]
PC of → *ji ju* 積聚, accumulation and collection, disease brought forth by the presence of parasites in the intestinal tract. *YYXS* 14: 治**蟲積**、食積、胎積、驚積，惡物、食傷，水精丹方, "To cure **worm accumulation**, food accumulation, fetal accumulation, fright accumulation, [the presence of] malign items, and harm caused by food, [use] the recipe for the elixir with *shui jing*".

Chong jie **蟲疥, bug *jie*-illness** [1]
PC identical with → *jie chuang* 疥瘡, *jie*-illness sores. *BCGM* SE *lang du* 狼毒 quotes *LSJYF*: 乾濕**蟲疥**：狼毒不拘多少，搗爛，以豬油、馬油調搽患處, "Dry and moist **bug *jie*-illness**: take any amount of *lang du* and grind to a pulp. Mix with lard and horse fat and apply externally to the ailing region".

Chong ju **蟲疽, bug impediment-illness** [2]
PC identical with → *chong chuang* 蟲瘡, bug sores. *SLBC* SE *xing* 杏：燒令烟盡，研如泥，綿裹，內女人陰中，治**蟲疽**, "Burn until all smoke has vanished. Grind to a mud-like consistency. Fill in a silk pouch and insert into the female yin (i.e. genital) part. This cures **bug impediment-illness**".

Chong lai **蟲癩, bug repudiation-illness** [3]

PC identical with → *lai* 癩, repudiation-illness. Because it was assumed already in ancient times that this disease is caused by bugs/worms, it was also called "bug repudiation-illness". *BCGM* SE *bai* 柏 quoting *TBC*: 療瘑疥及癩瘡良, "It is good in curing lair-illness, *jie*-illness, and repudiation-illness sores", writes: 療瘑疥及**蟲癩**良, "It is good in curing lair-illness, *jie*-illness, and **bug repudiation-illness**".

Chong ni **蟲䘌, hidden-worms infestation** [15] AN *ni chong* 䘌蟲.

PC identical with → *ni* 䘌, hidden worms. *PJF* 213: 聖湯，治下赤白痢，大孔**蟲䘌**生, "Decoction of sages. It cures red-white free-flux illness, and anal **hidden-worms infestation**".

Chong qu **蟲齲, worm decay of teeth** [1]

EA of bugs/worms eroding the teeth. *BCGM* Bai bing zhu zhi yao 百病主治藥：牙痛，有風熱，濕熱，胃火，腎虛，**蟲齲**, "Toothache may result from wind heat, moisture heat, stomach fire, kidney depletion, and **worm decay of teeth**".

Chong shang **蟲傷, injury caused by bugs/worms** [5] AN *zhu chong shang* 諸蟲傷, all types of injury caused by bugs/worms.

PC CD of all types of skin damage, sometimes affecting the condition of the entire body, resulting from an insect bite or poisonous sting. *RHZ* SE *shi yan* 食鹽：止風淚，邪氣，一切**蟲傷**瘡腫, "It stops wind tears, evil qi, and all types of **wounds caused by bugs/worms**, with sores and swelling". *BCGM* Bai bing zhu zhi yao. Zhu chong shang 百病主治藥 諸蟲傷 identifies the following creatures as *chong* 蟲: *she hui* 蛇虺, poisonous snake; *wu song* 蜈蚣, centipede; *feng chai* 蜂蠆, bee/wasp and scorpion; *zhi zhu* 蜘蛛, spider; *qu* 蠼螋, earwig; *can ci* 蠶蛓, silkworm; *qiu yin* 蚯蚓, earthworm; *wo niu* 蝸牛, snail; *she gong* 射工, "archer"; *sha shi* 沙虱, sand louse; *zhi* 蛭, leech; *lou gu* 螻蛄, mole cricket; *yi* 蟻, ant; *ying* 蠅, house-fly; *you yang* 蚰蜒, house-centipede. *BCGM* often combines the name of a bug/worm with the character *shang* 傷, e. g., *wu song shang* 蜈蚣傷, harm caused by a centipede; *you yang shang* 蚰蜒傷, harm caused by a house-centiped; *feng shang* 蜂傷, harm caused by bees, etc. The meaning of these terms is obvious; they do not have a separate entry in this dictionary.

Chong she **重舌, doubled tongue** [53]

PC with the growth underneath the tongue, mostly in children, of what appears like a second tongue. *ZBYHL* 30: 心脾有熱，熱氣隨脈波於舌本，血脈脹起，變生如舌之狀，在於舌本之下，謂之**重舌**, "When heart and spleen have heat and the heat qi following the vessels flows towards the base of the tongue, the blood vessels will distend and rise and assume a shape reminiscent of a tongue which is below the base of the [proper] tongue. One calls this '**doubled tongue**'".

Chong she shang **蟲蛇傷, injury caused by bugs/worms and snakes** [2]

PC identical with → *chong shang* 蟲傷, harm caused by bugs/worms. *RHZ* SE *wu lan* 吳藍：解毒藥、毒箭，金瘡，血悶，**蟲蛇傷**, "It dissolves the poison of pharmaceutical drugs, the poison of arrows, [heals] wounds inflicted by metal objects, blood heart-pressure, and **injury caused by bugs/worms and snakes**".

Chong shou shang **蟲獸傷, harm caused by bugs/worms and animals** [1]
PC CD of → 蟲傷, harm caused by bugs/worms, and → *zhu shou shang* 諸獸傷, harm caused by all types of animals. *BCGM* SE *xiong huang* 雄黃 quoting *RHZ*: 一切蛇蟲犬獸傷咬, "Harm from bites by all types of snakes, bugs/worms, dogs, and other animals", writes: 一切**蟲獸傷**, "All types of **harm caused by bugs/worms and animals**". *PJF* 306 has: 諸**蟲獸傷**門, "Division of all types of **harm caused by bugs/worms and animals**".

Chong tong **蟲痛, worm pain** [19]
PC CD of conditions of pain brought forth by the presence of *chong* 蟲, bugs/worms. These may be parasites, as in the case of pain resulting from worms in the heart and abdomen. These may also be worms identified as pathogenic agents in ancient beliefs, as in the case of pain resulting from teeth worms. *ZBYHL* 29: 若**蟲痛**，非針灸可瘥，敷藥蟲死，乃痛止, "If it is **worm pain**, neither needles nor moxa can bring a cure. One must apply medication to kill the worms, and the pain will end".

Chong xian **蟲癇, worm epilepsy** [2]
PC of → *xian* 癇, epilepsy, brought forth by bugs/worms. *BCGM* SE wu yi 蕪荑 quotes *DRF*: 小兒**蟲癇**：胃寒蟲上諸證，危惡與癇相似, "**Worm epilepsy** in children: all the pathological conditions of stomach cold and ascending worms are dangerous and malign and resemble those of epilepsy".

Chong xin teng **蟲心疼, worm heartache** [1]
PC identical with → *chong xin tong* 蟲心痛. *BCGM* Bai bing zhu zhi yao 百病主治藥：胡粉，葱汁丸服，治女人**蟲心疼**, "Ingestion of pills with *hu fen* and *cong zhi* cures **worm heartache** in women".

Chong xin tong **蟲心痛, worm heartache** [11] AN *chong xin teng* 蟲心疼.
PC CD of conditions of → *xin tong* 心痛, heartache, brought forth by the presence of worms, mostly these are → *hui chong* 蛔蟲, roundworms. *QJYF* 13: 九痛丸，治九種心痛，一**蟲心痛**, "The pills for nine types of pain. They cure nine types of heartache. The first is: **worm heartache".**

Chong xuan **蟲癬, bug *xuan*-illness** [4]
PC identical with → *xuan* 癬, *xuan*-illness a). *BCGM* SE *shui yin* 水銀 quoting *WTMY* 30: 疥癬癢痛不可忍者, "In the case of *jie*-illness and *xuan*-illness with unbearable itching and pain", writes: **蟲癬**瘙癢, "**Bug *xuan*-illness** with itching".

Chong ya **蟲牙, worm teeth** [29] AN *chong ya* 蚛牙.
PC identical with → *qu chi* 齲齒, decayed teeth. *PJF* 68: 雄黃散，治**蟲牙**痛, "The powder with *xiong huang* cures **worm teeth** with pain".

Chong ya **蚛牙, worm-borer teeth** [1] AN *feng chong ya tong* 風蚛牙痛, wind worm-borer teeth with pain.

PC identical with → *chong ya* 蟲牙, worm teeth. *RHZ* SE *shi dan* 石膽：治**蚛牙**，鼻內息肉, "It cures **worm-borer teeth** and tumorous flesh-growth in the nose".

Chong yang **蟲癢, worm itching** [3]

PC CD of conditions of itching brought forth by the presence of *chong* 蟲, bugs/worms. *QJYF* 18: 治大孔**蟲癢**方, "Recipe to cure anal **worm itching**".

Chong zhi **蟲痔, bug piles** [10]

PC of → *zhi chuang* 痔瘡, piles sores, with bugs/worms inside. The anus is moist and festers. In many cases erosion leads to punctuation with holes and the generation of fistulae. *QJYiF* 24: 以紙裹莨菪根，煻火燒熟，以蜜塗納下部中，一切**蟲痔**皆愈, "Wrap a *lang dang* root in paper, roast in a pit fire until done, smear with honey and insert from below. All types of **bug piles** will be cured".

Chou che **抽掣, convulsions** [5]

IS of jerking hands and feet. *KBBC* SE *huai jiao* 槐膠：治肝臟風，筋脈**抽掣**及急風口噤, "It cures wind in the liver depot, with **convulsions** of the sinews and vessels, and acute wind with clenched jaw".

Chou han **臭汗, malodorous sweating** [5]

IS of sweating accompanied by a rather strong odor. *MYBL* SE *yang qi shi* 陽起石：去**臭汗**，消水腫, "It ends **malodorous sweating**, and dissolves water swelling".

Chou ye **臭腋, malodorous armpit** [1]

PC identical with → *ye chou* 腋臭, armpit stench. *TBC* SE *chi tong xie* 赤銅屑：主丁腫惡瘡，驢馬脊瘡，**臭腋**，石上水磨取汁塗之, "To control pin-swelling and malign sores, sores on the back of donkeys and horses, and **malodorous armpits**, grind with water on a stone and apply the liquid to the [affected areas]".

Chu **搐, jerking** [p]

IS identical with → *chou che* 抽掣, convulsions. *RHZ* SE *chong tai yan* 重台根：治胎風，**搐**手足, "It cures fetal wind, and **jerking** of hands and feet".

Chu che **搐掣, jerking of hands and feet; convulsions** [1]

IS identical with → *chou che* 抽掣, convulsions. *TPSHF* 21: 治破傷風，身體拘急，手足**搐掣**，牙關急強，宜服羌活散方, "To cure wound wind, with the entire body cramping and being tense, **jerking of hands and feet**, and clenched jaw, the recipe to ingest the powder with qiang huo is advisable".

Chu huang shui **出黃水, discharge of yellow water** [18]

IS of a discharge of yellow liquid from local lesions resulting from pathological changes, or from locations where a topical medical treatment was applied. *QJYF* 5: 治小兒傷寒發黃…搗韭根汁澄清，取如大豆許，滴兒鼻中，即**出黃水**，瘥, "To cure children harmed by cold who turn yellow, … pound the roots of *jiu* and let the juice settle until the liquid is clear. Take an amount of the size of a soy bean and drop into the child's nose. This will cause a **discharge of yellow water**, and brings the cure".

***Chu jiang* 搐強, jerking with stiffness** [1]
IS of jerking hands and feet with muscles being stiff at the same time. *BCGM* SE *hu* 狐. LSZ: 肝燒灰，治風癇及破傷風，口緊**搐強**, "Liver burnt to ashes cures wind epilepsy and wound wind, with tight mouth and **jerking with stiffness**".

***Chu jing* 除驚, to eliminate fright** [3]
TA identical with → *zhi jing* 止驚, to stop fright. *MYBL* SE *shi hu* 石斛：逐皮膚邪熱疿氣，脚膝疼冷痹弱，定志**除驚**, "It expels from the skin evil heat and seething rash qi, and from the legs and knees pain, cold blockage, and weakness. It stabilizes the mind and **eliminates fright**".

***Chu li* 初痢, beginning free-flux illness** [1]
PC of → *li ji* 痢疾, free-flux illness, at its onset. *BCGM* SE *xian* 莧：利大小腸，治**初痢**, "It opens the passage through large and small intestine. It cures **beginning free-flux illness**".

***Chu nong* 出膿, discharge of pus** [29] AN *chu nong zhi* 出膿汁.
IS of a yellow-white liquid discharged from local lesions resulting from pathological changes. *ZBYHL* 31: 若不早**出膿**，膿食筋爛骨，則不可治也, "If there is no early **discharge of pus**, the pus will consume the sinews and make the bones rot. At this stage a cure will be impossible".

***Chu nong zhi* 出膿汁, discharge of pus** [2]
IS identical with → *chu nong* 出膿. *QJYF* 6: 治聤耳**出膿汁**方, "Recipe to cure *otitis media* with **discharge of pus**".

***Chu nuo* 搐搦, convulsions** [33]
IS of uncontrolled phases of jerking and immobility of the four limbs. *TPSHF* 83: 治小兒中風，筋脈拘急，項強，腰背硬，手足**搐搦**，發歇不定，羚羊角散方, "To cure children struck by wind, with sinews and vessels cramping and being tense, stiff nape, hardness of lumbar region and back, and with their hands and feet experiencing **convulsions** in irregular phases of outbreak and inactivity, [it is advisable to take] the recipe for the powder with *ling yang jiao*".

***Chu shui* 出水, discharge of water** [40]
IS of any abnormal discharge of liquids from the human body. This includes the discharge of liquids from the skin or mucous membranes, from lesions resulting from pathological changes, and also by way of spitting/vomiting, as well as large quantities of urine or watery stool. *ZBYHL* 23: 後六十日腫如裹水狀，如此可刺之。但**出水**，後乃有血，血出即除也, "Later, over a period of 60 days, a swelling develops resembling a water blister. At this point one may pierce it. At first, there is only a **discharge of water**. Later there will be blood. At the moment blood is discharged, remove [the needle]". Liquids discharged from lesions resulting from pathological changes are also called *chu zhi* 出汁. As the nature of the liquids discharged varies, authors have distinguished between *chu huang shui* 出黃水, discharge of yellow water, and *chu nong* 出膿, discharge of pus.

Chu zhi **出汁, discharge of liquid** [27] AN *zhi chu* 汁出; *liu shui* 流水, water flow; *shui yi* 水溢, water spill.

IS of a discharge of liquid from local sores resulting from pathological changes. A variant of → *chu shui* 出水, discharge of water. *QJYF* 5: 輕者臍不大腫，但出汁, "In mild cases, the umbilicus shows only a light swelling, but there is a **discharge of liquid**".

Chuan **喘, panting** [p] AN *qi chuan* 氣喘, *chuan ji* 喘急; *chuan ni* 喘逆, panting with [qi] counterflow; *shang qi* 上氣, rising qi.

① AN *chuan xi* 喘息. IS of rapid in- and exhalation, often accompanied by breathing difficulties. *SW* 22: 肺病者，**喘**咳逆氣，肩背痛, "In the case of a lung disease, one **pants** and coughs from qi moving contrary [to its regular course]. There is pain in the shoulders and the back".

② PC resulting from all types of causes with panting. *SW* 19: 其不及則令人**喘**, "If it is inadequate, this makes a person **pant**".

Chuan cu **喘促, panting** [26]

IS identical with → *chuan ji* 喘急①. *YXL* SE *xing ren* 杏仁：療肺氣咳嗽，上氣、**喘促**, "It cures lung qi cough, ascending qi, **panting**".

Chuan ji **喘急, panting** [73]

① AN *chuan cu* 喘促. IS identical with → *chuan* 喘①. *ZHF* 2: 治胸脅痞滿，心塞氣急，**喘急**方, "A recipe to cure obstacle-illness and a feeling of fullness in the chest and flanks, heart congestion and qi urgency, as well as **panting**".

② PC identical with → *chuan* 喘②. *ZBYHL* 47: 冷乳入腹，與胃氣相逆，則腹脹痛，氣息**喘急**, "When cold milk enters the abdomen and interacts with stomach qi, this will result in abdominal distension and pain, with breathing [changing to] **panting**".

Chuan ke **喘咳, panting with cough** [21]

① IS identical with → *chuan sou* 喘嗽①, panting with cough. *SW* 22: 肺病者，**喘咳**逆氣，肩背痛, "In the case of a lung disease, one **pants and coughs** from qi moving contrary [to its regular course]. There is pain in the shoulders and the back".

② IS identical with *chuan sou* 喘嗽②. *YXL* SE *zhi shi* 枳實：主上氣**喘咳**，腎內傷冷, " It controls rising qi and **panting with cough**, when the kidneys are harmed internally by cold".

Chuan man **喘滿, panting and fullness** [20]

IS of a hectic breathing associated with a feeling of depression and fullness. *SHL* 210: 鄭聲者，重語也，直視、譫語、**喘滿**者死, "Fading murmuring (lit: the [dissonant] sounds of [the music in the state of] Zheng) is repetitive, stuttering speech. Those who stare straight ahead, speak incoherently, **pant and experience a feeling of fullness**, they die".

Chuan ni **喘逆, panting with [qi] counterflow** [6]

① IS identical with → *chuan* 喘①, panting. *BJ* SE *jin cao* 藎草：主久咳，上氣**喘逆**, "It controls chronic cough, with ascending qi and **panting with [qi] counterflow**".

② PC identical with → *chuan* 喘②. *BCGM* Bai bing zhu zhi yao 百病主治藥：**喘逆**：古名咳逆上氣, "**Panting with [qi] counterflow**: In ancient times this was called 'cough with qi ascending contrary to its regular direction'".

***Chuan shi* 傳屍, corpse [evil] transmission** [59] AN *gu zheng lao* 骨蒸勞, exhaustion because of bone steaming; *fu lian* 伏連, hidden link.

PC of an infectious consumptive disease. The Song-era physician Chen Yan 陳言 believed it to be identical with → *lao zhai* 勞瘵, exhaustion consumption. *QJYiF* 20: RE *da jin ya san* 大金牙散, massive powder with *jin ya*: **傳屍**骨蒸病家合，佳, "All members of a household with patients suffering from **corpse [evil] transmission** and bone steaming should prepare [this medication]; very good".

***Chuan sou* 喘嗽, panting with cough** [39] AN *chuan ke* 喘咳.

① IS of → *ke sou* 咳嗽①, cough, together with → *chuan* 喘①, panting. *ZBYHL* 19: 肺之積，名曰息賁。在右肋下，覆大如杯，久不愈，令人洒淅寒熱，**喘嗽**, "Accumulations in the lung are called 'rapid breathing'. Below one's left flank there is something like an overturned cup. When this is not cured for a long time it causes that person to shiver and have alternating feelings of cold and heat, as well as **panting with cough**".

② PC identical with → *chuan* 喘②, panting, and → *ke sou* 咳嗽②, cough. *TPSHF* 46: 積年肺氣**喘嗽**，宜服含化密陀僧丸方, "For lung qi **panting with cough** that has lasted for years the recipe to ingest the 'pills with *mi tuo seng* that are to dissolve in the mouth' is advisable".

***Chuan tong* 穿痛, penetrating pain** [1]

IS identical with → *che tong* 徹痛. *PJF* SE *ren shen* 人參：五味子丸，治白濁及腎虛，兩腰及背脊**穿痛**, "Pills with *wu wei zi*, they cure white turbidity and kidney depletion, with **penetrating pain** in the two lumbar regions and the back".

***Chuan xi* 喘息, panting; to breathe** [45]

① IS identical with → *chuan* 喘①, panting. *BJ* SE *hai ge* 海蛤：主咳逆上氣，**喘息**煩滿, "It controls cough with qi ascending contrary to its regular direction, and **panting** with vexation and a feeling of fullness".

② PN of breathing. *BJ* SE *hai ge* 海蛤：心下結氣，不能**喘息**, "Bound qi below the heart. [Patients] cannot **breathe**".

***Chuang* 瘡, sores; wound** [p] AN *chuang bing* 瘡病, sores disease.

PC a) AD of → *chuang yang* 瘡瘍, sores and ulcers. *SHL* 312: 少陰病，咽中傷，生**瘡**，不能語言，聲不出者，苦酒湯主之, "In the case of diseases affecting the minor yin, if there is harm to the throat developing into **sores** so that one cannot speak, and no sound is emitted, the decoction with bitter wine will control it". b) CD of external harm inflicted on skin and flesh. *JGYL* Mj: 若身有**瘡**，被刀斧所傷 …, "If the body has a **wound** resulting from harm inflicted by means of a knife or axe, …". c) CD of all types of skin diseases. *ZBYHL* 35: 諸所癢處，以手搔之，隨手輦展，起赤皻瘰；痦瘰消已，生細粟**瘡**甚微, "Wherever there is an itching spot, if one scratches there with his hand, following the movement of the hand a line like a road and red folds will emerge. When the miliaria have vanished, very minute millet-grain-size **sores** will be generated".

***Chuang ban* 瘡瘢, sores scar** [2]

PC of a → *ban* 瘢, scar, left after having had sores or an ulcer. *ZHF* 2: 治得瘥後，**瘡瘢**紫黑，彌歲方減，此**惡毒**之氣, "If after one has achieved a cure there remain purple-black **sores scars** that vanish only after a full year, this is the qi of a malign poison".

***Chuang bing* 瘡病, sores disease** [3]

PC identical with → *chuang* 瘡, sores. *ZBYHL* 35: **瘡病**諸候, "All signs of **sores disease**".

***Chuang dou* 瘡痘, sores smallpox** [3]

PC CD of infectious rashes. *BCGM* SE *hong lan hua* 紅藍花 quoting *RMSQ*: 小兒瘡疹, "Sores papules in children", writes: 小兒**瘡痘**, "**Sores smallpox** in children".

***Chuang du* 瘡毒, sores with poison** [42]

① PC identical with → *du chuang* 毒瘡, poison sores. *QJYF* 25: 治馬嚙人及踏人，作**瘡毒**，腫熱痛方, "Recipe to cure **sores with poison**, associated with swelling, heat, and pain, resulting from a horse's biting or kicking a person".

② EA of → *du qi* 毒氣, poison qi, causing → *du chuang* 毒瘡，poison sores. *BCGM* Shi ji 十劑：引**瘡毒**自小便去者，則五葉藤、萱草根之屬，皆滑劑也, "To drain **sores with poison** by way of the passage of urine, *wu ye teng* and *xuan cao gen* are lubricating formulae".

***Chuang jie* 瘡疥, sores in general and *jie*-illness sores in particular** [85]

PC CD of → *chuang* 瘡, sores, and → *jie* 疥, *jie*-illness. *BCJJZ* SE *ji ji* 及已：今人多用以合**瘡疥**膏，甚驗, "Today's people often employ it to prepare ointments for **sores and *jie*-illness.** It is most effective".

***Chuang jie* 瘡癤, sores with pimples** [26]

PC identical with → *jie* 癤, pimples. *QJYF* 22: 治虛熱，消**瘡癤**方, "Recipe to cure depletion heat, and to dissolve **sores with pimples**".

***Chuang lai* 瘡癩, repudiation-illness; sores in general and repudiation-illness in particular** [4]

PC a) identical with → *lai* 癩, repudiation-illness. *BCGM* SE *han hao chong* 寒號蟲 quotes *ZXF*: 大風**瘡癩**：油調五靈脂末，塗之, "For massive wind, (i.e.) **repudiation-illness**, mix *wu ling zhi* powder with oil and apply externally". b) CD of → *chuang* 瘡, sores, and → *lai* 癩, repudiation-illness. *BCJJZ* SE *ling li jia* 鯪鯉甲：方用亦稀，惟療**瘡癩**及諸疰疾爾, "It is rarely used in recipes, and if so only for curing **sores in general, repudiation-illness in particular**, and all types of attachment-illness ailments".

***Chuang lou* 瘡漏, sores with leakage** [1]

PC identical with → *lou chuang* 漏瘡, leaking sores. *PJF* 306: 治犬咬成**瘡漏**方。用鍛石細研為末，以醋和塗瘡上, "Recipe to cure dog-bite wounds that have developed into **sores with leakage**. Use a forge stone ground to a fine powder, mix with vinegar and smear on the sores".

Chuang lou **瘡瘺, fistula** [14]

PC identical with → *lou chuang* 瘺瘡, fistula sores. *MYBL* SE *man li yu* 鰻鱺魚：主五痔，**瘡瘺**，殺諸蟲, "It controls the five types of piles, and **fistulas**, and it kills all types of bugs/worms".

Chuang ni **瘡䘌, hidden-worms sores** [2]

PC identical with → *ni chuang* 䘌瘡. *PJF* 130: 傷寒八九日至十餘日，大煩渴熱盛而三焦有**瘡䘌**者，多下, "When in the course of harm caused by cold from the eighth, ninth day to the tenth day [patients experience] massive vexation, thirst, an abundance of heat, and **hidden-worms sores** in the region of the triple burner, this is often accompanied by diarrhea".

Chuang nong **瘡膿, festering sores** [2]

PC identical with → *nong chuang* 膿瘡. *BJ* SE *ze lan* 澤蘭：金瘡，癰腫**瘡膿**, "Wounds inflicted by metal objects; obstruction-illnesses, swelling, and **festering sores**".

Chuang pao **瘡皰 sores with blisters** [3]

PC identical with → *pao* 皰, blisters. *HYBC* SE *mao xiang hua* 茅香花：主小兒遍身**瘡皰**，以桃葉同煮浴之, "To master **sores with blisters** covering a child's entire body, boil together with *tao* leaves and use the liquid for bathing".

Chuang shang shui du **瘡傷水毒, sores harmed by water poison** [1]

PC identical with → *chuang shang shui shi* 瘡傷水濕, sores harmed by water or moisture. *BCGM* SE *shang lu* 商陸 quotes *QJYiF*: **瘡傷水毒**：章陸根搗炙，布裹熨之，冷即易之, "**Sores harmed by water poison**: Take *zhang lu* root, pound to a pulp, and roast. Wrap in fabric and apply as a hot compress [to the sores]. Change when [the compress] has cooled".

Chuang shang shui shi **瘡傷水濕, sores harmed by water [or] moisture** [2]

PC of open sores having been affected by water/moisture bringing forth swelling, pain, and festering. *BCGM* SE *fen xi* 粉錫 quoting *QJYF* 瘡中水腫, "Sores struck by water with swelling", writes: **瘡傷水濕**, "**Sores harmed by water [or] moisture**".

Chuang shi **瘡蝕, sores with erosion** [4]

PC identical with → *shi chuang* 蝕瘡, erosion sores. *BCTJ* SE *shi liu huang* 石硫黄：本經所說功用，止於治**瘡蝕**，攻積聚冷氣，脚弱等, "The effects related by the *BJ* are restricted to a treatment of **sores with erosion**, to attacking accumulations and collections of cold qi, and [curing] weakness of one's legs".

Chuang tong **瘡痛, sores with pain** [2]

PC CD of → *chuang* 瘡, sores, conditions associated with excruciating pain. *QJYF* 22: 解心煩，止**瘡痛**, "It serves to resolve heart vexation, and it stops **sores with pain**".

Chuang tong **瘡癢, sores with itching** [6]
PC CD of → *chuang* 瘡, sores, conditions associated with itching as a major sign. *MYBL* SE *lou lu* 漏蘆：熱氣**瘡癢**，如麻豆，可作浴湯, "This can be used for a hot bath [to cure] heat qi **sores with itching** of the size of *ma dou*".

Chuang tou **瘡頭, the heads of sores** [9]
PI CD of the central spot or top of all types of → *chuang yang* 瘡瘍， sores and ulcers. In general it is from the heads of sores that suppuration occurs. *ZBYHL* 30: 一者，**瘡頭**烏而強凹；二者，**瘡頭**白而腫實, "The first is: the **heads of the sores** are black, with a hard indentation. The second is: the **heads of the sores** are white and swollen with matter".

Chuang tou **瘡根, the base of sores** [4]
① PI CD of the base of all types of → *chuang yang* 瘡瘍, sores and ulcers. *QJYF* 22: 以針刺瘡中心深至**瘡根**，並刺四畔令血出, "Pierce the center of the sores with a needle down into the **sores' base**, and pierce also on its four sides to let blood".
② PP CD of putrid tissues within all types of → *chuang yang* 瘡瘍, sores and ulcers. *TPSHF* 66: 出却**瘡根**，便用生肌膏藥封之, "Remove the **sores' base** and then use the 'ointment to grow muscles' to close it".

Chuang xuan **瘡癬, sores with *xuan*-illness** [25]
PC identical with → *xuan* 癬, *xuan*-illness. *QJYF* 12: **瘡癬**，先以布揩汁出後，取[耆婆萬病丸]酢和敷上, "**Sores with *xuan*-illness**: First use a piece of cloth to wipe the liquid off, and then mix the ['granny's pills for a myriad of of diseases'] with vinegar and apply externally".

Chuang yang **瘡瘍, sores and ulcers** [36] AD *chuang* 瘡, sores; *yang* 瘍, ulcer.
PC CD of → *kui yang* 潰瘍, festering ulcers, on skin and mucosa, associated with a red swelling. *BJ* SE *dang gui* 當歸：胃中熱氣，面赤，酒皰皶鼻，白癩赤癩，**瘡瘍**, "Heat qi in the stomach. The face is red. The nose has wine blisters and blotches. There is white repudiation-illness and red repudiation-illness, as well as **sores and ulcers**".

Chuang zhen **瘡疹, sores with papules** [14]
PC identical with → *dou chuang* 痘瘡, smallpox sores. *SJZL* 169 has a treatise on 小兒**瘡疹**, "Children's **sores with papules**"

Chuang zhi **瘡痔, sores in general and piles in particular** [9]
PC CD of → *chuang* 瘡, sores, and → *zhi* 痔, piles. *BJ* SE *ya zi* 牙子：主邪氣熱氣，疥瘙惡瘍，**瘡痔**，去白蟲, "It controls evil qi and heat qi, *jie*-illness, itching and malign abscesses, **sores in general and piles in particular**, and removes white bugs/worms".

Chuang zhong **瘡腫, sores with swelling** [73]
PC a) identical with → *chuang yang* 瘡瘍, sores and ulcers. *BCJJZ* SE *sheng qi* 生漆：外氣亦能使身肉**瘡腫**，自別有療法, "Qi from the outside may cause the body's flesh to develop **sores with swelling**. For this there is a separate therapeutic approach". b) Identical with → *zhong yang* 腫瘍, swollen ulcer. *MYBL* SE

hu ma 胡麻：生者摩**瘡腫**，生禿髮, "Fresh specimens rubbed on **sores with swelling** will lead to baldness".

Chui nai **吹奶, inflated breast** [18] AN *chui ru* 吹乳.

PC with milk blocked after delivery and the breasts turning red and swelling. *TPSHF* 81: 乳不時泄，蓄積在內，結成腫，壅閉乳道，致使津液不通，腐結疼痛，名曰**吹奶**。若不急治，腫甚成癰也, "When the milk does not flow in due time it collects internally to nodes generating a swelling. The passageway of the milk is thus blocked, so that the liquid fails to pass. This leads to putrid nodes and pain. It is called '**inflated breast**'. If this is not treated immediately, the swelling will be severe and turn into an obstruction-illness".

Chui ru **吹乳, inflated breast** [17]

PC identical with → *chui nai* 吹奶. *ZBYHL* 40: 熱食汗出，露乳傷風，喜發乳腫，名**吹乳**，因喜作癰, "If one has eaten hot food so that sweat leaves [the body], and if then the bare breast is harmed by wind, it will most likely develop breast swelling. This is called '**inflated breast**' because it tends to produce an obstruction-illness".

Chun bai **唇白, white lips** [2]

IS of lips with a red color that is much blander than normal. *ZBYHL* 17: **唇白**，齒齗生瘡, "**White lips**; the gums produce sores".

Chun dong **唇動, lip movement** [2]

IS of an uncontrolled trembling movement of the lips. *BCGM* Bai bingzhu zhi yao 百病主治藥：風則**唇動**或喎, "Wind causes the **lips to move**, or make [the mouth] be awry".

Chun gan **唇乾, desiccated lips** [4]

IS of either a feeling of dry mouth and lips, or an appearance of cracked lips. *ZBYHL* 36: 口噤**唇乾**，血為斷絕，腹滿不言，其人如醉，未死之間，為不可治, "Clenched jaw and **desiccated lips**. The bloodflow is interrupted. A feeling of abdominal fullness, and speechlessness. Such patients appear as if intoxicated, shortly prior to death. They cannot be cured".

Chun he **唇核, lip kernel** [1]

PC identical with → *chun sheng he* 唇生核, a kernel developing on the lips. *BCGM* Bai bing zhu zhi yao 百病主治藥 quoting from the SE *shi shi* 豕屎in the main text: 口唇生核, "Mouth and lips develop a kernel", writes: **唇核**：豬屎汁，溫服, "For **lip kernel**: The liquid of hog feces, to be ingested warm".

Chun jiao **唇焦, parched lips** [2]

IS of dry lips assuming a parched, black color. *ZBYHL* 4: 脾蒸，**唇焦**, "[Bone-] steaming because of spleen [depletion]: the **lips are parched**".

Chun jie **唇揭, peeling lips** [2]

IS with dry, peeling lips. *SW* 10: 多食酸，則肉胝䐢而**唇揭**, "If one consumes large quantities of sour [food], the flesh hardens and shows wrinkles and the **lips peel**".

Chun jin **唇噤, clenched lips** [1]

IS identical with → *kou jin* 口噤, clenched jaw. *BCGM* Bai bing zhu zhi yao 百病主治藥: Among the pathological conditions affecting the lips, *chun* 唇, an entry states *chun jin* **唇噤, clenched lips**.

Chun jin **唇緊, lip tightness** [8]

① IS of a tightness of flesh and muscles in the face with the mouth also being tight and difficult to open. *QJYF* 16: 汗出衄衄，口喎**唇緊**, "Sweating and nosebleed. Wry mouth and **tight lips**".

② AN *jin chun chuang* 緊唇瘡, tight lip sores. PC identical with → *jin chun* 緊唇, tight lips. *TPSHF* 36: 治**唇緊**面腫，宜用此方, "To cure **lip tightness** and facial swelling it is advisable to use this recipe".

Chun jin chuang **唇緊瘡, lip tightness with sores** [1]

PC identical with → *chun jin* 唇緊②, lip tightness. *PJF* 300: 治**唇緊瘡**疼。訶子肉、五倍子（各半兩）。右為細末，干貼唇上，立效, "To cure **lip tightness with sores** and pain: *He zi rou* and *wu pei zi*, one half *liang* each, are to be finely ground to be applied on the lips. Immediately effective".

Chun kou qing **唇口青, purple lips** [5]

PC with → *chun qing* 唇青, purple lips, as a major sign. *BJ* SE *qing xiang zi* 青葙子：子名草決明，療**唇口青**, "The seeds are called *cao jue ming*. They cure **purple lips**".

Chun kou qing bai **唇口青白, purple-pale lips** [1]

IS of dried lips assuming a pale, dark color. *TPSHF* 72: 婦人數年月水不通，面色萎黃，**唇口青白**, "Women who have failed to menstruate for several years develop a wilting-yellow complexion and have **purple-pale lips**".

Chun lie **唇裂, lip fissures** [8]

IS of dry lips that show cracks. *QJYF* 6: 甲煎唇脂，治**唇裂**口臭方, "Recipe to cure **lip fissures** and oral stench: lip fat with *jia* [aroma and others] boiled [to create a perfume]".

Chun qing **唇青, purple lips** [9]

IS of lips that have lost their usual red luster and have darkened instead. In severe cases they show a dark, purple coloring. *LS* 10: **唇青**，舌卷，卵縮, "**Purple lips**, curled tongue, contracted testicles".

Chun shen **唇沈, lip leakage** [2]

PC identical with → *jin chun* 緊唇, tight lips. *BCGM* Bai bing zhu zhi yao 百病主治藥：緊唇濕爛，乍瘥乍發，經年累月，又名**唇沈**, "Tight lips with festering. At times it heals and then develops again. This continues over months and years. Another name is '**lip leakage**'".

Chun sheng he **唇生核, a kernel developing on the lips** [2] AD *chun he* 唇核, lip kernel.

PC with a small swelling resembling a fruit pit growing on one's lip. *QJYF* 6: 治**唇生核**方，豬屎平量一升，以水投，絞取汁，温服之, "Recipe to cure a **kernel developing on the lips**: 1 *sheng* of hog feces is to be stirred with water. Strain the liquid and ingest it warm".

Chun zao **唇燥, dry lips** [4]

IS of dry lips that have lost their natural luster, in serious cases with fissures and bleeding. *ZHF* 4: 腰背強痛，心中虛悸，咽干**唇燥**, "Lower back and spine are stiff and ache. The heart is depleted and there is palpitation. The throat is desiccated and the **lips are dry**".

Ci **疵, blemish** [p]

PC of speckles on the skin. In general this is not associated with any abnormal sensation and has only aesthetic implications. *ZBYHL* 31: 若虛損，**疵**點變生, "In the case of a depletion harm, **blemishes**, i.e. speckles, develop".

Ci chuang **刺瘡, piercing sores** [4]

PC identical with → *hu niao ci zhuang* 狐尿刺瘡, sores resulting from being pierced by fox urine. *SLBC* SE *bai ma jing* 白馬莖：刺**瘡**，取黑駁馬尿熱浸, "For **piercing sores**: soak in hot urine taken from a dark colored horse".

Ci feng **刺風, piercing wind** [5]

PC of skin ailments brought forth by wind evil and associated with itching or pain or numbness. *ZBYHL* 2: **刺風**候, "Signs of **piercing wind**".

Ci teng **刺疼, piercing pain** [1]

IS identical with → *ci tong* 刺痛. *SJZL* 12: 治風氣凝滯，胸膈不快，身體**刺疼**，小乳香丸方, "Recipe 'for minor pills with *ru xiang*': to cure stagnating wind qi with an uncomfortable sensation in the region of the chest and abdomen and a **piercing pain** affecting the entire body".

Ci tong **刺痛, piercing pain** [61] AN *tong ci* 痛刺, *ci teng* 刺疼, *zhui tong* 錐痛, stabbing pain.

IS of an acute pain, with a feeling as if one had been pierced by something shaped like a needle or awl. *ZBYHL* 23: 卒然心腹**刺痛**，悶亂欲死, "Suddenly there is a **piercing pain** in the heart and abdominal region. One feels heart-pressure and disorder and wishes to die".

Ci zhang **刺脹, piercing distension** [4] AN *zhang ci* 脹刺, distension with [a feeling of] having been pierced.

IS of an uncomfortable feeling of distension as if having been hit or stabbed. *BCGM* SE *chu* 楮 quotes *WTMY*: 天行病後脹滿：兩脅**刺脹**，臍下如水腫，以構樹枝汁，隨意服之。小便利即消, "Distension and a feeling of fullness following disease sent by heaven: **piercing distension** in both flanks, below the navel this looks like an edema. Take the juice from the leaves of *gou shu* and ingest them at will. Once urination is stimulated [the distension] will be eliminated".

Cu bing **卒病, sudden disease** [4]

CD of all PC with a sudden onset. *QJYF* 12: 近病及**卒病**皆用多，積久病即少服, "It is much used for all new diseases and **sudden diseases**. For chronic diseases it is rarely ingested".

Cu bu de yu **卒不得語, sudden inability to speak** [4]

PC identical with → *feng yin* 風喑, wind muteness. *ZHF* 3: 治**卒不得語**方。以苦酒煮菰子，敷頸一周，以衣苞，一日一夕乃解，即瘥, "Recipe to cure

sudden inability to speak: Boil *gu zi* in bitter wine and apply this externally all around the nape. Then cover it with thick clothing which is to be taken off again after one day and one night. This brings the cure".

Cu chuang **醋瘡, vinegar sores** [1]
PC identical with → *zuo chuang* 酢瘡, acid sores. *BCSY* SE *chan si fu ren mai shang cao* 產死婦人冢上草：主小兒**醋瘡**, "It controls **vinegar sores** in children".

Cu e **卒惡, sudden [stroke by the] malign** [1]
PC identical with → *zhong e* 中惡, struck by the malign. *TBC* SE *ren shi* 人屎：主諸毒**卒惡**，熱黃悶欲死者, "It controls all types of poison and **sudden [stroke by the] malign**, with the appearance of heat, jaundice, and heart pressure to the extent that [the patient] wishes to die".

Cu e si **卒惡死, sudden [appearance of] death resulting from [being struck by] the malign** [1]
PC identical with → *cu zhong e si* 卒中惡死, "sudden [appearance of] death resulting from being struck by the malign". *BCGM* SE *shi* 豕：心血，治**卒惡死**，及痘瘡倒靨, "The blood from its heart...cures **sudden [appearance of] death resulting from [being struck by] the malign**, as well as inverted moles".

Cu feng **卒風**, sudden wind [stroke] [8]
PC identical with → *zhong feng* 中風, struck by wind. *QJYF* 18: 薑附湯…亦主**卒風**, "The decoction with *jiang* and *fu* [*zi*]...is also able to control **sudden wind [stroke]**".

Cu lin **卒淋, sudden dripping** [8]
PC of → *lin bing* 淋病, dripping disease, with a sudden onset. *QJYF* 21: **卒淋**，灸外踝尖七壯, "For **sudden dripping**, cauterize the tip of the external ankles seven times".

Cu re **卒熱, sudden heat** [8]
IS of a fever that develops all of a sudden. *TBC* SE *su* 粟：其米泔汁，主霍亂，**卒熱**, "The slop obtained by rinsing it controls cholera and **sudden heat**".

Cu shi yin sheng **卒失音聲, sudden loss of voice** [1]
PC identical with → *shi yin* 失音①, loss of voice. *BCGM* SE *xing* 杏 quotes *YZ*: **卒失音聲**：方同上, "For **sudden loss of voice**: the same recipe as listed above".

Cu si **卒死, sudden [appearance of] death** [46] AN *bao si* 暴死, *bao wang* 暴亡, *bao yao* 暴夭.
Serious PC with sudden loss of consciousness, and an appearance of being dead. Prognosis includes a possibility of revitalization, and of death. *LS* 49: 人不病**卒死**，何以知之, "If someone has not been ill and yet develops a **sudden [appearance of] death**, how can this be understood?"

Cu wu **卒忤, sudden hostility** [6]
PC identical with → *ke wu* 客忤, a visitor's hostility. *ZHF* 1: **卒忤**，停屍不能言, "In the case of **sudden hostility**, [a person appears like an] uninterred corpse, and cannot speak".

Cu xian **卒癇, sudden epilepsy** [3]
PC of a → *dian xian* 癲癇, peak-illness with epilepsy, which breaks out all of a sudden. *ZLBC* SE *lu feng fang* 露蜂房 quotes *YSCRF*: **卒癇**。蜂房大者一枚，水三升，煮令濃赤，以浴小兒, "For **sudden epilepsy**: boil one large homeycomb cell in three *sheng* of water until a thick, red liquid has formed. This is used to bathe the child".

Cu xin **醋心, vinegar center** [11] AN *suan xin* 酸心, sour center.
IS of a comparatively mild case of → *tun suan* 吞酸, sour swallowing. *TPSHF* 5: **醋心**嘔逆，宿食不消, "**Vinegar center** (i.e. stomach) with vomiting and adverse movement [of qi]. Food remains in the body overnight and fails to be digested".

Cu xin tong **卒心痛, sudden heartache** [25]
① IS of sudden → *xin tong* 心痛①, heartache. *JZBYHL* 9: 熱爭則**卒心痛**，煩冤善嘔, "When heat strikes this results in **sudden heartache**. One experiences vexation, a feeling of grievance and tends to vomit".
② AN *ji xin tong* 急心痛. PC of an acute experience of → *xin tong* 心痛②, heartache. *QJYF* 30: 凡**卒心痛**，汗出，刺大敦出血立已, "For all cases of **sudden heartache** with sweating, pierce the *da dun* [insertion hole] to let blood, and this will result in an instant cure".

Cu ya **卒瘂, sudden muteness** [1]
PC with a sudden onset of speech impairment or a very deep voice. *SLBC* SE *xing he ren* 杏核人：人患**卒啞**，取杏人三分，去皮尖，熬，別杵桂一分，和如泥，取李核大綿裹含，細細咽之, "When someone suffers from **sudden muteness** take three fen of *xing ren*, remove the skin and the tips, and heat. In addition, pound 1 *fen* of *gui*, and mix to generate a paste. Take an amount the size of a plum-pit and wrap in silk cloth. This is to be held in the mouth. Small amounts [of the drugs will be dissolved by one's saliva] and are to be swallowed".

Cu yan **卒魘, nightmare** [3]
PC identical with → *yan mei* 魘寐. *ZBYHL* 23: **卒魘**者，屈也，謂夢裏為鬼邪之所魘屈, "As for **nightmares**, this is 'to succumb'. That is to say, one is forced to succumb by demonic evil in one's dreams".

Cu yue bu zhi **卒噦不止, sudden retching that does not end** [4]
IS of sudden and unending dry retching. *MYBL* SE *pi pa ye* 枇杷葉：主**卒噦不止**，下氣, "It controls **sudden retching that does not end**, and makes the qi move downwards".

Cu yi cui si **卒縊垂死, sudden [appearance of] death from hanging** [1]
PC identical with → *zi yi si* 自縊死, [appearance of] death from hanging oneself. *BCGM* SE *ji* 雞 quotes *ZHF*: 卒縊垂死：心下猶温者，勿斷繩。刺雞冠血滴口中，以安心神, "For **sudden [appearance of] death from hanging**, when the region below the [victim's] heart is still warm, do not sever the rope. Pierce a cock's comb and drip the blood into [the victim's] mouth to calm his heart and spirit".

Cu yin **卒喑, sudden muteness** [1]

PC identical with → *bao yin* 暴喑, sudden muteness. *BCGM* Bai bing zhu zhi yao 百病主治藥：木通、菖蒲，並出音聲。小兒**卒喑**，麻油泡湯服, "*Mu tong* and *chang pu*, they both enable people to issue their voice. When children are affected by **sudden muteness**, add warm water to *ma you*, and have them ingest it".

Cu zhong 卒中, sudden stroke [3]

PC identical with → *zhong feng* 中風, struck by wind. *ZHBJF* 3: **卒中**，風癱，身體不自收，不能語，迷昧不知人, "In the case of **sudden stroke**, this is wind paralysis with an inability to pull in one's limbs at will, an inability to speak, and a mental confusion with an inability to recognize people".

Cu zhong **卒腫, sudden and violent swelling** [15]

IS of a sudden and violent swelling, either topical or affecting the entire body. *QJYF* 6: 舌**卒腫**，滿口溢出，如吹豬胞, "The tongue shows a **sudden and violent swelling**. It fills the mouth and [saliva] flows out. As if a pig bladder had been blown up".

Cu zhong e si **卒中惡死, sudden [appearance of] death resulting from being struck by the malign** [9] AN *cu e si* 卒惡死, sudden [appearance of] death resulting from [being struck by] the malign.

PC of sudden appearance of death resulting from being unexpectedly struck by the malign. *BCGM* SE *wu* 鶩 quoting *ZHF* 1: 救卒死，或先病痛，或常居寢臥，奄忽而絕，皆是中死, "For sudden [appearance of death] either following prior disease and pain, or after a normal life while asleep, with a sudden cut-off, these all are cases of a fatal strike", writes: **卒中惡死**, "**Sudden [appearance of] death resulting from being struck by the malign**".

Cu zhong feng **卒中風, sudden wind stroke** [1]

PC identical with → *zhong feng* 中風, struck by wind. *QJYF* 6 has a paragraph with the title: 治**卒中風**口噤不止, "To cure **sudden wind stroke**, with clenched jaw, not ending [by itself]".

Cuan shi **竄視, scurrying vision** [1] AN *mu cuan* 目竄, scurrying eyes.

IS of eyeballs making involuntary uncontrolled movements. *PJF* 87: 為僻，為**竄視**, "It causes unilateral paralysis; it causes **scurrying vision**".

Cun **皴, chapped skin** [p]

PC identical with *cun lie* 皴裂, chapped skin cracks. *QJYF* 22: 治手足**皴**痛方：煮茄根洗之, "Recipe to cure painful **chapped skin** on the hands and feet: Boil *qie gen* and [use the resulting liquid] to wash them".

Cun bai **寸白, inch-long white; tapeworm** [23]

EA, PC, AD of → *cun bai chong* 寸白蟲. *MYBL* SE *sang gen bai pi* 桑根白皮：利水道，去**寸白**, "It clears the water ways and removes **tapeworms**".

Cun bai chong **寸白蟲, inch-long white worm; tapeworm** [17] AD *cun bai* 寸白; *bai chong* 白蟲.

① EA of a white parasitic tapeworm in the intestinal tract of humans. *ZBYHL* 18: **寸白蟲**候：寸白者，九蟲內之一蟲也。長一寸而色白，形小褊，因腑臟虛弱而能發動, "The signs of **tapeworms**: tapeworms are one of the nine types of worms. They are one *cun* long, and their color is white. They are of a small and narrow physical shape. It is because of a depletion and weakness affecting the depots that they become active".

② PC brought forth by parasites in the intestinal tract. *BCJJZ* SE *fei shi* 榧實：食其子，療**寸白蟲**, "Ingestion of its seeds cures **tapeworm**[-disease]".

Cun bai chong bing **寸白蟲病, tapeworm disease** [3]
PC identical with → *cun bai chong* 寸白蟲②. *BCGM* SE *bing lang* 檳榔 quoting *QJYF* 治寸白蟲方, "Recipe to cure tapeworm [disease]", writes: **寸白蟲病**, "**tapeworm disease**".

Cun lie **皴裂, chapped skin cracks** [13] AD *cun* 皴; AN *jun lie* 皸裂; *cun zhu* 皴瘃; *jun zhu* 皸瘃, chapped skin and chilblains.
PC of painful, dry, chapped skin brought forth by exposure to cold or wind. *QJYF* 6: 治遠行唇口面**皴裂**方, "Recipe to cure lips, mouth, and face developing **chapped skin cracks** on a long journey".

Cun zhu **皴瘃, chapped skin and chilblains** [1]
PC identical with *cun lie* 皴裂, chapped skin cracks. *BCGM* SE *da mai* 大麥：苗冬月面目手足**皴瘃**，煮汁洗之, "When during the winter months the face, eyes, hands, and feet experience **chapped skin with chilblains**, boil the seedlings and wash [the skin] with the resulting liquid".

Cuo **痤, acne** [3]
PC of → *jie* 癤，pimples, brought forth by being affected by wind and moisture while sweating. *SW* 3: 汗出見濕，乃生**痤**疿, "When sweat flows and meets with moisture, this generates **acne** and seething rashes".

Cuo die sun shang **蹉跌損傷, injury from a fall** [1]
PC identical with → *die pu shang sun* 跌扑傷損. *BCGM* SE *lu* 鹿 quoting *QJYF*: 筋傷蹉跌, "The sinews are injured because of a fall", writes: **蹉跌損傷**, "**Injury from a fall**".

Cuo kou **撮口, pursed mouth** [30]
① IS of contracted lips, pursed like the mouth of a fish. *TPSHF* 85: 臍風**撮口**，天瘹驚風，並服此牛黄散方, "For navel wind with **pursed mouth**, [when the child suffers from] the hooked-up-by-heaven-illness fright wind, ingest this together with the recipe for the powder with *niu huang*".
② PC with pursed mouth as its main appearance, mostly seen in children. *WTMY* 35: 療小兒吃奶不穩，三日至七日以來，覺壯熱顏色赤，及鼻孔黄，即恐作**撮口**, "To cure children who have not been regularly breast-fed, since three to seven days, who feel very hot and have a red complexion, with their nostrils assuming a yellow color, this may turn into **pursed mouth**".

Cuo tong **撮痛, tugging pain** [5]
IS of a pain associated with a feeling as if one were being tugged. *WTMY* 7: 又療胸膈滿塞，心背**撮痛**，走注氣悶。宜服此柴胡湯方, "Also, to cure a feeling of fullness and blockage in the region of chest and diaphragm, with a **tugging pain** affecting the heart and back, and with qi pouring in and causing heart-pressure, the recipe to ingest the decoction with *chai hu* is advisable".

- D -

***Da bai yi* 大白蟻, big termites** [1]
PC with sounds in one's brain as its major sign. *BCGM* SE *ming* 茗 quoting *YFZY*: 頭內有蟲蛀響聲，名天白蟻。用茶子細末，吹入鼻中，效, "If in the head there is a ringing sound of insects boring, this is called 'heaven's termite'. Prepare a fine powder from *cha zi* and blow this into the nose. Effective", writes: 頭腦鳴響：狀如蟲蛀，名**大白蟻**, "Sounds in one's brain as if there were insects boring is called '**big termites**'". The term 大白蟻, "big termites", may simply be an erroneous writing of *tian bai yi* 天白蟻, "heaven's termite".

***Da bian bi* 大便閉, closure of major relief; constipation** [2]
IS identical with → *da bian mi* 大便秘①. *PJF* 143: 神聖自利膏，治傷寒及諸證**大便閉**, "The 'ointment by which gods and sages help themselves' cures harm caused by cold and all conditions of **constipation**".

***Da bian bi se* 大便閉澀, closure and roughness of major relief; constipation with roughness** [1]
IS identical with → *da bian mi* 大便秘①, constipation. *QXLF* 3 RE *sao feng san* 搜風散, powder to sweep away wind: 治風氣，中脘不利，**大便閉澀**, "It cures wind qi, with a blocked passage in the central duct and **constipation with roughness**".

***Da bian bu gu* 大便不固, major relief not firmly controlled; incontinence of stools** [1]
IS identical with → *yi shi* 遺屎, fecal incontinence. *SYDXF* 11: 治瘡疹漸黑，面陷，**大便不固**, "To cure sores and papules gradually assuming a dark color, when the face is sunken in, and [patients are] **incontinent of stools**".

***Da bian bu kuai* 大便不快, retarded major relief; prolonged defecation** [1]
IS of an extreme urgency to relieve oneself and yet the passage of stool is not smooth. *SJZL* 97: 治里急後重，**大便不快**，服炒桃仁法, "To cure abdominal cramps and a feeling of heavy pressure at one's behind, with **prolonged defecation**, [use the therapeutic] pattern of ingesting roasted *tao ren*".

***Da bian bu li* 大便不利, major relief impeded; stools do not pass freely** [2]
IS identical with → *bian nan* 便難, difficult defecation. *QJYF* 9: 胃中有宿食，**大便不利**方, "Recipe for food remaining in the stomach over night, with **stools not passing freely**".

***Da bian bu tong* 大便不通, major relief blocked; constipation** [28]
PC identical with → *da bian mi*. *ZBYHL* 9: 津液竭，則胃干，結熱在內，**大便不通**也, "When the body liquids are exhausted, the stomach is dry and bound heat forms inside. [This leads to] **constipation**".

***Da bian cu jie* 大便卒結, major relief suddenly bound; sudden constipation** [1]
PC of a → *da bian mi* 大便秘②, constipation that emerges all of a sudden, apparently not resulting from some previous pathological condition. *BCGM* SE *yang ti* 羊蹄 quoting *TPSHF*: 大便卒澀結不通, "Defecation is suddenly associ-

ated with roughness and nodes, and failure to pass", writes: 大便卒結, "**Sudden constipation**".

Da bian geng se **大便更澀, major relief changed to roughness; defecation changed to roughness** [1]

IS identical with → *bian nan* 便難, difficult defecation. *BCGM* SE *mu lian* 木蓮 quoting *YSJCF*: 大便急澀, "Defecation is urgent and rough", writes: **大便更澀**, "**Defecation has changed to roughness**", possibly a misreading of the character 急 as 更.

Da bian jian nan **大便艱難, major relief with difficulty; difficult defecation** [1]

IS identical with *bian nan* 便難, difficult defecation. *YSJCF* 3: 芎黃丸，治風熱壅盛，頭昏目赤，**大便艱難**, "Pills with *xiong huang* cure wind heat congestion, clouded head and red eyes, and **difficult defecation**". *BCGM* SE *tao* 桃 quoting *QJYF*: 大便難 writes: **大便艱難**, "**difficult defecation**".

Da bian jie **大便結, major relief bound; bound stools; constipation** [5]

IS identical with → *da bian mi* 大便秘①, constipation. *PJF* 135 RE po jie dan 破結丹, elixir to break through knottings: **大便結**，攻之不及，達之不可，以此主之, "In the case of **bound defecation** where attacks remain unsuccessful, and that cannot be reached, resorting to this [medication] will control it".

Da bian mi **大便秘, major relief closed; constipation** [5] AW *bian bi* 便閉, *bian mi* 便秘, *da bian bi* 大便閉; *bi se* 秘塞, *bi se* 閉塞; AN *da chang mi* 大腸秘, large intestine closure; *mi se* 秘澀, constipation roughness; *da bian jie* 大便結, bound stools; *da bian bu tong* 大便不通, constipation

① IS of various circumstances causing one's stool to harden und make defecation difficult. Also, defecation may be frequent with only small quantities discharged. *TPSHF* 8: 陽明病脅下堅滿，**大便秘**而嘔，口燥，宜柴胡湯, "For yang brilliance disease, when one has a feeling of hardness and fullness below the flanks, with **constipation** and vomiting, and a dry mouth, it is appropriate to take the decoction with *chai hu*".

② PC of diseases with constipation as their major sign. *BCGM* SE *xing* 杏 quotes [Li] Gao 杲：治**大便秘**，當分氣、血, "When treating **constipation** it is essential to distinguish between its association with qi and with blood".

Da bian nan **大便難, major relief with difficulty; difficult defecation** [2]

IS identical with *bian nan* 便難. *SHL* 181: 不更衣，內實，**大便難**, "They do not change clothes (i.e. they do not go to the toilet), have inner repletion and **defecation is difficult**".

Da bian nan se **大便難澀, major relief with difficulty and roughness; difficult and rough defecation** [1]

IS identical with *bian nan* 便難, difficult defecation. *BCGM* SE *ku gua* 甜瓜 quoting *TPSHF*: 大便有膿, "The stool carries pus", writes: **大便難澀**下膿, "**defecation is difficult and rough**, with a discharge of pus".

Da bian se **大便澀, major relief with roughness; rough defecation** [3]
IS identical with → *bian nan* 便難, difficult defecation. *ZBYHL* 12: 即是患黃，多**大便澀**, “Then this [person] suffers from jaundice, and often experiences **rough defecation**”.

Da bian se zhi **大便澀滯, major relief with roughness and sluggishness; rough and sluggish defecation** [2]
IS identical with → *bian nan* 便難, difficult defecation. *RMSQ* 4: 夫老人久病，**大便澀滯**不通者，可服神功丸、麻仁丸、四生丸則愈矣, “Now, when old people have a chronic disease, with **rough and sluggish defecation** or [stool] not passing at all, they may take the ‘wondrously effective pills’, or the pills with *ma ren* or the ‘pills with four unprocessed ingredients’ and will be cured”.

Da bian shuo **大便數, frequently repeated major relief; frequent defecation** [1]
IS of defecation with increased frequency. *QJYiF* 22: 小便不利，**大便數**而少, “Urination is impeded; **defecation is frequent** with small quantities”.

Da bian ying **大便硬, major relief with hardness; hard stools** [1]
IS of stools that are harder than normal and cannot be discharged easily. *SHL* 148: 心下滿，口不欲食，**大便硬**，脈細, “A feeling of fullness below the heart, loss of appetite, **hard stools**, and a subtle [movement in the] vessels”.

Da bian yong jie **大便壅結, major relief obstructed and bound; stools are obstructed and bound** [1]
PC identical with → *da bian mi* 大便秘②, constipation. *BCGM* SE shui yin fen 水銀粉 quoting *PJF*: 大腸壅結, “obstruction of the large intestine”, writes: **大便壅結, “Stools are obstructed and bound”.**

Da bian zao **大便燥, major relief with dryness; dry stools** [1]
IS of stools that are dry and cannot be discharged easily. *QJYiF* 19: 或已嘔吐，或**大便燥**，或復重下, “In some cases [patients] vomit, or they may have **dry stools**, or they repeatedly defecate”.

Da bing **大病, massive disease** [9]
PC CD of serious diseases with massive damage to a person’s body. The opposite of a → *xiao bing* 小病, minor disease. *SW* 13: 小病必甚，**大病**必死, “Minor diseases will be serious; **massive diseases** must end in death”.

Da chang bi se **大腸閟塞, closure of the large intestine** [2]
IS identical with → *da bian mi* 大便秘①, constipation. *BCGM* SE *ju* 橘 quotes *PJF*: **大腸閟塞**，陳皮連白，酒煮焙研末，每溫酒服二錢, “For **large intestine closure** take *chen pi* without discarding the white parts. Boil with wine, dry over fire, and grind to a powder. Each time ingest 2 *qian* with warm wine”.

Da chang feng **大腸風, wind [affecting the] large intestine** [1]
PC identical with *feng bi* 風秘, wind closure. *KBBC* SE *zhi ke* 枳殼：散留結胸膈痰滯，逐水，消脹滿、**大腸風**, “They disperse stagnating nodes with phlegm sluggishness in the chest and diaphragm, eliminate water, dissolve distension and fullness, and **wind [affecting the] large intestine**”.

Da chang huo 大腸火, fire [affecting the] large intestine [4]
PC of heat-type diseases affecting the large intestine. *ZZN* 1: 黄芩瀉**大腸火**, "*Huang qin* drains **fire [affecting the] large intestine**".

Da chang mi 大腸秘, tightness of the large intestine [1]
IS identical with → *da bian mi* 大便秘①, constipation. *BCYY* SE *xing he ren* 杏核仁：治肺燥喘熱，**大腸秘**，潤澤五臟, "They cure lung dryness with panting and fever, as well as **tightness of the large intestine**, and they moisten the five depots".

Da chang tuo 大腸脫, prolapse of the large intestine [2]
PC identical with → *tuo gang* 脫肛, prolapse of the rectum. *PJF* 5: 龍骨，甘，純陽。固**大腸脫**, "*Long gu*, sweet. Pure yang. It serves to stabilize a **prolapse of the large intestine**".

Da chang xue bi 大腸血閟, closure of the large intestine because of blood [2]
PC identical with → *xue mi* 血秘, tightness [of the large intestine] because of blood. *BCGM* SE *ju* 橘 quoting *ZZNYXF*: 大腸血閉 writes: **大腸血閟, closure of the large intestine because of blood.**

Da chang yong jie 大腸壅結, obstruction of the large intestine with nodes [1]
PC identical with → *da bian mi* 大便秘②, constipation. *PJF* 39: 粉糖丸，治**大腸壅結**不通, "Pills with powdered sugar cure **obstruction of the large intestine with nodes**, with no passage possible".

Da chuan 大喘, massive panting [4]
IS if of breathing with an obvious acceleration of frequency and expansion of depth. *SJZL* 卷27: 治陽毒傷寒，遍身壯熱，**大喘**上氣，燥悶，妙應湯方, "Recipe for the 'decoction with wondrous responses' to cure from yang poison and harm caused by cold, with strong heat affecting the entire body, **massive panting** with rising qi, restlessness and heart-pressure".

Da feng 大風, massive wind [131]
① EA; violent → *feng* 風, wind, evil. *SW* 3: 雖有**大風**苛毒，弗之能害, "Even though there is a **massive wind** [which is] a violent poison, it will be unable to harm that [person]".
② AN → *feng lai* 風癩, wind repudiation-illness ; *lai feng* 癩風, repudiation-illness wind. PC of a chronic, infectious skin disease with insensitive skin, red macules, festering swelling, and, in severe cases, loss of eyebrows, harm to the eyes, and collapse of the patient's nose. *SW* 55: 骨節重，鬚眉墮，名曰**大風**, "When the patient experiences his bones and joints to be heavy and the beard and eyebrows fall off, this is called **massive wind**". *BCGM* refers to numerous such pathological conditions, some of them possibly related to observations of leprosy, including *da feng wan bi* 大風頑痹, massive wind with persistent blockage; da feng chuang xian 大風瘡癬, massive wind with sores and xuan-illness; da feng mei fa tuo luo 大風眉髮脫落, massive wind with eyebrows falling off.

Da feng 大瘋, massive wind-illness [1]
PC identical with → *da feng* 大風, massive wind. *BCGM* SE *ma xian hao* 馬先蒿：**大瘋**癩疾：骨肉疽敗，眉須墮落，身體癢痛, "In the case of **mas-**

sive wind-illness and repudiation-illness: the bones and flesh develop impediment-illnesses and rot; the eyebrows and beard fall off. The entire body itches and is in pain".

***Da jie* 大疥, massive *jie*-illness** [1]
PC of → *jie chuang* 疥瘡, *jie*-illness sores, with festering, red-hot itching and painful lesions. *ZBYHL* 35: **大疥**者，作瘡，有膿汁，焮赤癢痛是也, "**Massive *jie*-illness** forms sores with festering. They are burning red, they itch, and they are painful".

***Da ke yin yin* 大渴引飲, Massive thirst with copious drinking** [4]
IS of severe thirst associated with the consumption of large quantities of liquid. *ZBYHL* 40: 壯熱，**大渴引飲**, "Strong [body] heat; [patients] experience **massive thirst and drink copiously**".

***Da kuang* 大狂, massive madness** [1]
IS of a more serious type of → *kuang luan* 狂亂, madness with confusion. *RHZ* SE *zhu gen* 苧根：治心膈熱，漏胎下血，產前後心煩悶，天行熱疾，大渴**大狂**, "It cures heat in the heart and diaphragm region, blood leaking from the uterus, vexation and a feeling of heart-pressure prior to and following delivery, heaven-sent heat illness, massive thirst and **massive madness**".

***Da lao* 大勞, massive exhaustion** [3]
① EA of excessive exhaustion. *ZHF* 2: 由**大勞**大熱交接，交接後入水所致, "This is brought forth if **massive exhaustion** and massive heat interact, and if after this interaction one enters a water (i.e. engages in sexual intercourse)".
② PC of a rather severe depletion exhaustion. *MYBL* SE *gou qi* 枸杞：補內傷**大勞**噓吸，堅筋骨, "Supplements internal harm that has led to **massive exhaustion** and difficult breathing. It strengthens sinews and bones".

***Da nü* 大衄, massive spontaneous external bleeding** [7]
PC of simultaneous bleeding from more than two and up to seven orifices. *ZBYHL* 48: 血失其常度，發溢漫行，乃至發於七竅，謂之**大衄**也, "When the blood exceeds its normal measure it will overflow, possibly through all the seven orifices. This is called '**massive spontaneous external bleeding**'".

***Da pu* 打撲, [injury from] a blow** [8]
PC identical with → *da pu shang sun* 打撲傷損, injury from a blow. *TPSHF* 67: 治**打撲**，頭破腦出，中風口噤方, "Recipe to cure **[injuries from] blows**, with the head broken open and brain protruding, wind stroke and clenched jaw".

***Da pu shang sun* 打撲傷損, injury from a blow** [18] AN *da pu sun shang* 打撲損傷; *sun shang da pu* 損傷打撲; *da shang* 打傷; *da sun* 打損; *ou shang* 毆傷; *da pu* 打撲, [injury from] a blow.
PC of bodily injuries received from being hit. *XSLSXDMF* RE *hei wan zi* 黑丸子, black pills: 治**打撲傷損**，驢馬跌墜，骨斷筋碎，百節疼痛, "It cures **injuries from blows**, [injuries resulting from] falling from a donkey or horse, bone fractures and ruptured sinews, with all joints aching".

Da pu sun **打撲損, injury from a blow** [2]

PC identical with → *da pu shang sun* 打撲傷損. *BCYY* SE *zi ran tong* 自然銅：今人**打撲損**，研極細，水飛過，同當歸、沒藥各半錢，以酒調，頻服，仍以手摩痛處, "For persons today with **injuries from blows**, grind extemely fine, conduct a water dispersion process to collect the finest particles floating on the surface. Then mix in wine with half a *qian* each of *dang gui* and *mo yao*, and ingest this repeatedly. Also, rub the aching locations with the hands".

Da pu sun shang **打撲損傷, injury from a blow** [4]

PC identical with → *da pu shang sun* 打撲傷損. *TPSHF* 67: 治**打撲損傷**後，止疼痛，補虛損，石斛丸方, "To cure the aftereffects of **injuries from blows**, to end pain, and to supplement depletion: [make use of] the recipe for the pills with *shi hu*".

Da re **大熱, massive heat** [140]

PC of extreme heat. Identical with → *re* 熱, heat. *SW* 28: 岐伯曰：所謂重實者，言**大熱**病，氣熱脈滿，是謂重實, "Qi Bo: As for the so-called 'doubled repletion', that is to say: a **massive heat** disease. [That is,] the qi is hot and the vessels are filled. That is called 'doubled repletion'".

Da shang **打傷, injury from a blow** [10]

PC identical with → *da pu shang sun* 打撲傷損. *QJYF* 25 Jin chuang 金瘡, "Wounds inflicted by metal objects": 燒乾梅為炭，搗末，敷之一宿即瘥，亦治**打傷**, "Roast plums until they are dry and turn into coal. Pound to a powder. Apply them externally over one night, and this will bring the cure. It also cures **injuries from blows**".

Da shui **大水, massive water; river** [15]

① PC of a more serious → *shui zhong* 水腫, water swelling, disease. *BJ* SE *gua di* 瓜蒂：主**大水**，身面四肢浮腫, "It controls **massive water**. The body, the face, and the four limbs are swollen".

② Inundation. *BCTJ* SE *yu xie* 玉屑：每歲五、六月**大水**暴漲，則玉隨流而至, "Each year during the 5th and 6th month there is a sudden and sharp rise of **massive water**. As a result, jade [pieces] are washed here".

③ River. *BCTJ* SE *long gu* 龍骨：此物出蜀中山澗**大水**中, "These items originate from mountain **rivers** in Sichuan".

Da sun **打損, injury from a blow** [5]

PC identical with → *da pu shang sun* 打撲傷損. *SLBC* SE *yi tang* 飴糖：主**打損**瘀血，熬令焦，和酒服之，能下惡血, "It controls stagnant blood [that has left the vessels] following an **injury from a blow**. Roast and ingest mixed with wine. It is capable of draining malign blood".

Da tong **大痛, massive pain** [9]

IS of an extremely violent pain. *QJYF* 16: 大建中湯，治心胸中大寒**大痛**, "Major decoction to fortify the center: to cure massive cold and **massive pain** in the heart and chest region".

Da tou bing **大頭病, massive head disease** [1]

PC identical with → *da tou feng* 大頭風, massive head wind. *SWBJQYBMJ* Lj: 夫**大頭病**者，是陽明邪熱太甚，資實少陽相火而為之也, "Now, as for '**massive head disease**', this is the result of excessive evil heat in the yang brilliance [conduits] lending strength to the minor yang minister fire".

Da tou feng **大頭風, massive head wind** [1]

PC of infectious diseases characterized by fever and an aversion to wind, as well as swelling and pain in front of and behind the ears. *PJF* 150 refers to *da tou feng* **大頭風, massive head wind**: 因傷寒感冒，瘟疫不正，天行毒氣，成大頭之病。憎寒壯熱，先從耳前後微腫疼痛，逐漸發腫，連咽喉頭項赤腫，名曰**大頭風**，又名洗頭雷風等。風腫病者形貌變異，大頭如栲栳大。其病傳染諸人, "Massive head disease is generated by harm caused by cold and an affection by the malign, by warmth-illness epidemics and improperness, and by poison qi sent by heaven. [Patients] hate cold and experience strong heat. At first there is a minor, painful swelling in front of the ears, gradually growing larger. It connects with the throat and the nape, which turn red and are swollen. This is called '**massive head wind**'. ...The patients assume a strange physical appearance; their head is big like a willow basket. This disease may be transmitted to other persons".

Da xiao bian bi **大小便閉, major and minor relief blocked; blocked defecation and urination** [16]

IS, PC CD of → *xiao bian bi* 小便閉, blocked urination, and → *da bian bi* 大便閉, blocked defecation. *QJYF* 17: **大小便閉**，小腹有氣結如斗大，脹滿, "**Defecation and urination are blocked**. There are bean-size qi nodes in the lower abdomen, with a feeling of distension and fullness".

Da xiao bian bi se **大小便閉澀, major and minor relief blocked and with roughness; defecation and urination are blocked or rough** [1]

IS identical with → *da xiao bian bu li* 大小便不利, defecation and urination do not pass freely. *BCGM* SE *ku zao* 苦棗 quoting *SXBC*: 大小便秘澀 writes: **大小便閉澀**, "**Defecation and urination are blocked or rough**".

Da xiao bian bu li **大小便不利, major and minor relief impeded; stools and urine do not pass freely** [8]

IS CD of → *xiao bian bu li* 小便不利, urination does not pass freely, and → *da bian bu li* 大便不利, stools do not pass freely. *ZBYHL* 42: 熱病，熱入大小腸，並令**大小便不利**也, "Heat disease. Heat enters the large and small intestines, and it causes **stools and urine not to pass freely**".

Da xiao bian bu tong **大小便不通, major and minor relief blocked; stools and urine fail to pass** [23]

IS, PC CD of → *xiao bian nan* 小便難, difficult urination, and → *da bian nan* 大便難, difficult defecation. *BJ* SE *yu pi* 榆皮：主**大小便不通**，利水道，除邪氣, "It controls **failure of stools and urine to pass**. It opens the water ways and eliminates evil qi".

Da xiao bian chi ru xue se **大小便赤如血色, major and minor relief red like blood; stools and urine are red like blood** [1]

IS of stools and urine assuming a red color like blood. *BCTJ* SE *hu huang lian* 胡黃連：治傷寒勞復，身熱，**大小便赤如血色**者, “It cures cases of harm caused by cold recurrence because of exhaustion, with a hot body and **stools and urine being red like blood**”.

Da xiao bian hua shuo **大小便滑數, major and minor relief smooth and frequent; smooth and frequent defecation and urination** [1]

IS of increased frequency of defecation and urination with their passage being difficult to control. *BCGM* SE *tian xiong* 天雄 quoting *HJJF san jian tang* 三建湯：大便滑泄, “Smooth outflow of stools”, writes: **大小便滑數**, “Smooth and **frequent defecation and urination**”.

Da xiao bian mi **大小便秘, major and minor relief blocked; stools and urine are blocked** [2]

IS, PC CD of → *xiao bian mi* 小便秘, blocked urine, and → *da bian mi* 大便秘, blocked stools. *ZBYHL* 14: 傷寒，**大小便秘**, “Harm caused by cold. **Stools and urine are blocked**”.

Da xiao bian nan **大小便難, major and minor relief with difficulty; difficult urination and defecation** [1]

IS CD of → *xiao bian nan* 小便難, difficult urination, and → *da bian nan* 大便難, difficult defecation. *ZBYHL* 6: 熱氣乘於大小腸，大小腸痞澀，故**大小便難**也, “When heat qi avails itself of the large and small intestines, then the large and small intestines have an obstacle-illness and passage is rough. Hence **urination and defecation are difficult**”.

Da xiao bian se **大小便澀, major and minor relief with roughness; defecation and urination are rough** [8]

IS CD of → *xiao bian se* 小便澀, urination is rough, and → *da bian se* 大便澀, defecation is rough. *ZBYHL* 46：熱搏水谷氣，蘊積成黃，蒸發於外，身疼膊背強，**大小便澀**，皮膚、面目、齒爪皆黃, “The heat pounds on the qi of water and grain. They accumulate and assume a yellow color. [Eventually, the heat] evaporates toward outside. The body aches; arms and back are stiff. **Defecation and urination are rough**. Skin, face and eyes, teeth and fingernails are all yellow”.

Da xiao bian shuo **大小便數, frequent major and minor relief; frequent defecation and urination** [2] AN *er bian pin shuo* 二便頻數.

IS of an increased frequency of defecation and urination. *QJYF* 26 SE huo 藿：宜腎，主**大小便數**, “Good for the kidneys. It controls **frequent defecation and urination**”.

Da xiao bian xue **大小便血, major and minor relief with blood; defecation and urination with blood** [11]

PC with blood leaving with stools and urine. *SJZL* 68: 治吐血及**大小便血**，三物湯方, “To cure blood spitting and **defecation and urination with blood**, [use] the recipe for the ‘Decoction with three items’”.

Da xiao chang bu tong **大小腸不通, large and small intestines are not passable** [1]
IS, PC identical with → *da xiao bu tong* 大小便不通, stools and urine fail to pass. *ZLBC* SE *xuan ming fen* 玄明粉 quotes *XJ*: 五藏秘澀，**大小腸不通**, "The five depots experience closure and roughness; **large and small intestines are not passable**".

Da xiao chang mi **大小腸秘, large and small intestine are blocked** [2]
IS identical with → *da xiao bian mi* 大小便秘, stools and urine are blocked. *ZLBC wei ling xian* 威靈仙 quotes *CYLHSF*: **大小腸秘**，服此立通, "When **large and small intestine are blocked**, to ingest this [medication] will immediately make them passable".

Da xiao chang re **大小腸熱, heat in the large and in the small intestine** [1]
CD of → *da chang re* 大腸熱, heat in the large intestine; → *xiao chang re* 小腸熱, heat in the small intestine. *BCGM* SE *zhi zi* 梔子 quotes *TYBC*: 本草言治**大小腸熱**, "The *BC* states: it cures **heat in the large and small intestine**".

Da xu **大虛, massive depletion** [2]
PC of a very serious variant of → *xu zheng* 虛證, depletion condition. *ZBYHL* 3: 寸關澀，無血氣，逆冷，是**大虛**, "If [the movement in the vessels] at the inch and gate sections is rough, and if [one feels] no blood and qi, with counterflowing cold, this is a **massive depletion**".

Dai bing **帶病, diseases [below] the belt; women's diseases** [1]
PC identical with → *dai xia bing* 帶下病, diseases below the belt. *BCYY* SE *ren ni* 人溺：產後温一杯飲，壓下敗血惡物。有飲過七日者，過多。恐久遠血藏寒，令人發**帶病**，人亦不覺, "Drinking a cup of warm [urine] following delivery pushes down rotten blood and other malign items. Drinking [warm urine] for more than seven days is excessive. It may cause [the patient] to accumulate cold in her blood over a long period of time, and this will cause her to develop **diseases [below] the belt**. People are not aware of this".

Dai ji **帶疾, ailments [below] the belt; women's ailments** [1]
PC identical with → *dai xia bing* 帶下病, diseases below the belt. *SXBC* SE *da ma ren* 大麻人：婦人多食發**帶疾**, "When women consume this in large quantities, they will develop **ailments [below] the belt**".

Dai lou **帶漏, leakage [from below the] belt** [2]
PC identical with → *lou dai* 漏帶. *HJJF* 5: 婦人宮臟冷，月水不調，赤白**帶漏**, "Cold in a woman's [fetal] palace and depots. Menstruation is irregular, with red and white **leakage [from below the] belt**".

Dai mai bing **帶脈病, belt vessel disease** [1]
PC associated with the belt vessel. *BCGM* SE *shao yao* 芍藥 quotes Wang Haogu 王好古：**帶脈病**苦腹痛滿，腰溶溶如坐水中, "A **belt vessel disease** entails suffering from abdominal pain and fullness. The lower back appears to float around as if one were sitting in water".

Dai xia **帶下, [diseases] below the belt** [p] AN *dai xia bing* 帶下病, diseases below the belt.

PC of an increased discharge of matter with an abnormal color, consistency, and odor from the vagina outside of the menstruation period, sometimes accompanied by illness signs affecting the entire body, sometimes appearing only topically. *SW* 60: 任脈為病，男子內結七疝，女子**帶下**瘕聚, "When the controlling vessel has a disease, in males [it causes] internal knottings and the seven elevation-illnesses. In females [it causes] **diseases] below the belt** and conglomeration-illness collections".

Dai xia bing **帶下病, diseases below the belt** [3]

PC identical with → *dai xia* 帶下, [diseases] below the belt. *BJ* SE *di yu* 地榆：主寒熱，鬼疰，中風，濕痹，女子**帶下病**，無子, "It controls alternating sensations of cold and heat, demon attachment-illness, wind stroke, moisture blockage, **diseases below the belt** in women, and childlessness".

Dai xia shi er bing **帶下十二病, twelve types of diseases below the belt** [1]

PC identical with → *dai xia bing* 帶下病, diseases below the belt. *MYBL* SE *yu quan* 玉泉：療婦人**帶下十二病**, "It cures the **twelve types of diseases below the belt** in women".

Dai xia shi er ji **帶下十二疾, twelve types of ailments below the belt** [2]

PC identical with → *dai xia bing* 帶下病, diseases below the belt. *BJ* SE *mu gou yin jing* 牡狗陰莖：除女子**帶下十二疾**, "It eliminates the **twelve types of ailments below the belt** in women".

Dai xia wu lou **帶下五漏, five types of leakage from below the belt** [1]

PC identical with → *wu se dai* 五色帶, [downflow of] five colors [from below] the belt. *BCGM* SE *di yu* 地榆 quoting *BJ*: 帶下病, "Diseases below the belt", writes: **帶下五漏, "Five types of leakage from below the belt"**.

Dai yan **戴眼, eyes turned upward** [1]

IS identical with → *shang shi* 上視, vision turned upward. *SW* 20: 足太陽氣絕者，其足不可屈伸，死必**戴眼**, "Those whose [movement of the] qi of the foot major yang [vessel] has been interrupted and who are unable to bend or stretch their feet, they will die with their **eyes turned upward**"

Dai zhi **代指, finger replacement** [21]

PC of → *chuang* 瘡, sores, conditions developing at the margins of one's fingernails with the edges being inflamed, swollen and painful. This will eventually result in festering and the formation of scabs, and finally the loss of the fingernail. *ZBYHL* 30: **代指**者，其指先腫，焮焮熱痛，其色不黯，然後方緣爪甲邊結膿，極者爪甲脫也, "In the case of **finger replacement**, the respective finger will swell at first. Then it becomes burning red with heat pain. The color is not bright. Next there develops bound pus at the edge of the nail. In extreme cases, the fingernail falls off".

Dan **疸, *dan*-illness; jaundice** [p]

PC identical with → *huang dan* 黃疸, yellow *dan*-illness. *BJ* SE *zhu* 术：主風寒濕痹，死肌，痙、疸, "It controls wind-cold-moisture blockage, muscle death, spasm, and ***dan*-illness**".

Dan **癉, solitary[-heat-]illness** [7]

① Identical with → *re* 熱, heat. *SW* 17: 熱氣留於小腸，腸中痛，**癉**熱焦渴則堅干不得出, "When heat qi stays in the small intestine, there is pain in the intestine. The heat of **solitary[-heat-]illness** burns and dries out [the intestine], and as a result [the stools] harden and are dry and cannot leave".

② PC identical with → *dan* 疸, as in *huang dan* 黃疸, yellow *dan*-illness. *SW* 19: 發**癉**，腹中熱，煩心出黃, "[The patient] develops **solitary[-heat-]illness** and has heat in the abdomen. The heart is vexed and the discharge is yellow".

Dan dan **膽癉, gallbladder solitary[-heat-]illness** [2]

PC of a bitter flavor in the mouth caused by gallbladder qi depletion. *SW* 47: 帝曰：有病…口苦者病名為何？何以得之？岐伯曰：病名曰**膽癉**, "[Huang] Di: Someone suffers from a bitter [taste] in his mouth. …What is the name of that disease? How did he get it? Qi Bo: The disease is named **gallbladder solitary[-heat-]illness**".

Dan du **丹毒, cinnabar poisoning** [79]

PC of skin ailments brought forth by heat poison, manifesting themselves as red rashes as if from burns, as if cinnabar had been pasted there. *ZBYHL* 31 Dan du bing zhu hou **丹毒**病諸候, "All signs of diseases of **cinnabar poisoning**": 人身體忽然焮赤，如丹塗之狀，故謂之丹。或發手足，或發腹上，如手掌大，皆風熱惡毒所為, "If the body suddenly turns red as if from burns, as if cinnabar had been applied, this is called *dan* 丹, cinnabar. Such [rashes] may develop on hands and feet, and on the abdomen. If the hands are swollen, this is caused by malign poison of wind and heat". *BCGM* refers to this also as → *dan zhong* 丹腫, cinnabar-red swelling; → *tian huo dan du* 天火丹毒, celestial fire cinnabar poisoning. As this ailment may occur in numerous variations, the term *dan du* 丹毒 includes variants such as *wu se dan du* 五色丹毒, multi-color cinnabar poisoning; *chi dan* 赤丹, red cinnabar [poisoning]; *bai dan* 白丹, white cinnabar [poisoning]; *chi you dan du* 赤游丹毒; red roaming cinnabar poisoning; *huo yan dan du* 火焰丹毒, cinnabar poisoning red like flaming; *ye huo dan du* 野火丹毒, wild fire cinnabar poisoning; *tian zao dan du* 天灶丹毒, celestial stove cinnabar poisoning; *huo zao dan du* 火灶丹毒, fire stove cinnabar poisoning; *yan huo dan du* 烟火丹毒, smoking fire cinnabar poisoning; *chan she dan du* 纏蛇丹毒, cinnabar poisoning like being twined by a snake; *huo dan* 火丹, fire cinnabar [poisoning].

Dan feng **膽風, gallbladder wind** [1]

PC of unbalanced depletion and repletion affecting the gallbladder channel, with dizziness and sleepiness. *SJZL* 42 RE *suan cao ren tang* 酸棗仁湯, decoction with *suan cao* kernels: 治**膽風**毒氣，虛實不調，昏困多睡, "It cures **gallbladder wind** with poison qi; unbalanced depletion and repletion, clouding with dizziness and sleepiness".

***Dan fu zhang* 單腹脹, solitary abdominal distension** [1]
PC identical with → *gu zhang* 鼓脹, drum-like distension. *DXZFXY* 3: 臌脹又名曰蠱，即所謂**單腹脹**也, "Another designation of drum-like distension is *gu*. This is the so-called **solitary abdominal distension**".

***Dan han* 但寒, pure cold** [3] AN *du han* 獨寒, solitary cold.
IS of one's solely having an aversion to cold without developing fever. *JGYL* Fj: 柴胡桂薑湯，治瘧寒多微有熱，或**但寒**不熱, "Decoction with *chai hu*, *gui*, and *jiang*: it cures malaria with much cold and little heat; in some cases [patients] experience **pure cold** with no fever".

***Dan huang* 疸黃, *dan*-illness with yellowness; jaundice** [2]
PC identical with → *huang dan* 黃疸, yellow *dan*-illness. *QJYF* 26: 主咳逆上氣，**疸黃**, "It controls cough with counterflow, (i.e.) rising qi, and **jaundice**".

***Dan ji* 疸疾, ailment of *dan*-illness** [6]
PC identical with → *huang dan* 黃疸, yellow *dan*-illness. *BCGM* SE *shi* 豕 quoting *ZHF* 疸病有五種, "There are five types of *dan*-disease", writes: 五種**疸疾**, "Five types of the **ailment of *dan*-illness".**

***Dan liu* 丹瘤, vermilion tumor** [6]
PC of a red kernel-type swelling without a head developing on the head, in the face, or at the throat. The tumor itself does not ache or itch, but is accompanied by fever with an aversion to cold and pain affecting head and body. *WKJY* Fj: 原夫此疾，古無方論，世俗通為**丹瘤**, "In ancient times there existed no recipe discourse for this ailment. It was commonly called '**vermilion tumor**'".

***Dan nüe* 癉瘧, solitary[-heat-]illness with malaria** [1]
PC identical with → *wen nüe* 温瘧, warmth malaria. *SW* 35: 其但熱而不寒者…名曰**癉瘧**, "When [the patient experiences] pure heat and no cold, ...[this disease] is named **solitary[-heat-]illness with malaria**".

***Dan re* 但熱, pure heat** [2] AN → *du re* 獨熱, solitary heat.
IS of fever in the absence of an aversion to cold. *SW* 35: 其**但熱**而不寒者…名曰癉瘧, "When [the patient experiences] **pure heat** and no cold, ...[this disease] is named solitary[-heat-]illness with malaria".

***Dan re* 膽熱, gallbladder heat** [7]
① PC of heat-type diseases affecting the gallbladder. *QJYF* 11: 肝生病，病實則**膽熱**, "When the liver generates disease, in the case of a repletion disease this will be **gallbladder heat**".
② EA bringing forth heat-type diseases in the gallbladder. *TPSHF* 3: 夫**膽熱**多睡者…皆積熱不除，肝膽氣實，故令多睡也, "When patients with **gallbladder heat** sleep a lot,. this is always because heat has accumulated and fails to disperse. The liver and the gallbladder have qi repletion. Hence this makes a person sleep a lot".

***Dan re* 丹熱, cinnabar heat** [3]
PC identical with → *chi dan* 赤丹, red cinnabar. *BCSY* SE *lan shi* 藍實：小兒**丹熱**，和水服之, "Cures **cinnabar heat** in children; ingest with water".

***Dan shi chong yan* 丹石衝眼, cinnabar [et al.] mineral [poison] rushes against the eyes** [1]

PC of a → *dan shi du fa* 丹石毒發, outbreak of cinnabar [et al.] mineral poisoning, with red, swollen and aching eyes. *BCGM* SE *bian xu* 萹蓄 quoting *SLBC*: 丹石發，衝眼目腫痛, "In case of an outbreak of cinnabar [et al.] mineral [poisoning, the poison] rushes against the eyes and causes them to swell and be painful", writes: 丹石衝眼, "**Cinnabar [et al.] mineral [poison] rushes against the eyes**".

***Dan shi du* 丹石毒, cinnabar [et al.] mineral poison** [22] AN *dan shi yao du* 丹石藥毒, cinnabar [et al.] mineral drug poison; *jin shi du* 金石毒, mineral substance poison; *jin shi yao du* 金石藥毒, mineral drug poison.

EA CD of all poisonous mineral drugs be they chemically refined or not. *YXL* SE *che qian zi* 車前子：壓丹石毒，去心胸煩熱, "To suppress **cinnabar [et al.] mineral poison** and to remove vexing heat from heart and chest".

***Dan shi du fa* 丹石毒發, outbreak of cinnabar [et al.] mineral poisoning** [7] AN *dan shi fa dong* 丹石發動, outbreak of cinnabar [et al.] mineral [poisoning]; *dan shi fa* 丹石發, outbreak of cinnabar [et al.] mineral [poisoning]; *dan shi yao fa* 丹石藥發, outbreak of cinnabar [et al.] mineral drug [poisoning]; *jin shi yao fa* 金石藥發, outbreak of mineral drug [poisoning]; *jin shi yao fa dong* 金石藥發動, outbreak of mineral drug [poisoning]; *jin shi fa dong* 金石發動, outbreak of mineral [drug poisoning].

PC CD of all types of poisoning resulting from an ingestion of medication based on differently toxic cinnabar [et al.] minerals. *WTMY* 31: 仙人煉絳雪，療一切病，肺氣積聚咳逆，嘔吐膿血，**丹石毒發**，天行時氣，一切熱病，諸黃膽等, "The immortals have a chemical process for preparing crimson color snow. It cures all diseases, including accumulations and collections of lung qi with cough and counterflow, vomiting pus and blood, **outbreaks of cinnabar [et al.] mineral poisoning**, heaven-sent seasonal qi, all types of heat disease, and all types of jaundice".

***Dan shi du feng* 丹石毒風, cinnabar [et al.] mineral poison wind** [1]

PC of a → *feng* 風②, wind, as poisoning by medication prepared from cinnabar [et al.] minerals. *YXL* SE *ning shui shi* 凝水石：寒水石，能壓**丹石毒風**，去心煩渴悶，解傷寒復勞, "*Han shui shi* is capable of suppressing **cinnabar [et al.] mineral poison wind**. It removes heart vexation with thirst and heart-pressure. It dissolves harm caused by cold and restores [those suffering from] exhaustion".

***Dan shi du li* 丹石毒痢, free-flux illness from cinnabar [et al.] mineral poisoning** [1]

PC of → *li ji* 痢疾, free-flux illness, brought forth by an accumulation of heat poison following the intake of *dan shi* 丹石. *BCGM* Bai bing zhu zhi yao 百病主治藥 quoting *SLBC* 猯：主服丹石勞熱患赤白痢, "It controls exhaustion heat with suffering from red and white free-flux illness resulting from the consumption of *dan shi*", writes 丹石毒痢, "Free-flux illness from **cinnabar [et al.] mineral poisoning**".

Dan shi fa **丹石發, outbreak of cinnabar [et al.] mineral [poisoning]** [5]
PC identical with → *dan shi du fa* 丹石毒發, outbreak of cinnabar [et al.] mineral poisoning. *SLBC* SE *bian xu* 萹蓄：**丹石發**，衝眼目腫痛，取根一握，洗。擣以少水，絞取汁服之, "For [treating an] outbreak of **cinnabar [et al.] mineral [poisoning]** rushing against the eyes and causing them to swell and ache, take a handful of the root, wash this, grind it with a little water, wring to obtain a juice and ingest this".

Dan shi fa dong **丹石發動, outbreak of cinnabar [et al.] mineral [poisoning]** [6]
PC identical with → *dan shi du fa* 丹石毒發, outbreak of cinnabar [et al.] mineral poisoning. *SLBC* SE *ji ni* 薺苨：**丹石發動**，取根食之尤良, "For [treating an] **outbreak of cinnabar [et al.] mineral [poisoning]**, eat the root. Very good".

Dan shi yao du **丹石藥毒, cinnabar [et al.] mineral drug poison** [2]
EA identical with → *dan shi du* 丹石毒, cinnabar [et al.] mineral poison. *RHZ* SE *feng* 蚌：壓**丹石藥毒**, "To suppress **cinnabar [et al.] mineral drug poison**".

Dan shi yao fa **丹石藥發 outbreak of cinnabar [et al.] mineral drug [poisoning]** [2]
PC identical with → *dan shi du fa* 丹石毒發, outbreak of cinnabar [et al.] mineral poisoning. *RHZ* SE *qu mai* 瞿麥：**丹石藥發**並眼目腫痛及腫毒，擣傅, "To [treat] an **outbreak of cinnabar [et al.] mineral drug [poisoning]** associated with swollen and aching eyes, and swelling [because of] poison, grind and apply externally".

Dan xu **膽虛, gallbladder depletion** [7]
PC of a depletion of gallbladder qi associated with fright palpitation and insomnia. *MJ* 2: **膽虛**，左手關上脈陽虛者，足少陽經也, "**Gallbladder depletion**: when the [movement in the] vessels at the gate section of the left hand shows a yang depletion, this is the leg minor yang conduit".

Dan yao du **丹藥毒, elixir drug poison** [2]
EA CD of the poison of mineral elixir medications. Their ingredients generally focus on cinnabar and mercury, as well as precious metals, and they are to be ingested following a chemical refinement process with the aim of achieving longevity. *SYDXF* 10: 用旋刺下羊血、雞鴨血熱服，兼解鼠莽毒及**丹藥毒**, "Ingest the hot blood that has been taken from a lamb, chicken or duck immediately after it was pierced, and this will dissolve the poison of *shu mang* and **elixir drug poison** alike".

Dan yu wo **但欲臥, one wishes nothing but to lie down/rest/sleep** [1]
IS identical with → *si wo* 嗜臥, a desire to lie down. *ZHF* 4: 治食過飽煩悶，**但欲臥**而腹脹方, "Recipe to cure overeating with vexation and heart-pressure, if one **wishes nothing but to lie down/rest/sleep** and feels abdominal distension".

Dan zhen **丹疹, cinnabar-red papules** [4]
PC identical with → *chi zhen* 赤疹, red papules. *YXL* SE *she xian* 蛇銜：能治**丹疹**, "It is able to cure **cinnabar-red papules**".

Dan zhong **丹腫, cinnabar-red swelling** [11]
PC identical with → *dan du* 丹毒, cinnabar poisoning. *QJYF* 5: 麻黃湯，治小兒**丹腫**, "Decoction with *ma huang* cures **cinnabar-red swelling** in children".

Dang xin tong **當心痛, pain exactly in the center** [2]

IS of pain exactly in the stomach pit. Note: *xin* 心, in the sense of center, is a reference here to the stomach. *ZZJ* Fj: 病甚則腹脅脹滿，吐逆不入食，**當心痛**，上下不通, "When the disease is serious this leads to distension and a feeling of fullness in the abdomen and flanks. Patients vomit with counterflow, and cannot eat. They experience **pain exactly in the center**, and there is no passage from above to below".

Dao chan **倒產, delivery of [a child in an] inverted position** [9]

PC identical with → *ni chan* 逆產, delivery of [a child in a] position contrary to normal. *SJZL* 159: 治難產，橫生**倒產**，困頓不省人事，聖功散方, "To cure difficult delivery, delivery of [a child in] a transverse position, and **delivery of [a child in an] inverted position**, and exhaustion to a degree that one fails to recognize others or items, [use] the recipe for the 'powder with sage-like achievements'".

Dao chuang shang shi **刀瘡傷濕, knife wounds harmed by moisture** [1] AD *shang shi* 傷濕, harm caused by moisture.

PC of festering and difficult-to-heal wounds brought forth by the impact of water/moisture on an open knife wound. *BCGM* SE *shi gao* 石膏 quotes *JDTF*: **刀瘡傷濕**，潰爛不生肌, "[To cure] **knife wounds harmed by moisture** with festering and an inability to generate muscles".

Dao han **盜汗, robber sweating** [82]

① IS of a profuse sweating during sleep that ends when one wakes up. *JGYL* Mj: 食已汗出，又身常暮臥**盜汗**出者，此勞氣也, "When [the patient] has finished eating and he begins to sweat, and if his body, at night while he is asleep, is regularly affected by **robber sweating**, [these are signs of] qi exhaustion".

② PC with robber sweating as major sign. *ZBYHL* 8: **盜汗**者，因眠睡而身體流汗也，此由陽虛所致, "As for **robber sweating**, if one has fallen asleep and sweat flows from the body, this results from a yang [qi] depletion".

Dao jian chuang **刀箭瘡, wounds inflicted by blades and arrows** [3]

PC of → *jin chuang* 金瘡, wounds inflicted by metal objects, specifically those that are caused by knives/swords and arrows. *RHZ* SE *mao xiang hua* 茅香花: 白茅香花塞鼻洪，傅久不合灸瘡，署**刀箭瘡**，止血並痛, "White *mao xiang hua* blockages nasal flood; apply it to sores resulting from cauterization that have not closed for a long time, and also smear it on **wounds inflicted by blades and arrows**".

Dao jian shang **刀箭傷, harm inflicted by blades and arrows** [1] AN *dao jian shang chuang* 刀箭傷瘡, wounds inflicted by blades and arrows.

PC of → *jin chuang* 金瘡, wounds inflicted by metal objects, specifically those that are caused by blades and arrows. *BCGM* SE *mei* 梅 quoting *RHZ*: 治刀箭，止血，研傅之, "Grind and apply it externally to cure blade and arrow [wounds], and to stop bleeding", writes: 治**刀箭傷**，止血，研爛傅之, "Grind to a pulp and apply it externally to cure **harm inflicted by blades and arrows**, and to stop bleeding".

Dao jian shang chuang **刀箭傷瘡, wounds inflicted by blades and arrows** [1]
PC identical with → *BHJJF*: **刀箭傷瘡**：香白芷嚼爛塗之, "For **wounds inflicted by blades and arrows**, chew *xiang bai zhi* to a pulp and apply this externally".

Dao jie **倒睫, inverted eyelashes** [25] AN *quan mao* 拳毛.
PC with → *jie mao dao ru* 睫毛倒入, intrusion of inverted eyelashes, as its major sign. *SJZL* 110: 治眼瞼緊急，**倒睫**拳攣，犀角芎藭散方, "Recipe for a powder with *xi jiao* and *xiong qiong* to cure tight eyelids and **inverted eyelashes** contracted like the fingers in a fist".

Dao sheng **倒生, birth of [a child in] an inverted position** [2]
PC identical with → *ni chan* 逆產, delivery of [a child in] a position contrary to normal. *QJYF* 2: 產難一服，橫生二服，**倒生**三服, "For difficult delivery, ingest one dose. For a birth of [a child in] a transverse position ingest two doses. For a **birth of [a child in] an inverted position** ingest 3 doses".

Dao yan **倒黶, inverted black mole** [17] AN *dao ye* 倒靨, inverted mole.
PC of → *dou chuang* 痘瘡, smallpox sores, which fail to develop a crust while the sores cave in and develop a purple-black color that is dry and has no luster. *XEWSZWLF* 8: 其候惡者，瘡變**倒黶**而黑陷, "Its malign signs are such that the sores change into an **inverted black mole** with a black cave".

Dao yan **倒靨, inverted mole** [5]
PC identical with → *dao yan* 倒黶, inverted black mole. *XEDZFL*, Lun dou zhen zhi fa 論痘診治法, "On diagnostic and therapeutic patterns for smallpox": 然**倒靨**、瀉、渴等症，若喜熱飲食，手足並冷，或不食嘔吐者，是為陽氣虛寒也，用辛熱之劑補之, "Now, in the case of conditions such as **inverted mole**, outflow, and thirst, when [patients] long for hot beverages and food, and if their hands and feet are all cold, in some cases they may not eat and rather vomit, this is a cold because of yang qi depletion. One employs acrid and hot preparations for supplementation".

Di er **底耳, low ear** [4]
PC with a strong stench and festering in the ears, sometimes accompanied by swelling and pain. *QJYF* 6: 治**底耳**方，黃礬燒，綿裹納耳中，不過二三日愈, "Recipe to cure **low ear**: roasted *huang fan* is wrapped in silk and inserted into the ear. A cure will be achieved at the latest within two or three days".

Di zhong hou feng **帝鍾喉風, throat wind affecting the uvula** [1]
PC with a swollen, painful uvula and difficulty in swallowing. *BCGM* SE *shi yan* 食鹽 quoting *PJF* 61: 帝鍾風，即喉間帝鍾長腫，有長數寸者, "Uvula wind refers to a swollen, extended uvula. Some are several *cun* long", writes: **帝鍾喉風**，垂長半寸, "**Throat wind affecting the uvula**, with a protrusion as long as half a *cun*".

Dian **癲, peak-illness** [p]
PC AD of → *dian ji* 癲疾, peak ailment. *BJ* SE *liu xu mao ti jia* 六畜毛蹄甲：主鬼疰蠱毒，寒熱驚癇，**癲**痓狂走, "It controls demon attachment-illness

and *gu poison*, cold and heat spells, fright and epilepsy, **peak-illness**, spasms, and crazy running".

***Dian* 顛, peak[-illness]; top** [p]

① PC identical with → *dian* 癲, peak-illness. *BCGM* SE *qiu shi* 秋石, fu fang 附方, attached recipes: 有人病**顛**腹鼓，日久加喘滿，垂困，亦服此而安也, "If someone suffers from **peak[-illness]** and abdominal drum, to which panting and a feeling of fullness are added after an extended period, as well as difficulties in sleeping, then have him ingest this too, and he will be calmed down".

② The uppermost part of a structure. *CJ* Lj: 茱萸出芳樹**顛**，鯉魚出洛水泉, "*Zhu yu* originates from the **top** of fragrant trees; *li yu* originates from the spring of the Luo river".

***Dian bing* 癲病, peak disease** [2]

PC identical with a *dian ji* 癲疾, peak ailment. *SW* 55: 月四五發，名曰**癲病**, "It breaks out four, five times a month. This is called **peak disease**".

***Dian dao* 顛倒, peak inversion; head first** [6]

① IS of mental or emotional derangement. *MYBL* SE *gen dang zi* 莨菪子：療癲狂風癇，**顛倒**拘攣, "It cures peak-illness with madness and wind epilepsy, as well as **peak inversion** with cramps and contraction".

② Inverted position of any item. *BCTJ* SE *xiong* 熊：好攀緣，上高木，見人則**顛倒**自投地而下, "They love to climb and move up high in trees. When they notice humans they throw themselves **head first** down to the ground".

***Dian ding tong* 巔頂痛, vertex pain** [1] AW *dian ding tong* 顛頂痛.

IS of → *tou tong* 頭痛①, headache, mainly affecting the top of the head. *ZZNYXF* Yong yao fan li 用藥凡例, "Guide to the use of pharmaceutical drugs": **巔頂痛**須用藁本, "For [a treatment of] **vertex pain** one should use *gao ben*".

***Dian ding tong* 顛頂痛, vertex pain** [1]

IS identical with → *dian ding tong* 巔頂痛, *BCGM* SE gao ben 藁本 quoting *YXQY ding dian tong* 頂巔痛, "Vertex pain", writes: *dian ding tong* **顛頂痛, "Vertex pain"**.

***Dian feng* 癜風, patches wind** [11]

PC identical with → *zi bai dian feng* 紫白癜風, purple and white patches wind. *BCGM* SE *qie zi* 茄子：燒灰，治口齒瘡䘌。生切，擦**癜風**, "Burned to ashes it will cure dental sores from hidden worms. Cut fresh specimens finely and rub on the **patches wind**".

***Dian ji* 顛疾, peak ailment** [1]

PC affecting the head. *SW* 47: 在母腹中時，其母有所大驚，氣上而不下，精氣並居，故令子發為**顛疾**也, "When [the fetus] is in the mother's abdomen and the mother is extremely frightened, the qi rises and does not move down. It takes residence together with the essence qi. Hence, this makes the child develop **peak-illness**".

***Dian ji* 癲疾, peak ailment** [21] AD *dian* 癲. AN *feng dian* 風癲; wind peak-illness; *dian bing* 癲病, peak disease.

PC a) of a mental disturbance of depression and unhappiness, with a calm attitude and little incentive to speak. *LS* 5: **癲疾**始生，先不樂, "When **peak ailment** begins [patients] at first are not joyful". b) Identical with a *dian xian* 癲癇, peak-illness with epilepsy. *ZHBJF* 5: 凡**癲疾**，發則仆地，吐涎沫, "When a **peak ailment** manifests itself [patients] fall to the ground. They spit saliva that is foam".

***Dian jing* 癲痙, peak-illness with spasms** [2]

PC CD of → *dian bing* 癲病, peak disease, and *jing bing* 痙病, spasms disease. *BJ* SE *liu chu mao ti jia* 六畜毛蹄甲：主鬼疰蠱毒，寒熱，**癲痙**狂走, "It controls demon attachment-illness and *gu poison*, cold and heat spells, as well as **peak-illness with spasms** and crazy running".

***Dian kuang* 癲狂, peak-illness and madness** [11]

PC of mental disturbance. Based on a patient's condition of silence or restlessness one may distinguish between the two types of → *dian* 癲, peak-illness, and → *kuang* 狂, madness. *LS* 22 has a chapter with the title Dian kuang **癲狂**：**癲**疾始生，先不樂，頭重痛…**狂**始發，少臥不飢，自高賢也，自辯智也，自尊貴也，善罵詈，日夜不休, "When **peak-illness** just begins, [patients] at first are not joyful, their head feels heavy and has pain. …When **madness** breaks out for the first time, [patients] do not lie down much and they have no appetite. They think of themselves as the greatest, wisest, and worthiest. They tend to insult and curse others, and this goes on day and night".

***Dian kuang* 顛狂, peak[-illness] and madness** [22]

PC identical with → *dian kuang* 癲狂, peak-illness and madness. *BCGM* SE *ting li* 葶藶 quoting *ZHF* 卒發癲狂, "Suddenly develops peak-illness and madness", writes: 卒發**顛狂**, "Suddenly develops **peak[-illness] and madness**".

***Dian quan* 顛犬, rabid dog** [1]

Identical with → *kuang quan* 狂犬, rabid dog. *SYDXF* 19: 雄黃為末，醋調塗，仍用酒服。凡為蛇傷及蜂蠆、蜈蚣、毒蟲、**顛犬**所傷，皆可用, "A powder prepared from *xiong huang* can be externally applied mixed with vinegar, and it can be taken internally together with wine. It can be used for all injuries caused by snakes, bees, scorpions, centipedes, poisonous bugs/worms, as well as **rabid dogs**".

***Dian xian* 癲癇, peak-illness with epilepsy** [60] AW *dian xian* 顛癇, peak[-illness] with epilepsy.

PC a) identical with → *xian* 癇, epilepsy. *QJYF* 14 lists 治**癲癇**瘈瘲方, "Recipes to cure **peak-illness with epilepsy** and clonic convulsions. b) CD of → *dian* 癲, peak-illness, and → *xian* 癇, epilepsy. *BJ* SE *fang kui* 防葵: [主]温瘧，**癲癇**，驚邪狂走, [It controls] "warmth malaria, **peak-illness with epilepsy**, fright evil and crazy running".

Dian xian 顛癇, peak[-illness] with epilepsy [2]
PC identical with → *dian xian* 癲癇, peak-illness with epilepsy. *BCGM* Bai bing zhu zhi yao 百病主治藥：雷丸，**顛癇**狂走, "*Lei wan* [cures] **peak[-illness] with epilepsy**, as well as crazy running".

Dian xie 癲邪, peak-illness evil [7]
PC identical with → *dian kuang* 癲狂, peak-illness and madness. *QJYF* 14: 其有種種形相，示表**癲邪**之端，而見其病，或有默默而不聲，或復多言而漫說, "It takes many different forms as a sign of the beginning of **peak-illness evil**. When the disease becomes manifest, in some cases [patients] are silent and do not use their voice; in other cases they speak again and again and their language is unrestrained".

Dian xie 顛邪, peak[-illness] evil [5]
PC identical with → *dian xie* 癲邪, peak-illness evil. *BCGM* SE *bai he* quoting *RHZ*: 安心定膽，益志，養五藏，治癲邪, "It pacifies the heart and stabilizes the gallbladder, benefits the mind, nourishes the five depots, and cures peak-illness evil", writes: 安心定膽，益志，養五藏，治**顛邪**, "It pacifies the heart and stabilizes the gallbladder, benefits the mind, nourishes the five depots, and cures **peak[-illness] evil**".

Diao teng 釣痛, pain as if being pulled with a hook [3]
IS of a violent pain associated with a sensation as if something were being intensely pulled on the affected location. *SYDXF* 12: 五苓散，治陰核氣結，腫大**釣痛**, "Powder with wu ling cures qi nodes in the testicles, with an enlargement resulting from a swelling and a pain as if one were pulled with a hook".

Diao xuan 掉眩, swaying and dizziness [5]
IS of head, body and extremities swaying, and a perception of → *xuan yun* 眩運, vertigo, affecting the head and the eyes. *SW* 74: 諸風**掉眩**，皆屬於肝, "All [diseases with] wind [causing] **swaying and dizziness**, without exception they are associated with the liver".

Diao yan 吊眼, hauled eyes [1]
IS identical with → *shang shi* 上視, vision turned upward. *BCGM* SE *dai zhe shi* 代赭石 quotes *RZZZF*: **吊眼**撮口，搐搦不定, "**Hauled eyes**, pursed mouth, and convulsions that cannot be stabilized".

Die jin 軼筋, twisted sinews [1]
IS identical with → *zhuan jin* 轉筋. *BJ* SE *kuo yu* 蛞蝓：主賊風喎僻，**軼筋**及脫肛，驚癇攣縮, "It controls [facial] wryness caused by robber wind, **twisted sinews** and prolapse of the rectum, as well as fright epilepsy with contractions".

Die ke shang sun 跌磕傷損, injury from a fall [1]
PC identical with → *die pu shang sun* 跌扑傷損. *BCGM* SE *niu* 牛 quotes *JBF*: **跌磕傷損**：黃牛屎炒熱封之，裹定即效, "For **injuries from falls**: Fry cattle excrement for hot external application. Wrap firmly. This will be effective".

Die pu 跌扑, [injury from a] fall; a fall [5]
① PC identical with → *die pu shang sun* 跌扑傷損, injury from a fall. *HJJF* 1 RE *zuo jing wan* 左經丸, pills to assist the conduits: **跌扑**閃肭，外傷內損，

並皆治之, "It cures **[injuries from] falls**, sprain, external and internal injuries alike".

② EA of losing one's balance and falling to the ground. *BCGM* SE *xiong qiong* 芎藭 quotes *SQF*: 因**跌扑**舉重，損胎不安, "Following a **fall** or having lifted something heavy, the fetus is injured and no longer calm".

Die pu shang sun **跌扑傷損, injury from a fall** [9] AN *die pu sun shang* 跌扑損傷; *cuo die sun shang* 蹉跌損傷; *die ke shang sun* 跌磕傷損; *die sun* 跌損; *die pu* 跌扑, [injuries resulting from] falls; *die pu zhe shang* 跌扑折傷, fractures and [further] injuries from falls; *die pu zhe shang* 跌仆折傷.

PC of bodily injuries resulting from a fall. *XSLSXDMF* RE *hei long san* 黑龍散, black dragon powder: 治**跌扑傷損**，筋骨碎斷，差爻出臼, "It cures **injuries from falls**, ruptured sinews and bone fractures, as well as dislocations".

Die pu sun shang **跌扑損傷, injury from a fall** [2]

PC identical with → *die pu shang sun* 跌扑傷損. *BCGM* SE *wu lian mei* 烏蘞莓 quotes *JBF*: **跌扑損傷**：五爪龍搗汁，和童尿、熱酒服之, "For **injuries from falls**: pound *wu gua long* to obtain the liquid. Mix with a boy's urine, and ingest with hot wine".

Die sun **跌損, injury from a fall** [1]

PC identical with → 跌扑傷損. *XSLSXDMF* Yi zhi zheng li bu jie ci di kou jue 醫治整理補接次第口訣：凡**跌損**，腸肚中污血，且服散血藥，如四物湯之類, "For all **injuries from falls**, with rotten blood inside the intestines and abdomen, one must ingest medication to disperse blood as, for example, the 'decoction with the four ingredients'".

Ding **丁, pin** [p]

PC AD of → *ding chuang* 丁瘡, pin sore. *QJYF* 22: 治十三種丁方, "Recipe to cure thirteen types of **pin**".

Ding **疔, pin-illness** [p]

PC AD of → *ding chuang* 疔瘡, pin-illness sores. *BCGM* SE *gou qi di gu pi* 枸杞地骨皮 quoting *QJYF* 22: 治十三種丁方, "Recipe to cure thirteen types of pin[-illness]", writes: 治十三種**疔**方, "Recipe to cure thirteen types of **pin-illness**".

Ding chuang **丁瘡, pin sores** [27] AD *ding* 丁, pin; *ding* 疔, pin-illness. AN *ding chuang* 疔瘡, pin-illness sores; *ding zhong* 丁腫, pin swelling; *ding zhong* 疔腫, pin-illness with swelling

PC CD of acute festering developing between skin and subdermal tissue, with its small size, deep-reaching root and hardness as major signs reminiscent of a pin. *ZBYHL* 31: 初作時，突起如丁蓋，故謂之**丁瘡**, "When it first becomes active it rises like a pinhead. Hence one speaks of '**pin sores**'".

Ding chuang **疔瘡, pin-illness sores** [58]

PC identical with → *ding chuang* 丁瘡, pin sores. *BCGM* SE *lu ci* 鸕鷀 quoting *RHZ*: 和脂油調丁瘡, "Mix with fat/oil to regulate pin sores", writes: 和脂油傅**疔瘡**, "Mix with fat/oil to apply externally to **pin-illness sores**".

Ding chuang zhong feng **疔瘡中風, pin-illness sores struck by wind** [1]
PC identical with → *zhu chuang zhong feng* 諸瘡中風, wind stroke via all possible sores. *BCGM* SE *lu* 驢 quotes *PJF*: **疔瘡中風**，腫痛，用驢屎炒，熨瘡上五十遍，極效, "To cure **pin-illness sores struck by wind** with swelling and pain use roasted donkey excrement as hot compresses to be externally applied on the sores 50 times. Extremely effective".

Ding du **疔毒, pin-illness poison** [12] AW *ding du* 丁毒, pin poison.
PC identical with → *ding* 疔, pin-illness *BCGM* SE *wu tou* 烏頭 quoting *PJF* 274: 冷疔瘡, "Cold pin-illness sores", and 緩疔, "Slow pin-illness", writes: **疔毒**, "**Pin-illness poison**".

Ding du **丁毒, pin poison** [3]
PC identical with → *ding du* 疔毒, pin-illness poison. *TBC* SE *jiang shi* 薑石：主熱豌豆瘡，**丁毒**等腫, "It controls swelling such as hot peas sores and **pin poison**".

Ding jie **疔瘑, pin-illness with pimples** [1]
PC CD of → *ding* 疔, pin-illness, and → *jie* 瘑, pimple. *BCGM* SE *xi er* 枲耳 quotes *JJF*: 萬應膏…治一切癰疽發背，無頭惡瘡，腫毒**疔瘑**, "The paste with a myriad of responses: It cures all obstruction- and impediment-illnesses with effusion of the back, malign sores without [pus] head, as well as swelling and poison associated with **pin-illness with pimples**".

Ding jing **定驚, to calm down fright** [5]
TA identical with → *zhi jing* 止驚, to stop fright. *HJJF* 10: 常服安神鎮心、**定驚**控痰, "Ingested regularly it pacifies the spirit and eases an [excited] heart; it **calms down fright** and discharges phlegm".

Ding ning **耵聹, earwax** [4]
PP of sticky matter in the ear cavity and of hard pits formed in the ear by dust and dirt having entered from outside. In severe cases this may blockage the ear duct and impair hearing ability. *LS* 24: 耳中有膿，若有干**耵聹**，耳無聞也, "There is pus in the ears. If it forms dry **earwax**, the ears can no longer hear".

Ding shi **叮螫, bite and sting** [6]
EA identical with → *shi ren* 螫人, to sting a person. *BCGM* SE *shi yan* 食鹽 quoting *QJYF* 25: 治蜂螫, "It cures [the suffering resulting from a] bee/wasp sting", writes: 蜂蠆**叮螫**, "**Bite and sting** by a bee/wasp and scorpion".

Ding tong **頂痛, vertex pain** [1]
IS identical with → *tou tong* 頭痛①, headache. *BCGM* SE *shi hu sui* 石胡荽：能上達頭腦而治**頂痛**目病, "It may ascend to reach the brain and cures **vertex pain** and eye diseases".

Ding xi **丁奚, pin-slave [condition]** [2] AN *fu gan* 腹疳, abdominal *gan*-illness.
PC of a severe type of → *pi gan* 脾疳, spleen *gan*-illness, affecting children. The appearance of patients with an enlarged abdomen, narrow neck, and consumption of muscles and flesh as characteristic signs is reminiscent of a pin. *MYBL* SE *zhi zhu* 蜘蛛：療小兒大腹**丁奚**, "It cures children suffering from **pin-slave [condition]** with an enlarged abdomen".

Ding yi **丁翳, pin shade** [2]
PC of → *mu yi* 目翳, eye shade, that resembles a nail because it is small and has a deep-reaching root. *TPSHF* 33: 睛上有翳如銀丁子頭，故謂之**丁翳**, "There is a shade on the eyeball resembling the head of a nail. Hence it is called '**pin shade**'".

Ding zhong **丁腫, pin swelling** [41]
PC a) identical with → *ding chuang* 丁瘡, pin sores. *QJYF* 22: 齊州榮姥丸，凡是**丁腫**皆用治之方, "The pills of grandma Rong from Qizhou: a recipe to treat all cases of **pin swelling**". b) Of pin sores with an obviously inflamed swelling and a root that cannot be felt by touching. *ZBYHL* 31: **丁腫**候，此由是丁瘡而帶焮腫，而無根者也, "Signs of **pin swelling**: This is an inflamed swelling resulting from pin sores, but without a root".

Ding zhong **疔腫, pin-illness with swelling** [65]
PC identical with → *ding zhong* 丁腫, pin swelling. *BCGM* SE *can* 蠶 quoting *MYBL* SE *bai jiang can* 白僵蠶：封丁腫, "Cover the pin swelling", writes: 封**疔腫**, "Cover the **pin-illness swelling**".

Dong bing **冬病, winter disease** [1]
CD of all PC that primarily have their onset in winter. *QJYF* and *PJF*: 胃而有石曰**冬病**, "When the stomach [movement in the vessels] is stone-like, this is called '**winter disease**'". *BCGM* Si shi yong yao li 四時用藥例, "Guide to drug use in the course of the four seasons": 春得秋病, 夏得**冬病**, 神而明之,機而行之,變通權宜,又不可泥一也, "If in spring one is affected by an autumn disease, if in summer one is affected by a **winter disease**, one must do everything to understand this, and act flexibly and do what is expedient. It would be wrong to cling to just one principle".

Dong chang ting chu **洞腸挺出, prolapse of the cavernous intestine** [1]
PC identical with → *tuo gang* 脫肛, prolapse of the rectum. *QJYF* 26: 豬洞腸，主**洞腸挺出**血多者, "A hog's intestinal cavity controls **prolapse of the cavernous intestine** with profuse bleeding". LSZ: 洞腸，廣腸也, "The 'cavernous intestine' is the 'wide intestine'".

Dong chuang **凍瘡, frost sores** [31]
PC of → *chuang* 瘡, sores, conditions resulting from cold harming the skin. *MYBL* SE *tu tou gu* 兔頭骨：腦，主**凍瘡**, "Its brain controls **frost sores**".

Dong li **洞痢, throughflux free-flux illness** [3]
PC of → *li ji* 痢疾, free-flux illness, with one's defecation difficult to control and carrying much white and less red mucous matter. *QJYF* 15: 駐車丸，治大冷**洞痢**腸滑，下赤白如魚腦，日夜無度，腹痛不可忍者方, "The 'Pills that bring a carriage to a halt' are a recipe to cure **throughflux free-flux illness** with massive cold and intestinal smoothness, a discharge of red and white matter resembling fish brain, occurring countless times during day and night, and going along with unbearable abdominal pain".

Dong si **凍死, [appearance of] death from freezing** [6]
PC of → *cu si* 卒死, sudden [appearance of] death, resulting from an extreme exposure to cold. *ZBYHL* 23: **凍死**一日猶可治，過此則不可治也, "**[Appear-**

ance of] death from freezing can be cured within one day; once this period has been exceeded it can no longer be cured".

Dong xia **洞下, throughflux discharge** [2]
PC identical with → *dong xie* 洞泄, vacating outflow. *QJYF* 3: 阿膠丸，治産後虛冷洞下, "Pills with *a jiao* cure depletion cold following delivery, with **throughflux discharge**".

Dong xie **洞泄, throughflux outflow** [7] AW *dong xie* 洞瀉; AN *dong xia* 洞下, throughflux discharge.
PC of outflow brought forth by an intake of cold through cold beverages, or a weakening of true yang qi, often resulting in thin and clear stools like water, with an uncontrollable quantity of discharges as its main characteristic. *SW* 4: 長夏善病**洞泄**寒中, "In late summer one tends to suffer from **throughflux outflow** and cold center".

Dong xie **洞瀉, throughflux outflow** [2]
PC identical with → *dong xie* 洞泄. *QJYF* 19: 若服冷藥過瘥而便**洞瀉**, "If one takes remedies of a cold nature beyond the point of recovery from a disease, this will cause **throughflux outflow** of stools".

Dong zhu xia li **洞注下痢, throughflux discharge with free-flux illness** [4]
PC of violent free-flux illness as if a hole was opened. *QJYF* 15 lists a 治少小**洞注下痢**方, "Recipe for curing children [suffering from] **throughflux discharge with free-flux illness**".

Dong zhu xia li **洞注下利, throughflux discharge with free-flux** [1]
PC identical with 洞注下痢. *BCGM* SE *chen lin mi* 陳廩米 quoting *QJYF* 15: 洞注下痢 writes: **洞注下利, "throughflux discharge with free-flux"**.

Dou **痘, smallpox** [p]
PC AD of → *dou chuang* 痘瘡, smallpox sores. *PJF* 44: 或鄰家有**痘**證，亦宜服, "If a neighbor has a **smallpox** condition, this too should be ingested".

Dou ban **痘瘢, smallpox scar** [2]
PC of → *ban* 瘢, scars, resulting from a smallpox. *BCGM* SE *huang ming jiao* 黄明膠：小兒**痘瘢**：黄明膠炒研末，温酒調服一錢匕, "[To cure] children with **smallpox scars**: Roast *huang ming jiao* and grind to a powder. Mix with warm wine and ingest a spoonful holding 1 *qian*".

Dou ban **豆瘢, bean scar** [2]
PC identical with → *dou ban* 痘瘢, smallpox scar. *BCGM* Bai bing zhu zhi yao 百病主治藥：密陀僧，人乳調塗**豆瘢**, "Apply *mi tuo seng* mixed with human milk to **bean scars**".

Dou chuang **痘瘡, smallpox sores** [137] AN *dou zhen* 痘疹, smallpox papules; *chuang zhen* 瘡疹, sores with papules; *ban dou* 瘢痘, smallpox with streaks; *ban chuang* 斑瘡, sores with streaks; *wan dou chuang* 豌豆瘡, pea[-size] smallpox sores; AD *dou* 痘, smallpox.
PC of a transmittable disease with skin papules appearing as blisters filled with water and pus. In general these designations refer to smallpox, including an in-

auspicious prognosis. However, they may also be used to refer to other types of infectious diseases with skin rashes and similar blisters. *PJF* 403: 消風散，治**痘瘡**或發或未發, "The 'powder to dissolve wind' cures **smallpox sores** that may or may not have opened".

***Dou ding* 痘疔, smallpox with pin-illness** [5]

PC identical with → *dou chuang* 痘瘡, smallpox sores. *XEDZFL* Lun dou zhen zhi fa 論痘疹治法, "On therapy patterns for smallpox papules": 毒甚，**痘疔**而不能發起, "[There are also cases] where the poison is extreme and yet the **smallpox with pin-illness** cannot emerge".

***Dou du* 痘毒, smallpox poison** [30]

① AN *dou zhen du* 痘疹毒, smallpox papules poison. EA of → *du qi* 毒氣①, poison qi, that brings forth → *dou zhen* 痘疹, smallpox papules. *XEDZFL si wei sheng ma ge gen tang* 四味升麻葛根湯：恐虛其表而**痘毒**不能托出也, "It is to be feared that the outer region is depleted and the **smallpox poison** cannot be discharged".

② PC of smallpox with extreme skin rashes, festering, serious swelling and massive purulence. *XEDZFL* Lun dou zhen zhi fa 論痘疹治法：一小兒**痘毒**，遍身腐潰，膿水淋漓, "When a child is affected by **smallpox poison**, its entire body will rot and fester, with massive flow of pus liquid".

***Dou feng chi yan* 痘風赤眼, smallpox wind-red-eye** [1]

PC identical with → *dou feng yan* 痘風眼, smallpox wind-eye. *BCGM* SE *chu sheng qi dai* 初生臍帶 quotes *HSF*: **痘風赤眼**：初生小兒臍帶血，乘熱點之，妙, "[To cure] **smallpox wind-red-eye**: Use the blood from the umbilical cord of a newborn as long as it is hot and drip it into [the affected eyes]. Miraculously effective".

***Dou feng yan* 痘風眼, smallpox wind-eye** [1]

PC of → *feng yan* 風眼, wind eye, i.e. a condition of inflamed eyes following exposure to wind, associated with a → *dou* 痘, smallpox, condition. *BCGM* Bai bing zhu zhi yao 百病主治藥, *yan mu* 眼目, Eyes: 小兒臍帶血並點**痘風眼**, "Blood from the umbilical cord of a child also to be poured into **smallpox-illness wind-eyes**".

***Dou fu ji* 豆腐積, accumulation of bean curd** [1]

PC of → *shi ji* 食積②, food accumulation, brought forth by an excessive consumption of food prepared from bean curd. *BCGM* SE *lai fu* 萊菔 quotes *BCHB*: 治**豆腐積**, "It cures **accumulations of bean curd**".

***Dou hou feng yan* 痘後風眼, wind-eye following smallpox** [1]

PC identical with → *dou feng yan* 痘風眼, smallpox wind-eye. *BCGM* SE *wei* 蝟 quotes *JiYF*: **痘後風眼**：發則兩瞼紅爛眵淚, "**Wind-eye following smallpox**: When it breaks out the two eyelids will turn red and fester, associated with gritty secretion and tearflow".

***Dou xian* 痘陷, smallpox groove** [2]

PC of → *dou chuang* 痘瘡, smallpox sores, with the smallpox poison sinking into the body and entering the blood, with smallpox sores and inverted moles, mental confusion, or qi depletion, white complexion, and noisy, urgent panting. *BCGM* SE *shi* 豕：頰骨：燒灰，治**痘陷**, "Its cheekbones: burned to ashes they cure **smallpox groove**".

Dou zhen **痘疹, smallpox papules** [34] AN *zhen dou* 疹痘.

PC identical with → *dou chuang* 痘瘡, smallpox sores. *XEDZFL Lun dou zhen zhi fa* 論痘疹治法, On therapy patterns for smallpox papules: 小兒**痘疹**未出已出之間，有類傷寒之狀，憎寒壯熱，身體疼痛, "When **smallpox papules** in children have not yet emerged and are about to emerge, this looks like harm caused by cold. They have an aversion to cold and are very hot. The entire body is in pain".

Dou zhen du **痘疹毒, smallpox papules poison** [1]

EA identical with → *dou du* 痘毒①, smallpox poison. *BCGM* SE *niu shi* 牛虱：預解小兒**痘疹毒**，焙研服之, "It serves to promptly resolve **smallpox papules poison** in children. Bake over a slow fire, grind, and have [the child] ingest it".

Du **毒, poison; poisoning** [p]

① PQ of harmful effects on the human organism exerted by pharmaceutical substances. *BJ Xu li* 序例, "Introductory guide": 無**毒**、有**毒**，斟酌其宜, "[For treatment] consider what is appropriate: [a substance] without **poison**, or [a substance] with **poison**".

② EA AD of → *du qi* 毒氣①, poison qi. *ZHF* 2: 治**毒**攻手足腫，疼痛欲斷方, "Recipe to cure **poison** attacking hands and feet and generating a swelling, with pain [so unbearable one wished life to be] severed".

③ PC of a) diseases generated by food poisoning. *JGYL* Lj: 諸**毒**病得熱更甚，宜冷飲之, "All diseases of [food] **poisoning** will be aggravated by heat. Hence it is advisable to have [patients] drink cold beverages". b) Contagious diseases. *ZHF* 2: 天行**毒**病，挾熱腹痛，下痢, "A heaven-sent **poison** disease, with heat below the arms and abdominal pain, as well as discharge with free-flux illness". c) AD of → *du qi* 毒氣②, poison qi. *ZHF* 5: 葛氏卒**毒**腫起急痛方, "Mr. Ge's recipe for sudden affliction with **poison** [qi] bringing forth swelling, and violent pain".

④ PE of poisoning a third organism. *MYBL* SE *yuan hua* 芫花：根：療疥瘡，可用**毒**魚, "The root. It cures *jie*-illness sores and can be used to **poison** fish".

⑤ Specific excretions. *ZHF* 2: 出錢飲汁，當吐**毒**出也, "Remove the coins and drink the liquid. [Patients] will vomit and thereby emit the **poison**".

⑥ Pharmaceutical substances or other matter with poison. *JGYL* Lj: 凡諸毒，多是假**毒**以投，無知時，宜煮甘草薺汁飲之, "Poisoning often results from some **poison** having been brought into [food, etc.]. If one is not sure he should drink a decoction made of *gan cao* and the juice of *ji*".

Du chi **妒齒, jealousy teeth** [2]

PP of teeth already eroded by bugs/worms. *BCGM* Bai bing zhu zhi yao 百病主治藥：地骨皮，**妒齒**已去，不能食物，煎水漱之, "When **jealousy teeth** are lost and one cannot eat anything, boil *di gu pi* in water and rinse [the mouth] with it".

***Du chuang* 毒瘡, poison sores** [52] AN *chuang du* 瘡毒, sores poison.

PC CD of all types of severe, local and heavily suppurating → *chuang* 瘡, sores. *TPSHF* 63: 治一切癰疽、發背、腦癰諸**毒瘡**，及奶癰疼痛，並宜用雄黃膏方, "Employ the recipe for an ointment with *xiong huang* to cure all types of **poison sores** including all obstruction-illnesses and impediment-illnesses, effusion of the back, and obstruction-illnesses affecting the brain, as well as painful obstruction-illnesses affecting the breast".

***Du feng* 毒風, poison wind** [48]

EA identical with → *feng du* 風毒, wind poison. *ZBYHL* 37: **毒風**之變，冷熱不同，故腠理發癩, "Changes resulting from [being affected by] **poison wind** include uneven alternating sensations of cold and heat. Hence the skin structures develop repudiation-illness". *BCGM* refers to numerous pathological conditions associated with poison wind: *du feng jiao qi* 毒風脚氣, poison wind with leg qi; *dan shi du feng* 丹石毒風, cinnabar [et al.] mineral poison wind; *dan du feng* 丹毒風, cinnabar poison wind; *du feng zhen bi* 毒風疹痹 poison wind with papules and blockage.

Du gu* 毒蠱, poison *gu [3]

EA PC identical with → *gu du* 蠱毒, *gu poison*. *BJ* SE *rong yan* 戎鹽：堅肌骨，去**毒蠱**, "It hardens muscles and bones, and eliminates **poison *gu***". *MYBL* SE *jin ya* 金牙：主鬼疰，**毒蠱**，諸疰, "It controls demon attachment-illness, **poison *gu***, and all [further] types of attachment-illness".

***Du han* 獨寒, solitary cold** [1]

IS identical with → *dan han* 但寒, pure cold. *SW* 20: **獨寒**者病, "If there is **solitary cold**, this is disease".

***Du han* 毒汗, sweating that eliminates poison** [2]

IS of sweating induced by the ingestion of medications for treating an illness. In general, once the sweating ends the disease should be cured too. *YXL* SE *bo he* 薄荷：發**毒汗**，破血，止痢，通利關節, "It causes **sweating that eliminates poison**, breaks through [stagnating] blood, ends free-flux illness, and makes joints move again".

***Du jing chuang* 妒精瘡, jealousy spirit sores** [2] AN *du jing yin chuang* 妒精陰瘡, jealousy spirit sores in the body's yin region.

PC of → *yin shi* 陰蝕, erosion in the genital region, developing at the glans penis of men and in the genital tract of women. *QJYF* 24: **妒精瘡**者，男子在陰頭節下，婦人在玉門內，並似甘瘡作臼, "As for '**jealousy spirit sores**', males have them below the glans penis section, females have them inside the jade gate. In all cases they resemble '*gan*[-illness] sores' forming an indentation".

***Du jing yin chuang* 妒精陰瘡, jealousy spirit sores in the body's yin region** [2]

PC identical with *du jing chuang* 妒精瘡, jealousy spirit sores. *BCGM* SE *huang fan* 黃礬 quoting *QJYF* 24: 妒精瘡, "Jealousy spirit sores", writes: **妒精陰瘡**, "**Jealousy spirit sores in the body's yin region**".

Du lai **毒癩, poison repudiation-illness** [1]

PC identical with → *lai* 癩, repudiation-illness. Because in former times it was believed that this disease is caused by some type of a poison, it was also called "poison repudiation-illness. *BCGM* SE *bai hua she* 白花蛇：主治癜風**毒癩**, "It controls the treatment of patches wind and **poison repudiation-illness**".

Du li **毒癘, poison epidemic** [3]

PC identical with → *wen yi* 瘟疫, warmth-illness epidemic. *BJ* SE *sheng ma* 升麻：it controls 時氣**毒癘**，頭痛寒熱, "**Poison epidemic** caused by seasonal qi, with headache and alternating sensations of cold and heat".

Du li **毒痢, poison free-flux illness** [16] AN *re du li* 熱毒痢, heat poison free-flux illness.

PC of → *li ji* 痢疾, ailment of free-flux illness, with blazing heat poison, apparent as vexation, thirst and fever, frequent free-flux illness-type defecation with pus and blood, abdominal pain and a feeling of heavy pressure at one's behind. *TPSHF* 18: 熱病**毒痢**，下膿血，腰臍下痛，宜服黃連散方, "For heat disease with **poison free-flux illness**, when one discharges pus and blood, with pain in the lower back and below the navel, the recipe to ingest the powder with *huang lian* is advisable".

Du qi **毒氣, poison qi** [127] AD *du* 毒, poison.

① EA a) of all infectious etiological agents. *MYBL* SE *xi jiao* 犀角：療傷寒溫疫，頭痛寒熱，諸**毒氣**, "It cures harm caused by cold and warmth epidemics, with headache and alternating sensations of cold and heat, as well as all types of **poison qi**. b) Of all types of poisonous matter or poisonous functions. *ZBYHL* 26: 凡豬肉本無毒，其野田間放，或食雜毒物而遇死者，此肉則有毒。人食之，則**毒氣**攻臟，故令人吐利，困悶不安, "Pork is originally not poisonous. However, when a pig is set free in the wilderness, it may be that it devours something poisonous and dies. In this case its meat is poisonous. If one consumes it, the **poison qi** will attack his depots and causes that person to vomit and have free-flux illness. He will feel uneasy and restless". c) Causing all types of lesions, swelling, and abscesses. *LS* 70: 此皆鼠瘻寒熱之**毒氣**也，留於脈而不去者也, "All these are **poison qi** [causing] mouse fistula and alternating sensations of cold and heat. [This poison qi] abides in the vessels and does not leave". d) Of all types of external causes of disease. *BJ* SE *shi dan* 石膽：主明目、目痛，金瘡，諸癇痙，女子陰蝕痛，石淋寒熱，崩中下血，諸邪**毒氣**，令人有子, "It controls clearing eyesight, aching eyes, wounds inflicted by metal objects, all types of epilepsy and spasm, painful erosion in the female genital region, stone dripping, and alternating sensations of cold and heat, collapsing center with a discharge of blood, all types of evil and **poison qi**. It helps people to have children". *BCGM* at various occasions speaks of *bai du qi* 百毒氣, the hundred poison qi; *zhu du qi* 諸毒氣, all types of poison qi; *gu du qi* 蠱毒氣, poison qi of *gu*; *re du qi* 熱毒氣, poison qi of heat; *leng du qi* 冷毒氣, poison qi of cold; *feng du qi* 風毒氣, wind poison qi; *e du qi* 惡毒氣, malign poison qi; *shang han du qi* 傷寒毒氣, poison qi of harm caused by cold; *zhu chong du qi* 諸蟲毒氣, poison qi of all types of bugs/worms, etc.

② PC manifesting itself as all types of red, painful and itching sores, swelling, and abscesses, sometimes with suppuration. *MYBL* SE *fu long gan* 伏龍肝：醋調，塗癰腫**毒氣**, "Mix with vinegar and smear on obstruction-illnesses with swelling, and [locations with] **poison qi**".

***Du re* 獨熱, solitary heat** [1]

IS identical with → *dan re* 但熱, pure heat. *TPSHF* 1: **獨熱**者，四肢俱熱，臟腑亦熱，其脈洪數，故曰**獨熱**, " '**Solitary heat**' is to say: the four limbs are all hot; the depots and palaces are hot too. And the [movements in the] vessels are vast and fast. Hence this is called '**solitary heat**' ".

***Du ru* 妒乳, jealousy breast** [20]

PC with milk blocked after delivery and the breasts turning red and swelling, being hot and painful, accompanied by fever. *ZHF* 5: 凡乳汁不得泄內結，名**妒乳**，乃急於癰, "Whenever the milk cannot flow off and forms nodes internally, this is called '**jealousy breast**'. This will quickly turn into an obstruction-illness".

***Du she shang* 毒蛇傷, harm caused by poisonous snakes** [1]

PC identical with → *she hui du* 蛇虺毒②, venomous snake poisoning. *PJF* 307: 蛇咬丹，治**毒蛇傷**, "The elixir for snake bites. It cures **harm caused by poisonous snakes**".

***Du she shang ren* 毒蛇傷人, harm caused to a person by poisonous snakes** [1]

PC identical with → *she hui du* 蛇虺毒②, venomous snake poisoning. *BCGM* Bai bing zhu zhi yao 百病主治藥：甘草，**毒蛇傷人**，目黑口噤，毒氣入腹，同白礬末，冷水服二錢, "For **harm caused to a person by poisonous snakes**, when the eyes are black and the jaws are clenched, with poison qi entering the abdomen, prepare a powder of *gan cao* with *bai fan* and ingest 2 *qian* with cold water".

***Du tong* 毒痛, poison-induced pain** [14]

IS of pain caused by poisoning or swelling with poison. *QJYF* 17: 治卒得屍疰，**毒痛**往來方, "Recipe to cure sudden corpse attachment-illness and **poison-induced pain** that comes and goes".

***Du yi* 毒疫, poison pestilence** [2] AN *yi du* 疫毒, epidemic poison.

PC identical with → *yi bing* 疫病, epidemic disease. *BJ* SE *mu xiang* 木香：主邪氣，辟**毒疫**温鬼, "It controls evil qi and sends off **poison pestilence** and warmth demons".

***Du yong* 肚癰, abdominal obstruction-illness** [1]

PC of → *yong* 癰, obstruction-illness, developing from the muscles of the abdominal wall. Prognosis of those festering to the outside is quite favorable; those festering towards the inside have a rather inauspicious prognosis. *XCWKJYF* Fu tie ri yao 敷貼熱藥：**肚癰**一證，十有九死, "Of persons with the condition of **abdominal obstruction-illness**, nine out of ten die".

***Du zhang* 肚脹, abdominal distension** [9]

IS identical with → *fu zhang* 腹脹①. *RHZ* SE *ma bian cao* 馬鞭草：通月經，治婦人血氣**肚脹**，月候不匀, "It makes the monthly period pass and cures women with **abdominal distension** resulting from blood and qi, with menstrual irregularity".

Du zhong **毒腫, poison swelling** [52]

PC identical with → *zhong du* 腫毒, swelling with poison. *ZHF* 5: 治癰疽妒乳諸**毒腫**方, "Recipes to cure all types of **poison swelling** associated with obstruction-illnesses and impediment-illnesses, and jealousy breast".

Duan chan **斷產, to cut birthing; to sterilize; sterility; to end pregnancy** [13]

① TA of severing a fertile woman's productive capacity so that she may lead a normal life and yet cannot become pregnant. *QJYF* 3: 婦人**斷產**方：蠶子故紙方一尺，燒為末，酒服之，終身不產, "Recipe to **sterilize** women: 1 square *chi* of old paper made from silkworm seeds is to be burned and made to powder. After it has been ingested with wine it will prevent [a woman] from having offspring for her entire life".

② TA of prematurely ending a pregnancy; abortion. *BCGM* SE *fuzi* 附子 quoting *WTMY* 34: 瘵妊身欲去之，並**斷產**方。…又方：附子二枚搗為屑，以淳苦酒和塗右足，去之大良， "Recipes to treat pregnant woman who wish to rid themselves of it, and also to **cut birthing**. …Further recipe: grind two pieces of *fu zi* to crumbs, mix with pure wine and apply to the right foot. Very good to remove it", writes: **斷產**下胎：生附子為末，淳酒和塗右足心，胎下去之。小品方. "**To cut birthing** and bring a fetus down: grind fresh *fu zi* to a powder, mix this with pure wine and apply to the sole of the right foot. Remove again once the fetus has been aborted. *Xiao pin fang*". The meaning of "abortion" conveyed by the use of *duan chan* 斷產in this *BCGM* quote is a departure from the meaning of "sterilization" conveyed by the original use of the term in the *WTMY*.

③ IS of infertility. *BCGM* SE *yin zhi* 印紙, quoting *BCSY*: 主令婦人斷產無子。剪有印處燒灰，水服之一錢匕，神效, "It is capable of cutting a woman's birthing resulting in that she will not have children. Cut out the location with the seal on it, burn it to ashes and ingest on *qian* on a spoon with water. Wondrously effective", from *Zhenglei bencao* 證類本草, SE *yin zhi* 印紙, writes: 婦人**斷產**無子，剪有印處燒灰，水服一錢匕，效。藏器, "If a woman's ability to give **birth is cut** and she has no children, cut out the location with the seal on it, burn it to ashes and ingest one *qian* on a spoon with water. Effective. [Chen] Cangqi". The meaning conveyed in this *BCGM* quote is opposite to the original meaning intended by the *Ben cao shi yi* as quoted in the *Zheng lei ben cao*.

Duan hu **短狐, short fox** [10]

EA identical with → *she gong* 射工①, archer. *ZHF* 7: 江南有射工毒蟲，一名**短狐**, "In the region south of the Yangzi there is a poisonous bug, the archer. Another name is '**short fox**'".

Duan jin **斷筋, ruptured sinew** [4] AN *jin duan* 筋斷, sinew rupture.

PC of a complete or partial rupture of a sinew as an injury caused from outside, resulting in the loss of its connecting function. *QJYF* 25: 治折骨**斷筋**方, "Recipe to cure bone fractures and **ruptured sinews**".

***Duan qi* 短氣, short of qi; panting** [27]

IS identical with a) → *chuan* 喘①, panting. *SW* 42: 肺風之狀，多汗惡風，色皏然白，時咳**短氣**, "The appearance of lung wind [is such]: [patients] sweat profusely and have an aversion to wind. Their [facial] color is a pale white. They often cough and are **short of qi**". b) → *qi duan* 氣短, short of qi. *BJ* SE *mai men dong* 麥門冬：胃絡脈絕，羸瘦**短氣**, "The [movement] in the stomach network vessel is interrupted. [Patients] are emaciated and **short of qi**".

***Dui kou* 對口, counter-orifice** [5] AN *fa nao* 發腦, opening-up of brain; *nao ju* 腦疽, brain-impediment-illness; *nao yong* 腦癰, brain-obstruction-illness.

PC of → *chuang* 瘡, sores, and → *ju* 疽, impediment-illness, developing, possibly as an abscess, in the center of the hairline above one's neck. Below this point is the *sheng ming zhong shu* 生命中樞, "central pivot of life". Hence the most serious conditions easily result from such an abscess. *WKJYF* Fj: 如治**對口**並腦疽，不必洗去舊藥，逐次添藥，恐動瘡口惹風也, "For treating **counter-orifice** and brain-impediment-illnesses one must not rinse off previously applied medication. Instead, one gradually adds additional medication, lest by irritating the opening of the sores wind is invited to enter it".

***Dun chong* 遁蟲, run-away bug** [1]

PC with a swollen and painful throat. *SHZBL* 3: 古方煎，治咽喉腫痛九種疾. 九般名：急喉閉、纏喉風、結喉、爛喉、重舌、木舌、**遁蟲**、蟲喋、飛絲入喉, "Among ancient recipes 'black dragon decoction' served to cure nine types of swollen and painful throat. The names of these nine types are: acute throat closure, throat-constricting wind, bound throat, festering throat, doubled tongue, wooden tongue, **run-away bug**, floating worm-borer, and flying silk threads entering the throat".

***Dun shi* 遁屍, run-away corpse [qi]** [12]

PC with recurrent heart pain and acute panting. *ZBYHL* 23: 心腹脹滿刺痛，氣息喘急，傍攻兩脅，上衝心胸，瘥後複發，停遁不消，故謂之**遁屍**也, "The heart and abdomen are distended with a feeling of fullness and piercing pain. Breathing is a hectic panting. In one's sides it affects both flanks. Above, it rushes against the heart and chest. Once it has healed it breaks out again. It may stop as if it had run away, but it has not dissolved. Hence it is called '**run-away corpse [qi]**'".

***Duo gu chuang* 多骨瘡, multiple bones sores** [1]

PC of → *gu ju* 骨疽, bone impediment-illness, with bone fracture and subsequent putrescence. *BCGM* SE *mi tuo seng* 密陀僧 quotes *SYSF*: 骨疽出骨：一名**多骨瘡**，不時出細骨, "Bone impediment-illness with [pieces of] bone coming out: another name is **multiple bones sores**. Fine pieces of bone appear every now and then".

***Duo meng* 多夢, frequent dreaming** [5]

IS of a restless sleep because of excessive dreaming. *ZBYHL* 38: 邪氣甚盛者，令人恍惚**多夢**, "An overabundance of evil qi makes people be absent-minded with **frequent dreaming**".

Duo mian **多眠, profuse sleeping** [7]

① IS identical with → *duo shui* 多睡, profuse sleeping. *SJZL* 175: 治小兒宿食不消，體熱**多眠**，嘔噦氣上，消谷丸方, "To cure children whose food remains in their body over night without being digested, whose body is hot with **profuse sleeping**, and who vomit with rising qi, [use] the recipe for the 'pills to digest grain'".

② PC of a disease with profuse sleeping.. *SHLZHRS* 85: **多眠**有四證, "[The disease of] **profuse sleeping** manifests itself in four conditions".

Duo shang **墮傷, damage from a fall** [2]

PC identical with → *zhui sun* 墜損. *BCTJ* SE *xing zhi* 杏枝：主**墮傷**，取一握，水一大升煮半，下酒三合，分再服，大效, "It controls **damage from a fall**. Take one handful and boil with one large *sheng* of water down to its half. Then pour 3 *ge* of wine into [the water], and ingest this in two portions. Very effective".

Duo shui **多睡, profuse sleeping** [21] AN *duo mian* 多眠; *hao mian* 好眠, a longing for sleep; *chang yu mian* 常欲眠, frequent desire to sleep; *xi mian* 喜眠, a tendency to sleep.

PC of constant weariness and a desire to sleep even though one sleeps much more than normal. *BCJJZ* SE *yu* 榆：初生莢人以作糜羹，令人**多睡**, "Prepare a thick soup from its pods as soon as they have emerged. It will cause **profuse sleeping**".

Duo tai **墮胎, to cause an abortion; spontaneous abortion** [62] AN *zhui tai* 墜胎.

① Any method to artificially and prematurely terminate a pregnancy. *BJ* SE *shui yin* 水銀：殺皮膚中虱，**墮胎**，除熱, "It kills lice in the skin, **causes abortion**, and eliminates heat". *BCGM* uses the term *duo tai* 墮胎 mostly in this sense.

② PC with a spontaneous premature termination of a pregnancy. *ZBYHL* 41: 婦人腎以系胞，妊娠而腰痛甚者，多**墮胎**也, "Because their kidneys are tied to the uterus, if women experience a severe pain in their lower back during pregnancy, this is often [a sign of an impending] **spontaneous abortion**".

Duo ti **多涕, profuse snivel** [3]

IS of profuse flow of snivel from the nose. *BJ* SE *du ruo* 杜若：風入腦戶，頭腫痛，**多涕**淚出, "When wind enters through the brain gate, the head will swell and ache, and there will be **profuse** release of **snivel** and tears".

Duo wang **多忘, forgetfulness** [15]

IS identical with → *jian wang* 健忘①. *JGYL* Lj: 胡荽久食之，令人**多忘**, "If *hu sui* is consumed over an extended period of time, it will cause **forgetfulness**".

Duo wo **多臥, much resting** [2] AN *dan yu wo* 但欲臥, exclusive desire to rest.

IS identical with → *si wo* 嗜臥, a desire to lie down. *ZHF* 4: 悲憂慘戚，**多臥**少起，久者積年, "Grief and worry are extreme. [Patients] **rest much** and they rarely rise. Long episodes may last for several years".

- E -

***E* 呃, hiccough** [6]

IS and PC AD of → *e ni* 呃逆, hiccough with counterflow [of qi]. *ZZYJ*: 咳逆為病，古為之噦，近為之**呃**, "The disease of cough with counterflow [of qi] was termed 'retching' in antiquity; it is called '**hiccough**' in more recent times".

***E bi* 惡痹, malign blockage** [1]

PC of a serious or difficult-to-cure blockage. *MYBL* SE *song zhi* 松脂：其赤者主**惡痹**, "Red ones master **malign blockage**".

***E bing* 惡病, malign disease** [9] AN *e ji* 惡疾, malign ailment; *e zheng* 惡症, malign condition; *e zheng* 惡證 malign condition; *e hou* 惡候.

PC of diseases with diverse illness signs and a bad prognosis. *QJYF* 5: 夫癇，小兒之**惡病**也，或有不及求醫而致困者也, "Now, epilepsy is a **malign disease** of children. There are cases where there is no time left to seek medical assistance and the disease develops into a fatal problem".

***E chuang* 惡瘡, malign sores** [462]

PC CD of all types of → *chuang yang* 瘡瘍, sores and ulcers, which are either extremely serious, accompany a lingering disease process, or have a bad prognosis. *BJ* SE *fan shi* 礬石：主寒熱，泄痢，白沃，陰蝕，**惡瘡**, "It controls alternating sensations of cold and heat, free-flux illness, white downpour, erosion in the genital region, and **malign sores**".

***E ci* 惡刺, malign piercing [9]**

① EA of cuts by sharp edges of poisonous herbs leading to swelling, pain, and putrefaction. *TPSHF* 68: 夫**惡刺**，是因毒蛇尿著草木，拂著人似刺扎，便腫痛肉爛, "**Malign piercing**: if a poisonous snake urinates on herbs or trees, and if one is pierced by this piece, this will result in swelling, pain, and putrefaction".
② PC identical with → *e ci zhuang* 惡刺瘡, sores resulting from malign piercing. *QJYF* 25: 治**惡刺**方：苦瓠開口，納小兒尿，煮兩三沸浸病上, "Recipe to cure [sores resulting from] **malign piercing**: Take a bitter gourd, open a hole, pour a child's urine into it. Heat until it boils two or three times, and apply to the sores".

***E ci chuang* 惡刺瘡, malign piercing sores** [4]

PC of sores, sometimes festering, brought forth by → *e ci* **惡刺**, malign piercing. *BCSY* SE *hu yan ke nei tu* 胡燕窠內土：又主**惡刺瘡**, "It also controls **malign piercing sores**".

***E du* 惡毒, malign poison** [29]

① EA capable of causing severe infectious diseases. *WTMY* 31: 主喉腫，邪氣**惡毒**入腹方, "Recipe to control throat swelling, and evil qi as well as **malign poison** entering the abdomen".
② PC a) appearing all over the body as violent → *du chuang* 毒瘡, poison sores. *ZHF* 2: 治得瘥後，瘡瘢紫黑，彌歲方減，此**惡毒**之氣, "If after one has achieved a cure there remain purple-black sore scars that vanish only after a full

year, this is the qi of a **malign poison**". b) CD of difficult-to-cure pathological conditions that assume serious manifestations and may appear in many different forms. *QJYF* 12: 但是一切**惡毒**無所不治方, "This is a recipe that is able to cure all types of **malign poison**".

E du feng **惡毒風, malign poison wind** [2]

① EA capable of bringing forth serious infectious diseases. *YXL* SE *ling yang jiao* 羚羊角：能治一切熱毒風攻注，中**惡毒風**，卒死昏亂不識人, "It is capable of curing all types of attack and influx of heat poison wind, when one was struck by **malign poison wind**, with sudden [appearance of] death, clouding with confusion, and a failure to recognize persons".

② PC of a sudden swelling with heat and pain. *RHZ* SE *ye zhu dan zhong huan* 野豬膽中黃：治鬼疰，癇疾及**惡毒風**, "To cure demon attachment-illness, epilepsy ailment, and **malign poison wind**".

E feng **惡風, malign wind** [15]

① EA identical with → *feng* 風, wind①. *SW* 17: 中**惡風**者，陽氣受也, "When one is struck by **malign wind**, the yang qi receives it".

② PC of a) → *feng* 風, wind②. *SW* 17: 來徐去疾，上虛下實，為**惡風**也, "When [the movement in the vessels] comes slowly and leaves hastily, with depletion above and repletion below, this is [being struck by] **malign wind**". b) Reference to → *da feng* 大風, massive wind. *ZBYHL* 2: **惡風**鬚眉墮落候, "Signs of the beard and eyebrows falling off because of **malign wind**".

E gui **惡鬼, malign demon** [11]

EA identical with → *gui xie* 鬼邪, demon evil. *BJ* SE *xiong huang* 雄黃：殺精物**惡鬼**，邪氣，百蟲毒, "It kills spirit beings, **malign demons**, evil qi, and the poison of all types of bugs/worms".

E hou **惡候, malign sign** [3]

PC identical with → *e bing* 惡病, malign disease. *SJZL* 5: 如中風髮直，面如桃花色，口眼俱閉，喉中作聲，汗出如油及汗出不流，多要下泄或瀉血者，並是**惡候**, "If one has been struck by wind, with one's hair standing up straight and the face assuming the color of peach blossoms, and both mouth and eyes closed, and sounds coming from the throat, sweat flowing like oil and sweat that appears but fails to flow, and if there is a tendency to discharge with outflow, and to defecate blood, all these are **malign signs**".

E ji **惡疾, malign ailment** [10]

PC a) identical with → *da feng* 大風, massive wind. *QJYF* 23: **惡疾**大風有多種不同, "**Malign ailment**, (i.e.) massive wind, assumes many different forms". b) Identical with → *e bing* 惡病, malign disease. *QJYF* 14 RE *tian men dong jiu* 天門冬酒, wine with *tian men dong*, cures 癲癇**惡疾**，耳聾頭風，四肢拘攣, "Peak-illness and epilepsy **malign ailments**, deafness and head wind, and the four limbs having cramps and contraction".

E jie **惡結, malign node** [1]

PC of sores and swelling resulting from stagnation and nodes formed of evil qi. *MYBL* SE *fang ji* 防己：散癰腫**惡結**, "It disperses obstruction-illnesses, swelling, and **malign nodes**".

E ju **惡疽, malign impediment-illness** [3]

PC CD of → *ju* 疽, impediment-illnesses, manifesting themselves as very serious conditions with an inauspicious prognosis. *QJYiF* 19: 露蜂房、亂髮、蛇皮，三味合燒灰，酒服方寸匕，日二。主諸**惡疽**、附骨癰，根在臟腑, "*Lu feng fang*, *luan fa* and *she pi*, these three substances are to be mixed and burned to ashes. They are to be ingested with wine, a dose of one square-inch size spoon twice per day to master all types of **malign impediment-illnesses**, and obstruction-illnesses attached to the bones, with a root in the depots and palaces".

E kou **鵝口, goose-mouth** [25] AN *e kou chuang* 鵝口瘡, goose-mouth sores; *e kou bai chuang* 鵝口白瘡, white goose-mouth sores.

PC of → *chuang* 瘡, sores, with a white layer covering the mucous membranes and top of the tongue in a child's mouth making it resemble a goose-mouth. *ZBYHL* 15: 小兒初生，口裏白屑起，乃至舌上生瘡，如鵝口裏，世謂之**鵝口**, "When in a newborn child a white scaling develops in the mouth eventually generating sores on its tongue so that it looks like the inside of a goose-mouth, this is generally called '**goose-mouth**'".

E kou bai chuang **鵝口白瘡, white goose-mouth sores** [2]

PC identical with → *e kou* 鵝口, goose-mouth. *BCGM* SE *ji* 雞 quotes *ZMML*: **鵝口白瘡**：雞肫黃皮為末，乳服半錢, "For **white goose-mouth sores**: prepare a powder from the yellow skin of a chicken gizzard and ingest one half *qian* with milk".

E kou chuang **鵝口瘡, goose-mouth sores** [7]

PC identical with → *e kou* 鵝口, goose-mouth. *RHZ* SE *lu jiao* 鹿角：小兒重舌，**鵝口瘡**，炙熨之, "When children have a heavy tongue with **goose-mouth sores**, press a heated [deer horn] on it".

E lai **惡癩, malign repudiation-illness** [1]

PC identical with → *lai* 癩, repudiation-illness. Because the appearance and the further course of this disease are very severe, it is also called 'malign repudiation-illness'". *QJYF* 12: 大風**惡癩**可二十服, "For massive wind, (i.e.) **malign repudiation-illness**, one may ingest twenty".

E li **惡痢, malign free-flux illness** [5]

PC of severe free-flux illness or free-flux illness lasting for an extended period of time. *SWBJQYBMJ* Mj RE *jiao zhu wan* 椒朮丸, pills with [*shu*] *jiao* and [*cang*] *zhu*: **惡痢**久不愈者，加桂, "For **malign free-flux illness** that fails to be healed for a long time, add *gui*".

E lu **惡露, malign dew** [16]

① Blood or turbid liquid (i.e. lochia) leaving from the birth canal after parturition. *ZHF* 8: *Yao zi yi wu fang* 藥子一物方, "the one-ingredient recipe with *yao zi*": 婦人難產後，腹中絞痛，及**惡露**不止, "For women who following a difficult delivery have a twisting pain in their abdomen and an unending outflow of **malign dew**".

② Turbid liquid. *WTMY* 29: 又療（諸瘡）若已中水及**惡露**、風寒，腫痛方, "A recipe to cure swelling and pain [of all types of sores] if they have been affected by water or **malign dew**, and wind cold".

***E meng* 惡夢, malign dream** [7]

IS of dreadful nightmares. *BCJJZ* SE *she xiang* 麝香：置頸間枕之，辟**惡夢**及屍疰鬼氣, "Place into the headrest under the neck. This will remove **malign dreams**, as well as corpse [qi] attachment-illness and demon qi".

***E meng ji* 惡夢悸, malign dream with palpitation** [2]

IS identical with → *jing meng* 驚夢, fright dream. *QJYF* 14: 主鬼氣注忤中惡，心腹痛，背急，氣喘，**惡夢悸**, "It controls demon qi influx and hostility, being struck by the malign with heartache and abdominal pain, a stiff back, panting with qi, and **malign dreams with palpitation**".

***E ni* 呃逆, hiccough with counterflow [of qi]** [20] AD *e* 呃, hiccough.

① IS of qi rushing upward from the abdomen, contrary to its normal direction, and leaving the body as hiccough with a very brief sound. *WSBJ* 12: 氣短促，**呃逆**不絕，不得安臥, "The qi [leaving] is very brief and urgent. [One experiences] **hiccough with a counterflow [of qi]** that does not end. One is unable to find rest and sleep".

② PC manifesting itself mainly as hiccough. *WSBJ* 12: 羌活附子湯，治**呃逆**, "Decoction with *jiang huo* and *fu zi* cures **hiccough with counterflow [of qi]**".

***E qi* 惡氣, malign qi** [135]

① EA GD of pathogenic evil that affects and harms the human organism either from outside or from within. *BJ* SE *chi jian* 赤箭：主殺鬼精物，蠱毒**惡氣**, "It controls the killing of demons and spirit beings, *gu poison*, and **malign qi**".

② A bad odor. *BCGM* SE *ban mao* 斑蝥：斑蝥人獲得之，尾後**惡氣**射出，臭不可聞, "When one has caught a *ban mao* it will shoot **malign qi** from behind its tail. The stench is unbearable".

***E rou* 惡肉, malign flesh** [64]

① PC of the growth of all types of unusual tissue on the body's outside. *ZHF* 5: **惡肉**病者，身中忽有肉，如赤小豆粒突出，便長如牛馬乳，亦如雞冠狀，亦宜服漏蘆湯，外可以燒鐵烙之, "Patients with **malign flesh** suddenly develop flesh protruding like some small red bean kernels on their body. They grow to the size of cow teats, or they may look like a cock's comb. One should ingest a decoction with *lou lu*. One can also cauterize them with a flatiron from outside".

② IS of tissue that has decayed within sores and abscesses, or that grows in an unusual way. *ZBYHL* 31: 凡癰膿潰之後，須著排膿藥，令熱毒膿血俱散盡。若有**惡肉**，亦敷藥食之, "Following suppuration of obstruction-illnesses one must apply pus medication to completely remove heat poison, pus, and blood. If there is **malign flesh**, one must externally apply medication to it to dissolve it".

***E she hui shang* 惡蛇虺傷, injury caused by the venom of a malign snake** [1]
PC identical with → *she hui shang* 蛇虺傷, harm caused by a venomous snake. *BCGM* SE *mu xiang* 木香 quotes *XZF*: 惡蛇虺傷：青木香不拘多少，煎水服，效不可述, "For **injury caused by the venom of a malign snake**: boil any amount of *qing mu xiang* in water and ingest. The effects are undescribable".

***E shui* 惡水, malign water/liquid; unclean water** [21]
① EA of all types of water/liquid that are polluted or are harmful and may bring forth disease for any reason. *SJZL* 133: 治皂莢水及**惡水**入瘡，熱痛不止，烏犀膏方, "To cure unending heat pain resulting from *zao jia* liquid and **malign water/liquid** having entered sores/wounds: recipe for an ointment with *wu xi*".
② General reference to all filthy, excreted matter, including matter that has been vomited, thin urine, excretions from the urinary duct, matter excreted from sores, pus, etc. In *QJYF* 12 following the listing of *lao po wan bing wan* 耆婆萬病丸, "granny's pills for a a myriad of of diseases", a commentary states: 平旦空腹酒服三丸，如梧子大，取微下三升**惡水**為良, "Ingest 3 pills of the size of *wu* seeds at dawn with wine on an empty stomach. It is best to use a mild dosage to drain three *sheng* of **malign water/liquid**".
③ Unclean water in the natural environment. *BCGM* SE *wen mu niao* 蚊母鳥：〔藏器曰〕此鳥大如雞，黑色。生南方池澤茹蘆中，江東亦多。其聲如人嘔吐，每吐出蚊一二升。夫蚊乃**惡水**中蟲，羽化所生，蚊雖是**惡水**中蟲羽化所生，然亦有蚊母吐之 "Cangqi: This bird is big like a chicken, and its color is black. It lives in the South in the marshes. East of the River are many too. They make sounds as if a human were vomiting. Each time they spit out one or two *sheng* mosquitos. Now, mosquitos are bugs found in **unclean water**. They come to life through a transformation of the feathers [of the mosquito mother bird]. Although mosqitos are bugs which come to life in unclean water through the transformation of feathers, they are also spat out by the 'mosquito mother' [bird]".

***E te* 呃忒, hiccough** [1]
IS identical with *e ni* 呃逆①, hiccough with counterflow [of qi]. *RMSQ* 4: 夫男子婦人咳逆，俗呼曰**呃忒**，乃陰陽不和也, "Now, regardless of whether males or females have cough with countermovement [of qi], it is commonly called **hiccough**. This is an imbalance of yin and yang".

***E wu* 惡物, malign item** [63]
① All types of excreted or secreted turbid, unclear items, including pus and blood, feces and urine, vomitus, items discharged from one's genital region, etc. *SHL* 233: 大豬膽一枚，瀉汁，和少許法醋，以灌穀道內，如一食頃，當大便出宿食**惡物**, "Take a large pig's gallbladder, pour the liquid out of it, fill in a small amount of vinegar and pour this into the anus. After the time it takes to have a meal, this will cause food remaining in the body over night and **malign items** to leave via defecation".
② Unclean items that must be discarded during a pharmaceutical processing of substances to be used as pharmaceutical drug. *QJYF* 19 SE *mi jiao* 麋角：曝乾淨擇，去**惡物**、粗骨皮及鎊不勻者, "Expose to the sun to dry them and se-

lect the clean parts. Remove **malign items**, coarse bone skin, and those parts that have not been evenly pounded".

E xin 惡心, **malign [feeling in the] center; nausea** [40]

IS of a feeling in the chest or abdomen of something rising contrary to its normal direction with an urge to vomit. This often entails that patients widely open their mouth as if they were vomiting. *ZHF* 4: 治人忽**惡心**不已方, "Recipes to cure persons suddenly experiencing a **malign [feeling in the] center** (i.e. stomach) that does not end".

E xuan 惡癬, **malign *xuan*-illness** [3]

PC of → *xuan* 癬, *xuan*-illness, that is difficult to cure and comes with severe local lesions. *PJF* 281: 又**惡癬**方：用紫背草入生明礬研細，敷二三次斷根, "Further recipe for **malign *xuan*-illness**: Add *zi bei cao* to fresh *ming fan* and grind to a fine powder. Externally apply two or three times to cut the root".

E xue 惡血, **malign blood** [136]

① PP a) of blood liquid that has left the conduits and decays there. *SW* 41: 得之舉重傷腰，衡絡絕，**惡血**歸之, "One gets this from an injury at the lower back which resulted from lifting something heavy. The transverse network vessel is ruptured and [all] the **malign blood** turns there. b) Identical with → *e lu* 惡露, malign dew, that is blood or turbid liquid leaving from the birth canal after parturition. *QJYF* 3: 凡產後七日內，**惡血**未盡，不可服湯, "For seven days following a delivery as long as the flow of **malign blood** has not ended one must not consume hot liquids". c) Of pus and blood. *QJYF* 22: 瀉後鋒針數針去**惡血**，氣針瀉其根，核上敷小豆末，取消為度, "After drainage is completed pierce with the sharp point needle several times to remove **malign blood**. By means of qi needling drain the root [of the problem]. Then apply a powder ground from small bones to the kernels on the skin until they have vanished".
② PC brought forth by decayed blood liquid stagnating in the body. *BJ* SE *shi liu huang* 石硫黃：主婦人陰蝕、疽痔、**惡血**, "It controls erosion in the female genital region, impediment-illnesses and piles, and **malign blood**".

E yang 惡癢, **malign itch** [3]

IS of a feeling of violent itching. *YXL* SE *jing tian* 景天：能治風疹**惡癢**, "It can cure wind papules and **malign itch**".

E yang 惡瘍, **malign ulcer** [3]

PC identical with → *e chuang* 惡瘡, malign sores. *BJ* SE *ya zi* 牙子：主邪氣熱氣，疥瘙**惡瘍**, "It controls evil qi, heat qi, *jie*-illness with itching, and **malign ulcers**".

E yi 呃噫, **hiccough** [9]

PC, IS identical with → *e ni* 呃逆, hiccough with counterflow [of qi]. *WSBJ* 12: 丁香柿蒂散，治諸種**呃噫**, "Powder with *ding xiang* and *shi di* cures all types of **hiccough**".

E zhang feng **鵝掌風, goose-palm wind** [4] AN *e zhang chuang* 鵝掌瘡, goose palm sores.

PC of the skin of syphilis patients breaking open, festering, and desiccating on the top and soles/palms of feet and hands. *WKZZ* 3, Yang mei chuang lun 楊梅瘡論, "Discourse on red bayberry sores": 手足皮膚枯槁，**鵝掌風**, "When the skin of hands and feet desiccates, this is **goose-palm wind**".

E zheng **惡症, malign condition** [2]

PC identical with → *e bing* 惡病, malign disease. *PJF* 169: 沉香海金沙丸，治一切積聚，痹濕，腫脹，肚大青筋，瘦，**惡症**, "Pills with *chen xiang* and *hai jin sha* cure all types of accumulation and collection, blockage with moisture, swelling and distension, large greenish sinews on the abdomen, emaciation, and **malign conditions**".

E zheng **惡證, malign condition** [3]

PC identical with → *e bing* 惡病, malign disease. *SYJYBZFL* 14: 不疼尤是**惡證**，不可不知, "If there is no pain this is an even more **malign condition**. One must know this".

E zhi **惡汁, malign sap** [8]

All types of excreted or secreted liquid, unclear items. *ZBYHL* 50: 凡癰癤，捻膿血不盡，而瘡口便合，其**惡汁**在里，雖瘥，終能更發，變成漏也, "Whenever one fails to completely squeeze pus and blood from obstruction-illnesses and pimples, and the wound closes, **malign sap** will remain inside. Although [the abscess appears to have been] healed, it may eventually break open again and start leaking".

E zhong **惡腫, malign swelling** [31]

PC of → *chuang* , 瘡 sores, with a topical swelling accompanied by putrefaction as its major sign. *WTMY* 30: 療**惡腫**，犀角湯方, "Recipe for a decoction with *xi jiao* to cure **malign swelling**".

E zhu **惡疰, malign attachment-illness** [2]

PC of extreme pain in the heart and abdomen that comes and goes with changing locations and does not heal. *WTMY* 7: E zhu xin tong fang san shou 惡疰心痛方三首, "Three recipes of **malign attachment-illness** and heartache": 又療心腹痛不可忍，似疰病者，或暴得**惡疰**攪刺欲死，桃仁大黃湯方, "Also, to heal unbearable pain in heart and abdomen resembling that of attachment-illness diseases, where in some cases one is suddenly afflicted with **malign attachment-illness** and a feeling of severe piercing that makes people wish to die, the recipe for a decoction with *tao ren* and *da huang* [is advisable]".

E zu **惡阻, malign obstruction** [6]

PC of frequent nausea and vomiting in the early stages of pregnancy. *QJYF* 2: 青竹茹湯，治妊娠**惡阻**，嘔吐不下食方, "Decoction with *qing zhu ru* is a recipe that cures **malign obstruction** during pregnancy with vomiting and an inability to swallow food".

E he **惡核, malign kernel** [7]

PC of → *jie he* 結核, nodular kernel, associated with a violent outbreak of a disease whereby suddenly many swellings develop accompanied by dryness and pain in the flesh and pain roaming through the entire body. If not treated immediately, this disease has an inauspicious prognosis. *BCJJZ* SE chen xiang 沉香：療**惡核**毒腫, "It cures **malign kernels** and poison swelling".

E lou **惡瘺, malign fistula** [1]

PC of very serious cases of → *lou* 瘺, fistula, with an inauspicious prognosis. *ZLBC* SE *hu yin jing* 狐陰莖 quotes *QJYF*: 治一切**惡瘺**中冷息肉, "To cure all types of **malign fistula**, cold in the center, and tumorous flesh-growths".

Er bian bi **二便閉, both [major and minor] relief closed; both defecation and urination are blocked** [2]

IS, PC CD of → *xiao bian bi* 小便閉, blocked urination, and → *da bian bi* 大便閉, blocked defecation. *BCGM* Bai bing zhu zhi yao 百病主治藥：蔓菁子油，**二便閉**，服一合, "*Man jing zi* oil: when **both defecation and urination are blocked** ingest 1 *ge*".

Er bian bu jin **二便不禁, both [major and minor] relief are uncontrolled; both defecation and urination are uncontrolled** [1]

IS of involuntary and uncontrollable passage of feces and urine. *BCGM* Zang fu xu shi biao ben yong yao shi 臟腑虛實標本用藥式：下寒則**二便不禁**，臍腹冷, "When the lower section is cold, **both defecation and urination are uncontrolled**. The navel and abdomen are cold".

Er bian bu li **二便不利, both [major and minor] relief impeded; both defecation and urination do not pass freely** [2]

IS identical with → *da xiao bian bu li* 大小便不利, stools and urine do not pass freely. *BCGM* SE *da huang* 大黃 quotes *QJYF*: 久患積聚，**二便不利**, "[Patients] chronically suffer from accumulation and collection. **Neither defecation nor urine pass freely**".

Er bian bu tong **二便不通, both [major and minor] relief blöocked; both defecation and urination fail to pass** [21]

IS, PC identical with → *da xiao bu tong* 大小便不通, blocked defecation and urination. *TPSHF* 58: **二便不通**，故為關格, " **Both defecation and urination fail to pass**. Hence there is 'barrier and resistance'".

Er bian pin shuo **二便頻數, both [major and minor] relief occur frequently; frequent defecation and urination** [1]

IS identical with → *da xiao bian shuo* 大小便數. *BCGM* SE *kui* 葵：今之治者，惟恐其大小**二便頻數**，泄其元氣，痘不起發, "Today's therapists simply fear its stimulation of **frequent defecation and urination** [assuming that it] drains the [patient's] original qi and fails to let the smallpox rise and break out".

Er gan **耳疳, *gan*-illness affecting the ear** [5] AN *gan er* 疳耳, *gan*-illness ear.

PC of → *gan chuang* 疳瘡, *gan*-illness sores, developing on the ear. *QXLF* 54: 陰蝕瘡、**耳疳**瘡，一切惡瘡皆治, "It cures all types of malign sores, such as erosion sores in the genital region and ***gan*-illness** sores **affecting the ears**".

***Er long* 耳聾, impaired hearing ability; deafness** [98] AD *long* 聾.

① IS of a significantly impaired hearing ability. *LS* 23: 熱病，身重骨痛，**耳聾**而好瞑, "In the case of heat disease, when the body feels heavy and the bones ache, and when [patients have an] **impaired hearing ability** and love to close their eyes".

② AN *long er* 聾耳; *long bi* 聾閉, deafness blockage. PC with impaired hearing ability/deafness as its major sign. *LS* 24: **耳聾**，取手小指次指爪甲上與肉交者，先取手，後取足, "For [treating patients with] **impaired hearing ability/deafness**, select [for piercing the location] where at the finger/toe next to the small finger/toe the nail meets the flesh. First take the hands, then take the feet".

***Er ming* 耳鳴, ringing in the ears** [31]

① IS of a sensation of a ringing sound in the ears. *LS* 33: 髓海不足，則腦轉**耳鳴**, "In case of insufficiency in the sea of marrow the brain will revolve and there is **ringing in the ears**".

② PC with ringing in the ears as its major sign. *SW* 28: 頭痛**耳鳴**，九竅不利，腸胃之所生也, "When the head aches and when there is a **ringing in the ears** and when the nine orifices are not freely passable, this is generated by the intestines and the stomach".

***Er yin bu tong* 二陰不通, the two yin [orifices] are not passable** [1]

IS, PC identical with → *da xiao bu tong* 大小便不通, blocked defecation and urination. *YXFM* 2: 下焦有濕熱，流入十二經，致**二陰不通**, "The lower burner has moisture heat which flows into the twelve conduits. Hence **the two yin [orifices] are not passable**".

***Er zhen* 兒枕, an infant's headrest** [p]

PC AD of → *er zhen tong* 兒枕痛, an infant's-headrest pain. *HYBC* SE *yan hu suo* 延胡索：破產後惡露及**兒枕**, "It breaks malign dew following delivery, and **an infant's headrest**".

***Er zhen tong* 兒枕痛, an infant's-headrest pain** [4] AD *er zhen* 兒枕, an infant's headrest; AN 血枕痛, blood headrest pain.

PC following delivery with swelling and lumps caused by stagnant blood (the "infant's headrest") in the abdominal region, accompanied by pain. *HYBC* SE *hu po* 琥珀：破癥瘕氣塊，產後血暈悶絕，**兒枕痛**等, "It breaks concretion-illness and conglomeration-illness [resulting in] qi lumps, blood dizziness and heart-pressure following delivery so severe that one wishes to die, as well as **an infant's-headrest pain**".

- F -

***Fa ban guai zheng* 發斑怪證, queer condition of macula appearance** [1]
PC identical with → *re du guai bing* 熱毒怪病, queer disease of heat poisoning. *BCGM* SE *hua shi* 滑石 calls this disease → *re du guai bing* 熱毒怪病, "Queer disease of heat poisoning". *BCGM* SE *fan shi* 礬石 calls the same disease **發斑怪證**, "**Queer condition of macula appearance**".

***Fa bei* 發背, effusion of the back** [159] AN *bei fa* 背發.
PC of → *yong* 癰, obstruction-illnesses, and *ju* 疽, impediment-illnesses, developing on one's back. As it was believed that the transporter holes of the five depots and six palaces are located on the back, conditions of obstruction-illnesses and impediment-illnesses there, often apparent as abscesses, were considered threatening. *ZHF* 5: 療奶發，諸癰疽**發背**, "To cure breast effusion, all types of obstruction-illnesses and impediment-illnesses with **effusion of the back**".

***Fa jia* 髮瘕, hair conglomeration-illness** [4]
PC of → *jia* 瘕, conglomerations, which form when someone inadvertently ingests hair. *YJWY* 20: 徐文伯以油為宮人吐**髮瘕**, "Xu Wenbo resorted to oil to have members of the palaces throw up **hair conglomeration-illness**".

***Fa jin* 發噤, clenched jaw** [4]
IS identical with → 口噤. *TPSHF* 82: 治小兒新生，**發噤**撮口，宜服鉤藤散方, "To cure **clenched jaw** and pursed mouth of newborn children, the recipe for ingesting the powder with *gou teng* is advisable".

***Fa nao* 發腦, brain effusion** [3]
PC identical with → *dui kou* 對口, counter-orifice. *TPSHF* 62: 治**發腦**，腫痛煩熱不可忍，黃耆散方, "To cure **brain effusion**, with unbearable swelling and pain, as well as vexing heat, [resort to] the recipe for the powder with *huang qi*".

***Fa re* 發熱, effusion of heat; fever** [184]
① AN *shen re* 身熱; *ti re* 體熱, body heat. IS of a personal uncomfortable feeling of dryness and heat, or a body temperature above normal. *SW* 74: 惡寒**發熱**如瘧, "[Patients have] an aversion to cold associated with **an effusion of heat**, resembling malaria".
② PE of pharmaceutical substances of a warm or hot thermo-quality that add to the yang qi and warmth in the body. *SW* 5: 氣薄則發泄，厚則**發熱**, "When the qi is weak, it brings forth outflow; when it is strong, it serves to **effuse heat**".

***Fa ru* 發乳, breast effusion** [5] AN *ru fa* 乳發.
PC of a grave → *ru yong* 乳癰, breast obstruction-illness, with local appearance and also severe headache and fever affecting the entire body. *ZBYHL* 卷 40: "凡**發乳**潰後，出膿血多，則腑臟虛燥，則渴而引飲, "Whenever after a **breast effusion** has opened there follows an emission of much pus and blood, this is a sign of depot and palace depletion and desiccation. As a result [patients] are thirsty and wish to drink".

***Fa yi* 發頤, jowl effusion** [2]

PC of → *yong* 癰, obstruction-illnesses, and → *ju* 疽, impediment-illnesses, developing behind the ear or on the cheeks. *XCWKJYF* Zong lun 總論：耳後一寸三分，至命之處，發之必死。故銳毒不治。銳毒者，銳其毒也，名曰**發頤**, "1 *cun* and 3 *fen* behind the ears is a vital point. When it is effused there, this means certain death. The reason is, the poison there is ferocious and difficult to cure. 'The poison is ferocious' means: the poison there is ferocious. This is called '**jowl effusion**'".

***Fa zheng* 髮癥, hair concretion-illness** [5]

PC of → *zheng* 癥, concretion-illness, which forms when someone inadvertently ingests hair. *ZBYHL* 19: **髮癥**候：有人因食飲內誤有頭髮，隨食而入成癥, "The signs of **hair concretion-illness**: Someone has hair from a head in his food or beverage. When consumed it forms a concretion-illness in [his body]".

***Fa zhi* 髮膩, greasy hair** [2]

IS of greasy, sticky hair that is difficult to comb. *BCGM* SE *huang da dou* 黃大豆：油，塗瘡疥，解**髮膩**, "The oil .. externally applied to sores and *jie*-illness it loosens **greasy hair**".

***Fan* 煩, vexation; uneasiness** [p]

IS AD of → *fan men* 煩悶, vexation with heart-pressure. *SW* 3: **煩**則喘喝，靜則多言, "If [the patient suffers from] **vexation**, he will pant with much noise; if he is at peace, he [nevertheless] speaks a lot".

***Fan chuan* 煩喘, vexation with panting** [4]

IS of rapid breathing associated with vexation and unrest. *SHZBL* 4: **煩喘**自汗，瘡不作黑厭，可治, "**Vexation with panting** and spontaneous sweating. If the sores do not develop a black dimple this can be cured".

***Fan du* 煩毒, vexation poison** [5]

IS of mental vexation caused by heat poison and ulcers with poison. *MYBL* SE *li shi* 理石：解**煩毒**，止消渴, "It resolves **vexation poison** and ends melting with thirst".

***Fan hua chuang* 反花瘡, reversed-blossoms sores** [10]

PC of → *chuang* 瘡, sores, conditions with a festering ulcer generating a flesh-growth assuming the shape of a flower. *ZBYHL* 35: 肉反散如花狀，因名**反花瘡**, "When the flesh reverses to spread in the shape of a flower, this is called '**reversed-blossoms sores**'". Original writing is *fan hua chuang* 翻花瘡, "tossed-flower sores".

***Fan hua e chuang* 反花惡瘡, reversed-blossoms malign sores** [12]

PC identical with → *fan hua chuang* 反花瘡, tossed-flower sores. *BCGM* SE *liu* 柳 quoting *TPSHF*: 反花瘡, "Reverse-flower sores", writes: **反花惡瘡**, "**Reversed-blossoms malign sores**".

***Fan hua zhi* 反花痔, reversed-blossoms piles** [2]

PC of → *zhi chuang* 痔瘡, piles sores, with the tumorous flesh-growths breaking open to all sides like blossoms. *BCGM* SE *mu gua* 木瓜 quoting *YXJC*: **反花痔瘡**：木瓜為末，以鱔魚身上涎調，貼之，以紙護住, "**Reversed-blossoms**

piles sores: grind *mu gua* to powder, mix with phlegm from the body of eels, and attach [to the piles]. Fix with paper". Original writing: *fan hua zhi* 翻花痔, "piles like blossoms turned inside out".

***Fan ke* 煩渴, vexation with thirst** [101]

IS of feeling a heart vexation and thirst in the mouth. *SHL* 26: 服桂枝湯，大汗出後，大**煩渴**不解，脈洪大者，白虎加人參湯主之, "If one has ingested the decoction with *gui zhi*, and after profuse sweating experiences massive **vexation with thirst** that cannot be resolved, with the movement in the vessels being vast and massive, this will be controlled by a decoction with *bai hu* to which *ren shen* has been added".

***Fan kuang* 煩狂, vexation with madness** [2]

IS identical with → *kuang fan* 狂煩, madness with vexation. *BJ* SE *lian shi* 楝實：主溫疾傷寒，大熱**煩狂**, "It controls warmth ailment and harm caused by cold, massive heat and **vexation with madness**".

***Fan luan* 煩亂, vexation with confusion** [14]

IS identical with → *men luan* 悶亂, heart-pressure with confusion. *SHL* 30: 陽明內結，譫語**煩亂**, "If yang brilliance [qi] forms internal nodes, [this results in] delirious speech and **vexation with confusion**".

***Fan man* 煩滿, vexation and [a feeling of] fullness** [55]

IS of a feeling of a vexed heart, of mental pressure and fullness. *SW* 34: 陰氣少而陽氣勝，故熱而**煩滿**也, "The yin qi is diminished and the yang qi dominates. Hence, [the body] is hot, and [the patient experiences] **vexation and [a feeling of] fullness**".

***Fan men* 煩懣, vexation and mental pressure** [7]

IS of a feeling of vexation developing into mental pressure. *BCGM* SE *gou* 狗 quoting *QJYiF* 單行白犬骨散，主產後煩悶不食方, "Recipe of a powder of a single substance, the bones of white dogs, for postpartum vexation and heart-pressure and an unwillingness to eat", writes: 產後**煩懣**不食者，白犬骨燒研，水服方寸匕, "In the case of postpartum **vexation and mental pressure** and an unwillingness to eat, roast and pulverize the bones of white dogs. Ingest 1 square-inch spoon full, with water".

***Fan men* 煩悶, vexation with heart-pressure** [111] AD *fan* 煩, vexation; AN *xin fan* 心煩, heart vexation; *fan xin* 煩心, vexed heart; *fan yu* 煩郁, vexation with pent-up [qi].

IS of an uncomfortable feeling of heat and pressure in the chest. *SW* 32: 熱爭則卒心痛，**煩悶**善嘔, "When the heat is fought [by the proper qi], [the patient] suddenly has a heartache. [He experiences] **vexation with heart-pressure** and has an urge to vomit".

***Fan mu* 反目, reverse eyes** [1]

IS identical with → *yan fan bu xia* 眼翻不下, eyes turned upward without coming down. *ZBYHL* 2: **反目**口噤，手足相引，身體皆熱, "**Reverse eyes,** clenched jaw; hands and feet are pulled in, the entire body is hot".

***Fan ou* 煩嘔, vexation with vomiting** [2]
IS of vomiting associated with signs of mental vexation. *ZBYHL* 11: 令人心下脹滿，氣逆**煩嘔**也, "It causes people to have a feeling of distension and fullness below the heart, with qi moving contrary to its normal direction and [patients experiencing] **vexation with vomiting**".

***Fan pi* 煩痞, vexation with obstacle-illness** [1]
IS of a feeling of distension and fullness together with vexation and heart-pressure. *SJZL* 69: 身體虛熱，胸中**煩痞**而口舌干也, "The entire body has depletion heat. There is **vexation with obstacle-illness** in the chest; the mouth and tongue are dry".

***Fan re* 煩熱, vexing heat** [168] AN re fan 熱煩, heat with vexation.
IS of a feeling of vexation and agitation in the heart, associated with heat. *BJ* SE *bei mu* 貝母：主傷寒**煩熱**, "It controls harm caused by cold, and **vexing heat**".

***Fan shi du* 礬石毒, alum mineral poison** [1]
EA of the poison of alum. *ZHF* 7: 中**礬石毒**，以大豆汁解之, "If struck by **alum mineral poison**, dissolve it with *da dou* juice".

***Fan teng* 煩疼, vexing pain** [10] AN *fan tong* 煩痛.
IS of pain accompanied by a feeling of vexation with heart-pressure. *SHL* 274: 太陰中風，四肢**煩疼**, "When the major yin is struck by wind, the four limbs will have **vexing pain**".

***Fan tong* 煩痛, vexing pain** [9]
IS identical with → *fan teng* 煩疼. *SHL* 146: 發熱，微惡寒，肢節**煩痛**, "Effusion of heat and a weak aversion to cold. The limbs and joints have a feeling of **vexing pain**".

***Fan wei* 反胃, turned over stomach** [212] AN *wei fan* 胃反, stomach turnover; *fan wei* 翻胃, upset stomach; *wei ni* 胃逆, stomach reflux.
PC with regurgitation of food as its major illness sign. *ZBYHL* 21: 向冬發寒熱及温病，食慾吐，或心中停飲不消，或為**反胃**, "By the time of winter, [patients] develop alternating sensations of cold and heat, and warmth disease. When they eat they have an urge to vomit. In some cases rheum remains in the center without digestion. In some cases [patients suffer from a] **turned over stomach**".

***Fan wei* 翻胃, upset stomach** [7]
PC identical with → *fan wei* 反胃, turned over stomach. *SJZL* 47: 治久患**翻胃**及小兒驚吐諸吐，田季散丸, "To cure all types of chronic vomiting, including [vomiting because of] an **upset stomach**, and children's vomiting because of fright, [use the] pills with *tian ji* powder".

***Fan xin* 煩心, vexed heart** [3]
IS identical with → *xin fan* 心煩, heart vexation. *SW* 17: 數則**煩心**，大則病進, "If it is frequent, the **heart is vexed**. If it is massive, a disease is advanced".

***Fan yu* 煩郁, vexation with pent-up [qi]** [3]
IS identical with → *fan men* 煩悶, vexation with heart-pressure. *ZBYHL* 12: 瘀熱與宿谷相搏，**煩郁**不得消, "Stagnant heat and undigested food strike at each other, bringing forth **vexation with pent-up [qi]** that cannot be dissolved".

***Fan zao* 煩燥, vexation and restlessness** [4]
IS identical with → *fan zao* 煩躁. 燥 is used erroneously as a homophone for 躁. *BCGM* SE *mu gua he* 木瓜核 quotes *TPSHF*: 霍亂，**煩燥**氣急，每嚼七粒，温水咽之, "For cholera, **vexation and restlessness** and qi urgency, chew seven kernels for each dose and swallow them with warm water".

***Fan zao* 煩躁, vexation with restlessness** [61]
IS of an uncomfortable feeling of vexation and heart-pressure accompanied by restlessness. *SHL* 29: 厥，咽中干，**煩躁**吐逆者，作甘草乾薑湯與之, "For [patients experiencing] recession, dryness in their throat, as well as **vexation with restlessness** and vomiting with counterflow [of qi], prepare a decoction with *gan cao* and *gan jiang* to offer to them".

***Fan zhang* 煩脹, vexation and distension** [3]
IS identical with → *zhang men* 脹悶, distension and heart-pressure. *PJF* 36: 厚朴飲，治胃反，兩脅**煩脹**，食不消化, "A drink with *hou pu* cures stomach turnover, **vexation and distension** in both flanks, and failure to digest food".

***Fan zhang* 反張, reversal strain; arched back rigidity** [6]
IS AD of → *jiao gong fan zhang* 角弓反張, arched reversal strain. *ZBYHL* 7: 搖頭，卒口噤，背直，身體**反張**, "The head shakes with a suddenly clenched jaw, the back is stiff with the body experiencing **reversal strain**".

***Fan zhong* 煩重, uncomfortable feeling of heaviness** [1]
IS of a feeling of extreme heaviness together with vexation and heart-pressure. *ZHF* 4: 四肢**煩重**，嘿嘿欲臥，食畢輒甚, "The four limbs experience **an uncomfortable feeling of heaviness**, [patients are] quiet and wish to lie down".

***Fang lao* 房勞, bedroom exhaustion** [13]
EA of excessive or inappropriate sexual intercourse. *ZBYHL* 46: 若乳母飲酒過度，醉及**房勞**，喘後乳者，最劇，能殺兒也, "If a breast-feeding mother drinks wine excessively, is intoxicated and experiences **chamber exhaustion**, pants and breast-feeds, this is very dangerous and may kill the child".

***Fei* 痱, seething rash** [4]
PC identical with → *re fei* 熱痱, heat with seething rash. *SJZL* 138: 熱氣內郁於皮腠之間， 輕則為**痱**，重則為痤也, "When heat qi enters and is pent-up internally in the region of the skin interstices, in light cases this is **seething rash**; in severe cases this develops into acne".

***Fei bao* 痱皰, seething rash with blisters** [1]
PC identical with → *re fei* 熱痱, heat with seething rash. *BCGM* SE *shi hui* 石灰 quotes *JXF*: 夏月**痱皰**：石灰煅一兩，蛤粉二兩，甘草一兩，研，撲之, "For **seething rash with blisters** during the summer months: [use] *shi hui*, heat prepared, 1 *liang*; *ge fen*, 2 *liang*; *gan cao*, 1 *liang*, all ground to a powder, to attack it".

Fei bing **肺病, lung disease** [22]

PC CD of all types of conditions where the seat of the disease is in the lung. *SW* 18: 秋胃微毛曰平，毛多胃少曰**肺病**, "When in autumn [one feels] stomach [qi together with] a slightly hair[-like movement in the vessels], that is called 'normal'. If [the movement is] mostly hair[-like] with diminished stomach [qi present], that is called '**lung disease**'".

Fei chuang **肥瘡, fat sores** [10]

PC of → *chuang* 瘡, sores, conditions that are relatively flat but fester with yellow-white pus. *QJYF* 22: 凡熱瘡起，便生白膿黃爛，瘡起即淺，但出黃汁名**肥瘡**, "Whenever heat sores emerge they may generate white pus and yellow festering. The sores that are flat and produce only yellow liquid are called '**fat sores**'".

Fei chuang **痱瘡, seething-rash sores** [4]

PC identical with *re fei* 熱痱, heat with seething rash. *TPSHF* 65: 夫盛夏之月, 人膚腠開, 易傷風熱水熱, 毒氣搏於皮膚, 則生痱瘡, "Now, in mid-summer months the skin interstices of man open, and one is easily harmed by wind heat and water heat. Where the poison qi strikes the skin **seething-rash sores** develop".

Fei fan **肺煩, lung vexation** [1]

PC of heart vexation brought forth by lung heat. *TYBC* SE *zhi zi* 梔子：故用梔子，以治**肺煩**, "Hence one resorts to *zhi zi* to cure **lung vexation**".

Fei feng **肺風, lung wind** [17]

PC of a lung affection by wind evil. *SW* 42: **肺風**之狀, 多汗惡風，色皏然白，時咳短氣, "The appearance of **lung wind** [is such]: [patients] sweat profusely and have an aversion to wind. Their [facial] color is a pale white. They often cough and are short of qi". *BCGM* refers to lung wind in the context of a loss of the lung's function to control breathing and to govern skin and body hair. E.g., *fei feng bi sai* 肺風鼻塞, lung wind with nasal congestion; *fei feng chuan cu* 肺風喘促, lung wind with hasty painting; *fei feng du chuang* 肺風毒瘡, lung wind with poison sores; *fei feng bai lai* 肺風白癩, lung wind with white repudiation-illness, and *fei feng mian chuang* 肺風面瘡, lung wind with facial sores.

Fei gan zhang **肺干脹, lung desiccation and distension** [1]

PC identical with → *fei qi gan zhang* 肺氣干脹, lung qi desiccation and distension. *BCGM* Bai bing zhu zhi yao 百病主治藥：豬胰，**肺干脹**喘急，浸酒服, "*Zhu yi*: In the case of **lung desiccation and distension** with urgent panting, ingest it steeped in wine".

Fei han **肺寒, lung cold** [8] AN → *fei leng* 肺冷.

PC of a cold-type disease with lung qi depletion brought forth by a depletion or weakness of yang qi. *QJYF* 8: 治**肺寒**方：炙肺俞百壯, "Recipe to cure **lung cold**: Cauterize the lung transporter 100 times".

Fei huan **痱緩, disablement with flaccidity** [1]

PC identical with → *feng fei* 風痱, wind disablement. *SJZL* 191: 此骨消則病**痱緩**, "In this case the bones dissolve, and this makes people suffer from **disablement with flaccidity**".

Fei huo **肺火, lung fire** [23]

PC and EA identical with → *fei re* 肺熱, lung heat. *SWBJQYBMJ* Lj: 石膏，瀉肺火, "*Shi gao* drains **lung fire**".

Fei ji **肺積, lung accumulation** [2]

PC identical with → *xi ben* 息賁, rapid breathing. *MJ* 8: 診得**肺積**脈浮而毛, "An examination finds a **lung accumulation** with a [movement in the] vessels that is at the surface and hair-like".

Fei ju **肺疽, lung impediment-illness** [2]

PC with blood spitting because of a heated lung that has resulted from drinking wine and an excessive consumption of hot, spicy food. *ZBYHL* 27: 吐血有三種…二曰**肺疽**…**肺疽**者，言飲酒之後，毒滿便吐, "There are three types of blood-spitting. ...Second: **lung impediment-illness** . ...[Blood-spitting because of] **lung impediment-illnesses**, that is to say: after one has drunk wine he is filled with poison and vomits [blood]".

Fei ke **肺咳, lung cough** [4] AN *fei sou* 肺嗽.

PC CD of cough brought forth by any evil qi clogging the lung. *SW* 38: 肺寒則外內合邪因而客之，則為**肺咳**, "When the lung is cold, both external and internal [cold evils] have merged. Subsequently, the [two cold] evils settle in the [lung]. This, then, causes **lung cough**".

Fei lao **肺勞, lung exhaustion** [5]

PC of a depletion exhaustion brought forth by exhaustion detrimentally affecting the lung. *ZBYHL* 3: **肺勞**者，短氣而面腫，鼻不聞香臭, "In the case of **lung exhaustion**, one is short of qi and the face is swollen. The nose is unable to distinguish between fragrant and foul odors". In earlier Chinese medical writings the scope of ailments covered by the term "lung exhaustion" appears to have been rather broad. In the *BCGM*, however, *fei lao* **肺勞** is mainly used in the sense of an infectious *fei lao chuan shi* 肺勞傳尸, lung exhaustion by corpse [evil] transmission, identifiable in retrospect as consumption/tuberculosis.

Fei leng **肺冷, lung cold** [1]

PC identical with → *fei han* 肺寒. *BCGM* SE *gan* 柑 quotes *KBBC*: 多食令人脾冷發痼癖, "Consumed in large quantities it causes spleen cold resulting in obstinacy-illness with aggregation-illness". To this LSZ added a statement: 令人肺冷生痰, "It causes **lung cold** and generates phlegm".

Fei nüe **肺瘧, lung malaria** [7]

PC of → *nüe ji* 瘧疾, malaria ailment, associated with illness signs of the lung conduits, such as much phlegm, heart cold, and a tendency to be frightened. *SW* 36: **肺瘧**者，令人心寒，寒甚熱，熱間善驚, "**Lung malaria**: it causes a person's heart to be cold. When it is very cold [it changes to] heat. While it is hot, [patients] tend to be frightened".

Fei qi **肥氣, fat qi** [4]
PC of pathological → *ji ju* 積聚, accumulation and collection, below the flanks brought forth by liver qi lumps. *LS* 4: 肝脈…微急為**肥氣**，在脅下若覆杯, "[The movement in the] liver vessels…If it is slightly hectic, this is [a sign] of **fat qi**. Below the flanks there is a feeling as if there were an overturned cup".

Fei qi gan zhang **肺氣干脹, lung qi desiccation with distension** [1]
PC of an urgent panting and counterflow of qi brought forth by a deficiency of yin and dryness. *BCTJ* SE *tun* 豚：主**肺氣干脹**喘急，潤五藏, "It controls **lung qi desiccation with distension**, urgent panting, and provides moisture to the five depots".

Fei re **肺熱, heat in the lung; lung heat** [68]
① PC of heat-type diseases affecting the lung. *SW* 32: **肺熱**病者右頰先赤, "In the case of the disease **heat in the lung**, the right cheek becomes red first".
② AN *fei huo* 肺火, lung fire. EA bringing forth heat-type disease in the lung. *TPSHF* 89: 夫小兒龜胸者，緣**肺熱**脹滿，致使胸高如龜, "When a child has a turtle chest (English equivalent: pigeon chest), this is because lung heat is filling it and making it distend. This leads to an elevation of the chest resembling the shape of a turtle".

Fei re gan **肥熱疳, obesity and heat *gan*–illness** [2]
PC of the initial stages of → *xiao er gan bing* 小兒疳病, *gan*-illness among children. *XEYZZJ* Fj: 大抵疳病當辨冷熱肥瘦。其初病者為**肥熱疳**，久病者為瘦冷疳, "On the whole, in the case of *gan*-illness one must distinguish between cold [*gan*], heat [*gan*], obesity [*gan*], and emaciation [*gan*]. [*Gan*-illness] in its early stages is **obesity and heat *gan***-illness. After some time this changes into an emaciation and cold *gan*-illness".

Fei shi **肺實, lung repletion** [8]
PC of a depletion of proper qi, with wind, cold, phlegm, heat etc., all types of pathogenic evil qi blocking the movement of lung qi, thereby causing cough, panting, and heart-pressure. *YXQY* Lj: 防風，氣溫味辛，療風通用，瀉**肺實**，散頭目滯氣, "*Fang feng*. Its qi is warm, its flavor is acrid. It can be employed to cure all types of wind. It drains **lung repletion**, and disperses sluggish qi in the head and eyes".

Fei shi **肺濕, lung moisture** [2]
EA of phlegm and moisture lodging in the lung. *DXXFYJ* 2: **肺濕**作喘，以甜葶藶研細末，棗肉為丸服之, "**Lung moisture** causes panting. [For treatment] ingest pills prepared from *tian ting li*, ground to a fine powder, and *zao rou*".

Fei shi **飛屍, flying corpse [qi]** [29]
PC with sudden outbreaks and frequently changing appearances that do not show a regular pattern. *ZHF* 8 RE *Bian Que xian shui wan* 扁鵲陷水丸, Bian Que's pills for immersion in water：腹內脹病，中惡邪氣，**飛屍**遊走，皆服二丸如小豆, "For a disease of abdominal distension, when one has been struck by malign and evil qi, and if **flying corpse** [**qi**] roves around, in all these cases ingest two pills the size of a small bean".

Fei sou **肺嗽, lung cough** [1]
PC identical with → *fei ke* 肺咳. *TPSHF* 46: 七曰**肺嗽**，嗽引頸項而唾涎沫是也, "The seventh is called '**lung cough**'. This is the case when the cough pulls on one's neck and one spits a foamy saliva".

Fei wei **肺痿, lung dysfunction** [81]
PC of a desiccation of lung lobes or feebleness with loss of function, resulting in a feeling of a pressed chest and panting, as well as spitting of turbid saliva with foam. *JGYL* Fj: 咳唾膿血，脈數虛者為**肺痿**，數實者為肺癰, "One coughs saliva with phlegm and blood. If the [movement in the] vessels is frequent and depleted, this is **lung dysfunction**. If it is frequent and replete, this is lung obstruction-illness".

Fei xu **肺虛, lung depletion** [30]
PC of lung depletion with an impediment of lung functions. *SW* 28: 氣虛者**肺虛**也，氣逆者足寒也, "A qi depletion is a **lung depletion**. When the qi moves contrary [to its regular course], the feet are cold".
Fei xu huo wang **肺虛火旺, lung depletion with strong fire** [1] EA, PM of a → *yin xu huo dong* 陰虛火動, yin depletion with excited fire, resulting from a unilateral insufficiency of lung yin. *BCGM* SE *ren shen* 人參 quotes LYW: 若**肺虛火旺**氣短自汗者，必用也, "If [patients suffering from] **lung depletion with strong fire** are short of qi and experience spontaneous sweating, it must be applied".

Fei xue **飛血, flying blood** [5]
IS of red vessels covering the white part of the eyeballs. *SJZL* 105: **飛血**者，謂赤脈散於白睛之上是也, " '**Flying blood**' is to say: red vessels are spread across the white parts of the eyeballs".

Fei yang **痱癢, seething-rash itching** [2]
PC identical with *re fei* 熱痱, heat with seething rash. *BCGM* SE *ting li* 葶藶 quoting *MYBL*: 身暴中風熱，痱癢 writes: 身暴中風熱，**痱癢**, "When the body is violently struck by wind heat [resulting in] **seething-rash itching**".

Fei yong **肺癰, lung obstruction-illness** [32] AN *fei yong* 肺壅, lung obstruction. PC of abscesses in the lung, with fever, chest pain, and vomiting of bad-smelling pus and blood. *JGYL* Fj: 咳而胸滿，振寒脈數，咽干不渴，時出濁唾腥臭久久吐膿如米粥者，為**肺癰**, "If someone coughs and has a feeling of fullness in his chest, shivers from cold and has a frequent [movement in the] vessels, with a dry throat and no desire to drink, occasional spitting of turbid saliva of a bad odor, and chronic vomiting of pus resembling rice gruel, this is a **lung obstruction-illness**".

Fei yong **肺壅, lung obstruction** [13]
PC identical with → *fei yong* 肺癰, lung obstruction-illness. *NJ* 56: 令人洒淅寒熱，喘咳，發**肺壅**, "They cause the [afflicted] person to shiver due to [alternating sensations of] cold and heat, and they make him cough and develop **lung obstruction**".

Fei zao **肺燥, lung dryness** [7]

PC brought forth by dryness evil harming the lung, or by heat harming lung liquid. *ZJSHL* 6: **肺燥**氣熱，以酸收之，以甘緩之, "**Lung dryness** and qi heat can be contained with sour flavor. Use sweet flavor to slow it down".

Fei zhang **肺脹, lung distension** [6]

PC of a chronic distension of the lung lobes and a failure to contract again, with heart-pressure and panting, coughing up of phlegm, and a purple color of lips and tongue. LS 35: **肺脹**者，虛滿而喘咳, "As for **lung distension**, it goes along with depletion and a feeling of fullness, as well as panting and cough".

Fei zhen **疿疹, seething-rash papules** [1]

PC identical with *re fei* 熱疿, heat with seething rash. *SJZL* 1: 炎暑流火，民病寒熱、瘡瘍、**疿疹**、癰痤，法宜調以辛温, "In the case of summerheat causing flowing fire [i.e. erysipelas], when people suffer from alternating sensations of cold and heat, ulcers, **seething-rash papules**, obstruction-illnesses and acne, this is to be corrected by means of acrid and warming [substances]".

Fei zi **疿子, seething-rash seeds** [3]

PC identical with *re fei* 熱疿, heat with seething rash. *TPSHF* 65: 其狀如湯之沸，輕者匝匝如粟粒，重者熱汗浸漬成瘡，因以為名。世呼為**疿子**也, "Its appearance is that of seething water. In minor cases [the skin] is filled with grain-like millet; in serious cases hot sweat soaks [the skin] and generates sores. Hence the name. It is commonly called **seething-rash seeds**".

Fen ci **粉刺, flour thorns; acne** [14] AN *feng ci* 風刺, wind thorns; *jiu ci* 酒刺, wine thorns.

PC of papules rising in the face like thorns. If squeezed they release a white powder resembling rice flour. *ZHBJF* 5, *liao chuang fang* 療瘡方, recipes to cure various sores: 最去面上**粉刺**, "Extremely suitable for removing facial **flour thorns**".

Fen hua chuang **粉花瘡, cosmetic-powder sores** [1]

PC CD of → *chuang* 瘡, sores, conditions developing in a woman's face. *BCGM* SE *ai* 艾 quotes *TYWF*: 婦人面瘡：名**粉花瘡**, "Sores in a woman's face are called '**cosmetic powder sores**'".

Fen lou **粉瘤, powder tumor** [3]

PC of a mildly red tumor that is soft and, after being opened with a needle, releases a white substance like a fatty paste or powder. Elsewhere it is said that this tumor grows in the face. *RMSQ* 8: 在手背為膠瘤，在面者為**粉瘤**, "Those developing on the back of the hand are 'glue tumors'. Those in the face are '**powder tumors**'".

Fen yu **膹郁, rushing and pent-up [qi]** [4] AW *fen yu* 憤郁, anger with pent-up [qi].

IS of a feeling of pressure and fullness in the chest region, with qi moving upwards contrary to its proper direction. *SW* 74: 諸氣**膹郁**，皆屬於肺, "All types of **rushing and pent-up** qi are associated with the lung".

***Fen yu* 憤郁, anger with pent-up [qi]** [1]
IS identical with and presumably erroneous writing of → *fen yu* 膹郁, rushing and pent-up [qi]. *BCGM* Zang fu xu shi biao ben yao shi 臟腑虛實標本用藥式：肺本病：諸氣**憤郁**，諸痿喘嘔, "The lung… its own diseases: All types of **anger with pent-up [qi]**, all types of dysfunction, panting, and vomiting".

***Fen zi* 粉滓, dregs** [17]
PC identical with → *gan zeng* 皯黵, dermal dark spots. *QJYF* 6: 治面**粉滓**方，熬礬石以清酒和敷之，不過三上, "Recipe to cure facial **dregs**: Heat *fan shi* and apply together with clear wine. Do not apply onto [the skin] more often than three times".

***Feng* 風, wind** [p]
① AN *feng qi* 風氣, wind qi; *feng xie* 風邪, wind evil. EA. **Wind** moves and changes its strength and direction frequently. Therefore disease signs that have this particular quality are often attributed to wind intrusion. *SW* 42: **風**者，善行數變, "**Wind** tends to move and undergoes frequent changes". **風**者，百病之長也，至其變化乃生他病也, "**Wind** is the chief [cause] of the one hundred illnesses. When it comes to changes and transformations, other diseases result".
② AN *feng bing* 風病, wind disease; *feng ji* 風疾, wind ailment; *feng zheng* 風證, wind condition; *feng qi* 風氣, wind qi. PC resulting from wind intrusion, with principal signs including an aversion to wind, heat spells, and sweating. In some instances associated with shaking and shivering, convulsions, confusion, or abnormal skin sensitivity. *SW* 42: 風之傷人也，或為寒熱，或為熱中，或為寒中，或為癘風，或為偏枯，或為**風**也, "When wind harms a person, it may cause cold and heat; or it may cause a heated center; or it may cause a cold center; or it may cause *li*-wind; or it may cause unilateral withering; or it may cause **wind**". *SW* 74: 諸**風**掉眩，皆屬於肝, "Without exception, all [diseases with] **wind** [causing] swaying and dizziness are associated with the liver".

***Feng bi* 風秘, wind closure** [14]
PC of → *bian pi* 便秘，constipation, brought about by intestinal and stomach dryness and a depletion of body liquids. The notion of wind causing intestinal dryness is associated with the observation that wind in nature disperses moisture. *WTMY* 27: 若是**風秘**，自依後服大黃等五味丸, "In the case of **wind closure**, it is advisable to ingest pills with *da huang* and further ingredients, altogether five substances, as listed below".

***Feng bi* 風閉, wind closure** [4]
PC identical with *feng bi* 風秘. *PJF* 295: 能消丸治五痔腫痛，下血不止，或營衛滯澀，身體疼痛，大便**風閉**不通, "The 'pills able to dissolve' cure the five types of piles with swelling and pain, unending discharge of blood, with in some cases the camp and guardian [qi] being sluggish and rough, the entire body being in pain, and defecation failing to pass because of **wind closure**".

***Feng bi* 風痹, wind blockage** [102]
PC of → *bi bing* 痹病, blockage diseases, resulting mostly from an intrusion of wind evil. *ZBYHL* 1: 風寒濕三氣合而為痹，風多者為**風痹**, "If the three qi of

wind, cold and moisture jointly [enter the body] they will cause a blockage, and if most of it is wind, it is a **wind blockage**".

Feng bi qi **風痹氣, wind-blockage qi** [1]
PC identical with → *feng bi* 風痹, wind blockage. *BCGM* SE *bao* 鴇 quotes *YSZY*: 補益虛人，去**風痹氣**, "It supplements persons with a depletion, and it removes **wind-blockage qi**".

Feng bing 風病， **wind disease** [60]
PC brought about by wind. *ZBYHL* 1: **風病** … 血氣俱虛，風邪併入, "**Wind disease**…when both blood and qi are depleted, wind evil enters". *BCGM* mentions many kinds of **wind disease** such as *feng bing ma mu* 風病麻木, **wind disease** with [numbness like] hemp and logs, *feng bing luan ji* 風病攣急, **wind disease** with tension, and *feng bing tan huan* 風病癱瘓, **wind disease** with paralysis.

Feng chi **風齒, wind teeth** [1] AN *chi feng* 齒風, tooth wind; *kou chi feng* 口齒風, mouth and tooth wind.
PC identical with → *feng ya* 風牙, wind teeth. *ZBYHL* 29: **風齒**候，頭面有風，陽明之脈虛，風乘虛隨脈流入於齒者，則令齒有風, "Signs of **wind teeth**: if head and wind have wind, and if the yin brilliance vessels are depleted, wind avails itself of this depletion and follows the vessels to flow through that person to his teeth. This causes the teeth to have wind".

Feng chi **風赤, wind redness** [6]
PC identical with → *chi feng yan* 赤風眼, red wind-eye. *TPSHF* 32 RE *qing xiang zi wan* 青葙子丸, pills with *qing xiang zi*: 治眼**風赤**，昏暗淚出, "They cure eyes with **wind redness**, clouding with dim vision and tearflow".

Feng chi lan yan **風赤爛眼, wind red festering eye** [3] AN *chi lan yan* 赤爛眼, red festering eye.
PC identical with → 風眼, wind eye. *BCGM* Bai bing zhu zhi yao 百病主治藥眼目：五倍子主**風赤爛眼**研傅之, "*Wu pei zi* controls **wind red festering eyes**. Grind and apply externally".

Feng chi yan **風赤眼, wind red eye** [12] AN *chi feng yan* 赤風眼, red wind eye. AD *feng chi* 風赤, wind redness.
PC of → *feng yan* 風眼, wind eye, with apparent redness and swelling. *TPSHF* 32 RE *xi jiao san* 犀角散, powder with *xi jiao*: 治**風赤眼**，澀痛淚出, "It cures **wind red eye**, with roughness, pain, and tearflow".

Feng chong **風蟲, wind and/or bugs/worms** [67]
① EA of → *feng xie* 風邪, wind evil, and/or bugs/worms causing tooth diseases. *WTMY* 22 RE *Cui shi liao ya teng fang* 崔氏療牙疼方, Mr. Cui's recipe to cure toothache: 齒痛不問**風蟲**，無不瘥, "Effective for toothache regardless whether it was caused by **wind and/or bugs/worms**".
② PC brought about by **wind and/or bugs/worms**. *PJF* 70: 地骨皮湯，治牙齒風蟲, "A decoction with *di gu pi* cures teeth afflicted by **wind and/or bugs/worms**". *BCGM* uses *feng chong* 風蟲 mainly to refer to tooth diseases.

***Feng chong ya tong* 風蟲牙痛, wind worm-borer teeth with pain** [1]
PC identical with → *chong ya* 蟲牙, worm-borer teeth. *RHZ* SE *mang cao* 莽草：**風蟲牙痛**，喉痹，亦濃煎汁含後淨漱口, "For **wind worm-borer teeth with pain** and throat blockage: here, too, it is to be boiled down to a thick liquid that is to be held in the mouth. After that the mouth is to be carefully rinsed clean again".

***Feng chu* 風搐, wind convulsions** [6]
PC of → *feng jing* 風痙, wind spasms, characterized by stiffness and convulsions of body and limbs. *BCGM* SE *zhu ti* 鯠鮧：治婦人產難，產後**風搐**, "It cures difficult delivery and postpartum **wind convulsions**".

***Feng chuang* 風瘡, wind sores** [54]
PC of festering and oozing, aching and/or itching skin papules brought forth by wind evil, moisture and heat. *TPSHF* RE *zao yu fang* 澡浴方, recipe for bathing: 治遍身熱毒**風瘡**, "It cures heat poison and **wind sores** affecting the entire body".

***Feng ci* 風刺, wind thorns** [6]
PC identical with *fen ci* 粉刺, flour thorns. *SJZL* 137: 治諸癬，並面上**風刺**方, "Recipe to cure all types of *xuan*-illness, and also facial **wind thorns**".

***Feng dan* 風丹, wind cinnabar-red bolus** [3]
PC a) of → *dan du* 丹毒, cinnabar poisoning, with a slowly spreading red swelling developing on a crimson halo. b) CD of red heat papules brought forth by heat poison. *WTMY* 24: 救急療熱毒**風丹**並發背，犀角膏方, "The recipe for the ointment with *xi jiao* to bring urgent relief and cure **wind cinnabar-red bolus** [caused by] heat poison".

***Feng dian* 風癲, wind peak-illness** [11]
PC identical with a *dian ji* 癲疾, peak ailment. *ZHBJF* 3 quotes *JXF*: 已生蠶紙作灰，酒水任下，瘥。療**風癲**也, "Prepare ashes from paper with hatched silkworm eggs and ingest with wine or water. This will bring the cure. It heals **wind peak-illness**".

***Feng dian* 風顛, wind peak[-illness]** [1]
PC identical with → *feng dian* 風癲, wind peak-illness. *BCGM* SE *tian men dong* 天門冬 quotes *WTMY* RE *feng dian fang* 風癲方， recipe for wind peak-illness, as: **風顛**發作：則吐，耳如蟬鳴，引脅牽痛。天門冬去心皮，曝搗為末。酒服方寸匕，日三服, "When **wind peak[-illness]** breaks out, [patients] spit and their ears experience sounds like those of cicadas. Pain affects the flanks. [For treatment use] *tian men dong*, with heart and skin removed. Dry under the sun and pound to a powder. Ingest 1 square-inch spoon with wine three times a day".

***Feng du* 風毒, wind poison** [100]
EA CD of → *feng* 風, wind, and → *du* 毒, poison, resulting in a pathogenic evil qi including the characteristics of both. *ZBYHL* 30: 喉痹是**風毒**之氣客於咽喉之間, "Throat blockage results from the qi of **wind poison** settling in the region of throat and wind pipe". *BCGM* refers to numerous pathological conditions

associated with wind poison: *feng du jiao qi* 風毒脚氣, wind poison with leg qi; *feng du chuang zhong* 風毒瘡腫, wind poison with sores and swelling; *feng du luo li* 風毒瘰癧, wind poison and scrofula with pervasion-illness; *feng du chi mu* 風毒赤目, wind poison with red eyes.

***Feng fei* 風痱, wind[-caused] disablement** [1] AW 風疿.

PC of an inability to move one arm at will, with mental clarity maintained, caused by wind stroke. *ZBYHL* 1: **風痱**之狀，身體無痛，四肢不收，神智不亂，一臂不隨者, **風痱**也。時能言者可治，不能言者不可治, "The signs of **wind[-caused] disablement**: When the body is entirely free of pain, with an inability to pull in the four limbs, and with no mental confusion, and if one is unable to move one arm at will, this is **wind[-caused] disablement**. Those [patients] who at times can speak, they can be cured. Those who cannot speak, they cannot be cured".

***Feng fei* 風疿, wind[-caused] disablement** [1]

PC identical with → *feng fei* 風痱. *BCGM* SE *gou* 狗 quoting *MYBL mu gou yin jing* 牡狗陰莖：齒…主癲癇寒熱，卒風痱, "The teeth …control peak-illness with epilepsy, alternating sensations of cold and heat, and sudden wind disablement", writes: 癲癇寒熱，卒**風疿**, "Peak-illness with alternating sensations of cold and heat, and sudden **wind[-caused] disablement**". 疿 may simply be an erroneous writing of 痱.

***Feng gan* 風疳, wind *gan*-illness** [12]

PC of swollen and painful gums brought about by wind heat poison, with loose teeth festering, emitting both pus and blood, and lips and cheek swollen and painful. *TPSHF* 34: 臟腑壅滯，久積風熱 … 則令齒齦浮腫，動搖脫落，損爛，膿血俱出，蟲蝕齒根，口內常臭，面色青黄，唇頰腫痛者，則是**風疳**之候也, "When the depots and palaces experience obstruction with [qi] sluggishness and wind heat accumulates over an extended time, ...the gums will be inflated. The teeth will be loose and fall out. There will be festering, emitting both pus and blood. Bugs/worms gnaw on the dental roots. The mouth has a persistent stench. The facial complexion is greenish-yellow. Lips and cheeks are swollen and painful. These are the signs of **wind *gan*-illness**".

***Feng gou* 風狗, rabid dog** [7]

Identical with → *kuang quan* 狂犬. *BCGM* SE *chu ji* 槜雞 quotes *TYWF*: **風狗**咬傷：不治即死, "If a wound caused by a **rabid dog's** bite is not treated, [the patient] will die".

***Feng han* 風寒, wind cold** [160]

EA CD of → *feng* 風, wind, and → *han* 寒， cold, resulting in a pathogenic evil qi including the characteristics of both. *SW* 35: 瘧者，**風寒**之氣不常也, "As for malaria, this is an irregular [presence] of the qi of **wind and cold** [in the body]". *BCGM* refers to numerous pathological conditions associated with wind cold: *feng han ke ni* 風寒咳逆, wind cold with cough and counterflow [of qi]; *feng han shi bi* 風寒濕痹, wind cold with moisture blockage; feng han tou tong 風寒頭痛, wind cold with headache.

Feng han bi **風寒痹, wind cold blockage** [1]
PC of → *bi bing* 痹病, blockage disease, brought forth jointly by wind and cold evil, with pain affecting the entire body. *BCGM* SE *sang chai huo* 桑柴火：能助藥力，除**風寒痹**諸痛, "It is capable of supporting the strength of [other] medications. It eliminates all types of pain associated with **wind cold blockage**".

Feng han shi **風寒濕, wind, cold and moisture** [34]
CD of wind, cold, and moisture. EA simultaneously referring to → *feng xie* 風邪, wind evil, → *han xie* 寒邪, cold evil, and → shi xie 濕邪, moisture evil. *SW* 43: **風寒濕**三氣雜至，合而為痹也, "When the three qi **wind, cold, and moisture** arrive together, they merge and cause a blockage".

Feng han shi bi **風寒濕痹, wind, cold and moisture blockage** [27]
PC of → *bi bing* 痹病, blockage disease, jointly caused by the three qi wind, cold and moisture, with the joints of one's limbs aching and experiencing swelling and distension. In extreme cases this leads to an inability to move. *BJ* SE *wan jiao* 蔓椒：主**風寒濕痹**，歷節疼, "It controls **wind, cold and moisture blockage**, with severe pain in the joints".

Feng han shi qi **風寒濕氣, wind, cold, and moisture qi** [2]
EA of the three evil qi → *feng* 風, wind, → *han* 寒, cold, and → *shi* 濕, moisture, that together may cause a disease. *SW* 43: 六腑亦各有俞，**風寒濕氣**中其俞，而食飲應之, 循俞而入，各舍其腑也, "Of the six palaces, too, each has its [respective] transporters. When **wind, cold, and moisture qi** strike these transporters and if food and beverages correspond to them, they enter via the transporters and each [qi] lodges in its respective palace".

Feng huan **風緩, wind sluggishness** [5]
PC of legs without strength, in severe cases not moving according to one's will. *QJYF* 25: **風緩**湯. . 治脚弱，舉體痹不仁，熱毒氣入臟，胸中滿塞不通，食即嘔吐方, "The decoction for **wind sluggishness**: a recipe to cure weakness of one's legs, blockage with numbness in the entire body, qi of heat poison entering the depots, fullness and blockage in the chest. If one eats, the food is thrown up again".

Feng huo **風火, wind and fire** [5]
EA identified as simultaneous appearance of → *feng* 風, wind, and → *huo* 火, fire. *SW* 68: 燥熱相臨，**風火**相值, "Dryness and heat come down on each other. **Wind and fire** come into contact".

Feng huo zheng **風火證, wind and fire condition** [1]
PC brought about by → *feng* 風, wind and → *huo* 火, fire. *BCGM* SE *ren ru* 人乳 quotes *HSYT*: 治**風火證**，養老尤宜, "It cures **wind and fire condition**, and is particularly well-suited for nourishing old people".

Feng ji **風疾, wind ailment** [60]
PC a) AN *da feng* 大風, massive wind; *e feng* 惡風, malign wind. Identical with *da feng*, 大風, massive wind. *ZBYHL* 2: 體癢搔之，漸漸生瘡，經年不瘥，即成**風疾**, "The body itches and if it is scratched it will gradually generate sores. If this is not healed over a period of years, **wind ailment** will result". b) Brought

about by wind. *BCGM* mentions many kinds of wind ailment such as *feng ji luan ji* 風疾攣急 wind ailment with tension, *feng ji dan du* 風疾丹毒, wind ailment with cinnabar poisoning, and *tian diao feng ji* 天吊風疾, wind ailment with [eyeballs] hauled by heaven.

***Feng jin* 風噤, wind lockjaw** [4] AN *jin feng* 噤風, lockjaw wind.
PC of a *feng jing* 風痙, wind spasms, characterized by clenched jaw and a pursed mouth that is difficult to open. *MYBL* SE *mu dan* 牡丹：除時氣頭痛，客熱，五勞，勞氣，頭、腰痛，**風噤**，癲疾, "It eliminates seasonal qi with headache, visitor heat, the five types of exhaustion, exhaustion qi, head and lumbar pain, **wind lockjaw**, and the ailment of peak illness".

***Feng jing* 風痙, wind spasms** [19] AW *jing* 痙. AN *ci* 痓, spasms; *jing feng* 痙風, spasms wind; *jing bing* 痙病, spasms disease. Depending on the actual status of a patient further designations are *feng chu* 風搐; wind convulsions; *feng jin* 風噤, wind lockjaw.
PC characterized by stiffness of the body, lockjaw, and convulsions. *ZBYHL* 1: 風痙者，口噤不開，背強而直, "As for **wind spasms**, the jaws are clenched and the mouth does not open; the back is stiff and straight".

***Feng ju* 風疽, wind impediment-illness** [3]
PC of festering flat abscesses emerging out of a swelling resulting from contractions of blood vessels. Usually they cannot be cured over an extended period of time. *ZBYHL* 33: 腫起，流之血脈而攣曲疾痛，所以發瘡歷年，謂之**風疽**, "A swelling rises and the blood vessels passing through it contract and are bent, with pain. If, as a result, sores develop and stay for years, they are called '**wind impediment-illness**'".

***Feng jue* 風厥, wind and recession** [1]
PC of → *jue* 厥, recession, brought about by liver qi transformed into wind. *SW* 7: 二陽一陰發病，主驚駭背痛，善噫善欠，名曰**風厥**, "When the second yang and the first yin develop a disease, it is responsible for shock and back pain. [Patients] tend to belch; [patients] tend to yawn. This is called '**wind and recession**'". WB commentary: 肝氣為風，腎氣陵逆，既風又厥，故名**風厥**, "Liver qi becomes wind. The kidney qi rises contrary to its proper direction. This, then, is a situation of wind [presence] and [kidney qi] recession. Hence this is called **wind and recession**".

***Feng jue* 風蹶, wind fall** [1]
PC of painful lower back and knees. Possibly AW of → *feng jue* 風厥, wind and recession. *BCTJ* SE *hai tong pi* 海桐皮：古方多用浸酒治**風蹶**, "Steeped in wine often used in ancient recipes to cure **wind fall**".

***Feng kuang* 風狂, wind madness** [9] AD *kuang* 狂, madness.
PC of psychic derangement manifesting itself as senseless movements and irregular outbursts of joy and anger. *ZBYHL* 2: 皆由血氣虛, 受風邪，致令陰陽氣相併所致，故名**風狂**, "Whenever wind evil is received in a situation of blood and qi depletion, this causes yin and yang qi to unite. Hence this is called **wind madness**".

Feng lai **風癩, wind repudiation-illness** [9] AN *lai feng* 癩風, repudiation-illness wind.

PC identical with → *da feng* 大風②, massive wind. *BJ* SE *huang qi* 黄耆: *da feng lai ji* 大**風癩**疾, massive **wind repudiation-illness**. *BCGM* Bai bing zhu zhi yao 百病主治藥, Zhu chuang, *shang* 諸瘡上：丁瘡、惡瘡、楊梅瘡、**風癩**、疥癬、熱瘡、瘑瘡、手瘡、足瘡、胻瘡, "Pin sores, malign sores, red bayberry sores, **wind repudiation-illness**, *jie-* and *xuan*-illness, heat sores, lair-illness sores, hand sores, feet sores, and shin sores".

Feng lan yan **風爛眼**, wind festering eye [2]

PC of identical with → l*an xian feng yan* 爛弦風眼, festering [eyelid] rim with wind eye. *BCGM* SE tong qing 銅青 quoting Xu Zhicai 徐之才 writes: 主**風爛眼**，淚出, "It controls wind festering eye, with tearflow".

Feng lao **風勞, wind exhaustion** [13]

PC of → *xu lao* 虛勞, depletion exhaustion, brought forth by wind evil availing itself of a body in a state of depletion. *ZBYHL* 6: 本患**風勞**而服散石，**風勞**未盡，石勢因發，解石之後，體尚虛羸，故猶挾**風勞**也, "If someone originally suffered from **wind exhaustion** and then ingests a mineral longevity elixir, before the **wind exhaustion** is completely eliminated; the effects of the mineral will already manifest themselves. After the [effects of the] mineral have been resolved, the [patient's] body remains in a state of depletion and emaciation. Hence it is still plagued by **wind exhaustion**".

Feng lei **風淚, wind tears** [3]

PC of tearflow not caused by emotional excitement. *ZBYHL* 28: 風熱在內乘肝，其氣外衝於目，故見**風淚**出, "If heat avails itself of the liver in [the body's] interior, its qi will rush to the eyes. Hence one sees **wind tears** appear".

Feng lei **風羸, wind emaciation** [1]

PC identical with *feng xu* 風虛, wind [intruding into a state of] depletion. *FKJYMF* 1: 酈縣菊水, 太尉胡廣久患風羸, 常飲此水後, 疾遂瘳, "*Ju* water from Li county: officer Hu Guang suffered from **wind emaciation** for a long time. After he had regularly consumed this liquid, his ailment was cured".

Feng lei yan **風淚眼**, wind-tears eyes [1]

PC of → *feng yan* 風眼, wind eye, with apparent tearflow. *BCGM* SE *yang* 羊 quoting *YXL*: 膽點眼中，主赤障，白膜，風淚, "[Its] bile dropped into the eyes will control red screens, white membranes, and wind tears", writes: 點赤障、白翳、**風淚眼**, "Drop into red screens, white shades, and **wind-tears eyes**".

Feng leng **風冷, wind cold** [40]

EA identical with → *feng han* 風寒. *ZBYHL* 2: **風冷**客於關戶之間，所以失聲也, "**Wind cold** settles in the throat. Hence one loses the voice". *BCGM* refers to the following pathological conditions associated with wind cold: *feng leng bi tong* **風冷**痹痛, wind cold with blockage and pain; *feng leng shi yin* **風冷**失音, wind cold with loss of voice; *feng leng jiao qi* **風冷**脚氣, wind cold with leg qi.

Feng li **風癘, wind epidemics** [3]

PC identical with → *li feng* 癘風, epidemics wind. *BCGM* SE *lian ou* 蓮藕 quotes *TPSHF*: 遍身**風癘**荷葉三十枚，石灰一斗，淋汁合煮。漬之，半日乃出。數日一作，良, "For **wind epidemics** affecting the entire body: 30 lotus leaves are to be boiled with the 1 *dou* of strained *shi hui* liquid. Steep the [body in the liquid] for half a day and then remove it. Do this once every few days. Good [effect]".

Feng li **風瀝, wind pervasion-illness** [2]

PC identical with → *luo li* 瘰瀝, scrofula with pervasion-illness. *BCTJ* SE guan bian shan 關邊山：主風熱上壅，喉咽腫痛及項上**風瀝**, "It controls obstructions resulting from wind and heat in the upper sections, as well as swollen, painful throat and **wind pervasion-illness** on the nape".

Feng lou **蜂瘺, bee fistula** [4]

PC of → *lou* 瘺, fistula, with swelling developing on one's neck at three or four, or four or five places. In severe cases the entire chest is swollen. Eventually the swelling opens to fester and develop into fistula with the appearance of obstruction-illnesses. When healed to close at one place they will once again effuse at another place. *ZBYHL* 34: **蜂瘺**者，由飲食勞倦，渴乏多飲流水，即得蜂毒，流入於臟。其根在脾。出發於頸項，歷歷三四處，或累累四五處蜂台，或發胸前俱腫，以潰生瘡，狀如癰形，瘥而復移, "The origin of **bee fistula** lies in one's food and exhaustion. If someone is tired and thirsty and often drinks running water, and then is affected by the poison of bees, this will flow into the depots. From its root in the spleen it effuses at the front and back of the neck. Either at three or four places, or at four or five places, resembling a wild honeycomb. Or it may effuse in front of the chest which then is entirely swollen. When it festers it develops into sores of the appearance of obstruction-illnesses. After being healed it re-appears somewhere else".

Feng lou chuang **風漏瘡, wind-leakage sores** [1]

PC identical with → *leng lou chuang* 冷漏瘡, cold-leakage sores. *BCGM* SE *lou lan zi* 漏籃子 quotes *RZZZF*: **風漏瘡**年久者，復其元陽，當用漏籃子輩，加減用之。如不當用而輕用之，又恐熱氣乘虛變移結核，而為害尤甚也, "For **wind-leakage sores** that have lasted for years, to restore the original yang [qi] one must resort to items like *lou lan zi*. The amounts may vary. If it is used haphazardly where it must not be used, the heat qi may avail itself of the depletion and form nodular kernels, resulting in very serious harm".

Feng luan **風攣, wind contraction** [2]

PC, brought forth by wind evil, of hands and feet contracted, with difficulties to walk. *BJ* SE *yan fang* 雁肪：主**風攣**，拘急偏枯，氣不通利, "It controls **wind contraction**, cramping and tension with unilateral withering, and impediments of qi flow".

Feng ni **風逆, wind counterflow** [1]

PC of four limbs swollen and difficulties in moving. *SJZL* 193: **風逆**四肢腫，復溜主之, "In the case of **wind counterflow** the four limbs are swollen. [Needling the] *fu liu* [insertion hole] controls this".

Feng nüe **風瘧, wind-*nüe*** [2]

PC of → *nüe*-disease that breaks out in autumn in persons who took in wind in summer when they longed for cold. *SW* 4: 夏暑汗不出者，秋成**風瘧**, "If in summer [despite] summerheat no sweat leaves [the body], this generates **wind-*nüe*** in autumn".

Feng pi **風僻, wind wryness** [2]

PC identical with → *pian feng* 偏風, unilateral wind. *FKJYMF* 5: 甘草湯，治**風僻**積年不瘥，手脚枯細, "Decoction with *gan cao* cures **wind wryness** that has continued for several years without being healed; hands and legs have withered and are thin".

Feng qi **風氣, wind qi** [110]

① EA: *SW* 10: **風氣**循風府而上，則為腦風, "**Wind qi** that moves up along the wind palace, it becomes brain wind".

② PC brought about by wind. *ZBYHL* 2: **風氣**者，由氣虛受風故也…有冷有熱，冷則厥逆，熱則煩惋。其因風所為，故名**風氣**, "As for [pathological conditions of] **wind qi**, they arise because of a qi depletion that has taken in wind... There are those associated with cold and those associated with heat. Cold results in recession with counterflow; heat results in vexation with sighing. Because they are caused by wind, they are called **wind qi**".

③ A climatic condition. *BCYY*, Xu li 序例: mentions wind qi as one of the five qi generating the flavors, from which emerge the ten thousand things: **風氣**散，故其味可用以收, "**Wind qi** dissipates. Hence the flavor [it generates] may be used to contract [what is dissipated]".

Feng qi **風臍, wind navel** [1]

PC of oozing from the navel region of newborns. *WTMY* 36: 古今錄驗療小兒**風臍**汁出，甘草散方, "The *GJLY* heals **wind navel** with liquid excretion by means of the recipe for the powder with *gan cao*".

Feng qu **風齲, wind tooth-decay** [1] AN *feng zhu* 風蛀, wind bug-attachment.

PC of tooth ache brought about by wind-heat, with swollen gums emitting pus. *ZBYHL* 29: 風氣客之，結搏齒間，與血氣相乘，則齦腫。熱氣加之，膿汁出而臭，侵食齒齦，謂之齲齒，亦曰**風齲**, "If wind qi settles there, it will form knottings between the teeth, which are then availed of by blood and qi. As a result, the gums will swell. If heat qi is added, pus will leave, and there is a strong stench. This is called 'decaying teeth'; another designation is '**wind tooth-decay**'".

Feng quan **風犬, mad dog** [3]

Identical with → *kuang gou* 狂犬, rabid dog. 風犬: possibly AW of 瘋犬. *BCGM* SE *chu ji* 㹀雞 quotes *JJF*: **風犬**咬毒：膽礬末傅之立愈, "For the poison from a bite by a **mad dog**, apply powderized *dan fan* to it. This will bring an immediate cure".

***Feng re* 風熱, wind and heat** [340]
EA CD of → *re* 熱, heat, and → *feng* 風, wind, with the latter dominating. *SW* 71: 故**風熱**参布，云物沸騰, "Hence **wind and heat** unite and spread; cloudy things surge [as if] boiling". *ZBYHL* 9 identifies heat-ulcer disease as **風熱**所為也, "caused by **wind and heat**". *BCGM* refers to numerous pathological conditions associated with wind and heat: *feng re tou tong* 風熱頭痛, wind and heat with headache; feng re chuang zhen 風熱瘡疹, wind and heat with sores and papules; feng re ke sou 風熱咳嗽, wind and heat with cough.

***Feng sao* 風瘙, wind itching** [34] AN *feng yang* 風癢, *feng sao yang* 風瘙癢
PC of wind evil or wind cold entering the skin, with the skin itching, or the emergence of skin papules, as major signs. *ZBYHL* 2: **風瘙**身體隱疹候：邪氣客於皮膚，復逢風寒相折，則起風瘙疹…身體為癢, "Signs of **wind itching** with hidden macules on the entire body: Evil qi settles in the skin. When there it meets with wind cold again, resulting in mutual damage, then wind itching will emerge with papules. .. The body itches".

***Feng sao yang* 風瘙癢, wind itching** [34]
PC identical with → *feng sao* 風瘙. *ZBYHL* 2: **風瘙癢**候：此由游風在於皮膚…遇熱則瘙癢, "Signs of **wind itching**. This [condition] results from wind roaming in the skin. .. When it meets with heat, then this causes itching".

***Feng shang* 風傷, wind harm** [3]
PC of harm brought forth by wind evil. *MYBL* SE *e shi* 惡實：主明目，補中，除**風傷**, "It is in control of clearing the eyes, supplementing the center, and eliminating **wind harm**".

***Feng shi* 風濕, wind and moisture** [200]
① EA CD of → *feng* 風, wind, and → *shi* 濕, moisture, with their merger resulting in a pathogenic evil qi including the characteristics of both. *JGYL* Fj: **風濕**相搏，骨節疼煩, "When **wind and moisture** clash with each other, the joints of the bones will be in discomforting pain".
② PC brought about by wind [and] moisture with fever and body pain. *JGYL* Fj: 一身盡疼，發熱，日晡所劇者，名**風濕**, "If the entire body is in pain and effuses heat with an intensity reaching a peak between 3 to 5 in the afternoon, this is called **wind moisture**". *BCGM* refers to numerous pathological conditions associated with wind moisture, such as *feng shi bi tong* 風濕痹痛, wind moisture with blockages and pain; *feng shi bu ren* 風濕不仁, wind moisture with insensitivity; *feng shi chuang* 風濕瘡, wind moisture with sores.

***Feng shi* 風屍, wind[-type] corpse [qi]** [3]
PC whereby a patient has a feeling of a heavy and numb body, brought forth by being affected by wind cold. *ZBYHL* 23: **風屍**者，在人四肢，循環經絡，其狀淫躍去來，沉沉默默，不知痛處，若衝風則發是也, "**Wind[-type] corpse [qi]** travels in one's four limbs through the conduits and network vessels. It is as if something were coming and going with wild leaps, deep insideand

without a sound. One cannot identify a specific region that hurts. It breaks out whenever one is affected by wind".

Feng shi bi **風濕痹, wind and moisture blockage** [26]
PC of the two qi wind and moisture jointly causing → *bi bing* 痹病, blockage disease, with the joints of one's limbs aching and experiencing swelling and distension. In extreme cases this leads to an inability to move. *BJ* SE *yi yi ren* 薏苡人：主筋急拘攣，不可屈伸，**風濕痹**, "It controls sinew tightness and cramps and contraction, with an inability to bend or stretch, [conditions associated with] **wind and moisture blockage**".

Feng shi chuang **風濕瘡, wind and moisture sores** [3]
PC of → *chuang* 瘡, sores, brought forth jointly by wind and moisture evil. *MYBL* SE *song ye* 松葉：主**風濕瘡**, "It controls **wind and moisture sores**".

Feng shi qi **風濕氣, wind and moisture qi** [5]
① EA of the two evils → *feng* 風, wind, and → *shi* 濕, moisture, together causing a disease. *ZBYHL* 1: 人腠理虛者，則由**風濕氣**傷之, "When the interstitial structures of man are depleted, they will be the starting points of his being harmed by **wind and moisture qi**".
② PC brought forth jointly by the two evils wind and moisture. *PJF* 92: 搜風順氣丸，治**風濕氣**，口眼喎斜，大便結澀, "The 'pills to wipe off wind and smoothen the path of qi' cure **wind and moisture qi**, slanted mouth and eyes, as well as a rough passage of bound stools".

Feng shi xuan **風濕癬, wind and moisture *xuan*-illness** [1]
PC identical with → *gan shi xuan* 乾濕癬, dry [*xuan*-illness] and moist *xuan*-illness. *KBBC* SE *wu pei zi* 五倍子：**風濕癬**瘡，瘙癢膿水, "Sores of **wind and moisture *xuan*-illness**, they itch and contain liquid pus".

Feng shui **風水, wind and water** [29]
PC of → *shui zhong* 水腫, edemata, brought forth by wind that harms a body while it is sweating. It is often accompanied by aching joints and an aversion to wind. *SW* 61: 腎汗出逢於風，內不得入於臟腑，外不得越於皮膚，客於玄府，行於皮里，傳為胕腫，本之於腎, 名曰**風水**, "When sweat leaves the kidneys and encounters wind, internally it cannot enter the depots and palaces and externally it cannot transgress beyond the skin. It settles in the dark palaces and moves inside the skin. Its transmission leads to *fu*-swelling. This is based in the kidneys. The name is **wind and water**".

Feng su **風粟, wind millet** [2]
PC of facial skin papules of either virid or yellow-red color, covered, dark, rough, and aching. *BCGM* SE *shao shang sha* 杓上砂：面上**風粟**，或青或黃赤，隱暗澀痛, "Facial **wind millet**, sometimes virid, sometimes yellow-red. [They may be] dormant and invisible, with roughness and aching".

Feng tan **風痰, wind phlegm** [110]
EA of a pathogenic qi resulting from a combination of → *feng* 風, wind, and → *tan* 痰, phlegm, with the latter being brought about by the former. *ZBYHL* 20: **風痰**相結，上沖於頭，即令頭痛, "When **wind [and] phlegm** unite,

they rise to rush against the head, and this causes headache". *BCGM* refers to numerous pathological conditions associated with wind phlegm, such as *feng tan xuan yun* 風痰眩運, wind phlegm with dizziness; *feng tan ke sou* 風痰咳嗽, wind phlegm with cough; *feng tan ma mu* 風痰麻木, wind phlegm with [the numbness of] hemp and logs.

***Feng tan* 風癱, wind paralysis** [3] AN → *tan huan feng* 癱瘓風, wind paralysis.
PC of hands and feet not moving according to one's will, as may result from all possible causes. *ZHBJF* 3: 卒中**風癱**，身體不自收, "In the case of being suddenly struck by **wind**, resulting in **paralysis**, one is unable to contract one's body".

***Feng tong* 風痛, wind pain** [37]
PC of various types of pain brought about by wind evil. *MYBL* SE *xiong qiong* 芎藭：主脅**風痛**, "It controls **wind pain** in the flanks". *BCGM* refers to numerous pathological conditions of wind pain, such as *tou mian feng tong* 頭面風痛, head and face wind pain; *gu jie feng tong* 骨節風痛, bone joints wind pain; *gu cao feng tong* 骨槽風痛, bone socket wind pain. *Feng tong* 風痛, wind pain, is not to be confused with → tong feng 痛風, pain wind, which may be caused by various pathogenic qi and is called "wind" because of its mobile nature in the body.

***Feng tou* 風頭, wind head** [22]
PC identical with → *tou feng* 頭風, head wind. *BJ* SE *xin yi* 辛荑：主五藏身體寒熱，**風頭**腦痛, "It controls cold and heat spells in the five depots and the entire body, and **wind head** with aching brain".

***Feng wai* 風喎, wind wryness** [2]
PC with → *kou wai* 口喎, wryness of the mouth, brought forth by wind evil stroke. *BCGM* Bai bing zhu zhi yao 百病主治藥 quoting *YSJCF* 1: a recipe 治口眼喎斜, "To cure wryness of mouth and eyes", writes: 白附子…**風喎**，同僵蠶、全蠍研末，酒服, "*Bai fu zi*…[cures] **wind wryness**. Powderize together with dead silkworms and complete scorpions, and ingest with wine".

***Feng wan ji ji* 風頑急疾, acute wind ailment that has become stubborn** [1]
PC CD of → *feng* 風②, wind, diseases that began with an acute onset and then turned difficult to heal. *BCGM* SE *wu tou* 烏頭：自非**風頑急疾**，不可輕投, "If it is not an **acute wind ailment that has become stubborn**, it must not be resorted to lightheartedly".

***Feng wen* 風温, wind and warmth** [8]
PC brought about by wind and heat. *SW* 71: 岐伯曰：**風温**春化同，熱曛昏火夏化同, "Qi Bo: **Wind and warmth** agree with the transformations [evoked by] spring. Heat, the red-yellow [color of] dusk, and fire agree with the transformations [evoked by] summer".

***Feng wu* 風忤, wind hostility** [1]
PC identical with → *ke wu* 客忤, visitor's hostility. *BCGM* SE *jiu* 韭 quoting *JGYL*: 卒死客忤, "Sudden [appearance of] death because of a visitor's hostility", writes: **風忤**邪惡, "**Wind hostility**, evil and malign [qi]".

Feng xian **風涎, wind drool** [15]

① EA of a pathogenic qi resulting from a combination of → *feng* 風, wind, and → *xian* 涎, drool, with the generation of the latter stimulated by the former. *BCTJ* SE *lu* 蘆：此藥大吐上膈**風涎**, "This drug [cures] massive spitting of **wind drool** from above the diaphragm".

② PC of wind drool blocking the interior of the chest, leading to mental pressure, and fainting with unconsciousness. *SZZF* 2: 風氣一蒸，痰涎並起，而上填塞胸中，即使人悶倒無知…此名之曰**風涎**, "As soon as wind qi steams, both phlegm and drool emerge and rise, leading to a blockage in the chest. This causes that person to experience heart pressure, to fall to the ground, and to lose his conscience…This is called **wind drool**".

Feng xian **風癇, wind epilepsy** [50]

PC of → *xian* 癇, epilepsy, resulting from the effects of wind evil. *ZBYHL* 45: **風癇**者，因衣厚汗出，而風入為之, "**Epilepsy** is caused if one sweats because one wears thick clothing, and wind enters [via the perspiration holes]".

Feng xie **風邪, wind evil** [80]

EA of wind entering the human organism and causing a disease. Because it enters where it does not belong it is termed "evil". *ZBYHL* 1: 血氣俱虛，**風邪**併入，在於陽則皮膚緩，在於陰則腹里急, "When blood and qi are depleted, **wind evil** enters both. When it settles in the yang [section], the skin will be relaxed. When it settles in the yin [section], the skin will be tight". *BCGM* frequently mentions "**wind evil**" as entering the brain, the depots, and the bone marrow, as passing into the heart, and as attacking the eyes to eventually cause a disease, as well as therapeutic strategies such as eliminating, or dissipating wind evil.

Feng xie **風泄, wind outflow** [2]

PC of → *xie xie* 泄瀉, outflow, brought forth by wind evil. *SWBJQYBMJ* Mj: 厥陰**風泄**，以風治風，小續命湯、消風散主之, "For **wind outflow** from the ceasing yin [conduits] use wind to cure wind. The 'small decoction to prolong life' and the 'powder to dissolve wind' control this".

Feng xu **風虛, wind [intrusion into a state of] depletion** [82]

① EA of wind evil intruding into the human body when its qi and blood are in a state of depletion. *ZBYHL* 3: **風虛**者，百病之長。勞傷之人，血氣虛弱，其膚腠虛疏，風邪易侵, "**Wind [intrusion into a state of] depletion** is the most important disease of all. When a person is harmed by exhaustion, when blood and qi are depleted and weak, and the skin structures are depleted and wide open, wind evil easily intrudes".

② PC resulting from wind evil intruding into a person whose qi and blood are in a state of depletion. *ZBYHL* 4: 依經為之，引肺中氣，去**風虛**病，令人目明, "It acts along the conduits. It pulls the qi from the lung and removes the disease of wind [intrusion into a state of] depletion". *BCGM* refers to numerous pathological conditions associated with wind [intrusion into a state of] depletion, such as *feng xu jiu bi* 風虛久痹, chronic blockage because of wind [intrusion into a state of] depletion; feng xu xuan yun 風虛眩運, dizziness because of wind [intrusion into a state of] depletion; feng xu han re 風虛寒熱, alternating sensations of cold and heat because of wind [intrusion into a state of] depletion.

***Feng xuan* 風眩, wind dizziness** [41] AW 風旋

PC, brought forth by wind evil, of dizziness in the head and eyes. *ZBYHL* 37: **風眩**，是體虛受風，風入於腦也…循脈引於目系，目系急，故令眩也，"**Wind dizziness** results from wind being received by a body in a state of depletion, with the wind then entering the brain. .. It moves along the vessels and pulls on the eye[-brain] connection. Then the eye[-brain] connection is tight, and this causes dizziness".

***Feng xuan* 風癬, wind *xuan*-illness** [16]

PC of → *xuan* 癬, *xuan*-illness a), with a circular outer edge and local numbness. *ZBYHL* 2: **風癬**，是惡風冷氣客於皮，折於血氣所生。亦作圓文匡郭，但抓搔頑痹，不知痛癢, "**Wind *xuan*-illness**. In this case malign wind and cold qi have settled in the skin. [The disease] is generated because of harm inflicted upon blood and qi. It too develops a circular edge. However, when scratched it is numb, and one fails to feel pain or itching".

***Feng ya* 風牙, wind tooth** [20] AN *feng chi* 風齒; *chi feng* 齒風, tooth wind; *kou chi feng* 口齒風, mouth and tooth wind.

PC of toothache and exposure of tooth roots brought about by → *feng xie* 風邪, wind evil. *SJZL* 120 RE *mang cao san fang* 莽草散方, recipe for the powder with *mang cao*: 治**風牙**疼, "It cures **wind-tooth** ache".

***Feng yan* 風眼, wind eye** [44]

PC of red and festering canthi and eyelids brought about by harm caused to the eyes by heat. *ZBYHL* 28: 風熱之氣傷於目，而眥瞼皆赤爛，見風彌甚，世亦云**風眼**, "In the case of harm to the eyes by the qi of wind and heat, and if all the canthi and eyelids are red and fester, and if this condition worsens if one encounters wind, this is commonly called **wind eye**". *BCGM* distinguishes, on the basis of different appearances and presumed etiologies, between → *feng chi yan* 風赤眼, wind red eyes; → *feng lan yan* 風爛眼, festering eyes because of wind; → *feng lei yan* 風淚眼, tearful eyes because of wind; → *lan xian feng yan* 爛弦風眼, festering [eyelid] rim with wind eye; → *tai chi feng yan* 胎赤風眼; fetal redness wind eye; → *dou feng yan* 痘風眼, smallpox-induced wind eye; → *xue feng yan* 血風眼, bleeding wind eye.

***Feng yang* 風癢, wind itching** [18] AN *feng sao* 風瘙; *feng sao yang* 風瘙癢.

PC identical with → *feng sao* 風瘙. *ZBYHL* 2: **風癢**候：邪氣客於肌肉，則令肌肉虛，真氣散去，又被寒搏皮膚，外發腠理，閉毫毛…故肉癢也, "Signs of **wind itching**: When evil qi settles in the muscles and in the skin, then this causes muscles and skin to be depleted. The true qi disperses. If then the skin is struck by cold again, [the evil qi seeks] to effuse through the interstitial structures. [However,] the finest hair is closed [by the evil qi, and the evil qi cannot effuse]. .. Hence the flesh itches".

Feng yi **風翳, wind shade** [3] AN *feng zhang* 風障, wind screen.

PC of impaired vision with the dark parts of the eyes obstructed by an excrescence. *QJYF* 6: 治風翳方. 取死豬鼻燒灰，治下篩，日一，向日，水服方寸匕, "Recipes to cure **wind shade**. Take the nose of a dead pig and burn it to ashes. Pass them through a sieve. Once a day face the sun and ingest one square inch spoon".

Feng yin **風喑, wind silence** [2]

PC, brough forth by wind evil, of aphasia. *QJYF* 14: 凡**風喑**、暴屍厥及鬼魘不寤，皆相似, "All cases of **wind silence**, sudden corpse[-like condition because of qi] recession, and demonic nightmares with an inability to sleep resemble each other".

Feng yong **風壅, wind obstruction** [7]

PC PM referring to obstructions caused by wind qi. *TPSHF* 45 RE *xi jiao san* 犀角散, powder with *xi jiao*: 治脚氣, 春夏防發，稍覺**風壅**氣滯，臟腑不通，心神煩悶，脚膝時疼，宜服犀角散方, "Cures leg qi, prevents outbreaks in spring and autumn. There is a slight sensation of **wind obstruction** and qi sluggishness. The depots and palaces are no longer penetrable. Heart and spirit experience vexation with pressure. Legs and knees hurt at times. In such cases the recipe to ingest the powder with *xi jiao* is appropriate".

Feng you dan zhong **風游丹腫, wind roaming cinnabar swelling** [2]

PC identical with → *chi you dan du* 赤游丹毒, red roaming cinnabar poison. *TBC* SE *yun tai* 芸薹：主**風游丹腫**，乳癰, "It controls **wind roaming cinnabar swelling**, and obstruction-illnesses on the breast".

Feng zao **風燥, wind dryness** [1]

EA a combination of → *feng* 風, wind, and → *zao* 燥, dryness, resulting in a pathogenic evil qi including the characteristics of both. *SW* 71: **風燥**火熱勝復更作, "**Wind [and] dryness**, fire and heat dominate and return to revenge, and are active alternately".

Feng zhang **風障, wind screen** [2]

PC identical with → *feng yi* 風翳, wind shade. *PJF* 75 quoting *LML*: 枸杞方，亦治暴赤眼，**風障**赤膜, "The recipe with *gou qi* also cures sudden red eyes, and **wind screen** with a red membrane".

Feng zhen **風疹, wind papules** [43] AN *feng zhen* 疹風, papules wind; *yin zhen* 癮疹, dormant papules.

PC, brought forth by wind evil, of eruptive skin papules of different sizes, accompanied by unbearable itching. If scratched they rise further. *QJYF* 22: 風邪客於肌中…**風疹**瘙癢，皆由於此, "Wind evil has settled in the skin. .. as a result **wind papules** and itching develop".

Feng zheng **風證, wind conditions** [3]

PC brought about by evil wind. *ZBYHL* 13: 脚氣而挾風毒，毒少風多，則**風證**偏見, "When there is leg *qi* together with wind poison, and when the poison is little and the wind much, this is a situation where **wind conditions** appear". *BCGM* SE *wu tou* 烏頭, quotes *QKMY*: 一切**風證**，不問頭風痛風，黃

鴉吊脚風痹, "All **wind conditions**, including head wind, pain wind, yellow crow hoisting legs, and wind blockage".

***Feng zhi* 風痔, wind piles** [2]

PC → *zhi* 痔, piles, with irregular episodes of swelling and pain. *BCGM* SE *can* 蠶 quotes *SJF*: **風痔**，腫痛發歇不定者是也, "**Wind piles** are those with irregular episodes of swelling and pain".

***Feng zhong* 風腫, wind swelling** [28]

PC of a swelling brought forth by wind, with neither head nor root. The swelling is extreme, as if something had been inflated. There is no reddening and no pain. *ZBYHL* 28: 腫而因風所發，故謂之**風腫**, "A swelling emerging because of wind. Hence one calls it '**wind swelling**' ". *BCGM* lists numerous conditions associated with 'wind swelling', such as *tou mian feng* zhong 頭面風腫, wind swelling on the head and face, and *feng zhong sao yang* 風腫瘙癢, wind swelling with itching.

***Feng zhu* 風蛀, wind with bug-attachment** [2]

PC of toothache brought forth by → *feng chong* 風蟲, wind bugs/worms. *PJF* 68 RE *bi ba san* 蓽茇散, powder with *bi ba*: 治**風蛀**牙疼不可忍者, "It cures **wind with bug-attachment** with unbearable toothache".

***Feng zhu* 風疰, wind attachment-illness** [7]

PC of a pain erratically moving through the body and skin for an extended period of time without healing. *BJ* SE *yuan qing* 芫青：主蠱毒，**風疰**，鬼疰，墮胎, "It controls *gu* poison, **wind attachment-illness**, demon attachment-illness, and may cause abortion".

***Fu bi* 腹痹, abdominal blockage** [5]

PC identical with → *xiao fu bi* 小腹痹, lower abdominal blockage. *BCGM* SE *da ma* 大麻 quoting *WTMY* 19: 脚氣上，脚腫小腹痹, "Leg qi, upper [section]: the feet are swollen with lower abdominal blockage", writes: 脚氣**腹痹**, "Leg qi and **abdominal blockage**".

***Fu da* 腹大, abdominal enlargement** [32] AN *fu gu da* 腹鼓大, drum-like enlargement of the abdomen; *fu gu* 腹鼓, abdominal drum.

IS of a distended and enlarged abdominal region. *SW* 22: 腎病者，**腹大**脛腫，喘咳身重, "In the case of a kidney disease, the **abdomen is enlarged** and the shins are swollen. [The patient] pants and coughs and the body feels heavy".

***Fu dou chuang* 麩豆瘡, bran-beans sores** [1]

PC identical with → *xiao er fu dou* 小兒麩豆, children's bran-beans. *YBC* SE *zhen zhu* 真珠：治兒子**麩豆瘡**入眼, "It cures children's **bran-beans sores** entering the eyes".

***Fu feng* 浮風, floating wind** [10]

PC a) identical with → *feng yang* 風癢, wind itching. *YXL* SE *bai hua she* 白花蛇：主治…**浮風**瘾疹, "It cures … **floating wind** and dormant papules". b) Feeling of nausea brought forth by wind evil that has settled in the stomach. *KBBC* SE *cheng zi pi* 橙子皮：食之去胃中**浮風**, "Eating this removes **floating wind** from the stomach".

***Fu feng* 膚風, skin wind** [1] AD *pi fu feng* 皮膚風.
PC CD of → *pi zhen* 皮疹, skin papules; *chuan zhong* 瘡腫, sores and swelling; *tuo xie* 脫屑, desquamation, and *sao yang* 瘙癢, itching. *BCGM* Bai bing zhu zhi yao 百病主治藥：鼠粘子，除**膚風**，利小便, "*Shu zhan zi* serves to remove **skin wind** and facilitates urination".

***Fu gan* 腹疳, abdominal *gan*-illness** [2]
PC identical with → *ding xi* 丁奚, pin-slave [condition]. *BCTJ* SE *zhi zhu* 蜘蛛：小兒**腹疳**者，燒熟啖之, "Burn it and feed it to children with **abdominal *gan*-illness**".

***Fu gen* 腐根, rotten roots** [1]
PC of the fourth stage of → *zou ma ya gan* 走馬牙疳, running horse dental *gan*-illness. *HYKY* 18: 重則齒自脫落，名曰**腐根**, "In severe cases the teeth fall out by themselves. This is called '**rotten roots**'".

***Fu gu* 腹鼓, abdominal drum** [1]
IS identical with → *fu da* 腹大, abdominal enlargement. *BCGM* SE *qiu shi* 秋石 quotes *SYL*: 有人病顛**腹鼓**，日久加喘滿，垂困，亦服此而安也, "If someone suffers from peak[-illness] and **abdominal drum**, to which after an extended period are added panting and a feeling of fullness, as well as difficulties to sleep, have him ingest this also, and he will be calmed down".

***Fu gu ju* 附骨疽, bone-attached impediment-illness** [10]
PC of → *ju* 疽, impediment-illness, developing at a depth close to the bones. Skin and flesh tissue at the affected location are tense and painful, and there is only a small chance of festering towards the outside. Movement is incapacitated. *QJYF* 22: 凡附骨疽者，以其無破，附骨成膿，故名**附骨疽**, "As for all impediment-illnesses that are attached to a bone, because they do not break and develop pus while they are attached to a bone they are called '**bone-attached impediment-illnesses**'".

***Fu gu teng tong* 附骨疼痛, pain attached to the bones** [1]
IS of a feeling of pain deep in the body and its extremities. *YXL* SE *ling yang jiao* 羚羊角：主中風筋攣，**附骨疼痛**, "It controls wind stroke with sinew cramps, and **pain attached to the bones**".

***Fu gu yong* 附骨癰, bone-attached obstruction-illness** [1]
PC identical with → *fu gu ju* 附骨疽, bone-attached impediment-illness. *MYBL* SE *lu feng fang* 露蜂房：主諸惡疽，**附骨癰**，根在臟腑, "It controls all types of malign impediment-illnesses and **bone-attached obstruction-illnesses**, whose roots are in the depots and palaces". *BCGM* Bai bing zhu zhi yao 百病主治藥 quotes this as 惡疽、附骨疽，根在臟腑, "Malign impediment-illnesses and bone-attached impediment-illnesses, whose roots are in the depots and palaces". Elsewhere in the *BCGM*, SE *lu feng fang* 露蜂房, the *MYBL* is quoted as follows: 治惡疽、**附骨癰**，根在臟腑, "It cures malign impediment-illnesses, and **bone-attached obstruction-illnesses** whose roots are in the depots and palaces".

Fu huo **伏火, hidden fire, to subdue fire** [29]

① PC of the body being affected by depletion heat following a deeply-penetrating invasion by fire heat. *SJZL* 186: 治一切冷氣**伏火**，太陽丹方, "Recipe for a major yang elixir. Cures all types of cold qi and **hidden fire**".

② TA of treating fire heat by means of pharmaceutical substances of a cold nature. *BCGM*, Bai bing zhu zhi yao 百病主治藥：其證莖盛不衰，精出不止，多發消渴癰疽。**伏火**解毒, "With its condition being a persistent erection and continuous emission of essence, and frequent outbreak of melting with thirst and obstruction-illnesses and impediment-illnesses, [employ the approach] to dissolve poison by **subduing fire**".

③ PTP to prepare pharmaceutical substances. Refers to the approaches applied by alchemists to decrease the "fire poison" of mineral substances. *BCGM* SE *dan sha* 丹砂 quotes *QXZ*: 丹砂**伏火**，化為黃銀, "If *dan sha*'s **fire is subdued** it is transformed to yellow silver".

Fu jia **伏瘕, hidden conglomeration-illness** [4]

PC of a → *jia* 瘕, conglomeration-illness, lying deeply hidden in the abdomen. *MYBL* SE *yin chen hao* 茵陳蒿：除頭熱，去**伏瘕**, "It eliminates heat in the head, and it removes **hidden conglomeration-illness**".

Fu leng **腹冷, abdominal cold** [12]

① IS of a feeling of cold in the abdomen. *QJYF* 13: 羊肉當歸湯，治**腹冷**絞痛方, "The decoction with *yang rou* and *dang gui*: a recipe to cure **abdominal cold** and twisting pain".

② PC of cold-type abdominal diseases. *SLBC* SE *jun da* 莙薘：先患**腹冷**，食必破腹, "If one first suffered from **abdominal cold**, eating it will destroy the abdomen".

Fu lian **伏連**, hidden link [10]

PC identical with → *chuan shi* 傳屍, corpse [evil] transmission. *WTMY* 13: 傳屍之疾…內傳五臟，名之**伏連**, "The ailment of corpse [evil] transmission, when it is transmitted internally to the five depots, it is called **hidden link**".

Fu liang **伏梁, hidden beam** [19] AN *xin ji* 心積, heart accumulation.

PC of → *ji* 積, accumulation, associated with the heart. It is shaped like a lower arm. Below it rises from the navel; above it reaches to below the heart. It is accompanied by vexation. In serious cases patients spit blood. They cannot be cured for an extended period of time. NJ 56: 心之積，名曰**伏梁**，起臍上，大如臂，上至心下。久不愈，令人病煩心, "An accumulation in the heart is called '**hidden beam**'. It rises from above the navel and is as large as a lower arm. It extends upward to below the heart and lasts a long time without healing. It makes the [afflicted] person suffer from a feeling of vexation in his heart".

Fu ming **腹鳴, abdominal sounds** [12]

IS identical with → *chang ming* 腸鳴①, intestinal sounds. *WTMY* 39: **腹鳴**濯濯，若中有水聲, "[It cures] **abdominal sounds** with a wash-out. It sounds as if there were water in [the abdomen].

***Fu nei zhong ming* 腹內鐘鳴, a bell ringing in the abdomen** [1]

PC identical with → *tai ti* 胎啼, fetal cry. *FRDQLF* 15: 治孕婦**腹內鐘鳴**。用鼠窟前后土為細末，研麝香，酒調下二錢，其疾立愈, "To cure **a bell ringing in a** pregnant woman's **abdomen** use a fine powder prepared from the soil surrounding a rat hole, grind *she xiang*, and ingest 2 *qian* of [these two ingredients] mixed with wine. The ailment will be healed immediately".

***Fu qi* 浮氣, floating qi** [4]

① IS identical with → *fu zhong* 浮腫, floating swelling. *HYBC* SE *yue wang yu suan* 越王余筭：主水腫**浮氣**，結聚宿滯不消，腹中虛鳴，並宜煮服之, "It controls water swelling and **floating qi**, nodular collections that abide, are sluggish and fail to be dissolved, and depletion rumble in the abdomen. For all this it is advisable to boil and ingest it".

② EA identical with → *zhi qi* 滯氣①, sluggish qi. *BCGM* SE *su* 蘇 quotes *BCHB*: 紫蘇熟水第一，以其能下胸膈**浮氣**也, "*Zi su* maceration is best because it is able to make **floating qi** in the chest and diaphragm descend".

***Fu qi* 伏氣, deep-lying qi** [4]

EA of evil qi lying deeply inside the body without having caused a disease yet. *SHL* Ping mai fa 平脈法：假令舊有**伏氣**，當須脈之, "If someone has had **deep-lying qi** for a long time, this must [be examined] through [the movement] in his vessels".

***Fu re* 伏熱, hidden heat** [26]

PC of the body being affected by repletion heat following its invasion by heat evil. *ZBYHL* 7: **伏熱**在胃，令人胸滿, "When **hidden heat** is present in the stomach, this causes a feeling of fullness in one's chest".

***Fu re* 浮熱, floating heat** [13]

PC of heat situated in the upper/outer sections of the human body, or in the skin. *MYBL* SE *wu you* 屋游：主**浮熱**在皮膚, "It controls **floating heat** in the skin".

***Fu ren bing* 婦人病, women's diseases** [2]

PC CD of all types of gynecological and also internal diseases affecting women. *ZBYHL* 38: **婦人病**之有異於丈夫者，或因產後臟虛受寒，或因經水往來，取冷過度，非獨關飲食失節，多挾有血氣所成也, "**Women's diseases** differ from those of males because having given birth their depleted depots may receive cold, or in the course of periodic menstruation they may be excessively affected by cold. [Their diseases] are not related to immoderate eating and drinking; they often emerge because of [their personal] blood and qi [conditions]".

***Fu ren san shi liu ji* 婦人三十六疾, 36 types of women's ailments** [1] AN *nü ren san shi liu ji* 女人三十六疾; *fu ren xia jiao san shi liu ji* 婦人下焦三十六疾, 36 types of ailments affecting the lower burner in women.

PC CD of all types of diseases associated with gynecology and obstetrics. *QJYF* 4: 白石脂丸，治**婦人三十六疾**, "Pills with *bai shi zhi* cure **36 types of women's ailments**".

***Fu ren xia jiao san shi liu ji* 婦人下焦三十六疾, 36 types of ailments affecting the lower burner in women** [1]

PC identical with → *fu ren san shi liu ji* 婦人三十六疾, 36 types of women's ailments. *QJYF* 2: 承澤丸，治**婦人下焦三十六疾**, "The 'pills upholding moisture' cure **36 types of ailments affecting the lower burner in women**".

***Fu ren xue mai bu tiao* 婦人血脈不調, disharmony in a woman's blood vessels** [1]

PC identical with → *yue shui bu tiao* 月水不調, menstrual irregularity. *RHZ* SE *jing san leng* 京三棱：治**婦人血脈不調**，心腹痛，落胎, "It cures **disharmony in a woman's blood vessels**, pain in heart and abdomen, and premature birth".

***Fu she shang* 蝮蛇傷, harm caused by a pallas pit viper** [2]

PC of → *she hui du* 蛇虺毒②, venomous snake poisoning, resulting from a pallas pit viper bite. *BCGM* SE *bai zhi* 白芷：夷堅志所載治**蝮蛇傷**之方，亦制以所畏也，而本草不曾言及, "The recipes listed in the *YJZ* for curing **harm caused by a pallas pit viper** also seek to overpower [such harm] by using items that are feared [by a pallas pit viper]. They have not been mentioned in *ben cao* [literature]".

***Fu shi* 伏屍, hidden corpse [qi]** [12]

PC of a heart pain and hectic panting that cannot be healed over many years with the patient oscillating between periods of wellbeing and recurring breakouts. *BJ* SE *tian men dong* 天門冬：主諸暴風濕偏痹，強骨髓，殺三蟲，去**伏屍**, "It controls all types of sudden wind moisture with unilateral blockage, strengthens bones and marrow, kills the three types of bugs/worms, and removes **hidden corpse [qi]**".

***Fu shi du fa* 服石毒發, outbreak of poisoning after ingesting [stalactite] mineral** [2]

PC identical with → *ru shi fa* 乳石發, outbreak of stalactite mineral [poisoning]. *BCGM* SE *wan dou* 豌豆 quoting *WTMY* 38: 一切石發, "All outbreaks of mineral [poisoning]", writes: **服石毒發**, "**Outbreak of poisoning after ingesting [stalactite] mineral**".

***Fu shu* 伏暑, hidden summerheat** [19]

① PC resembling heatstroke manifesting itself in late autumn and winter with high fever, vexation and restlessness, vomiting, diarrhea and exhaustion. *SJZL* 34: 治**伏暑**吐逆，小香薷湯方, "The small recipe for a decoction with *xiang ru* to cure **hidden summerheat** with vomiting and counterflow".

② EA of summerheat qi lying hidden in the body without immediately manifesting itself in a disease, and possibly breaking out in autumn or winter. *JSF* Zhu shu men 諸暑門：二氣丹，治**伏暑**傷冷，二氣交錯, "The 'elixir for the two qi' cures an interlock of the two qi of **hidden summerheat** and harm caused by cold".

***Fu shui* 伏水, hidden water/liquid** [2]

EA of water evil abiding in the human body. *QJYF* 7: 小黄酒，治風虚痰癖，四肢偏枯，兩脚弱，手不能上頭。或小腹縮痛，脅下攣急，心下有**伏水**, "Ordinary yellow wine cures wind depletion with phlegm aggregation-illness, unilateral withering of any of the four limbs, weakness of both legs, inability to raise the hands above the head, in some cases with a contracting pain, cramps and tightness below the flanks, and the presence of **hidden water** below the heart".

***Fu yi* 浮翳, floating shade** [14]
PC of → *mu yi* 目翳, eye shade, that is very small and floats loosely on the surface. *QJYF* 6: 治目風淚出，**浮翳**多膿，爛眥方, "Recipe to cure eye wind with a release of tears, **floating shade** with much pus, and festering canthi".

***Fu yi* 膚翳, dermal shade** [21] AN *yin fu* 淫膚, excessive skin; *mu fu* 目膚, eye skin. PC identical with → *mu yi* 目翳. *ZBYHL* 28: **膚翳**者，明眼睛上有物如蠅翅者即是, "A '**dermal shade**': These are items on the clear eye resembling fly wings".

***Fu yin* 伏飲, hidden rheum** [1]
PC of → *yin* 飲②, rheum, disease with rheum, stagnating below the heart and a feeling of fullness in the chest, vomiting, alternating sensations of cold and heat, as well as vertigo. *SJZL* 63: 然又有五飲…沉伏於內曰**伏飲**, "Further, there are five types of rheum…The type that lies hidden inside is called '**hidden rheum**'".

***Fu yu* 怫鬱, anger with pent-up [qi]** [7]
EA and IS identical with → *yu* 郁, pent-up [qi]; depression. *ZHF* 4: 谷疸者，食畢頭旋，心**怫鬱**不安而發黃, "In the case of grain *dan*-illness, following a meal, [patients] develop head spinning, their heart experiences **anger with pent-up [qi]** and restlessness, and they develop a yellow complexion".

***Fu zang leng* 腹臟冷, cold in the abdominal depots** [1]
IS identical with → *fu leng* 腹冷, abdominal cold. *RHZ* SE gan jiang 乾薑：治轉筋吐瀉，**腹臟冷**, "It cures twisted sinews with vomiting and diarrhea, and **cold in the abdominal depots**".

***Fu zhang* 腹脹, abdominal distension** [126]
① IS of a) an uncomfortable feeling of fullness and pressure in the abdominal region. *SW* 19: 脈盛，皮熱，**腹脹**，前後不通，悶瞀，此謂五實, "An abounding [movement in the] vessels, a hot skin, an **abdominal distension**, [defecation and urination at one's] front and behind are not passable; mental and physical pressure, these are called the five repletions". b) AN *du zhang* 肚脹; *lu zhang* 臚脹, the abdominal wall is distended. A concrete distension and massive swelling of the abdominal region. *TPSHF* 19: 治乾霍亂，不吐不瀉，**腹脹**如鼓，心胸痰壅，宜服此方, "To cure dry cholera, when one neither vomits nor has diarrhea, and if there is drum-like **abdominal distension**, with the heart and chest congested by phlegm, it is advisable to ingest this recipe".
② PC with abdominal distension. *ZBYHL* 15: 脾氣盛，為形有餘，則病**腹脹**, "When spleen qi abounds, one's physical appearance has an excess. This leads to the disease of **abdominal swelling**".

***Fu zhong* 浮腫, surface swelling** [106]
IS identical with → *zhong* 腫, swelling. *SW* 38: 使人多涕唾而面**浮腫**，氣逆也, "This makes a person develop plenty of snivel and spittle; the face has **surface swelling** [because of] qi moving contrary [to its regular course]". In the *BCGM*,

fu zhong 浮腫 refers to an edematose swelling affecting the entire body, as in *si zhi mian mu fu zhong* 四肢面目浮腫, "the four limbs, face, and eyes have surface swelling", and it also refers to topical swelling of an inflammatory type, as in *zeng qi xun mian fu zhong* 甑氣熏面浮腫, "Facial surface swelling following exposure to the qi from a steamer".

Fu zhong **胕腫, *fu*-swelling** [7]
IS of an → *shui zhong* 水腫, edematose swelling, with surface swelling of the entire body. *SW* 61: 上下溢於皮膚，故為**胕腫**, "Above and below it spills into the skin; hence, [this] leads to ***fu*-swelling**".

Fu zhong er ku **腹中兒哭, an infant crying in the abdomen** [2]
PC identical with → *tai ti* 胎啼, fetal cry. *FRLFBY* 15: "治孕婦**腹中兒哭**，用川黃連濃煎汁，母常呷之, "To cure **an infant crying in a** pregnant woman's **abdomen** use *chuan huang lian* boiled to a concentrated sap. Let the mother ingest this repeatedly".

- G -

***Ga qi* 呷氣, creaking qi** [2]
PC identical with → *xiao chuan* 哮喘, roaring panting. *BCGM* SE *niu* 牛：牛喉嚨治**呷氣**、反胃，皆以類相從也, "That the throat of an ox cures **creaking qi** and a turned-over stomach is always because like follows like".

***Ga sou* 呷嗽, creaking cough** [5] AN *ya sou* 呀嗽.
PC of a cough, resulting from phlegm stagnating in the region of the chest and diaphragm, with a creaking sound in the throat. *ZBYHL* 14: 其胸膈痰飲多者，嗽則氣動於痰，上搏喉咽之間，痰氣相擊，隨嗽動息，呼呷有聲，謂之**呷嗽**, "When much phlegm rheum is present in the region of the chest and diaphragm, cough will stimulate the phlegm to move. It ascends into the throat where the phlegm and qi strike each other. Just as the cough is active or not [patients] will breathe with a creaking sound. This is called '**creaking cough**'".

***Gan* 皯, gloom** [p] AW *gan* 奸.
PC identical with → *mian gan* 面皯, facial gloom. *TPSHF* 40: 治面上瘡及**皯**，易容膏, "The ointment to modify one's appearance, it cures sores and **gloom** on the face".

***Gan* 奸, gloom** [p]
PC identical with → *gan* 皯. *WTMY* 32: 文仲療**奸**，令人面皮薄如蕣花方, "Wenzhong's recipe to cure **gloom**. It makes one's facial skin thin like a *shun* flower".

***Gan* 疳, *gan*-illness; sweets-illness** [p] AN *gan ji* 疳疾, *gan*-ailment; *gan bing* 疳病, *gan*-disease; *gan qi* 疳氣, *gan*-illness qi; *gan shou* 疳瘦, *gan*-illness with emaciation.
PC of a chronic malnutrition disease resulting from various causes that harm the spleen and stomach and disturb their functions. The major sign is physical depletion, weakness, and emaciation. It may assume numerous different manifestations, each of which has a specific designation. Until the Tang, this was generally considered a disease affecting adults and children alike. Beginning with the Song, this gradually developed into a disease diagnosed in children only. *ZBYHL* 4: 蒸盛，過傷內則變為**疳**, "Excessive steaming harming the interior will change into ***gan*-illness**".

***Gan bing* 疳病, *gan*-disease** [11]
PC identical with → *gan* 疳, *gan*-illness. *QJYiF* 24: 試法，先指琢其脊上兩邊，若逐指即起如粟者，即是**疳病**，若不起者，非是疳也, "The method to test this is as follows: One palpitates both sides of the spine with one finger. If, when one lifts the finger, something as small as a grain of millet rises, this is ***gan*-disease**. If nothing rises, this is not a *gan*-illness".

***Gan chong* 疳蟲, *gan*-illness worm/bug; *gan*-illness [caused by] worms/bugs** [20]
① EA of worms causing all types of → *gan* 疳, *gan*-illness. *QJYF* 6：治**疳蟲**蝕鼻生瘡方, "Recipe to cure ***gan*-illness worms/bugs** eroding the nose and generating sores".

② PC of → *gan* 疳, *gan*-illness, caused by worms/bugs in the intestinal tract. *RHZ* SE *yang ti* 羊蹄：葉治小兒**疳蟲**, "The leaves cure ***gan*-illness worms/bugs** in children".

***Gan chuang* 疳瘡, *gan*-illness sores** [49] AN *gan shi* 疳蝕, *gan*-illness with erosion; *gan shi* 疳濕, *gan*-illness with moisture.

PC in a broad sense of *gan* 疳, *gan*-illness, with festering ulcers. In severe cases this includes various pathological conditions of ulcers affecting adults. In a narrow sense it refers to ulcers developing on a human body and its four extremities because of a → *gan* 疳, *gan*-illness. Depending on whether they develop at the eyes, the ears, the mouth, the nose or in the genital region they are given different names. *QJYF* 5: 治小兒**疳瘡**方：以豬脂和胡粉敷之，日五六度, "Recipe to cure **gan-illness sores** in children: smear lard with *hu fen* [on the sores], five or six times a day".

***Gan dan huo* 肝膽火, liver fire and gallbladder fire** [3]

CD of → *gan huo* 肝火, liver fire, and → *dan huo* 膽火, gallbladder fire. *BCGM* Bai bing zhu zhi yao 百病主治藥：脅痛有**肝膽火**, "When the flanks ache, this is because of **liver fire and gallbladder fire**".

***Gan dan xin huo* 肝膽心火, liver fire, gallbladder fire, and heart fire** [2]

CD of → *gan huo* 肝火, liver fire, → *dan huo* 膽火, gallbladder fire, and → *xin huo* 心火, heart fire. *BCGM* Bai bing zhu zhi yao 百病主治藥：黃連平**肝膽心火**, "*Huang lian* soothes **liver fire, gallbladder fire and heart fire**".

***Gan dan xin pi huo* 肝膽心脾火, liver fire, gallbladder fire, heart fire, and spleen fire** [1]

CD of → *gan huo* 肝火, liver fire, → *dan huo* 膽火, gallbladder fire, → *xin huo* 心火, heart fire, and → *pi huo* 脾火, spleen fire. *BCGM* Bai bing zhu zhi yao 百病主治藥：黃連，瀉**肝膽心脾火**，退客熱, "*Huang lian* drains **liver fire, gallbladder fire, heart fire, and spleen fire**; it removes visitor heat".

***Gan er* 疳耳, ear affected by *gan*-illness** [2]

PC identical with → *er gan* 耳疳, ear *gan*-illness. *BCGM* SE *hu* 鵠 quotes *TXF*: **疳耳**出膿：用天鵝油調草烏末，入龍腦少許，和傅立效, "When an **ear affected by *gan*-illness** produces pus mix *tian e* oil with *cao wu* powder. Add a little *long nao*. Mix and apply externally. Instantly effective".

***Gan fen* 乾糞, dry stool** [1]

SEC identical with → *zao shi* 燥屎, dry stool. *TPSHF* 58: 治**乾糞**塞腸症，腸脹痛不通方, "To cure the condition of **dry stool** that blocks the intestines, [use] the 'recipe for an intestinal distension with pain and blocked passage'".

***Gan feng* 肝風, liver wind** [23]

① EA and PM of wind diseases such as swaying and dizziness brought forth by internal harm. *KTYL* Fj: 小兒吸受外邪，先傷肺經，起自寒熱、氣粗，久延漸入心胞絡，雖有微汗，而痰多、鼻煽、煩躁、神昏，切忌妄投辛香金石重劑，以致陰液消亡，熱勢愈熾，正氣愈虛，**肝風**陡動，則肢掣目竄，痙厥生矣，慎勿誤認驚風, "When children inhale external evil, this will initially harm the lung conduits. [The disease] manifests itself as alternating spells of cold and heat and qi roughness. After some time it will enter the network of the heart. There will be mild sweating associated with much phlegm, flaring nostrils, and vexation with irritation, as well as mental confusion. At this time one must under no circumstances prescribe acrid and fragrant [substances] as well as heavy medication such as mineral [drugs], lest the yin body liquids should become completely exhausted. This would let the power of heat [qi] become stronger and stronger associated with an increasing depletion of proper qi. As a result the **liver wind** is vigorously stimulated resulting in a contraction of the four limbs, scurrying eyes, spasm and recession. This must not be misinterpreted as fright wind".

② PC of a liver affection by wind evil. *SW* 42: **肝風**之狀，多汗惡風，善悲，色微蒼，嗌乾，善怒，時憎女子, "The appearance of **liver wind** [is such]: [patients] sweat profusely and have an aversion to wind. They tend to be sad. Their [facial] color is slightly greenish. When the throat is dry, they tend to be angry. At times they hate women".

***Gan gu* 疳痼, *gan*-illness with obstinacy-illness** [1]

PC identical with → *gan ji* 疳積, *gan*-illness with accumulation. *SLBC* SE *shi yu* 鰣魚：稍發**疳痼**, "It may cause an outbreak of a ***gan*-illness with obstinacy-illness**".

***Gan hui* 疳蛔, *gan*-illness [caused by] roundworm** [6]

PC of → *gan* 疳, *gan*-illness, caused by → *hui chong* 蛔蟲, roundworms. *RHZ* SE *bai bu gen* 百部根：治**疳蛔**及傳屍、骨蒸勞，殺蛔蟲、寸白、蟯蟲, "It cures ***gan*-illness [caused by] roundworms** and corpse [evil] transmission, as well as bone steaming with exhaustion; it kills roundworms, tapeworms, and pinworms".

***Gan huo* 肝火, liver fire** [9]

PC and EA identical with → *gan re* 肝熱, liver heat. *DXXF* 1: 人中白瀉**肝火**, "*Ren zhong bai* drains **liver fire**".

***Gan huo luan* 乾霍亂, dry cholera** [21]

PC of → *huo luan* 霍亂, cholera, including abdominal fullness with twisting pain, shortness of breath, and mental confusion in the absence of vomiting and diarrhea. *ZBYHL* 22: 但腹滿，煩亂，絞痛，短氣，其腸胃先挾實，故不吐痢，名為**乾霍亂**也, "If one suffers only from abdominal fullness, mental confusion, twisting pain, and shortness of qi, intestines and stomach cling to their matter. Hence there is neither vomiting nor free-flux illness. This is called **dry cholera**".

***Gan ji* 疳疾, *gan*-ailment** [21]

PC identical with → *gan* 疳, *gan*-illness. *RHZ* SE *dai zhe* 代赭：止吐血，鼻衄，腸風，痔瘺，月經不止，小兒驚癇，**疳疾**，反胃, "It ends bloodspitting, nosebleed, intestinal wind, piles and fistulas, incessant menstruation, fright epilepsy in children, ***gan*-ailment**, and turned over stomach".

Gan ji 疳魃, _gan_-illness [caused by] jealousy-demon [1]

PC identical with *xiao er ji bing* 小兒魃病, jealousy-demon disease in children. *BCGM* SE *ru zhi* 乳汁：有孕之乳，謂之忌奶，小兒飲之吐瀉，成**疳魃**之病, "Breast-milk of pregnant women is called 'taboo breast-milk'. When children drink it they will vomit and have diarrhea. This develops into the disease of '**_gan_-illness [caused by] jealousy-demon**'".

Gan ji 疳積, _gan_-illness with accumulation [8] AN *gan gu* 疳痼, *gan*-illness with obstinacy-illness.

PC of → *gan* 疳, *gan*-illness, that is associated with → *ji* 積, accumulations. In general this condition is associated with an emaciated body, desiccated hair, an enlarged abdomen and greenish sinews. *XEYZZJ* Lj: 牛黄丸，治小兒**疳積**, "Pills with *niu huang* cure **_gan_-illness with accumulation** in children".

Gan jiao qi 乾脚氣, dry leg qi [0]

PC of those cases of → *jiao qi* 脚氣, leg qi, where the legs are desiccated and emaciated, painful, and not swollen. *TPSHF* 45: 治**乾脚氣**，風毒搏於脚膝，皮內乾枯，脚脛漸細，骨中疼痛, "To cure **dry leg qi**. Wind poison has struck at the legs and knees. The interior of the skin has dried up. Gradually the legs and shins shrink. Inside the bones one feels pain".

Gan jie 乾結, desiccated and nodular [3]

IS of a desiccation of matter secreted internally or discharged externally. *SYDXF* 12: 身熱，手足清冷，皮燥，大便**乾結**, "The body is hot, hands and feet are cold. The skin is dry. The stools are **desiccated and nodular**".

Gan jing 肝驚, liver fright [1]

PC of a → *jing feng* 驚風, fright wind, associated with depletion heat. *BYCY* 2: 亦有**肝驚**，虛熱而生風者，當審其氣血有餘不足而治之, "There are also cases of **liver fright** with depletion heat generating wind. One must examine whether qi and blood have a surplus or are insufficient, and treat this accordingly".

Gan ke 乾咳, dry cough [2]

IS identical with → *zao ke* 燥嗽. *WTMY* 10: 羚羊角飲，主肺熱，胸背痛，時時**乾咳**，不能食方, "Drink with *yang ling jiao*, a recipe to control lung heat, chest and back pain, frequent **dry cough**, and inability to eat".

Gan ke sou 乾咳嗽, dry cough [1]

IS identical with → *zao ke* 燥嗽. *DXXF* 2: **乾咳嗽**難治，此系火郁之證, "**Dry cough** is difficult to cure. It is one of the conditions associated with pent-up fire".

Gan lao 肝勞, liver exhaustion [3]

PC of a depletion exhaustion brought forth by exhaustion detrimentally affecting the liver. *ZBYHL* 3: **肝勞**者，面目乾黑，口苦，精神不守，恐畏不能獨臥，目視不明, "In the case of **liver exhaustion**, the face and the eyes turn dry and dark. The mouth has a bitter taste. The essence and spirit are not guarded. One is fearful and cannot sleep alone. Vision is obscured".

Gan lao 疳勞, _gan_-illness with exhaustion [4]

PC of obstructed nutrition among children experiencing tidal fever and emaciation with their spleen and stomach being in a state of depletion weakness. *LXJ*

Fj: 孩子無故肚大項細，四肢消瘦，筋脈骨節弛緩，是小來少乳，嚼食與吃，早成骨熱疳勞, "Without apparent reason children develop an enlarged abdomen and a narrow nape. Their four limbs are emaciated; the sinews, vessels, and joints slacken. This is because they have been weaned early and were offered food to chew instead. Hence they early develop bone heat and ***gan*-illness with exhaustion**".

***Gan li* 疳痢, *gan*-illness with free-flux illness** [50]

PC of a prolonged free-flux illness among children that cannot be cured and is accompanied by damage to the spleen and stomach. It is apparent as a fading yellow complexion, emaciation of the muscles and body, robber sweat and strong fever of the type seen in the case of *gan*-disease. *WTMY* 25 療積年**疳痢**羸瘦，面色痿黃方, "Recipe to heal ***gan*-illness with free-flux illness** with emaciation and a complexion of dysfunction with jaundice lasting for years".

***Gan mao* 感冒, affection by the malicious** [2]

PC of an affection by an external evil with fever and an aversion to cold, headache and body pain, blocked nose and flow of snivel, itching in the throat and cough. *HJJF* 2: 大抵**感冒**，古人不敢輕發汗者，止由麻黃能開腠理，用或不能得其宜，則導泄真氣，因而致虛，變生他證, "In general, in the case of an **affection by the malicious**, the ancients did not dare to lightheartedly cause them to sweat. As *ma huang* is able to open the interstitial structures, inadequate use may cause an outflow of true qi and subsequently cause a depletion, which in turn will generate further pathological conditions".

***Gan ni* 疳䘌, sweets-illness with hidden worms** [28] AN *gan ni* 甘䘌.

PC of → *ni* 䘌, hidden worms, disease brought forth by frequent consumption of sweet items, with the teeth turning black and rotting, or ulcers developing in the anal and genital areas, and festering with stench. *ZBYHL* 18: **疳䘌**候：人有嗜甘味多，而動腸胃間諸蟲，致令侵食腑臟，此猶是䘌也, "The signs of **sweets-illness with hidden worms**: When someone consumes large amounts of sweet items, and thereby excites all types of worms in the region of intestines and stomach, this causes them to enter and consume the depots and palaces. This is the same as hidden worms".

***Gan ni* 甘䘌, hidden worms brought forth by a consumption of sweets** [1]

PC identical with → *gan ni* 疳䘌, *gan*-illness with hidden worms. *BCSY* SE *da hong xia zha* 大紅蝦鮓：主飛屍，蛔蟲，口中**甘䘌**, "It controls flying corpse [qi], roundworms, and **hidden worms** in the mouth **brought forth by the consumption of sweets**".

***Gan nüe* 肝瘧, liver malaria** [3]

PC of → *nüe ji* 瘧疾, malaria ailment, associated with illness signs of liver qi such as a greenish complexion, and a tendency to sigh. *SW* 36: **肝瘧**者，令人色蒼蒼然，太息, "**Liver malaria**: it lets a person's complexion become greenish. [Patients] take deep breaths".

***Gan ou* 乾嘔, dry vomiting** [35]
IS of a sound of vomiting without any matter being thrown up. *SHL* 12: 傷寒表不解，心下有水氣，**乾嘔**，發熱而咳, "If harm caused by cold has not been resolved in the exterior, there is water and qi below the heart, **dry vomiting**, an effusion of heat, and cough".

***Gan pao* 皯皰, [facial] gloom and blisters** [11]
PC CD of → *mian gan* 面皯, facial gloom, and → *mian pao* 面皰, facial blisters. *BJ* SE *xiong zhi* 熊脂：寒熱羸瘦，頭瘍白禿，面**皯皰**, "Alternating sensations of cold and heat with emaciation, head ulcers and baldness, facial **gloom and blisters**".

***Gan pao* 鼾皰, [facial] gloom and blisters** [3]
PC CD of → *mian gan* 面鼾, facial gloom, and → *mian pao* 面皰, facial blisters. *YXL* SE *gao ben* 藁本：通血，去頭風，**鼾皰**, "It makes blood flow and eliminates head wind with **[facial] gloom and blisters**".

***Gan qi* 疳氣, *gan*-illness qi** [19]
PC identical with → *gan* 疳, *gan*-illness. *HYBC* SE *a le bo* 阿勒勃：子療小兒**疳氣**, "The seeds cure ***gan*-illness qi** in children".

***Gan re* 疳熱, *gan*-illness with heat** [12] AN *re gan* 熱疳, heat-type *gan*-illness.
PC of → *gan* 疳, *gan*-illness, associated with an inner abundance of depletion heat in children. *YXL* SE *qing dai* 青黛：能解小兒**疳熱**消瘦, "Able to dissolve ***gan*-illness with heat** with emaciation in children".

***Gan re* 肝熱, heat in the liver; liver heat** [16]
① AN *gan huo* 肝火, liver fire. PC of heat-type diseases affecting the liver. *SW* 32: **肝熱**病者左頰先赤, "In the case of **liver heat** disease, the left cheek becomes red first".
② EA bringing forth heat-type disease in the eyes. *BCGM* emphasizes the latter with 16 references, all related to eye disease. E.g. *BCGM* SE *huang lian* 黄連：況眼疾本於**肝熱**，肝與心為子母。心火也，肝亦火也，腎孤臟也，人患一水不勝二火。豈可久服苦藥，使心有所偏勝，是以火救火，其可乎, "Also, eye afflictions originate from **heat in the liver**. The relationship between the liver and heart is that of a son and mother. The heart is fire; the liver, too, is fire. The kidneys are an orphan depot. When a person suffers from a situation where one water cannot overcome two fires, how could it be right to ingest bitter medication? This would make the heart dominate unilaterally, that is, one would rescue [the patient] from fire by means of fire. How could this be?".

***Gan se* 乾澀, desiccated and rough** [2]
EA of a depletion of body liquids and dryness, and hence causes in the birth canal a roughness that cannot be smoothed, which in turn brings about difficult births, the inability of a dead fetus to pass down, or constipation. *ZBYHL* 43: 穢露早下，致子道**乾澀**，產婦力疲，皆令難也, "If water breaks too early this may make the birth canal **desiccated and rough**, so that giving birth requires strength and is tiring. All this makes [birth] more difficult".

***Gan shi* 疳蝕, *gan*-illness with erosion** [24]
PC identical with → *gan chuang* 疳瘡, *gan*-illness sores. *TBC* SE *fei lian* 飛廉：用葉莖及根，療**疳蝕**，殺蟲, "One makes use of its leaves, stem and root to cure ***gan*-illness with erosion**. It kills worms".

***Gan shi* 疳濕, *gan*-illness with moisture** [2]
PC identical with → *gan chuang* 疳瘡, *gan*-illness sores. *ZBYHL* 50: **疳濕**之病…其上蝕者，則口鼻齒齦生瘡；其下蝕者，則肛門傷爛，皆難治, "The disease of ***gan*-illness with moisture**. ...If the erosion affects the upper body parts, sores develop at the mouth, the nose, the teeth, and the gums. In case it affects the lower body parts, the anus will be harmed and festers. All these conditions are difficult to cure".

***Gan shi er xuan* 乾濕二癬, the two types of dry and moist *xuan*-illness** [1]
PC identical with → *gan shi xuan* 乾濕癬, dry and moist *xuan*-illness. *TBC* SE *dong bi tu* 東壁土：此土摩**乾濕二癬**，極有效也, "Smear this soil on **the two types of dryness and moisture *xuan*-illness**. The effect is extraordinary".

***Gan shi jiao qi* 乾濕脚氣, dry and moist leg qi** [4]
PC CD of → *gan jiao qi* 乾脚氣, dry leg qi, and → *shi jiao qi* 濕脚氣, moist leg qi. *SLBC* SE *yi yi ren* 薏苡仁：去**乾濕脚氣**，大驗, "It eliminates **dry and moist leg qi**. Very effective".

***Gan shi xuan* 乾濕癬, dry and moist *xuan*-illness** [1]
PC CD of → *gan xuan* 乾癬, dry *xuan*-illness, and *shi xuan* 濕癬, moist *xuan*-illness. *WTMY* 30 lists **乾濕癬**方一十五首, "15 recipes for **dry and moist *xuan*-illness**".

***Gan shou* 疳瘦, *gan*-illness with emaciation** [10]
PC identical with → *gan* 疳, *gan*-illness. *YXL* SE *chan chu* 蟾蜍：小孩子**疳瘦**者，空心一丸, "For children suffering from ***gan*-illness with emaciation**, one pill on an empty stomach".

***Gan shui* 疳水, *gan*-illness water** [2]
PC of *gan*-illness where the entire body is swollen and the skin has turned yellow. *YYXS* 32: 小兒腫滿一如吹，只為風邪與氣為。若見皮膚熟李樣，此名**疳水**定無疑, "When children are completely swollen as if inflated, this can have been brought forth only by wind evil and qi. If the skin appears like ripe plums, this is definitely ***gan*-illness water**".

***Gan tong* 乾痛, desiccation and pain** [3]
IS identical with → *zao tong* 燥痛, dryness and pain. *TBC* SE *zuo ye he cao* 昨葉何草：主口中**乾痛**，水穀血痢，止血, "It controls **desiccation and pain** in the mouth, bloody free-flux illness of solid and liquid food; it stops bleeding".

***Gan xie* 疳瀉, *gan*-illness outflow** [7] AW *gan xie* 疳泄.
PC of outflow brought forth by → *gan* 疳, *gan*-illness. This is a diarrhea associated with yellow complexion, emaciation and loss of hair, as well as an enlarged abdomen because of [the child patient's] having eaten soil. *HYBC* SE *wu yi* 蕪荑：孩子**疳瀉**，得訶子、豆蔻良, "For ***gan*-illness outflow** in children take *he zi* and *dou kou liang*".

Gan xie **疳泄, *gan*-illness outflow** [3]

PC identical with → *gan xie* 疳瀉. *BCGM* Bai bing zhu zhi yao 百病主治藥 quoting *HYBC* SE *wu yi* 蕪荑：小兒疳瀉writes: 小兒**疳泄**, "Children's ***gan*-illness outflow**".

Gan xu **肝虛, liver depletion** [35]

PC of liver depletion with an impediment of liver functions. *SW* 76: **肝虛**、腎虛、脾虛，皆令人體重煩冤, "**Liver depletion**, kidney depletion, spleen depletion, all [these conditions] make a person's body become heavy; they [cause feelings of] vexation and grievance".

Gan xuan **乾癬, dry *xuan*-illness** [1]

PC of → *xuan* 癬, *xuan*-illness, with a dry, itching skin. If scratched it sheds a white scaling. *ZBYHL* 35: **乾癬**，但有匡郭，皮枯索，癢，搔之白屑出是也, "**Dry *xuan*-illness**: it has just one outer wall, the skin is dried up, it itches, and when scratched it sheds a white scaling".

Gan xue qi **乾血氣, desiccated blood and qi** [7]

PC of a feeling of abdominal lumps and → *bi jing* 閉經, blocked menstruation, resulting from an internal stagnation of blood flow. *SWBJQYBMJ* Lj RE *hong hua san* 紅花散, powder with *hong hua*: 月事不調，遠年**乾血氣**，皆治之, "When the monthly affair is irregular, and if [a woman has suffered from] **desiccated blood and qi** for many years, all this is cured by it".

Gan yan **疳眼, *gan*-illness eye** [5] AN *yan gan* 眼疳, ocular *gan*-illness.

PC of → *gan* 疳, *gan*-illness, together with itching eyes that are red, fester and develop ulcers, or sometimes grow a shade, with harm inflicted to the eyes. *TPSHF* 89: 治小兒雀目及**疳眼**，宜服煮肝石決明散方, "To cure sparrow eye and ***gan*-illness eye** in children, the recipe to ingest the powder with cooked liver and *shi jue ming* is advisable".

Gan yue **乾嘔, dry retching** [2]

IS identical with → *yue* 嘔, retching. *BCGM* SE *ban xia* 半夏 quoting *WTMY* 傷寒病嘔, "Harm caused by cold disease, retching". writes: 傷寒**乾嘔**, "Harm caused by cold, **dry retching**".

Gan yu **肝鬱, pent-up liver [qi]** [1]

EA of mental blockage with liver qi accumulation. *DXSJ* Mj: 怒氣大逆，**肝鬱**木盛, "Anger makes qi massively rise contrary to its regular direction; there is **pent-up liver [qi]** and an abundance of wood [qi]".

Gan zao **肝燥, liver dryness** [8]

PC brought forth by a loss and depletion of liver blood. *MYZZ* 4: 前症若因腎虛陰火而**肝燥**者，宜用六味地黃丸，生腎水，滋肝血, "If the conditions described above are associated with **liver dryness** brought forth by kidney depletion and yin fire, it is advisable to use the pills with the six ingredients including *di huang* to generate kidney water which in turn will provide moisture to the liver blood".

***Gan zeng* 皯䵳, dermal dark spots** [33] AN *gan zeng* 奸䵳; *que ban* 雀斑, sparrow speckles; *que luan ban* 雀卵斑, sparrow egg speckles; *fen zi* 粉滓, dregs; *mian yun* 面䵳, facial speckles; AD *zeng* 䵳, speckles.

PC of numerous dark spots appearing on one's face. *QJYF* 6: 治人面**皯䵳**黑，膚色粗陋，皮厚狀丑方, "Recipe for thick skin and an unsightly appearance to cure facial **dermal dark spots**, associated with coarse and crude skin".

***Gan zeng* 奸䵳, dermal dark speckles** [4]

PC identical with → 皯䵳. *ZLBC* SE *gu yang jiao* 羖羊角 quotes *ZHF*: 療面多**奸䵳**如雀卵色。以羖羊膽一枚，酒二升，合煮三沸以塗拭之，日三度，差, "To cure numerous **dermal dark speckles** in one's face with the color of sparrow eggs, take 1 *gu yang* gallbladder and heat with 2 *sheng* of wine three times until boiling. Then apply externally three times daily. This will bring the cure".

***Gan zhi* 疳痔, *gan*-illness and piles** [2]

PC CD of → *gan* 疳, *gan*-illness, and → *zhi* 痔, piles. *BCGM* SE *qiu* 楸 quoting *BCSY*: 傅惡瘡疽瘺，癧腫疳野雞病, "Externally apply to malign sores, impediment-illnesses, fistula, obstruction-illnesses, swelling, *gan*-illness and chicken disease". writes: 惡瘡疽瘺，癧腫**疳痔**, "Malign sores, impediment-illnesses, fistula, obstruction-illnesses, swelling, ***gan*-illness and piles**".

***Gang jing* 剛痙, hard spasms** [1]

PC of → *jing bing* 痙病, spasms disease, with the special characteristic of fever without sweating and an aversion to cold. *JGYL* Fj: 太陽病，發熱無汗，反惡寒者，名曰**剛痙**, "If someone suffers from a major yang disease, with an effusion of heat but without sweating and with an abnormal aversion to cold, this is called '**hard spasms**'".

***Gao dan* 膏癉, pasty *dan*-illness** [1]

PC of patients drinking little and yet passing urine copiously. *ZLBC* SE *qin jiao* 秦椒 quotes *SHLY*: 治**膏癉**，其人飲少小便多方, "Recipe to cure **pasty *dan*-illness**. Persons afflicted with this drink little while they discharge urine copiously".

***Gao lin* 膏淋, pasty dripping** [14]

PC of → *lin bing* 淋病, dripping disease, with urine appearing turbid like water in which rice has been washed or oily like a fatty paste. *ZBYHL* 14: **膏淋**者，淋而有肥，狀似膏, "**Pasty dripping**, this is dripping urine with fat; it has the appearance of a paste".

***Ge bing* 膈病, occlusion disease** [2]

PC identical with → *ge qi* 膈氣, occlusion qi. *SJZL* 62: 五種雖殊，其為**膈病**則一, "The five types may be different, but they all alike constitute occlusion disease".

***Ge pi* 膈痞, diaphragm obstacle-illness** [2] AN *ge yong* 膈壅, diaphragm obstruction.

IS of a feeling of distension, fullness, and congestion in the chest and diaphragm region. *BCGM* SE *yang* 羊 quoting *DNBS* 治老人胸滿痞塞，食飲不下, "To cure old people with fullness and blockage in their chest who are unable to pass down food and beverages". writes: 老人**膈痞**，不下飲食, "When old people have a **diaphragm obstacle-illness** they are unable to pass down beverages and food".

Ge qi **膈氣, occlusion qi** [39] AD *ge* 膈; AN *ge zhong* 膈中, occluded center; *ge bing* 膈病, occlusion disease.

PC of a → *ye ge* 噎膈, gullet occlusion, a disease situated in the chest and diaphragm region with a sensation of an obstacle in the chest, heart-pressure, and pain, and a failure of beverages and food to move through a blocked esophagus. *ZBYHL* 13: 陰陽不和，而腑臟生病，結於胸膈之間，故稱為**膈氣**, "When yin and yang are out of harmony, and depots and palaces generate a disease, this leads to [qi] nodes in the region of the chest and diaphragm. Hence this is called **occlusion qi**".

Ge re **膈熱, diaphragm heat** [13]

① PC of heat-type diseases affecting the regions above and below the diaphragm. *XMLF* 9 *run fei san* 潤肺散, powder to moisten the lung: 治小兒**膈熱**, "It cures **diaphragm heat** in children".

② IS of heat in the regions above and below the diaphragm. *XMLF* 4: „眩悸**膈熱**，坐臥不寧, "[Patients experience] dizziness, palpitation, **diaphragm heat**, and are unable to sit or lie calmly".

Ge xiao **膈消, diaphragm melting** [2]

PC identical with → *shang xiao* 上消①，upper melting. *SWBJQYBMJ* Xiao ke lun: 上消者上焦受病，又謂之**膈消**病也。多飲水而少食，大便如常，或小便清利，知其燥在上焦也, "In the case of 'upper melting' the upper burner has been affected by a disease. It is also called *ge xiao bing* 膈消病, disease of **diaphragm melting**. [Patients] drink a lot of water, and eat little. Defecation is normal. In some cases urine is clear and passes freely. This indicates that the upper burner is affected by dryness".

Ge xiao wu du **歌笑無度, excessive singing and laughing** [1]

IS of a mental disturbance with patients singing and laughing beyond normality. *SYXJ* SE *hu* 狐：治驚癎，神情恍惚，語言錯謬，**歌笑無度**, "It cures fright with epilepsy, absent-mindedness, muddled and delirious language, as well as **excessive singing and laughing**".

Ge ye **膈噎, occluded gullet** [2]

PC identical with *ye ge* 噎膈, gullet occlusion. *JSF* Ou tu fan wei ge ye men 嘔吐翻胃噎膈門：陰陽平匀，氣順痰下，**膈噎**之疾無由作矣, "When yin and yang are balanced, when the qi follows its proper course and phlegm moves downwards, the ailment of **occluded gullet** has no cause from which it could emerge".

Ge yong **膈壅, diaphragm obstruction** [1]

IS identical with → *ge pi* 膈痞, diaphram obstacle-illness. *SJZL* 59: 治熱盛夢泄，怔忪恍惚，**膈壅**舌乾，清心丸方, "To cure abounding heat with dream efflux, panicking with absent-mindedness, and **diaphragm obstruction** with a dry tongue, [ingest] the recipe for pills to clear the heart".

Ge zhong **膈中, occluded center** [2]

PC identical with → *ge qi* 膈氣, occlusion qi. *LS* 4: (脾脈) 微急為**膈中**，食飲入而還出, "When [the movement in the vessels associated with the spleen] is slightly urgent, this is [the disease of] **occluded center**. Food and beverages enter [the throat] and are thrown out again".

Geng **哽, choking [on a foreign object stuck] in the gullet** [p]

① AN *geng* 鯁, fishbone stuck in the throat.
PC identical with → *geng yan* 哽咽. *WTMY* 8: 又療食**哽**方，鷹糞燒灰存性，"Another recipe to cure food **choking**: roast eagle feces to ashes while retaining its nature".
② EA of choking caused by a foreign object stuck in the throat. *WTMY* 8: 禮云'魚去乙'，謂其頭間有骨如乙字形者，**哽**入不肯出故也, "The *Li* [*ji*] states: 'From a fish remove the *yi*.' That is to say, in its head it has a bone shaped like the character *yi*. It is the reason of **choking**, as it enters [the throat] but does not leave it".

Geng **鯁, choking; fishbone stuck in the throat** [p]

① PC identical with → *geng* 哽①, choking on food stuck in the gullet. *SJZL*124: 治一切**鯁**，萞麻丸方：萞麻仁、細麴。右二味等分研細，用沙糖和丸如皂子大，以綿裹含之，痰出立效, "Recipe for pills with bi ma to cure all types of **choking**: *bi ma* seeds, yeast of best quality. Grind equal amounts of these two items to a fine powder and use granulated sugar to prepare pills the size of *zao* [jia] seeds. Wrap them in silk floss and have [the patient] hold them in his mouth. Once he emits phlegm there will be an immediate effect".
② EA of foreign objects causing choking. *ZHF* 6: 小嚼薤白令柔，以繩系中，持繩端，吞薤到**鯁**處，引之，**鯁**當隨出, "Chew the white part of a scallion a bit until it has softened. Then tie a string around it and, holding the end of the string, swallow the scallion until it has reached the location where the **object is stuck in the throat**. Then pull it out again, and the **object stuck in the throat** will follow it and be released".

Geng gu **哽骨, choking from a bone** [1]

PC identical with → *gu geng* 骨哽. *BCGM* SE *qian guang shi* 鉛光石：主**哽骨**, "It controls **choking on a bone**".

Geng yan **哽咽, choking [on a foreign object stuck] in the gullet** [28] AD *geng* 哽.

PC of choking caused by a foreign object stuck in the throat. *WTMY* 8: 療骨**哽咽**不得下飲食方, "Recipe to cure **choking** on a bone stuck **in the gullet** causing an inability to ingest beverages and food".

Geng yan **鯁咽, choking on a fishbone stuck in the gullet** [3]

PC of → *geng yan* 哽咽, choking, caused by a fishbone stuck in the throat. *BCGM* SE *yi tang* 飴糖 quoting *ZHF* 魚骨哽在喉中, "Choking on a fishbone stuck in the throat". writes: 魚骨**鯁咽**, "**Choking on a fishbone stuck in the gullet**".

***Geng ye* 哽噎, choking from gullet occlusion** [5]

① PC of an uncomfortable feeling of distension and pain in the throat and esophagus blocked by some item. *BJ* SE *lou gu* 螻蛄：主產難，出肉中刺，潰癰腫，下**哽噎**，解毒，除惡瘡, "It controls difficult birth, eliminates thorns from one's flesh, opens obstruction-illnesses and swelling; brings down **choking from gullet occlusion**, dissolves poison, and removes malign sores".

② IS identical with → *ye sai* 噎塞②, gullet occlusion with blockage. *BCGM* SE *tuan* 猯 quoting *WTMY* 28: 胸中忽然或哽入咽，怵怵如蟲行, "Suddenly in the chest there may be choking because [something] has entered the throat. This is as startling as if bugs/worms were moving there". writes: 胸中**哽噎**，怵怵如蟲行, "**Choking from gullet occlusion** in the chest; this is as startling as if bugs/worms were moving there".

***Gong tong* 攻痛, beating pain** [4]

IS of pain accompanied by a sensation as if one had been beaten. *WTMY* 23: 文仲療喉中卒毒**攻痛**方, "Wenzhong's recipe for curing a **beating pain** brought forth suddenly by poison in the throat".

***Gou xian* 狗癇, dog epilepsy** [1]

PC of a → *dian xian* 癲癇, peak-illness with epilepsy, which, at the time of its outbreaks, makes the patient's four limbs twitch, accompanied by his making sounds that resemble the barking of dogs. *SJZL* 171: **狗癇**即狗吠, "**Dog epilepsy**, that is, barking [like a] dog".

Gu* 蠱, *gu [p]

① EA PC AD of → *gu du* 蠱毒, *gu poison*. *ZHF* 7: 人有養蓄**蠱**以病患…欲知蠱與非蠱，當令病患唾水中，沉者是，浮者非， "Someone has raised a ***gu*** to have [a third person] suffer from a [*gu*-]disease. …If one wishes to know whether it indeed is *gu* or not, one has the patient spit into water. If the spittle sinks into the depth, it is [*gu*]; if it floats on the surface, it is not".

② IS identical with → *gu zhang* 蠱脹， *gu*-distension. *SJZL* 191: 男子如**蠱**，女子如妊娠, "In males it appear like ***gu***; in females it appears like a pregnancy". The most ancient form of the character *gu* 蠱 shows three worms/snakes in a vessel. Some people who are after the belongings of others are said to bring all possible poisonous snakes/worms/bugs into a vessel and bury it for 100 days. When the vessel is opened again, the most poisonous creature has survived by devouring all the others. This, then, is the *gu*, the manifestation of a spirit requiring a human host to proliferate. Those who manage to bring this creature into someone else's food so that the *gu*-spirit may use that person as its host, they will be rewarded by the spirit with the riches of that person.

***Gu* 瞽, blind** [5]

PC AD of → *shi ming* 失明, loss of vision. *QJYF* 27: 以明鑒給矇**瞽**，以絲竹娛聾夫, "They provide the illiterate and **blind** with a bright mirror, and they amuse the deaf with musical instruments".

Gu bi 骨痹, bone blockage [2]

PC of a → 痹① a), blockage disease, resulting from an intrusion of wind, cold, and moisture into the bones, resulting in discomfort and pain in one's skeletal structure, and a feeling of heaviness in the limbs, which cannot be raised. *SW* 55: 病在骨，骨重不可舉，骨髓酸痛，寒氣至，名曰**骨痹**, "When the disease is in the bones, [with the patient experiencing his] bones being so heavy that he cannot lift them and the bones and marrow are sore and in pain, [this results] from extreme cold qi. [The disease] is named **bone blockage**".

***Gu bing* 故病, old disease** [2]

PC identical with → *su ji* 宿疾, abiding ailment. *BCGM* Xu li 序例：**故病**未已，新病復起, "The **old disease** has not ended yet, and a new disease arises already".

***Gu cao feng* 骨槽風, bone socket wind** [3]

PC of festering gums eventually harming the premolar teeth. *TPSHF* 34 RE *ding xiang san* 丁香散, powder with *ding xiang*: **骨槽風**，膿血不止, "**Bone socket wind**, with unending pus and blood flow".

***Gu cao lao chou* 骨槽勞臭, bone socket exhaustion stench** [1]

PC of bones in the tooth sockets rotting and emitting pus and foul stench, with no cure possible for an extended period of time. *HYBC* SE *ding xiang* 丁香：主風疳䘌，**骨槽勞臭**, "It controls wind *gan*-illness with hidden bugs/worms and **bone socket exhaustion stench**".

***Gu chuang* 骨瘡, bone sores** [1]

PC identical with → *gu ju* 骨疽, bone impediment-illness. *BCGM* SE *shui she* 水蛇：小兒**骨瘡**：海上方詩云：小兒骨痛不堪言，出血流膿實可憐, "**Bone sores** among children: A poem in the *Hai shang fang* states: The pain in the bones of children is undescribable; blood flow and putrescence are truly pitiable".

***Gu dan* 穀疸, grain *dan*-illness** [8] AN *gu huang* 穀黃, grain jaundice; *shi huang* 食黃, food jaundice

PC of → *huang dan* 黃疸, yellow *dan*-illness, resulting from a consumption of inappropriate beverages and food. *JGYL* Mj: 穀氣不消，胃中苦濁…身體盡黃，名曰**穀疸**, "The qi of grain is not dissolved and there is a turbidity in the stomach. ...The entire body is yellow. This is called '**grain *dan*-illness**'".

***Gu du* 蠱毒, *gu* poison; *gu* poisoning** [240] AD *gu* 蠱. AN *du gu* 毒蠱, poisonous *gu*; *gui gu* 鬼蠱, demon-*gu*; *gu qi* 蠱氣, *gu*-qi.

① EA assumed – since ancient times – to be a type of poison emitted by certain worms/snakes with an ability to produce varying changes, eventually leading to illness, in a person who has taken it in by means of wine or food. *ZHF* 7: 療飲中**蠱毒**，令人腹內堅痛，面目青黃，淋露骨立，病變無常方, "Recipe to heal unusual pathological changes such as ***gu* poison** taken in by a drink, with the result that this person feels hardening and pain in his abdomen, with his face and eyes turning greenish-yellow, [sweat] dripping [like] dew drops, and an emaciation to the bones".

② AN *gu zhu* 蠱疰, *gu*-attachment-illness; *zhong gu* 中蠱, *gu*-stroke; *gu ji* 蠱疾, *gu*-ailment. PC of abdominal fullness with accumulations, pain and emaciation brought forth by ***gu* poison**, in some cases with blood spitting, and blood in the stool and urine. The illness takes many different forms. *ZHF* 7: 療**蠱毒**下血方, "Recipe for curing ***gu* poisoning** with discharge of blood".

Gu feng **骨風, bone wind** [2]

PC of swollen and painful knees, calves, and feet, with difficulties in bending and stretching one's legs. *BCTJ* SE *shui ying* 水英：丈夫、婦人無故兩脚腫滿，連膝脛中痛，屈伸急強者，名**骨風**, "If men or women without apparent cause experience swelling of both feet, with pain reaching into the calves and knees, and bending and stretching [are hampered by] stiffness, this is called '**bone wind**'".

Gu geng **骨哽, choking on a bone** [62] AW *geng gu* 哽骨; *gu geng* 骨鯁; *gu geng* 骨骾.

PC of an animal bone stuck in the throat and causing choking, with major signs including throat closure with pain, inability to swallow, and an inability to dislodge the bone. *WTMY* 8: 療食諸肉**骨哽**方，白雄雞左右翮大毛各一枚燒末，水服一刀圭也, "Recipe to cure **choking on a bone** when eating meat: burn one feather of the left and right wings of a white rooster to a powder and ingest with water the amount one can scoop up with a knife's blade. Excellent".

Gu geng **骨鯁, choking on a bone** [27]

PC identical with → 骨哽. *ZHF* 6: 療**骨鯁**，仍取所余者骨，左右手，反覆擲背後，立出, "To cure **choking on a bone**: Take the remaining bones and with the left and right hand repeatedly throw them behind your back. [The bone stuck in the throat] will appear immediately".

Gu geng **骨骾, choking on a bone** [1]

PC identical with → *gu geng* 骨哽. *BCGM* SE *sang du chong* 桑蠹蟲 quotes *YLQF*: 咽喉**骨骾**：桑木上蟲糞，米醋煎呷, "For **choking on a bone** in the throat: boil the droppings from bugs/worms on a mulberry tree with rice and vinegar, and sip".

Gu huang **穀黄, grain jaundice** [2]

PC identical with → *gu dan* 穀疸, grain *dan*-illness. *YXL* SE *bai xian pi* 白鮮皮：主解熱黄、酒黄、急黄、**穀黄**、勞黄等, "It controls dissolution of heat jaundice, wine jaundice, acute jaundice, **grain jaundice**, and exhaustion jaundice".

Gu huang **食黄, food jaundice** [6]

PC identical with → *gu dan* 穀疸, grain *dan*-illness. *TPSHF* 55: 治**食黄**，腹中結燥，茅根散方, "To cure **food jaundice**, with abdominal nodes and dryness, [use the] recipe for the powder with *mao gen*".

Gu ji **故疾, abiding ailment** [2]

PC identical with → *su ji* 宿疾. *BCYY* SE *shu mi* 稷米：然發**故疾**，只堪為飯, "However, as it brings forth **abiding ailments**, it may only be used for [ordinary] food".

Gu ji **痼疾, ailment of obstinacy-illness** [31]
PC a) identical with → *su ji* 宿疾, abiding ailment. *MYBL* SE *fang feng* 防風：叉尾者，發**痼疾**, "Those with a forked 'tail' bring forth **ailments of obstinacy-illness**". b) CD of stubborn ailments that are difficult to heal. *MYBL* SE *dan shen* 丹參：去心腹**痼疾**, "It removes **ailment of obstinacy-illness** from heart and abdomen".

Gu ji **蠱疾, *gu*-ailment** [2]
PC identical with → *gu du* 蠱毒②, *gu poison*. *PJF* 174: 治誤食頭髮如**蠱疾**者，右用雄黃研細，水飛過，酒調服，吐出惡物乃愈, "To cure something resembling ***gu*-ailment** following mistaken consumption of human hair. [For these indications listed] above, one uses finely ground *xiong huang*, refined with water, and ingests it mixed with wine. [Patients] will vomit the malign items and this is the cure".

Gu jie **蠱疥, *gu jie*-illness** [1]
PC identical with → *jie chuang* 疥瘡, *jie*-illness sores. *TBC* SE *gou she cao* 狗舌草：主**蠱疥**瘙瘡，殺小蟲, "It controls itching and sores associated with ***gu jie*-illness**, and it kills small bugs/worms".

Gu jie feng **骨節風, bone-joints wind** [9]
PC, brought forth by wind evil, of pain in one's joints and difficulties to move. *BCSY* SE *mi hou tao* 獼猴桃：主**骨節風**，癱緩不隨, "It controls **bone-joints wind** and paralysis".

Gu ju **骨疽, bone impediment-illness** [21]
PC of → *ju* 疽, impediment-illness, developing at a bone or in the vicinity of bones, with the opening of the sores festering for a long time without closing to heal. In some cases such abscesses appear healed and will break open again. Also, together with the pus they release bits and pieces. *ZBYHL* 32: **骨疽**膿出不可止者，出碎骨, "When in the case of **bone impediment-illness** pus leaves without end, it will emit fragments of bones".

Gu lao **穀勞, grain exhaustion** [1]
EA of immoderate eating and drinking. *BCGM* SE *nie mi* 糵米：**穀勞**嗜臥，飽食便臥，得穀勞病, "**Grain exhaustion** and a desire to lie down: If one has eaten to fullness and lies down immediately, he is affected by grain exhaustion disease".

Gu lao bing **穀勞病, food exhaustion disease** [1]
PC brought forth by immoderate eating and drinking, as well as depletion weakness of the spleen and stomach, with a feeling of heavy limbs and a desire to sleep, especially after meals. *ZHF* 4: 治飽食便臥，得**穀勞病**，令人四肢煩重，嘿嘿欲臥，食畢輒甚方, "Recipe to cure **food exhaustion disease** brought forth by eating to fullness followed by immediate rest. It makes a person have an uncomfortable feeling of heaviness of his four limbs. [Patients] are quiet and wish to lie down".

Gu leng **痼冷, obstinacy-illness cold** [14] AN → *chen han* 沉寒, deep-seated cold.
PC brought forth by cold evil abiding deep in the body for an extended period of time. *QJYF* 16: 治心腹**痼冷**，百治不瘥方, "Cures **obstinacy-illness cold** in the heart and abdominal region; a recipe for all types of treatments [of diseases] that otherwise cannot be cured".

Gu li **骨立, emaciation to the bones** [11]
IS of the skeleton becoming visible and a skinny physical appearance as a consequence of extreme emaciation. *ZHF* 7: 療飲中蠱毒，令人腹內堅痛，面目青黃，淋露**骨立**，病變無常方, "Recipe to heal unusual pathological changes such as *gu* poison taken in a drink, with the result that this person feels hardening and pain in his abdomen, with his face and eyes turning greenish-yellow, [sweat] dripping [like] dew drops, and an **emaciation to the bones**".

Gu li **蠱痢, *gu* free-flux illness** [6]
PC of → *li ji* 痢疾, free-flux illness ailment, with pus and blood, including pieces of coagulated blood looking like chicken or duck liver. *SJZL* 77: 凡下痢膿血間雜瘀黑有片，如雞鴨肝，與血皆下者，**蠱痢**也, "Whenever discharge with free-flux illness shows pus and blood mixed with pieces of black coagulates looking like chicken or duck liver that are discharged together with the blood, this is ***gu*** **free-flux illness**".

Gu qi **蠱氣, *gu*-qi** [6]
EA PC identical with → *gu du* 蠱毒, *gu poison*. *MYBL* SE *jiao yu pi* 鮫魚皮：主**蠱氣**，蠱疰方用之, "It controls ***gu*-qi**; in recipes for *gu*-attachment-illness one makes use of it". *RHZ* SE *chun* 蓴：解百藥毒並**蠱氣**, "It dissolves all types of pharmaceutical poisons and also ***gu*-qi**".

Gu re **痼熱, obstinacy-illness heat** [3] AW → *gu re* 固熱, obstinate heat.
PC of heat-type illnesses that have deeply penetrated the human body and continue for long without being cured. *MYBL* SE *li he ren* 李核仁：實，味苦，除**痼熱**, "The fruit has a bitter flavor; it eliminates **stubborn heat**".

Gu re **固熱, obstinate heat** [1]
PC identical with → *gu re* 痼熱, obstinacy-illness heat. *MYBL* SE *fan shi* 礬石：除**固熱**在骨髓, "It eliminates **obstinate heat** in the bone marrow".

Gu re **骨熱, bone heat** [18]
IS of an uncomfortable feeling of vexing heat in the bones and joints. *QJYF* 19: 腰背強急，體重**骨熱**, "Lower back and spine are stiff and tense. The body feels heavy and has **bone heat**".

Gu ruan **骨軟, bone softness** [3]
PC identical with → *ruan jiao* 軟脚, soft legs. *BCGM* SE *he shou wu* 何首烏 quotes *JYF*: **骨軟**風疾，腰膝疼，行步不得, "In the case of **bone softness** wind ailment, the lumbar region and the knees ache, and one is unable to walk".

Gu sui **骨碎, compound fracture** [4]
PC of → *gu zhe* 骨折, bone fracture, with the bone(s) broken to many pieces. *QJYF* 25: 治腕折，四肢**骨碎**, "To cure wrist fracture, and **compound fracture** of any of the four extremities".

Gu tong **鼓痛, drum[-like distension] with pain** [2]
IS identical with → *zhang tong* 脹痛, distension with pain. *MYBL* SE *ren shen* 人參：療腸胃中冷，心腹**鼓痛**，胸脅逆滿, "It cures cold in stomach and intestines, **drum[-like distension] with pain** in the region of heart and abdomen, as well as [qi] moving contrary to its normal direction and causing a feeling of fullness in chest and flanks".

Gu wei **骨痿, bone dysfunction** [6]
IS of a dysfunction disease brought forth by kidney depletion and internal heat, sometimes with heat evil having harmed the kidneys, and an internal wasting away of yin essence and bone marrow. *SW* 44: 腎氣熱，則腰脊不舉，骨枯而髓減，發為**骨痿**, "When the kidney qi is hot, the lower back and the spine cannot be raised. The bones dry and the marrow decreases. This develops into **bone dysfunction**".

Gu xu **骨虛, bone depletion** [1]
PC of pain in the bones and teeth associated with a depletion of bone marrow. *ZBYHL* 29: 齒者，骨之所終，髓之所養，髓弱**骨虛**，風氣客之，則齒齼, "Teeth are the end of bones. They are nourished by marrow. When the marrow is weak, and the **bones are depleted**, and when wind qi enters to reside there, the teeth will have a feeling as if exposed to sour flavor".

Gu zei **穀賊, grain intrusion** [10]
PC of swelling and pain in the gullet resulting from an inadvertent ingestion of awns or spikes of cereals. *TPSHF* 35: 禾裹有短穗而強澀者是也。誤作米而食之，則令喉裏腫結不通，致風熱氣衝於喉間，與血氣相搏，則生腫結，如食飲，疼痛妨悶，故謂之**穀賊**, "When standing grain is bound, this includes those short spikes that are stiff and rough. If in the preparation of rice they are mistakenly included they cause swelling and nodes in the gullet, blocking passages through it. This leads to a rush of wind and heat qi into the gullet which clashes with blood and qi there. This generates swelling and nodes. Drinking and eating causes pain. [The gullet] is sealed and [patients experience] heart-pressure. Hence one calls this '**grain intrusion**'".

Gu zhang **鼓脹, drum[-like] distension** [34]
① AN *gu zhang* 蠱脹, *gu*-distension; *shui zhang* 水脹, water distension; *shui gu* 水蠱, water *gu*. PC of an abdominal distension and big upswell brought forth by stagnant water qi accumulating in the abdomen. *SW* 40: 黃帝問曰：有病心腹滿，旦食則不能暮食，此為何病？岐伯對曰：名為**鼓脹**, "Huang Di: "Someone suffers from [the following]: the heart and abdomen are full [to the extent that] if one has had breakfast, one cannot eat in the evening. Which disease is that". Qi Bo responded: "The name is **drum[-like] distension**".
② IS of a feeling of abdominal distension and extreme fullness. *ZBYHL* 4: 體熱如火，煩躁無汗，心腹**鼓脹**，食即欲嘔，小便如血，大便秘澀, "The body is hot like fire, with vexation, but no sweating. Heart and abdomen have **drum[-like] distension**. When one eats one has an urge to vomit. The urine resembles blood. Defecation is blocked and rough".

Gu zhang **蠱脹, *gu*-distension** [5]
PC identical with → *gu zhang* 鼓脹①. *SJZL* 72: 治虛積食氣，**蠱脹**水氣，年深癥癖，五食丸方, "To cure depletion with food qi accumulation, ***gu*-distension**, and water qi, as well as long-term concretion-illness and aggregation-illness, the recipe for the 'pills with the five victuals' [is appropriate]".

Gu zhe **骨折, bone fracture** [9]
PC of a comminuted or complete bone fracture, with pain, swelling, purple coloring, functional impairment, deformity and sounds of bones rubbing against each other. *WTMY* 29: 救急療**骨折**，接令如故，不限人畜也方, "Recipe for treating humans and animals in emergency cases of **bone fractures** restoring the same condition as before".

Gu zheng **骨蒸, bone steaming** [126]
① PC of an infectious consumptive disease with a development of vexing heat in the afternoon. The Song-era physician Chen Yan 陳言 assumed that it is identical with → *lao zhai* 勞瘵, exhaustion consumption. *ZBYHL* 4: **骨蒸**，其根在腎，旦起體涼，日晚即熱，煩躁，寢不能安，食無味，小便赤黃，忽忽煩亂，細喘無力，腰疼，兩足逆冷，手心常熱, "**Bone steaming**: its root lies in the kidneys. In the morning, when [the patient] rises, the body is cool. In the evening it is hot. [Patients] experience vexation and if they lie down they cannot find rest. Food appears to have no flavor; the urine is red-yellow. Every now and then the vexation turns into disorder. [Patients] pant mildly with no strength. Their lower back aches. The two feet are cold with countermovement [of qi], and the palms are often hot".
② IS of heat and vexation with a feeling as if this originated in the bones. *QJYF* 10: 茵陳丸，治急黃，熱氣**骨蒸**，兩目赤脈方, "Pills with *yin chen*, a recipe to cure acute jaundice and heat qi with **bone steaming**, with red vessels in both eyes".

Gu zheng lao **骨蒸勞, exhaustion because of bone steaming** [4]
PC identical with → *chuan shi* 傳屍, corpse [evil] transmission. *RHZ* SE *huang qi* 黃芪：治血及煩悶熱毒，**骨蒸勞**, "It cures [ailments associated with] blood as well as vexation and heart-pressure associated with heat poison, and also **exhaustion because of bone steaming**".

Gu zhu **蠱疰, *gu*-attachment-illness** [11]
EA PC identical with → *gu du* 蠱毒, *gu poison*. *BJ* SE *wei mao* 衛茅：除邪，殺鬼毒**蠱疰**, "It eliminates evil. It kills *gu* poison and ***gu*-attachment-illness**". *QJYF* 17: 治鬼疰、**蠱疰**，毒氣變化無常方, "Recipe to cure abnormal changes resulting from poison qi such as demon attachment-illness and ***gu*-attachment-illness**".

Gu zui **穀嘴, grain mouth** [1]
PC identical with → *mian pao* 面皰, facial blister. *BCGM* Bai bing zhu zhi yao 百病主治藥：(面）皰是風熱，即**穀嘴**, "[Facial] blisters are [a sign of] wind heat; this is [the so-called] **grain mouth**".

Guai bing **怪病, queer disease** [10] AN *qi bing* 奇病, strange disease; *qi ji* 奇疾, strange ailment; *guai ji* 怪疾, queer ailment; *yi ji* 異疾, unusual ailment; *guai zheng* 怪證, queer condition; *guai zheng* 怪症.

PC CD of rarely seen diseases with odd signs. *YXGM* 21: 水丸梧子意須斟，除驅**怪病**安心志, "Water pills [the size of] *wu zi* must be considered. They eliminate queer diseases and calm heart and mind". *BCGM* quotes its data on "**queer disease**". mostly from the *QJF*.

Guai zheng **怪證, queer condition** [1]

PC identical with → *guai bing* 怪病, queer disease. *BCGM* SE *gou* 狗：此亦**怪證**，取狗之血腥，以引其蟲耳, "This, too, is a **queer condition**. Make use of the fishy smell of dog blood to draw away these bugs/worms".

Guan ge **關格, blockade** [36]

PC of an inability to pass stools and urine resulting from an irregularity of the qi dynamics in the organism. This may be accompanied by vomiting. *ZBYHL* 14: **關格**者，大小便不通也, "**Blockade**, this is when defecation and urination fail to pass".

Guan jie bu tong **關節不通, joints are not passable** [1]

IS of an impairment of the movement of the joints. *SLBC* SE *ma zi* 麻子：治**關節不通**，髮落，通血脈, "It cures **impassable joints** and loss of hair; it penetrates blood vessels".

Guan jie ji **關節急, tension of the joints** [1]

IS of difficulties in bending or stretching the joints accompanied by uncomfortable contraction. *BCSY* SE *chun* 蓴：常食發氣，令**關節急**，嗜睡, "Consumed regularly it makes people emit qi, causes **tension of the joints**, and makes people sleepy".

Guan jie zhong **關節重, the joints feel heavy** [3]

IS of a feeling of unbearable heaviness in the joints, and a sensation of fatigue when one starts moving. *MYBL* SE *gou ji* 狗脊：女子傷中，**關節重**, "For women harmed in their center, with their **joints feeling heavy**".

Gui bei **龜背, turtle back** [7]

PC of children with a congenital convex bend in their spinal column giving their back an elevated appearance like that of a turtle. *TPSHF* 89：治小兒**龜背**，宜服麻黄丸方, "To cure **turtle back** in children the recipe to ingest the pills with *ma huang* is advisable".

Gui bing **鬼病, demonic disease** [5]

PC identical with → *gui mei* 鬼魅②, demonic seduction-specters. *ZBYHL* 2: 脈有表無裏，邪之祟上得**鬼病**也, "The movement in the vessels appears on the outside, not inside. [The patient] was affected by a **demonic disease** resulting from a curse issued by the evil".

Gui bing **龜病, turtle disease** [2]

PC of a swelling in the abdominal region with a solid lump resembling → *bie zheng* 鱉癥, "turtle[-shaped] concretion-illness". *PJF* 174: 人間**龜病**不能言，

肚裏生成硬似磚, "When someone has the **turtle disease** and cannot speak, a hardening resembling a brick develops in his abdomen".

Gui da **鬼打, demonic hit** [7]

PC identical with → *gui ji* 鬼擊, demon assault. *QJYF* 20: 倉公散，主猝**鬼打**，鬼排，鬼刺，心腹痛，吐下血便，死不知人, "Cang gong's powder controls sudden **demon hit**, demon push, demon stabbing, with cardiac and abdominal pain, vomiting and defecation with blood, death[-like unconsciousness] and inability to recognize people".

Gui e qi **鬼惡氣, malign demon qi** [1]

EA identical with → *gui xie* 鬼邪, demon evil. *BCGM* SE *ai* 艾 quoting *YXL*: 除鬼氣, "It removes demon qi". writes: 治一切**鬼惡氣**, "It cures all types of **malign demon qi**".

Gui fei **鬼痱, demon[-caused] disablement** [1] AW *gui pai* 鬼排.

PC identical with → *gui da* 鬼打, demonic hit; → *gui ji* 鬼擊, demonic assault. *QJYF* 12: 倉公散，治卒鬼擊、**鬼痱**、鬼刺，心腹痛如刺, "Cang gong's powder cures sudden demonic assault, **demon[-caused] disablement**, and demonic stabbing, with a pain in the heart and abdomen as if one had been stabbed".

Gui gu **鬼蠱, demon *gu*** [4] EA

PC identical with → *gu du* 蠱毒, *gu* poison. *BJ* SE *shi yan* 食鹽：主殺**鬼蠱**邪疰毒氣, "It controls killing of **demon *gu***, evil attachment-illness, and poison qi". *MYBL* SE *chang you* 常山：療**鬼蠱**往來，水脹，洒洒惡寒, "It cures **demon *gu*** that comes and goes, with edema, shivering and an aversion to cold".

Gui ji **鬼擊, demonic assault** [23] AN *gui da* 鬼打, demonic hit; *gui pai* 鬼排, demonic push.

PC with sudden twisting pain in the heart and abdomen, sometimes associated with bleeding, sometimes with sudden unconsciousness. *BJ* SE *bai ji* 白及 RE *fei shi zou ma tang* 飛屍走馬湯, decoction for flying corpse [qi resembling] a running horse: 主癰腫惡瘡敗疽，傷陰死肌，胃中邪氣，賊風**鬼擊**, "It controls obstruction-illnesses, swelling, malign sores, rotting impediment-illnesses, harmed yin, dead muscles, evil qi in the stomach, robber wind and **demonic assault**".

Gui jiao **鬼交, intercourse with demons** [19]

PC of males and females dreaming of sexual intercourse with emission of essence. *QJYF* 27: 男不可無女，女不可無男…強抑鬱閉之，難持易失，使人漏精尿濁，以致**鬼交**之病, "For men to be without a woman, that is impossible. For women to be without a male, that is impossible. ...If [sexual desire] is pent-up with force, it will be difficult to hold and easy to lose. As a result, essence/semen will drip and urine will be turbid. In the end this leads to the disease of **intercourse with demons**".

Gui jing wu **鬼精物, demon spirit being** [9]

EA identical with → *gui xie* 鬼邪, demon evil. *BJ* SE *she xiang* 麝香：主辟惡氣，殺**鬼精物**，温瘧蠱毒，癇痓，去三蟲, "It controls the elimination of malign qi, kills **demon spirit beings**, [cures] warmth malaria, *gu poison*, epilepsy and spasms, and removes the three bugs/worms".

***Gui kuang* 鬼狂, demonic madness** [1]

PC CD of → *gui zhu* 鬼疰, demon attachment-illness, and → *kuang xie* 狂邪, madness evil. *BCGM* Bai bing zhu zhi yao 百病主治藥 quoting *MYBL* SE *ban tian he* 半天河：鬼疰狂邪氣, "[It cures] demon attachment-illness, madness evil qi". writes: **鬼狂**, "**demonic madness**".

***Gui mei* 鬼魅, demonic seduction-specters** [41] AN *xie mei* 邪魅, evil seduction-specter; *gui qi* 鬼氣, demon qi; *gui du* 鬼毒, demon poison.

① AN *gui xie* 鬼邪demon evil. EA capable of bringing forth sudden violent diseases, strange diseases and recurring diseases believed to be associated with the activity of demons by people since antiquity. *ZBYHL* 40: 若陰陽調和，則臟腑強盛，風邪**鬼魅**不能傷之, "If yin and yang are balanced, then the depots and palaces are strong and flourish. Wind evil and **demonic seduction-specters** are unable to cause harm".

② AN *gui bing* 鬼病, demon disease. PC of sudden violent or unusual or recurrent natures that are difficult to explain. Hence since antiquity there is a belief that such conditions are caused by demonic intrusion. *MYBL* SE *huang huan* 黃環：主蠱毒鬼疰**鬼魅**，邪氣在藏中，除咳逆寒熱, "It controls *gu poison*, demon attachment-illness, and **demonic seduction-specters**, with evil qi situated in the depots, and removes cough with [qi] moving contrary to its proper direction, as well as alternating sensations of cold and heat".

***Gui mi* 鬼迷, deception by a demon** [1]

PC identical with → *gui mei* 鬼魅②, demonic seduction-specters. *BYXF* 17 RE *shen xian jie du wan bing wan* 神仙解毒萬病丸, pills of the immortals that dissolve poison [and cure] a myriad of of diseases: 驚死，**鬼迷**，未隔宿者，並冷水磨灌下, "[For patients] with [an appearance of] death because they were frightened and have succumbed to **deception by a demon**, if this has not continued over night yet, grind [these pills] with cold water and force [the patient] to drink this".

***Gui nue* 鬼瘧, demonic malaria** [19]

PC of → *nue ji* 瘧疾, malaria, that continues for a long time unhealed, with irregular phases of outbreak and inactivity. *BJ* SE *yuan hua* 芫花：主咳逆上氣，喉鳴喘，咽腫，短氣，蠱毒，**鬼瘧**, "It controls cough with qi rising contrary to its proper direction of flow, noisy panting in the throat, gullet swelling, shortness of qi, *gu poison*, and **demonic malaria**".

***Gui pai* 鬼排, demon push** [7]

PC identical with → *gui ji* 鬼擊, demon assault, and → *gui fei* 鬼痱, demon disablement. *ZBYHL* 23: 鬼擊者…一名為**鬼排**，言鬼排觸於人也, "Another name of 'demon assault' is '**demon push**'. That is to say, a demon has given a human person a push".

Gui qi 鬼氣, demon qi [63] EA

PC identical with → *gui mei* 鬼魅, demonic seduction-specters. *ZBYHL* 23: 客邪**鬼氣**卒急傷人，入於腑臟，使陰陽離絕, "When visiting evil and **demon qi** suddenly harm man, they enter the depots and palaces and cause [the balance of] yin and yang [qi] to break". *WTMY* 13 RE *yan nian tao nu tan* 延年桃奴湯，decoction to extend one's years with dried peaches that have remained on the trees over winter: 主伏連**鬼氣**, "It controls hidden link and **demon qi**".

Gui shi tou 鬼舐頭, head licked by a demon [6]

PC of one's hair on the head falling out in small amounts. The skin on the skull is bald but has no color or glossiness, and there is neither pain nor itching. *ZBYHL* 27: 髮禿落，肌肉枯死，或如錢大，或如指大，髮不生，亦不癢，故謂之**鬼舐頭**, "Loss of hair. Muscle flesh dries up and dies. In some cases [the region affected is] as large as a coin. In some cases as large as a finger. No hair grows there, and it does not itch. Hence this is called '**head licked by a demon**'".

Gui sui 鬼祟, cursed by a demon [5]

EA identical with → *gui xie* 鬼邪, demon evil. *QJYF* 24: 語聲不出，短氣欲死，飲食不下，吐逆上氣，去來無常，狀如**鬼祟**, "[The patient] is unable to speak. He experiences shortness of qi and wishes to die. He can neither drink nor eat. He vomits with counter-movement of qi. This comes and goes without any regularity. The appearance resembles that of being **cursed by a demon**".

Gui tai 鬼胎, demon fetus [10]

PC of → *zheng jia* 癥瘕, concretion-illness and conglomeration-illness, assuming an appearance of pregnancy, with blocked menses and abdominal distension. *TPSHF* 77: 治婦人經脈不通，癥塊脹滿，腹有**鬼胎**方, "Recipe to cure women with a blockage of conduit vessels, concretion-illness lumps with distension and a feeling of fullness, and a **demon fetus** in the abdomen".

Gui wu 鬼忤, demon hostility [1]

PC identical with → *ke wu* 客忤, visitor's hostility. *QJYF* 11: 蜥蜴丸，治癥堅水腫、蜚尸、遁尸、百注、尸注、骨血相注，惡氣**鬼忤**，蠱毒、邪氣往來, "Pills with skink cure concretion-illness hardness and water swelling, gadfly corpse [qi], run-away corpse [qi], the hundred influxes, corpse [qi] influx, mutual influx between bones and blood, malign qi and **demon hostility**, *gu* poison, and evil qi that come and go".

Gui xie 鬼邪, demon evil [8] AN *e gui* 惡鬼, malign demon; *jing wu* 精物, spirit being; *gui jing wu* 鬼精物, demon spirit being; *yang gui* 殃鬼, calamitous demon; *bai jing lao wu* 百精老物, all types of ancient spirit beings; *gui e qi* 鬼惡氣, demonic malign qi; *gui sui* 鬼祟, demon curse.

EA identical with → *gui mei* 鬼魅①, demonic seduction-specters. *ZHF* 1: 五尸之中尸注，又挾諸**鬼邪**為害也, "Among the five corpse [evils is] corpse influx, it also comprises all harm caused by **demon evil**".

Gui xiong 龜胸, turtle chest [1]

PC of children with a congenital forward bend in their spinal column giving their chest an elevated appearance like a turtle. *TPSHF* 89: 小兒**龜胸**者，緣肺

熱脹滿，致使胸高如龜，"The reason for a **turtle chest** in children is a distension and fullness resulting from lung heat causing the chest to arch like a turtle".

***Gui yan* 鬼魘, demonic nightmare** [1]

PC of bad dreams forced upon people by a demon-mare. *QJYF* 25: 治**鬼魘**不悟方，伏龍肝為末，吹鼻中，"Recipe to cure **demonic nightmares** and unconsciousness: grind *fu long gan* to a powder, and blow into [the patient's] nose".

***Gui yao* 臀腰, lumbar sprain** [6]

PC of an acute pain of a lower lumbar sprain. *ZBYHL* 5: **臀腰**者，謂卒然傷損於腰而致痛也，"**Lumbar sprain** is to say: a sudden harm inflicted on one's lower back resulting in pain".

***Gui yong* 潰癰, festering obstruction-illness; causing the festering of obstruction-illnesses** [7]

① PC identical with → *yong chuang* 癰瘡, obstruction-illness sores b). *BJ* SE *liu hua* 柳華：實，主**潰癰**，逐膿血，"Their fruits master **festering obstruction-illnesses**, they eliminate pus and blood".

② TA of eliminating pus from festering obstruction-illnesses. *BCGM* SE *ji* 雞：翅翮形銳而飛揚，乃其致力之處，故能破血消腫，**潰癰**下哽，"The shafts of the feathers are pointed and serve to enable flying. These are locations where utmost strength is required. Hence they are able to break through blood and to dissolve swelling. They **cause the festering of obstruction-illnesses**, and make items move down that are stuck in one's gullet and cause choking".

***Gui yu* 鬼語, demon speech** [1]

IS of uncontrolled and irregular language behavior with mental confusion. *WTMY* 34: 廣濟療產後血暈，心悶不識人，或神言**鬼語**，氣欲絕方，"Recipe for qi [flow] that is about to be discontinued: provides encompassing help in the case of postpartum mental confusion, heart pressure, and an inability to recognize persons, with [patients] sometimes [expressing themselves with] spirit language and **demon speech**".

***Gui zhu* 鬼疰, demon attachment-illness** [92] AD *zhu* 疰, attachment-illness. AN *gui zhu* 鬼注, demon influx; *zhu bing* 疰病, attachment-illness disease; *zhu ji* 疰疾, attachment-illness ailment; *shi zhu* 屍疰, corpse [qi] attachment-illness; *xie zhu* 邪疰, evil attachment-illness; *zhu qi* 疰氣, attachment-illness qi.

PC of a slowly developing infectious weakness. The Song dynasty physician Chen Yan 陳言 and others believed that this is → *lao zhai* 勞瘵, exhaustion consumption. *QJYF* 1: 夫療寒以熱藥，療熱以寒藥，飲食不消以吐下藥，**鬼疰**蠱毒以蠱毒藥，癰腫瘡瘤以瘡瘤藥，風濕以風濕藥，風勞氣冷各隨其所宜，"Now, when healing cold with hot medication, when healing heat with cold medication, when failure to digest beverages and food is [healed] with medications inducing vomiting and discharge, when **demon attachment-illness** and *gu* poison is [healed] with medication for *gu* poison, and when obstruction-illness swelling, sores and tumors are [healed] with medication for sores and tumors, when wind moisture is [healed] with wind moisture medication, for wind exhaustion and qi cold, in all instances one must follow what is appropriate".

SYJYBZFL 10: 夫骨蒸、殗殜、復連、屍疰、勞疰、蟲疰、毒疰、熱疰、冷疰、食疰、**鬼疰**等，皆曰傳屍者，以疰者，注也，病自上注下，與前人相似，故曰疰, "Now, [diseases] such as…corpse attachment-illness, exhaustion attachment-illness, bug/worm attachment-illness, poison attachment-illness, heat attachment-illness, cold attachment-illness, food attachment-illness, **demon attachment-illness**, the fact that they are termed 'corpse [qi] transmissions' is because *zhu* 疰，'attachment-illness', is *zhu* 注, 'influx'. The disease is an influx from above to below, and appears similar to [its appearance in] previously [affected] persons. Hence it is called *zhu* 疰".

***Gui zhu* 鬼注, demon influx** [5]

PC identical with → *gui zhu* 鬼疰, demon attachment-illness. *QJYF* 1: 屍注、**鬼注**病者，葛云，即是五屍之中屍注，又挾諸鬼邪為害也, "In view of the diseases corpse [qi] influx and **demon influx**, Ge says: these are examples of corpse [qi] influx among the five 'corpse [qi' conditions]. They also refer to all types of suffering inflicted by demon evil". *ZBYHL* 24: 注之言住也，言其連滯停住也。人有先無他病，忽被鬼排擊，當時或心腹刺痛，或悶倒地，如中惡之類，其得瘥之後，餘氣不歇，停住積久，有時發動，連滯停住，乃至於死。死後注易傍人，故謂之**鬼注**, "*Zhu* 注, influx, stands for *zhu* 住, to stay with; to be attached to. That is to say the [disease] stays with one/is attached [to a patient] for an extended period of time. When someone originally had no other disease and then was suddenly attacked by a demon, his heart and abdomen may experience a piercing pain. Or he experiences heart-pressure and falls to the ground, as if struck by the malign. After this has been cured, there may be additional qi that have not been knocked off. They stay long, and at times they break out. This continues for an extended period of time until [the patient] dies. After he has died, [these qi] flow over into a bystander. Hence one refers to '**demon influx**'".

***Gui zhu xin tong* 鬼疰心痛, heartache because of demon attachment-illness** [2]
AD *zhu xin tong* 疰心痛，heartache from [demon] attachment-illness.

PC of sudden → *xin tong* 心痛, heartache, acquired in the wilderness as a result of → *gui zhu* 鬼疰, demon attachment-illness. *WTMY* 31: 療諸毒疰氣，心腹脹滿，大小便不通，**鬼疰心痛**, "It cures all types of poison and [demon] attachment-illness qi, distension and a feeling of fullness in the heart and abdomen, failure of defecation and urination to pass, as well as **heartache because of demon attachment-illness**".

***Guo* 瘑, lair-illness** [16]

PC AD of → *guo chuang* 瘑瘡, lair-illness sores. *ZBYHL* 35: 風氣多者，其**瘑**則乾燥, "If there is much wind qi, the **lair-illness** [sores] will be dry".

***Guo chuang* 瘑瘡, lair-illness sores** [20] AD *guo* 瘑, lair-illness.

PC of sores affecting both hands and feet, with pain and itching and gradual extension. In some cases crumbs are shed off. *ZBYHL* 35: 多著手足間，遞相對，如新生茱萸子，痛癢，抓搔成瘡，黄汁出，浸淫生長，拆裂，時瘥時劇，變化生蟲，故名**瘑瘡**, "They often affect hands or feet, moving from one to the next. The appearance is that of young *zhu yu* seeds. [Hands and feet] are painful and itch. If scratched they develop sores, emitting yellow liquid. [Skin lesions] soaked [with pus and/or liquid] spread and grow, and develop cracks. They may recede for a while and then be violent again. Eventually their transformation generates bugs/worms. Hence they are called **lair-illness sores**".

***Guo jie* 瘑疥, lair-illness and *jie*-illness** [10]
PC CD of → *guo chuang* 瘑瘡, lair-illness sores, and → *jie chuang* 疥瘡, *jie*-illness sores. *YXL* SE *shi hui* 石灰：治瘑疥，蝕惡肉，不入湯服, "It cures **lair-illness and *jie*-illness** and erodes malign flesh. Must not be ingested as a decoction".

- H -

***Ha ma wen* 蛤蟆瘟, frog warmth-illness** [2] AW → *ha ma wen* 蝦蟆瘟.
PC identical with → *zha sai* 痄腮, mumps. *BCMQ* SE *chan chu* 蟾蜍：病患面赤項頸大者，名**蛤蟆瘟**, "If someone suffers from a red face and enlarged neck, this is called **frog warmth-illness**".

***Ha ma wen* 蝦蟆瘟, frog warmth-illness** [1]
PC identical with → *ha ma wen* 蛤蟆瘟, frog warmth-illness. *DXSJ* Mj: **蝦蟆瘟**，風熱也，宜服車前葉汁, "**Frog warmth-illness**: this is wind and heat. One should ingest the juice prepared from *che qian* leaves".

***Hai shui shang lie* 海水傷裂, skin cracks as damage caused by ocean water** [1]
PC of injured, cracked and painful skin brought forth by ocean salt water. *BCGM* SE *jiu* 酒 quotes *SLQL*: **海水傷裂**：凡人為海水咸物所傷，及風吹裂，痛不可忍, "**Skin cracks as damage caused by ocean water**: whenever wind blows into the skin cracks of a person injured by salty matter in ocean water, the pain is unbearable".

***Han* 寒, cold** [p]
① AN *leng* 冷; *han qi* 寒氣, cold qi; *han leng* 寒冷, cold; *leng qi* 冷氣, cold qi; *han xie* 寒邪. EA capable of causing cold-type disease. *SW* 72: **寒**淫於內，治以甘熱, "If **cold** has encroached upon the interior, this is treated with sweet [flavor] and hot [qi]".
② AN *han leng* 寒冷, cold; *leng qi* 冷氣, cold qi; *han bing* 寒病, cold disease; *han ji* 寒疾, cold ailments; *leng bing* 冷病, cold disease; *leng ji* 冷疾, cold ailment; *leng zheng* 冷證. PC of unilateral dominance of yin and cold brought forth by different causes. *SW* 5: 陰勝則**寒**, "When the yin dominates, there is **cold**".
③ AN cold condition; *shen leng* 身冷, bodily cold; *ti han* 體寒, bodily cold. IS of a low temperature in the external parts of the body, or of a subjectively felt cold. *SW* 5: 身常清，數栗而**寒**, "The body is permanently cool. One shivers frequently and feels **cold**".
④ AN *leng* 冷. PQ referring to one of the four types of qi in pharmaceutical substances. *BJ* Xu li 序例：［藥］有**寒**、熱、温、涼四氣, "[Drugs] have the four qi of **cold**, heat, warmth, and coolness".
⑤ TA of treating disease with pharmaceutical substances of a cold and cool nature. *SW* 74: 熱者**寒**之, "Treat heat with **cold**".

***Han ban* 汗斑, sweat macule** [9]
PC identical with → *li yang feng* 瀝瘍風, pervasion-illness with ulcers wind. *PJF* 112: 治紫白癜癬、**汗斑**，用蒼耳葉勤擦, "To cure purple and white patches and *xuan*-illness, and **sweat macules**, use the leaves of *cang er* for frequent rubbing [on the affected skin]".

***Han bi* 寒痹, cold blockage** [6] AN *bi han* 痹寒， blocking cold.
PC of → *bi bing* 痹病, blockage disease, brought forth mostly by cold evil, with pain affecting the entire body and numbness of skin. *LS* 6: **寒痹**之為病也，留

而不去，時痛而皮不仁, "When a **cold blockage** generates a disease that stays for a long time and does not disappear, this will eventually cause pain and numbness of the skin".

Han bing **寒病, cold disease** [1]

PC identical with → *han* 寒, cold②. *SW* 74: 言熱未已，**寒病**復始, "They say: The heat has not ended yet, [but] a **cold disease** sets in as well".

Han chan **寒顫, trembling from cold** [2]

IS identical with → *zhen han* 振寒, shaking from cold. *TPSHF* 23 RE *fang feng san* 防風散, powder with *fang feng*: 治風虛多汗，惡風**寒顫**, "It cures wind [intruding into a state of] depletion with much sweating, aversion to wind and **trembling from cold**".

Han chuan **寒喘, cold panting** [1]

PC of panting brought forth by cold evil. *BYXF* 5: 治**寒喘**五味子湯, "Decoction with five ingredients to cure **cold panting**".

Han chuang **寒瘡, cold sores** [2] AN *miao jing chuang* 貓睛瘡, cat eyes sores; *miao yan jing chuang* 貓眼睛瘡.

PC of sores on body and face with luster but without pus and blood, irregular episodes of pain and itching, and a lack of appetite. *SYDXF* 10: 面上及遍身生瘡似貓兒眼，有光彩，無膿血，但痛癢不常，飲食減少，冬則遍脛，名曰**寒瘡**, "The entire body and the face develop sores reminiscent of cat eyes. They have luster but no pus or blood. They ache and itch in irregular intervals, and [patients] drink and eat less and less. In winter they cover the entire shins. This is called '**cold sores**'".

Han hou **寒齁, cold snore** [3]

PC of → *hou* 齁, snore, brought forth by cold evil. *BCGM* Bai bing zhu zhi yao 百病主治藥：石胡荽，**寒齁**擂酒服, "*Shi hu sui*, for **cold snore** pound and ingest with wine".

Han hua **寒滑, cold smoothness; cold [and] smoothing** [9]

① PC identical with → *leng hua* 冷滑①. *PJF* 208: **寒滑**，氣泄不固，故形質下脫, "**Cold smoothness**: the qi flows out and cannot be stabilized. Hence one's material body loses substance".

② PQ identical with → *leng hua* 冷滑②, cold [and] smoothing. *QJYF* 26: 凡瓜，味甘，**寒滑**，無毒, "All melons have a sweet flavor, **cold [and] smoothing** [nature], and no poison".

Han ji **寒疾, cold ailment** [3]

PC identical with → *han* 寒, cold②. *SW* 69: 地積堅冰，陽光不治，民病**寒疾**於下, "The earth accumulates solid ice. Yang light does not govern. People suffer from **cold ailment** in the lower sections".

Han ji **寒積, cold accumulation** [3]

EA identical with → *ji leng* 積冷, accumulated cold. *ZBYHL* 17: 由腸虛而**寒積**，故冷痢久不斷也, "Because of intestinal depletion followed by **cold accumulation**, long and unending cold free-flux illness results".

Han jia **寒瘕, cold conglomeration-illness** [2] AN *leng jia* 冷瘕.
PC of → *jia* 瘕, conglomeration-illness, brought forth by accumulations of evil cold qi. *YXL* SE *yang qi shi* 陽起石：能暖女子子宮久冷，冷癥**寒瘕**, "It is able to provide warmth to a uterus that has been cold over a long time, with cold concretion-illness and **cold conglomeration-illness**".

Han lao **寒勞, cold exhaustion** [1]
PC identical with → *leng lao* 冷勞. *PJF* 351 lists *sheng jiang dang gui yang rou tang* 生薑當歸羊肉湯, decoction with *sheng jiang*, *dang gui*, and *yang rou*: 治產後身腹中有激痛及**寒勞**不足, "It cures violent abdominal pain following delivery, as well as **cold exhaustion** and [qi] insufficiency".

Han leng **寒冷, cold** [12]
① EA identical with → *han* 寒①, cold . *SHL* 380: 所以然者，胃中**寒冷**故也, "This is so because of the presence of **cold** in the stomach".
② PC identical with → *han* 寒②. *MYBL* SE *shu jiao* 蜀椒：除六腑**寒冷**，傷寒温瘧, "It removes the **cold** from the six palaces, and [serves to cure] harm caused by cold, and warmth malaria".
③ IS identical with → *han* 寒③. *TBC* SE *luan jing* 欒荊：濕痹**寒冷**疼痛, "Moisture-blockage with **cold** and pain".
④ PQ identical with → *han* 寒④. *BCJJZ* SE *ji xue cao* 積雪草：方藥亦不用，想此草當**寒冷**爾, "It is not made use of in pharmaceutical recipes because it is thought to be of a **cold** quality".

Han li **寒痢, cold free-flux illness** [4]
PC identical with → *leng li* 冷痢. *BCGM* SE *xiao mai* 小麥 quoting *WTMY*: recipe for *leng li* 冷痢, "Cold free-flux illness". writes: **寒痢**白色，炒麵每以方寸匕入粥中食之, "**Cold free-flux illness** of white color; add a square-inch-sized spoon full of fried noodles to a congee and [have the patient] consume it".

Han li **寒利, cold free-flux; cold [and] disinhibiting** [3]
① PC identical with → *leng li* 冷利①, cold free-flux. *PJF* 128: 芍藥之酸，通**寒利**腹中痛, "The sour nature of *shao yao* cures **cold free-flux** and abdominal pain".
② PQ identical with → *leng li* 冷利②, cold and disinhibiting. *BCGM* SE *qie* 茄 quotes *SSB*: 茄性**寒利**，多食必腹痛下利, "*Qie*, its nature is **cold [and] disinhibiting**. If one consumes large amounts abdominal pain and free-flux discharge will be inevitable".

Han nüe **寒瘧, cold malaria** [11]
① PC of malaria with alternating sensations of cold first and then heat, or with only sensations of cold and no feeling of heat. *SW* 35: 先寒而後熱也，病以時作，名曰**寒瘧**, "[The patient] is cold first and hot afterwards. The disease is active in a [specific] time [of the year]. It is called **cold malaria**".
② IS of a type of aversion to cold and shivering resembling cold malaria. *BCTJ* SE *ta gan* 獺肝：五藏及肉皆寒，惟肝温。主…四肢**寒瘧**，虛汗客熱, "The five depots and the meat are all cold. Only the liver is warm. It controls...**cold malaria** affecting the four limbs, depletion sweating with visitor heat".

Han ou 寒嘔, cold vomiting [3]
PC of → *ou tu* 嘔吐, vomiting, brought forth by stomach cold. *PJF* 206: 病者胃中寒，心下淡淡，四肢厥冷，食即嘔吐，名曰**寒嘔**, "Patients have cold in their stomach, liquid gurgles below the heart, the four limbs are affected by recession with cold. Food is thrown up again. This is called **cold vomiting**".

Han pi 寒澼, cold wash-out [5]
PC identical with → *han pi* 寒癖, cold aggregation-illness. *Pi* 澼 is an erroneous writing of *pi* 癖 in the *BCGM*; e.g., SE *ba dou* 巴豆 quotes *QJYF*: **寒澼**宿食：不消，大便閉塞。巴豆仁一升，清酒五升，煮三日三夜，研熟，合酒微火煎令可丸如豌豆大。每服一丸，水下。欲吐者，二丸, "**Cold wash-out** and food remaining in the body over night: Failing digestion and blocked stools. *Ba dou* kernels, 1 *sheng*, are to be boiled with clear wine, 5 *sheng*, for three days and three nights. Check whether they are thoroughly done. Then boil with wine over s small fire until they can be formed to pills the size of garden peas. Each dosis is one pill, to be ingested with water. [Patients] with an inclination to vomit [ingest] two pills".

Han pi 寒癖, cold aggregation-illness [2] AW *han pi* 寒澼.
① AN *leng pi* 冷癖. PC of painful → *pi* 癖, aggregation-illness, resulting from liquids and cold qi stagnant accumulations in the costal region being affected by further cold. *ZBYHL* 20: 水飲停積，肋下弦強是也。因遇寒即痛，所以謂之**寒癖**, "Beverages accumulate, and this is shown by a feeling of tense strings below the ribs. When this is affected by cold, pain results. Hence one calls this condition '**cold aggregation-illness**'".
② IS of a passage of thin white urine following the intake of medication in the course of a treatment of **cold aggregation**. *ZHF* 1: 須取汁，清旦服，至日晡令盡。其間當下諸**寒癖**。訖，作白粥漸食之, "Take the juice and consume it in the early morning. By late afternoon this should be finished. In the course [of this treatment] one should purge all **cold aggregation-illnesses**. When this process has come to an end, prepare a white gruel for slow consumption".

Han pi 寒痞, cold obstacle-illness [1]
PC of → *pi* 痞, blockages, brought forth by nodes of cold evil qi. *PJF* 218 RE *jiao gan dan* 交感丹, elixir of sympathy: 中則**寒痞**，飲食減少, "In their center [patients have a] **cold obstacle-illness**, they drink and eat less and less".

Han qi 寒氣, cold qi [24]
① CC *SW* 5: **寒氣**生濁，熱氣生清, "**Cold qi** generates turbidity; heat qi generates clarity".
② EA identical with → *han* 寒①, cold. *SW* 43: 痛者，**寒氣**多也，有寒故痛也, "In the case of pain, much **cold qi** is present. [Because] there is cold, hence there is pain".
③ IS identical with → *wu han* 惡寒, aversion to cold. *BJ* SE *qin pi* 秦皮：主風寒濕痹，洗洗**寒氣**，"Controls wind cold moisture blockage. Eliminates **cold qi**".

④ PQ identical with *han* 寒, cold④. *BCGM* SE *cha* 茶; in his discussion of the effects of tea leaves, LSZ states: 温飲則火因**寒氣**而下降, "If drunk warm the fire will follow the **cold qi** and descend".

Han re **寒熱, cold and heat; cold or hot** [574] AN *leng re* 冷熱.

① CD of → *han* 寒, cold, and → *re* 熱, heat. CC of cold and heat. *LS* 66: 風雨**寒熱**，不得虛邪，不能獨傷人, "Wind, rain, **cold, and heat** are unable to harm a person by themselves as long as they cannot act as a depletion evil".

② Cold and heat qualities of pharmaceutical substances. *ZLBC* Fj Xuli shang 序例上 quotes *BJ*: 藥有酸咸甘苦辛五味，又有**寒熱**温涼四氣, "Pharmaceutical substances may have one of the five flavors: sour, salty, sweet, bitter, acrid. Also, the four qi include **cold, heat,** warmth and coolness".

③ EA identified as cold and heat. *SW* 71: **寒熱**内賊，其病益甚, "**Cold or heat** would cause internal injuries. The illness [you try to heal] will become even more severe".

④ PC of having cold and/or heat. *SW* 3: 因於露風，乃生**寒熱**, "If subsequently one exposes himself and is affected by wind, this will generate **cold and heat**". *BCGM* Bai bing zhu zhi yao 百病主治藥identifies as pathological conditions of cold and heat those of external affection and internal harm such as *huo yu* 火郁, pent-up fire; *xu lao* 虛勞, depletion exhaustion; *nüe* 瘧, malaria; *chuang* 瘡, sores; *luo li* 瘰癧, scrofula with pervasion-illness.

⑤ PC of an aversion to cold with fever. *LS* 26: 淅淅身時**寒熱**, "The body shivers and alternately experiences **cold and heat**".

⑥ Temperatures assigned to items. *LS* 71: 必先明知十二經脈之本末，皮膚之**寒熱**, "It is essential to first know the begin and end of the twelve conduits, and whether the skin is **cold or hot**".

Han re feng bi **寒熱風痹, cold, heat and wind blockage** [5]

PC of the three qi wind, cold, and heat jointly causing → *bi bing* 痹病, blockage disease, with the joints of one's limbs aching and experiencing swelling and distension. In extreme cases this leads to an inability to move. *MYBL* SE *bian qing* 扁青：去**寒熱風痹**, "It removes **cold, heat and wind blockage**".

Han re guai bing **寒熱怪病, queer disease of alternating sensations of cold and heat** [1]

PC of an unusual disease with alternating sensations of cold and heat continuing for several days, eventually resulting in a stone-like hardening of the four extremities, and emaciation progressing daily. *BCGM* SE *hua shi* quotes *QJF*: 寒熱不止，數日四肢堅如石，擊之似鐘磬聲，日漸瘦惡, "Alternating sensations of cold and heat that do not end. After several days the four limbs turn as hard as stone. If one strikes them, there is a sound like that produced by the chimestone of a bell. Emaciation increases day by day". LSZ calls this: **寒熱怪病**, "**Queer disease of alternating sensations of cold and heat**".

Han re nüe **寒熱瘧, cold and heat malaria** [3]

PC identical with → *nüe* 瘧, malaria. *ZBYHL* 11: **寒熱瘧**候：夫瘧者，風寒之氣也, "Signs of **cold and heat malaria**: As for malaria, it is the qi of wind and cold".

***Han re nüe ji* 寒熱瘧疾, cold and heat malaria ailment** [5]
PC identical with → *nüe* 瘧, malaria. *SJZL* 191: 陽溪二穴…治…**寒熱瘧疾**, "The two *yang xi* insertion holes [serve to] cure the **ailment of cold and heat malaria**".

***Han re tong* 寒熱痛**, cold [pain] and heat pain [4]
IS CD of → *han tong* 寒痛, cold pain, and → *re tong* 熱痛, heat pain. *BJ* SE *rou cong rong* 肉蓯蓉：除莖中**寒熱痛**, "Removes **cold [pain] and heat pain** from the penis".

***Han re xian* 寒熱癇, cold [epilepsy] and heat epilepsy** [1]
PC CD of → *han xian* 寒癇, cold epilepsy, and → *re xian* 熱癇. *MYBL* SE *gui gai* 鬼蓋：主小兒**寒熱癇**, "Controls **cold [epilepsy] and heat epilepsy** in children".

***Han re bi* 寒熱痹, cold [blockage] and heat blockage** [3]
PC CD of → *han bi* 寒痹, cold blockage, and → *re bi* 熱痹, heat blockage. *QJYF* 30: 消濼，主**寒熱痹**，頭痛, "The *xiao luo* [needle insertion hole] controls **cold [blockage] and heat blockage**, as well as headache".

***Han shan* 寒疝, cold elevation-illness** [29]
PC of a) AN *leng shan* 冷疝. A swollen and painful scrotum brought forth by cold evil as a type of → *shan* 疝, elevatipn-illness. *ZJJYJ* 9: **寒疝**，陰挺出，偏大腫，腹臍痛， "**Cold elevation-illness**: The testicles protrude, with a unilateral enormous swelling. The abdominal region of the umbilicus is in pain". b) an acute and ferocious abdominal pain brought forth by cold evil. *JGYL* Fj: **寒疝**，繞臍痛。若發則白津出，手足厥冷，其脈沉緊, "**Cold elevation-illness**: pain around the navel. When it develops, a white liquid leaves. Hands and legs are affected by recession and cold. The [movement in the] vessels is deep insideand tight".

***Han shi* 寒濕, cold and moisture; cold-moisture** [103]
① EA CD of → han 寒, cold, and → shi 濕, moisture as causes of disease. *SW* 55: 名曰肌痹，傷於**寒濕**, "This is called muscle blockage. [It results from] harm caused by **cold and moisture**".
② AN *shi leng* 濕冷, moisture and cold. PC brought forth by cold and moisture. *SW* 71: 寒濕之氣，持於氣交，民病**寒濕**, "The qi of cold and moisture are held in [the sphere of] qi interaction. People suffer from **cold and moisture**". *BCGM* lists numerous diseases associated with cold and moisture, such as *han shi bi* 寒濕痹, cold-moisture blockage; *han shi sou* 寒濕嗽, cold-moisture cough; *han shi xie* 寒濕泄, cold-moisture diarrhea; *han shi jiao qi* 寒濕脚氣, cold-moist leg qi.

***Han shi* 汗濕, sweating with moisture** [1]
IS of constant topical sweating resulting in continuous moisture. *ZBYHL* 4: 腎榮於陰器，腎氣虛，不能制津液，則**汗濕**, "The kidneys nourish the genital organ. When the kidney qi is depleted, they are unable to control the body liquids. This results in **sweating with moisture**".

Han shi bi **寒濕痹, cold and moisture blockage** [5]

PC of the two qi cold and moisture jointly causing → *bi bing* 痹病, blockage disease, with the joints of one's limbs aching and experiencing swelling and distension. In extreme cases this leads to an inability to move. *BJ* SE *wang sun* 王孫：主五藏邪氣，**寒濕痹**，四肢疼酸，膝冷痛, "It controls evil qi affecting the five depots, **cold and moisture blockage**, with the four limbs aching and the knees being cold and painful".

Han shi feng bi **寒濕風痹, cold, moisture and wind blockage** [2]

PC of the three qi cold, moisture and wind jointly causing → *bi bing* 痹病, blockage disease, with the joints of one's limbs aching and experiencing swelling and distension. In extreme cases this leads to an inability to move. *BJ* SE *qin jiao* 秦艽：主寒熱邪氣，**寒濕風痹**，肢節痛, "It controls cold and heat evil qi, **cold, moisture and wind blockage**, and aching limbs and joints".

Han shi jie xiong **寒實結胸, cold repletion with bound chest** [5]

PC of → *jie xiong* 結胸, bound chest, brought forth by cold evil. *SHL* 141: **寒實結胸**，無熱證者，與三物小陷胸湯， "In the case of **cold repletion with bound chest** without signs of heat apply the 'minor decoction sinking into the chest with three items'".

Han shi qi **寒濕氣, cold and moisture qi** [1]

EA of → *han* 寒, cold, and → *shi* 濕, moisture, together causing a disease. *ZBYHL* 8: 此由**寒濕氣**不散，瘀熱在於脾胃故也, "The reason is that **cold and moisture qi** fail to disperse. Stagnant heat is blocked in the spleen and stomach".

Han sou **寒嗽, cold cough** [20] AN *leng sou* 冷嗽

PC of → *ke sou* 咳嗽, cough, brought forth by cold evil. *TPSHF* 46: **寒嗽**，因飲冷食寒，注入於胃，從肺脈上，氣內外合，因之而嗽是也, "**Cold cough**: This is because the cold of beverages and the cold of food have poured into the stomach. The [cold] qi rises by way of the lung vessel. Inner and outer [cold] meet. Hence cough results".

Han tan **寒痰, cold and phlegm** [21]

① AN *leng tan* 冷痰. EA CD of → *han* 寒, cold, and → *tan* 痰, phlegm as causes of disease. *YXL* SE *yuan hua* 芫花：利五藏**寒痰**, "It discharges **cold and phlegm** from all five depots".

② AN *tan leng* 痰冷, phlegm and cold. PC brought forth by cold and phlegm. *YXQY* Fj: 半夏，氣微寒，味辛平，治**寒痰**, "*Ban xia*, its qi is slightly cold; its flavor is acrid-balanced. It cures **cold and phlegm**".

Han tong **寒痛, cold pain; to be cold and painful** [9]

IS identical with → *leng tong* 冷痛. *SW* 63: 繆傳引上齒，齒唇**寒痛**，視其手背脈血者去之, "If [the evil] is transmitted misleadingly and pulls on the upper teeth and if the teeth and lips are **cold and painful**, find out which vessels on the back of the hand have blood and remove it.

Han xie **寒邪, cold evil** [14]

EA identical with → *han* 寒①, cold. *SW* 71: 民避**寒邪**，君子周密, "The people avoid the **cold evil**; the gentleman [stays in a] firmly closed [house]".

Han xie **寒泄, cold outflow** [4]
PC identical with → *leng xie* 冷泄. *BJ* SE *gu yang jiao* 羖羊角：主青盲，明目，殺疥蟲，止**寒泄**, "It controls green blindness, clears the eyes, kills *jie*-illness bugs/worms, and stops **cold outflow**".

Han xin **寒心, cold heart** [1]
IS identical with → *xin han* 心寒, the heart has cold. *BJ* SE *xing he ren* 杏核仁：主…**寒心**，賁豚, "It controls…**cold heart** and running piglet".

Han xue **寒血, cold blood** [5]
EA identical with → *leng xue* 冷血. *MYBL* SE *tu si zi* 菟絲子：主口苦燥渴，**寒血**為積, "It controls a bitter taste in the mouth, with dryness and thirst, and **cold blood** forming accumulations".

Han xue **汗血, to sweat blood** [4]
PC identical with → *xue han* 血汗, blood sweat. *ZBYHL* 27: **汗血**候：肝藏血，心之液為汗。言肝心俱傷於邪，故血從膚腠而出也, "Signs of **sweating blood**: The liver stores the blood. The liquid associated with the heart is sweat. That is to say, if the liver and heart are simultaneously affected by evil, blood will leave through the dermal interstices".

Han yin **寒飲, cold rheum** [1] AN *leng yin* 冷飲.
EA of cold beverages as causes of disease. *ZBYHL* 7: 此中有**寒飲**，不可吐也，當温之, "In this case, [patients] have **cold rheum** in their center. One must not make them vomit. Rather one should apply a warming therapy".

Han yu **寒郁, pent-up cold** [3]
EA of accumulation nodes of stagnating cold evil. *BCGM* SE *fu zi* 附子 quotes *DSZY*: 卮子降濕熱，烏頭破**寒郁**, "*Zhi zi* brings moisture and heat down; *wu tou* breaks open **pent-up cold**".

Han zhang 寒脹, **cold distension** [3]
PC of an abdominal distension brought forth by cold. *LSMC* Fj: 多食寒涼，及脾胃久虛之人，胃中寒則脹滿，或藏寒生滿病，以治**寒脹**，中滿分消湯主之, "If one consumes much cold and cool [food/beverages] and if such people have intestinal and stomach depletion over an extended period of time, the cold in the stomach will cause distension and a feeling of fullness. In some cases, the abiding cold will cause a fullness disease. To cure such **cold distension**, the 'decoction for separating and dissolving cases of central fullness' will control this".

Han zhong **寒腫, cold swelling** [1] AN *zhong han* 腫寒， swelling with cold.
IS of a swelling that is accompanied by a feeling of cold. *MYBL* SE *wu zei yu gu* 烏賊魚骨：腹痛環臍，陰中**寒腫**, "Abdominal pain surrounding the navel. **Cold swelling** in the yin (i.e. genital) region".

Han zhong 寒中, **cold center** [15] AN → ***zhong han*** **中寒, central cold.**
PC of intestinal sounds and abdominal pain with diarrhea brought forth by intestinal and stomach depletion and weakness. *SW* 4: 長夏善病洞泄**寒中**, "In late summer [patients] tend to suffer from vacating diarrhea and **cold center**".

***Hao mian* 好眠, a longing for sleep** [6]

IS identical with → *duo shui* 多睡, profuse sleeping. *ZBYHL* 20: 其為病也，胸脅脹滿，水穀不消，結在腹內兩肋，水入腸胃，動作有聲，體重多唾，短氣**好眠**, "When this results in a disease, the chest and the flanks experience distension and a feeling of fullness. Water and grain are no longer dissolved and form nodes in both flanks in the abdomen. The water that flows into the intestines and the stomach makes sounds when [the body] moves it. The body feels heavy with much saliva. [Patients are] short of qi and have **a longing for sleep**".

***Hao ou* 好嘔to be prone to vomit** [2]

IS identical with → *xi ou* 喜嘔. *QJYF* 18: 白蟲在脾中為病，令人**好嘔**, "When white bugs/worms are in one's liver and cause a disease, this causes that person to **be prone to vomit".**

***Hao yan* 好魘, to be prone to have nightmares** [1]

PC identical with → *yan mei* 魘寐, nightmare. *BCSY* SE *wa zeng* 瓦甑：**好魘**及無夢，取火燒死者灰，著枕中、履中即止, "For **proneness to nightmares** and the absence of dreams: take the ashes of an incinerated corpse and deposit it in a headrest or in a shoe. This will stop it".

***He* 核, kernel** [p]

① PS of the hard kernel in a fruit that contains the nutlet. *BJ* SE *rui he* 蕤核：主心腹邪結氣，明目, "*Rui* **kernels**. They control evil and bound qi in heart and abdomen, and clear the eyes".

② PC of swelling or strange items shaped like a kernel and developing anywhere on the body. Sometimes one has a sensation as if some passage were blocked by an item resembling a kernel. *MYBL* SE *xuan shen* 玄參：下水，止煩渴，散頸下**核**, "It drains water, ends vexation with thirst, and disperses **kernels** below the neck".

***He bing* 合病, joint disease** [2]

PC in the course of harm caused by cold condition affecting the six conduits, when two or sometimes three conduits simultaneously receive evil which leads to disease. *SHL* 268: 三陽**合病**，脈浮大，上關上，但欲眠睡，目合則汗, "When the three yang [conduits] have a **joint disease**, the [movement in the] vessels is at the surface and massive. [The movement] rises to above the 'gate'-section. One only desires to sleep. When one closes the eyes, sweating sets in".

***He hou* 齁齁, roaring panting** [4]

PC identical with → *hou chuan* 齁喘. *PJF* 163: 夫治哮呴嗽者，一名**齁齁**，涎在咽喉間，令人喘嗽不寧, "Now, to cure roaring cough, another name is '**roaring panting**'. There is saliva in the throat that makes people pant and cough and not find rest".

***He qian xuan chuang* 荷錢癬瘡, lotus germ-bud *xuan*-illness sores** [1]

PC identical with → *qian xuan* 錢癬, coin[-size] *xuan*-illness. *BCGM* SE *mu jin* 木槿 quotes *JYF*: **荷錢癬瘡**：巴豆仁三個，連油杵泥，以生絹包擦，日一二次，三日痊好, "For **lotus germ-bud *xuan*-illness sores**: 3 kernels of *ba dou* are to be pounded with their own oil until they form a pulp. This is wrapped in a cloth made from raw silk to rub [the afflicted region] once or twice daily. After three days a complete cure will be achieved".

***He xi feng* 鶴膝風, crane knee wind** [2] AN *xi feng* 膝風, knee wind; *feng jiao ruan* 風脚軟， wind-induced leg weakness.

PC of swelling and pain of the knee, and shrinking of the lower leg, with difficulties in bending and stretching, and a lack of strength to walk. *SJZL* 8: 治脚膝風，俗名**鶴膝風**，乾蠍丸方, "Recipe for pills with dried scorpions to cure leg and knee wind, commonly called '**crane knee wind**'".

***He yu zhi ji* 河魚之疾, river fish ailment** [2]

PC of → *pi shi* 脾濕, spleen moisture, brought forth by extended immersion in water. *LBLY* Fj: 水母…性暖，治**河魚之疾**, "*Shui mu*...its nature is warm. It cures **river fish ailment**".

***He zhong* 核腫, kernel swelling** [2]

① IS of swollen testicles. *YXL* SE *hai zao* 海藻：療疝氣下墜疼痛，**核腫**, "It cures elevation-illness qi that has sunken [into the testicles] and creates pain with **kernel swelling**".

② PC identical with → *zhong he* 腫核, swelling with kernels. *BCGM* SE *mao* 貓 quotes *ZHF*: 治鼠瘺**核腫**，或已潰出膿血者，取貓肉如常作羹，空心食之，云不傳之法也, "To cure mouse fistula with **kernel swelling**, and also those cases which have opened to release pus and blood, take cat meat and prepare an ordinary thick soup to be consumed on an empty stomach. This is a method that is not supposed to be transferred to others".

***Hei ban* 黑斑, black macule** [6]

① IS of black → *ban* 斑①, macules, developing on the skin. *ZLBC* SE *ai ye* 艾葉quotes *SHLY*: 治婦人妊娠七月，若傷寒壯熱，赤斑變為**黑斑**，溺血, "To cure women in their seventh month of pregnancy, if they have been harmed by cold and have a high fever, with red macules developing into **black macules**, and blood in their urine".

② PC of black macules or chunks appearing on one's face that neither ache nor itch. *BCGM* SE *xi er* 枲耳 quotes *ZXF*: 面上**黑斑**：蒼耳葉焙為末，食後米飲調服一錢，一月愈, "**Black macules** on the face: Bake *cang er* leaves over a slow fire and prepare a powder. After meals ingest 1 *qian* mixed with the liquid obtained by boiling rice. A cure will be achieved within one month".

***Hei dan* 黑疸, dark *dan*-illness** [10]

PC of a long-lasting → *huang dan* 黃疸, yellow *dan*-illness, where the proper qi has weakened, and the yellow complexion has darkened. *JGYL* Mj: 酒疸下之，久久為**黑疸**, "If one treats *dan* illness [caused by] wine by purgative means, after some time it will turn into **dark *dan*-illness**".

***Hei gan* 黑皯, gloom** [10] AW 黑皯.

PC identical with → *mian gan* 面皯, facial gloom. *BJ* SE *nü wei* 女萎：久服去面**黑皯**，好顏色, "If ingested for an extended period of time it will remove facial **gloom** and improve one's complexion".

Hei gan **黑皯, gloom** [3]
PC identical with → *mian gan* 面皯, facial gloom. *MYBL* SE *da dou huang juan* 大豆黃卷：去**黑皯**，潤澤皮毛, "It removes **gloom** and returns glossiness to skin and hair".

Hei huang **黑黃, dark jaundice** [2]
PC identical with → *hei dan* 黑疸, dark *dan*-illness. *PJF* 196: **黑黃**，病人身面黑黃, "**Dark jaundice**: the patient's body and facial complexion is dark yellow".

Hei yi **黑翳, black membrane** [2]
PC of a → *mu yi* 目翳, eye shade, with a black/dark speckled membrane. *WTMY* 21: 療眼**黑翳**覆瞳子膚起方, "Recipe to cure eyes with a **black/dark membrane** rising as a skin in front of the pupil".

Hei zhi **黑痣, black mole** [3] AN *yan zi* 黶子; *hei zi* 黑子, black spot.
PC of black aax 痣, mole. Such moles emerge when wind evil and blood qi strike each other. They differ from ordinary moles. *ZBYHL* 31: **黑痣**者，風邪搏於血氣，變化所生也, "**Black moles** develop through a transformation caused by wind evil clashing with blood and qi".

Hei zi **黑子, black spot** [21]
PC identical with → *hei zhi* 黑痣, black mole. *ZBYHL* 31: 面及體生黑點為黑痣，亦云**黑子**, "When black stains develop on one's face or body, these are black moles. Another name is '**black spot**'".

Heng chan **橫產, transverse delivery** [3]
PC identical with → *heng sheng* 橫生, transverse birth. *ZBYHL* 43: **橫產**，由初覺腹痛，產時未至，驚動傷早，兒轉未竟，便用力產之，故令橫也, "A **transverse delivery** results from one's first feeling abdominal pain. Then, although the due date is not reached yet, [the woman] is nervous and moves and harms [the fetus because it is too] early. The turning of the child remains incomplete, and [the woman] uses force to give birth to it. Hence it assumes a transverse position".

Heng chuang **胻疮, shin sores** [3]
PC identical with → *lian chuang* 臁疮, shank sores. *QJYF* 22: 在腨胫间喜生疮，中水恶露寒冻不瘥，经年成骨疽，亦名**胻疮**. "There is a tendency for sores to develop in the region of the calves and shins. If they are subjected to water, malign dew, and freezing, and if this is not healed, in the course of a year this develops into a bone impediment-illness. It is also called **shin sores**". *BCGM* Bai bing zhu zhi yao 百病主治药：胻疮，即**臁疮**, "**Shin sores** are shank sores".

Heng ju **胻疽, shin impediment-illness** [2]
PC of → heng chuang 胻疮, shin sores. *BCGM* SE shi 豕 quoting *QJYF* 22: 在腨胫间喜生疮，中水恶露寒冻不瘥，经年成骨疽，亦名胻疮, "There is a tendency for sores to develop in the region of the calves and shins. If they are subjected to water, malign dew, and freezing, and if this is not healed, after several years this develops into a bone impediment-illness. It is also called 'shin sores'". writes: **胻疽**青爛：生於胻脛間，惡水淋漓，經年瘡冷，敗為深疽青黑，好肉虛腫，百藥不瘥，或瘥而復發, "**Shin impediment-illnesses** with a blu-

ish-green and festering color develop in the region of the shin. Bad water leaks from them. In the course of a year the sores become cold and rot and turn into a deep-lying impediment illness with greenish-blue to black color. [What is left of] good flesh is hollow and swollen. No medication will achieve a cure. If it appears cured, it will break out again".

***Heng ni* 橫逆, [birth of a child] in a transverse postion and in a position contrary to normal.** [4]
PC CD of → *heng sheng* 橫生, transverse birth, and → *ni sheng* 逆產, delivery [of a child in] a position contrary to normal. *QJYF* 2: 亦治**橫逆**生者, "They also cure births [of a child] in a **transverse postion and and in a position contrary to normal**".

***Heng sheng* 橫生, birth [of a child] in a transverse position** [24] AN *heng chan* 橫產, delivery [of a child] in a transverse position.
PC of → *nan chan* 難產, difficult birth, of a baby from a breech presentation, with the child entering the birth canal with the buttocks or feet first. *MYBL* SE *wu gou xue* 烏狗血：主產難**橫生**，血上搶心者, "It controls difficult birth and **birth [of a child] in a transverse position**, as well as rising blood knocking at the heart".

***Hong beng* 紅崩, red collapse** [1]
PC identical with → *chi beng* 赤崩. *BCGM* SE *zhan* 氈quotes *HSF*: 氈燒灰，酒服二錢，白崩用白氈，**紅崩**用紅氈, "Burn felt to ashes and ingest two *qian* with wine. For **white collapse** take white felt; for red collapse take red felt".

***Hong han* 紅汗, red sweat** [1]
PC identical with → *xue han* 血汗, blood sweat. *SYDXF* 7: 黃耆建中湯，治汗出污衣…病名**紅汗**, "The 'decoction with *huang qi* to build up the center' cures sweating that soils one's clothing. ...This disease is called '**red sweat**'".

***Hong li* 紅痢, red free-flux illness** [4]
PC identical with → *chi li* 赤痢. *SYDXF* 17 RE *du shen wan* 獨神丸, pills with a single wondrous ingredient: **紅痢**，生地黃、春茶煎湯嚼下, "For **red free-flux illness**, chew [the pills] and swallow them with a decoction of *sheng di huang* with tea harvested in the early spring".

***Hong zhong* 紅腫, red and swollen** [8]
IS identical with → *chi zhong* 赤腫. *SYDXF* 16: 傷寒病安後，眼目疼痛**紅腫**, "After harm caused by cold disease has been healed, the eyes are painful, **red and swollen**".

***Hong zhong* 洪腫, vast swelling** [5]
IS of a conspicuous → *fu zhong* 浮腫, surface swelling. *JGYL* Mj: 風氣相擊，身體**洪腫**，汗出乃愈, "When wind and qi hit each other, the body develops a **vast swelling**. It is cured when sweat leaves the body".

***Hou* 齁, roaring** [4]
PC AD of → *hou chuan* 齁喘, roaring panting. *YXL* SE *yu bai pi* 榆白皮：能主利五淋，治不眠，療**齁**, "It is able to master and set free the five types of dripping. It cures insomnia. It heals **roaring**".

Hou bi **喉痹, throat blockage** [215]

CD of PCs with a swollen, painful, and obstructed throat that, in severe cases, does not even let liquids enter and impairs breathing. *SW* 7: 一陰一陽結，謂之**喉痹**, "First yin and first yang nodes are called '**throat blockage**'". References in the *BCGM* to throat blockage include some diseases of the mouth and the tongue.

Hou bi **喉閉, throat closure** [14]

① PC identical with → *hou bi* 喉痹, throat blockage. *TBC* SE *di bu rong* 地不容：主解蠱毒，止煩熱，辟瘴癘，利**喉閉**及痰毒, "It controls the dissolution of *gu* poison, stops vexing heat, eliminates miasmatic epidemics, opens **throat closure** and [drains] phlegm poison".

② IS of muscle spasm making drinking impossible. *PJF* 376: 開關散，治嬰孩小兒驚風癇疾，**喉閉**，牙關緊急, "Powder that opens barriers. It cures fright wind epilepsy ailment of newborns and children, with **throat closure**, and clenched jaw".

Hou bing **喉病, throat disease** [1]

PC CD of diseases affecting the throat. *BCGM* Bai bing zhu zhi yao 百病主治藥：白礬…同鹽，點一切**喉病**, "*Bai fan*…with salt: swab on all **throat diseases**".

Hou chuan **齁喘, roaring panting** [14] AD *hou* 齁; AN *hou he* 齁鮯, *he hou* 鮯齁.

PC identical with *xiao chuan* 哮喘. *YS* 4: 信州老兵女三歲，因食鹽蝦過多，遂得**齁喘**之疾, "The three-year-old daughter of an old soldier in Xinzhou ate too much salt and too many shrimps. As a result she developed the ailment of **roaring panting**".

Hou feng **喉風, throat wind** [18] CD of

PCs with mouth, tongue, and throat swelling and pain. *SJZL* 122: 治一切**喉風**閉塞咽喉諸疾，去毒丸方, "The recipe for 'pills to remove poison' cures all types of **throat wind** closing the throat". The diseases alluded to by the terms throat wind, *hou feng* 喉風, and throat blockage, *hou bi* 喉痹, are basically identical. Throat wind signifies a swift onset of the disease. The name throat blockage is meant to focus attention on the closure of the throat. *BCGM* regularly makes use of both these terms indiscriminately. Thus, 九種喉痹, nine types of throat blockage, includes *ji hou feng* 急喉風, acute throat wind, and *chan hou feng* 纏喉風, throat-constricting wind. Also, it uses terms such as *ji hou feng bi* 急喉風痹, acute throat wind blockage, and *ma hou bi feng* 馬喉痹風, throat blockage wind [as fast as a galloping] horse.

Hou feng ji zheng **喉風急證, acute condition of throat wind** [1]

PC identical with → *ji hou feng* 急喉風, acute throat wind. *BCGM* SE *shan dou gen* 山豆根 quotes *XCWKJYF*: **喉風急證**：牙關緊閉, 水穀不下, "**Acute condition of throat wind**: tightly closed jaws; water and grain fail to move down".

***Hou he* 齁鮯, roaring panting** [5]

PC identical with → *hou chuan* 齁喘, roaring panting. *BCTJ* SE *shi xian* 石莧：土人與甘草同服，治**齁鮯**及吐風涎, "The locals ingest it together with *gan cao* to cure **roaring panting** and spitting of wind drool".

***Hou lou* 喉瘺, throat fistula** [1]

PC of → *lou* 瘺, fistula, developing at the throat. *BCGM* SE *gou ju* 枸橘 (leaves): 又治**喉瘺**，消腫導毒, "They also cure **throat fistula**. They dissolve the swelling and eliminate the poison".

***Hou ming chuan* 喉鳴喘, chirp-panting throat** [1]

IS of hectic, difficult breathing with chirping sounds emitted from the throat. *BJ* SE *yuan hua* 芫花：主咳逆上氣，**喉鳴喘**，咽腫短氣, "It controls cough with counterflow and rising qi, **chirp-panting throat**, swollen throat, and shortness of qi".

***Hou se* 喉塞, throat obstruction** [2] AN *hou zhong se* 喉中塞.

PC with an impassable throat that makes ingesting beverages and food difficult. *BCGM* SE *wo niu* 蝸牛 quoting *SJZL* 122: 治咽喉閉塞不通, "To cure throat obstruction and impassability". writes: **喉塞**口噤, "**Throat obstruction** and clenched jaw".

***Hou she zhu ji* 喉舌諸疾, all types of ailments of the throat and the tongue** [1]

PC CD of diseases affecting the throat and the tongue. *BCGM* SE *she tui* 蛇蛻：治驚癇、癜駁、**喉舌諸疾**, "To cure fright epilepsy, patches and variegations, and **all types of ailments of the throat and the tongue**".

***Hou xiao* 齁哮, roaring panting** [1]

PC identical with → *xiao chuan* 哮喘. *BCGM* SE *mao* 貓quotes *ZXF*: **齁哮**痰咳：貓糞燒灰，砂糖湯服一錢, "**Roaring panting** and phlegmy cough: Burn cat feces to ashes. Ingest 1 *qian* with rock sugar decoction".

***Hou xing* 喉腥, bad odor in the throat** [5]

IS of a feeling as if there were a bad-smelling object in the throat. *HJJF* 1: 肺熱**喉腥**，脾熱口甜，膽熱口苦, "Lung heat and **bad odor in the throat;** spleen heat and a sweet flavor in the mouth; gallbladder heat and a bitter flavor in the mouth".

***Hou yan bi* 喉咽閉, throat closure** [1]

IS identical with → *yan hou bi se* 咽喉閉塞. *BJ* SE *fei lian* 蜚蠊：破積聚，**喉咽閉**，內寒無子, "It breaks through accumulations and collections, **throat closure** and [cures] internal cold with childlessness".

***Hou zhong* 後重, a feeling of heavy pressure at one's behind** [21] AN *xia zhong* 下重.

IS of an urge to defecate but when one actually tries to relieve oneself nothing is discharged. *MYBL* SE *bai la* 白蠟：療久泄，**後重**，見白膿, "It heals prolonged outflow and flush, **a feeling of heavy pressure at one's behind**, with an appearance of white pus".

***Hou zhong qi sai* 喉中氣塞, qi blockage in the throat** [1]

IS of difficult breathing, as if there were an obstacle in the throat blocking the passage of qi. *BCYY* SE *ha jie* 蛤蚧：**喉中氣塞**，胸鬲噎痛，蛤蚧、阿膠、

生犀角、鹿角膠、羚羊角一兩；除膠外，皆為屑，次入膠，分四服, "[For curing] **qi blockage in the throat**, with choking and pain in the region of chest and diaphragm: 1 *liang* each of *ha jie*, *a jiao*, fresh *xi jiao*, *lu jiao* glue, and *ling yang jiao*. Except for the glues, work all items into crumbs and one by one add them to the glues. Divide into four portions and ingest".

Hou zhong se **喉中塞, throat obstruction** [1]
PC identical with → *hou se* 喉塞. *BCSY* SE *xuan gou gen* 懸鉤根：取莖燒為末服之，亦主**喉中塞**也, "Roast the stem, grind to a powder, and ingest this. It also controls **throat obstruction**".

Hou zhong sheng rou **喉中生肉, flesh growth in the throat** [1]
PC identical with → *yang sheng xi rou* 咽生瘜肉, the throat grows tumorous flesh. *ZLBC* SE *shi yan* 食鹽 quotes *SZRSJ*: 主卒**喉中生肉**，以綿裹箸頭柱鹽揩，日六七度易, "To control sudden **flesh growth in the throat**: Swab with salt using the tips of chopsticks wrapped in silk cloth. Change six, seven times daily".

Hou zhong si wu **喉中似物, a sensation as if there were an object in the throat** [1]
PC identical with *mei he ge qi* 梅核膈氣, plum-pit occlusion qi. *ZLBC* SE *bai rang he* 白蘘荷 quotes *HShF*: 治**喉中似物**，吞吐不出，腹脹羸瘦, "It cures **a sensation as if there were an object in the throat** that cannot be swallowed and cannot be thrown out. The abdomen is distended with emaciaton".

Hou zhong shui ji ming **喉中水雞鳴, water fowl chirping in the throat** [1]
IS of hectic, difficult breathing, with sounds emitted from the throat similar to the chirping of water fowl. *WTMY* 10: 療上氣咳嗽，**喉中水雞鳴**，唾膿血腥臭，麻黃湯方, "To cure rising qi with cough, **water fowl chirping in the throat**, spitting of pus and blood with a malodorous stench: the recipe for a decoction with *ma huang*".

Hou zhong xing chou **喉中腥臭, malodorous stench from within the throat** [2]
AN *hou zhong xing qi* 喉中腥氣, malodorous qi from within the throat.
PC with a malodorous stench emitted by the throat that the patient himself is able to perceive. LSZ suggests that this is brought forth by lung heat. *BCGM* SE *huang qin* 黃芩quoting LTY: 黃芩之苦寒，能瀉火補氣而利肺，治**喉中腥臭**, "The bitter and cold nature of *huang qin* is capable of draining fire and supplementing qi and of setting free the lung function. It cures **malodorous stench from within the throat**".

Hou zhong xing qi **喉中腥氣, malodorous qi from within the throat** [1]
PC identical with → *hou zhong xing chou* 喉中腥臭, malodorous stench from within the throat. *BCGM* Bai bing zhu zhi yao 百病主治藥：知母、黃芩，並瀉肺熱，**喉中腥氣**, "*Zhi mu* and *huang qin*, they both serve to drain lung heat and **malodorous qi from within the throat**".

Hou zi **瘊子, wart** [2]
PC identical with → *you* 疣. *BCYY* SE *ku cai* 苦菜：葉如苦苣，更狹，其綠色差淡，折之白乳汁出，常常點**瘊子**，自落, "The leaves resemble those of *ku ju* but are even narrower. Their green color is weaker. When broken they will

release a white milk juice. If this is repeatedly dropped on a **wart**, it will fall off by itself".

Hu chou **胡臭, barbarian stench** [30] AN *hu chou* 狐臭, fox odor

PC of a distinct odor originating in the armpits or from other parts of the body. *QJYF* 24: 有天生**胡臭**，有為人所染臭者, "There is [one's own] natural **barbarian stench**, and there is stench that is acquired from another person".

Hu chou **狐臭, fox stench** [6]

PC identical with → *hu chou* 胡臭, barbarian stench. *ZHF* 6: 療身體及腋下**狐臭**方, "Recipe to cure **fox stench** from the body and armpits".

Hu ci chuang **狐刺瘡, sores resulting from fox piercing** [1]

PC identical with → *hu niao ci zhuang* 狐尿刺瘡, sores resulting from fox urine piercing. *BCSY* SE *yi xue zhong chu tu* 蟻穴中出土：取七枚如粒，和醋搽**狐刺瘡**, "Take seven grain-size portions, mix with vinegar and apply to the **sores resulting from fox piercing**".

Hu ci niao chuang **狐刺尿瘡, sores resulting from a fox's piercing urine** [1]

PC identical with → *hu niao ci zhuang* 狐尿刺瘡, sores resulting from fox urine piercing. *BCGM* SE *qu* 曲 quotes *GJLY*: **狐刺尿瘡**：曲末和獨頭蒜，杵如麥粒，納瘡孔中，蟲出愈, "**Sores resulting from a fox's piercing urine**: pound yeast powder and a single clove of garlic to the size of wheat grain and insert into the opening of the sores. When a bug has left it will be healed".

Hu huo **狐惑, fox and delusion** [5]

PC of putrid flesh and festering ulcers in the throat and private parts brought forth by moisture, heat, and bug poison. *JGYL* Fj: **狐惑**之為病，狀如傷寒，默默欲眠，目不得閉，臥起不安。蝕於喉為惑，蝕於陰為狐, "In its appearance the disease **fox and delusion** resembles harm caused by cold. Patients are quiet and wish to sleep. But they cannot close their eyes. Both when lying down and rising they find no peace. If the lesion is in the throat, this is 'delusion'; if it is in one's genital parts, this is 'fox'".

Hu jia **狐瘕, fox conglomeration-illness** [3]

PC of conglomerations formed as a result of a frightening event or other mental harm experienced during menstruation. It is often associated with mental problems. *WTMY* 34: **狐瘕**者，婦人月水當日數來，而反悲哀自恐，若以遠行，逢暴風疾雨，電雷驚恐, "As for '**fox conglomeration-illness**', [its causes are as follows]: When a woman's period arrives on time in large quantities, and if still she is plagued by sorrow or spontaneous fear, or if she travels a long way and encounters violent wind and torrential rain, and is terrified by lightning and thunder".

Hu mei **狐魅, fox seduction-specter** [9]

PC of a psychiatric problem with mental instability and use of strange language. It was believed that this is caused by fox demons or hostile magic. *SLBC* SE *hu yin jing* 狐陰莖：**狐魅**狀候，或叉手有禮見人，或於靜處獨語，或裸形見人，或祗揖無度，或多語，成緊合口，叉手坐，禮度過，常尿屎亂放，此之謂也, "The signs of **fox seduction-specter**: patients may display rituals of reverence [without being in an appropriate situation]. Or they speak to themselves in quiet places. Or they expose themselves to others undressed. Or they excessively bow with their hands clasped. Or they are talkative. Or their mouth is firmly closed. They sit with their hands laid together, perform the rites excessively, and they frequently pass urine and defecate in a disorderly way. This is what that means".

***Hu niao chuang* 狐尿瘡, fox urine sores** [4]
PC identical with → *hu niao ci zhuang* 狐尿刺瘡, sores resulting from fox urine piercing. *BCGM* SE *liao* 蓼 quoting *BCSY*: 搗傅狐刺瘡, "Pound and apply to the fox piercing sores". writes: 搗爛，傅**狐尿瘡**, "Pound until mashed and apply to the **fox urine sores**".

***Hu niao ci* 狐尿刺, fox urine piercing** [4]
① EA of poisonous substances left on herbs and trees by all types of poisonous bugs/snakes/insects. *QJYF* 25: 治因瘡腫痛劇者，數日死；或中風寒，或中水，或中**狐尿刺**主之方, "To cure those who experience excruciatingly painful sores and swelling and will die within a few days. Apply recipes that help control being struck by wind cold, by water, and by **fox urine piercing**.
② PC identical with → *hu niao ci zhuang* 狐尿刺瘡. *QJYiF* 20: 諸螳螂之類，盛暑之時多有孕育，著諸物上，必有精汁，其汁乾久則有毒，人手觸之不王相之間，則成其疾，名曰**狐尿刺**，日夜磣痛，不識眠睡，百方治之不瘥, "When they breed at the time of abounding summerheat, all types of mantis attach themselves to various items, where they leave their sperm liquid. When this liquid has dried for some time it will be poisonous. When someone touches it with his hand he will develop this ailment without noticing it. It is called '**fox urine piercing**'. A gritty pain is felt day and night, and one cannot sleep".

***Hu niao ci chuang* 狐尿刺瘡, sores resulting from being pierced by fox urine** [8]
AN *hu niao ci* 狐尿刺, fox urine piercing; *hu ci chuang* 狐刺瘡, sores resulting from fox piercing; *ci chuang* 刺瘡, piercing sores; *hu niao chuang* 狐尿瘡, sores resulting from fox urine; *hu ci niao chuang* 狐刺尿瘡, sores resulting from the piercing urine of foxes.
PC CD of → *chuang* 瘡, sores, conditions resulting from touching poisonous substances left on herbs and trees by all types of poisonous bugs/snakes/insects. *MYBL* SE *lu feng fang* 露峰房：水煮，洗**狐尿刺瘡**, "Boil in water and use to wash **sores resulting from being pierced by fox urine**".

***Hu shan* 狐疝, fox elevation-illness** [4]
PC of → *shan* 疝, elevation-illness, with a sudden swelling and pulling pain affecting the scrotum, and with alternating appearance and disappearance of the swelling. *QJYF* 30: **狐疝**走上下，引小腹痛, "**Fox elevation-illness** moves up and down. The pain pulls on the lower abdomen". The image of a "fo". implies a feeling of an item erratically moving in the body.

Hu xi yu jue **呼吸欲絕, breathing on the verge of interruption** [3]
IS of difficult breathing as if it were not to continue. *MYBL* SE *bai qian* 白前：主上氣衝喉中，**呼吸欲絕**, "It controls rising qi rushing into the throat, with **breathing on the verge of interruption**".

Hu zhong **忽腫, sudden and violent swelling** [2]
IS identical with → *cu zhong* 卒腫. *TPSHF* 9: 下焦有熱，則熱氣衝陰，陰頭**忽腫**，便溺不得，乃至生瘡, "When the lower burner is affected by heat, the heat qi will rush against the penis. As a result, the glans penis shows a **sudden and violent swelling**. Urination is impossible. This will develop into sores".

Hua li **滑利, smooth free-flux; to stimulate smoothness and free flow** [12]
① PC identical with → *hua xie* 滑泄①, smooth outflow. *SJZL* 45：臟腑**滑利**，水穀不消，脹滿腸鳴, "**Smooth free-flux** from the depots and palaces. Liquid and solid food are not digested. A feeling of distension and fullness, and intestinal sounds".
② PE of moistening and smoothening to enable passage. Identical with *hua xie* 滑泄②, smooth outflow. *MYBL* SE *yu pi* 榆皮：主腸胃邪熱氣，消腫。性**滑利**, "It controls heat evil qi in the intestines and the stomach. It dissolves swelling. Its nature is **to stimulate smoothness and free flow**".

Hua li **滑痢, smooth free-flux-illness** [6]
PC identical with → *hua li* 滑利①, smooth free-flux. *PJF* 38: 夏月不宜吃豬肉、冷水，恐致**滑痢**不止, "In summer one should not eat pork or drink cold water, lest one contract **smooth free-flux-illness** that will not end".

Hua tai **滑胎, to smoothen fetal [passage]** [12]
TA of using all types of pharmaceutical drugs with a lubricating ability to smoothen the passage through an aperture so as to assist a woman in giving birth. *QJYF* 2 lists: **滑胎**令易產方, "Recipes **to smoothen fetal [passage]** and ease delivery".

Hua xie **滑泄, smooth outflow; to smoothen outflow** [18] AW *hua xie* 滑瀉.
① PC of an uncontrollable → *xie xie* 泄瀉, outflow. *TPSHF* 26：RE *ban gan san* 拌肝散, powder to assist the liver: 治脾勞虛冷，大腸**滑泄**, "It cures spleen exhaustion with depletion cold, and **smooth outflow** from the large intestine".
② PE of opening and smoothening passages. *BCYY* SE *xie* 薤：千金治肺氣喘急，用薤白，亦取其**滑泄**也, "The *QJ*[*YF* states]: To cure panting and rapid lung qi, use *xie bai*. This is also to resort to its [ability to] **smoothen outflow**".

Hua xie **滑瀉, smooth outflow** [5]
PC identical with → *hua xie* 滑泄①, smooth outflow. *QXLF* 13: 治臟腑**滑瀉**, "To cure **smooth outflow** from the depots and palaces".

Hua xuan **花癬, flowery *xuan*-illness** [1]
PC identical with → *xuan* 癬, *xuan*-illness a). *HYBC* SE *hai hong dou* 海紅豆：主人黑皮䵟黷，**花癬**，頭面游風, "It controls blackened skin and dermal dark spots, **flowery *xuan*-illness**, as well as roaming wind in the head and face".

***Hua yi* 花翳, flowery shade** [3]
PC of → *mu yi* 目翳, eye shade, with many white dots resembling date flowers and fish scales. *TPSHF* 6: 治眼生**花翳**，龍腦散方, "Recipe for the powder with *long nao* to cure eyes developing **flowery shades**".

***Huai zheng* 壞證, condition following malpractice** [2] Difficult to cure
PC of various sorts resulting from a mistaken treatment of harm caused by cold. *SYJYBZFL* 4: 其如**壞證**治法，除各見本門外，編集於後, "As for therapeutic approaches to cure **conditions following malpractice**, in addition to all those documented in the respective sections, there is additional data compiled below". *SHL* calls them 壞病, diseases resulting from malpractice.

***Huai zi bu ru* 懷子不乳, pregnant with no prospect of breast-feeding** [2]
PC identical with → *nan chan* 難產, difficult birth. *PJF* 328: 治婦人**懷子不乳**, "To cure women who are **pregnant with no prospect of breast-feeding**".

***Huan* 瘓, right side paralysis** [p]
PC AD of → *tan huan* 癱瘓②, paralysis. If a → *tan huan* 癱瘓, paralysis, affects one's right side, the abbreviation is *huan* 瘓. *HJJF* 1: 乳香應痛丸，治一切風氣，左癱右**瘓**，口眼喎斜，半身不遂，語言謇澀, "The 'pills with *ru xiang* that respond to pain' cure all types of wind qi, left side paralysis, **right side paralysis**, with mouth and eyes assuming an awry position, and one half of the body not following one's will. The [patient's] language is hampered".

***Huan* 緩, relaxed; to slacken; to relax** [p].
① AN *zong chi* 縱弛; *chi huan* 弛緩; *zong huan* 縱緩; *huan ruo* 緩弱; *ju huan* 拘緩. IS of a slackening and weakening of limbs and joints so that even though one may still be able to raise the four extremities one depends on physical assistance, such as a cane, to move. *ZBYHL* 2: 四肢頑痹，支節火燃，心裏懊熱，手足俱**緩**, "The four limbs are affected by stubborn blockage. The joints feel as if on fire. The heart feels regret and heat. Hands and feet **slacken**"...
② PuQ AD of *huan mai* 緩脈, relaxed movement in the vessels. *SW* 18: **緩**而滑曰熱中, "If [the movement in the vessels] is **relaxed** and smooth, this is called: 'heated center'".
③ TA AD of *huan ji* 緩急, to relax tensions, and *huan zhong* 緩中, to relax the center. *SW* 22: 肝苦急，急食甘以**緩**之, "When the liver suffers from tensions, quickly consume sweet [flavor] to **relax** [these tensions]".

***Huan bing* 緩病, slow disease** [1]
CD of PCs with a slow onset and a slow further development. *BCGM* SE *da huang* 大黄 quoting *YSZL* 14: 滾痰丸…一切無病之人, 遍身筋骨等處平白疼痛, 不能名狀者, 每服七八十丸, "The pills to remove phlegm. ...In all those cases where a healthy has pain all over the body and all the time, involving sinews, bones, etc. without being able to give the signs a name, each time ingest 70 to 80 pills". writes: 滾痰丸…**緩病**七八十丸, "The pills to remove phlegm. ...For **slow diseases** [ingest] 70 to 80 pills

***Huan ji* 緩急, tight; to relax tension; relaxed or urgent; slow and acute; critical** [14]

① IS of a stiffness and tension of the joints and sinews, with the term *huan* 緩, slack, as opposite to *ji* 急, stiff, tense, remaining meaningless. *BJ* SE *gou ji* 狗脊: 主腰背強，關機**緩急**, "It controls stiffness of the lumbar region and back; as well as joints and muscles that are **tight**".

② TA of employing pharmaceutical substances of sweet-sour flavor to resolve and eliminate tension and pain. *YXQY* Lj: 甘能**緩急**，淡能利竅, "Sweet flavor is able **to relax tension**; bland flavor is able to make orifices passable".

③ Refers to sequence and speed of therapies. 指次序先後與速度快慢. *SW* 74: 氣有多少，病有盛衰，治有**緩急**, "The qi is present in different quantities, the disease [qi] may abound or be weak, the treatment may be **relaxed or urgent** (depending on what is to be treated first: acute signs or basic disease)".

④ Refers to the critical or stable status of a disease. *ZBYHL* 42: 云有**緩急**，緩者延引日月，急者止在旦夕, "It is said that there are **slow and acute episodes**. Slow episodes continue for days or even months; acute episodes reach their end within one day".

⑤ Refers to a critical situation only, with the term *huan* 緩, slow, relaxed, as opposed to *ji* 急, critical, remaining meaningless. *JGYL* Fj: 胸痹，**緩急**者，薏苡附子散主之, "Chest blockage. **Very critical** cases can be controlled by the powder with *yi yi* and *fu zi*".

***Huan ju* 緩疽, chronic progressive impediment-illness** [2]

PC CD of → *ju* 疽, impediment-illnesses, with nodular swelling and deep-reaching pain where the erosion of tissue and festering slowly progress and the prognosis is inauspicious. *ZBYHL* 33: 以其結腫積久，而肉腐壞遲，故名**緩疽**, "As its nodular swelling collects over an extended period of time, and because the flesh rots away completely one calls this '**chronic progressive impediment-illness**'".

***Huan ruo* 緩弱, relaxed; to slacken** [8]

① IS identical with → *huan* 緩①. *QJYF* 8: 偏枯、冷痹，**緩弱**疼重, "Hemilateral withering; cold blockage; **slackening**, pain and a feeling of heaviness".

② PC identical with → *jiao qi* 脚氣, leg qi. *TBC* SE *e shi* 惡實: 根，主牙齒疼痛，勞瘧，脚**緩弱**，風毒癰疽, "The root: it controls toothache, exhaustion malaria, **slackening** of the legs, and wind poison with obstruction- as well as impediment-illnesses".

***Huan yi* 幻翳, illusory shade** [1]

PC identical with → *mu yi* 目翳. *ZZNYXF* 2: 青白色**幻翳**遮睛, "An **illusory shade** of greenish-white color covers the eyeball".

***Huan zhong* 緩中, to relax the center** [8]

TA of employing pharmaceutical substances of sweet-sour flavor to regulate the spleen and stomach, and to ease abdominal pain and vomiting in situations of spleen and stomach tightness. *MYBL* SE *shao yao* 芍藥: 主通順血脈，**緩中**, "It works by making the blood vessels smoothly penetrable, and **relaxes the center**".

***Huang* 黄, jaundice** [p]
PC identical with → *huang dan* 黄疸, yellow *dan*-illness. *ZBYHL* 12: 若其人眼睛澀疼，鼻骨疼，兩膊及項強，腰背急，即是患**黄**, "If this person's eyes feel rough and are painful, if the nasal bone aches, if both arms and the nape of the neck are stiff, and if the back and the lumbar region are tight, [this person] suffers from **jaundice**".

***Huang bing* 黄病, jaundice** [29]
PC identical with → *huang dan* 黄疸, yellow *dan*-illness. *ZHF* 4: 治卒發黄膽諸**黄病**, "To cure a sudden outbreak of yellow gallbladder, all types of **jaundice**".

***Huang dan* 黄癉, yellow *dan*-illness; jaundice** [1]
PC identical with → *huang dan* 黄疸. *BCGM* SE *niu* 牛 quoting *TBC* 消渴黄疸, "Melting with thirst and yellow *dan*-illness". writes: 消渴**黄癉**, "Melting with thirst and **yellow *dan*-illness**".

***Huang dan* 黄疸, yellow *dan*-illness; jaundice** [157] AD *huang* 黄, *dan* 疸; AN *huang bing* 黄病, yellow disease ; *huang ji* 黄疾, yellow ailment ; *dan ji* 疸疾, *dan*-ailment ; *dan huang* 疸黄, *dan*-illness with yellowness. Rare: *huang dan* 黄癉.
PC with a yellow coloring of eyes, the body, and urine. *SW* 28: **黄疸**暴痛，癲疾厥狂，久逆之所生也, "**Yellow *dan*-illness**, violent pain, peak-illness, and recession with madness, they are generated by [qi] moving contrary [to its regular course] for a long time". LSZ: **黄疸**有五，皆屬濕熱, "There are five types of **yellow *dan*-illness**. All of them are associated with moisture and heat".

***Huang du* 黄毒, yellow poisoning** [12]
PC identical with → *huang dan* 黄疸, yellow *dan*-illness; jaundice. *TBC* SE *gan lan* 甘藍: 治**黄毒**者，作菹，經宿漬色黄，和鹽食之, "To cure **yellow poisoning**, prepare pickled vegetables, let them soak overnight until they turn yellow, and eat them with salt".

***Huang han* 黄汗, yellow sweat** [11]
PC associated with sweat of a yellow color resembling cypress juice that stains one's garments. *JGYL* Mj: **黄汗**之為病…汗沾衣，色正黄如柏汁, "The disease of **yellow sweat**… The sweat stains the garments. Its color is truly yellow like cypress juice".

***Huang hu* 恍惚, absent-mindedness** [50]
IS of unstable spirit and thoughts; the heart palpitates and cannot calm down. *SHL* 88: 汗家，重發汗，必**恍惚**心亂, "If a patient who has sweated is made to sweat again, this will inevitably result in **absent-mindedness** and mental confusion".

***Huang ji* 黄疾, jaundice** [7]
PC identical with → *huang dan* 黄疸, yellow *dan*-illness; jaundice. *BCGM* SE *huang qi* 黄耆 quoting *ZHF* 4: 酒疸者，心懊痛，足脛滿，小便黄, "In the case of wine *dan*-illness one experiences annoyance with pain in the heart and a feeling of fullness in legs and shins. The urine is yellow". writes: 酒疸**黄疾**：心下懊痛，足脛滿，小便黄, "In the case of wine *dan*-illness with **jaundice** one

experiences annoyance with pain in the heart and a feeling of fullness in legs and shins. The urine is yellow".

***Huang ji* 黄積, yellow accumulation** [2]

PC of → *shi ji* 食積, food accumulation with a fading, yellow complexion resulting from inadequate digestion. *BCGM* SE *shu* 秫：粘滯，易成**黄積**病，小兒不宜多食, "It is sticky and blocking, and easily generates **yellow accumulation** disease. Children must not eat much of it".

***Huang lan chuang* 黄爛瘡, yellow-festering sores** [4]

PC of shallow *chuang* 瘡, sores, conditions from which drips a yellow liquid as major sign. *QJYF* 5: 治小兒**黄爛瘡**方：四交道中土、灶下土。右二味各等分，為末敷之, "Recipe to cure **yellow-festering sores** among children: soil from a crossroad, soil from below a kitchen stove. Take equal portions of these two items, prepare a powder, and apply it externally".

***Huang shou* 黄瘦, yellow emaciation** [23]

① IS of an emaciated body assuming a withered-yellow complexion. *ZHF* 7: 食菹菜誤吞水蛭，蛭啖臟血，腸痛，漸**黄瘦**, "If one inadvertently takes in leeches when consuming cabbage, these leeches will feed on the blood of the depots, [resulting in] intestinal pain and a gradual development of **yellow emaciation**".

② PC with withered-yellow complexion as its major pathological sign. *ZBYHL* 47: 其病腹大頸小，**黄瘦**是也, "Patients suffer from an enlarged abdomen and a smaller nape, with **yellow emaciation**".

***Huang shui chuang* 黄水瘡, yellow water sores** [5]

PC of sores that appear as scabies in the beginning, and are filled by yellow water after a little while. Identifiable as impetigo. *WKJYF* Lj: 香疥藥，治風癬瘡、**黄水瘡**、疥瘡、牛皮癬瘡, "'Fragrant *jie*-illness medication' cures wind *xuan*-illness sores, **yellow water sores**, *jie*-illness sores, and ox-hide *xuan*-illness sores".

***Huang shui fei chuang* 黄水肥瘡, yellow water fat sores** [2]

PC identical with → *huang shui chuang* 黄水瘡, yellow water sores. *BCGM* SE *hu yan ke tu* 胡燕窠土 quoting *PJF* 299: 麝香散，治頭生惡瘡, "Powder with *she xiang* cures malign sores on the head". writes: **黄水肥瘡, "Yellow water fat sores"**.

***Huang shui fei chuang* 黄水肥瘡, yellow water fat sores** [2]

PC identical with → *huang shui chuang* 黄水瘡, yellow water sores. *BCGM* SE *hu yan ke tu* 胡燕窠土 quoting *PJF* 299: 麝香散，治頭生惡瘡，"Powder with *she xiang* cures malign sores on the head". writes: **黄水肥瘡**，燕窠土一分，麝香半分，研傅之, "For **yellow water fat sores**, take soil obtained from a swallow's nest, 1 *fen*, and *she xiang*, ½ *fen*, grind to power, and apply externally".

***Huang shui mian chuang* 黄水面瘡, yellow water facial sores** [1]

PC of → *huang shui chuang* 黄水瘡, yellow water sores, in the face. *BCGM* SE *tao* 桃：寒食節桃花，為末，水調内服，治**黄水面瘡**, "Consume a powder from peach blossoms of the Cold Food Festival, mixed with water. This is to cure **yellow water facial sores**".

***Huang shui nong chuang* 黃水膿瘡, yellow water pus sores** [2]
PC identical with → *huang shui chuang* 黃水瘡, yellow water sores. *BCGM* SE *fen xi* 粉錫 quotes *SZRF*: **黃水膿瘡**：官粉煆黃、松香各三錢，黃丹一錢，飛礬二錢，為末，香油二兩，熬膏傅之, "**Yellow water pus sores**: *Guan fen* heated until it turns yellow, *song xiang*, 3 *qian* each; *huang dan*, 1 *qian*; *fei fan*, 2 *qian*, powderized; *xiang you*, 2 *liang*. Boil until an ointment is generated, and apply".

***Huang zhang* 黃脹, yellow distension** [1]
IS of yellow complexion and abdominal distension. *BCGM* Bai bing zhu zhi yao 百病主治藥：豭豬項肉，酒積**黃脹**，同甘遂服, "The meat of *jia zhu* nape: ingest together with *gan sui* [to cure] wine accumulation and **yellow distension**".

***Huang zhong* 黃腫, yellow swelling** [23]
IS of a) → *shui zhong* 水腫, edematose disease, with a swelling covering the entire body and the skin assuming a yellow complexion. *JGYL* Mj: 裏水者，一身面目**黃腫**，其脈沉，小便不利, "If water is inside the entire body, the face and the eyes assume a **yellow swelling**. The [movement in the] vessels is in the depth. Urine fails to flow freely". b) → *huang dan* 黃疸, yellow *dan*-illness, with superficial distension of the skin and at the same time the body, face and eyes assuming a yellow complexion. *SJZL* 35: 治痰逆多時，久瘧不瘥，及面目四肢**黃腫**，蜀漆丸方, "To cure phlegm frequently moving against its proper direction, malaria that has not been cured for anextended period of time, as well as **yellow swelling** of face, eyes, and the four limbs, [take the] recipe for pills with *shu qi*". c) → *shi ji* 食積, food accumulations, with a slight yellow coloring of the body's skin together with a swelling of face and legs. *PJF* 23: 丹砂丸，治宿食不消，及治厭食，遍身**黃腫**，多年不瘥, "Pills with *dan sha* cure food that has remained in the body overnight and failed to be digested, and also aversion to food, with a **yellow swelling** covering the entire body for many years without cure".

***Hui* 蛔, roundworm** [p]
EA, PC identical with → *hui chong* 蛔蟲. *BCTJ* SE *bian xu* 萹蓄：葛洪小兒**蛔**方，煮汁令濃，飲之即差, "Ge Hong's recipe for **roundworms** in children: Boil the sap until it is concentrated. Drinking it will bring the cure".

***Hui bing* 蛔病, roundworm disease** [1]
PC identical with → *hui chong* 蛔蟲②, roundworm. *BCGM* SE *zhu* 豕 quoting *QJYF* 小兒羸瘦有蛔蟲, "Children with emaciation have roundworms". writes: 小兒**蛔病**羸瘦, "Children with **roundworm disease** and emaciation".

***Hui chong* 蛔蟲, roundworm** [65]
① AD *hui* 蛔. AN *chang chong* 長蟲, longworm. EA of a lengthy parasite present in the intestinal tract of humans. *BCJJZ* SE *ai ye* 艾葉：汁又殺**蛔蟲**, "The juice also kills **roundworms**".
② AD *hui* 蛔. AN *hui bing* 蛔病, roundworm disease. PC brought forth by roundworm parasites in the intestinal tract. *JGYL* Mj: **蛔蟲**之為病，令人吐涎，心痛發作有時, "When **roundworms** cause a disease, this makes people vomit saliva. [Patients experience] heartache at regular intervals".

③ PS prepared from the body of roundworms. *QJYF* 6: 以**蛔蟲**燒為末敷之, "Apply a powder prepared from burned **roundworms**".

Hui jue **蛔厥, roundworm with recession** [6]

PC of → *hui chong* 蛔蟲②, roundworm, disease with the major signs of abdominal pain and agitation. The four extremities are cold because of [yang qi] recession. Sometimes roundworms are vomited. *JGYL* Mj: **蛔厥**者，烏梅丸主之, "**Roundworm with recession**: the pills with *wu mei* will control this".

Hui nu **恚怒, rage** [6]

① EA of an irritation of one's sentiments resulting from vehement hatred and annoyance lasting for an extended period of time. *MYBL* SE *bi jie* 萆薢：傷中**恚怒**，陰痿失溺, "[It cures] harm to the center caused by **rage**, dysfunction of the yin [member, i.e. penis] and involuntary loss of urine".

② PC brought forth by ①. *YD* SE *jie geng* 桔梗：得牡蠣、遠志，療**恚怒**, "With *mu li* and *yuan zhi* it cures **rage**".

③ IS of fury/rage/extreme anger. *MYBL* SE *fu shen* 茯神：止驚悸，多**恚怒**善忘, "It ends palpitation with fear, frequent **rage**, and a tendency to be forgetful".

Hui tong **蛔痛, roundworm pain** [10]

PC CD of conditions of abdominal pain brought forth by → *hui chong* 蛔蟲, roundworms. *BCGM* SE *han hao chong* 寒號蟲 quotes *JiXF*: 小兒**蛔痛**：五靈脂末二錢，白礬火飛半錢。每服一錢，水一盞，煎五分，温服。當吐蟲出，愈, "**Roundworm pain** in children: *wu ling zhi* powder, 2 *qian*; *bai fan* sublimate, ½ *qian*. Each dose to be ingested is 1 *qian*. Place in a bowl of water and boil down to one half. To be ingested warm. This will remove the worms by vomiting. This is the cure".

Hui xin tong **蛔心痛, roundworm heartache** [2]

PC of conditions of → *xin tong* 心痛, heartache, brought forth specifically by roundworms. *SLBC* SE *bai you ma* 白油麻：治**蛔心痛**，傅一切瘡疥癬，殺一切蟲, "It cures **roundworm heartache**. Apply on all types of sores, *jie*-illness, and *xuan*-illness. It will kill all types of worms/bugs".

Hun **昏, clouding; dim vision; functional disturbance** [p]

① IS a) of mental confusion, in extreme cases: coma. *SW* 70: 其病**昏**惑悲忘, "Its illnesses are **clouding**, sadness, and forgetfulness". b) Of dim-sightedness; dim vision. *QJYF* 6: 年至四十，即漸眼**昏**, "When one has reached the age of 40, gradually **dim vision** sets in".

② Functional disturbance. *JYBC* SE *shu mi* 黍米：**昏**五藏，令人好睡, "Must not be consumed for long as it **disturbs the functions** of the five depots. It gives people good sleep".

Hun'an **昏暗, dim vision** [20]

IS identical with → *mu hun* 目昏. *QJYF* 6: 肝中有風熱，令人眼**昏暗**, "When there is wind heat in the liver, this makes the eyes experience **dim vision**".

Hun dao **昏倒, clouding with fall** [2]

IS of a fall resulting from loss of consciousness. *BCGM* SE *ren shen* 人參 quoting *JBF*: 一小兒七歲，聞雷即**昏倒**，不知人事，此氣怯也, "There was a child of seven years. When it heard thunder it had a **clouding and fell** to the ground, and was unconscious. This is a case of qi timidity".

Hun hua **昏花, clouding with flowery vision** [4]

IS of dim-sightedness. *RZTJYF*, section *Xian bu* 羨補：四神丸，治腎經虛損，眼目**昏花**, "The 'pills with the four wondrous [ingredients]' cure depletion harm of the kidney, and **clouding with flowery vision** of the eyes".

Hun huang **昏恍, clouding with absent-mindedness** [1]

IS of absent-mindedness and instability of one's spirit, despite basic mental clarity. *WTMY* 14: 手足不隨，精神**昏恍**, "The hands and feet do not follow one's will. The essence spirit is **clouded with absent-mindedness**".

Hun huo **昏霍, clouding with disorder** [1]

IS of a deranged mental state. Patients may sing or laugh uncontrolled, exiting a normal frame of behavior or mental state. *BCGM* SE *yin xing* 銀杏 quotes *RYBC*: 小兒食多**昏霍**，發驚引疳, "When children consume large amounts of it, this will result in **clouding with disorder**. It causes fright and *gan*-illness".

Hun kuang **昏狂, clouding with madness** [3]

IS CD of → *shen hun* 神昏, spirit clouding, and → *feng kuang* 風狂, wind madness. *BCGM* SE *wu bo mu* 烏柏木 quotes *SJZL*: 暗疔**昏狂**，瘡頭凸紅, "Hidden pin-illness and **clouding with madness**. The heads of the sores stick out and are red".

Hun kui **昏憒, muddle-headedness** [10] AN *shen hun* 神昏, spirit clouding.

IS of mental confusion with a failure to engage in a normal dialogue; in extreme cases with lethargy and a failure to respond to calls. *ZBYHL* 1: 令人懈惰，精神**昏憒**, "It causes indolence with **muddle-headedness**".

Hun luan **昏亂, clouding with disorder; state of turmoil** [3]

① IS CD of → *hun kuei* 昏憒, muddle-headedness, with → *kuang luan* 狂亂, madness with disorder. *YXL* SE *ling yang jiao* 羚羊角：中惡毒風，卒死**昏亂**不識人, "To be struck by the malign and poison wind [results in] sudden [appearance of] death, with **clouding with disorder** and a failure to recognize persons".

② PM in the sense of *hun luan* 混亂, confusion. *BCBS* SE *dang gui* 當歸：氣血**昏亂**者，服之即定, "When those whose qi and blood are in a **state of turmoil** ingest it, it will stabilize them".

Hun mang **昏盲, clouding with blindness** [3]

IS CD of → *mu mang* 目盲, blindness, and → *mu hun* 目昏, visual clouding. *BCGM* Bai bing zhu zhi yao 百病主治藥：有赤目傳變，內障**昏盲**, "There are red eyes that worsen, with internal screen, and **clouding with blindness**".

Hun mao **昏瞀, clouding with dim vision** [7]

IS of mental confusion. *BCYY*, introduction, final part: 此胃中有結熱，故**昏瞀**不省人, "In this case there is bound heat in the stomach. Hence [patients] experience **clouding with dim vision** and a failure to recognize people".

***Hun mao* 昏冒, clouding with indistinct vision** [4]

IS identical with → *hun mao* 昏瞀, clouding with dim vision. *SJZL* 5: 中風**昏冒**，涎潮氣壅, "Wind stroke and **clouding with indistinct vision.** Saliva billows [from the throat], and the qi is obstructed".

***Hun mao* 昏耄, clouding with senility** [4]

IS of decrease of mental faculties due to old age, with dim vision. *RHZ* SE *yin yang huo* 淫羊藿：老人**昏耄**，中年健忘, "Old people display **clouding with senility**; middle aged persons are forgetful".

***Hun men* 昏悶, clouding with heart-pressure** [8]

IS of an uncomfortable feeling of vertigo, vexation and heart-pressure. *TPSHF* 5: 心膈煩熱，頭目**昏悶**, "The heart and diaphragm experience vexing heat; the head and the eyes experience a **clouding with heart-pressure**".

***Hun mi* 昏迷, clouding with confusion** [15]

IS of a complete loss of mind. *TPSHF* 78: 頭目旋運，神志**昏迷**，四肢煩亂，不知人事, "The head and eyes revolve. The spirit mind has a **clouding with confusion**. The four extremities experience vexation and disorder. [Patients are] unable to recognize persons or items".

***Hun mu* 昏目, visual clouding** [5]

PE causing one to experience a → *mu hun* 目昏, visual clouding. *TYBC* SE *ze xie* 澤瀉：本經云久服明目，扁鵲云多服**昏目**，何也, "The *BJ* says: 'Ingested over a long time it clears the eyes'. Bian Que says: 'If consumed in large quantities it causes **visual clouding**'. Now, why is that".

***Hun sai* 昏塞, clouding and blockage** [6]

IS of slowed down thinking with an obvious decrease of one's faculty of memory. *ZBYHL* 35: 人神采**昏塞**，身體沉重, "A person's spirit experiences **clouding and blockage**; the body feels very heavy".

***Hun se* 昏澀, clouding with roughness** [3]

IS of an uncomfortable feeling of dryness in the eyes with dim-sightedness. *TPSHF* 31: 治骨蒸，五心煩熱，眼目**昏澀**，肢節酸疼，不能飲食，宜服升麻散方, "To cure bone steaming, vexing heat affecting the five centers (i.e. the two palm centers, the two food sole centers, the abdominal center), **clouding with roughness** in the eyes, sour pain in one's limbs and joints, failure to drink and eat, the recipe to ingest the powder with *sheng ma* is advisable".

***Hun teng* 昏痛, clouding with pain** [2]

IS of pain in the eyes accompanied by an inability to see things clearly. *YXL* SE *gou qi* 枸杞：主患眼風障，赤膜**昏痛**，取葉擣汁注眼中，妙, "It controls suffering from wind screen in the eye, red membrane and **clouding with pain**. Take the leaves, pound them to get a juice, and pour this into the eyes. Miraculously effective".

***Hun xuan* 昏眩, clouding with giddiness** [3]

IS of an uncomfortable feeling with vertigo and blurred vision. *TPSHF* 3: 治膽虛冷，精神不守，頭目**昏眩**，恆多恐畏，宜服酸棗仁散方, "To cure gallbladder depletion with cold, instability of essence spirit, **clouding with giddi-**

ness affecting head and eyes, permanent fear, the recipe to ingest the powder with *suan zao* kernels is advisable".

***Hun yun* 昏運, clouding with dizziness** [5]

IS of an uncomfortable feeling of head and eyes being dizzy. *SJZL* 34: 治傷暑，胸膈躁悶，**昏運**倒仆欲死，解毒散方, "To cure harm caused by summerheat, agitation and pressure in the region of the chest and diaphragm, **clouding with dizziness** and falling as if one were to die: [apply] the recipe for the 'powder to dissolve poison'".

***Huo* 蜮, *huo*-bug** [9]

EA identical with → *she gong* 射工①, archer. *ZHF* 7: 江南有射工毒蟲，一名短狐，一名**蜮**, "In the region south of the Yangzi there is a poisonous bug, the archer. Other names are 'short fox' and ***huo*-bug**". *BCGM* SE *xi gui chong* 溪鬼蟲：蜮，音或，„蜮 is read *huo*". According to ancient sources, this is a turtle-shaped being with three legs, living on the bottom of streams. It is said to hold sand in its mouth and spout it at humans who fall ill as a result.

***Huo* 火 fire** [p]

① A group of pharmaceutical substances added to *materia medica* by *BCGM* as *huo bu* 火部, "fire section". including 11 different fires, e.g., *ai huo* 艾火, "**fire** of the moxa herb". *BCGM*, *huo bu* 火部：火之用其至矣哉, "The usefulness of **fire** is extreme".

② Physiological term referring to those yang qi in the human organism that have a warming, nourishing, and stimulating function. *SW* 5: 少**火**生氣, "A small **fire** generates qi".

③ AN *huo bing* 火病, fire disease. PC of exuberant yang qi manifesting itself as dryness, heat, shock, sores, redness and swelling. *SW* 74: 諸躁狂越，皆屬於**火**, "All [cases of] overexcitement and jumping in madness, without exception they are associated with **fire**".

④ AN *huo qi* 火氣, fire qi; *huo xie* 火邪, fire evil. EA able to bring forth fire disease, similar to heat-type diseases they flame upward. *SW* 74: **火**淫所勝，平以酸冷, "When **fire** [as the qi controlling heaven] encroaches upon what it dominates, this is balanced with sour [flavor] and cold".

***Huo ban* 火瘢, fire scar** [2]

PC of a → *ban* 瘢, scar, resulting from burns. *BCGM* SE *gou* 狗 quotes *TPSHF*: 眉髮**火瘢**不生者，蒲灰，以正月狗腦和敷，日三，則生, "For a **fire scar** that does not let the eyebrows grow again: *pu* ashes are to be externally applied together with a dog's brain taken in a year's first month. After three days, they will grow". Possibly this is a modified quote that in fact originates from *QJYF* 13: 治眉毛鬢髮為火燒瘡瘢毛不生方：蒲灰以正月狗腦和敷，即生, "Recipe for scars of sores resulting from burns with eyebrows and hair on the temples failing to grow again: *pu* ashes are to be externally applied together with a dog's brain taken in a year's first month".

***Huo biao re chuang* 火飆熱瘡, fire flame heat sores** [1]
PC identical with → *re chuang* 熱瘡, heat sores. *BCSY* SE *huo shi* 活師：主**火飆熱瘡**及疥瘡，並搗碎傅之, "It controls **fire flame heat sores**, as well as *jie*-illness sores. For all these conditions alike, pound to small pieces and apply externally".

***Huo bing* 火病, fire disease** [11]
PC identical with → *huo* 火③, fire. *DXXF* 2: 吐血，**火病**也, "Blood-spitting is [a sign of] **fire disease**".

***Huo chuang* 火瘡, fire sores** [19]
PC of ulcerating sores brought forth by → *tang huo shang* 湯火傷, harm caused by boiling water and fire. *BJ* SE *qing lang gan* 青琅玕：主身癢，**火瘡**, "It controls body itching, **fire sores**". *BCGM* has many alternative designations, such as → *tang huo chuang* 湯火瘡, boiling water and fire sores; → *tang huo shang chuang* 湯火傷瘡, wounds caused by boiling water and fire; → *tang huo zhu chuang* 湯火灼瘡, sores following scorching by boiling water and fire; → *huo zhu chuang* 火灼瘡, sores following scorching by fire; → *zhuo chuang* 灼瘡, scorching sores; → *tang huo shang zhuo chuang* 湯火傷灼瘡, sores following harm from scorching by boiling water and fire; → *tang huo shao chuang* 湯火燒瘡, sores following burns by boiling water and fire; → *re huo zhuo lan chuang* 熱火灼爛瘡, festering sores following scorching by heat and fire; → *huo lan chuang* 火爛瘡, festering fire sores; → *huo zhuo lan chuang* 火灼爛瘡, festering sores following scorching by fire; → *huo yang* 火瘍, fire ulcers; → *huo shao chuang* 火燒瘡, sores following burns by fire; → *huo shao cheng chuang* 火燒成瘡, sores generated by burns with fire; → *huo he du chuang* 火赫毒瘡, burning fire poison sores; → *huo liao cheng chuang* 火燎成瘡, sores generated by burns with fire.

***Huo dan* 火丹, fire cinnabar** [10]
PC of → *dan du* 丹毒, cinnabar-red poison, displaying a color like fire that rushes through the skin, spreading with great speed. *QJYF* 22: 治小兒**火丹**赤如朱走皮中方, "Recipe to cure **fire cinnabar** among children as if vermilion were running through the skin".

***Huo he du chuang* 火赫毒瘡, sores generated by burning fire poison** [2]
PC identical with → *huo chuang* 火瘡, fire sores. *BCGM*, Bai bing zhu zhi yao 綱目 百病主治藥, Zhu chuang 諸瘡; *re chuang* 熱瘡：枸杞葉塗**火赫毒瘡**, "The leaves of *gou qi* are to be applied externally to **sores generated by burning fire poison**".

***Huo huang* 火黄, fire jaundice** [2]
PC identical with → *re huang* 熱黄, heat jaundice. *TPSHF* 55: **火黄**者，遍身如火色, "In the case of **fire jaundice** the entire body has the color of fire".

***Huo jing* 火驚, fire fright** [3]
PC identical with → *jing re* 驚熱, fright heat. *BCSY* SE *zhen shao mu* 震燒木：主**火驚**失心，煮服之, "Controls **fire fright** with loss of heart [wind]; to be ingested boiled".

Huo jue **火厥, fire recession** [1]

PC identical with → *re jue* 熱厥, heat recession. *BCGM* Bai bing zhu zhi fang yao 百病主治藥：卒厥：有屍厥、氣厥、**火厥**、痰厥、血厥, "Sudden recession includes corpse[-like condition because of qi] recession, qi recession, **fire recession**, phlegm recession, and blood recession".

Huo ke **火咳, fire cough** [1]

PC identical with → *re ke* 熱咳, heat cough. *RMSQ* 3: 少氣善咳，亦**火咳**也, "If someone is short of qi and tends to cough, this, too, is **fire cough**".

Huo lan chuang **火爛瘡, festering fire sores** [5]

PC identical with → *huo chuang* 火瘡, fire sores. *WTMY* 29: **火爛瘡**方，丹參細切，以羊脂煎成膏，敷瘡上, "Recipe for **festering fire sores**: a fine cut of *dan shen* is prepared with lamb fat to a paste to be applied to the sores".

Huo liao cheng chuang **火燎成瘡, sores generated by burns from fire** [1]

PC identical with → *huo chuang* 火瘡, fire sores. *BCGM* SE *xiao mai* 小麥 quotes *QJF*: **火燎成瘡**：炒麵，入巵子仁末，和油傅之, "For **sores generated by burns from fire**: mix parched flour with *zhi zi ren* powder, add oil, and apply externally".

Huo luan **霍亂, cholera** [403]

PC of an acute disease with vomiting, diarrhea, and abdominal pain. It may also include a feeling of fullness in the abdomen with a twisting pain, short breath, and mental confusion, in the absence of vomiting and diarrhea. The former is also called *shi huo luan* 濕霍亂, moisture cholera; the latter is also called *gan huo luan* 乾霍亂, dry cholera. *SW* 69: 民病飧泄**霍亂**，體重腹痛, "People suffer from outflow of [undigested] food and **cholera**. The body is heavy; the abdomen is painful". The etiology of cholera is complex, and includes all possible types of internal harm and affection from the outside. *BCGM* Bai bing zhu zhi yao 百病主治藥：**霍亂**有濕熱、寒濕，並七情內傷、六氣外感, "**Cholera** includes moisture-heat, cold-moisture, as well as internal harm by the seven emotions, and affection from outside by any of the six qi".

Huo qi **火氣, fire qi** [28]

① CC identical with → *re qi* 熱氣, heat qi. *SW* 36: 喜見日月光**火氣**乃快然, "[Patients] love to see the light of sun and moon. [Exposure to] **fire qi** makes them happy".

② PE generated by pharmaceutical drugs or other therapies. Identical with → *re qi* 熱氣， heat qi. *BCGM* SE *shen zhen huo* 神針火：凡在筋骨隱痛者，針之，**火氣**直達病所，甚效, "In all cases of latent pain in sinews and muscles, needle the [affected region]. The [resulting] **fire qi** will proceed directly to the location of the disease. This is very effectiv"..

③ EA identical with → *huo* 火, fire. *BCGM* SW *wu wei zi* 五味子：又黃昏嗽乃**火氣**浮入肺中，不宜用涼藥，宜五味子、五倍子斂而降之, "Also, for cough at the time of dusk watch, which is **fire qi** floating into the lung, it is not appropriate to use cooling medication. *Wu wei zi* is appropriate. *Wu wei zi* collects [the fire qi] and moves it down".

④ The qi of burning fire. *QJYF* 6: 熏衣香方…以微火燒之，以盆水納籠下，以殺**火氣**, "Recipe to fumigate clothing with aromatic substances. …Burn [the ingredients] with a small fire. Place a bowl of water underneath the basket to counteract the **fire qi**".

***Huo re* 火熱, fire and heat** [16]
DC CD of → *huo* 火, fire, and → *re* 熱, heat. *SW* 74: 寒氣大來，水之勝也，**火熱**受邪，心病生焉, "When cold qi arrives massively, that is a domination of water [qi]. **Fire and heat** receive evil [qi]. Heart diseases emerge from this". *BCGM* Bai bing zhu zhi yao 百病主治藥 lists pathological conditions brought about by fire and heat: **火熱**：有鬱火、實火、虛火，氣分熱、血分熱、五臟熱、十二經熱, "**Fire and heat** include pent-up fire, repletion fire, depletion fire, heat in the qi section, heat in the blood section, heat in the five depots, heat in the twelve conduits".

***Huo re sou* 火熱嗽, fire-heat cough** [1]
PC identical with → *re ke* 熱咳, heat cough. *BCYYBY* SE *wu wei zi* 五味子. **火熱嗽**必用之, "Is to be used for **fire-heat cough**".

***Huo shao cheng chuang* 火燒成瘡, sores generated by burns from fire** [3]
PC identical with → *huo chuang* 火瘡, fire sores. *XPF* 10: 治**火燒成瘡**方。白糖燒灰粉之, 即燥，易瘥, "Recipe to cure **sores generated by burns from fire**: Burn *bai tang* to ashes and apply them externally. This will dry them. A cure is easily achieved".

***Huo shao chuang* 火燒瘡, sores following burns from fire** [4]
PC identical with → *huo chuang* 火瘡, fire sores. *QJYF* 25: 治**火燒瘡**方：死鼠頭一枚，以臘月豬膏煎，令消盡，以敷, "Recipe to cure **sores following burns from fire**: one head of a dead rat is to be boiled with lard from the 12th month until completely dissolved. This is to be applied".

***Huo sou* 火嗽, fire cough** [1]
PC identical with → *re ke* 熱咳, heat cough. *DXZFXY* 1: **火嗽**者，有聲痰少，面赤, "In the case of **fire cough**, [the cough] makes sounds, and there is little phlegm. The face is red".

***Huo tan* 火痰, fire phlegm** [1]
Identical with → *tan huo* 痰火, phlegm fire. *BCGM* SE *ban xia* 半夏 quotes *HSYT*: 痰分之病，半夏為主…治**火痰**以薑汁、竹瀝或荊瀝和之, "To cure diseases associated with phlegm, *ban xia* is the top substance. …To cure **fire phlegm** add *jiang zhi*, *zhu li* or *jing li*".

***Huo xie* 火邪, fire evil** [16]
EA identical with → *huo* 火, fire. *SHL* 114: 到經不解，必清血，名為**火邪**, "Once it reaches the conduit without having been resolved, one must cool the blood. This is called **fire evil**".

***Huo yan* 火眼, fire eye** [8]
PC of seasonally prevalent eye diseases characterized by red and hot eyeballs that are swollen and painful. *ZLBC* SE *ai ye* 艾葉 quotes *DMF*: 治**火眼**, "It cures **fire eye**".

Huo yan dan du **火焰丹毒, flaming cinnabar poison** [6] AN → *huo yan dan zhong* 火焰丹腫, flaming cinnabar swelling.

PC of → *dan du* 丹毒, cinnabar red poison, starting from the head and generating a dark red complexion. *BCGM* SE *zhi zi* 梔子 quoting *HSF* from *ZLBC:* 治火丹毒，搗和水調傅之, "To cure flaming cinnabar poison, pound and apply externally mixed with water". writes: **火焰丹毒**：梔子搗和水塗之, "For **flaming cinnabar poison**, pound *zhi zi*, add water and apply it externally".

Huo yan dan zhong **火焰丹腫, flaming cinnabar swelling** [1]

PC identical with → *huo yan dan du* 火焰丹毒, flaming cinnabar poison. *BCGM* quoting *BCTJ*: 火焰丹毒, "Flaming cinnabar poison". writes: **火焰丹腫, "Flaming cinnabar swelling"**.

Huo yan re chuang **火焱熱瘡, flaming heat sores** [1]

PC identical with → *re chuang* 熱瘡, heat sores. *BCSY* SE *hai zao* 海藻：搗傅小兒赤白游疹，**火焱熱瘡**, "Pound to pulp and apply on white roaming papules in children, as well as **flaming heat sores**".

Huo yang **火瘍, fire ulcers** [1]

PC of ulcerating sores brought forth by → *tang huo shang* 湯火傷, harm caused by boiling water and fire. *BJ* SE *huang qin* 黃芩：主…惡瘡、疽、蝕、**火瘍**, "It controls…malign sores, *dan*-illness, erosion, **fire ulcers**".

Huo yu **火郁, pent-up fire** [29] AN *yu huo* 鬱火; *re yu* 熱郁, pent-up heat.

PC of internal fire heat being oppressed and yang qi being restrained. *SW* 71: 火郁發之, "When the **fire [qi] is pent-up**, effuse it". LSZ identifies numerous ailments as associated with **pent-up heat**, as for example, → *tan yin* 痰飲, phlegm rheum; → *ke ni* 咳逆, cough with counter-movement; → *fei wei fei yong* 肺痿肺癰, lung dysfunction and lung obstruction-illnesses; → *han re bing* 寒熱病, cold and heat spells disease; → *ke sou xue* 咳嗽血, blood cough; → *xin fu tong* 心腹痛, heart-abdomen pain.

Huo zao dan du **火灶丹毒, fire stove cinnabar poison** [1]

PC of → *dan du* 丹毒, cinnabar poison, starting from the two feet and displaying a red color resembling a burning fire. *BCGM* quoting *YSCRF*: 灶丹, "Stove cinnabar". writes: **火灶丹毒, "Fire stove cinnabar poison"**.

Huo zhuo chuang **火灼瘡, sores resulting from scorching fire** [2]

PC identical with → *huo chuang* 火瘡, fire sores. *YXL* SE *shi yan* 食鹽：兼主**火灼瘡**, "It also controls **sores resulting from scorching fire**".

Huo zhuo lan chuang **火灼爛瘡, festering sores following scorching by fire** [2]

PC identical with → *huo chuang* 火瘡, fire sores. *WTMY* 29: 千金墮**火灼爛瘡**方，榆白皮熟嚼封之，瘥, "Recipe worth thousands in gold for **festering sores following scorching by fire**: *yu bai pi* is to be thoroughly boiled, then chewed and used to cover [the sores]. This brings the cure".

- J -

***Ji* 悸, palpitation** [p]

① IS identical with → *xin ji* 心悸①, heart palpitation. *JGYL* Fj: 虛勞裏急，**悸**，衄，腹中痛, "Depletion exhaustion with internal tensions, **palpitation**, nosebleed, and abdominal pain".

② EA of very strong emotional stimulus of fear. *XTS* 202 (Sun Ti zhuan 孫逖傳): 宿為華州刺史，因**悸**病瘖, "While he served as governer of Hua zhou he experienced **palpitation** and turned mute as a result".

***Ji* 積, accumulation** [p]

PC CD of lumps forming in chest and abdomen that are fixed and cannot be moved, with pain at a specific location. It was believed that these lumps were generated by the five depots. *NJ* 55: **積**者，陰氣也，其始發有常處，其痛不離其部，上下有所終始，左右有所窮處, "**Accumulations** [consist of] yin qi. They stay where they developed in the first place. The pain [they cause] does not leave this section. Their upper and lower [extensions are clearly marked by] the end and beginning; to the left and to the right locations where they subside [are clearly defined]".

***Ji bing* 急病, acute disease** [7]

CD of PCs with a sudden onset and a rapid development. *TPSHF* 82: 一曰撮口，二曰著噤，三曰臍風，皆是**急病**, "The first is called 'pursed mouth'. The second is called 'inability to speak'. The third is called 'navel wind'. All these are **acute diseases**".

***Ji bing* 繼病, transmission disease** [3]

PC transmitted from a suckling to a second child in the womb of the suckling's mother, and possibly also into another pregnant woman's womb. Identical with → *ba bing* 魃病, drought-demon disease. *JYBC* SE *bo lao* 伯勞：毛，主小兒**繼病**, "Its hair controls **transmission disease** in children".

***Ji chuang* 肌瘡, muscle sores** [5]

PC of → *chuang* 瘡, sores, conditions mentioned prior to the *BCGM* only in *MYBL* and *TBC*. Neither causes nor appearances of these sores are mentioned. Hence the meaning of this term remains unclear. *MYBL SE wa* 蛙：主小兒赤氣，**肌瘡**，臍傷, "It controls children's red qi, **muscle sores**, and umbilical injury".

***Ji gan* 急疳, acute *gan*-illness** [13]

PC of → *gan chuang* 疳瘡, *gan*-illness sores, characterized by a swift eruption, a severe nature, and rapid development, mostly affecting the face, the mouth, and the nose. This condition includes → *zou ma ya gan* 走馬牙疳, running horse dental *gan*-illness. *QJYiF* 24: 又**急疳**，食鼻口，數日盡，欲死方, "Further recipe for **acute *gan*-illness** which eats the nose and mouth and ends after several days when one is about /wishes to die".

Ji gou **積垢, accumulated filth** [5]

EA PM of heavy and turbid evil accumulating in the body, such as phlegm turbidity and abiding food which in turn may bring forth further disease. *JFFH*: 砒丹巴硇，毒熱類聚，劑成丸藥，其氣凶暴，其體重滯，**積垢**雖行，毒氣未過, "If substances like *pi* [*shuang*], *dan*, *ba* [*dou*], and *nao* [*sha*] – [i.e. substances representing] one-sided collections of poison heat - are used to prepare pills for medication, their qi is extremely violent, and their material consistency is heavy and sluggish. Even though one may be able to move the **accumulated filth**, its poison qi cannot be overcome".

Ji guan zhi **雞冠痔, cock's comb piles** [1]

PC of → *zhi chuang* 痔瘡, piles sores, that resemble the shape of a cock's comb. *PJF* 295: **雞冠痔**三十年者, "[To cure] **cock's comb piles** that have a history of thirty years".

Ji hou bi **急喉痹, acute throat blockage** [8] AN *ji hou bi feng* 急喉痹風, acute throat blockage wind; *ji hou zhong bi* 急喉腫痹, acute throat swelling with blockage; *ji hou bi* 急喉閉, acute throat closure; *zou ma hou bi* 走馬喉痹, running horse throat blockage; *ma hou bi* 馬喉痹, throat blockage [as fast as a running] horse.

PC of → throat blockage, *hou bi* 喉痹, with a sudden onset of a visibly swollen throat, and the occlusion of the throat possibly resulting in a blockage of breathing as major sign. *YXL* SE *fan shi* 礬石：生含咽津，治**急喉痹**, "By holding unprocessed [*fan shi*] in the mouth, and swallowing the resulting [saliva] liquid, one treats **acute throat blockage**".

Ji hou bi **急喉閉, acute throat closure** [1]

PC identical with → *ji hou bi* 急喉痹, acute throat blockage. *TPSHF* 35: 治咽喉風毒及**急喉閉**腫痛，下湯飲不得，宜用龍腦丸方, "To cure throat wind poison and **acute throat closure** with swelling and pain, when it is impossible to ingest a decoction, it is advisable to use the recipe for the pills with *long nao*".

Ji hou bi feng **急喉痹風, acute throat blockage wind** [1]

PC identical with → *ji hou bi* 急喉痹, acute throat blockage. *BCGM* SE *xuan shen* 玄參 quotes *TPSHF*: **急喉痹風**：不拘大人小兒。玄參、鼠粘子半生半炒各一兩，為末，新水服一盞立瘥, "For **acute throat blockage wind**, regardless of whether adults or children are concerned: Prepare a powder from 1 *liang* each of *xuan shen* and *shu zhan zi*, one half raw, the other half roasted, and ingest with one bowl of fresh water. This will bring an immediate cure".

Ji hou feng **急喉風, acute throat wind** [3]

PC identical with → *ji hou bi* 急喉痹, acute throat blockage. *BCGM* SE *zao jia* 皂莢 quoting *SHZBL* 3: 九般名：急喉閉、纏喉風、結喉、爛喉、重舌、木舌、遁蟲、蟲喋、飛絲入喉, "The names of nine types: acute throat closure, throat-constricting wind, bound throat, festering throat, doubled tongue, wooden tongue, run-away bug, floating worm-borer, and flying silk threads entering the throat", writes: 其方治九種喉痹：**急喉風**、纏喉風、結喉、爛喉、遁蟲、蟲喋、重舌、木舌、飛絲入口, "This recipe cures nine types of throat blockage: **acute throat wind**, throat-constricting wind, bound throat, festering throat, run-away bug, floating bug, doubled tongue, wooden tongue, and flying silk threats entering the throat".

***Ji hou feng bi* 急喉風痹, acute throat wind blockage** [1]
PC identical with → *ji hou bi* 急喉痹, acute throat blockage. *BCGM* SE *can* 蠶: **急喉風痹**，王氏博濟如聖散, "For **acute throat wind blockage**: Mr. Wang's sage-like recipe for ubiquitous assistance".

***Ji hou zhong bi* 急喉腫痹, acute throat swelling and blockage** [1]
PC identical with → *zou ma hou bi* 走馬喉痹, running horse throat blockage. *BCGM* SE *deng zhan you* 燈盞油 quoting *PJF* 61: 急喉腫閉最堪憂, "Acute throat swelling and closure causing extreme anxiety", writes: **急喉腫痹**最堪憂, "**Acute throat swelling and blockage** causing extreme anxiety".

***Ji huang* 急黃, acute jaundice** [18]
PC of an acute and severe variation of → *huang dan* 黃疸, yellow *dan*-illness. *ZBYHL* 12: 卒然發黃，心滿氣喘，命在頃刻，故云**急黃**也, "There is a sudden outbreak of jaundice, with a feeling of fullness in the heart and qi panting. Life is jeopardized. Hence this is called '**acute jaundice**'".

***Ji jiang* 脊強, stiff spine** [8]
IS of stiff back with difficulties to move. *SW* 60: 督脈為病，**脊強**反折, "When the supervisor vessel has a disease, [this causes] a **stiff spine** bent backwards".

***Ji jiang* 急強, tense and stiff** [3] AW *jiang ji* 強急, stiff and tense
IS of hardening of the body, limbs and bones with cramps and a feeling of tightness. Bending and stretching are difficult. *SLBC* SE *ling yang* 羚羊：治筋骨**急強**，中風, "It cures **tension and stiffness** of the sinews and bones, as well as being struck by wind".

***Ji jie* 積結, accumulation with nodes** [4]
PC identical with → *jie ji* 結積, nodular accumulation. *BCTJ* SE *ju you* 橘柚：青橘，主氣滯，下食，破**積結**及膈氣方用之, "*Qing yu* is used in recipes to master qi sluggishness, make food pass down, and crush **accumulation with nodes**, as well as occlusion qi".

***Ji jing* 急驚, acute fright** [23] AN → *ji feng* 急風, acute wind.
PC AD for → *ji jing feng* 急驚風, acute fright wind. *XEYZZJ* Lj: **急驚**，因聞大聲或大驚而發搐，發過則如故，此無陰也, "**Acute fright**: convulsions resulting from a loud sound or massive fright. After an outbreak this returns to normal. The reason is an absence of yin".

***Ji jing feng* 急驚風, acute fright wind** [6] AN → *ji jing* 急驚, acute fright.
PC of a rather brief and violent development of → 驚風, fright wind, with fever. *TPSHF* 85 RE *xiong huang wan* 雄黃丸, pills with *xiong huang*: 治小兒**急驚風**，牙關緊急，筋脈抽掣，腰背強硬，口內多涎, "They cure **acute fright wind** in children, with clenched jaw, shrunken sinews and vessels, a stiff lumbar region and back, and much spittle in the mouth". *BCGM* has mostly 急驚, acute fright, for 急驚風, acute fright wind.

***Ji ju* 積聚, accumulation and collection** [147] AN *jie ju* 結聚, nodular collection. PC CD of → *ji* 積, accumulation, and → *ju* 聚, collection. In many cases the two form one pair; in some cases there may be slight differences between the two. *LS* 46: 人之善病腸中**積聚**者，何以候之, "When a person tends to have the disease of **accumulation and collection** in his intestines, how can this be diagnosed?"

Ji lao* 急勞, *acute exhaustion [9]
PC of an acute state of → *xu lao* 虛勞, depletion exhaustion, with apparent internal heat. *TPSHF* 27: **急勞**，四肢煩熱，百節酸疼，口乾心躁，小便黃赤，不欲飲食, "**Acute exhaustion**: the four limbs are affected by vexing heat. All joints ache. The mouth is dry and the heart is restless. The urine is yellow-red. [Patients] have no appetite".

***Ji lao* 積勞, accumulating exhaustion** [2]
EA of a recurrent, long-term → *lao juan* 勞倦, exhaustion to fatigue. *ZHF* 4: 凡男女因**積勞**虛損，或大病後不復，常苦四體沉滯，骨肉疼酸， "Whenever males and females following an **accumulating exhaustion** experience a state of depletion detriment, or if after a massive disease they have not yet recovered, they will continuously suffer from sluggish [qi] deep in their four extremities, with their bones and flesh being in pain".

***Ji leng* 積冷, accumulated cold** [24]
① AN *leng ji* 冷積.cold accumulation; *jie leng* 結冷, bound cold; *han ji* 寒積, cold accumulation; *ting han* 停寒, stagnant cold; *chen han* 沉寒, deep-seated cold. EA of accumulated cold. *ZBYHL* 3: 瘕病者，皆由久寒**積冷**，飲食不消所致也, "All cases of conglomeration-illness disease are brought forth by chronic cold and **accumulated cold**, leaving beverages and food undigested".
② PC brought forth by the EA accumulated cold. *ZBYHL* 20: 此患由血氣衰少，腑臟虛弱，故令風冷之氣獨盛於內，其冷氣久積不散，所以謂之久寒**積冷**也, "This ailment results from weakness and deficiency of blood and qi, and of depletion and weakness of the depots and palaces. This causes a singular internal abundance of wind cold, and the cold qi will accumulate over an extended period of time without dispersing. Hence one calls this chronic cold and **accumulated cold**".

***Ji li* 積痢, accumulation free-flux illness** [13]
PC of → *li ji* 痢疾, free-flux illness, associated with harm caused by long-time food accumulations that cannot be healed for an extended period of time, with alternating phases of activity and dormancy. *XEWSZWLF* 11: **積痢**，謂有積傷為痢，浸久，或瘥而復發也, "**Accumulation free-flux illness**, that is to say: One is harmed by [food] accumulations, and this develops into free-flux illness. It lasts long. Sometimes it appears cured and then breaks out again".

***Ji man* 急滿, tightness and fullness** [5]
IS identical with → *man ji* 滿急, fullness and tightness. *ZBYHL* 18: 病成翻大小便不通，頭項滿痛，小腹**急滿**，起坐不安, "The disease develops into a failure to defecate and urinate. A feeling of fullness and pain in head and neck, of

tightness and fullness in the lower abdomen. Patients are not at peace, both when they are up and when they sit down".

Ji man jing feng **急慢驚風, acute and slow fright wind** [12]
PC CD of → *ji jing feng* 急驚風, acute fright wind, and → *man jing feng* 慢驚風, slow fright wind. Sometimes used to designate all types of → *jing feng* 驚風, fright wind. *XEYZZJ* Lj: 龍腦散治**急慢驚風**, "The powder with *long nao* cures **acute and slow fright wind**".

Ji nü **肌衄, spontaneous muscle bleeding** [1]
PC identical with → *xue han* 血汗, blood sweat. *PJF* 190: 治**肌衄**及腿上血出，用胎髮燒作灰敷之即止, "To cure **spontaneous muscle bleeding** and bleeding from the legs, burn the hair of a fetus to ashes and apply this externally. This will end [the bleeding]".

Ji nüe **積瘧, accumulation malaria** [3]
PC identical with → *shi nüe* 食瘧, food malaria. *PJF* 179, RE *suan* bing wan 蒜餅丸, pills with *suan* cake: 大概**積瘧**有驗, "They may be effective to cure **accumulation malaria**".

Ji pi **積癖, accumulation aggregation-illness** [4] AN *pi ji* 癖積.
PC identical with → *pi* 癖, aggregation-illness. *MYBL* SE *lang du* 狼毒：主脅下**積癖**, "It controls **accumulation aggregation-illness** below the flanks".

Ji qi **悸氣, palpitating qi** [3]
PC with fright, fear and heart palpitation. *BJ* SE *jie geng* 桔梗：主胸脅痛如刀刺，腹滿腸鳴幽幽，驚恐**悸氣**, "It controls pain as if stabbed with a knife in chest and flanks, a feeling of abdominal fullness, intestinal sounds as if from a distance, and if one is terrified with **palpitating qi**".

Ji qi **積氣, accumulated qi** [24]
① EA of pathological qi halting and accumulating at any place in the body. *SW* 10: 有**積氣**在中，時害於食，名曰心痹, "**Accumulated qi** in the center. Occasionally this is harm caused by food. It is called heart blockage".
② PC brought forth by accumulated qi. *SW* 64: 滑則病狐疝風，澀則病少腹**積氣**, "If [the vessels] are smooth, the disease is fox[-type] elevation-illness wind. If they are rough, the disease is **accumulated qi** in the lower abdomen".

Jie qi **結氣, bound qi** [113]
① EA of pathological qi halting and congealing at any place in the body. *JGYL* Lj: 婦人之病，因虛、積冷、**結氣**，為諸經水斷絕, "The diseases of females are such that because of depletion, accumulated cold, and **bound qi** the passage of the monthly period is blocked".
② PC brought forth by bound qi. *BJ* SE *ku shen* 苦參：主心腹**結氣**，癥瘕積聚，黃疸, "It controls **bound qi** in the region of heart and abdomen, concretion-illness and conglomeration-illness, accumulation and collection, as well as yellow *dan*-illness".

Ji re **積熱, accumulated heat** [60]
① EA identified as accumulated heat. *ZHF* 7: 飲酒**積熱**，遂發黃, "If consumption of wine leads to **accumulated heat**, this will bring forth yellowing".

② PC brough forth by accumulated heat as etiological agent. *BJ* SE *xiao shi* 消石：主五藏**積熱**, "It controls **accumulated heat** in the five depots".

Ji re 肌熱**, muscle heat** [21]

PC of a patient feeling dryness and heat in the outer sections of the flesh/muscles or of a third person sensing heat when touching this region with his hand. *SJZL* 87: 治熱勞，**肌熱**煩躁，面紅頰赤，人參湯方, "To cure heat exhaustion, **muscle heat** with vexation and agitation; red face, red cheeks: recipe for a decoction with *ren shen*".

Ji re li 積熱痢**, accumulated heat free-flux illness** [2]

PC identical with → *re li* 熱痢, heat free-flux illness. *BCGM* Bai bing zhu zhi yao 百病主治藥：冬瓜葉，**積熱痢**，拖麵食, "[To cure] **accumulated heat free-flux illness** with *dong gua* leaves, consume them coated with flour". Also: 柴胡，**積熱痢**，同黃芩，半水半酒煎服, "[To cure] **accumulated heat free-flux illness** with *chai hu*, ingest after boiling together with *huang qin* in [a liquid consisting of] half water half wine". *BCGM* further has 積熱下痢, accumulated heat discharge free-flux illness, and 積熱瀉痢, accumulated heat outflow free-flux illness.

Ji re xia li 積熱下痢**, accumulated heat discharge free-flux illness** [1]

PC identical with → *re li* 熱痢, heat free-flux illness. *BCGM* SE *chai hu* 柴胡 quotes *JJF*: **積熱下痢**：柴胡、黃芩等分，半酒半水煎七分，浸冷，空心服之, "For **accumulated heat free-flux illness**: Boil equal amounts of *chai hu* and *huang* qi in [a liquid consisting of] one half wine and one half water down to 70%. Wait until it has cooled down and ingest on an empty stomach".

Ji re xie li 積熱瀉痢**, accumulated heat outflow free-flux illness** [1]

PC identical with → *re li* 熱痢, heat free-flux illness. *BCGM* SE *dong gua* 冬瓜：**積熱瀉痢**：冬瓜葉嫩心，拖麵煎餅食之, "For **accumulated heat outflow free-flux illness**: *dong gua* leaves with a tender heart are to be dragged through flour, boiled to form cakes and consumed".

Ji rou ji 肌肉急**, muscle-flesh tension** [1]

IS of an uncomfortable feeling of contraction of tight muscles making it difficult to stretch the body. *WTMY* 38: 下焦虛熱，骨節煩疼，**肌肉急**, "The lower burner has depletion heat. The bones and joints experience vexing pain. The **muscle-flesh is tense**".

Ji shou 肌瘦**, muscle-flesh emaciation** [10]

IS of an emaciation of muscles and flesh. *TPSHF* 79: 治產後惡血稽留，經久未消，致月水不通，面色萎黃，臍腹疼痛，**肌瘦**無力，益母草子散方, "To cure malign blood retained without dissolving for an extended period after having given birth, with a failure of menses to pass, a wilting-yellow complexion, navel and abdominal pain, **muscle-flesh emaciation** and physical weakness, the recipe for the powder with *yi mu cao* seeds [is advisable]".

Ji tan 積痰**, accumulated phlegm** [5]

EA identical with → *tan ji* 痰積①, phlegm accumulation. *DXXF* 5: 又方，治**積痰**傷經不行，夜則妄語, "An additional recipe. It cures **accumulated phlegm** harming the conduits and closing their passage. At night [patients] use absurd language".

***Ji teng* 急疼, sudden violent pain** [2]
IS identical with *ji tong* 急痛. *WTMY* 23: 廣濟療喉痹**急疼**，悶妨不通方, "Recipe from the *GJF* to cure throat blockage with **sudden violent pain**, and heart-pressure with a feeling of uneasiness and blockage".

***Ji tong* 急痛, sudden violent pain** [44] AN *ji teng* 急疼, *teng ji* 疼急
IS of a pain that emerges suddenly and is violent. *LS* 10: 食不下，煩心，心下**急痛**, "[Patients] are unable to eat. They experience vexation in their heart, and a sudden **violent pain** in the region below their heart".

***Ji xia* 雞瘕, chicken conglomeration-illness** [2]
PC of conglomeration brought forth by the consumption of chicken eggs that fail to be digested. It was believed that the failure to digest chicken eggs resulted in the forming of lumps in the shape of fledglings. Hence the designation of this condition. *BCTJ* SE *su* 蘇：蘇主**雞瘕**, "*Su* controls **chicken conglomeration-illness**".

***Ji xian* 雞癇, chicken epilepsy** [2]
PC of a → *dian xian* 癲癇, peak-illness with epilepsy, which, at the time of its outbreaks, lets the patient's four limbs twitch, accompanied by a shaking head and the body arching back, with spontaneous shaking. *QJYF* 5: **雞癇**之為病，搖頭反折，喜驚自搖, "The disease of **chicken epilepsy**: the head shakes and [the body] arches back, with a tendency to be frightened and exhibit spontaneous shaking".

***Ji xin tong* 急心痛, acute heartache** [5]
PC identical with → *cu xin tong* 卒心痛②, sudden heartache. *PJF* 335: 治婦人**急心痛**，用南康真蛤粉為末細，炒赤，以酒調熱服愈, "To cure **acute heartache** in women prepare a fine powder from genuine *ge fen* from Nankang and roast until it has assumed a red color. Mix with wine and ingest heated. This will bring the cure".

***Ji xue* 積血, accumulated blood** [22]
PC brought forth by blood accumulations resulting from stagnant blood. *LH* 6: 食血之蟲死，而**積血**之病癒, "Once the bug consuming one's blood has died, the disease of '**accumulated blood**' is healed".

***Ji yan* 雞眼, chicken eye; corn** [6]
PC identical with → *rou ci* 肉刺, flesh thorn, corn. *SJZL* 138: 肉刺者，生於足指間，形如硬胝，與肉相附，隱痛成刺，由靴履急窄，相磨而成，俗呼為**雞眼**是也, "Flesh thorns grow between the toes. Their appearance is hard and callous. They are attached to the flesh, and form painful, deep-reaching thorns. They develop when boots or shoes are too narrow. They are commonly called '**chicken eyes**'".

***Ji ying* 急硬, tension and hardness** [2]
IS of a loss of regular flexibility of any body part with cramps and a feeling of tightness and hardening. *BCSY* SE *tian zhong luo* 田中螺：小腹**急硬**，小便

赤澀，脚手浮腫, "Lower abdominal **tension and hardness**. Urine is red and rough. The legs and hands are swollen".

Ji zhao feng **雞爪風, chicken's claw wind** [1]

PC, brought forth by wind heat, of convulsions experienced by women following delivery. *XMLF* 3: 產後風熱搐搦，俗謂**雞爪風**, "Wind heat convulsions following delivery are commonly called **chicken's claw wind**".

Ji zheng **積癥, accumulation concretion-illness** [1]

PC identical with → *zheng ji* → 癥積, concretion-illness accumulation. *BCGM Bai bing zhu zhi yao* 百病主治藥：硇砂，噎膈吐食，有**積癥**，用之神效, "*Nao sha* is wondrously effective if applied for gullet occlusion and vomiting of food, when there is a **accumulation concretion-illness**".

Ji zhi **積滯, accumulation and sluggishness** [61]

① EA PM of cold, phlegm rheum, beverages and food and other pathogenic qi residing and accumulating in the body, rather than leaving the human body, and possibly generating further diseases in turn. *TPSHF* 28: 夫虛勞癥瘕病者，皆由久寒**積滯**，冷飲食不能消化所致也, "Now, as for diseases such as depletion exhaustion, concretion-illness and conglomeration-illness, they all result from cold **accumulation and sluggishness** over an extended period of time and a failure to digest cold beverages and food". *BCGM* Bai bing zhu zhi yao 百病主治藥 identifies vomiting, diarrhea, free-flux illness, and the passing of blood with urine and defecation as resulting from accumulation and sluggishness.

② PC brought forth by accumulation and sluggishness of pathogenic qi. *TPSHF* 5: 治脾臟冷氣**積滯**，醋心嘔逆，宿食不消，腹臟虛鳴，時時疼痛，宜服吳茱萸丸方, "To cure **accumulation and sluggishness** of cold qi in the spleen depot, as well as heartburn with vomiting and counterflow, food remaining in the body over night without being digested, depletion sounds in abdominal depots, and frequent pain, the recipe to ingest the pills with *wu zhu yu* is advisable".

Ji zhong **積腫, accumulation swelling** [1]

PC of → *zhong ji* 腫疾, swelling ailment, brought forth by accumulations of phlegm and food. *BCGM* Bai bing zhu zhi yao 百病主治藥：諸腫，有風腫，熱腫，水腫，濕腫，氣腫，虛腫，**積腫**，血腫, "All types of swelling include wind swelling; heat swelling; water/edematose swelling; moisture swelling; qi swelling; depletion swelling; **accumulation swelling**; blood swelling".

Ji zhong chuan xi **肌中竄鼷, mice scurrying in the muscles** [1]

PC identical with → *ji zhong shu xi* 肌中鼠鼷, mice in the muscles. *BCGM* Bai bing zhu zhi yao 百病主治藥 quoting *ma dao* 馬刀 monograph: 肌中鼠鼷, "Mice in the muscles", writes: **肌中竄鼷, "Mice scurrying in the muscles"**.

Ji zhong shu xi **肌中鼠鼷, mice in the muscles** [1] AN *ji zhong chuan xi* 肌中竄鼷, mice scurrying in the muscles.

PC of two or three smooth → *luo li* 瘰癧, scrofula with pervasion-illness, that grow in a row in the muscles. They have not opened to fester yet and are movable with the skin. *BCGM* SE *ma dao* 馬刀 quoting *MYBL*: 肌中鼠鼷 writes: **肌中鼠鼷, "Mice in the muscles"**.

***Jia* 瘕, empty[-lumps]-illness; conglomeration-illness** [p]

PC of painful abdominal nodes/lumps that sometimes move and sometimes do not move in accordance with the movement of the body's qi. *ZBYHL* 19: 瘕病者，由寒温不適，飲食不消，與臟氣相搏，積在腹内，結塊**瘕**痛，隨氣移動是也。言其虛假不牢，故謂之為**瘕**也, "In the case of a **conglomeration-illness** disease, cold and warmth are out of sorts; beverages and food remain undigested and clash with the qi of the depots. This leads to abdominal accumulations, nodular lumps and painful **conglomeration-illness** that follow the qi in its movement. As these are empty entities (*xu jia* 虛假) without hard substance one speaks of **瘕** [to signify the meaning of '**empty-lumps-illness**']".

***Jia jie* 痂疥, crust with *jie*-illness** [3]

PC of → *jie chuang* 疥瘡, *jie*-illness sores, that have opened to fester and have formed a crust. *BJ* SE *xiong huang* 雌黃：主惡瘡，頭禿，**痂疥**, "It controls malign sores, baldness on the head, and **crust with *jie*-illness**".

***Jia jing shang han* 夾驚傷寒, fright related harm caused by cold** [2]

PC of children suffering from → *shang han* 傷寒, harm caused by cold, together with high fever and fright. *YYXS* 10: **夾驚傷寒**候：渾身壯熱，心躁發渴，睡裏多驚, "Signs of **fright related harm caused by cold**: the entire body is very hot. The heart is restless, and one develops thirst. While sleeping [patients] are often frightened".

***Jia ju* 甲疽, nail impediment-illness** [16]

PC of → *chuang* 瘡, sores, that develops either to the side of or below the fingernails, with red swelling, heat and pain, and emitting pus or water. In some instances a red flesh protrusion emerges, and the fingernail is raised. *ZBYHL* 35: 甲疽之狀，瘡皮厚，甲錯剝起是也, "The appearance of **nail impediment-illness**: The skin around the sores is thick and flaky, and slightly elevated".

***Jia tong* 嫁痛, marriage pain** [2]

PC of injury inflicted on a woman's outer genital parts following crude and violent sexual intercourse. *QJYF* 3: 治**嫁痛**單行方：大黃十八銖，取好酒一升，煮三沸，頓服之佳, "Single substance recipe to cure **marriage pain**: boil 18 *zhu* of *da huang* in 1 *sheng* of good wine. Let it boil 3 times. Ingesting it will have a good effect".

***Jia xuan* 痂癬, crusts with *xuan*-illness** [2]

PC of → *xuan* 癬, *xuan*-illness a), with a lesion developing a crust. *BJ* SE *shu yang quan* 蜀羊泉：主頭禿惡瘡，熱氣，疥瘙**痂癬**蟲, "It controls baldness on the head with malign sores, heat qi, *jie*-illness with itching; crusts with ***xuan*-illness**, and bugs/worms".

***Jia yang* 痂瘍, crust ulcers** [4]

PC CD of all → *chuang yang* 瘡瘍, sores and ulcers, developing as if a scar had been crushed. *MYBL* SE *chi he* 赤赫：主**痂瘍**，惡敗瘡, "It controls **crust ulcers**, and malign decay sores".

***Jia yin shang han* 夾陰傷寒, sexuality related harm caused by cold** [3
PC of a type of → *shang han* 傷寒, harm caused by cold, where a person first followed his lust and then was affected by cold evil, with the result of yang weakness and an abundance of yin. *BCGM* SE *ren shen* 人參 quotes *SHYY*: **夾陰傷寒**，先因欲事，後感寒邪，陽衰陰盛，六脈沉伏，小腹絞痛，四肢逆冷，嘔吐清水，不假此藥，無以回陽, "**Sexuality related harm caused by cold**: A person first followed his lust and then was affected by cold evil, with the result of yang weakness and yin abundance. The movements in the six vessels are deep inside and subdued. The lower abdomen has a twisting pain. The four limbs have counterflow with cold. [Patients] vomit clear water. If one does not take recourse to this drug, there is no other way to have the yang return".

***Jian du* 箭毒, arrow poison** [11] AN *zu du* 鏃毒, arrowhead poison.
EA of wounds generated by poison smeared on an arrowhead. *ZLBC* SE *xiong huang* 雄黃：又方：治**箭毒**. 搗為末傅之，沸汁出愈, "Another recipe: To cure **arrow poison**. Pound [*xiong huang*] to powder and apply externally. When juice appears with bubbles as if boiling, [the patient] is cured".

***Jian ji* 堅積, hard accumulation** [19]
PC of → *ji* 積, accumulations, which are hard and stable and difficult to cure. *BJ* SE *shao yao* 芍藥：主邪氣腹痛，除血痹，破**堅積**，寒熱疝瘕, "It controls evil qi with abdominal pain. It eliminates blood blockage. It crushes **hard accumulations**, alternating sensations of cold and heat, and elevation-illness with conglomeration-illness. LSZ: **堅積**之病，非平和之藥所能取捷, "**Hard accumulation** is a disease that cannot be overcome by medication with a balanced and harmonious nature".

***Jian man* 堅滿, hardness and fullness** [8]
IS of an uncomfortable feeling of fullness in a region that, when pressed, feels hard. *SW* 74: 厥陰之復，少腹**堅滿**，裏急暴痛, "When the ceasing yin [qi] takes revenge, the lower abdomen **hardens and** [has a feeling of] **fullness**. There is internal tightness and violent pain".

***Jian pi* 堅癖, hard aggregation-illness** [6]
PC of difficult-to-cure, painful lumps in the region of flanks and abdomen formed by stagnating phlegm rheum and blood that fail to dissipate. *JGYL* Lj: 婦人經水閉不利，臟**堅癖**不止，中有乾血，下白物，礬石丸主之, "When menstruation is blocked and when there is a **hard aggregation-illness** of dried blood in the depots that does not end, with the passing down of white matter, this is controlled by pills with *fan shi*".

***Jian ri nüe* 間日瘧, every-other-day malaria** [1]
PC of → *nüe ji* 瘧疾, malaria ailment, with outbreaks every second day. *ZBYHL* 11: **間日瘧**候. 間日而作也, "The appearance of '**every-other-day malaria**' is such that its outbreaks occur every other day".

***Jian tong* 堅痛, hardening with pain** [7] AN *ying tong* 硬痛.

IS of pain together with a local hardening. *SW* 60: 缺盆骨上切之**堅痛**如筋者灸之, "Cauterize the location above the broken basin bone which, when squeezed, feels **hard and generates pain** as if it were a sinew".

***Jian wang* 健忘, forgetfulness** [45] AW *shan wang* 善忘, *xi wang* 喜忘, *duo wang* 多忘.

① IS of bad memory. *QJYF* 19: 無比薯蕷丸，治諸百損方. …**健忘**，加遠志一兩, "Unparalleled pills with *shu yu*, they are a recipe to cure all types of injury... In the case of **forgetfulness**, add 1 *liang* of *yuan zhi*".

② PC of a disease with forgetfulness as its main sign. *QJYF* 14: 治**健忘**方：天門冬、遠志、茯苓、乾地黃, "Recipe for treating **forgetfulness**: *tian men dong*, *yuan zhi*, *fu ling*, *gan di huang*".

***Jian zhang* 堅脹, hardness and distension** [3] AN *zhang jian* 脹堅, distension with hardness.

IS of an uncomfortable feeling of distension associated with an abdomen that appears hard when pressed. *QJYF* 12: 筋極則拘攣，小腹**堅脹**，心痛，膝寒冷，四肢骨節皆疼痛, "If the sinews are affected to an extreme, they will cramp and contract. The lower abdomen feels **hard and distended**. The heart aches, the knees are cold. The bones and joints of the four limbs are all in pain".

***Jian zheng* 堅癥, hard concretion-illness** [3]

PC identical with → *zheng jian* 癥堅, concretion-illness hardness. *BJ* SE *ma lu* 馬陸：主腹中大**堅癥**，破積聚, "It controls large **hardness concretion-illness** in the abdomen, and breaks open accumulations and collections".

***Jiang ji* 強急, stiff and tense** [1]

IS identical with → *ji jiang* 急強, tense and stiff. *BCGM* SE *xi'er* 枲耳 quoting *ZHF:* 骨節皆強，筋急, "Bones and joints are all stiff; the muscles are tense", writes: 骨節**強急**, "Bones and joints are **stiff and tense**".

***Jiang tong* 強痛, stiffness with pain** [4] AN *tong jiang* 痛強, pain with stiffness.

IS of pain accompanied by a hardening of muscle tissue. *ZHF* 4: 小腹拘急，腰背**強痛**，心中虛悸，咽乾唇燥，面體少色, "Cramps and tension in the lower abdomen. **Stiffness with pain** affecting the lumbar region and the back. Depletion and palpitation in the heart. Dry throat and parched lips. Face and body have a pale complexion".

***Jiang ying* 強硬, stiffness** [4]

IS of a specific part of the body turning stiff making any movement rather uncomfortable. *TPSHF* 6: 治肺臟中風，心胸氣促，項背**強硬**，皮膚不仁，麻黃散方, "To cure a lung depot struck by wind with agitated qi in the heart and chest, **stiffness** of the nape and back, and numbness of the skin, the recipe [to ingest] the powder with *ma huang* [is advisable]".

***Jiang zhi* 強直, rigidity** [21]

IS of stiffness and straightness of the limbs and trunk. *SW* 74: 諸暴**強直**，皆屬於風, "All [cases of] sudden **rigidity** are associated with wind".

Jiang zhong **強腫, stiff and swollen** [1]
IS identical with → *zhong jiang* 腫強, swollen and stiff. *BCGM* Bai bing zhu zhi yao 百病主治藥：醋，小兒舌**強腫**，和飴含之, "Vinegar: children with a **stiff and swollen** tongue should hold it in their mouth together with *yi*".

Jiao bi **脚痹, leg blockage** [11]
PC of → *bi* 痹① a), blockage, affecting legs and feet. *MYBL* SE *song jie* 松節：主百節久風，風虛，**脚痹**疼痛, "It controls chronic wind in the hundred joints, wind [intruding into a state of] depletion, and **leg blockage** with pain".

Jiao chang **交腸, communicating bowels** [2]
PC of a severe rupture, received during delivery, in a woman's lower abdomen resulting in the discharge of feces through her urinary tract. *SYDXF* 10: 婦人小便中出大糞，名**交腸**, "When a woman discharges feces together with her urine, this is called '**communicating intestines**'".

Jiao chang sha **絞腸沙, twisting-intestines sand** [9] AN *jiao chang sha* 攪腸沙.
PC identical with → *gan huo luan* 乾霍亂, dry cholera. *QXLF* 2: 有一證，心腹絞痛，冷汗出，脹悶欲絕，俗謂之**絞腸沙**, "There is a condition of a twisting pain in the heart and abdomen, cold sweat leaving the body, with a feeling of distension and heart-pressure that makes one wish to die. This is commonly called '**twisting-intestines sand**'".

Jiao chang sha **攪腸沙, annoying-intestines sand** [4]
PC identical with → *jiao chang sha* 絞腸沙, twisting-intestines sand. *ZBZZZS* 3: 乾霍亂，忽然心腹脹滿攪痛，欲吐不吐，欲瀉不瀉，躁亂憒憒無奈，俗名**攪腸沙**者是也, "Dry cholera: a sudden feeling of distension and fullness in heart and abdomen, with annoying pain. One wishes to vomit but does not. One has an urge to defecate but fails to defecate. [Patients] are extremely confused. This is commonly called '**annoying-intestines sand**'".

Jiao ci **疞刺, flatulent painful piercing** [4]
IS of a pressing pain in the abdomen together with a feeling as if pierced. *HJJF* 6: 心腹諸疾，**疞刺**切痛, "All illnesses affecting heart and abdomen, and all types of **flatulent painful piercing** and cutting pain."

Jiao feng **脚風, leg wind** [5]
PC CD of pain, cramps, and lack of strength in the lower limbs. *QJYF* 17: 青丸，主**脚風**，皮肉身體諸風方, "Virid pills: a recipe to master **leg wind**, and all types of wind affecting skin, flesh and the entire body".

Jiao gong fan zhang **角弓反張, arched reverse strain; arched back rigidity; opisthotonos** [20] AD *fan zhang* **反張, arched strain**
IS of the body being bent backwards because of contracting muscles. *ZHF* 3: 身體**角弓反張**，四肢不隨, "The body shows **arched back rigidity**; the four limbs do not follow [one's will]".

Jiao gu bu kai **交骨不開, the interlocking bones fail to open** [2]
PC of a → *nan chan* 難產, difficult birth, because of a woman's narrow pelvis. *SYDXF* 14: 治產五七日不下垂死者，及矮小女子**交骨不開**者, "It cures cases where a child has died during birth and has failed to descend for as long as five

or seven days, as well as when an undersized woman's **interlocking bones fail to open**".

Jiao jian **脚趼, callous legs** [1]

PC identical with → *zu jian* 足趼, callous feet. *BCGM* SE *xiao mai* 小麥 quotes *HSF*: 遠行**脚趼**成泡者，水調生麵塗之, "For **callous legs** developing blisters after a long walk, mix fresh [*xiao mai*] flour with water and apply externally".

Jiao long bing **蛟龍病, flood dragon disease** [2] AN *jiao long zheng* 蛟龍症, flood dragon condition.

PC with blue hands and abdominal fullness and an unbearable pain. *JGYL* Lj: 春秋二時，龍帶精入芹菜中，人偶食之為病。發時手青腹滿，痛不可忍，名**蛟龍病**, "In the two seasons of spring and autumn, dragons place their essence/semen into celery. If a person happens to consume such plants, this will result in blue hands and abdominal fullness, and unbearable pain. It is called '**flood-dragon disease**'". LSZ refutes the claim that flood dragons can deposit their essence/semen in celery plants, and wonders whether this could be semen of lizards or snakes.

Jiao long zheng **蛟龍症, flood-dragon condition** [5]

PC identical with → *jiao long bing* 蛟龍病, flood-dragon disease. *BCGM* SE *jiao long* 蛟龍 quoting *JGYL*: 蛟龍病, "Flood-dragon disease", writes: **蛟龍症**, "**Flood-dragon condition**".

Jiao qi **脚氣, leg qi** [242] AN *jiao ruo* 脚弱, leg weakness.

PC of legs being painful and weak. They may be swollen, or dried up and emaciated. In serious cases the functioning of the heart and spleen is impaired. *ZHF* 3: **脚氣**之病，先起嶺南，稍來江東，得之無漸, "The disease '**leg qi**' originated from Lingnan; it has gradually reached the region east of the Yangzi. The onset is rather sudden". Etiology and appearance of this disease vary. *BCGM* Bai bing zhu zhi yao 百病主治藥：**脚氣**：有風濕、寒濕、濕熱、食積, "**Leg qi** includes wind-moisture, cold-moisture, moisture-heat, and food accumulation". Basically one can distinguish between → *gan jiao qi* 乾脚氣, dry leg qi, and → *shi jiao qi* 濕脚氣, moist leg qi.

Jiao ruo **脚弱, leg weakness** [27]

① PC identical with → *jiao qi* 脚氣, leg qi. *ZHF* 3 lists 治風毒**脚弱**痹滿上氣方, "Recipes to cure wind-poison, **leg weakness**, blockage-fullness, and rising qi".

② IS of weak legs making walking difficult. *QJYF* 7: 患嘔吐而復**脚弱**，余診之，乃告為脚氣, "[The patient] suffered from vomiting and also **leg weakness**. I examined him and identified it as leg qi".

Jiao she **嚼舌, tongue chewing** [3]

IS of inadvertent gnawing on the tip of one's own tongue. *ZBYHL* 26: 病發時嗇嗇惡寒，頭微痛，乾嘔，背迫急，口噤不覺，**嚼舌**，大小便秘澀, "When the disease develops, one shivers and has an aversion to cold. There is a mild headache, associated with dry vomiting. The back is tight, the jaws are clenched and [the patient] loses consciousness. [Patients] **chew their tongue**; defecation and urination are impaired and rough".

***Jiao tong* 疞痛, flatulent pain** [10]

IS of a pressing pain in the abdomen. *JGYL* Lj: 婦人懷妊，腹中**疞痛**，當歸芍藥散主之, "When women in the course of pregnancy have a **flatulent pain** in the abdomen, this is mastered by the powder with *dang gui* and *shao yao*."

***Jiao tong* 絞痛, twisting pain** [30] AN *jiao tong* 攪痛, annoying pain.

IS of a violent pain affecting the internal organs, with a sensation as if they were pressed by wringing. *ZHF* 1: 治寒疝來去，每發**絞痛**方, "Recipe to cure cold elevation-illness that comes and goes. Whenever it breaks out it comes with **twisting pain**".

***Jiao tong* 攪痛, annoying pain** [1]

IS identical with → *jiao tong* 絞痛, twisting pain. *QJYF* 15: 桃花丸，治下冷，臍下**攪痛**方, "Pills with *tao hua*, a recipt to cure cold in the lower parts, and **annoying pain** below the navel".

***Jie* 疥, *jie*-illness** [p]

PC AD of → *jie chuang* 疥瘡, *jie*-illness sores. *ZBYHL* 50: **疥**候：疥瘡，多生手足指間，染漸生至於身體，癢，有膿汁, "The signs of ***jie*-illness**: *jie*-illness sores often grow in the region of fingers and toes, from where they gradually infect the body itself. They itch, and they contain pus liquid".

***Jie* 癤, pimple** [p] AN *jie zi* 癤子; *chuang jie* 瘡癤, pimple sores; *jie zhong* 癤腫, pimple swelling.

PC CD of acute festering developing as a mild condition in a small dermal region. *ZBYHL* 32: 腫一寸至二寸，**癤**也, "When the swelling extends over one to two inches, these are **pimples**".

***Jie chang* 截腸, severed intestine** [2]

PC identical with → *tuo gang* 脫肛, prolapse of the rectum. *SYDXF* 10: 大腸頭出寸余，痛苦，直候乾，自退落。又出，名為**截腸**病, "When the end of the large intestine protrudes a *cun* or more, with pain, and when, after its protruding part has dried and fallen off by itself, another section appears, this is called the '**severed intestine**' disease".

***Jie chong* 疥蟲, *jie*-illness bug** [8]

① EA of small bugs capable of causing *jie*-illness sores. *BJ* SE *lü ru* 蔄茹：主蝕惡肉，敗瘡死肌，殺**疥蟲**, "It controls the erosion of malign flesh and of dead muscles in rotten flesh, and it kills ***jie*-illness bugs/worms**".

② PC identical with → *chong jie* 蟲疥, bug *jie*-illness. *MYBL* SE *xiong huang* 雄黄：療**疥蟲**，𧏾瘡，目痛，鼻中息肉, "It cures ***jie*-illness bugs/worms**, hidden worm infestation sores, eye pain, and tumorous flesh-growth in the nose".

***Jie chuang* 疥瘡, *jie*-illness sores** [26] AD *jie* 疥; AN *sao jie* 瘙疥, itching *jie*-illness; *chong jie* 蟲疥, bug *jie*-illness.

PC of → *chuang* 瘡, sores, brought forth by "*jie*-illness bugs/worms". It often occurs between fingers and toes and has itching. In some cases it may fester. *ZBYHL* 50: **疥瘡**，多生手足指間，染漸生至於身體，癢，有膿汁, "***Jie*-illness**

sores often grow between fingers and toes, from where they gradually infect the body itself. They itch, and they contain pus liquid".

Jie du **癤毒, pimples with poison** [8]

PC identical with → jie 癤, pimples. *SYJYBZFL* 14: 遠志酒，治一切癰疽發背**癤毒**, "Wine with *yuan zhi* cures all types of obstruction- and impediment-illnesses with effusion of the back, and **pimples with poison**".

Jie he **結核, nodular kernels** [37]

① PC a) identical with → *luo li jie he* 瘰癧結核, nodular kernels of scrofula with pervasion-illness. *QJYF* 5: 治小兒無故寒熱，強健如故，而身體頸項**結核**瘰癧, "To cure alternating and seemingly unfounded sensations of cold and heat among children, and return their strength to normal, as well as **nodular kernels** of scrofula with pervasion-illness affecting the body and the front and back of the neck". b) Of any other swelling between skin and flesh reminiscent of fruit kernels. *TPSHF* 35: 治癭氣**結核**，瘤瘤腫硬，宜服松蘿丸方, "To cure **nodular kernels** of goiter qi, and pimples that are swollen and hard, the recipe to ingest pills with *song luo* is advisable".

② IS of a swelling reminiscent of fruit kernels between skin and flesh. *ZBYHL* 50: 其狀作**結核**，在皮肉間，三兩個相連累也, "As its external appearance it develops **nodular kernels** in the region of skin and flesh, two or three in a line".

Jie hou **結喉, bound throat** [1]

PC with swelling and pain in the throat following an attachment-illness of evil qi there as the major sign. *SHZBL* 3: 黑龍煎，治咽喉腫痛九種疾…急喉閉、纏喉風、**結喉**、爛喉、重舌、木舌、遁蟲、蟲喋、飛絲入喉, "'Black dragon decoction' cures nine types of ailments of swollen and aching throat … acute throat closure, throat-constricting wind, **bound throat**, festering throat, doubled tongue, wooden tongue, runaway bug, floating worm-borer, flying silk threads entering the throat".

Jie ji **結積, nodular accumulation** [7] AN *ji jie* 積結 accumulation and nodes.

PC identical with → *ji* 積, accumulation. *BCJJZ* SE *shui zhi* 水蛭：楚王食寒菹，所得而吞之，果能去**結積**，雖曰陰佑，亦是物性兼然 "When the king of Chu consumed cold pickled vegetables, they were infested with [leeches] with the result that he swallowed them. They were indeed able to rid him of **nodular accumulation**. Although someone said that this was a case of numinous protection, it was also brought forth by the nature of that item [leeches]".

Jie jia **結瘕, nodular conglomeration-illness** [4]

PC identical with → *xue jia* 血瘕, blood conglomeration-illness. *BCSY* SE *shi ci mu gen pi* 石刺木根皮：主破血，因產血不盡**結瘕**者, "It controls the crushing of blood that has not left [a woman's body] completely after delivery, [forming] **nodular conglomeration-illness**".

Jie jin **結筋, bound sinews** [2]

PC of cramped sinews brought forth by wind cold, with local hardening but without red swelling. *ZBYHL* 22: 十二經之筋皆起於手足指，而絡於身也。體虛者，風冷之氣中之，冷氣停積，故結聚，謂之**結筋**也, "The sinew paths begin in the fingers and toes and they wind around the body. When the body in a condition of depletion is struck by the qi of wind cold, the cold qi accumulates and forms nodular collections. This is called **bound sinews**".

***Jie jing* 截驚, to cut fright** [2]

TA identical with → *zhi jing* 止驚, to stop fright. *BCGM* SE *gan jiao* 甘蕉 quotes *WSZX* : 小兒**截驚**：以芭蕉汁、薄荷汁煎匀，塗頭頂, "To **cut fright** in children: Boil equal parts of *ba jiao* sap and *bo he* sap and smear on the crown of the head".

***Jie ju* 結聚, nodular collection** [17]

① EA PM of all types of pathogenic evil halting and collecting inside the body. *ZBYHL* 20: 經久不瘥，乃**結聚**成形, "If not cured for an extended period of time, **nodular collections** assume shape".

② PC identical with → *ji ju* 積聚, accumulation and collection. *ZBYHL* 19: 小口微出氣十二通，以除**結聚**, "Close the mouse except for a tiny opening and blow out qi twelve times. This will eliminate **nodular collections**".

***Jie lai* 疥癩, *jie*-illness with repudiation-illness; *jie*-illness and repudiation-illness** [15]

PC a) of → *lai* 癩, repudiation-illness, that is similar to papules and *xuan*-illness, with itching skin. *QJYiF* 21: **疥癩**者，狀如癬瘙，身體狂癢，十年成大患, "***Jie*-illness with repudiation-illness** appears similar to *xuan*-illness with itching. The body is maddened by the itching. Over a period of ten years this develops into massive suffering". b) CD of → *jie* 疥, *jie*-illness, and → *lai* 癩, repudiation-illness, referring to various types of skin ailments. *RHZ* SE *bi ma zi* 蓖麻子：瘡痍**疥癩**亦可研傅, "Ground to a powder it may also be externally applied to sores, wounds, ***jie*-illness, and repudiation-illness**".

***Jie lou* 疥瘺, *jie*-illness and fistula** [2]

PC CD of → *jie* 疥, *jie*-illness, and → *lou* 瘺, fistula. *BJ* SE *shui yin* 水銀：主**疥瘺**，痂瘍，白禿, "It controls ***jie*-illness and fistula**, crust ulcers, and white baldness".

***Jie lu* 解顱, open skull** [16] AN *lu jie* 顱解.

PC of children whose fontanel fails to close until they have reached a certain age. *ZBYHL* 48: **解顱**者，其狀小兒年大，囟應合而不合，頭縫開解是也, "As for '**open skull**', its appearance is such that children that have reached an advanced age and whose fontanel should have closed but has not, leaving the crevice of the fontanel open".

***Jie mao dao ruo* 睫毛倒入, intrusion of inverted eyelashes** [1]

IS of curled eyelashes with their ends pointing inward and rubbing the cornea, resulting in a feeling of roughness, pain and flow of tears. *BCGM* SE *shi hu* 石斛 quotes *XZF*: **睫毛倒入**：川石斛、川芎藭等分，為末。口內含水，隨左右嗃鼻，日二次, "For **intrusion of inverted eyelashes**: Powderize equal amounts of *chuan shi hu* and *chuan xiong qiong*. Hold water in the mouth and inhale [the powder] through the [left or right] nostril depending on whether it is the left or the right [eyelash], twice daily".

***Jie nüe* 截瘧, to interrupt malaria** [11]

TA applied to prevent an expected outbreak of malaria. *SYDXF* 11: 通神餅，**截瘧**有功, "The 'spirit-like cake' has the effect to **interrupt malaria**".

***Jie nüe* 痎瘧, epidemic malaria** [2] AN *yao nüe* 妖瘧, goblin malaria.

PC possibly identical with → *lao nüe ji* 老瘧, chronic malaria, with irregular outbreaks. *NJ* 56: **痎瘧**，連歲不已, "Accumulations in the liver are called 'fat qi'. They are located below the ribs on the left and resemble a cup turned upside down. They have a head and foot, and they last a long time without healing. They make the [afflicted] person develop a cough with counterflow [of qi], and **epidemic malaria** that fails to end, even after years".

***Jie nüe* 痎瘧, *jie*-illness with malaria** [8]

PC identical with → *nüe ji* 瘧疾, malaria. *SW* 3: 夏傷於暑, 秋為**痎瘧**, "If one has been harmed in summer by summerheat, in autumn this causes ***jie*-illness with malaria**".

***Jie re* 結熱, bound heat** [29] AN *re jie* 熱結, heat nodes.

① EA of repletion evil brought about by evil heat that has intruded into the body where it blocks the qi mechanism or coagulates with other types of evil qi. *ZBYHL* 46: 熱入腹內，與腑臟之氣相結，謂之**結熱**, "When heat enters the abdomen and ties up with the qi of the depots and palaces, this is called '**bound heat**'". ② PC of blocked depot qi brought about by the etiological agent mentioned under ①, with blocked urine and stools, panting, fullness, and spitting because of [qi] moving contrary to its normal course. *MYBL* SE *da yan* 大鹽：主胃腸**結熱**，喘逆, "It controls **bound heat** in stomach and intestines, with panting [because of qi] moving contrary to its normal course".

***Jie sao* 疥瘙, *jie*-illness with itching** [18] AN *sao jie* 瘙疥, itching *jie*-illness.

PC identical with → *jie chuang* 疥瘡, *jie*-illness sores. *BJ* SE *shi hui* 石灰：主疽瘍，**疥瘙**，熱氣，惡瘡, "It controls impediment-illness ulcers, ***jie*-illness with itching**, heat qi, and malign sores".

***Jie tan* 結痰, bound phlegm** [4] AN *wan tan* 頑痰, stubborn phlegm; *lao tan* 老痰, chronic phlegm.

EA of sticky → *tan* 痰①, phlegm, nodes that fail to leave the body easily. *MYBL* SE *rui he* 蕤核：主目腫眥爛，齆鼻，破心下**結痰**痞氣, "It controls swollen eyes with festering canthi, and nasal congestion, and it breaks through **bound phlegm** and obstacle-illness qi below the heart".

***Jie tong* 結痛, nodes with pain** [6]

IS of a painful sensation brought forth by an accumulation of cold, heat, blood, qi, phlegm, or water in the body. *BJ* SE *fu ling* 茯苓：主胸脅逆氣，憂恚驚邪恐悸，心下**結痛**, "It controls qi moving contrary to its regular direction in chest and flanks, palpitation resulting from worrying, rage, fright, and fear, as well as **nodes with pain** below the heart".

***Jie xiong* 結胸, bound chest** [35]

PC brought forth by internal evil qi "binding" the chest, with the chest and abdomen experiencing distension, hardening and pain to a degree that one does not wish to apply pressure. As this disease often occurs following harm caused by cold, it is also called → *shang han jie xiong* 傷寒結胸, bound chest following harm caused by cold. *SHL* 134: 陽氣內陷，心下因硬，則為**結胸**, "If yang qi gets stuck internally resulting in a hardening below the heart, this is called **bound chest**". As the qi that may congeal differ, *BCGM* has → *re shi jie xiong* 熱實結胸; bound chest because of heat repletion; → *han shi jie xiong* 寒實結胸, bound chest because of cold repletion; → *tan qi jie xiong* 痰氣結胸, bound chest because of phlegm qi; → *liu qi jie xiong* 留氣結胸, bound chest because of residing qi; → *xue jie xiong* 血結胸, bound chest because of blood.

***Jie xuan* 疥癬, *jie*-illness and *xuan*-illness** [91] AN *xuan jie* 癬疥, *xuan*-illness and *jie*-illness.

PC CD of →*jie* 疥, *jie*-illness, and → *xuan* 癬, *xuan*-illness. *BJ* SE *ban mao* 斑貓：主寒熱，鬼疰，蠱毒，鼠瘺，**疥癬**，惡瘡, "It controls alternating sensations of cold and heat, demon attachment-illness, *gu* poison, mouse fistula, ***jie*-illness and *xuan*-illness**, as well as malign sores".

***Jie xue* 結血, bound blood** [6]

EA PM brought forth by stagnant blood that congeals to nodes and may in turn generate further diseases. *TBC* SE *nao sha* 硇砂:主積聚，破**結血**、爛胎，止痛下氣, "It controls accumulations and collections, breaks through **bound blood,** destroys (i.e. aborts) a fetus, stops pain and causes qi to move downward".

***Jie zao* 結燥, binding dryness** [2]

IS identical with → *zao jie* 燥結, dryness node. *BCGM* SE *da ma* 大麻 quotes Chen Shiliang 陳士良：利大腸風熱，**結燥**及熱淋, "It makes the large intestine passable again when it is affected by wind and heat, [and cures] **binding dryness** and heat dripping".

***Jie zhi* 結滯, nodular and sluggish [qi]** [13]

① *EA, PM* identical with → *ji zhi* 積滯①, accumulation and sluggishness. *ZBYHL* 6: 將適失宜，脾胃虛弱者，石勢**結滯**，乘於脾胃，致令脾胃氣不和，不勝於穀，故氣逆而嘔, "If the balance in nourishment is missed and the spleen and stomach are depleted and weak, the force of the mineral forms **nodes and is sluggish**, and avails itself of the spleen and stomach. This in turn causes an imbalance in the qi of the spleen and stomach which is no longer capable of transforming the grain. Hence the qi moves contrary to its regular direction and this results in vomiting".

② PC identical with → *ji zhi* 積滯②, accumulation and sluggishness. *WTMY* 38: 療熱氣**結滯**，經年數數發方, "Recipe to heal **nodular and sluggish** heat qi which appears again and again over many years".

***Jie zhong* 癤腫, pimple swelling** [2]

PC identical with → *jie* 癤, pimple. *WTMY* 24: 主**癤腫**方：生椒末、麴末、釜月下土末之，以大酢和敷之, "Recipe to master **pimple swelling**: fresh [*shu*] *jiao* powder, *qu* powder and powderized soil taken from underneath a cooking cauldron, mix with a large quantity of vinegar and apply this externally".

***Jie zi* 癤子, pimple** [3]

PC identical with → *jie* 癤. *QJYF* 22: 治**癤子**方：凡癤無頭者，吞葵子一枚，不得多服, "Recipe to cure **pimples**: For all pimples without [pus] head, swallow one *kui* seed. One need not ingest much of this".

***Jin chuang* 金瘡, sores inflicted by means of metal objects** [327] AN *jin chuang* 金創;, wounds inflicted by means of metal objects; *dao jian chuang* 刀箭瘡, wounds inflicted by knives and arrows.

PC CD of all types of bodily injuries inflicted by means of metal items, including fresh wounds not yet infected, and also long-lasting open sores that have an inflammation. *BJ* SE *xie* 薤：主**金瘡**瘡敗, "It controls **sores inflicted by means of metal [weapons/utensils]** and sores decay".

***Jin chuang* 金創, wounds inflicted by means of metal objects** [4]

PC of → *jin chuang*, wounds inflicted by means of metal objects, that are of recent origin. *MYBL* SE *bai ma jing* 白馬莖：屎，名馬通，微温。主婦人崩中，止渴及吐下血，鼻衄，**金創**止血, "Dung is called *ma tong*; it is slightly warm. It controls collapsing center of females, ends thirst and both the spitting and discharge of blood, nosebleed, and stops bleeding in case of **wounds inflicted by means of metal objects**."

***Jin chuang zhong feng* 金瘡中風 wind stroke via wounds inflicted by metal objects** [11] AN *jin chuang de feng* 金瘡得風, wind obtained through wounds inflicted by metal objects.

PC identical with → *po shang feng* 破傷風, wound wind. *WTMY* 29: 必效療**金瘡中風**，角弓反張者方, "It will certainly cure **wind stroke via wounds inflicted by metal objects** and also arched reverse strain".

***Jin chuang zhong feng* 金創中風, wind stroke via wounds inflicted by metal objects** [1]

PC identical with → *po shang feng* 破傷風, wound wind. *ZLBC* SE *ge gen* 葛根 quotes *ZYGLF*: **金創中風**，痓欲死者，取生根四大兩切，以水三升煮取一升，去滓分温四服, "For [treating] those who suffer from **wind stroke via wounds inflicted by metal objects** with spasms to the extent that they are about to die, cut four large *liang* (PUU: equivalent to 3 *liang* of later centuries) of fresh roots and boil in 3 *sheng* of water down to 1 *sheng*. Remove the dregs and ingest warm in four portions".

***Jin chun* 緊唇, tight lips** [10] AN *jin chun chuang* 緊唇瘡, tight lips sores; *chun jin* 唇緊, tight lips; *shen chun* 沛唇, leaking lips; *chun shen* 唇沛, lip leakage.

PC with lips growing sores, as well as swelling, distension, festering, fissures and pain. *ZBYHL* 30: 風邪寒濕之氣搏於瘡，則微腫濕爛，或冷或熱，乍瘥乍發，積月累年，謂之**緊唇**, "When the sores are struck by the qi of wind evil, cold and moisture, they will develop a slight swelling with moist festering which may be cold or hot; it may appear to heal and then develops again. This continues for months and even years, and is called '**tight lips**'".

***Jin chun chuang* 緊唇瘡, tight lips sores** [2]
PC identical with → *jin chun* 緊唇, tight lips. *TBC* SE *ni bai yin* 溺白垽：燒研末，主**緊唇瘡**, "Burned and ground to powder it controls **tight lip sores**".

***Jin duan* 筋斷, sinew rupture** [4]
PC identical with → *duan jin* 斷筋, ruptured sinew. *QJYF* 11: **筋斷**折痛不可忍, "**Sinew rupture** with unbearable pain".

***Jin feng* 噤風, lockjaw wind** [8]
PC identical with → *feng jin* 風噤, wind lockjaw. *BCGM* SE *qiao weng* 雀瓮 quoting *TPSHF* 82: 小兒撮口及發噤, "Children have cursed lips and develop lockjaw", writes: 撮口**噤風**, "Cursed lips and **lockjaw wind**".

***Jin gu feng* 筋骨風, sinews and joints wind** [5]
PC, brought forth by wind evil, of aching joints and sinews. *YXL* SE *suan zao* 酸棗：酸棗人，主**筋骨風**, "*Suan zao* kernels control **sinews and joints wind**".

***Jin han* 筋寒, sinew cold** [1]
PC of sinew cramps with pain brought forth by cold evil. *BQSYZJYLJ*, Yi bai er shi xue yü long ge 一百二十穴玉龍歌, The Jade Dragon's Song on the 120 holes: 臂細無力轉動難，**筋寒**骨痛夜無眠, "The arms are lean and have no strength; it is difficult to move them. The **sinews** are **cold**, the bones ache and one cannot sleep at night".

***Jin ji* 緊急, tightness and tension; violent** [2]
① IS of tightening and hardening, and of difficulties to bend and stretch in general. *HJJF* 5: 腰胯沉重，百節酸疼，項筋**緊急**, "The lower back feels heavy. All the joints ache. The sinews of the nape are **tight**".
② Refers to the violent nature of an illness or to a violent effect of a medication. *BCGM* SE *chanchu* 蟾蜍：每用一錠，井華水服。如瘡勢緊急，五七錠, "Each application 1 tablet. Ingest with well effulgence water (PUU: clear water drawn from a well in the early morning hours). In the case of **violent** sores take five to seven tablets".

***Jin ji* 筋急, sinew tension** [32]
IS of a difficulty to stretch the sinews, accompanied by uncomfortable contraction. *SW* 10: 多食辛，則**筋急**而爪枯, "If one consumes large quantities of acrid [food], the **sinews become tense** and the nails dry".

***Jin kou li* 禁口痢, clenched jaw with free-flux illness** [12] AW *jin kou li* 噤口痢.
PC of → *li ji* 痢疾, free-flux illness, accompanied by an inability to eat, with food that has just been eaten being thrown up again. *SYDXF* 6: 真料參苓白朮散，治**禁口痢**，食飲不下, "The powder with genuine ingredients [*ren*] *shen* and [*fu*] *ling* and *bai zhu* cures **clenched jaw with free-flux illness** with an inability to drink and eat".

***Jin kou li* 噤口痢, clenched jaw with free-flux illness** [6]
PC identical with → *jin kou li* 禁口痢. *DXXF* 2: **噤口痢**者，胃口熱甚故也, "**Clenched jaw with free-flux illness** is caused by extreme heat in the upper stomach opening".

***Jin luan* 筋攣, sinew contraction** [21]

IS of bending resulting from contracted sinews making it difficult to stretch the body. *BJ* SE *da dou huang* 大豆黃：主濕痹，**筋攣**，膝痛, "It controls moisture blockage, **sinew contraction**, and pain in the knees".

***Jin mai ju jue* 筋脈沮絕, sinews and vessels are worn out and severed** [1]

IS of a slackening and loss of strength with an inability to move following a destruction of sinews. *BCGM* Wu wei yi ji 五味宜忌 quoting *SW* 3: 筋脈沮馳, "Sinews and vessels are worn out", writes: **筋脈沮絕**, "**Sinews and vessels are worn out and severed**".

***Jin nu rou* 筋弩肉, sinew tumorous flesh-growth** [1]

PC identical with → *nu rou* 弩肉, tumorous flesh-growth. *HYBC* SE *ke* 珂：主消翳膜及**筋弩肉**，並刮點之, "It is in control of dissolving shade membranes and **sinew tumorous flesh-growths**. Do both smear and drop [liquid] on them".

***Jin ren fu shang* 金刃斧傷, injury inflicted by metal [objects, such as] blade and hatchet** [1]

PC of → 金瘡, sores inflicted by metal objects, resulting from the impact of a blade or hatchet. *BCGM* SE *li* 栗 quotes *BHJJF*: **金刃斧傷**：用獨殼大栗研傅, "For **injury inflicted by metal [objects, such as] blade and hatchet**, use the largest chestnut kernel, grind it and apply externally".

***Jin ren jian shang* 金刃箭傷, injury inflicted by metal [objects, such as] blade and arrow** [1]

PC identical with → *dao jian shang* 刀箭傷, harm inflicted by blade and arrow. *BCGM* SE *san qi* 三七：**金刃箭傷**、跌扑杖瘡，血出不止者，嚼爛塗，或為末摻之，其血即止, "For **injury inflicted by metal [objects, such as] blade and arrow**, as well as wounds from falls and being hit with a rod, with unending bleeding, chew to a pulp and apply externally, or prepare a powder to be inserted into the wound, and the bleeding will end immediately".

***Jin ren jian zu shang* 金刃箭鏃傷, injury inflicted by metal [objects, such as] blade and arrowhead** [1]

PC identical with → *dao jian shang* 刀箭傷, harm inflicted by blade and arrow. *BCGM* SE *hua ru shi* 花乳石 quoting *HJJF* 8: 花蕊石散，治一切**金刃箭鏃傷**中及打撲傷損, "The powder with *hua rui shi* cures all types of **injury inflicted by metal [objects, such as] blade and being struck by an arrowhead** as well as injuries from blows and falls".

***Jin ren shang* 金刃傷, injury inflicted by metal [objects, such as a] blade** [1]

PC identical with → *jin chuang* 金瘡, wounds inflicted by metal objects. *SJZL* 139: 治**金刃傷**破見骨，中風口噤，豆淋酒方, "Recipe for a wine made by straining beans to cure **injury inflicted by metal [objects, such as a] blade** where the [wound is] open and the bones are visible, as well as wind stroke with clenched jaw".

Jin ren shang chuang **金刃傷瘡, wounds inflicted by metal [objects, such as a] blade** [2]
PC identical with → *jin chuang* 金瘡, wounds inflicted by metal objects. *BCGM* SE *sang* 桑 qotes *ZYJYGLF*: **金刃傷瘡**：新桑白皮燒灰，和馬糞塗瘡上，數易之, "For **wounds inflicted by metal [objects such as a] blade**: Burn fresh *sang bai pi* to ashes, mix with horse dung for external application on the wound. Replace several times".

Jin ren shang sun **金刃傷損, injury inflicted by metal [objects, such as a] blade** [1]
PC identical with → *jin chuang* 金瘡, wounds inflicted by metal objects. *BCGM* SE *xiang lu hu*i 香爐灰：跌扑**金刃傷損**，罨之，止血生肌, "Used to foment **injuries obtained by** falls and **metal [objects, such as a] blade** it will end the bleeding and generate muscle-flesh".

Jin ren suo shang **金刃所傷, injury inflicted by metal [objects, such as a] blade** [3]
PC identical with → 金瘡, wounds inflicted by metal objects. *TPSHF* 68: 凡**金刃所傷**，不令著風即瘥矣，"For all **injury inflicted by metal [objects, such as a] blade** applies: if one does not allow them to be affected by wind they will heal".

Jin sai chuang **金腮瘡, metal cheek sores** [2]
PC of → *chuang* 瘡, sores, conditions that develop on one's cheeks. In the beginning they appear like rice grains. In extreme cases they fester and pierce through the cheeks. *SJZL* 132: 治大人小兒蝕透腮頰，初生如米豆，名**金腮瘡**, "To cure erosions piercing through the cheeks of adults and children. In the beginning they appear like rice grains. They are called '**metal cheek sores**'".

Jin shi du **金石毒, mineral substance poison** [5]
EA identical with → *dan shi du* 丹石毒, cinnabar [et al.] mineral substance poison. *BCTJ* SE *shi she* 石蛇：尤能解**金石毒**，以左盤者良, "In particular it is capable of dissolving **mineral substance poison**. Those coiled up to the left are good".

Jin shi fa dong **金石發動, outbreak of mineral [drug poisoning]** [1]
PC identical with → *dan shi du fa* 丹石毒發, outbreak of cinnabar [et al.] mineral poisoning. *BCTJ* SE *gan jiao gen* 甘蕉根：俚醫以治時疾, 狂熱及消渴, **金石發動**躁熱, 並可飲其汁, "Common physicians use this to cure seasonal ailments, madness heat and melting with thirst, **outbreaks of mineral [drug poisoning]** with restlessness and heat. For all these it is advisable to drink its juice".

Jin shi yao du **金石藥毒, mineral drug poison** [6]
EA identical with → *dan shi du* 丹石毒, cinnabar [et al.] mineral substance poison. *RHZ* SE *hei dou* 黑豆：制**金石藥毒**, "It controls **mineral drug poison**".

Jin shi yao fa **金石藥發, outbreak of mineral drug [poisoning]** [1]
PC identical with → *dan shi du fa* 丹石毒發, outbreak of cinnabar [et al.] mineral poisoning. *BCTJ* SE *mai men dong* 麥門冬：又主**金石藥發**, "It also controls **outbreaks of mineral drug [poisoning]**".

Jin shi yao fa dong **金石藥發動, outbreak of mineral drug [poisoning]** [1]

PC identical with → *dan shi du fa* 丹石毒發, outbreak of cinnabar [et al.] mineral poison. *RHZ* SE *pu sa shi* 菩薩石：解藥毒、蠱毒，及**金石藥發動**作癰疽渴疾, "It dissolves the poison of medication and *gu* poison, and the **outbreak of mineral drug [poisoning]** causing obstruction-illness, impediment-illness as well as thirst ailment/diabetes".

Jin tong **緊痛, tightening with pain** [1]

IS of pain accompanied by a feeling of pressure and strain. *TPSHF* 88: 治小兒痃氣，兩脅下**緊痛**，羸瘦，鱉甲丸方, "Recipe for pills with *bie jia*: to cure string-illness qi in children, with a **tightening with pain** below both flanks and emaciation".

Jin wei **筋痿, sinew dysfunction** [4]

PC a) of a dysfunction disease brought forth by an insufficiency of yin-blood and an internal flourishing of liver heat, resulting in a withering of sinews and vessels. *BJ* SE *hu zhang* 虎掌：主心痛，寒熱，結氣積聚，伏梁，傷**筋痿**拘緩, "It controls heart pain, cold and heat spells, bound qi and accumulations and collections, hidden beams, as well as ailments such as **sinew dysfunction** and cramps. b) Identical with → *yin wei* 陰痿②, dysfunction of the yin [member, i.e. penis]. *SW* 44: 思想無窮，所願不得，意淫於外，入房太甚，宗筋弛縱，發為**筋痿**, "When pondering is without limits, when one does not get what one had longed for, when [lewd] sentiments flow unrestrained to the outside and when one enters the [women's] chambers excessively, the basic sinew slackens. This develops into **sinew dysfunction**".

Jin xue **近血, nearby bleeding** [1]

PC of bleeding where the location of the bleeding is inside the rectum near the anus. The bleeding occurs first and defecation afterwards. The blood has a fresh red color. *WTMY* 6: 先見血後便轉，此為**近血**, "If one sees blood first and this changes to defecation afterwards, this is '**nearby bleeding**'".

Jin yi **筋溢, sinew copiousness** [2]

IS identical with → *jin ruan* 筋軟, sinew softness. *MYBL* SE *bai pu xi* 敗蒲席：主**筋溢**、惡瘡, "It controls **sinew copiousness** and malign sores".

Jin yin **噤喑, clenched jaw with muteness** [2]

IS of muteness resulting from a → *kou jin* 口噤, clenched jaw. *BCGM* SE *fu zi* 附子 quoting *QJYiF*: 口噤不開, "Clenched mouth that fails to open", writes: **噤喑, "Clenched jaw with muteness".**

Jin yin chuang **浸淫瘡, sores soaked [with pus and/or liquid]** [7] AN *jin yin e chuang* 浸淫惡瘡, malign sores soaked [with pus and/or liquid]; *jin yin du chuang* 浸淫毒瘡, poison sores soaked [with pus and/or liquid].

PC of → *chuang* 瘡, sores, conditions that itch at first and are painful later. They fester with liquid seeping from them. The liquid disperses into ever wider areas and, in serious cases, affects the entire body. *ZBYHL* 35: **浸淫瘡**…初生甚小，先癢後痛而成瘡，汁出，侵潰肌肉；浸淫漸闊，乃遍體, "**Sores soaked [with pus and/or liquid]** ... in the beginning they are very small. There is an itch first, then a swelling and eventually there are sores, with liquid seeping from them and intruding into muscles and flesh. The region affected by the soaking gradually widens until it covers the entire body".

***Jin yin du chuang* 浸淫毒瘡, poison sores soaked [with pus and/or liquid]** [3]
PC identical with → *jin yin chuang* 浸淫瘡, sores soaked [with pus and/or liquid]. *BCGM* SE *ji yu* 鯽魚quotes *TPSHF*: 或腫痛，或赤癢，上下周匝，煩毒欲死，此**浸淫毒瘡**也。生鯽魚切片，和鹽搗貼，頻易之, "When it is swollen and painful, or red and itches, covering everything from top to bottom, with fierce vexation bringing people close to death, these are **poison sores soaked [with pus and/or liquid]**. Cut raw *ji yu* to pieces and pound with table salt to a pulp [and apply externally]. Frequently change it".

***Jin yin e chuang* 浸淫惡瘡, malign sores soaked [with pus and/or liquid]** [4]
PC identical with → *jin yin chuang* 浸淫瘡, sores soaked [with pus and/or liquid]. *QJYF* 19: 胡麻生嚼塗小兒頭瘡及**浸淫惡瘡**，大效, "Fresh *hu ma* is to be chewed to be externally applied to head sores and **malign sores soaked [with pus and/or liquid]** in children".

***Jin yu* 金郁, pent-up metal [qi]** [3]
PC of lung qi accumulation forming nodes and failing to move. *SW* 71: **金郁**泄之, "In the case of **pent-up metal [qi]**, drain it".

***Jing* 痙, spasms** [p] AW 痓
① IS of a contraction of sinews/muscles and stiffness of neck and back, as well as convulsions of hands and feet. *LS* 23: 九曰, 熱而**痙**者死, "The ninth item: ‚those who have fever and **spasms**, they will die'".
② PC of → *jing bing* 痙病, spasms disease. *BJ* SE *mu dan* 牡丹：主寒熱，中風，瘛瘲，**痙**，驚癇邪氣, "It controls [alternating sensations of] cold and heat, wind stroke, clonic spasms, **spasms**, fright epilepsy – [such] evil qi".

***Jing* 痓, spasms** [p]
① IS identical with → *jing* 痙①. *SW* 45: 發喉痹，嗌腫，**痓**，治主病者, "It develops into a throat block, a swollen throat region, and a **spasms**. Treat the [conduit] controlling the disease".
② PC identical with → *jing* 痙②. *JGYL* Fj:太陽病，發熱，脈沉而細者，名曰**痓**, "If someone suffers from major yang disease, effuses heat, and displays a movement in the vessels that is in the depth and fine, then this is **spasms**". In ancient Chinese medical literature, the two characters 痓 and 痙 had identical meanings and were used interchangeably.

***Jing* 驚, fright** [p]
① The emotion of fright. *SW* 21:凡人之**驚**恐恚勞動靜，皆為變也, "Whenever a person is **frightened**, fearful, angry, or overworked, whether one is active or quiet, all this causes changes".
② EA AD of → *jing bu* 驚怖, horror. *SW* 47:此得之在母腹中時，其母有所大**驚**，氣上而不下，精氣並居，故令子發為顛疾也, "It is acquired in the mother's abdomen. When the mother is extremely **frightened**, the qi rises and

does not move down. It takes residence together with the essence qi. Hence, this makes the child develop a peak ailment".

③ IS a) AD of → *shan jing* 善驚, a tendency to be frightened. *SW* 30: 聞木音則惕然而**驚**, "When he hears the sound of wood, he is scared and **frightened**". b) Identical with → *jing chu* 驚搐, fright convulsion. *QJYF* 5: 因壯熱，便四肢攣掣，**驚**，乃成癇疾, "It is because of strong heat that the four limbs contract, [patients] experience **fright**, and this generates epilepsy ailment".

④ PC AD of *jing feng* 驚風, fright wind. *XEYZZJ* Lj: 剪刀股丸，治一切驚風，久經宣利，虛而生**驚**者, "Pills with *jian dao gu* cure all types of fright wind, when one has applied, over an extended period of time, dissipating and disinhibiting [medication] resulting in the depletion and generation of **fright**".

***Jing bi* 經閉, menstrual blockage** [22] AN *yue bi* 月閉; *xue bi* 血閉, [menstrual] blood blockage; *yue jing yu bi* 月經瘀閉; *yue shui bu tong* 月水不通.

PC of a failure of menstruation to begin in a young woman at the age of puberty, or a ceasing of menstruation for more than three months in a woman who is not pregnant. *QJYF* 4: 牡蠣丸，治**經閉**不通，不欲飲食方, "Pills with *mu li*: a recipe to cure **menstruation that is blocked** and fails to pass, with an unwillingness to drink and eat".

***Jing bing* 經病, menstrual disease** [1] AN *yue jia bing* 月家病 menstruant's disease.

PC CD of all types of diseases associated with menstruation. *NKBW* 6: 夫婦人病，多是月經乍多乍少，或前或後，時發疼痛，醫者一例呼為**經病**, "Now, women's diseases are often associated with either an excessive or a minimal monthly period, or with its early or belated arrival. Often this causes pain. Physicians summarize all [these conditions] with the term '**menstrual disease**'".

***Jing bing* 痙病, spasms disease** [3]

PC identical with → *feng jing* 風痙, wind spasms. *JGYL* Fj: 獨頭動搖，卒口噤，背反張者，**痙病**也, "If only the head sways, and suddenly there is clenched jaw with the back arched backwards, this is **spasms disease**".

***Jing bu* 驚怖, to be horrified** [8]

EA of a frightening experience strong enough to cause pathological changes in a person. *ZBYHL* 45: 驚癇者，因**驚怖**大啼乃發, "Fright epilepsy will break out when [a person] was **horrified** and cries out loudly".

***Jing bu si* 驚怖死, [appearance of] death from being horrified** [1]

PC identical with → *jing si* 驚死. *BCGM* Bai bing zhu zhi yao 百病主治藥：醇酒，**驚怖死**，俗名嚇死，灌之, "For **[appearance of] death from being horrified,** commonly called '[appearance of] death from intimidation', unmixed wine is to be forcibly instilled [into the patient]".

***Jing bu tiao* 經不調, menstrual irregularity** [1]

PC identical with → *yue shui bu tiao* 月水不調. *NKBW* 16: 補陰丸，治婦人百疾，或**經不調**，或崩中漏不止, "The pills to supplement yin, they cure all types of women's disease, **menstrual irregularity**, or collapsing center with incessant leaking".

Jing bu zhi 經不止, **incessant menstruation** [2]
PC identical with → *yue shui bu zhi* 月水不止. *BCGM* Bai bing zhu zhi yao 百病主治藥：蓮房，**經不止**，燒研，酒服, "Receptacles of *lian*: In the case of **incessant menstruation**, roast and grind them and ingest [the powder] with wine".

Jing chu 驚搐, **fright convulsion** [6] AN *jing zhi* 驚掣.
IS of mental instability associated with convulsions affecting the four limbs. *TPSHF* 85: 五臟多熱，夜間**驚搐**, "The five depots have much heat; at night [these patients] experience **fright convulsion**".

Jing chu 精出, **seminal emission** [8]
IS of an ejaculation of sperma unrelated to sexual intercourse. *YXL* 14: 主鬼交**精出**, "It controls **seminal emission** during intercourse with a demon".

Jing chuang 脛瘡, **lower leg sores** [2]
PC identical with → *lian chuang* 臁瘡, shank sores. *BCTJ* SE *ma chi xian* 馬齒莧:武在西川，自苦**脛瘡**焮癢不可堪，百醫無效, "Wu himself, when he was in Sichuan, suffered from a **lower leg sore**. It was inflamed and itched unbearably. No physician was able to cure this".

Jing cuan 驚竄, **[eyeballs] scurrying because of fright** [3]
IS of mental restlessness, with scurrying eyes and an inability to freely move. *BYTY* 1: 發熱飲湯，抽搐乏力，**驚竄**切牙，合面而睡者，屬心經虛熱, "When they effuse heat and are thirsty, have twitching and lack of strength, with the [**eyeballs] scurrying because of fright**, and when they press their teeth upon each other, and sleep with their face turned upwards, this is associated with a heart conduit depletion heat".

Jing dan 痙疸, **spasms with *dan*-illness** [2]
PC CD of → *jing* 痙, spasms, and → *dan* 疸, *dan*-illness. *BJ* SE *zhu* 术：主風寒濕痹，死肌, **痙疸**, "It controls blockage resulting from a presence of wind, cold, and moisture, as well as dead muscles, and **spasms with *dan*-illness**".

Jing feng 驚風, **fright wind** [69] AN *xiao er jing xian* 小兒驚癇, fright epilepsy among children.
PC of children characterised by jerking and arched back rigidity, eyeballs turned upward, and twitching hands and legs. *XEYZZJ* Lj RE *she xiang wan* 麝香丸, "pills with *she xiang*": 治小兒慢驚、疳等病…**驚風**，發搐眼上, "They cure diseases of children such as chronic fright and *gan*-illness. …**Fright wind** causing convulsions and eyes turning upward". *BCGM* distinguishes between → *ji jing feng* 急驚風, acute fright wind; → *man jing feng* 慢驚風; slow fright wind; → *wu sha jing feng* 烏紗驚風, black gauze fright wind; → *tian diao jing feng* 天吊驚風, heaven-hauled fright wind; → *tai feng* 胎風, fetal wind; → *tai jing* 胎驚, fetal fright.

Jing feng 痙風, **spasms wind** [8]
PC identical with → *feng jing* 風痙, wind spasms. *BCGM* Bai bing zhu zhi yao 百病主治藥：鴨涎，小兒**痙風**反張，滴之, "Duckling saliva: when children suffer from **spasms wind** and arched back, drip it".

***Jing hai* 驚駭, shock** [5]

IS of extreme fear. *SW* 3: "俞氣化薄，傳為善畏，及為**驚駭**, "The qi of the transporters is transformed and strikes [the depots]. Its transmission [in the organism] causes a tendency to be frightened and the [patient] is **shocked**".

***Jing han* 莖寒, penile cold** [2]

IS identical with *yin zhong han* 莖中寒, cold in the penis. *BCGM* Bai bing zhu zhi yao 百病主治藥 SE *tu si zi* 菟絲子：主**莖寒**，精自出，溺有餘瀝, "It controls **penile cold**, and spontaneous emission of essence. Following urination, a remnant will drip off spontaneously".

***Jing han* 精寒, seminal cold** [5]

IS identical with → *jing leng* 精冷. *QJYiF* 19: 人參丸，主百病三蟲，疝瘕成魚、鱉、蝦蟆，令人面目枯，無潤澤，**精寒**，勞瘦方, "The pills with *ren shen* are a recipe to control the one hundred diseases and the three types of bugs/worms, elevation-illness and conglomeration-illness forming [inside the body objects shaped like] fish, turtle and frog, and causing the human face and eyes to dry up and lack glossiness. [They also cure] **seminal cold**, exhaustion and emaciation".

***Jing hou bu tiao* 經候不調, menstrual irregularity** [6]

PC identical with → *yue shui bu tiao* 月水不調. *QJYF* 4: 小五石澤蘭丸，治婦人勞冷虛損，飲食減少，面無光色，腹中冷痛，**經候不調**, "The small pills with the five mineral substances and *ze lan* cure women suffering from exhaustion cold and depletion harm. They drink and eat little. Their facial complexion has lost its glossiness. They feel cold and pain in their abdomen, and they experience **menstrual irregularity**".

***Jing hou bu tong* 經候不通, menstrual blockage** [2]

PC identical with → *yue shui bu tong* 月水不通. *SJZL* 151:治婦人**經候不通**，已經三兩月者，鱉甲湯方, "To cure **menstrual blockage** that has already lasted for two or three months, [use] the recipe for the decoction with *bie jia*".

***Jing hua* 精滑, smooth flow of essence/semen** [11] AN *jing zi chu* 精自出, spontaneous seminal emission; *jing yi zi chu* 精溢自出, *jing liu* 精流, seminal flow; *shen hua* 腎滑, smooth [flow from the] kidneys

PC of emissions of seminal fluid, in males independently of erotic dreams, in severe cases with continuous leakage even while awake. *TPSHF* 14: 腎氣乏弱，**精滑**，夜夢泄，宜服薯蕷散方, "In the case of kidney qi feebleness; **smooth flow of essence/semen**, (i.e.) wet dreams, the recipe to ingest the powder with *shu yu* is advisable".

***Jing huo* 驚惑, fright delusion** [1]

IS of mental unrest and confused thinking. *YXQY* Mj: 惡寒戰慄，**驚惑**悲笑，譫妄, "Aversion to cold with shivering, **fright delusion** with [alternating episodes of] grief and laughing, delirium".

***Jing ji* 痙疾, spasms ailment** [4]

PC identical with → *jing bing* 痙病, spasms disease. *BCGM* SE *ling yang* 羼羊：治子癇痙疾, "It cures infant's epilepsy and **spasms ailment**".

Jing ji **驚悸, fright palpitation** [83]

① IS of a feeling of nervousness and fear, or restlessness with a pounding heart following an experience of fright, as well as without such external stimulus. *BJ* SE *ren shen* 人參：止**驚悸**，除邪氣，明目, "It stops **fright palpitation**, eliminates evil qi, and clears the eyes".

② PC with fright palpitation. *BJ* SE *bai shi* 柏實：主**驚悸**，安五藏，益氣，除風濕痹, "It controls **fright palpitation**, calms the five depots, increases qi, and eliminates wind moisture blockage".

Jing jiang **痙強, spasms with stiffness** [1]

IS of → *jing* 痙, spasms, with the special characteristic of muscle stiffness. *QJYF* 3: 四石湯，治產後卒中風，發疾口噤瘛瘲，悶滿不知人，並緩急諸風毒痹，身體**痙強**，及挾胎中風，婦人百病方, "The recipe with four minerals cures sudden wind stroke following delivery, with an immediate appearance of clenched jaw, clonic spasms, heart-pressure, a feeling of fullness and an inability to recognize people, as well as all types of more or less severe blockages brought forth by wind poison, and **spasms with stiffness** affecting the entire body, wind stroke affecting the fetus and the one hundred diseases of women".

Jing jing **驚痙, fright with spasms** [1]

PC CD of → *meng yan* 夢魘, nightmare, and → *jing* 痙, spasms. *BCGM* Bai bing zhu zhi yao 百病主治藥 quoting *MYBL*: 殺鬼精物，溫瘧蠱毒癇痙，去三蟲，除邪，令人無夢魘, "It kills demonic and spiritual beings, warmth malaria, *gu* poison, epileptic and other spasms, eliminates the three types of bugs/worms, removes evil, and makes a person have no nightmares", abbreviates this lengthy indication and simply writes: **驚痙**邪氣, "**Fright with spasms** and evil qi".

Jing kong **驚恐, terrified** [8]

EA identical with → *jing bu* 驚怖, horrified. *SW* 21: 有所**驚恐**，喘出於肺, "When [the patient] is **terrified** for some reason, the [resulting] panting originates from the lung".

Jing ku **驚哭, fright crying** [2]

IS identical with → *jing ti* 驚啼. *YXL* SE *zha chan* 蚱蟬：主治小兒**驚哭**不止, "It controls unending **fright crying** in children".

Jing kuang **驚狂, fright with madness** [7]

IS and PC CD of → *jing* 驚, fright, and → *kuang* 狂, madness. *TBC* SE *fang kui* 防葵：久服主邪氣**驚狂**之患, "Ingested over a long time it controls suffering from evil qi and **fright with madness**".

Jing leng **莖冷, penile cold** [3]

IS identical with *yin zhong han* 莖中寒, cold in the penis. *MYBL* SE *shi long rui* 石龍芮：補陰氣不足，失精**莖冷**, "It supplements insufficient yin qi, loss of essence/semen, and **penile cold**".

Jing leng **精冷, seminal cold** [5] AN → *jing han* 精寒.

IS of male semen being clear, watery and cold as ice. *QJYF* 12 RE *zi ge wan* 紫葛丸, pills with *zi ge* 紫葛：羸瘦無力，弱房少精，**精冷**, ...所錄諸病，皆紫葛

丸治之, "Emaciation and lack of strength, loss of potency and small quantities of ejaculate; **seminal cold**, … the pills with *zi ge* cure all the diseases listed above".

Jing li **驚痢, fright free-flux-illness** [1]
PC of → *li ji* 痢疾, free-flux illness, in children brought forth by fright. The feces is a mucous liquid of virid color. *RHZ* SE *jia ya* 家鴨：補虛，消熱毒，利小腸，止**驚痢**, "It supplements depletion, dissolves heat poison, stimulates the passage through the small intestine, and ends **fright free-flux-illness**".

Jing liu **精流, essence/semen flow** [3]
PC identical with → *jing hua* 精滑, smooth flow of essence/semen. *KBBC* SE *bu gu zhi* 補骨脂：主五勞七傷，風虛冷，骨髓傷敗，腎冷**精流**, "It controls the five types of exhaustion and seven types of harm, wind [intruding into a state of] depletion cold, injured bone marrow, and kidney cold with **essence/semen flow**".

Jing lou **精漏, essence/semen leakage** [1]
PC identical with → *yi jing* 遺精, involuntary loss of essence/semen. *PJF* 33: 四妙丹，治元氣久虛及小腸腎余，膀胱疝氣，五淋白濁，精滑**精漏**, "The elixir with the four miraculous [ingredients]. It cures long-term depletion of original qi and surplus in the small intestine and kidneys, elevation-illness qi in the bladder, as well as the five types of dripping with white turbidity, smooth flow of essence/semen, and **essence/semen leakage**".

Jing luo bu tong **經絡不通, impassability of conduits and network [vessels]** [2]
PC identical with → *yue shui bu tong* 月水不通, menstrual blockage. *HYBC* SE *su fang mu* 蘇方木：產後惡露，不安怯起，衝心腹中攪痛及**經絡不通**, "[It cures] post-partum lochia causing [the woman] to be restless and striking against the heart and abdomen where it causes an annoying pain, as well as **impassability of conduits and network [vessels]**".

Jing mai bu tiao **經脈不調, conduit vessels irregularity; menstrual irregularity** [2]
PC identical with → *yue shui bu tiao* 月水不調, menstrual irregularity. *NKBW* 49: 紫桂丸，補益血海，治衝任氣虛，**經脈不調**, "The 'purple pills with *gui*' serve to supplement the sea of blood to cure qi depletion in the throughway and controller [vessels], as well as **conduit vessels irregularity**".

Jing mai bu tong **經脈不通, impassability of conduit vessels** [9]
PC identical with → *yue shui bu tong* 月水不通, menstrual blockage. *YXL* SE *mu dan* 牡丹：治女子**經脈不通**，血瀝腰疼, "It cures **impassability of conduit vessels**, blood dripping, and lower back pain".

Jing mai bu yun **經脈不勻, irregular passage through the conduit vessels** [1]
PC identical with → *yue shui bu tiao* 月水不調, menstrual irregularity. *RHZ* SE *dan shen* 丹參：止血崩帶下，調婦人**經脈不勻**, "It ends blood collapse with discharge from below the belt, and regulates **irregular passage through the conduit vessels** of women".

Jing mai bu zhi **經脈不止, incessant passage through conduit vessels** [1]
PC identical with → *yue shui bu zhi* 月水不止，incessant menstruation. *RHZ* SE *ma lin* 馬藺:治婦人血氣煩悶，產後血運並**經脈不止**，崩中帶下, "Cures

in women vexation and heart-pressure resulting from [stagnant] blood and qi, blood[-induced brain] movements following delivery, and **incessant passage through conduit vessels**, as well as collapsing center with discharge from below the belt".

Jing mai ni xing **經脈逆行, counterflow in the conduit vessels** [3]
PC identical with → *yue jing ni xing* 月經逆行, menstrual counterflow. *BCGM* SE *jiu* 韭 quotes [Zhu] Zhenheng 震亨：主吐血唾血，衄血尿血，婦人**經脈逆行**, "It controls spitting of blood, saliva with blood, nosebleed, and urine with blood. In females **counterflow in the counduit vessels**".

Jing mei **精魅, spirit seduction-specter** [13] EA
PC identical with → *gui mei* 鬼魅, demonic seduction specters. *BJ* SE *dan sha* 丹砂：主身體五藏百病，養精神，安魂魄，益氣明目，殺**精魅**邪惡鬼, "It controls all types of diseases in the human body and its five depots, nourishes the spirit, pacifies *hun* and *po* souls, increases qi and clears the eyes, kills **spirit seduction-specters**, as well as evil and malign demons". *MYBL* SE *bai tian gong* 敗天公：主鬼疰**精魅**, "It controls demon attachment-illness and **spirit seduction-specters**".

Jing meng **驚夢, fright dream** [2] AN *jing yan* 驚魘, startled by nightmare demons. IS of waking up in fright because of an encounter with something frightening in a dream. *MYBL* SE *ling yang jiao* 羚羊角：除邪氣**驚夢**, "It eliminates evil qi and **fright dreams**".

Jing qi **驚氣, fright qi** [18]
① EA identical with → *jing xie* 驚邪, fright evil①. *MYBL* SE *wu zei yü gu* 烏賊魚骨:**驚氣**入腹，腹痛環臍, "**Fright qi** enters the abdomen. [This results in] abdominal pain around the umbilicus".
② PC identical with → *jing xie* 驚邪②. *BJ* SE *mi wu* 蘼蕪：主咳逆，定**驚氣**, "It controls cough with counterflow, and stabilizes **fright qi**".

Jing re **驚熱, fright heat** [28] AN → *re jing* 熱驚; heat fright; *huo jing* 火驚, fire fright.
PC of → *jing feng* 驚風, fright wind, in children brought forth by heat evil. *WTMY* 3 RE *yin chen wan* 茵陳丸, pills with *yin chen*: 時氣、傷寒、痎瘧、小兒**驚熱**欲發癇，服之無不瘥, "If ingested for treating seasonal qi, harm caused by cold, malaria, and **fright heat** among children with a tendency to develop epilepsy, [these pills] will be effective in all instances".

Jing shen cuo za **精神錯雜, jumbled essence spirit** [1]
IS of mental derangement. *BCGM* SE *ren dong* 忍冬quoting *ZBYHL* 23: 舉身沉重，精神雜錯，恆覺昏謬, "The body feels very heavy. The essence spirit is jumbled. One has a constant feeling of clouding and muddle-headedness", erroneously identifies this as a *ZHF* passage and writes: **精神錯雜, "Jumbled essence spirit"**.

Jing shui bu duan **經水不斷, incessant menstruation** [1]
PC identical with → *yue shui bu zhi* 月水不止. *PJF* 334: 治**經水不斷**，當歸、芍藥、熟地黄、川芎、厚朴、枳實各等分，上㕮咀，酒水同煎服, "To

cure **incessant menstruation**, [take] equal portions of *dang gui*, *shao yao*, *shou di huang*, *chuan xiong*, *hou pu*, and *zhi shi*. Chew these ingredients to pieces, boil them with wine and water, and ingest this".

Jing shui bu li **經水不利, impeded menstruation** [4] AN *yue shui bu li* 月水不利; *yue jing bu li* 月經不利; *nü jing bu li* 女經不利; *yue xin se zhi* 月信澀滯; *jing shui ning se* 經水凝澀.

PC of a → *jing bing* 經病, menstrual disease, with menstrual blood being discharged in small quantities only and lacking free flow. *JGYL* Lj: **經水不利**，少腹滿痛, "**Impeded menstruation**, with a feeling of fullness and pain in the lower abdomen".

Jing shui bu tiao **經水不調, menstrual irregularity** [7]

PC identical with → *yue shui bu tiao* 月水不調. *SJZL* 150: 治婦人風虛勞冷，四肢困倦，面色萎黃，**經水不調**，飲食減少, "To cure female wind [intruding into a state of] depletion exhaustion cold, fatigue of the four limbs, wilting-yellow complexion, **menstrual irregularity**, minimal ingestion of beverages and food".

Jing shui bu tong **經水不通, menstrual blockage** [2]

PC identical with → *yue shui bu tong* 月水不通. *SJZL* 151:治婦人**經水不通**，腰腹刺痛，拘倦少力, "To cure women with **menstrual blockage**, a piercing pain in the lumbar and abdominal region, as well as cramps with fatigue and a lack of strength".

Jing shui bu zhi **經水不止, incessant menstruation** [8]

PC identical with → *yue shui bu zhi* 月水不止. *YXZC* 7: 柴胡調經湯，治**經水不止**，其色鮮紅, "The 'decoction with *chai hu* to regulate menstruation' cures **incessant menstruation** with a fresh red color".

Jing shui guo duo **經水過多, excessive menstruation** [3] AN *yue jing tai guo* 月經太過; *yue shui guo duo* 月水過多; *yue xin lai duo* 月信來多.

PC of → *jing bing* 經病, menstrual disease, with the amount of menstrual blood discharged vastly exceeding normal levels. *ZBYHL* 40: 婦人**經水過多**，亡津液者，亦大便難也, "In the case of **excessive menstruation**, when women lose body liquid, they will also have difficulties defecating".

Jing shui ku **經水枯, desiccation of menstrual liquid** [1]

PC identical with → *xue ku* 血枯, blood desiccation. *BCGM* 40, SE *mai men dong* 麥門冬quotes [Zhang] Yuan su 元素：主血妄行及**經水枯**，乳汁不下, "It controls disorderly passage of blood and **desiccation of menstrual liquid**, as well as failure to produce breast milk".

Jing shui ning se **經水凝澀, impeded menstruation** [1]

PC identical with → *jing shui bu li* 經水不利. *BCGM* SE *zi jing* 紫荊：婦人血氣疼痛，**經水凝澀**, "Blood and qi pain in women, and **impeded menstruation**".

Jing shui shi lai shi duan **經水適來適斷, menstruation that is sometimes regular, sometimes interrupted** [1]

PC of → *yue shui bu tiao* 月水不調, menstrual irregularity, with menstruation that sometimes arrives in due time, and fails to arrive at others. *FRDQLF* 14: **經水適來適斷**，病後勞復，餘熱不解，宜服黃龍湯, "For **menstruation that is sometimes regular, sometimes interrupted**, and if it returns after a disease episode, when [the woman] is in a state of exhaustion, with remnant heat not dissolved, it is advisable to ingest the decoction with *huang long*".

Jing si **驚死, [appearance of] death from fright/shock** [4] *AN jing bu si* 驚怖死; *xia si* 嚇死, [appearance of] death from intimidation.

PC of → *cu si* 卒死, sudden [appearance of] death, resulting from an unforeseen and violent experience of fright/shock. *QXLF* 69 RE *zhu du tong zhi fang* 諸毒通治方, recipe to cure all types of poison: **驚死**、鬼迷死,未隔宿者,並冷水磨灌下, "For **[appearance of] death from fright/shock** and [appearance of] death from demonic enchantment that have not lasted overnight yet, grind together with cold water and forcibly instill into [the patient]".

Jing tan **驚痰, fright phlegm** [4]

EA of phlegm aggregation brought forth by fright. *YXRM* 5: 汗吐下溫俱從緩，免動**驚痰**與蛔蟲, "[Therapeutic approaches of] causing sweating, vomiting, purging, and warming are to be conducted with mild strength only, lest one should activate **fright phlegm** or roundworms".

Jing ti **驚啼, fright crying** [25] AN *jing ku* 驚哭.

IS of children suddenly waking up and crying as if frightened. *BJ* SE *ling li jia* 鯪鯉甲：主五邪**驚啼**, "It controls the five types of evil [qi] and **fright crying**".

Jing ti **驚惕, fearfulness** [1]

IS identical with → *jing ji* 驚悸①, fright palpitation. *MYBL* SE *long dan* 龍膽：益肝膽氣，止**驚惕**, "It adds to one's liver and gallbladder qi, and stops **fearfulness**".

Jing tong **痙痛, spasms with pain** [1]

PC CD of → *tong zheng* 痛證, pain condition, and → *jing bing* 痙病, spasms disease. *BJ* SE *di yu* 地榆：主婦人乳**痙痛**，七傷，帶下病, "It controls **spasms with pain** in a woman's breast, the seven types of harm, and diseases below the belt".

Jing tou han **莖頭寒, glans penis cold** [2]

IS identical with *yin zhong han* 莖中寒, cold in one's penis. *MYBL* SE *yang qi shi* 陽起石：療男子**莖頭寒**，陰下濕癢, "It cures male **glans penis cold**; wetness and itching down in the private parts".

Jing tu **驚吐, fright vomiting** [2]

PC of vomiting brought forth by having been frightened. *SJZL* 47: 治久患翻胃及小兒**驚吐**諸吐, "To cure all types of vomiting, including [vomiting because of] an upset stomach lasting for a long time, and children's **vomiting because of fright**".

Jing tuo **精脫, involuntary tossing of seminal fluid** [2]
PC identical with → *tuo jing* 脫精. *WSBJ* 15: 治陽虛陰盛，**精脫**，淫樂脛痠, "[To cure] yang depletion and yin flourishing, **involuntary tossing of seminal fluid**, and painful shins following excessive [sexual] joy".

Jing wei **莖痿, penile dysfunction** [2] AN *jing wei* 莖萎, penile wilting.
PC identical with → *yin wei* 陰痿, dysfunction of the yin [member, i.e. penis]. *QJYF* 26: 馬心，主喜忘。肺，主寒熱**莖痿**, "A horse's heart controls forgetfulness; its lung controls alternating sensations of cold and heat and **penile dysfunction**".

Jing wei **莖萎, penile wilting** [2]
PC identical with → *yin wei* 陰痿, dysfunction of the yin [member, i.e. penis]. *BCGM* SE *bai bi* 敗筆 quoting *YXL*: 治男子交婚之夕莖痿 writes: 治男子交婚之夕**莖萎**, "It cures males with **penile wilting** on the wedding night".

Jing wu **精物, spirit being** [11]
EA identical with → *gui xie* 鬼邪, demon evil. *BJ* SE *xiong huang* 雄黃：殺**精物**惡鬼，邪氣，百蟲毒, "It kills **spirit beings**, malign demons, evil qi, and the poison of all types of bugs/worms".

Jing wu **驚忤, frightened by [a demon's] hostility** [12]
PC of sudden loss of speech, or a condition of being frightened or experiencing fright epilepsy, believed to be caused by a hostile demon. *BCJJZ* SE *sheng ma* 升麻：取葉挼作小兒浴湯，主**驚忤**, "One takes the leaves and rubs them to prepare a hot bath for children. It controls their being **frightened by [a demon's] hostility**".

Jing xian **驚癇, fright epilepsy** [247]
PC a) CD of → *jing* 驚, fright, and → *xian* 癇, epilepsy. *BJ* SE *long chi* 龍齒：主小兒、大人**驚癇**, "It controls **fright epilepsy** in children and adults". *MYBL* SE *long chi* 龍齒:小兒五**驚**、十二**癇**, "The five types of **fright** and twelve types of **epilepsy** in children". b) Identical with → *xian* 癇, epilepsy, resulting from a frightening experience. *ZBYHL* 45: **驚癇**者，因驚怖大啼乃發, "**Fright epilepsy** develops someone was horrified and cries out loudly".

Jing xie **驚邪, fright evil** [25] AN *jing qi* 驚氣, fright qi.
① EA identical with → *jing bu* 驚怖, horrified. *BJ* SE *fu ling* 茯苓：主胸脅逆氣，憂恚、**驚邪**、恐悸，心下結痛, "It controls counterflow qi in chest and flanks, sorrow and rage, **fright evil**, fear, and nodes with pain below the heart".
② PC caused by being frightened. *BJ* SE *fang kui* 防葵：咳逆，温瘧，癲癇，**驚邪**狂走, "Cough with counterflow, warmth malaria, peak-illness with epilepsy, **fright evil** and mad walking".

Jing xie **精泄, involuntary outflow of seminal fluid** [3]
PC identical with → *yi jing* 遺精. *BCGM* SE *ba ji tian* 巴戟天 quoting *YXL*: 鬼交泄精，writes: 鬼交**精泄**, "**Involuntary outflow of seminal fluid** during intercourse with a demon".

Jing xu **精虛, essence depletion** [3]

PC of depletion with insufficiency of that matter which constitutes the human body and maintains life and reproductive functions. *WTMY* 38: 氣能致精，氣散則**精虛**, "The qi is able to collect essence. When the qi disperses then this results in **essence depletion**".

Jing xue bu tong **經血不通, menstrual blockage** [1]

PC identical with → *yue shui bu tong* 月水不通. *HJJF* 9: 婦人、室女**經血不通**，煎紅花酒下, "Women and virgins with **menstrual blockage** should ingest it boiled in *hong hua* wine".

Jing xue bu zhi **經血不止, incessant menstruation** [6]

PC identical with → *yue shui bu zhi* 月水不止. *SJZL* 152: 治婦人**經血不止**，心多驚恐，紫石英湯方, "To cure women with **incessant menstruation**, with the heart being very terrified, [use] the recipe for the decoction with *zi shi ying*".

Jing xue ni xing **經血逆行, menstrual counterflow** [1]

PC identical with → *yue jing ni xing* 月經逆行. *DXXF* 5: **經血逆行**，或血腥，或吐血，或唾血，用韭菜汁服效, "For **menstrual counterflow**, which may be associated with reeking of blood, spitting of blood, or saliva with blood, use the juice of chives. Its ingestion is effective".

Jing yan **驚魘, startled by nightmare demons** [1]

PC of sudden awaking from a nightmare with palpitation and panic. *QJYF* 14: 大定心湯，治心氣虛悸，恍惚多忘，或夢**驚魘**，志少不足方, "The 'decoction to massively calm down an [excited] heart' is a recipe to cure heart qi depletion [resulting in] palpitation, absent-mindedness with frequent forgetfulness, or being **startled**, in one's dreams, **by nightmare demons**, with mental deficits".

Jing yi zi chu **精溢自出, spontaneous seminal emission** [3]

IS of → *jing hua* 精滑, smooth flow of essence/semen, in males independently of erotic dreams, in severe cases with a continuous leaking even while they are awake". *YXL* SE *tu si zi* 菟絲子： " 夜夢鬼交，**精溢自出**, "At night they dream of intercourse with demons and experience **spontaneous seminal emission**".

Jing yin **驚喑, fright wordlessness** [2]

IS of children who can no longer speak following a frightful experience. *BCGM* SE *wu yi* 蕪荑 quotes *QYXJ*: 嬰孩**驚喑**：風后失音不能言, "**Fright wordlessness** in children: Loss of voice and inability to speak after a wind [stroke]".

Jing zhi **痙直, spasms with straightness** [2]

IS of → *jing* 痙, spasms, with the special characteristic of severe muscle stiffness causing the entire body to be straight and unable to bend. *ZBYHL* 1: 卒然身體**痙直**者，死也, "Those whose entire body is suddenly affected by **spasms with straightness**, they will die".

Jing zhi **驚掣, fright convulsion** [2]

IS identical with → *jing chu* 驚搐. *QJYF* 5:龍膽湯，治嬰兒出腹，血脈盛實，寒熱溫壯，四肢**驚掣**, "Decoction with *long dan* cures children with an abdominal protrusion, full and repleted blood vessels, with alternating sensations of cold and heat, a temperature of strong warmth, and **fright convulsion** affecting the four limbs".

Jing zhong han **莖中寒, cold in the penis** [4] AN → *jing leng* 莖冷; penile cold; → *jing han* 莖寒; → *jing tou han* 莖頭寒; the glans penis is cold.

IS of cold in the penis. *MYBL* SE *tu si zi* 菟絲子：主**莖中寒**，精自出, "It controls **cold in the penis** and spontaneous emission of essence".

Jing zi chu **精自出, spontaneous emission of essence** [6]

PC identical with → *jing hua* 精滑, smooth flow of essence/semen. *MYBL* SE *tu si zi* 菟絲子：主莖中寒，**精自出**, "It controls cold in the penis with **spontaneous emission of essence**".

Jiu ban **灸瘢, cauterization scar** [1]

PC of a → *ban* 瘢, scar, resulting from moxibustion applied directly to the skin. *QJYF* 5: 見其故**灸瘢**，便知其先疾之也, "When one sees these old **cauterization scars**, it is immediately apparent which earlier ailments this [patient had suffered from]".

Jiu bao zha bi **酒皰皻鼻, wine-blister sediment nose** [1]

PC identical with → *jiu zha* 酒皻, wine sediments. *BCGM* SE *zhi zi* 卮子 quotes *BJ*: 五內邪氣，胃中熱氣，面赤**酒皰皻鼻**，白癩赤癩瘡瘍, "[To cure] the five internal evil qi, heat qi in the stomach, a red face with **wine-blister sediment nose**, white repudiation-illness, red-repudiation illness, sores and ulcers".

Jiu bi zha **酒鼻皻, wine nose sediments** [1]

PC identical with → *jiu zha* 酒皻, wine sediments. *BCGM* SE *shan zhu yu* 山茱萸：暖腰膝，助水臟，除一切風，逐一切氣，破癥結，治**酒鼻皻**, "It warms the lower back and knees, assists water depots, removes all types of wind, expels all types of qi, breaks through conglomeration-illness nodes, and cures **wine nose sediments**".

Jiu bie **酒鱉, wine turtle** [5]

PC of → *bie jia* 鱉瘕, turtle[-shaped] conglomeration-illness, caused by excessive consumption of wine. *RZZZF* 1: 猶有所謂血鱉、氣鱉、**酒鱉**者，又不可不知也, "Furthermore there are the so-called 'blood turtle', 'qi turtle', and '**wine turtle**'. One must know them".

Jiu bing **酒病, wine disease** [11]

PC CD of all types of conditions resulting from excessive consumption of wine. *QJYF* 25: 治**酒病**方：葱白、豉各二升, "Recipe to cure **wine disease**: *cong bai* and *chi*, two *sheng* of each".

Jiu bing **久病, chronic disease** [30]

PC that has lasted for an extended period of time. The opposite of → *xin bing* 新病, new disease. *SW* 17: 征其脈與五色俱奪者，此**久病**也, "If it is verified that both the [movement in the] vessels and the five complexions are lost, it is a **chronic disease**".

***Jiu chuang* 久瘡, chronic sores** [2]

PC CD of → *chuang* 瘡, sores, conditions lasting for long without being cured. *ZBYHL* 35: 諸**久瘡**者，內熱外虛，為風濕所乘，則頭面身體生瘡。其臟內熱實氣盛，熱結肌肉，其熱留滯不歇，故瘡經久不瘥, "For all types of **chronic sores** the following applies. There is inner heat associated with external depletion. Wind and moisture avail themselves [of this depletion] and as a result head, the face and entire body develop sores. Heat abounds in the depots as repletion qi. The heat combines with the muscles and the flesh. The heat abides and does not abate. Hence the sores do not heal for a long time".

***Jiu chuang* 灸瘡, cauterization sores** [34]

PC of → *chuang* 瘡, sores, conditions resulting from burning inflicted by means of moxa cauterization. *ZBYHL* 35: **灸瘡**，膿潰以後，更焮腫急痛, "**Cauterization sores**: once the festering has ended they turn into inflamed swelling with acute pain".

***Jiu ci* 酒刺, wine thorns** [1]

PC identical with → *fen ci* 粉刺, flour thorns. *PJF* 51 *wu shen yuan* 五參圓：治去**酒刺**面瘡, "It cures and removes facial sores of **wine thorns**".

***Jiu dan* 酒疸, *dan*-illness [caused by] wine** [31] AN *jiu huang* 酒黃, jaundice [caused by] wine.

PC of → *huang dan* 黃疸, yellow *dan*-illness, resulting from an excessive consumption of wine/alcoholic beverages. *JGYL* Mj: 心中懊憹而熱，不能食，時欲吐，名曰**酒疸**, "[Patients] experience annoyance in their heart and are hot. They cannot eat, and at times wish to vomit. This is called '***dan*-illness [caused by] wine**'".

***Jiu dian* 久癲, chronic peak-illness** [2]

PC of → *dian ji* 癲疾, peak-illness, that cannot be cured over an extended period of time. *BCGM* SE *ren bao* 人胞 quotes *LSJYF*: **久癲**失志：氣血弱者。紫河車治淨，爛煮食之, "If [a patient] suffers from **chronic peak-illness** and has lost his mind, and if qi and blood are weak, cleanse a human placenta carefully, boil into a pulp, and eat it".

***Jiu du* 酒毒, wine poison; wine poisoning** [96]

① EA The harmful effects of wine/alcolholic beverages on the human body. *ZBYHL* 26: 飲酒過多，**酒毒**漬於腸胃, "If one consumes excessive amounts of wine, the **wine poison** will soak the intestines and stomach".

② PC brought forth by the poison in wine after excessive wine consumption. *TPSHF* 40: 治**酒毒**，木蘭皮膏方, "Recipe for a paste with *mu lan* bark to cure **wine poisoning**".

***Jiu feng* 酒風, wine wind** [3]

PC of a hot and sluggish body with heavy perspiration, an aversion to wind and short breath, brought forth by excessive consumption of alcoholic beverages. *SW* 46: 有病身熱解惰，汗出如浴，惡風少氣，此為何病？岐伯曰：病名曰**酒風**, "Someone suffers from [the following]: his body is hot and sluggish. Sweat leaves [his body] as if he had taken a bath. He has an aversion to wind and is short of qi. Which disease is that? Qi Bo: The disease is called **wine wind**".

Jiu feng **久風, long-lasting wind** [6]
PC identical with → *wan feng* 頑風, stubborn wind. *QJYF* 8: 蠻夷酒治**久風**枯攣, "Wine of the Man and Yi [southern tribes] cures **long-lasting wind** and desiccation with contractions".

Jiu gan **久疳, chronic *gan*-illness** [2]
PC of a chronic and incurable → *gan* 疳, *gan*-illness. *XEWSZWLF* Fj: 二香青蟾丸，治**久疳**積熱, "The 'pills with the two fragrances and virid toad' cure **chronic *gan*-illness** with heat accumulation".

Jiu han **久寒, chronic cold** [7]
① EA identical with → *jiu leng* 久冷. *ZBYHL* 3: 瘕病者，皆由**久寒**積冷，飲食不消所致也, "All cases of conglomeration-illness disease are brought forth by **chronic cold** leading to accumulated cold which leaves beverages and food undigested".
② PC identical with → *jiu leng* 久冷. *BC* SE *bai shi ying* 白石英：主胸膈間**久寒**, "It controls **chronic cold** in the region between the chest and diaphragm".

Jiu huang **酒黃, wine jaundice** [9]
PC identical with → *huang dan* 酒疸, *dan*-illness [caused by] wine. *YXL* SE *bai xian pi* 白鮮皮：主解熱黃、**酒黃**、急黃、穀黃、勞黃等, "It controls dissolution of heat jaundice, wine **jaundice**, acute jaundice, grain jaundice, and exhaustion jaundice".

Jiu ji **久積, accumulation over a long period; lasting accumulation** [17]
① EA PM of an accumulation persisting in the body for an extended period of time which then may bring forth further disease that is difficult to cure. *ZBYHL* 20: 冷氣**久積**不散，所以謂之久寒積冷也, "When cold qi **accumulates over a long period** and fails to dissipate, it is called cold accumulating for long".
② PC of → *ji* 積, accumulation, lasting for an extended period of time. *BCYY* SE *qian dan* 鉛丹：治瘧及**久積**皆用, "They served to cure all cases of malaria and **lasting accumulation**".

Jiu ji **酒積, wine accumulation** [22]
PC of → *shi ji* 食積, food accumulation, resulting from an excessive consumption of wine, often accompanied by a yellow facial complexion with depletion swelling, a distended, swollen abdomen, as well as vomiting and diarrhea. *HJJF* 3: **酒積**面黃，四肢虛腫，行步不能, "**Wine accumulation** with a yellow face, depletion swelling of the four limbs, and an inability to walk".

Jiu ke **久咳, chronic cough** [32]
PC identical with → *jiu sou* 久嗽. *SW* 38: 五臟之**久咳**，乃移於六腑, "If the **coughing** of [any of] the five depots **extends over a long time**, it is transmitted to [one of] the six palaces".

Jiu leng **久冷, chronic cold** [24] AN *jiu han* 久寒.
① EA of cold evil staying in the body for a long time. *QJYF* 16: 胃反朝食暮吐，食訖腹中刺痛，此由**久冷**, "If a person suffers from stomach turnover in

that what he eats in the morning will be vomited in the evening, and has a piercing pain when the food reaches the stomach, this is because of **chronic cold**".
② PC of a → *han bing* 寒病, cold disease, which fails to heal over an extended period of time. *QJYF* 15: 治久冷，或痢不痢, "Cures **chronic cold**, with and without free-flux illness".

Jiu li **久痢, prolonged free-flux illness** [120]
PC of → *li ji* 痢疾, free-flux illness, that lasts for an extended period of time without being healed. *ZBYHL* 17: 虛損不復，遂連滯涉引歲月，則為**久痢**也, "If one fails to recover from a depletion injury, which then continues for months and years, this becomes **prolonged free-flux illness**".

Jiu li **酒痢, wine free-flux illness** [12]
PC of → *li ji* 痢疾, free-flux illness, brought forth by excessive consumption of wine with an accumulation of heat poison. It is often accompanied by high fever and a discharge of blood. *HJJF* 6: 腸風黑散，治榮衛氣虛，…大便鮮血，臍腹疼痛，裏急後重，或肛門脫出，或久患**酒痢**, "Black powder for intestinal wind cures camp and guardian qi depletion, … Stools with fresh blood. Pain in the region of the navel and abdomen. An inner feeling of urgency and a feeling of heavy pressure at the behind. In some cases with prolapse of the rectum, in some cases with a prolonged suffering of **wine free-flux illness**".

Jiu lou **九瘺, nine types of fistula** [1]
PC identical with → *jiu lou* 九漏, nine types of leakage. *QJYF* 26: 去癩疾，諸**九瘺**，心腹痛, "To remove repudiation ailments, all **nine types of fistula**, and pain in the heart and abdomen".

Jiu lou **久漏, long-term leakage** [3]
PC of → *lou chuang* 漏瘡, leaking sores, that fail to heal over an extended period of time. *PJF* 293: **久漏**方，上用九孔蜂房炙黃為末，以臘月豬脂研敷，候收汁，以真龍骨、降真香節細末，入少許乳香，內瘡孔中, "Recipe for **long-term leakage**: [For the indications listed] above, roast a wild honeycomb with nine holes until yellow and powderize. Then grind with lard from the 12th month and apply externally. Wait until [the sores] have absorbed the liquid. Then prepare a fine powder of genuine *long gu* and *jiang zhen xiang*, and add a small amount of *ru xiang*. This is to be put into the holes of the sores".

Jiu lou **九漏, nine types of leakage** [6]
PC CD of numerous different types of → *lou chuang* 漏瘡, leaking sores, developing from → *luo li* 瘰癧, scrofula with pervasion-illness, breaking open to fester. *QJYF* 22: 夫**九漏**之為病，皆寒熱瘰癧在於頸腋者, "Now, the diseases of **nine types of leakage**, they all are connected with alternating sensations of cold and heat and scrofula with pervasion-illness at the neck and in the armpits". LSZ: **九漏**，雖有九名，皆取象耳，但分部位可也, "The **nine types of leakage**, although they have nine different designations, are all alike. It is only according to their location that they may be distinguished".

Jiu nüe **久瘧, lasting malaria** [46]

PC of → *nüe ji* 瘧疾, malaria ailment, that is not cured within three years. *MYBL* SE *zhi mu* 知母：療傷寒，**久瘧**，煩熱, "It cures harm caused by cold, **lasting malaria**, and vexing heat".

Jiu pao **酒皰, wine blister** [1]

PC identical with → *jiu zha* 酒皻, wine sediments. *BJ* SE *zhi* 梔子：面赤**酒皰**皻鼻，白癩赤癩, "A red face with **wine blisters** and a sediments nose, white repudiation-illness, and red repudiation-illness".

Jiu pi **酒癖, wine aggregation-illness** [5]

PC of → *pi* 癖, aggregation-illness, of wine and other beverages that collect below the flanks and fail to dissipate if, after excessive consumption of wine, one continues to ingest much liquid. Its major sign is an acute pain below the flanks. *ZBYHL* 20: **酒癖**者，因大飲酒後，渴而引飲無度，酒與飲俱不散，停滯在於脅肋下，結聚成癖，時時而痛, "As for **wine aggregation-illness**, if after one has drunk much wine he further drinks excessively, the wine and the other beverages fail to dissipate and remain in the region below the flanks. There they form an aggregation-illness of nodular collections which often cause pain".

Jiu re **久熱, lasting heat** [3]

PC associated with heat-type illnesses that continue for an extended period of time without being cured. *MYBL* SE *mang xiao* 芒消：主五藏積聚，**久熱**、胃閉, "It controls accumulations and collections in the five depots, **lasting heat**, and stomach closure".

Jiu re **酒熱, wine heat** [1]

EA of heat type diseases resulting from the impact of alcohol on the human body. *ZBYHL* 26: 往往有腹背穿穴者，是**酒熱**毒氣所為, "If a person frequently experiences holes piercing through [the skin] on the abdomen and on the back, this is caused by the poison qi of **wine heat**".

Jiu re li **久熱痢, chronic heat free-flux illness** [1]

PC of → *re li* 熱痢, heat free-flux illness, which remains uncured for an extended period of time. *ZBYHL* 17: **久熱痢**候：此由腸虛熱積，其痢連滯，故久不瘥也, "Signs of **chronic heat free-flux illness**: This results from intestinal depletion with heat accumulation. This free-flux illness drags on slowly. Hence it remains uncured for a long time".

Jiu sou **久嗽, chronic cough** [46] AN *jiu ke* 久咳, *lao sou* 老嗽.

PC of → *ke sou* 咳嗽②, cough, which is chronic and cannot be cured. *ZBYHL* 14: 諸**久嗽**不已，三焦受之, "In all cases of **chronic cough** that does not end, [the disease] has been received by the triple burner".

Jiu tuo **臼脫, dislocation** [1]

PC identical with *tuo jiu* 脫臼. *BCGM* SE *di huang* 地黃 quoting *LSh*: 許元公過橋墮馬，右臂**臼脫**, "Xu Yuangong fell from his horse when he crossed a bridge and suffered a **dislocation** of his right arm".

***Jiu xie* 久泄, prolonged outflow** [30] AW *jiu xie* 久瀉.

PC of a → *xie xie* 泄瀉②, outflow, lasting for an extended period of time. *MYBL* SE *sang er* 桑耳：其黄熟陳白者，止**久泄**, "Those that are yellow and ripe, and then have been left for some time until they turn white, they end **prolonged outflow**".

***Jiu xie* 久瀉, prolonged outflow** [7]

PC identical with → *jiu xie* 久泄. *TPSHF* 59: 治老人**久瀉**不止，訶黎勒散方, "To cure old people suffering from a **prolonged outflow** that will not end, use the recipe for the powder with *he li lei*".

***Jiu xu* 久虛, chronic depletion** [3]

PC of depletion lasting for a long time without cure. *QJYF* 4: 鍾乳澤蘭丸，治婦人**久虛**羸瘦、弱甚, "The pills with *zhong ru* and *ze lan* cure females with **chronic depletion** and emaciation, and who are extremely weak".

***Jiu zha* 酒皶, wine sediments** [11]

PC identical with → *jiu zha* 酒齇. *BCGM* Bai bing zhu zhi yao 百病主治藥, Mian 面：白斂同杏仁研塗，去粉滓**酒皶**, "Grind *bai lian* and *xing ren* and apply externally. This will remove dregs and **wine sediments**".

***Jiu zha* 酒齇, wine sediments** [32] AD *zha* 齇; AN *bi zha* 鼻齇, nose sediments; *chi zha* 赤齇, red sediments; *zha chi* 齇赤, sediments redness; *zha pao* 齇皰, sediments blisters; *chi bi* 赤鼻, red nose; *zha liu* 齇瘤, sediments tumor; *jiu zha bi* 酒齇鼻, wine sediments nose; *jiu zha feng* 酒齇風, wine sediments wind; *jiu pao* 酒皰, wine blisters; *zha pao* 皻皰, sediments blisters; *pi pao* 皶皰, sediments blisters.

PC with major signs of a swollen, red nose with papules that may, when squeezed, release white sediments. The condition flares up again and again until evetually the nose has increased in size and has assumed a red color. *ZBZZZS* 8, Qi qiao men, xia 七竅門下：鼻赤，一名**酒齇**鼻，乃血熱入肺也，肺氣通於鼻，鼻為清氣出入之道路，多飲酒人，邪熱熏蒸肺葉，伏留不散，故見於鼻，或肺素有風熱，雖不飲酒，其鼻亦赤，謂之**酒齇**，蓋俗名也, "Nasal redness is also called '**wine sediments**' nose. This is an influx of blood into the lung. The lung qi corresponds with the nose. The nose is the clear qi's path of exit and entry. Persons who drink much wine have evil heat steaming their lung lobes. It remains dormant there and fails to dissipate. Hence this manifests itself at the nose. In other cases, the lung persistently has wind heat. Even though one does not drink wine, the nose is red nevertheless. When this is called '**wine sediments**' this is so because it is a commonly used designation". *BCGM* SE *mu lan* 木蘭 quoting *BJ*: 面熱赤皰酒皶writes: 面熱赤皰**酒齇**, "The face is hot, with red blisters and **wine sediments**". In ancient medical literature, the character 齇 appears in various forms. E.g., *ZBYHL* has 酒皶；*QJYF* has 酒皻；*BCSY* and *RHZ* have 酒齇; *TPSHF* has 酒皻. *BCGM* mostly writes 酒齇, or its abbreviation 齇. *BCGM* has many related pathological terms, including *jiu zha chi bi* 酒齇赤鼻, wine sediments red nose; *jiu zha bi* 酒齇鼻, wine sediments nose; *jiu biz ha* 酒鼻齇, wine nose sediments; *bi shang zha bao* 鼻上齇皰, sediment blisters on the nose; *bi wai zha liu* 鼻外齇瘤, sediment tumor outside the nose; *jiu bao zha bi* 酒皰齇鼻, wine blister sediment nose; *bi zha* 鼻齇, nose sediments; *zha* 齇,

sediments; *zha bao* 齇皰, nasal sediment blister; *jiu zha feng* 酒齇風, nose sediments wind; *jiu zha* 酒齇, wine sediments; *chi zha* 赤齇, red sediments; *bi zha* 鼻齇, nose sediments; *jiu zha* 酒皶, wine sediments; *jiu zha chi bi* 酒皶赤鼻, wine sediments red nose; *chi zha* 赤皶, red sediments; *bi zha* 鼻皶, nose sediments; *chi bi* 赤鼻, rednose.

Jiu zha bi **酒齇鼻, nose with wine sediments** [1]
PC identical with → *jiu zha* 酒齇, wine sediments. *BCGM* SE *yu* •榆：煎汁，洗**酒齇鼻**, "Boil [the leaves] to obtain a liquid and use it to wash a **nose with wine sediments**".

Jiu zha chi bi **酒齇赤鼻, red nose with wine sediments** [2]
PC identical with → *jiu zha* 酒齇, wine sediments. *BCGM* SE *shi yan* 食鹽 quotes *RZZZF*: **酒齇赤鼻**：白鹽常擦之，妙, "**Red nose with wine sediments**: continuously rub it with white salt. Miraculous".

Jiu zha chi bi **酒皶赤鼻, red nose with wine sediments** [3]
PC identical with → *jiu zha* 酒齇, wine sediments. *BCGM* Bai bing zhu zhi yao 百病主治藥：龍腦香酥和，塗**酒皶赤鼻**, "A mixture of *long nao xiang* with butter is to be smeared on a **red nose with wine sediments**".

Jiu zha feng **酒齇風, nose sediments wind** [1]
PC identical with → *jiu zha* 酒齇, wine sediments. *BCGM* SE *ju* 橘 quotes *BCYY*: 治**酒齇風**鼻赤。炒研，每服一錢，胡桃肉一個，擂酒服，以知為度, "To cure **nose sediments wind** and nasal redness, burn and grind it. Each time ingest 1 *qian*".

Jiu zha feng **酒齇風, wine sediments wind** [1]
PC identical with → *jiu zha* 酒齇, wine sediments. *BCGM* SE *ju* 橘 quoting *BCYY* SE *hu tao* 胡桃：酒楂風 writes: **酒齇風**, "**Wine sediments wind**".

Jiu zhi **酒痔, wine piles** [5]
PC of → *zhi chuang* 痔瘡, piles sores, growing as a painful swelling to the side of the anus and opening following the consumption of wine, with the blood released being of a light red color. *ZBYHL* 34: **酒痔**，肛邊生瘡，亦有血出, "**Wine piles** are sores growing to the side of the anus. They bleed too".

Jiu zhi **久痔, chronic piles** [3]
PC of → *zhi chuang* 痔瘡, piles sores, which fail to heal over an extended period of time. *TPSHF* 60: 夫**久痔**者，由臟腑久積風虛熱毒，流注於大腸，乃成斯疾也, "Now, as for **chronic piles**, this ailment forms when heat poison from the depots and palaces – resulting from a long-term collection of wind [intruding into a state of] depletion – then flows into the large intestine".

Jiu zhong **酒腫, wine swelling** [3]
PC of → *bie jia* 鱉瘕, turtle[-shaped] conglomeration-illness, and → *fou zhong* 浮腫, surface swelling, caused by excessive consumption of wine. *PJF* 192: 香附子，治**酒腫**腹腫，脾虛發腫, "*Xiang fu zi* cures **wine swelling**, abdominal swelling, and spleen depletion resulting in swelling".

***Ju* 聚, collection** [p]

PC CD of formless qi collections in the chest and abdomen. Their upper and lower extensions vary. Associated pain does not occur at a well-defined location. It was believed that such collections were generated by the six palaces. *NJ* 55: **聚**者，陽氣也，其始發無根本，上下無所留止，其痛無常處, "**Collections** [consist of] yang qi. In the beginning they develop without roots. They move upward and downward and do not remain in a specific place. The pain [they cause] has no permanent location".

***Ju* 疽, impediment-illness; corruption-illness** [p]

PC CD of acute, festering abscesses developing within the skin, reaching into the depth and showing a scattered appearance of several tips of putrescence on the skin. The affected skin appears thick and its color is tender. This may be accompanied by conditions affecting the entire body, including a severe aversion to cold and fever. *LS* 81: 熱氣淳盛，下陷肌膚，筋髓枯，內連五藏，血氣竭，當其癰下，筋骨良肉皆無餘，故命曰**疽**, "In the case of pure, flourishing heat qi, the skin and muscles will cave in; the sinews and the marrow dry. This then combines internally with the five depots whose blood and qi is exhausted. As a result, underneath an obstruction-illness the sinews, the bones and good flesh, they all vanish. Hence this is called '**corruption-illness**'". The term *ju* 疽 appears to have been associated with two different meanings, based on the etymology of the character 且 giving **疽** its meaning. 且, it appears from the pronunciation of *ju* 疽, is borrowed from *ju* 沮, which has two meanings: one is "impediment", the other is "corruption; to diminish". The definition provided by *LS* 81, quoted here, appears to refer to an illness associated with a "corruption" of tissue. In the *BCGM* the use of the term may have been associated with the meaning of "**impediment-illness**".

***Ju huan* 拘緩, relaxed; to slacken** [4]

IS modified version of → *huan* 緩①. *BJ* SE *hu zhang* 虎掌：寒風濕痹，四肢**拘緩**不收, "In the case of cold wind moisture blockage, the four limbs **slacken** and cannot be contracted".

***Ju ji* 拘急, cramps with tension** [29] AN *ju luan* 拘攣, cramps with contraction.

IS of pain and lack of mobility brought forth by shrinkage of muscles and sinews as well as convulsions of the stomach and intestines. *BJ* SE *gen dang zi* 莨菪子：主齒痛出蟲，肉痹**拘急**, "It controls toothache and extracts [tooth] bugs/worms, as well as flesh blockage and **cramps with tension**".

***Ju ji* 疽疾, ailment of impediment-illness** [2]

PC, CD of conditions of → *yong* 癰, obstruction-illnesses, and → *ju* 疽, impediment-illnesses. *JYBJF* Lun fu bu huan jin zheng qi san 論服不換金正氣散：**疽疾**將安之際，合多服加料十全湯，以補其氣血，使易生肌肉故也, "When the **ailment of an impediment-illness** comes close to being healed, it is advisable to consume large quantities of the 'decoction with added ingredients that is always successful' to supplement the [patient's] qi and blood. The reason is that this will easily generate new muscles and flesh".

***Ju juan* 拘倦, stiff and weary** [2]
IS of sinews, vessels, and muscle tissue being tense and weary. *SJZL* 15: 療偏正頭痛，解身體**拘倦**, "It heals lateral and frontal headache, and it resolves a body's **stiffness and weariness**".

***Ju lou* 疽瘺, impediment-illness with fistula** [4]
PC CD of → *ju* 疽, impediment-illness, and → *lou* 瘺, fistula, or of impediment-illness that opens to fester and develops into a fistula. *ZLBC* SE *yang lu mu* 楊櫨木：主**疽瘺**惡瘡，水煮葉汁洗瘡，立差, "It controls **impediment-illness with fistula** and malign sores. When the sores are washed with the liquid obtained from boiling the leaves with water, this will bring an immediate cure".

***Ju luan* 拘攣, cramps with contraction** [45]
IS of contracted sinews and muscles with a bent body that is unable to stretch. *SW* 63: 邪客於足太陽之絡，令人**拘攣**背急，引脅而痛, "When an evil has settled in the network [vessels] of the foot major yang [conduits], it makes the [affected] person have a **cramp with contraction** and a tense back, creating pain pulling into the flanks".

***Ju shi* 疽蝕, impediment-illness erosion** [4]
PC CD of → *ju* 疽, impediment-illnesses, that fester and at the same time develop open sores of the type of an ulcer. *BJ* SE *lang du* 狼毒：主咳逆上氣，破積聚飲食，寒熱水氣，惡瘡，鼠瘺，**疽蝕**，鬼精蠱毒, "It controls cough with qi rising contrary to its regular course, breaks accumulations and collections of beverages and food, [controls] cold and hot water qi, malign sores, mouse fistula, **impediment-illness erosion**, as well as demon's essence [that is] *gu* poison".

***Ju tong* 拘痛, cramps with pain** [5]
IS identical with → *luan tong* 攣痛. *WTMY* 19: 六生散，療急風痹，身軀**拘痛**方, "Powder with the six raw ingredients: recipe to cure acute wind blockage, and **cramps with pain** affecting the entire body".

***Ju tou* 疽頭, head of an impediment-illness** [1]
PI CD of the central elevation or tip of → *yong* 癰, obstruction-illness, and *ju* 疽, impediment-illness. It is from here that the pus is discharged. *BCGM Bai bing zhu zhi yao* 百病主治藥：**疽頭**凹黑，(蕎麥)煮食即起, "When the **head of an impediment-illness** is sunken in and black, eat boiled [*qiao mai*] and it will rise".

***Ju zhi* 舉痔, raised piles** [1]
PC identical with → *shu zhi* 鼠痔, mouse piles. *HJJF* 8: 穀道四面弩肉如奶，名**舉痔**, "When the path of grain (i.e. the anus) is aligned on all four sides with tumorous flesh-growths resembling breast nipples, this is called '**raised piles**'".

***Jue* 蹶, lameness** [3]
PC, with *jue* 蹶 used for *que* 瘸, dysfunction/lameness, to refer to an impaired ability to walk. *MYBL* SE *bao yu* 鮑魚：主墜墮，骽**蹶**，踠折，瘀血: "It controls [injuries from] falls, **lameness** of the legs, fractures, and stagnant blood [that has left the vessels]".

Jue chan **絕產, barred from offspring; infertility** [3]

PC identical with → *jue yun* 絕孕①, barred from pregnancy. *MYBL* SE *hu yin jing* 狐陰莖：主女子**絕產**，陰癢, "It controls female **infertility**, and vaginal itching".

Jue jin **絕筋, severed sinew** [2]

PC of an injury resulting in completely ruptured sinews, identical with → *duan jin* 斷筋. *BJ* SE *di huang* 地黃：主折跌**絕筋**, "It controls fractures from falls, with **severed sinews**".

Jue nüe **厥瘧, recession malaria** [2]

PC of a → *han nüe* 寒瘧, cold malaria, that manifests itself with cold spells only and no heat, and a darkened complexion. *PJF* 198: 寒而不熱，面色黑者，名為**厥瘧**, "If [patients] experience cold spells without fever, and if their complexion is black, that is called **recession malaria**".

Jue qi **厥氣, receding qi** [2]

EA of qi moving in disorder, contrary to its regular direction. It may cause all kinds of disease. *SW* 5: 暴怒傷陰，暴喜傷陽。**厥氣**上行，滿脈去形, "Violent anger harms the yin; violent joy harms the yang. **Receding qi** moves upwards; it fills the vessels and leaves the physical appearance".

Jue yang **絕陽, severed yang** [7] AN *nei jue* 內絕, internal severance; *yang dao jue shang* 陽道絕傷, harm of yang path severance.

PC CD of conditions with blocked sexual potency of male adults as a major sign. *ZLBC* SE *rou cong rong* 肉蓯蓉 quotes *RHZ*: 治男**絕陽**不興，女絕陰不產, "It cures in males a **severed yang** with an inability to achieve erection; in females a severed yin with an inability to have offspring".

Jue yin **絕陰, severed yin; childlessness** [6]

PC identical with → *jue yun* 絕孕①, barred from pregnancy. *RHZ* SE *rou cong rong* 肉蓯蓉：治男絕陽不興，女**絕陰**不產, "It cures in males a severed yang with an inability to achieve erection; in females a **severed yin** with an inability to have offspring".

Jue yin bing **厥陰病, ceasing yin disease** [5]

PC in a later phase of harm caused by cold disease when, in the body's dynamics, the yang is weakened and the yin has waned, with ceasing counterflow (i.e. cold) in the four limbs, or ceasing [yang qi, i.e. cold] and heat alternating with each other, or cold and heat intermingling with each other as frequently seen signs. *SW* 31: 十二日**厥陰病**衰，囊縱，少腹微下，大氣皆去，病日已矣, "On the twelfth day, the **disease in the ceasing yin [conduits]** weakens. The scrotum slackens, and the lower abdomen moves down slightly. Large [quantities of] qi depart. The disease reaches its end within a day".

Jue yin tou tong **厥陰頭痛, ceasing yin headache** [2]

PC of headache resulting from cold affecting the ceasing yin liver [conduit], with qi rising contrary to its proper direction and striking the top of the head. This is accompanied by dry vomiting and the spitting of saliva with foam. *SJZL* 24: 厥

陰頭痛一證，治以吳茱萸湯者是也, "The condition of ceasing yin headache is to be treated with the decoction with *wu zhu yu*".

***Jue yun* 絕孕, barred from pregnancy** [12]

① AN *bu yun* 不孕, infertility; *jue yin* 絕陰, barred yin; *jue chan* 絕產, barred from offspring.

PC with an inability, in the course of a marriage, to become pregnant over an extended period of time. *BJ* SE *zi shi ying* 紫石英：女子風寒在子宮，**絕孕**十年無子, "A woman with wind cold in her uterus, so that she has been **barred from pregnancy** and has had no child for ten years".

② An inability to become pregnant after → *duan chan* 斷產, sterilization. *BCGM* SE *ling ling xiang* 零陵香 quotes *YLJY*: 婦人斷產：零陵香為末，酒服二錢。每服至一兩，即一年**絕孕**, "For sterilization of a woman: Grind *ling ling xiang* to a powder, and ingest 2 *qian* with wine. Each time her dose should reach 1 *liang*. This will make her be **barred from pregnancy** for one year".

***Jun ca* 皸拆, chapped skin cracks** [1]

PC identical with → *jun lie* 皸裂. *TBC* SE *bai ji* 白及：山野人患手足**皸拆**者，嚼以塗之有效, "When people living in the wilderness suffer from **chapped skin cracks** on their hands and feet chew this and apply it externally, it is effective".

***Jun che* 皸坼, chapped skin crack** [1]

PC identical with → *jun lie* 皸裂. *BCSY* SE *tie ruo* 鐵爇：金瘡，毒物傷皮肉，止風水不入，入水不爛，手足**皸坼**, "In the case of wounds inflicted by metal objects, and poisonous matter harming the skin, it prevents wind and water from entering. Also, [when the wound is] put into water it will not rot. [It furthermore cures] **chapped skin cracks** on the hands and feet".

***Jun lie* 皸裂, chapped skin cracks** [10]

PC identical with → *cun lie* 皴裂. *ZBYHL* 30: 言冬時觸冒風寒，手足破，故謂之**皸裂**, "That is to say, in winter one encounters malicious wind cold causing the hands and feet to break open. Hence this is called '**chapped skin cracks**'".

***Jun zhu* 皸瘃, chapped skin and chilblain** [2]

PC identical with → *cun lie* 皴裂, chapped skin cracks. *BCGM* SE *zhe gu* 鷓鴣 quoting *BCTJ*: 膏手可以已瘴瘃，令不龜裂, "The ointment is able to end chapped skin cracks on the hands lest turtle [shell] cracks should develop", writes: 塗手**皸瘃**，令不龜裂, "When hands with **chapped skin and chilblain** are washed with it it will prevent the emergence of turtle [shell] cracks".

- K -

***Ka xue* 喀血, to spit blood** [43]

① IS of blood from the lung being emitted through the mouth. This may or may not be accompanied by cough. *SJZL* 48: 肺氣盛實，其氣上蒸，發嗽多痰，心胸煩躁，往往**喀血**, "The lung qi abounds to repletion. This qi rises like steam and coughs up much phlegm. The heart and chest experience vexation and restlessness. [Patients] again and again **spit blood**".

② PC with blood spitting. *SJZL* 68: 如患**喀血**，用前件藥末一兩，鄆州蛤粉二兩, "If someone suffers from **blood spitting**, take 1 *liang* powder of the pharmaceutical substance mentioned before plus 2 *liang* of *ge fen* from Yunzhou".

***Ke* 咳, cough** [p]

① IS identical with → *ke sou* 咳嗽①. *SW* 3: 秋傷於濕，上逆而**咳**，發為痿厥, "If one has been harmed in autumn by moisture, [the qi] rises contrary [to its regular course] and one **coughs**. This develops into a dysfunction with receding [qi]".

② PC identical with → *ke sou* 咳嗽②. *SW* 38: 五臟六腑皆令人**咳**，非獨肺也, "The five depots and six palaces, they all [may] make a person **cough**, not only the lung".

***Ke han* 客寒, visitor cold** [7]

EA of cold evil affecting the human body from outside. *WTMY* 37: 未有外熱能入於內而成其腫，皆由表虛**客寒**所搏, "External heat is unable to enter the interior and to generate such a swelling. [Such a swelling] is always caused by the pouncing of **visitor cold** taking advantage of an outer depletion".

***Ke ji* 渴疾, thirst ailment; diabetes** [16]

PC identical with → *xiao ke* 消渴, melting with thirst; diabetes. *SXBC* SE *da qing* 大青：葉似茶葉，可以作湯，療**渴疾**, "The leaves resemble tea leaves. They are suitable for preparing decoctions and are able to cure **thirst ailment**".

***Ke lao* 咳勞, cough exhaustion** [1]

PC of depletion exhaustion with cough. *BCGM* Bai bing zhu zhi yao 百病主治藥：鬼臼，**咳勞**, "*Gui jiu* [cures] **cough exhaustion**".

***Ke leng* 客冷, visitor cold** [1]

EA identical with → *ke han* 客寒. *WTMY* 36: 療小兒**客冷**白痢方, "Recipe to cure **visitor cold** and white free-flux illness in children".

***Ke ni* 咳逆, cough with counterflow [of qi]** [140]

① IS identical with a) → *e ni* 呃逆①, hiccough with counterflow of qi. *ZBYHL* 13: 寒膈之為病，心腹脹滿，**咳逆**，腹上苦冷，雷鳴，繞臍痛，食不消, "The disease of cold occlusion: distension and a feeling of fullness in the center (i.e. stomach) and abdomen. **Cough with counterflow [of qi]**. An uncomfortable feeling of cold above the abdomen. Thunderous sounds [in the abdomen]. Pain winding around the navel. Food is not digested". b) → *ke sou* 咳嗽①, cough. *JGYL* Fj: 肺癰，胸滿脹，一身面目浮腫，鼻塞清涕出，不聞香臭酸辛，**咳逆**上氣，喘鳴迫塞，葶藶大棗瀉肺湯主之, "Lung obstruction-illness, a feeling of fullness and distension in the chest; the surface of the entire body, the face and the eyes are swollen; the nose is blocked with clear snivel leaving. One cannot distinguish aromatic odors from stench, and sour from acrid flavor. **Cough with counterflow of qi**. Noisy panting pressing against a blockade: The decoction with *ting li* and *da zao* to drain the lung controls it".

② PC identical with a) *e ni* 呃逆②, hiccough with counterflow [of qi]. *BJ* SE *li lu* 藜蘆：主蠱毒，**咳逆**，泄痢，腸澼, "It controls *gu* poison, **cough with counterflow** [of qi], outflow and free-flux illness, intestinal flush". b) *ke sou* 咳嗽②, cough. *ZBYHL* 14: **咳逆**者，是咳嗽而氣逆上也, "**Cough with counterflow** [of qi] is a cough with adversely rising qi". LSZ: "In the Ming era, *ke ni* **咳逆**, **cough with counterflow** [of qi], mostly referred to *e ni* 呃逆, hiccough with counterflow [of qi], while the term *chuan ni* 喘逆served to express the ancient meaning of *ke sou shang qi* 咳嗽上氣, cough with rising qi". In ancient sources quoted in the *BCGM*, the term *ke ni* 咳逆 refers to *ke sou* 咳嗽, cough.

***Ke nong xue* 咳膿血, cough with pus and blood** [3]

IS of cough followed by a spitting of pus and phlegm. *YXZC* 2: 天門冬膏，治血虛肺燥，皮膚折裂，及肺痿**咳膿血**證, "Paste with *tian men dong*: It cures blood depletion and lung dryness, with cracking skin and lung dysfunction and **cough with pus and blood**".

***Ke re* 客熱, visitor heat** [61]

① EA identified as heat evil intruding into the human organism from outside. *ZBYHL* 39: 外熱加之，非腑臟自生，故云**客熱**也, "If heat from outside is added to it, this is not generated by the depots and palaces themselves. Hence one speaks of '**visitor heat**'".

② PC identical with → *re* 熱, heat. *SHL* 122: 脈乃數也，數為**客熱**, "In this case the movement in the vessels is frequent. A frequent [movement in the vessels] signals **visitor heat**".

***Ke sou* 咳嗽, cough** [335] AD *ke* 咳; *sou* 嗽. AN *ke ni* 咳逆, a cough with counterflow [of qi]; *sou ni* 嗽逆.

① IS. A reflex reaction of the respiratory apparatus provoked by some stimulus. *JGYL* Mj: 留飲者，脅下痛引缺盆，**咳嗽**則輒已, "In the case of abiding rheum, there is pain below the flanks that pulls on the 'broken bowl'; when [patients] **cough** this will end soon".

② PC of cough. *SW* 5: 秋傷於濕，冬生**咳嗽**, "If he is harmed by moisture in autumn, he will develop a **cough** in winter".

***Ke wu* 客忤, visitor's hostility** [69] AN *zu wu* 卒忤, sudden hostility; *gui wu* 鬼忤, demon hostility; *wu e* 忤惡, the hostile and the malign.

PC of a sudden twisting pain, encountered while outside one's home, in the heart and abdomen, with heart-pressure and shortness of qi, in severe cases leading to loss of consciousness, explained as resulting from the hostile acts of demons "visiting" the human body. *ZHF* 1: **客忤**者，中惡之類也，多於道間、門外得之，令人心腹絞痛脹滿，氣衝心胸，不即治，亦殺人, "**Visitor's hostility** is an example of a stroke by the malign. One is often affected by this while away from home. It causes a twisting pain in the heart and abdomen, and a feeling of distension and fullness. Qi rushes against the heart and chest. If it is not cured immediately, it will kill that person".

***Ke wu si* 客忤死, [appearance of] death from a visitor's hostility** [1] AD *wu si* 忤死, [appearance of] death from hostility.

PC of → *cu si* 卒死, sudden [appearance of] death. *ZHF* 1 lists: 救卒**客忤死**方, "Recipes to rescue from a sudden **[appearance of] death from a visitor's hostility**".

***Ke wu tian diao* 客忤天吊, hauled-by-heaven following visitor's hostiliy** [4]

PC identical with → *tian diao jing feng* 天吊驚風, heaven-hauled fright wind. *RHZ* SE *lu* 驢：乳治小兒癇，**客忤天吊**，風疾, "Its milk cures epilepsy in children, **hauled-by-heaven following visitor's hostility**, as well as wind ailments".

***Ke xue* 咳血, to cough up blood** [17] AN *sou xue* 嗽血.

① AN *ke sou xue* 咳嗽血. IS of blood coughed up from within the lung. *ZBYHL* 9: 七曰**咳血**衄血，汗不出，出不至足者死, "On day seven, patients who **cough up blood** and have a nosebleed, and who do not sweat or do not sweat sufficiently, they will die".

② PC of the coughing up of blood. *JSF* Xue bing men 血病門：**咳血**一證，不嗽者易治，兼嗽者為難愈，為肺傷故也, "The condition of '**coughing up of blood**', those who do not cough, they are easy to cure; those who have [a normal] cough at the same time, are difficult to cure. The reason is that their lung has been harmed".

***Ke xue* 客血, visitor blood** [2]

PI identical with → *yue xue* 瘀血①, stagnant blood [that has left the vessels]. *MYBL* SE *dang gui* 當歸：溫中止痛，除**客血**內塞, "It warms the center and ends pain. It eliminates **visitor blood** [causing] internal blockages".

***Ke yi* 咳噫, hiccough** [4]

IS identical with → *e ni* 呃逆①, hiccough with counterflow [of qi]. *ZLBC* SE *sheng jiang* 生薑 quotes *WTMY*: 久患**咳噫**，連咳四五十聲, "Long-term suffering from **hiccough** is a cough sounding 40 to 50 times".

***Kong nao sha* 控腦砂, grit impacting the brain** [1]

PC identical with → *bi yuan* 鼻淵, nasal deep-source [outflow]. *YXZC* 5: 鼻中時時流臭黃水，甚者腦亦時痛，俗名**控腦砂**, "There is a frequent flow of malodorous yellow water from within the nose. In severe cases the brain aches from time to time. This is commonly called '**grit impacting the brain**'".

***Kou bi gan* 口鼻疳, oral and nasal *gan*-illness** [1]

PC identical with → *bi gan* 鼻疳, nasal *gan*-illness. *BCGM* Zhu bing zhu zhi yao 諸病主治藥 quoting *QJYiF*: 急疳食鼻口, "Acute *gan*-illness eats the nose and mouth", writes: 口鼻疳, "Oral and nasal *gan*-illness".

***Kou chi bing* 口齒病, mouth and tooth diseases** [2]

PC identical with → *kou chi zhu bing* 口齒諸病, all types of diseases of the mouth and the teeth. *BCGM* SE *yun tai* 芸薹 quoting *SLBC* 發口瘡齒痛, "Develops mouth sores and a toothache", writes: 發瘡及**口齒病**, "Develops sores and **mouth and tooth diseases**".

Kou chi gan **口齒疳, oral and dental *gan*-illness** [2]

PC identical with → *kou gan* 口疳, oral *gan*-illness. *TPSHF* 87: 唇口癢痛，牙齒峭黑，舌上生瘡，腦中乾熱，齦肉赤爛，頰腫齒疼，熱毒熏蒸，口多臭氣，故曰**口齒疳**也, "The lips and mouth itch and ache. The teeth become pointed and turn black. Sores develop on the tongue. There is heat in the chest. The flesh of the gums turns red and rots. The cheeks are swollen, and the teeth ache. Heat poison steams. Much qi with a bad odor comes from the mouth. Hence this is called '**oral and dental *gan*-illness**'".

Kou chi zhu bing **口齒諸病, all types of mouth and tooth diseases** [2] AN *kou chi bing* 口齒病, oral and dental diseases.

All PC of the oral cavity and the teeth. *BCGM* SE *peng sha* 蓬砂：陰㿉骨哽，惡瘡及**口齒諸病**, "For yin (i.e. scrotal) prominence-illness, choking with a bone stuck in the throat, malign sores, and **all types of mouth and tooth diseases**".

Kou chou **口臭, malodorous mouth** [23]

① AN *kou chou qi* 口臭氣, malodorous qi from the mouth; *kou zhong qi chou* 口中氣臭, malodorous qi in the mouth. PC of bad breath. *BCJJZ* SE *xi xin* 細辛：人患**口臭**者，含之多效, "When someone suffers from a **malodorous mouth**, holding this in the mouth is often effective".

② IS of bad breath. *ZBYHL* 30: **口臭**，由五臟六腑不調，氣上胸膈, "**Malodorous mouth** is the result of an imbalance of the five depots and six palaces, with qi rising into the chest and diaphragm".

Kou chou qi **口臭氣, malodorous qi from the mouth** [2]

PC identical with → *kou chou* 口臭②. *MYBL* SE *dou kou* 豆蔻：主溫中，心腹痛，嘔吐，去**口臭氣**, "It controls warming the center, heart and abdominal pain, and vomiting, and eliminates **malodorous qi from the mouth**".

Kou chuang **口瘡, mouth sores** [119]

PC of → *chuang* 瘡, sores, developing on the tongue, cheeks or upper palate with one or several light yellow or greyish festering spots, repeatedly erupting with a burning pain . *MYBL* SE *da qing* 大青：主療時氣，頭痛，大熱，**口瘡**, "It controls the cure of [ailments resulting from] seasonal qi, headache, massive heat, and **mouth sores**".

Kou chun shun dong **口唇瞤動, mouth and lips shiver** [1]

IS of lips displaying involuntary uncontrolled trembling or pulsating movements. *BCGM* Bai bing zhu zhi yao 百病主治藥：風濕入脾，**口唇瞤動**, "When wind and moisture enter the spleen, the **mouth and lips will shiver**".

Kou gan **口乾, desiccated mouth** [61]

IS of an uncomfortable feeling of dryness in the mouth. *SW* 31: 病一日則巨陽與少陰俱病，則頭痛**口乾**而煩滿, "If the disease is in its first day, the great yang [conduit] and the minor yin [conduit] both have the disease. As a result, the head aches, the **mouth is desiccated**, and there is vexation and a feeling of fullness".

Kou gan **口疳, oral *gan*-illness** [12] AN *kou chi gan* 口齒疳, oral and dental *gan*-illness.

PC of → *gan chuang* 疳瘡, *gan*-illness sores, affecting the mouth, the tongue and the gums with ulcers that fester and bleed and have a bad stench . *WTMY* 飛廉：療䘌齒，及**口疳**蟲食，紫藍灰方, "Recipe with *zi lan hui* to cure hidden worms teeth and **oral *gan*-illness** resulting from worms eating".

Kou jin **口噤, clenched jaw** [135] AW 口禁.

IS of lockjaw with an inability to open the mouth. *JGYL* Fj: 獨頭動搖，卒**口噤**，背反張者，痙病也, "When the head shakes, with a suddenly **clenched jaw**, and the spine is arched backwards, this is spasms disease". The *BCGM* at three locations erroneously refers to *kou jin* 口噤 as 口禁.

Kou jin **口禁, clenched jaw** [3]

IS AW of → *kou jin* 口噤. A writing error. *BCGM* SW *rou cong rong* 肉蓯蓉：破傷風病：**口禁**身強。肉蓯蓉切片晒乾，用一小盞，底上穿定，燒烟於瘡上熏之，累效, "It breaks illnesses of harm caused by wind with **clenched jaw** and a stiff body. Cut *rou cong rong* into pieces and dry them under the sun. Take a small bowl and pierce some [of the *rou cong rong*] through a hole in the bottom where it is fixed. Then roast [this] and fumigate [the wound] with the smoke. This is often effective".

Kou jin **口緊, tight mouth** [7]

IS identical with → *kou jin* 口噤, clenched jaw. *BCGM* SE *hu* 狐：肝燒灰，治風癇及破傷風，**口緊**搐強, "Liver burnt to ashes cures wind epilepsy and wound wind, with **tight mouth** and jerking with stiffness".

Kou jin feng **口噤風, clenched jaw wind** [1]

PC identical with → *feng jin* 風噤, wind lockjaw. *BCGM* SE *niu* 牛：齝草…療反胃霍亂，小兒**口噤風**, "The cud...cures turned over stomach, cholera, and **clenched jaw wind** in children".

Kou ku **口苦, bitter taste in the mouth** [8]

① IS of a perception of bitterness in the mouth unrelated to the normal sensation following the ingestion of bitter beverages or food. *SW* 47: **口苦**者病名為何？何以得之, "A **bitter taste in the mouth**, what is the name of that disease? How did he get it?"

② PC of a bitter taste in the mouth. *ZBYHL* 3: 東向坐，仰頭不息五通，以舌撩口，漱滿，二七咽。治**口苦**乾燥, "Sit facing east. Raise the head and do not breathe for as long as five breaths would take. Stroke the mouth internally with the tongue until it is filled with saliva. Swallow this two times seven times. This cures **bitter taste in the mouth** with dryness".

Kou li **口戾, slanted mouth** [1]

IS identical with → *kou wai* 口喎, wryness of the mouth. *BCGM* SE *kuo yu* 蛞蝓：喎，苦乖切，**口戾**也, "[The term] 喎, [pronounced *kuai* out of] *k*[*u*] and [*g*]*uai*, has the meaning of '**slanted mouth**'".

***Kou mi* 口糜, oral rice gruel** [5] AN *kou she chuang mi* 口舌瘡糜, gruel-type sores affecting the mouth and tongue.

PC of a → *kou chuang* 口瘡, mouth sores, with the mucous membrane in the oral cavity breaking up in pieces and festering extremely, in serious cases assuming the appearance of rice gruel. *SJZL* 117: 治小腸熱脹，**口糜**生瘡，柴胡澤瀉湯方, "To cure heat distension of the small intestines, and **oral rice-gruel** developing into sores, [use] the recipe for a decoction with *chai hu* and *ze xie*".

***Kou mu shun dong* 口目瞤動, mouth and eyes shiver** [1]

IS of the lips and eyes displaying involuntary unconcontrolled trembling or pulsating movements. *YLFQS*: 食治老人中風，**口目瞤動**，煩悶不安，牛蒡餺飥方, "Recipe with *niu bang bo tuo* for a dietary treatment of old people being struck by wind, with **mouth and eyes shivering**, vexation and heart-pressure that fail to subside".

***Kou nei re chuang* 口內熱瘡, heat sores in the mouth** [2] AN → *kou zhong re chuang* 口中熱瘡.

PC of heat-type → *kou chuang* 口瘡, sores in the mouth. *BCSY* SE *gu wen qian* 古文錢：含青錢，又主**口內熱瘡**, "Includes copper. Also, it controls **heat sores in the mouth**".

***Kou nei rou qiu* 口內肉球, flesh balls in the mouth** [1]

PC of a growth of flesh balls as redundancies in the mouth. *BCGM* SE *she* 麝 quotes *QJF*: **口內肉球**：有根如綫五寸余，如釵股，吐出乃能食物，捻之則痛徹心者，麝香一錢研水服之，日三，自消, "**Flesh balls in the mouth**: They have thread-like roots of a length of 5 *cun* or longer, as if a hairpin had been inserted. When they are spit out, [the patient] can eat food again. If twisted with two fingers they cause a pain that goes right into the heart. Grind 1 *qian* of *she xiang* with water and ingest this three times a day, and they will dissolve by themselves".

***Kou pi* 口僻, slanted mouth** [7]

IS identical with → *kou wai* 口喎, wryness of the mouth. *LS* 13: 卒**口僻**，急者目不合, "In the case of suddenly **slanted mouth**, if it is critical, the eyes do not close".

***Kou pian* 口偏, slanted mouth** [3]

IS identical with → *kou wai* 口喎, wryness of the mouth. *QJYF* 8: 風著人面，引**口偏**著耳, "When wind attaches itself to the human face, it pulls the **mouth slanted** towards one of the ears".

***Kou she cu chai* 口舌粗拆, rough and cracked mouth and tongue** [1]

IS of a rough and cracked surface of the tongue. *BCTJ* SE *cu lin zi* 醋林子：不可多食，令人**口舌粗拆**, "One must not eat much of it lest it cause a **rough and cracked mouth and tongue**".

***Kou shi chuang mi* 口舌瘡糜, gruel-type sores affecting the mouth and tongue** [1]

PC identical with → *kou mi* 口糜, oral rice-gruel. *BCGM* SE *hu zhang tian nan xing* 虎掌天南星：治驚癇，口眼喎斜，喉痹，**口舌瘡糜**, "It cures fright epilepsy, wry mouth and slanted eyes, throat blockage, and **gruel-type sores affecting the mouth and tongue**".

***Kou tian* 口甜, sweet taste in the mouth** [1]
PC with a perception of sweetness in the mouth unrelated to the normal sensation following the ingestion of sweet beverages or food as major sign. *HJJF* 1: 薄荷煎丸…治肺熱喉腥，脾熱**口甜**，膽熱口苦, "Pills with *bo he* decoction... cure lung heat with a fishy throat stench, spleen heat with a **sweet taste in the mouth**, and gallbladder heat with a bitter taste in the mouth".

***Kou tu qing shui* 口吐清水, spitting of clear water** [5]
IS of frequent spitting of clear and thin liquid. *SJZL* 99: 治九蟲動作，腹中刺痛，**口吐清水**，面色黑黃，及蟲心痛者，石榴枝湯方, "To cure activities of the nine bugs/worms, with piercing pain in the abdomen, **spitting of clear water**, a black-yellow complexion, as well as bug heart pain: [use the] recipe for a decoction with *shi liu* twigs".

***Kou wai* 口喎, wryness of the mouth** [26] AD *wai* 喎; wryness; AN *kou li* 口戾, slanted mouth; *kou pi* 口僻; *kou pian* 口偏.
IS of the edges of the mouth being slanted on one side. *QJYF* 8: 治卒中風**口喎**方, "Recipe to cure sudden wind stroke with **wryness of the mouth**".

***Kou xun* 口蕈, mouth fungus** [1]
PC identical with → *kou zhong sheng xun* 口中生蕈, fungus growth in the mouth. *BCGM* SE *qie* 茄：治血淋下血，血痢陰挺，齒䘌**口蕈**, "It cures blood dripping, blood discharge, bloody free-flux illness, yin (i.e. testicle) protrusion, teeth with hidden worms, and **mouth fungus**".

***Kou zhong qi chou* 口中氣臭, malodorous qi in the mouth** [1]
PC identical with → *kou chou* 口臭②. *BCGM* SE *fan shi* 礬石quotes *SSB*: **口中氣臭**：明礬入麝香為末，擦牙上, "For **malodorous qi in the mouth**, add *ming fan* to *she xiang* and prepare a powder to rub the teeth with".

***Kou zhong re chuang* 口中熱瘡, heat sores in the mouth** [1]
PC identical with → *kou nei re chuang* 口內熱瘡. *BCSY* SE *gu jin hui* 故錦灰：故錦燒作灰，主小兒**口中熱瘡**, "Ancient brocade burnt to ashes controls **heat sores in the mouth** of children".

***Kou zhong sheng xun* 口中生蕈, fungus growth in the mouth** [2] AN *kou xun* 口蕈.
PC of the growth of fungus-like substance in the mouth. *BCGM* SE *fan shi* 礬石quotes *ZXF*: **口中生蕈**：用醋漱口, "For **fungus growth in the mouth** rinse the mouth with vinegar".

***Kou zhong xian shui* 口中涎水, saliva water filling the mouth** [1]
IS of larger than normal quantities of saliva in the mouth. *ZLBC* SE *wei ling xian* 威靈仙 quotes *CYLHSF*: 宣通五藏，腹內宿滯，心頭痰水，膀胱宿膿，**口中涎水**, "It passes through the five depots, and [relieves people of] sluggish [food] remaining in the abdomen overnight, of phlegm water [in the chest] on top of the heart, of pus lodging in the bladder, and of **saliva water filling the mouth**".

Ku bi **枯痹, desiccation blockage** [2]

PC of → *bi* 痹① a), blockage, with limbs and body assuming an altered appearance of desiccation and emaciation. *BCTJ* SE *yin yu* 茵芋quotes Hu Qia 胡洽：治賊風，手足**枯痹**，四肢拘攣。茵芋酒主之, "To cure robber wind, with hands and feet affected by **desiccation blockage**, and the four limbs having cramps and contractions, wine with *yin yu* will control this".

Ku shou **枯瘦, withered and emaciated** [3]

IS of a desiccation of the body and limbs brought forth by extreme emaciation. *ZBYHL* 3: 久不已，令人羸瘠**枯瘦**, "If it does not heal over an extended period of time, it causes a person to be thin and lean, **withered and emaciated**".

Ku zao **枯燥, withered and dry** [9]

① IS of shrivelling dry skin and muscles/flesh losing their functions. *BCJJZ* SE *chi xiao dou* 赤小豆：小豆性逐津液，久服令人**枯燥**矣, "The nature of soybeans is to expel liquids. If consumed for long it will make people appear **withered and dry**".

② Appearance of items that have lost their liquid elements. *BCJJZ* SE *zhi mu* 知母：葉至難死，掘出隨生，須**枯燥**乃止, "The leaves do not easily die. If plucked they still live. Only if they have been made to **wither and dry**, do they stop further growth".

Ku zhu **哭疰, weeping [demon's] attachment-illness** [1]

PC of a chronic sadness with weeping that does not end by itself, and is brought forth by hearing someone else weep, or develops spontaneously out of one's own weeping. *QJYF* 17: 治**哭疰**方：梳齒間刮取垢，水服之, "Recipe for treating **weeping [demon's] attachment-illness**: scratch the filth from between the teeth of a comb, and consume this with water".

Kuang **狂, crazy; madness** [p]

① PC identical with → *feng kuang* 風狂, wind madness. *SW* 40: 灸之則喑，石之則**狂**, "When the [patient] is cauterized, he will turn mute; when he is [treated with] stones, he will become **crazy**".

② IS identical with → *kuang luan* 狂亂, madness with confusion. *SW* 79: 二陰二陽皆交至，病在腎，罵詈妄行，巔疾為**狂**, "When the second yin arrives all intertwined with the second yang, the disease is in the kidneys. [The patient] voices insults, making absurd movements. [He suffers from] peak-illness and is **crazy**".

Kuang ban **狂斑, madness with macules** [2]

PC CD of → *zhan kuang* 譫狂, incoherent language and madness, and → *fa ban* 發斑, appearance of macula. *BCGM* SE *da qing* 大青 quotes *ZZFu*: 陽毒則**狂斑**煩亂, "Yang poisoning results in **madness with macules**, and vexation with confusion".

Kuang bing **狂病, madness disease** [4]

PC identical with → *feng kuang* 風狂, wind madness. *MYBL* SE *jia zhu rou* 豭豬肉：味酸，冷。療**狂病**, "Sour flavor; cold; heals the **disease of madness**".

Kuang dang 狂盪, madness with restlessness [1]
IS identical with → *kuang luan* 狂亂, madness with confusion. *SXBC* SE *ku zao* 苦棗：主傷寒熱伏在臟腑，**狂盪**煩滿, "It controls harm caused by cold, with heat hiding in the depots and palaces, **madness with restlessness**, and vexation with a feeling of fullness".

Kuang dian **狂癲, madness and peak-illness** [4]
PC identical with → *dian kuang* 癲狂, peak-illness and madness. *MYBL* SE *niu huang* 牛黃：療小兒百病，諸癇熱，口不開，大人**狂癲**, "It cures all types of diseases of children, all types of epilepsy with heat, and inability to open the mouth, and in adults **madness and peak-illness**".

Kuang dian **狂顛, madness and peak[-illness]** [6]
PC identical with → *dian kuang* 癲狂, peak-illness and madness. *BCGM* SE *fu long gan* 伏龍肝 quotes *QJF*: **狂顛**謬亂不識人，伏龍肝末，水服方寸匕，日三服, "In the case of **madness and peak[-illness]**, when [patients] are confused and do not recognize others, ingest *fu long gan* powder, one square inch-sized spoon, with water three times a day".

Kuang fan **狂煩, madness with vexation** [6]
IS CD of → *kuang luan* 狂亂, madness with confusion, and → *fan zao* 煩躁, vexation with restlessness. *BJ* SE *lu jian* 鹵鹼：主大熱消渴**狂煩**, "It controls massive heat, melting with thirst, and **madness with vexation**".

Kuang gou **狂狗, rabid dog** [3]
Identical with → *kuang quan* 狂犬, rabid dog. *WTMY* 40: **狂狗**咬人，每至七日即合一發, "When a **rabid dog** bites a person, [the resulting disease] will break out after seven days".

Kuang huo **狂惑, madness with delusion** [5]
IS identical with → *kuang luan* 狂亂, madness with confusion. *BJ* SE *bai wei* 白微：主暴中風，身熱肢滿，忽忽不知人，**狂惑**, "It controls sudden wind stroke with the body being hot and the limbs having a feeling of fullness. Suddenly one fails to recognize people. **Madness with delusion**".

Kuang jiao **狂叫, crazy shouting** [3]
IS of people shouting meaninglessly with a loud voice as if they were crazy. *RHZ* SE *bai he* 百合：癲邪啼泣，**狂叫**驚悸, "Peak-illness evil, weeping tears, **crazy shouting**, palpitation with fright".

Kuang jing **狂痙, madness with spasms** [4]
PC CD of → *kuang* 狂, madness, and → *jing* 痙, spasms. *BJ* SE *niu huang* 牛黃：主驚癇寒熱，熱盛**狂痙**, "It controls fright epilepsy with alternating sensations of cold and heat, as well as plenty of heat with **madness and spasms**".

Kuang luan **狂亂, madness with confusion** [16]
IS of an abnormal psychic state including meaningless activity, confused language, and uncontrolled emotions of joy and anger. *JGYL* Lj: 菜中有水莨菪，葉圓而光，有毒，誤食之，令人**狂亂**, "Among the vegetables is *shui lang dang*. Its leaves are circular and glossy, and it is poisonous. If inadvertently one consumes it, he will develop **madness with confusion**".

***Kuang men* 狂悶, madness with heart-pressure** [3]
IS CD of → *kuang luan* 狂亂, madness with confusion, and → *fang men* 煩悶, vexation with heart-pressure. *RHZ* SE *dan shen* 丹參：頭痛赤眼，熱温**狂悶**, "Headache with red eyes, heat, warmth, and **madness with heart-pressure**".

***Kuang nüe* 狂瘧, madness malaria** [2]
PC of → *nüe ji* 瘧疾, malaria ailment, associated with illness signs of heat, madness and restlessness. *BCGM* SE *zi shen* 紫參 quotes Wang Haogu 王好古：主**狂瘧**瘟瘧, "It controls **madness malaria** and warmth malaria".

***Kuang quan* 狂犬, rabid dog** [20]
Refers to rabid dogs, and also to humans that have been bitten by rabid dogs and have therefore been affected themselves by rabid dog disease. *QJYF* 22 *wu ma gao* 烏麻膏：**狂犬**蟲狼六畜所傷不可識者, "If someone has been harmed by **rabid dogs**, bugs/worms, wolves, or the six domestic animals, and if one does not know [which of these animals caused the injury]".

***Kuang re* 狂熱, madness with heat** [5]
IS identical with *re kuang* 熱狂, heat with madness. *YXL* SE *bei zi* 貝子：治傷寒**狂熱**, "It cures harm caused by cold, and **madness with heat**".

***Kuang ti* 狂啼, madness with crying** [1]
IS of uncontrollable crying with loud voice as if in a state of madness. *BCSY* SE *la xue* 臘雪：小兒熱癇**狂啼**，大人丹石發動, "In children it cures heat with epilepsy, and **madness with crying**; in adults excitement brought forth by a consumption of cinnabar [et al.] mineral substances".

***Kuang wang* 狂妄, madness with absurd behavior** [3]
IS of an abnormal psychic state of one's emotions running unreasonably high, with excessive self-centeredness and self-confidence. *SW* 70: 其病笑，瘧，瘡瘍，血流，**狂妄**，目赤, "Its illnesses are laughing and malaria, sores and ulcers, blood flow, **madness and absurd behavior**, as well as red eyes".

***Kuang xie* 狂邪, madness evil** [12]
① PC identical with → *feng kuang* 風狂, wind madness. *MYBL* SE *bai xiong ji rou* 白雄雞肉：主下氣，療**狂邪**，安五藏, "It controls by making qi descend. It cures **madness evil**. It pacifies the five depots".
② IS identical with → *kuang luan* 狂亂, madness with confusion. *MYBL* SE *xuan shen* 玄參：主暴中風、傷寒，身熱支滿，**狂邪**忽忽不知人, "It controls sudden wind stroke, harm caused by cold, with a hot body and a feeling of fullness in the limbs. [Patients] have a **madness evil** and no longer recognize others".

***Kuang yan* 狂言, crazy language** [18]
IS of confused and rude language lacking logic and reason. *LS* 22: **狂言**、驚、善笑、好歌樂、妄行不休者，得之大恐, "**Crazy language**, fright, a tendency to laugh, an inclination to sing and be joyous, and unending absurd movements, one gets this after having been severely frightened".

***Kuang yi* 狂易, madness with altered [behavior]** [5]
IS identical with → *kuang luan* 狂亂, madness with confusion. *BJ* SE *qiang lang* 蜣螂：主小兒驚癇，瘈瘲，腹脹，寒熱，大人癲疾**狂易**, "In children it

controls fright epilepsy, tugging with convulsion, and abdominal distension. In adults, peak-illness ailments and **madness with altered [behavior]**".

Kuang yu **狂語, crazy language** [4]
IS identical with → *kuang yan* 狂言. *ZBYHL* 25: 心腹煩亂，不食而**狂語**, "Vexation and confusion in the heart and abdomen; rejection of food; **crazy language**".

Kuang yue **狂越, jumping in madness** [5]
IS identical with → *kuang luan* 狂亂, madness with confusion. *SW* 74: 諸躁**狂越**，皆屬於火, "All [cases of] overexcitement and **jumping in madness**, without exception they are associated with fire".

Kuang yun **狂運, madness with dizziness** [1]
IS CD of → *kuang* 狂, madness, and → *xuan yun* 眩運, dizziness. *RHZ* SE *bai he* 百合：治產後血**狂運**, "It cures bleeding and **madness with dizziness** after delivery".

Kuang zao **狂躁, madness with restlessness** [12]
IS of an extreme state of agitation, close to wind disease and madness. *TPSHF* 84: 心神**狂躁**，身熱如火，頭痛煩渴，眠臥不得, "The spirit of the heart displays **madness with restlessness**. The body is as hot as fire. Headache, vexation, and thirst. One cannot lie down to sleep".

Kuang zou **狂走, crazy walking** [29]
IS of disorderly walking without destination, without caring about being tired, and without considering perils. *BJ* SE *fang kui* 防葵：温瘧，癲癇，驚邪**狂走**, "Warmth malaria, peak-illness with epilepsy, fright evil with **crazy walking**".

Kuangji **狂疾, madness ailment** [1]
PC identical with → *feng kuang* 風狂, wind madness. *NJ* 59: **狂疾**之始發，少臥而不飢，自高賢也，自辨智也，自倨貴也，妄笑好歌樂，妄行不休是也, "When the **ailment of madness** breaks out for the first time, [patients] do not lie down much and they have no appetite. They think of themselves as the greatest, wisest, and worthiest. They laugh without meaning, and they love to sing and be joyful. Their endless movements make no sense".

Kui cao **潰槽, bursting trough** [1]
PC of the second stage of → *zou ma ya gan* 走馬牙疳, running horse dental *gan*-illness, with the signs of the first stage → *peng sha* **崩砂**, collapsing sand, and in addition festering and decaying teeth and gums. *HYKY* 18: 盛則齦爛，名曰**潰槽**, "When it has gained strength, the gums will rot. This is called '**bursting trough**'".

Kui ji **瘣疾, demonic ailment** [2]
PC identical with → *yin tuo* 陰脫, yin prolapse. *SYDXF* 15: 磁石散，治子宮不收，名**瘣疾**, "Powder with *ci shi* cures a uterus that fails to recede. This is called '**demonic ailment**'".

***Kui xu* 虧虛, deficient and depleted** [1]

PC identical with → *xu* 虛②, depletion. *SJZL* 88: 內傷於肺，陽氣**虧虛**，故呼吸微弱, "Internally the lung was harmed. The yang qi is **deficient and depleted**. Hence breathing is weak".

***Kui yang* 潰瘍, festering ulcer** [7]

PC of → *chuang yang* 瘡瘍, ulcerous sores, that have opened to fester. *SJZL* 133: 周官瘍醫掌腫瘍、**潰瘍**、金瘍、折瘍, "Among the Zhou officials, the physician responsible for ulcers took care of swollen ulcers, **festering ulcers**, ulcers inflicted by metal [objects], and ulcers resulting from fractures".

***Kun juan* 困倦, fatigue** [5]

IS of a feeling of spiritual and physical fatigue. *SJZL* 13: 夜夢驚恐，精神**困倦**, "If during the night one has terrifying dreams, his essence spirit will be **fatigued**".

- L -

***La li* 蠟梨, polished pear** [2]
PC identical with → *bai tu* 白禿, white baldness. *BCGM* SE *zhu du chong* 竹蠹蟲：小兒**蠟梨**頭瘡，取慈竹內者，搗和牛溺塗之, "For **polished pear** and head sores of children, take those found in *zi*-bamboo, pound with ox urine, and smear it [on the lesion]".

***La li* 臘梨, preserved pear** [2]
PC identical with → *bai tu* 白禿, white baldness, resembling the appearance of a preserved pear. *BCGM* SE *fei zao jia* 肥皂莢 quoting *PJF*: 大人小兒禿刺黎溜膿, "For adults and children with baldness, *la-li* (i.e. a phonetic transliteration of 臘梨, *la li*, with two characters meaning, among other things, "cut and black") and beginning putrescence", writes: **臘梨**頭瘡：不拘大人小兒, "**Preserved pear** and head sores, regardless of whether adults or children are affected".

***Lai* 癩, *lai*-illness; repudiation-illness** [p] AN *chuang lai* 瘡癩, sores of repudiation-illness; *lai chuang* 癩瘡, repudiation-illness sores; *lai ji* 癩疾， ailment of repudiation-illness; *lai bing* 癩病, disease of repudiation-illness; *e lai* 惡癩, malign repudiation-illness; *du lai* 毒癩, poison repudiation-illness; *chong lai* 蟲癩, bug repudiation-illness.
PC identical with → *da feng* 大風②, massive wind. *ZBYHL* 37: **癩**病，是賊風入百脈，傷五臟，連注骨髓俱傷，而發於外，使眉睫墮落，皮肉生瘡，筋爛節斷，語聲嘶破。而毒風之變，冷熱不同，故腠理發**癩**，形狀亦異, "**Repudiation-illness** results from robber wind entering the one hundred vessels, harming the five depots, flowing into the bones and their marrow and harming all [these structures]. When it then dissipates towards the outside, it causes the eyebrows and eyelashes to fall off and generates sores in the skin and flesh. The sinews decay, the joints are severed, and language is hoarse and broken. Because the poison wind undergoes changes, [the appearances of the disease] differ according to whether there is cold or heat. Hence the interstitial structures develop **repudiation-illness**. The physical appearance [of those afflicted] looks rather strange".

***Lai bing* 癩病, disease of repudiation-illness** [2]
PC identical with → *lai* 癩, repudiation-illness . *ZHF* 5: **癩病**方，初覺皮膚不仁，或淫淫苦癢如蟲行，或眼前見物如垂絲，或癮疹赤黑，此即急療, "Recipes for **the disease of repudiation-illness**. At first there is a feeling of numbness in the skin. In some cases [patients have a feeling] as if there was something [in their skin]. They suffer from an itch as if bugs/worms were moving [in the skin]. In some cases one sees items like drooping silk threads in front of the eyes. In some cases there is a tendency to develop red and black dormant papules. These [conditions] must be cured quickly".

***Lai chuang* 癩瘡, repudiation-illness sores** [6]
PC a) identical with → *lai* 癩, repudiation-illness. *QJYF* 12: **癩瘡**，先以酢泔洗後，取藥和豬脂敷之, "**Repudiation-illness sores**: First wash [the lesions]

with vinegar and the slop from rinsing rice. Then take the remedies, mix with lard and apply externally". b) Identical with → *tu chuang* 禿瘡, baldness sores. *BCGM* SE *mu fu rong* 木芙蓉quotes *YXJC*: 頭上**癩瘡**：芙蓉根皮為末，香油調傅。先以松毛、柳枝煎湯洗之, "For **repudiation-illness sores** on the head: prepare a powder from the bark of the root of *fu rong*, mix with *xiang you* and apply externally. Before this [treatment, the lesion] is to be washed with a decoction made from pine nedles and willow twigs".

Lai feng **癩風, repudiation wind** [6]
PC identical with → *feng lai* 風癩, wind repudiation-illness. *BCGM* SE *ban xia* 半夏: quotes *SJZL*: **癩風**眉落，生半夏、羊屎燒焦，等分為末，自然薑汁日調塗, "[For treating] **repudiation wind** with eyebrows falling off: burn equal amounts of fresh *ban xia* and sheep droppings and powderize, and externally apply mixed with natural ginger juice daily".

Lai ji **癩疾, ailment of repudiation-illness** [14]
PC identical with → *lai* 癩, repudiation-illness. *BJ* SE *shi hui* 石灰：主疽瘍疥瘙，熱氣，惡瘡，**癩疾**，死肌墮眉, "It controls impediment-illness ulcers, *jie*-illness with itching; heat qi, malign sores, and the **ailment of repudiation-illness** with dead muscles and eyebrows falling off".

Lan chi yan **爛赤眼, festering red eye** [3]
PC identical with → *mu chi lan* 目赤爛, eye festering and redness. *BCGM* Bai bing zhu zhi yao 百病主治藥：守宮糞，塗**爛赤眼**, "The excrements of geckos are to be smeared on **festering red eyes**".

Lan chuang **爛瘡, festering sores** [27]
PC a) CD of open → *chuang* 瘡, sores, conditions with localized erosion. *ZHF* 5: 赤龍皮湯，洗諸敗**爛瘡**方, "The decoction with *chi long pi* is used to wash all types of decaying **festering sores**". b) Identical with → *biao chuang* 熛瘡, flaming-heat sores. *QJYF* 5: 小兒瘡初起，熛漿似火瘡，名熛瘡，亦名**爛瘡**, "When sores in children start to emerge, they are flaming red with a thick liquid resembling fire sores. They are called flaming-heat sores; they are also called **festering sores**".

Lan dou **爛痘, festering smallpox** [5]
PC of → *dou chuang* 痘瘡, smallpox sores, with festering skin rash. *CSXZ* 28: 蟬花散，治**爛痘**生疽蟲, "Powder with *chan hua* cures impediment-illness bugs/worms generated by **festering smallpox**".

Lan hou **爛喉, festering throat** [1]
PC of a festering throat. *SHZBL* 3: 黑龍煎，治咽喉腫痛九種疾…急喉閉、纏喉風、結喉、**爛喉**、重舌、木舌、遁蟲、蟲喋、飛絲入喉, "Decoction with *hei long* cures nine types of ailments of swollen and aching throats…acute throat closure, throat-constricting wind, bound throat, **festering throat**, doubled tongue, wooden tongue, run-away bug, floating worm-borer, and flying silk threads entering the throat".

Lan xian **爛弦, festering [eyelid] rim** [10]
PC AD of → *lan xian feng yan* 爛弦風眼, festering [eyelid] rim with wind eye. *WSYJF* 7: 用銅青、白堊粉、五倍子為末。熱湯泡，閉目熱洗，冷再熱洗之，**爛弦**者最效, "Prepare a powder from *tong qing*, *bai e fen* and *wu pei zi* and heat to boiling. Wash the closed eyes with the hot liquid. When [the liquid] is cold heat it again to wash the [eyes]. For **festering [eyelid] rim** this is most effective".

Lan xian feng chi **爛弦風赤, festering [eyelid] rim with wind redness** [1]
PC identical with → *lan xian feng yan* 爛弦風眼, festering [eyelid] rim with wind eye *BCGM* Bai bing zhu zhi yao 百病主治藥quoting main text of SE *huang lian* 黃連：爛弦風眼, "Festering [eyelid] rim with wind eye", writes: **爛弦風赤**, "**Festering [eyelid] rim with wind redness**".

Lan xian feng chi yan **爛弦風赤眼, festering [eyelid] rim with wind red eyes** [1]
PC identical with → *lan xian feng yan* 爛弦風眼, festering [eyelid] rim with wind eye. *BCGM* SE *yang* 羊quotes *YJZ*: 二百味草花膏，治**爛弦風赤眼**, "The paste with the 200 herbal flowers cures **festering [eyelid] rim with wind red eyes**".

Lan xian feng yan **爛弦風眼, festering [eyelid] rim with wind eye** [14] AN *lan xian feng chi* 爛弦風赤, festering [eyelid] rim with wind redness; *lan xian feng chi yan* 爛弦風赤眼, festering [eyelid] rim with wind red eyes; *feng lan yan* 風爛眼, wind festering eye
PC of a → *feng yan* 風眼, wind eye, with apparent festering of the eyelids. *BCGM* SE *shui yin fen* 水銀粉 quoting *TPSHF* 32: 眼赤爛， "Eyes, red and festering", writes: **爛弦風眼**, festering [eyelid] **rim with wind eye**".

Lan yong **爛癰, festering obstruction-illness** [1]
PC identical with → *yong chuang* 癰瘡, obstruction-illness sores b). *BCGM* Bai bing zhu zhi yao 百病主治藥：地骨皮，洗**爛癰**, "With *di gu pi* rinse **festering obstruction-illnesses**".

Lan zhang **嵐瘴, hazy miasma** [4]
EA identical with → *zhang qi* 瘴氣, miasmatic qi ①. *RHZ* SE *shi yan* 石燕：御風寒，**嵐瘴**，温疫氣, "Controls wind cold, **hazy miasma**, and warmth epidemic qi".

Lang lou **狼瘺, wolf fistula** [1]
PC of → *lou* 瘺, fistula, initially developing as swelling in the neck. Later on this moves to the broken bowl region (supraclavicular fossa) where it opens to fester, and also it moves upward to link up with the ears. They ache and release pus. *TPSHF* 66: 治**狼瘺**發於頸耳，疼痛出膿水，空青散方, "For treating **wolf fistula** developing at the neck and the ears, which ache and release pus, [use] the recipe for the powder with *kong qing*".

Lao **勞, exhaustion; fatigued** [885] AW 癆.
① PC AD of → *xu lao* 虛勞, depletion exhaustion. *SW* 74: 勞者温之, "That which is **fatigued**: warm it".

② EA of any excessive exhaustion of physical or mental powers, as well as of subtle matter in the human organism, including excessive sexual intercourse, uncontrolled eating and drinking. Also, physical and mental exhaustion that may bring forth a wide range of pathological conditions. *SW* 39: **勞**則喘息汗出，外內皆越，故氣耗矣, "**Exhaustion** causes panting breath and sweat to leave [the body]. Both outside and inside [the limits] are exceeded. Hence, the qi is wasted".

③ Hard work to exhaustion. *BCGM* SE *su* 粟 quotes *JMYS*: 任性返道，**勞**而無獲, "If one acts self-willed and opposes the Way, he will have worked hard to **exhaustion** and yet remains without result".

***Lao* 癆, exhaustion-illness; fatigued** [5]

PC identical with → *lao* 勞①, exhaustion. *SYSS* Shi yao zong lun 十藥總論: 予師用藥治**癆**，如羿之射，無不中的, "My teacher used pharmaceutical drugs to cure **exhaustion-illness**. It was as if Yi had shot an arrow: there was none that did not hit the target".

***Lao bing* 勞病, exhaustion disease** [4]

PC identical with → *xu lao* 虛勞, depletion exhaustion. *TPSHF* 56 RE *ta gan wan* 獺肝丸, pills with otter liver: 治**勞病**，轉疰相染, "They cure **exhaustion disease** and [prevent] a further transmission".

***Lao chong* 勞蟲, exhaustion bug** [19] AN *lao zhai chong* 勞瘵蟲, exhaustion consumption bug; *zhai chong* 瘵蟲, consumption bug.

EA of a bug capable of causing exhaustion. *RHZ* SE *zao jia* 皂莢：通關節，除頭風，消痰，殺**勞蟲**，治骨蒸, "It penetrates joints, eliminates head wind, dissolves phlegm, kills **exhaustion bugs/worms**, cures bone steaming".

***Lao dan* 勞疸, dan-illness [caused by] exhaustion** [2] AN *lao huang* 勞黃, exhaustion jaundice.

PC of *dan*-illness brought forth by exhaustion. *ZHF* 4: 疸病有五種，謂黃膽，穀疸，酒疸，女疸，**勞疸**也, "There are five types of the disease '*dan*-illness': They include yellow bile; *dan*-illness [caused by] grain; *dan*-illness [caused by] wine; *dan*-illness caused by [exhaustion with] women; and ***dan*-illness caused by exhaustion**". In the *BCGM*, *lao dan* 勞疸 mostly refers to *dan*-illness attributed to sexual exhaustion, to spleen exhaustion, and to food exhaustion.

***Lao fa* 勞乏, exhaustion resulting in fatigue** [9]

① IS identical with *lao juan* 勞倦, exhaustion to being tired. *TBC* SE *bo he* 薄荷：人家種之，飲汁發汗，大解**勞乏**, "This [herb] is cultivated by man. Drinking its juice makes people sweat. It massively resolves **exhaustion that has resulted in fatigue**".

② PC identical with → *xu lao* 虛勞, depletion exhaustion. *YXL* SE *chai hu* 茈胡：能治熱勞，骨節煩疼，熱氣，肩背疼痛，宣暢血氣，**勞乏**羸瘦, "It is able to cure heat exhaustion, an uncomfortable feeling of pain in the bones and joints, pain in the shoulders and back. It stimulates the passage of blood and qi. [It further cures] **exhaustion resulting in fatigue** and emaciation".

***Lao feng* 勞風, exhaustion wind** [1] AN → *xu lao feng* 虛勞風, depletion exhaustion wind.

PC of cough and expectoration of phlegm brought about by wind harm caused by wind in a state of exhaustion. *SW* 10: 唾出若涕，惡風而振寒，此為**勞風**之病, "What is spat resembles snivel [from the nose. The patient] has an aversion to wind and shakes from cold. This is the disease of **exhaustion-wind**".

***Lao feng* 老風, old wind** [2]

PC identical with → *wan feng* 頑風, stubborn wind. *MYBL* SE *mi wu* 蘼蕪：主身中**老風**，頭中久風，風眩, "It controls **old wind** in the body, long-lasting wind in the head, and wind dizziness".

***Lao fu* 勞復, recurrence because of exhaustion**[48]

PC of a renewed outbreak of a serious disease because the patient, after it was healed in the first place, overly exhausted himself too early, did not eat and drink appropriately, and failed to be cautious in his sexual activity. *SHL* 393: 大病瘥後**勞復**者，枳實梔子豉湯主之, "When a massive disease that has been cured undergoes a **recurrence because of exhaustion**, this is to be controlled by means of a decoction with *zhi shi*, *zhi zi*, and *gu*". Cases of recurrence resulting from an inadequate diet are called *shi fu* 食復, recurrence because of food. Cases of a recurrence resulting from immoderate sexual activity are called *nü lao fu* 女勞復, recurrence because of exhaustion from [intercourse with] women. *BCGM* has *shang han lao fu* 傷寒勞復, recurrence, because of exhaustion, of harm caused by cold; *da bing hou lao fu* 大病後勞復, recurrence, because of exhaustion, following a massive disease; *shi xing bing hou lao fu* 時行病後勞復, recurrence, because of exhaustion, following seasonally prevalent diseases; *tian xing lao fu* 天行勞復, epidemic recurrence because of exhaustion; and *du bing chu qi shou lao shang shi zhi fu* 篤病初起受勞傷食致復, recurrence of a serious disease following exhaustion and harm caused by food received at the moment the patient rose for the first time again.

***Lao huang* 勞黃, exhaustion jaundice** [2]

PC identical with → *lao dan* 勞疸, exhaustion with *dan*-illness. *ZBYHL* 12: 額上黑，微汗出，手足中熱，薄暮發，膀胱急，四肢煩，小便自利，名為**勞黃**, "If at dusk the forehead is darkened, with slight sweating, and heat affecting hands and feet, the bladder cramps, the four limbs vexed, and urine flows by itself, this is called '**exhaustion jaundice**'".

***Lao ji* 勞極, exhaustion to the extreme** [15]

PC of a state of → *xu lao* 虛勞, depletion exhaustion, that is an apparent state of kidney depletion. *BJ* SE *a jiao* 阿膠：**勞極**，洒洒如瘧狀，腰腹痛，四肢酸疼，女子下血，安胎"[It cures] **exhaustion extreme;** [patients] shiver as if they suffered from malaria. Their lower back and abdomen ache. Their four limbs are painful. Women lose blood. It pacifies a fetus".

***Lao ji* 勞疾, exhaustion ailment** [5]

PC identical with → *xu lao* 虛勞, depletion exhaustion. *ZBYHL* 3 lists a *dao yin fa* 導引法, therapeutic method of guiding and pulling: 治頸、脊、腰、脚痛，

勞疾, "It cures pain in the neck, the spine, the lower back, and the legs, as well as **exhaustion ailment**".

***Lao juan* 勞倦, exhaustion to being tired** [12]

① EA of extreme exhaustion, including excessive physical and mental exertion. *SW* 62: 有所**勞倦**，形氣衰少，穀氣不盛，上焦不行，下脘不通, "When one experiences **exhaustion to being tired** and when the qi of the physical appearance is weak and diminished and when the grain qi does not abound, the upper burner does not move [its qi] and the lower [stomach] duct is blocked".
② AN *ti juan* 體倦, physical fatigue.
IS of weariness brought forth by extreme exhaustion. *ZBYHL* 1: 極力左右振兩臀，不息九通，愈臀痛**勞倦**, "Shake your behind with utmost force. Do so nine times and this will cure pain in the buttocks and **exhaustion to being tired**".

***Lao jue* 勞絕, exhaustion cut** [1]

PC identical with → *lao ji* 勞極, exhaustion to the extreme. *BJ* SE *bai jiao* 白膠：主傷中**勞絕**，腰痛羸瘦, "It controls harm to the center and **exhaustion cut**, lower back pain and emaciation".

***Lao ke* 勞渴, exhaustion thirst** [2]

PC of thirst brought forth by exhaustion detriment affecting the body liquids. *BCSY* SE *jing jie* 荊芥：去邪，除**勞渴**，出汗，除冷風，煮汁服之, "It drives away evil, eliminates **exhaustion thirst**, causes sweating, eliminates cold wind. Boil the juice and ingest it".

***Lao ke* 勞咳, exhaustion cough** [7]

PC identical with → *lao sou* 勞嗽. *YXL* SE *kuan dong hua* 款冬花：主療肺氣心促急，熱乏**勞咳**，連連不絕，涕唾稠粘, "It controls the cure of lung qi and heart palpitation, heat, weariness, and **exhaustion cough** that continues without ending. Snivel and saliva are thick and sticky".

***Lao li* 勞力, exhaustion of physical strength** [2]

EA of excessive physical exertion or of an inappropriate sudden use of one's strength. *ZBYHL* 8: 言語思慮則勞神，梳頭澡洗則**勞力**，勞則生熱, "Speaking and pondering causes mental exhaustion. Combing and bathing lead to **exhaustion of physical strength**. When exhaustion sets in heat is generated".

***Lao li* 勞痢, exhaustion free-flux illness** [6]

PC of a free-flux illness resembling depletion exhaustion, whereby long-lasting free-flux illness harms the proper qi. *TBC* SE *yang shen* 羊腎：羊腎合脂為羹，療**勞痢**甚效, "A soup prepared from lamb kidneys and fat is very effective in curing **exhaustion free-flux illness**".

***Lao lin* 勞淋, exhaustion dripping** [2]

PC of strangury that has been brought forth by exhaustion harming the kidney qi, and that breaks out when one is affected by further exhaustion. *ZBYHL* 14: **勞淋**者，謂勞傷腎氣，而生熱成淋也, "As for **exhaustion dripping**, that is to say, the kidney qi was harmed by exhaustion. As a result, heat develops and dripping".

Lao long 勞聾, exhaustion deafness [1]

PC of deafness brought forth by a depletion of kidney qi. *TPSHF* 36: 夫**勞聾**者，是腎氣虛乏故也, "Now, as for **exhaustion deafness**, the reason is a depletion of kidney qi".

Lao long 老聾, chronic deafness [2]

PC of → *er long* 耳聾②, deafness, lasting for a very long time. *ZHF* 6 SE *shu dan* 鼠膽：治三十年**老聾**, "It cures **chronic deafness** that has lasted for thirty years".

Lao men 勞悶, exhaustion heart-pressure [2]

IS of a feeling of weariness, vexation, and heart-pressure. *HYBC* SE *wa na qi* 膃肭臍：主五勞七傷，陰痿少力，腎氣衰弱虛損，背膊**勞悶**，面黑精冷，最良, "It controls the five types of exhaustion and seven types of harm. Yin [i.e. penis] dysfunction and loss of strength; kidney qi weakness and depletion detriment; **exhaustion heart-pressure** affecting the region of one's back and arms, with a dark face and cold essence. It is excellent".

Lao nue 勞瘧, exhaustion malaria [17] AN *lao zhang* 勞瘴, exhaustion miasma; *nue lao* 瘧勞, malaria exhaustion.

PC of a malaria that has not been cured for a long time and leaves people in a state of external and internal depletion, and that breaks out following even a slight exhaustion. *ZHF* 3: **勞瘧**積久，眾治不瘥, "**Exhaustion malaria** accumulates over an extended period of time, when all treatments have failed".

Lao nüe 老瘧, chronic malaria [9]

PC of → *nüe ji* 瘧疾, malaria ailment, that has not been cured and has turned into a chronic malaria that may continue for thirty years. *ZHF* 3 lists **老瘧**久不斷者, "**Chronic malaria** that cannot be ended for a long time".

Lao qi 勞氣, qi exhaustion [14]

PC identical with → *xu lao* 虛勞, depletion exhaustion. *MYBL* SE *mu dan* 牡丹：除時氣頭痛，客熱，五勞，**勞氣**, "It eliminates seasonal qi causing headache; visitor heat; the five types of exhaustion; **qi exhaustion**".

Lao re 勞熱, exhaustion heat [39] AW → *re lao* 熱勞, heat exhaustion.

PC of depletion heat brought forth by yin depletion. *ZBYHL* 28: 若腑臟**勞熱**，熱氣乘於肝，而衝發於目，則目熱而澀也，甚則赤痛, "When the palaces and depots have **exhaustion heat**, the heat qi will avail itself of the liver and rush to effuse in the eyes. As a result, the eyes feel hot and rough. In extreme cases, they will be red and ache".

Lao shang 勞傷, exhaustion harm [17]

PC identical with → *xu lao* 虛勞, depletion exhaustion. *BJ* SE *wu wei zi* 五味子：主益氣，咳逆上氣，**勞傷**羸瘦, "It controls the increase of qi, cough with qi rising contrary to its proper flow, **exhaustion harm**, and emaciation".

Lao shou 勞瘦, exhaustion emaciation [25] AW 癆瘦.

PC of → *xu lao* 虛勞, depletion exhaustion, with emaciation of one's physical appearance. *QJYiF* 19: 令人面目枯，無潤澤，精寒**勞瘦**, "It causes a person's face and eyes to wither and lose all their luster and moisture. His essence will be cold, and there is **exhaustion emaciation**".

***Lao shou* 癆瘦, exhaustion-illness with emaciation** [1]
PC identical with *lao shou* 勞瘦. *BCGM* Bai bing zhu zhi yao 百病主治藥 quoting *RHZ* SE *luo bo* 蘿卜：治**勞瘦**咳嗽, "It cures exhaustion with emaciation and cough", writes: 治**癆瘦**咳嗽, "It cures **exhaustion-illness with emaciation** and cough".

***Lao sou* 勞嗽, exhaustion cough** [15] AN *lao ke* 勞咳.
PC of cough brought forth by → *xu lao* 虛勞, depletion exhaustion. *TPSHF* 14: 治傷寒後肺萎**勞嗽**，涕唾稠粘，日晚即發寒熱，面色或赤，心肋妨滿，宜服獺肝圓方, "It cures lung wilting and **exhaustion cough** following harm caused by cold. Snivel and spittle are thick and pasty. In the evening [patients] experience cold and hot spells. Their complexion sometimes turns red. The region of heart and ribs has a feeling of blockage and fullness. In such cases the recipe to ingest the pills with otter liver is advisable.

***Lao sou* 老嗽, chronic cough** [3]
PC identical with → *jiu sou* 久嗽. *BCSY* SE *qu yu* 鴝鵒：臘月得者，主**老嗽**, "Those gathered during *la*-months control **chronic cough**".

***Lao sun* 勞損, exhaustion detriment** [38] AW 癆損.
PC identical with → *xu lao* 虛勞, depletion exhaustion. *ZBYHL* 4: 夫**勞損**之人，體虛，易傷風邪, "Now, people affected by **exhaustion detriment**, their body is depleted and hence easily harmed by wind evil".

***Lao sun* 癆損, exhaustion-illness detriment** [1]
PC identical with → *lao sun* 勞損, exhaustion detriment. *BCGM* SE *fu pen zi* 覆盆子 quoting *KBBC* 療勞損風虛，補肝明目, "It cures exhaustion detriment and wind [intruding into a state of] depletion, supplements the liver and clears the eyes", writes: 療**癆損**風虛，補肝明目, "It cures **exhaustion-illness detriment** and wind [intruding into a state of] depletion, supplements the liver and clears the eyes".

***Lao tan* 勞痰, exhaustion phlegm** [2]
PC of → *tan yin* 痰飲, phlegm rheum, brought forth by → *xu lao* 虛勞, depletion exhaustion, or phlegm rheum accompanied by depletion exhaustion. *RYJY* RE *er chen tang* 二陳湯, decoction with two matured ingredients: 夫二陳湯內有半夏，性煨烈，若風痰、寒痰與食痰則相宜；若**勞痰**、吐血、鼻血、瀉血、尿血、血崩，皆不可用, "Now, the ingredients of *er chen tang*include *ban xia*. Its nature is heating and fierce. In the case of wind phlegm, cold phlegm, and food phlegm [this medication] is appropriate. In the case of **exhaustion phlegm**, blood spitting, nosebleed, blood in the stools, blood in the urine, and blood collapse, it must never be used".

***Lao tan* 老痰, chronic phlegm** [5]
① EA identical with → *jie tan* 結痰, bound phlegm. *ZYMZ* 2: **老痰**，即結痰，頑痰，堅結膠固，吐咯難出, "**Chronic phlegm** is identical to bound phlegm

and stubborn phlegm. It is as hard as glue. It is difficult to emit through vomiting or cough".

② PC of matter in the throat that can neither be coughed up nor be swallowed down. *DXXF* 2: 喉中有物咯不出，咽不下，此是**老痰**, "If there is matter in the throat that can neither be coughed up nor be swallowed down, this is '**chronic phlegm**'".

Lao xin **勞心, heart exhaustion** [3]

PC of a → *xu lao* 虛勞, depletion exhaustion, brought forth by exhaustion detriment affecting the heart. *PJF* 188: **勞心**者，補益其心志, "In the case of **heart exhaustion**, supplement that person's heart/mind".

Lao xue **老血, old blood** [22]

① EA identical with → *su xue* 宿血①, residual blood. *MYBL* SE *she gan* 射干: 療**老血**在心脾間，咳唾，言語氣臭, "It cures **old blood** in the region between heart and spleen, coughing up of spittle, as well as bad odor emitted when one speaks".

② PC identical with → *su xue* 宿血②, residual blood. *MYBL* SE *bi jie* 萆薢: 主傷中恚怒，陰痿失溺，關節**老血**, "It controls harm to the center with rage and anger, dysfunction of the yin [member, i.e. penis] with loss of urine, as well as **old blood** in the joints".

Lao ya jing **老鴉驚, old-crow fright** [1]

PC of → *jing feng* 驚風, fright wind, with a loud cry and subsequent loss of consciousness. *BCGM* SE *shi suan* 石蒜 quotes *WRXXEF*: 小兒驚風：大叫一聲就死者，名**老鴉驚**, "When someone makes one loud cry and then dies, this is called '**old-crow fright**'".

Lao yi **勞役, exhaustion from labor** [9]

EA of excessive physical exertion. *ZBYHL* 21. 風邪傷於腑臟，而血氣虛弱，又因**勞役**，大汗之後，或經大下，而亡津液, "Wind evil has harmed the palaces and depots, and has left blood and qi in a state of depletion weakness. Also, following **exhaustion from labor**, after massive sweating or because of massive menstruation, the body liquids have been lost".

Lao zhai **勞瘵, exhaustion consumption** [34] AW 癆瘵; AD 瘵, AN *zhai ji* 瘵疾, consumption ailment; *xu zhai* 虛瘵, depletion consumption; *lei zhai* 羸瘵, emaciation consumption; *pi zhai* 疲瘵, weariness consumption; *zhai zhu* 瘵疰, consumption attachment-illness; *chuan shi* 傳屍, corpse [evil] transmission.

PC of infectious → *xu lao* 虛勞, depletion exhaustion. *SJZL* 93: 凡欲取下**勞瘵**藥，先服温中平補五臟四神湯， "Whenever one intends to use drugs to end exhaustion consumption one should first ingest the 'decoction with the four wondrous ingredients' that warms the center, and levels and supplements the five depots".

Lao zhai **癆瘵, exhaustion-illness with consumption** [1]

PC identical with → *lao zhai* 勞瘵, exhaustion consumption. *SJZL* 37: 治寒熱往來，久成**癆瘵**，地骨皮湯方, "To cure alternating sensations of cold and heat that, if lasting for an extended period of time, generate **exhaustion-illness with consumption**, [use] the recipe for the decoction with *di gu pi*".

***Lao zhai chong* 勞瘵蟲, exhaustion consumption bugs/worms** [3]
EA identical with → *lao chong* 勞蟲, exhaustion bug. *BCGM* SE *shui ta* 水獺：足…為末酒服，殺**勞瘵蟲**。時珍, "Grind…its feet…to a powder and ingest with wine. It will kill **exhaustion consumption bugs/worms**. [L] SZ".

***Lao zhang* 勞瘴, exhaustion miasma** [1]
PC identical with → *lao nue* 勞瘧, exhaustion malaria. *BCTJ* SE *tu hong shan* 土紅山：治**勞瘴**甚佳, "It is very good for curing **exhaustion miasma**".

***Lao zheng* 勞證, exhaustion condition** [1]
PC identical with → *xu lao* 虛勞, depletion exhaustion. *TPSHF* 48 lists *liu huang wan* 硫黃丸, pills with sulphur: 治積聚氣，多年不消，變成**勞證**, "They cure accumulated and collected qi that has failed to dissolve for many years and has transformed into an **exhaustion condition**".

***Lao zhu* 勞疰, exhaustion attachment-illness** [3]
PC identical with → *lao zhai* 勞瘵, exhaustion consumption. *SYJYBZFL* 10: 夫骨蒸、殗殜、伏連、屍疰、**勞疰**、蟲疰、毒疰、熱疰、冷疰、食疰、鬼疰等，皆曰傳屍者, "Now, bone steaming, progressive calamity, hidden link, corpse [evil] attachment-illness, **exhaustion attachment-illness**, bug attachment-illness, poison attachment-illness, heat attachment-illness, cold attachment-illness, food attachment-illness, and demon attachment-illness; all these are examples of corpse [evil] transmission".

***Lei chan* 羸顫, emaciation with shivering** [1]
IS of an uncontrolled shivering movement of the entire body because of depletion and weakness. *RHZ* SE *yin yu* 茵芋：治一切冷風，筋骨怯弱**羸顫**, "It cures all types of cold wind, and weakness of the sinews and bones, as well as **emaciation with shivering**".

***Lei kun* 羸困, emaciation with weariness** [3]
IS of an emaciated body associated with a feeling of weariness. *MYBL* SE *hu ma* 胡麻：傷寒、温瘧大吐後，虛熱**羸困**, "Depletion heat and **emaciation with weariness** after massive vomiting following harm caused by cold and warmth malaria".

***Lei lie* 羸劣, emaciation with degradation** [2]
PC identical with → *xu lei* 虛羸, depletion and emaciation. *ZBYHL* 38: 暴病**羸劣**，飲食未調, "[The patient] suddenly contracted the disease of **emaciation with degradation**. His beverages and food were not balanced".

***Lei ming* 雷鳴, thunderous sounds** [10]
IS a) identical with → *chang ming* 腸鳴①, intestinal sounds. *YXL* SE *da ji* 大戟：下惡血癖塊，腹内**雷鳴**, "It moves down aggregation-illness lumps of malign blood, as well as **thunderous sounds** in the abdomen". b) Identical with → *hou ming chuan* 喉鳴喘, noisy panting in the throat. *BJ* SE *xing he ren* 杏核人：主咳逆上氣**雷鳴**, "It controls cough with counterflow, rising qi and **thunderous sounds**". This meaning is attested in the *BCGM* only once.

***Lei ruo* 羸弱, emaciation with weakness** [12]

PC identical with → *xu lei* 虛羸, depletion and thinness. *ZHF* 4: **羸弱**，加甘草二兩，並長將息, "For **emaciation with weakness** add *gan cao*, two *liang*, and let the patient rest for an extended period of time."

***Lei shou* 羸瘦, emaciation with thinness, lean** [67]

① PC identical with → *xu lei* 虛羸, depletion and emaciation. *BJ* SE *mai men dong* 麥門冬：主心腹結氣，腸中傷飽，胃絡脈絕，**羸瘦**短氣, "It controls bound qi in the heart and abdomen, harm in the intestines resulting from overeating, interruption of the movement in the stomach network vessels, **emaciation with thinness** and shortness of qi".

② IS of physical emaciation. *SW* 47: 所謂無損不足者，身**羸瘦**，無用鑱石也, "As for the so-called 'do not diminish an insufficiency', when the body is **lean**, do not employ the chisel stone".

***Lei sun* 羸損, emaciation detriment** [1]

PC identical with → *xu sun* 虛損, depletion detriment. *RHZ* SE *fang feng* 防風：五勞七傷，**羸損**盜汗，心煩體重，能安神定思, "The five types of exhaustion and the seven types of harm; **emaciation detriment**, and robber sweat, heart vexation and a feeling of a heavy body. It is able to pacify the spirit and to stabilize thoughts".

***Lei tou feng* 雷頭風, thundering head wind** [16]

PC of → *tou feng* 頭風, head wind, characterized by headache together with lumps rising in the face and/or sounds in the head. *SWBJQYBMJ* 2: **雷頭風**附：夫治雷頭者，諸藥不效，為與證不相對也, "**Thundering head wind**, attachment: Now, for curing thundering head [wind], all pharmaceutical drugs remained without effect. They simply failed to match this condition".

***Lei zhai* 羸瘵, emaciation with consumption** [1]

PC identical with *lao zhai* 勞瘵, exhaustion consumption. *PJF* 233: 外觸風寒，內傷氣血，表裏受病，陰陽相搏，久而不瘳，遂成**羸瘵**, "If on the outside one is struck by wind and cold, and if inside qi and blood are harmed, the outside and inside are affected by disease; yin and yang strike each other. If this is not cured for an extended period of time, it will result in **emaciation with consumption**".

***Lei zi* 瘰子, cluster-illness seeds** [2]

IS of small pimple-like swellings rising from the skin, without the latter changing its color. *BCGM* SE *tao* 桃quotes *TPSHF*: 面上粉刺：**瘰子**如米粉, "Facial flour thorns: these are the **cluster-illness seeds** resembling ground rice".

***Leng* 冷, cold** [p]

① EA identical with → *han* 寒①, cold. *JGYL* Lj: 婦人之病，因虛積**冷**結氣，為諸經水斷絕, "The diseases of women are such that because of depletion they accumulate **cold** [which in turn causes] bound qi. This interrupts their monthly period".

② IS identical with → *han* 寒, cold③. *SHL* 148: 傷寒五六日，頭汗出、微惡寒、手足**冷**, "If harm caused by cold lasts for five, six days, the head will sweat, one has a slight aversion to cold, and the hands and feet are **cold**".
③ PQ identical with → *han* 寒, cold④. *SW* 74: 火淫於內，治以咸**冷**, "If fire has encroached upon the interior, this is treated with salty [flavor] and **cold** [qi]".
④ Low temperature of items. *SW* 35: 頭痛如破，渴欲**冷**飲, "His head aches as if it [were about to] burst. He is thirsty and longs for **cold** beverages".

***Leng bai chuang* 冷敗瘡, cold decay sores** [1]
PC identical with → *leng lou* 冷瘺, cold fistulas. *BCGM* SE *li yü* 鱧魚 quotes *MYBL*: 腸及肝主治**冷敗瘡**中生蟲, "Its intestines and liver control the therapy of bugs/worms growing in **cold decay sores**".

***Leng bi* 冷閉, cold closure** [3]
PC identical with → *leng mi* 冷秘, cold tightness. *BCGM* Bai bing zhu zhi yao 百病主治藥：半夏，辛能潤燥，主**冷閉**，同硫黄丸服, "*Ban xia*, acrid, is able to moisten that which is dried up. It controls **cold closure**. Consume together with the pills with *liu huang*".

***Leng bi* 冷痹, cold blockage** [17]
PC brought forth jointly by a joint invasion, of a condition of yang depletion, of wind and cold evil with aching joints, swelling and distension, and in serious causes impairment of mobility. *QJYF* 7: 腎氣虛弱，臥冷濕當風得之。不時速治，喜流入脚膝，或為偏枯**冷痹**，緩弱疼重, "If the kidney qi is depleted and weak, and if one lies down in a cold and moist place and happens to be affected by wind, this must be treated very soon. [The wind] tends to flow into the legs and knees. In some cases it generates hemilateral withering with **cold blockage**, slackening, weakness, pain and a feeling of heaviness".

***Leng bing* 冷病, cold disease** [14]
PC identical with → *han* 寒, cold②. *ZBYHL* 6: 人多疑**冷病**, "People often suspect they suffer from **cold disease**".

***Leng bing qi* 冷病氣, cold disease qi** [1]
PC identical with → *han* 寒, cold②. *SLBC* SE *ji mi* 稷米：孟詵云：稷，益諸不足。山東多食。服丹石人發熱，食之熱消也。發三十六種**冷病氣**, "Meng Shen: *Ji* augments all insufficiencies. In Shandong they often consume it. People who have ingested elixir minerals effuse heat. When they consume [*ji*], the heat is dissolved. It develops 36 types of **cold disease qi**".

***Leng chuang* 冷瘡, cold sores** [3]
PC of → *chuang* 瘡, sores, which do not ache or itch and cannot be cured for an extended period of time. *ZBYHL* 35: 冷氣入於瘡，令血澀不行，其瘡則頑，令不知痛癢，亦經久難瘥，名為**冷瘡**, "When cold qi enters the sores, the cold blood cannot move freely. As a result the sores become stubborn. They neither ache nor itch, and are incurable for a long time. They are called **cold sores**".

***Leng dai* 冷帶, cold discharge**, [2]
PC of → *dai xia* 帶下, discharge from below the belt, brought forth by depletion cold in the lower burner. The color of the discharge is usually white. *PJF* 329: 冷

帶雜下，多因下焦不固，內挾風冷得之, "**Cold discharge** of varying [color] is often caused by an instable condition of the lower burner. One may get it if one holds wind cold in the body".

***Leng feng* 冷風, cold wind** [26]

EA identical with → *feng leng* 風冷, wind cold. *ZBYHL* 21 refers to a gymnastics as being capable of: 除腹肚**冷風**, "eliminating **cold wind** from the abdomen". *BCGM* refers to the following pathological conditions associated with cold wind: *leng feng wan bi* 冷風頑痹, cold wind with stubborn blockage; *leng feng tan huan* 冷風癱緩, cold wind with paralysis and slackening; *leng feng ma bi* 冷風麻痹, cold wind with hemp[-like numbness] blockage.

***Leng feng shi qi* 冷風濕氣, cold, wind, and moisture qi** [1]

PC brought forth jointly by the three evils → *feng* 風, wind, → leng, 冷, cold, and → *shi* 濕, moisture. *HRXT* 2: **冷風濕氣**，以生薑湯調下, "For **cold, wind and moisture qi** ingest mixed with a decoction of *sheng jiang*".

***Leng gan* 冷疳, cold *gan*-illness** [3]

PC of pediatric → *gan* 疳, *gan*-illness, characterized by a long duration with emaciation and weakness. *XEYZZJ* FJ: 大抵疳病當辨冷熱肥瘦。其初病者為肥熱疳，久病者為瘦**冷疳**, "Generally speaking, *gan*-illness may be divided into the four types of cold [*gan*-illness], heat [*gan*-illness], fat [*gan*-illness], and emaciation [*gan*-illness]. At the onset of the disease [patients] have the fat and heat type of *gan*-illness; when it has lasted for a long time it changes into the emaciation and **cold** types of ***gan*-illness**".

***Leng han* 冷汗, cold sweating** [9]

IS of sweating with both the skin and the sweat being cold. *QJYF* 8: 遺矢便利，**冷汗**出, "[Patients] will experience free-flux defecation, and **cold sweating**".

***Leng hua* 冷滑, cold smoothness; cold [and] smoothing** [12]

① PC of stools outflow and incontinence brought forth by harm caused by cold and yang depletion with cold in the depots. *TPSHF* 40: 治**冷滑**，下痢不禁，虛羸，縮砂丸方, "Recipe for pills with *suo sha* to cure **cold smoothness**, discharge with free-flux illness and incontinence, as well as depletion with emaciation".

② PQ of substances of a cold nature and a smoothing and disinhibiting effect on stools and urination. *BCJJZ* SE *luo kui* 落葵：葉惟可蒸鮓，性**冷滑**, "The leaves can be steamed to be prepared as vegetables with salted ground rice and other condiments. Their nature is **cold [and] smoothening**".

***Leng ji* 冷疾, cold ailment** [7]

PC identical with → *han* 寒, cold②. *QJYiF* 3, SE *wu tou* 烏頭：主食不下，心腹**冷疾**, "It controls [a condition in which] food fails to move down, when the center and abdomen have a **cold ailment**".

***Leng ji* 冷積, cold accumulation** [14]

① EA identical with → *ji leng* 積冷, accumulated cold. *SJZL* 57: 有**冷積**不散，乍間乍甚，為久久腹痛者, "If there is **cold accumulation** which fails to disperse, which sometimes intermits and then is extreme again, and causes abdominal pain over a long time".

② PC identical with → *ji leng* 積冷, accumulated cold. *QJYF* 28: 關上脈襜襜大，而尺寸細者，其人必心腹**冷積**, "If a person's movement in the vessels is expanded and massive in his gate section, while it is fine in his foot-long section, he must have a **cold accumulation** in his center and abdomen".

***Leng jia* 冷瘕, cold conglomeration-illness** [2]

PC identical with → *han jia* 寒瘕. *YXL* SE *bie jia* 鱉甲：能主宿食，癥塊，痃癖氣，**冷瘕**勞瘦, "It is able to control food remaining in the body overnight, concretion-illness lumps, string-illness and aggregation-illness qi, **cold conglomeration-illness**, and exhaustion with emaciation".

***Leng jie* 冷結, cold knottings** [1]

EA identical with → *ji leng* 積冷, accumulated cold. *QJYF* 1: 須灸而不與灸之者，令人**冷結**重凝, "If cauterization is required but fails to be applied, this leads to **cold knottings** with heavy coagulation".

***Leng lao* 冷勞, cold exhaustion** [20] AN *han lao* 寒勞.

PC of → *xu lao* 虛勞, depletion exhaustion, with yang depletion and internal cold. *TPSHF* 28: 夫**冷勞**之人，氣血枯竭，表裏俱虛，陰陽不和，精氣散失，則內生寒冷也，皆由臟腑久虛, "Now, people with **cold exhaustion**, their qi and blood are withered and dried up; their outer and inner sections are depleted. Yin and yang do not harmonize. Their essence qi dissipates. As a result they have cold in their interior. The reason is always that their depots and palaces have experienced depletion for an extended period of time".

***Leng lao li* 冷勞痢, cold exhaustion free-flux illness** [1]

PC of → *leng li* 冷痢, cold free-flux illness, continuing for long without cure and leaving the body exhausted and emaciated. *SJZL* 77: 治氣痢不瘥，疲劣變成**冷勞痢**，烏梅丸方, "Recipe for pills with *wu mei* to cure qi free-flux illness that has not been cured, with exhaustion and emaciation resulting in **cold exhaustion free-flux illness**".

***Leng lei* 冷淚, cold tears** [9]

IS of frequent tearflow without swelling of the eyes. The tearflow increases when the eyes face wind. *QJYF* 6: 治目中風，**冷淚**出，眥赤癢，乳汁煎方, "To cure wind in the eyes with a flow of **cold tears**, when the canthi are red and ache, [use] the recipe with boiled human milk".

***Leng li* 冷利, cold free flow; cold [and] disinhibiting** [32]

① PC of → *xia li* 下利, free-flux illness, brought forth by harm caused by cold following an affection with cold. *QJYF* 26: 豕腎，除**冷利**，理腎氣，通膀胱, "Hog kidney: ends **cold free flow**; orders kidney qi; penetrates the bladder".

② PQ of pharmaceutical substances of a cold nature that are able to promote the passage of stools and urine. *BCJJZ* SE *che qian* 車前：子，性**冷利**, "Seeds: their nature is **cold [and] disinhibiting**".

***Leng li* 冷痢, cold free-flux illness** [35]
PC of → *li* 痢, free-flux illness, brought forth by cold evil, with the outflow being either entirely white, or mostly white with some traces of red. *ZHF* 4: 若**冷痢**者，加赤石脂、龍骨，即便愈也, "In the case of **cold free-flux illness**, add *chi shi zhi* and *long gu*, and this will bring an immediate cure".

***Leng lian* 冷臁, cold shanks** [1]
PC identical with → *lian chuang* 臁瘡, shank sores. *BCGM* Bai bing zhu zhi yao 百病主治藥 quoting *JYZF lian chuang* 臁瘡, "Shank sores", writes: *leng lian* 冷臁, "**Cold shanks**".

***Leng lin* 冷淋, cold dribble** [2]
PC of → *lin* 淋, dribble condition, brought forth by depletion cold of kidney qi and characterized by a feeling of shivering with cold prior to urination. *TPSHF* 58: 夫**冷淋**者，由臟腑虛冷。其狀，先寒顫然後尿是也, "Now, as for **cold dribble**, it is caused by depletion cold of the depots and palaces. Its characteristic sign is as follows. First one shivers with cold, and then urinates".

***Leng lou* 冷瘺, cold fistulas** [2]
PC of → *leng chuang* 冷瘡, cold sores, with an unending flow of pus, that do not heal for an extended period of time. *ZBYHL* 34: 瘡得風冷，久不瘥，因成瘺，膿汁不絕，故為**冷瘺**也, "When sores are affected by wind and cold and do not heal for a long time, they will form fistulas with unending flow of pus. Hence these are **cold fistulas**".

***Leng lou* 冷漏, cold drip** [2]
PC identical with → *leng lou* 冷瘺, cold fistulas. *TPSHF* 61: **冷漏**，瘡口膿水常出，經年不乾者, "**Cold drip**: the openings of the sores continuously emit pus and liquid; they do not dry out for years".

***Leng lou chuang* 冷漏瘡, cold leakage sores** [1] AN → *feng lou chuang* 風漏瘡, wind leaking sores.
PC identical with → *leng lou* 冷瘺, cold fistulas. *BCGM* SE *lou lan zi* 漏籃子：主惡痢，**冷漏瘡**, "It controls malign free-flux illness and **cold leakage sores**".

***Leng lu chuang* 冷露瘡, cold dew sores** [1]
PC identical with → *leng lou* 冷瘺, cold fistulas. *PJF* 274: **冷露瘡**，用細茶同藿葉一處煮，一般燒灰，油調，照瘡大小，攤在葉上，貼之, "[To cure] **cold dew sores**, take fine tea leaves and boil them with leaves of pulse plants. Then burn them in a pan to ashes, and mix them with oil. Put this on a leaf the size of the sores and attach it".

***Leng ma* 冷麻, cold and numb** [2]
IS of numbness accompanied by a feeling of cold. *TPSHF* 23: 治腰脚疼痛。攣急不得屈伸，及腿膝**冷麻**，牛膝丸方, "To cure pain in the lower back and legs, when the fists are cramped and one is unable to either bend or stretch [his fingers], and when the thighs and knees are **cold and numb**, [use] the recipe for pills with *niu xi*".

***Leng mi* 冷秘, cold tightness** [3]
PC of → *bian mi* 便秘, constipation, brought forth by either cold evil or a condition of yang depletion with depot cold. *SJZL* 97: 下焦虛冷，窘迫後重，是謂**冷秘**, "When the lower burner is affected by depletion and cold, with a feeling of anal pressure, this is called **cold tightness**".

***Leng nong* 冷膿, cold pus** [10]
IS of greenish-white pus liquid. LSZ believes cold pus that stays in the body is able to cause lower back pain. *RHZ* SE *qian niu zi* 牽牛子：取腰痛，下**冷膿**, "It eliminates lower back pain, and purges **cold pus**".

***Leng pi* 冷澼, cold flush** [1]
PC AW of → *leng pi* 冷癖, cold aggregation-illness. *BCGM* Bai bing zhu zhi yao 百病主治藥：硫黃，**冷澼**在脅，咳逆上氣, "*Liu huang* [cures] **cold flush** in the flanks, and cough with qi rising in counter-movement".

***Leng pi* 冷癖, cold aggregation-illness** [4] AW *leng pi* 冷澼, cold flush.
PC identical with *han pi* 寒癖①. *ZHF* 4: 腹中**冷癖**，水穀癥結，心下停痰，兩脅痞滿, "[To cure] **cold aggregation-illness** in the abdomen, with water and grain forming hidden-illness nodes, halting phlegm below the heart. In both flanks there is an obstacle-illness and a feeling of fullness".

***Leng qi* 冷氣, cold qi** [239]
① EA identical with → *han* 寒①, cold. *ZBYHL* 14: 因乘風取涼，**冷氣**卒傷於肺，即發成嗽, "Because [this person] was intruded by wind and adopted a state of coolness, the **cold qi** caused sudden harm to the lung. This in turn generated cough".
② PC identical with → *han* 寒, cold②. *ZHF* 4: 短氣，心胸滿，心下堅，**冷氣**也，此疾有十許方，"[When a person experiences] shortness of qi/breath, fullness of the heart and chest, as well as hardenings below his heart, this is [a condition of] **cold qi**. For this ailment there are more than ten recipes".

***Leng qi li* 冷氣痢, cold qi free-flux illness** [1]
PC identical with → *leng li* 冷痢, cold free-flux illness. *PJF* 256: **冷氣痢**，風冷，乾薑湯下, "For **cold qi free-flux illness** and wind cold, ingest it with a decoction with *gan jiang*".

***Leng re* 冷熱, cold and heat; cold or hot** [71]
CD of 冷 and 熱. CC, PQ, EA, IS. PC identical with → *han re* 寒熱, cold and heat; cold or hot. *ZHF* 1: 心腹痛皆宿結冷熱所為, "Pain in the heart and abdominal region, this is always caused by bound **cold and heat** having settled there".

***Leng re li* 冷熱痢, cold and heat free-flux illness** [9]
PC CD of → *leng li* 冷痢, cold free-flux illness, and → *re li* 熱痢, heat free-flux illness. *ZBYHL* 17: 夫**冷熱痢**者…冷熱相乘，其痢乍黃乍白是也, "In the case of **cold and heat free-flux illness**, …cold and heat act upon each other. The stools are sometimes yellow, sometimes white".

Leng shan **冷疝, cold elevation-illness** [1]
PC identical with → *han shan* 寒疝①, cold elevation-illness. *HYXS* Lj: **冷疝**腹痛，氣滯不和, "In the case of **cold elevation-illness** the abdomen aches, and the qi flow is sluggish and unbalanced".

Leng sou **冷嗽, cold cough** [2]
PC identical with → *han sou* 寒嗽. *QJYF* 18: 杏仁煎，治**冷嗽**上氣，鼻中不利方, "Decoction with *xing ren*: a recipe to cure **cold cough** with rising qi and a blocked nose".

Leng tan **冷痰, cold and phlegm** [26]
① EA identical with → *han tan* 寒痰①, cold and phlegm. *YXL* SE *wu tou* 烏頭：能治惡風憎寒，濕痹逆氣，**冷痰**包心, "It is capable of curing aversion to wind and a hatred of cold, moisture blockage and counterflow qi, as well as **cold and phlegm** that enclose the heart".
② PC identical with → *han tan* 寒痰②, cold and phlegm. *ZBYHL* 20: **冷痰**者…吞酸氣逆，四肢變青，不能食飲也, "In the case of **cold and phlegm** … one experiences acid regurgitation with qi counterflow. The four limbs assume a greenish-blue color. [Patients] cannot eat or drink".

Leng tong **冷痛, cold pain; to be cold and in pain** [88] AN *han tong* 寒痛, cold pain; *leng teng* 冷疼.
IS of pain accompanied by a feeling of cold. *BJ* SE *wang sun* 王孫：主五藏邪氣，寒濕痹，四肢疼酸，膝**冷痛**, "It controls evil qi in the five depots, cold-moisture blockage, sour pain in the four limbs, and **cold pain** in the knees".

Leng tu **冷吐, cold vomiting; cold spitting** [8]
① PC identical with → *han ou* 寒嘔. *PJF* 26: 丁附散，治**冷吐**，翻胃, "Powder with *ding* and *fu*, to cure **cold vomiting** and upset stomach".
② TA of letting patients gargle with a liquid medication to cure ailments affecting the oral cavity. The patient is requested to hold a warm or hot liquid medication in his mouth until it has cooled down, then he is supposed to spit it out. *QJYF* 6: 治齒間血出方。以苦竹葉濃煮之，與鹽少許，寒温得所，含之，**冷吐**, "Recipe to cure intradental bleeding: Boil bitter bamboo leaves to a thick liquid, and add a little salt. When it is not too cold and not too warm hold it in the mouth until it has **cooled** down, then **spit** it out".

Leng xi rou **冷息肉, cold tumorous flesh-growth** [1]
PI of pale redundant flesh within a → *lou* 瘺, fistula, that is very cold if touched. *ZLBC* SE *hu yin jing* 狐陰莖 quoting *QJYF*: 治一切惡瘺中**冷息肉**, "To cure all types of **cold tumorous flesh-growths** in malign fistula".

Leng xie **冷泄, cold outflow** [11]
PC of → *xie xie* 泄瀉, outflow, brought forth by an affection with cold. *SW* 74: 飲食不下，舌本強，食則嘔，**冷泄**腹脹, "Beverages and food do not descend. The base of the tongue is stiff. What is eaten is thrown up again. [Patients suffer from] **cold outflow** and a distended abdomen".

***Leng xie* 冷瀉, cold outflow** [4]
PC identical with → *leng xie* 冷泄. *WTMY* 37: 五香丸，療心腹鼓脹**冷瀉**, "Pills with five aromatic ingredients heal drum-like distention of the heart and abdomen, and **cold outflow**".

***Leng xuan* 冷痃, cold string-illness** [1]
PC of a feeling of painful string-illness qi resulting from cold that affects older accumulations of evil cold in the abdomen. *WTMY* 12 RE *jie geng fang* 桔梗丸方, recipe for pills with *jie geng*: 療**冷痃**癖氣, "It heals **cold string-illness** with aggregation-illness qi".

***Leng xuan pi* 冷痃癖, cold string-illness with aggregation-illness** [2]
CD of → *leng xuan* 冷痃, cold string-illness, and → *leng pi* 冷癖, cold aggregation-illness. *YXL* SE *tian liao zi* 天蓼子：主**冷痃癖**氣塊，女子虛勞, "It controls qi lumps of **cold string-illness and aggregation-illness**; in women: depletion exhaustion".

***Leng xue* 冷血, cold and blood** [5] AN *han xue* 寒血.
EA resulting from a merging of cold evil with stagnant blood. *ZBYHL* 42: 由挾寒冷宿血在胞而有胎，則**冷血**相搏，令胎不長, "If a woman holds cold and residual blood in her womb and becomes pregnant, **cold and blood** will strike each other. As a result, the fetus cannot grow".

***Leng yue* 冷噦, cold retching** [2]
IS of dry retching appearing as major illness sign of a pathological condition brought forth by drinking water when one has been affected by a warmth disease with heat and fever. *SHZBL* 5: 温病有熱，飲水，暴**冷噦**，茅根葛根湯, "If in the case of warmth disease with fever one drinks water and then experiences violent **cold retching**, [this is to be treated] with a decoction with *mao gen* and *ge gen*".

***Leng yin* 冷飲, cold rheum; cold beverage** [23]
① EA identical with → *han yin* 寒飲, cold drink. *ZBYHL* 42: 妊娠腹滿者，由腹內宿有寒冷停飲，挾以妊娠，重因觸冷，則**冷飲**發動, "When a pregnant woman has a feeling of abdominal fullness, this is because cold beverages have stayed in her abdomen for an extended period of time. If in addition to the pregnancy, there is yet another exposure to cold, **cold rheum** will be activated [to cause the feeling of fullness]".
② Designation of cold beverages, and of the consumption of such beverages. *SW* 35: 頭痛如破，渴欲**冷飲**, "His head aches as if it [were about to] burst. He is thirsty and longs for **cold beverages**".

***Leng zhang* 冷瘴, cold miasma** [2]
PC of → *zhang nüe* 瘴瘧, miasmatic malaria, with a feeling of both extreme cold and fever. *ZNZN* Fj: **冷瘴**，其症惡寒發震發熱, "**Cold miasma**. Its pathological signs include an aversion to cold, shaking, and an effusion of heat".

***Leng zhang* 冷脹, cold distension** [2]
① PC of drum-like distension brought forth by cold. *SLBC* SE *wei rou* 蝟肉：此豬多食苦參，不理**冷脹**，只理熱風水脹, "These pigs eat much *ku shen*.

[Hence their meat] is not capable of regulating **cold distension**; it is able only to regulate distensions because of heat, wind, and water".
② IS of a distension that develops accompanied by a feeling of cold or cold. *QJYF* 4: *qin di li* 秦荻梨：主心腹**冷脹**, "Controls **cold distension** of the heart and abdominal region".

***Leng zheng* 冷證, cold condition** [1]
PC identical with → *han* 寒, cold②. *SYDXF* 12: 蒜丸，治**冷證**腹痛, "Pills with *suan* cure **cold condition** and abdominal pain".

***Leng zheng* 冷癥, cold concretion-illness** [5]
PC of → *zheng* 癥, concretion-illness, brought forth by cold evil and stagnant blood. *YXL* SE *yang qi shi* 陽起石：能暖女子子宮久冷，**冷癥**寒瘕, "It is able to provide a uterus with warmth that has been affected by cold over a long time, with **cold concretion-illness** and cold conglomeration-illness".

***Leng zhi* 冷滯, cold sluggish [discharge]; cold sluggishness** [7]
PC of a) → *zhi xia* 滯下, sluggish discharge, with the color of the discharge being mostly white. *QJYF* 15: 治中結陽丸，斷**冷滯**，下赤白青色如魚腦，脫肛出，積日腹痛，經時不斷者方, "The pills that regulate the center and bind yang [qi]: they end **cold sluggish** discharge of a red-white-greenish color reminiscent of fish brain, with prolapse of the rectum, and abdominal pain over several days that does not end during menstruation". b) Of all diseases constituting a long-term stagnation in the organism of cold items such as wind, phlegm, qi, blood, and pus in the body. *QJYF* 12: 胞中瘀血**冷滯**, "Stagnant blood with **cold sluggishness** in the uterus". *TPSHF* 44: 腎臟風虛**冷滯**, "Kidney depot wind [intruding into a state of] depletion and **cold sluggish [discharge]**". *TPSHF* 50: 五膈氣脾胃**冷滯**, "The five types of occlusion qi with **cold sluggishness** in the spleen and stomach. *TPSHF* 51: 心膈**冷滯**痰飲嘔逆, "Cold sluggishness of phlegm rheum in the heart and diaphragm with vomiting and counterflow". *PJF* 286 refers to flesh with white pus and diminished blood as: 瘡口**冷滯**, "**Cold sluggishness** in the opening of sores".

***Li* 癘, illness affecting many; epidemic; *li*[-wind]** [7]
PC a) identical with → *wen yi* 瘟疫, warmth-illness epidemic. *QJYF* 15: 臟腑傷痾，隨時受**癘**, "When the depots and palaces are harmed by an *a*-illness, they will subsequently be affected by an **epidemic**". b) identical with → *da feng* 大風 massive wind②. *SW* 42: **癘**者，有榮氣熱胕，其氣不清，故使其鼻柱壞而色敗，皮膚瘍潰, "In case of ***li*[-wind]**, the camp qi is hot and rots. This qi is not clear. Hence, it makes the nasal column decay and ruins the complexion. The skin has ulcers and festers".

***Li* 痢, free-flux illness; diarrhea** [p]
① PC AD of → *li ji* 痢疾, free-flux illness ailment. *ZBYHL* 17: 其**痢**而赤白者，是熱乘於血，血滲腸內則赤也；冷氣入腸，搏於腸間，津液凝滯則白也；冷熱相交，故赤白相雜, "If in the case of **free-flux illness** [the feces] has a red and white color, heat has availed itself of the blood. As soon as the blood seeps into the intestines [the feces assumes] a red color. When cold enters

the intestines, it throbs in the intestines. The body liquids coagulate and their movement is sluggish; [the feces assumes] a white color. Cold and heat interact. Hence red and white mix with each other".

② IS a) identical with *xie xie* 泄瀉①, outflow. *ZHF* 8: 若積聚堅結，服四丸，取**痢**, "In the case of accumulations and collections, hardenings and formation of nodes, ingest four pills. This will cure **free-flux illness**". b) Of a discharge of pus and blood. *BCGM* Li Dongyuan sui zheng yong yao fan li 李東垣隨證用藥凡例：先**痢**後便，黃檗為君，地榆佐之。先便後**痢**，黃芩為君，當歸佐之, "If there is **free-flux illness** first, followed by [normal] defecation, *huang bo* will be the ruler [drug in the recipe], *di yu* will assist it. If there is [normal] defecation first, followed by **free-flux illness**, *huang qin* serves as the ruler, assisted by *dang gui*".

Li **利, free flow; to enable free flow; to regulate; to benefit** [p]

① IS a) identical with → *xie xie* 泄瀉①, outflow. *SHL* 34: 太陽病，桂枝證，醫反下之，**利**遂不止, "If in the case of major yang disease, which is a *gui zhi* condition, the physician inappropriately drains it, this causes unending **free flow**". b) designation of various normal physiological functions, identical with the meaning of *tong li* 通利, "free flow".*SHL* 59: 大下之後，復發汗，小便不**利**者，亡津液也。勿治之，得小便**利**，必自愈, "If after a massive discharge and repeated sweating urine does not **flow freely**, this is because of a loss of body liquids. This must not be treated. To obtain a **free flow** of urine, [the organism] will heal itself".

② PC identical with → *xie xie* 泄瀉②, outflow. *SHL* 159: 此**利**在下焦，赤石脂禹餘糧湯主之, "This is a **free flow** from the lower burner. The decoction with *chi shi zhi* and *yu yu liang* will control it".

③ TA of a) stimulating urination and defecation as well as discharge of pathological matter, such as cold pus, phlegm accumulations, as well as extravascular blood. *SHL* 179: 少陽陽明者，發汗、**利**小便已，胃中燥、煩、實、大便難是也, "In cases where the minor yang and yang brilliance [conduits are affected] if one has induced sweating and **stimulated the free flow** of urine, this is a condition with dryness in the stomach, vexation, repletion, and difficult defecation". b) regulating or strengthening the functions and constitution of the organism, including *li wei* 利胃，**regulate** stomach functions; *li fei* 利肺, **regulate** lung functions; *li shui dao* 利水道, **enable free flow** in the passage ways of water; *li xue mai* 利血脈, **enable free flow** in blood vessels; *li er mu* 利耳目, **strengthen the functions** of the ears and eyes; *li qiao* 利竅, open orifices; *li ren* 利人, **benefit** humans; *li lao ren* 利老人, **benefit** old people, etc. *SW* 40: 以五丸為後飯，飲以鮑魚汁，**利**腸中及傷肝也, "Five pills are to be taken before meals; they are to be swallowed with abalone liquid. They **clear** the intestines and the center, and they reach a harmed liver".

Li **瘰, pervasion-illness** [p]

PC identical with → *luo li* 瘰癧, scrofula with pervasion-illness. *SYDXF* 19: 海菜丸，治**癧**生於頭項上交接, "Pills with edible seaweed. They cure **pervasion-illness** developing where the head and nape meet".

***Li chuang* 瀝瘡, pervasion-illness sores** [3]

PC identical with → *luo li* 瘰癧. *BCGM* SE *shang lu* 商陸 quoting *WTMY* 23: 療瘰癧方, "Recipe to cure scrofula", writes: 項上**瀝瘡**, "**Pervasion-illness sores** on the nape".

***Li feng* 癘風, epidemic wind** [14]

PC identical with → *da feng* 大風, massive wind. *SW* 42: 鼻柱壞而色敗，皮膚瘍潰，風寒客於脈而不去，名曰**癘風**, "It causes the nasal column to decay and ruins the complexion. The skin has ulcers and festers. If wind and cold settle in the vessels and do not leave, this is called '**epidemic wind**'". *BCGM* occasionally has → *feng li* 風癘, wind epidemics.

***Li feng* 痢風, free-flux illness wind** [1]

PC of → *li ji* 痢疾, ailment of free-flux illness, in its final stage when patients suffer from aching and dysfunctional legs. *BCGM* SE *gu sui bu* 骨碎補 quoting *ZZYJ*: 痢後風 ，因痢後下虛，不善調將，或多行，或房勞，或感外邪，致兩脚酸軟，若痛若痹，遂成風痢, "Wind after free-flux illness: If after a free-flux illness the lower [body section] is depleted and not well harmonized and nourished, or if one has walked much, or if he has taxed himself in the women's quarters, or if he was affected by an external evil, so that both legs are sore and soft, with sensations of pain and blockage, this generates wind free-flux illness", writes: 遂成**痢風**, "This generates **free-flux illness wind**".

***Li hun* 離魂, *hun*-soul departure** [4]

PC of persons believing to see their own physical appearance. *QJF*: 人自覺自形作兩人，並臥，不別真假。不語，問亦無對。乃是**離魂**, "If someone believes he and his physical appearance are two persons, who lie down side by side, and if he is unable to distinguish between real and false, does not speak, and when asked fails to answer, this is a case of ***hun*-soul departure**".

***Li ji* 痢疾, ailment of free-flux illness** [29] AD *li* 痢; AN *chang pi* 腸澼, intestinal flush; *zhi xia* 滯下, sluggish discharge; *xia li* 下痢, discharge with free-flux illness; *li xia* 痢下, free-flux illness discharge; *xie li* 泄痢, free-flux illness; *xie li* 瀉痢, free-flux illness; *pi xie* 澼泄, flushing outflow.

PC of abdominal pain, with internal cramps and a feeling of heavy pressure at one's behind. Patients excrete a mucous liquid with pus and blood. The frequency of defecation grows while the amount passed decreases. *YXL* SE *hong dou kou* 紅豆蔻：去宿食，温腹腸，吐瀉**痢疾**, "It removes food that remains in the body overnight. It warms abdomen and intestines. [It cures] spitting with outflow, as well as the **ailment of free-flux illness**". *BCGM* speaks of *shi xing li ji* 時行痢疾, seasonally active ailment of free-flux illness; *jin kou li ji* 禁口痢疾, clenched jaw with the ailment of free-flux illness; *xiu xi li ji* 休息痢疾, resting ailment of free-flux illness; *chi bai li ji* 赤白痢疾, ailment of red and white free-flux illness; *wu se li ji* 五色痢疾, ailment of five-colors free-flux illness.

***Li ji* 裏急, internal tension** [21]

IS of a) intra-abdominal cramps with an uncomfortable feeling of pain. *JGYL* Lj: 暮即發熱，少腹**裏急**, "Heat effuses at sunset, and there is a feeling of **internal**

tension in the lower abdomen". b) a feeling of an urge to defecate. *XMLF* 10: 泄瀉膿血，四肢沉重，臍腹疼痛，**裏急**，夜起頻並, "Outflow with pus and blood, the four limbs feel very heavy. Pain in the region of navel and abdomen. **Internal tension** [urges people to defecate] several times during the night".

***Li ji hou zhong* 裏急後重, internal tension and pressure behind** [17]
IS of a very uncomfortable abdominal pain with a frequent urge to defecate, and while there is a feeling of a heavy load having arrived at the anus, defecation is impossible because there is nothing left. *NJ* 57: 大瘕泄者，**裏急後重**，數至圊而不能便，莖中痛, "In the case of a massive conglomeration-illness with outflow, one feels **internal tension and pressure** behind. One goes to the latrine frequently and is still unable to pass stools. Pain is felt in the penis".

***Li jie* 歷節, pervading joints [wind]** [21]
PC identical with → *li jie feng* 歷節風, pervading joints wind. *JGYL* Fj: 病**歷節**，不可屈伸，疼痛，"If one suffers from **pervading joints [wind]** he cannot bend and stretch, and is in pain".

***Li jie feng* 歷節風, pervading joints wind** [21]
PC of → *tong feng* 痛風, pain wind, characterized by spontaneous sweating, shortness of qi/breath, aching joints, and difficulties in bending and stretching. *ZBYHL* 2: **歷節風**之狀，短氣，白汗出，歷節疼痛不可忍，屈伸不得是也，"The signs of **pervading joints wind** are shortness of qi, release of white sweat (i.e. cold sweat, or spontaneous sweat), an unbearable pain pervading the joints, as well as an inability to bend and stretch".

***Li qi* 癘氣, epidemic qi** [1]
EA identical with → *yi qi* 疫氣, epidemic qi. *ZHF* 2: 其年歲中有**癘氣**兼挾鬼毒相注，名為溫病, "In the middle of that year **epidemic qi** and demonic poison merge with each other. This is called warmth disease".

***Li shui* 裏水, internal water** [1]
PC of → *shui zhong* 水腫, water swelling, disease with the body being swollen and turning yellow, a deep movement in the vessels, and anuria. *JGYL* Mj: **裏水**者，一身面目黃腫，其脈沉，小便不利, "In the case of **internal water**, the complete body, including the face and eyes, is yellow and swollen. The [movement in the] vessels is in the depth, and urine cannot be passed freely".

***Li xia* 利下, free flow discharge** [21]
① PC identical with → *xie xie* 泄瀉②, outflow. *BCGM* SE *wo niu* 蝸牛：面上赤瘡，鼻上酒齇，久**利下**脫肛, "[It cures] red sores on one's face, wine sediments on the nose, chronic **free flow discharge** and prolapse of the rectum".
② PE of increased urination and defecation, including diarrhea or discharge of various body matters, following the intake of medications. *TPSHF* 11: 分溫二服，如人行五七里再服。當**利下**惡物, "Ingest two dosages, warm. Ingest the second dosage after the time it takes a person to walk five to seven *li*. This will cause **free flow discharge** of malign items".

Li xia **痢下, free-flux illness discharge** [25]
PC identical with *xia li* 下痢, discharge with free-flux illness. *QJYF* 15: 治**痢下**久不瘥神驗方, "Wondrously effective recipe to cure **free-flux illness discharge** that fails to heal over an extended period of time".

Li xu **裏虛, interior depletion** [3], AN *nei xu* 內虛.
PC brought forth by depletion weakness of qi and blood in the depots and palaces. *SHL* 214: 明日又不大便，脈反微澀者，**裏虛**也，為難治, "The next day, if there is again an inability to defecate, but the [movement in the] vessels is faint and rough, this is **interior depletion**. This is difficult to cure".

Li xue **痢血, free-flux illness with blood** [12]
PC a) identical with → *xue li* 血痢, bloody free-flux illness. *WTMY* 25: 熱毒**痢血**，其痢行數甚，數痢出不多，腹中刺痛, "In the case of **free-flux illness with blood** resulting from heat poison, the frequency of free-flux illness is greatly increased, while the amount discharged is not large. There is piercing pain in the abdomen". b) Identical with → *bian xue* 便血, stools with blood. *MYBL* SE *bai ye* 柏葉：主吐血、衄血、**痢血**、崩中, "It controls blood spitting, nosebleeds, **free-flux illness with blood**, and collapsing center".

Li xue yao tong **瀝血腰痛, trickling blood and lumbar pain** [2]
PC identical with → *xue li yao tong* 血瀝腰痛. *YXL* SE *dang gui* 當歸：主女人**瀝血腰痛**, "It controls **trickling blood and lumbar pain** of females".

Li yang **癧瘍, pervasion-illness with ulcer** [18]
PC identical with → *li yang feng* 癧瘍風, pervasion-illness with ulcer wind. *ZBYHL* 31: **癧瘍**者，人有頸邊、胸前、掖下自然斑剝，點相連，色微白而圓，亦有烏色者，亦無痛癢，謂之癧瘍風, "**Pervasion-illness with ulcer**: when someone has macules with interconnected dots at the sides of the neck, on the chest, and in the armpits, that appear to have come by themselves, are white and round, occasionally black, and neither itch nor ache, this is called pervasion-illness with ulcer wind". *BCGM*: **癧瘍**是汗斑，癜風是白斑片，赤者名赤疵, "**Pervasion-illness with ulcer** manifests itself as sweat macules. Patch wind appears as white macule flakes. Red ones are called red blemishes".

Li yang feng **癧瘍風, pervasion-illness with ulcer wind** [19] AD *li yang* 癧瘍, pervasion-illness with ulcer
PC of white macules and dots appearing on the skin in the neck, on the chest, and below the armpits, without itching or pain. *ZBYHL* 31: 人有頸邊、胸前、掖下自然斑剝，點相連，色微白而圓，亦有烏色者，亦無痛癢，謂之**癧瘍風**, "If someone has macules with interconnected dots at the sides of the neck, on the chest, and below the armpits, that appear to have come by themselves, are white and round, occasionally black, and neither itch nor ache, this is called **pervasion-illness with ulcer wind**".

Li yi **癘疫, epidemic** [1]
PC identical with → *wen yi* 瘟疫, warmth-illness epidemic. *BCTJ* SE *ta gan* 獺肝 RE *ta gan wan* 獺肝丸, pills with otter liver: 諸鬼毒**癘疫**等, "[They cure] all types of **epidemics** caused by demonic poison".

Li zi **瘰子, pervasion-illness seeds** [5]

PC identical with → *luo li* 瘰癧, scrofula with pervasion-illness. *BCSY* SE *tie ruo* 鐵爇：項邊**癧子**，以桃核燒熏, "[For treating] **pervasion-illness seeds** at the side of the nape, burn with peach kernels for steaming".

Lian chuang **臁瘡, shank sores** [49] AN *heng chuang* 胻瘡, shin sores; *jing chuang* 脛瘡, lower leg sores.

PC of chronic ulcerous conditions developing on the front side of the shinbone. *SSLF* 7: 治遠年裏外**臁瘡**不差, "To cure chronic inner and outer **shank sores** that do not heal".

Lian mei **煉眉, tempered eyebrows** [2]

PC identical with → *lian mei chuang* 煉眉瘡, tempered eyebrows sores. *BCGM* Bai bing zhu zhi yao 百病主治藥：諸瘡下：頭瘡、軟癤、禿瘡、**煉眉**, "All types of sores, final section: head sores, soft pimples, baldness sores, **tempered eyebrows**".

Lian mei chuang **煉眉瘡, tempered eyebrow sores** [2] AD *lian mei* 煉眉, tempered eyebrows.

PC identical with → *mei chuang* 眉瘡, eyebrow sores. *BCGM* SE *gan guo* 甘鍋：主**煉眉瘡**、湯火瘡，研末，入輕粉少許傅之, "To control **tempered eyebrow sores** and hot water burns, grind [it] to a powder, add a little *qing fen* and apply this externally".

Lian yin chuang **煉銀瘡, tempered-silver sores** [1]

PC identical with → *mei chuang* 眉瘡, eyebrow sores. *WKJY* Lj: 治小兒面湮瘡，俗云煉銀**瘡**者，是母受胎之日，食酸辣及邪味過度，多生此瘡, "To cure facial clog-up sores in children. This is commonly called '**tempered-silver sores**'. When a mother, on the day she conceives the child, eats too much sour and peppery food or bad substances, [the child] is likely to develop these sores".

Lian yin xuan **煉銀癬, tempered-silver *xuan*-illness** [1]

PC identical with → *mei chuang* 眉瘡, eyebrow sores. *BCGM* Bai bing zhu zhi yao 百病主治藥：煉眉，即**煉銀癬**, "Tempered eyebrows, this is identical with **tempered-silver *xuan*-illness**".

Liang gan shang han **兩感傷寒, dual-affection harm caused by cold** [1]

PC of a type of → *shang han* 傷寒, harm caused by cold brought forth by cold evil affecting all yin and yang conduits in the inner and outer sections of the human body. *SHBZG* 1: 傷寒熱甚雖不死，**兩感傷寒**漫料理, "If the case of harm caused by cold heat is extreme one still does not die. In the case of **dual-affection harm caused by cold** one must proceed slowly to handle this".

Lin **淋, dripping** [p] AN *lin bing* 淋病, dripping disease; *lin ji* 淋疾, dripping ailment; *lin zheng* 淋證, dripping condition.

PC of a frequent urge to urinate, with the urine dribbling and failing to completely leave the body. The urinary tract is rough and painful, the lower abdomen is hard, tense and aches. *JGYL* 13: **淋**之為病，小便如粟狀，小腹弦急，痛引臍中, "The disease of **dripping**: the urine appears like millet. The lower abdomen is as tense as a string. The pain pulls on the navel".

***Lin bi* 淋閉, dripping [resulting from] blockage** [12] AW 淋閟, dripping [resulting from] closure.

PC a) CD of → *lin bing* 淋病, dripping disease, and → *long bi* 癃閉, protuberance-illness with blockage. *BJ* SE *shi long chu* 石龍蒭：心腹邪氣，小便不利**淋閉**, "[To cure] evil qi in the heart and abdomen, inhibited urine flow, with **dripping [resulting from] blockage**". b) Occasionally used for female amenorrhea. *BCGM* SE *niu xi* 牛膝 quotes *BCF*: 萬病丸：治婦人月經**淋閉**，月信不來, "The pills for a myriad of diseases: They cure a woman's menstrual **dripping [resulting from] blockage**, and complete failure of the monthly period to arrive".

***Lin bi* 淋閟, dripping [resulting from] closure** [5]

PC identical with → *lin bi* 淋閉 a). *BCGM* SE *can* 蠶：下焦熱痛**淋閟**，消腫毒, "[It cures] heat pain in the lower burner with **dripping [resulting from] closure**. It dissolves swelling and poison".

***Lin bing* 淋病, dripping disease** [4]

PC identical with → *lin* 淋, dripping. *JGYL* 13: 消渴小便利**淋病**脈證並治, "It cures [movements in the] vessels and pathological conditions of melting with thirst, uninhibited flow of urine, and **dripping disease** alike".

***Lin ji* 淋疾, dripping ailment** [19]

PC identical with → *lin* 淋, dripping. *WTMY*38: 石氣流入膀胱，作其**淋疾**, "Stone qi flows into the urinary bladder where it generates the **dripping ailment**".

***Lin jie* 淋結, nodes leading to dripping** [5]

IS of failure of urine to pass associated with a feeling of distension and fullness in the lower abdomen. *MYBL* SE *ge shang ting chang* 葛上亭長：主蠱毒鬼疰，破**淋結**積聚，墮胎, "It controls *gu* poison and demon attachment-illness; it breaks through **nodes leading to dripping**, as well as accumulations and collections. It causes abortion".

***Lin li* 淋瀝, dripping** [52]

① AN *lin lu* 淋露[sweat]dripping [like] dew drops. IS of various types of rough and trickling discharge, such as *xiao bian* 小便, urine; *jing xue* 經血, menstrual blood; *bai dai* 白帶, white [discharge from below the] belt; *e lu* 惡露, lochia; *bai jing* 敗精, vanquished essence/semen; *bian xue* 便血, urine with blood, etc. *ZBYHL* 14: 數而且澀，則**淋瀝**不宣，故謂之為淋, "If [urination is] frequent and rough, [the liquid] **drips** and is not drained completely. Hence one calls it 'dripping'".

② PC of various ailments with dripping as their major sign. *BJ* SE *bai xian* 白鮮：主頭風，黃疸，咳逆，**淋瀝**，女子陰中腫痛, "It controls head wind, yellow *dan*-illness, cough with qi counterflow, **dripping**, and painful swelling in the private parts of females".

***Lin li* 淋漓, dripping** [8]

IS of discharges, be it vomiting, excretions, or any seeping via the skin, leaving the body in small amounts only with interruptions and failure of complete evacuation. *QJYF* 4: 胞門不閉，**淋漓**去血，經逾日月不止, "The gate of the bladder is not closed, through **dripping** it loses blood. This continues for days and months without end".

***Lin long* 淋癃, dripping and protuberance-illness** [1]
PC referring to → *lin* 淋, dripping. *BCGM* SE *xun lu xiang ru xiang* 熏陸香乳香 quoting *SYDXF* RE *ru shi san* 乳石散, powder with *ru shi*: 治血淋及五淋, "It cures blood dripping and the five types of dripping", writes: **淋癃**溺血, "**Dripping and protuberance-illness** with blood in the urine".

***Lin lou* 淋漏, dripping leakage** [2]
PC identical with → *lou xia* 漏下, leaking discharge. *QJYF* 30: 大泉、照海，主不字，陰暴出，**淋漏**，月水不來, "The [insertion of a needle at the holes called] *da quan* and *zhao hai* controls inability to have a child, sudden uterine prolapse, **dripping leakage**, and failure of the monthly period to arrive".

***Lin lu* 淋露, [sweat] dripping [like] dew drops** [16]
IS a) identical with → *lin li* 淋瀝①, dripping. *BJ* SE *mu xiang* 木香：強志，主**淋露**, "It strengthens the mind, and controls **dripping [like] dew drops**". b) A manifestation of depletion and exhaustion. *LS* 73: 審其所在，寒熱**淋露**，以輸異處, "Find out the whereabouts [of the disease]. Because cold and heat and [sweat] **dripping [like] dew drops** [may be situated at different locations] their transportation holes are in different places".

***Lin lu* 林露, forest dew** [1]
IS erroneous writing of → *lin lu* 淋露, dripping [like] dew drops b). *BCGM* SE *ji ni* 薺苨：蠱毒腹痛，面目青黃，**林露**骨立, "*Gu* poison with abdominal pain; the face and eyes green-yellow; **forest dew** and bones visible under the skin". The phrase 骨立 appears in the *BCGM* four times; the writing 林露骨立 appears once, presumably as a scribal error.

***Lin mi* 淋秘, dripping with blockage** [1]
PC identical with → *long lin* 癃淋, protuberance-illness and dripping. *PJF* 214 has a section 小便**淋秘**, "Urinary **dripping with blockage**".

***Lin se* 淋澀, dripping with roughness** [13]
IS of a feeling of roughness in the urinary tract and inhibited urination. *QJYF* 3: 葵根湯，治產後**淋澀**方, "Decoction with *kui gen* is a recipe to cure **dripping with roughness** following delivery".

***Lin ti* 鱗體, scaly body** [1] AN *tai gou* 胎垢, fetal filth; *she ti* 蛇體, snake body.
PC of newborns with a coarse skin throwing off scraps like the scales of a snake. *XEWSZWLF* 20: **鱗體**者，謂皮膚之上，如蛇皮鱗甲之狀, "A '**scaly body**' is to say: an appearance of scales, like a snake, on the skin".

***Lin tong* 淋痛, dripping with pain** [17]
IS identical with → *se tong* 澀痛 a), roughness and pain. *ZBYHL* 38: 二者陰中**淋痛**, "The second [type of pain] is **dripping with pain** in [a female's] private parts".

***Lin zhuo* 淋濁, dripping turbidity** [1]
PC identical with → *zhuo lin* 濁淋, turbid dripping. *YXRM* 4: 蒸下則見遺精、**淋濁**、泄瀉、腰痛、脚酸、陰物自強等證, "If the lower body section is steamed, this will bring forth conditions such as involuntary loss of essence/semen, **dripping turbidity**, outflow, painful lumbar region, sore legs, and a spontaneous stiffening of the yin item (i.e. male member)".

***Liu* 瘤, tumor** [p]
PC of soft topical swellings in the skin that neither itch nor are painful. In the beginning they may be the size of a plum; gradually they grow larger. *ZBYHL* 31: **瘤**者，皮肉中忽腫起，初如梅李大，漸長大，不痛不癢，又不結強, "**Tumors**: suddenly a swelling rises in the skin. In the beginning it is the size of a plum. Gradually it grows larger. It does not ache, and it does not itch. Also, it does not turn into unyielding nodes".

***Liu du* 流毒, flowing poison** [3]
EA of → *du qi* 毒氣, poison qi, moving between organs or other regions in the body and causing illness. *SJZL* 142: 血痔者，肺熱**流毒**也, "Bleeding piles are [caused by] **flowing poison** of lung heat".

***Liu fu nüe* 六腑瘧, six types of palace malaria** [1]
PC erroneous writing of → *liu jing nüe* 六經瘧, six types of conduit-specific malaria. *BCGM* Bai bing zhu zhi yao 百病主治藥：五臟瘧、**六腑瘧**、勞瘧、瘧母, "Five types of depot malaria; **six types of palace malaria**, exhaustion malaria, malaria mother".

***Liu gou* 留垢, remnants of filth** [3]
PP of pathological matter remaining in the body, identical with → *su gou* 宿垢, overnight filth. *TYBC ze xie* 澤瀉：**留垢**，即胞中陳積物也, "'**Remnants of filth**', that is items collecting in the bladder for an extended time".

***Liu ji* 六極, six types of extreme [exhaustion]** [4]
PC CD of extreme depletion detriment conditions of the human body, its essence, qi, and/or blood. *BJ* SE *sang gen bai pi* 桑根白皮：主傷中，五勞**六極**，羸瘦，崩中脈絕，補虛益氣, "It controls central harm; the five types of exhaustion and **six types of extreme [exhaustion]**; emaciation; collapsing center and interrupted vessel [movement]. It supplements depletion and increases qi".

***Liu ji* 六急, the six types of tension** [2]
PC CD of tension and stiffness of vessels and sinews and impeded movement. *BJ* SE *gan qi* 乾漆：安五藏，五緩**六急**，風寒濕痹, "It pacifies the five depots, the five types of slackening and **the six types of tension**, as well as wind cold moisture blockage".

***Liu jie* 留結, abiding node** [9]
① EA PM of all types of pathogenic evil stagnating in the body. *BYHL* 31: **留結**不散，謂之為瘤, "When **abiding nodes** fail to dissipate, this is called 'tumor'".
② AN *pi jie* 痞結, obstacle-illness node. PC caused by abiding nodes. *YD* SE *ba dou* 巴豆：主痰飲**留結**，利水穀, "It controls phlegm rheum and **abiding nodes**; and it frees the passage of water and grain (i.e. liquid and solid food)".

***Liu jing nüe* 六经疟, six types of conduit-specific malaria** [1]
PC CD of → *nüe ji* 瘧疾, malaria ailment, differently affecting the foot yin and yang conduits. *SW* 36 lists different malaria conditions such as *zu tai yang zhi nüe* 足太陽之瘧, foot major yang malaria; *zu shao yang zhi nüe* 足少陽之瘧, foot minor yang malaria; *zu yang ming zhi nüe* 足陽明之瘧, foot yang brilliance malaria; *zu tai yin zhi nüe* 足太陰之瘧, foot major yin malaria; *zu shao yin zhi nüe* 足少陰之瘧, foot minor yin malaria; *zu jüe yin zhi nüe* 足厥陰之瘧, foot ceasing yin malaria. *QXLF* 12: 素問論**六經瘧**, "The *Su wen* discusses **six types of conduit-specific malaria**".

***Liu jing tou tong* 六經頭痛, six types of conduit-specific headache** [1]
PC CD of → *tai yang tou tong* 太陽頭痛, major yang headache; → *yang ming tou tong* 陽明頭痛, yang brilliance headache; → *shao yang tou tong* 少陽頭痛, minor yang headache; → *shao yin tou tong* 少陰頭痛, minor yin headache; *tai yin tou tong* 太陰頭痛, major yin headache; → *jue yin tou tong* 厥陰頭痛, ceasing yin headache. *BCGM* Li Dong yuan sui zheng yong fan li 李東垣隨證用藥凡例 quoting Li Dongyuan's 李東垣*YYXF*: 如頭痛須用川芎 writes: **六經頭痛**須用川芎, "For [a cure of] the **six types of conduit-specific headache** one must use *chuan xiong*".

***Liu pi* 留澼, abiding flush** [3]
PC identical with → *liu pi* 留癖, abiding aggregation-illness. *BCGM* Bai bing zhu zhi yao 百病主治藥 quoting *BJ* SE *rao hua* 蕘花：腸胃中留癖, "Abiding aggregation-illness in the intestines and the stomach", writes: 腸胃**留澼**, "**Abiding flush** in the intestines and the stomach", and elsewhere: 腸中**留澼**, "**Abiding flush** in the intestines".

***Liu pi* 留癖, abiding aggregation-illness** [2] AW *liu pi* 留澼, abiding flush.
PC of a swelling resulting from rheum remaining in the body, collecting and dispersing at irregular intervals, which is difficult to cure. *BJ* SE *rao hua* 蕘花：蕩滌腸中**留癖**，飲食寒熱邪氣，利水道, "It purges from the intestines **abiding aggregation-illness**, beverages and food, cold and heat, and evil qi".

***Liu qi jie xiong* 留氣結胸, bound chest because of abiding qi** [2]
PC identical with → *xiong bi* 胸痹, chest blockage. *BCTJ* SE *ren shen* 人参：張仲景治胸痹，心中痞堅，**留氣結胸**, "Zhang Zhongjing [applies it] to cure chest blockage, obstacle-illness and hardening in the heart, and **bound chest because of abiding qi**".

***Liu qing shui* 流清水, clear water flow** [3]
IS of large quantities of clear and thin liquid flowing from the mouth. *BCGM* SE *bi ba* 蓽茇 quotes *XQF*: 胃冷，口酸，**流清水**，心下連臍痛, "The stomach is cold, the mouth has a sour [taste], **clear water flow**, pain between the heart and navel".

***Liu qing ti* 流清涕, clear snivel flow** [4] AD *qing ti* 清涕
IS of a profuse flow of clear, water-like snivel. *TPSHF* 37: 治肺虛，外傷風冷，致鼻塞，常**流清涕**，頭目昏疼，四肢不利，服訶黎勒散方, "To cure lung depletion and harm caused by wind cold from the outside resulting in a stuffed

nose and permanent **clear snivel flow**, as well as headache and visual clouding, and the four limbs not functioning properly, [use] the recipe for an ingestion of the powder with *he li lei*".

Liu re **留熱, abiding heat** [15] AN *yu re* 餘熱, residual heat; *yi re* 遺熱, left-over heat.

PC of a → *re bing* 熱病, heat disease, brought about by → *shang han*, 傷寒, harm caused by cold, where the evil heat stays on in the organism despite treatment. Also, of repeated fever brought about by exhaustion or food. *BJ* SE *yan lü* 庵蕳：主五藏瘀血，腹中水氣，臚脹**留熱**, "It controls stagnant blood in the five depots, water qi in the abdomen, as well as distension and **abiding heat**".

Liu shi **留濕, abiding moisture** [4] AN *shi zhi* 濕滯, sluggish moisture.

EA of moisture evil having settled in the organs and conduits. *HJJF* 3 RE *shou zhong jin wan* 守中金丸, gold pills that guard the center: 又治脾胃**留濕**，體重節痛，面色萎黄，肌肉消瘦, "In addition they cure **abiding moisture** in the spleen and stomach, a feeling of bodily heaviness, aching joints, wilting-yellow complexion, as well as emaciation".

Liu shi er zhong feng **六十二種風, sixty two types of wind** [2]

DC *BCTJ* SE *hong lan hua* 紅藍花：張仲景治**六十二種風**，兼腹內血氣刺痛, "Zhang Zhongjing treated the **62 types of wind** along with blood [stasis] and qi [stagnation causing] piercing pain in the abdomen".

Liu shui **流水, water flow** [144]

① IS identical with *chu zhi* 出汁, discharge of liquid. *SJZL* 1: 民病腹滿，身重，濡泄，寒瘍**流水**, "People suffer from a feeling of abdominal fullness. The body feels heavy. They have outflow and **water flow** from cold ulcers".

② PS of water freely flowing in nature. *BJ* SE *yun mu* 雲母：東**流水**為雲母所畏，煉雲母用之，與諸水不同，即其效也, "**Water flowing** eastward is feared by *yun mu*. Use it for refining *yun mu*. It is unlike any other type of water. Hence its effectiveness".

Liu tan **留痰, abiding phlegm** [1]

EA identical with → *ting tan* 停痰, halting phlegm. *YXL* SE *han fang ji* 漢防己：散**留痰**，主肺氣嗽喘, "It disperses **abiding phlegm**, and it controls lung qi cough and panting".

Liu xian **流涎, saliva flow; drooling** [13]

① IS of constant flow of saliva from the mouth. *WTMY* 17: 或口乾舌燥，或**流涎**出口, "In some cases the mouth is dry and the tongue is desiccated, and in other cases there may be **saliva flow** from the mouth".

② PC of drooling. *YYXS* 6: 温胃散，治脾冷**流涎**, "The powder to warm the stomach, it cures spleen cold and **drooling**".

Liu xian **六癇, six types of epilepsy** [1]

PC of → *xian ji* 癇疾, epilepsy ailment, classified into six categories based on pecularities in their appearances and their similarities with certain domestic animals. *BCGM* SE *long chi* 龍齒：六畜齒治**六癇**，皆比類之義也, "Resorting to teeth from the six types of domestic animals to cure the **six types of epilep-**

sy is always based on the idea that [patient appearance and animal appearance] constitute one category".

***Liu xue* 留血, residual blood** [16]

① EA identical with → *su xue* 宿血①. *BJ lu er* 鹿茸：角，主惡瘡癰腫，逐邪惡氣，**留血**在陰中, "The horns master malign sores, obstruction-illnesses and swelling; they eliminate evil and malign qi, as well as **residual blood** in the yin [i.e. male member]".

② PC identical with → *su xue* 宿血②. *YXL* SE *fei lian* 飛廉：主**留血**, "It controls **residual blood**".

***Liu yin* 留飲, abiding rheum** [31]

① EA of → *yin* 飲, rheum, stagnating and accumulating in the body and causing disease. *BJ* SE *da huang* 大黃：破癥瘕積聚，**留飲**宿食，蕩滌腸胃，推陳致新, "It breaks through concretion-illness and conglomeration-illness, accumulations and collections, **abiding rheum** and food remaining in the body overnight, and purges the intestines and stomach. It eliminates that which is old and lets that which is new arrive".

② PC a) CD of all types of rheum diseases brought forth by rheum abiding in the body. *YXL* SE *dong kui zi* 冬葵子：霜葵生食，動五種**留飲**, "*Kui* that has been exposed to frost if consumed fresh will activate the five types of **abiding rheum**". b) Of → *yin* 飲②, rheum, disease brought forth by rheum abiding below the heart. *JGYL* Mj: **留飲**者，脅下痛引缺盆，咳嗽則輒甚, "In the case of **abiding rheum**, there is pain below the flanks that pulls into the broken basin. When [the patient] coughs [the pain] always becomes severe".

***Liu yin* 流飲, flowing rheum** [1]

PC of → *yin* 飲② , rheum, disease brought forth by rheum flowing into the region of intestines and stomach, with the seeping into this region producing sounds. In some cases urination is blocked, and there is shortness of qi. In other cases this goes along with depletion and distension. *ZBYHL* 20: 水流走於腸胃之間，漉漉有聲，謂之**流飲**, "When water flows into the region of the intestines and stomach, with the seeping producing sounds, this is called '**flowing rheum**'".

***Liu ying* 瘤癭, tumorous goiter** [4]

PC identical with → *ying liu* 癭瘤, goiter tumor. *YXL* SE *hai ge* 海蛤：主治項下**瘤癭**, "It controls the treatment of **tumorous goiter** below the nape".

***Liu you* 瘤疣, tumorous wart** [2]

PC CD of → *liu* 瘤, tumor, and → *you* 疣, wart. *BCGM* SE *cao zhi zhu* 草蜘蛛：**瘤疣**：用稻上花蜘蛛十餘，安桃枝上，待絲垂下，取東邊者捻為綫系之。七日一換，自消落也, "For **tumorous warts**: Take at least ten spiders from the blossoms of paddy rice and place them on peach twigs. Wait until they have created threads that hang down. Take those on the eastern side and twist them to strings and wind them around the [tumor or wart]. Change after seven days. They will dissolve and fall off by themselves".

Liu yu **六郁, the six types of pent-up [matter in the organism]** [7]
PC CD of → *qi yu* 氣鬱, pent-up qi; → *shi yu* 濕郁, pent-up moisture; → *tan yu* 痰郁, pent-up phlegm; → *re yu* 熱郁, pent-up heat; → *xue yu* 血郁, pent-up blood; and → *shi yu* 食郁, pent-up food. *DXXF* 3: 傳化失常，**六郁**之病見矣, "When transmission and transformation do not continue as normal, the diseases of any of **the six types of pent-up [matter in the organism]** will appear".

Liu zhu **流注, influx** [14]
① PM of evil qi moving around in, and erratically entering, various parts of the human body. *JGYL* Fj RE *jiu tong wan* 九痛丸, pills for nine types of pain: 又治連年積冷，**流注**心胸痛, "They also cure cold accumulations over several years, as well as **influx** with pain in the heart and chest".
② PC of sores with pus in deep-lying regions of the human body. *WKJY* Mj: 一弱人，**流注**內潰，出敗膿五六碗, "A weak person with **influx** and internal festering emitted five to six bowls of pus".

Liu zhuo ti **流濁涕, turbid snivel flow** [2]
IS of a profuse flow of turbid, pus-like snivel. *SJZL* 180: 治小兒肺傷冷，鼻**流濁涕**，前胡橘皮湯方, "Recipe for a decoction with *qian hu* and *ju pi* to cure children whose lung has been harmed by cold, with **turbid snivel flow**".

Liu zui **瘤贅, tumor reduncancy** [7] AN *zui liu* 贅瘤.
PC identical with → *liu* 瘤, tumor. *BCSY* SE *bo luo hui* 博落回：主惡瘡癭根，**瘤贅**，瘜肉，白癜風, "It controls malign sores and [eliminates] goiter to its root, **tumor redundancy**, tumorous flesh-growths, and white patches wind".

Long **癃, protuberance-illness** [p] AN *long ji* 癃疾, ailment of protuberance-illness.
PC a) AN *long bi* 癃閉, protuberance-illness with closure; *long se* 癃澀, protuberance-illness with roughness; *bi long* 閉癃, closure with protuberance-illness; *long jie* 癃結, nodes of protuberance-illness. Passing of urine in small amounts; in serious cases passage is completely inhibited. *LS* 63: 膀胱之胞薄以懦，得酸即縮卷，約而不通，水道不通，故**癃**, "The urinary bladder is thin and weak. When it is affected by sour flavor it shrinks so much that it is almost impassable. The water tracts are impassable. Hence this results in **protuberance-illness**". b) Identical with → *lin* 淋, dripping. *SW* 23: 膀胱不利為**癃**, "When the urinary bladder is impassable, this is '**protuberance-illness**'".

Long **聾, deafness** [p]
IS, PC identical with → *er long* 耳聾. *SW* 49: 所謂浮為**聾**者，皆在氣也, "As for the so-called '[a movement] near the surface is [a sign of] **deafness**', [that is to say: The reason] always lies with the qi".

Long bi **癃閉, protuberance-illness with closure** [12]
PC identical with → *long* 癃 a), protuberance-illness. *BJ* SE *hua shi* 滑石：女子乳難，**癃閉**，利小便, "[It cures] female lactation problems, as well as **protuberance-illness with closure**, and stimulates urination".

Long bi **聾閉, deafness blockage** [18]
PC identical with → *er long* 耳聾②, deafness. *BCGM* SE *chang pu* 菖蒲 quoting *ZHF*, SE *shui su* 水蘇 quoting *SLBC*, and SE *bi ma* 蓖麻quoting *QJYF*, and SE

mu xiang 木香quoting *WTMY*: *er long* 耳聾, "deafness", always writes: 耳卒**聾閉**, "Ears with sudden **deafness blockage**".

Long er **聾耳, deaf ears** [1]

PC identical with → *er long* 耳聾②, deafness. *ZLBC* SE *gua lou gen* 栝樓根 quotes *ZHF*: 治二三年**聾耳**方：栝樓根三十斤細切之，以水煮，用釀酒如常法，久久服之, "Recipe for **ears that have been deaf** for two to three years: Prepare a fine cut of 30 *jin* of *gua lou* root, boil in water, and prepare a [medicinal] wine from this according to the usual method. Ingest for a very long time".

Long ji **癃疾, ailment of protuberance-illness** [1]

PC identical with → *long* 癃, protuberance-illness. *BCGM xi luo* 犀洛 quoting *MYBL* 主癃, "It controls protuberance-illness", writes: 主**癃疾**, "It controls the **ailment of protuberance-illness**".

Long jie **癃結, protuberance-illness nodes** [1]

PC identical with → *long* 癃 a), protuberance-illness. *BJ* SE *qu mai* 瞿麥：主關格，諸**癃結**，小便不通, "It controls blockage and repulsion, all types of nodes associated with **protuberance-illness**, with blocked urination".

Long lin **癃淋, protuberance-illness and dripping** [4]

PC CD of → *long* 癃, protuberance-illness, and → *lin* 淋, dripping. *BCGM* SE *mu xiang* 木香：膀胱氣不化則**癃淋**, "Failure of the urinary bladder qi to transform results in **protuberance-illness and dripping**". The main feature of "protuberance-illness" is *xia jiao qi bi* 下焦氣閉, a blockage of the qi of the lower burner; the main features of "dripping" are distinguished as → *re lin* 熱淋, heat dripping; → *qi lin* 氣淋, qi dripping; → *xu lin* 虛淋, depletion dripping; → *gao lin* 膏淋, pasty dripping; and → *sha shi lin* 沙石淋, sand and stone dripping.

Long ming **聾鳴, deafness and ringing** [3]

PC identical with → *ming long* 鳴聾, ringing in the ears and deafness. *QJYF* 6: 治耳**聾鳴**，汁出，皆由腎寒，或一二十年不瘥方, "Recipe to cure **deafness and ringing** in the ears with release of liquid. All such conditions result from kidney cold. In some instances a cure is not achieved for ten to twenty years".

Long se **癃澀, protuberance-illness with roughness** [1]

PC identical with → *long* 癃 a), protuberance-illness. *BCGM* SE *mu gua* 木瓜 quoting *LS* 水道不行故癃, "The water tracts are not passable. Hence this is protuberance-illness", writes: 水道不利而**癃澀**, "**Protuberance-illness with roughness** whereby the water tracts are not freely passable".

Lou **漏, leakage** [p]

① PC of various types that have continuous seepage of liquid as their common sign. a) Identical with → *lou chuang* 漏瘡, leaking sores; fistula. *ZBYHL* 50: 時發寒熱，仍膿血不止，謂之**漏**也, "At times [patients] develop alternating sensations of cold and heat. This goes along with unending festering and bleeding. One calls this '**leakage**'". b) Identical with → *lou jing* 漏精, leaking essence/semen. *BCGM* SE *ren gui* 人傀：**漏**者，精寒不固，常自遺泄也, "In the case of '**leakage**', one's essence/semen is cold and unstable. It often flows off spontaneously". c) Identical with → *lou xia* 漏下, "leaking discharge". *ZBYHL* 38: 血非時而下，淋瀝不斷，謂之**漏**, "When blood flows down any time, and when there is continuous dripping, this is called '**leakage**'. d) Later stage in the development of → *zhi chuang* 痔瘡, piles sores, with recurrent bleeding over an extended period of time as a major sign. *DXXF* 2: 諸痔久不愈，必至穿穴為**漏**矣, "All cases of piles that do not heal over an extended period of time will develop holes and eventually turn into **leakage**". e) Identical with → *jiu lou* 九漏, nine types of leakage. *QJYF* 23: 凡項邊、腋下先作瘰癧者，欲作**漏**也, "All cases that begin as scrofula pervasion-illness to the side of the nape or in the armpits may eventually turn into **leakage**".

② PI: the opening of leaking sores where pus is emitted. *QJYF* 23: 搗生商陸根，捻作餅子如錢大，厚三分，安**漏**上, "Grind fresh *shang lu* root and knead into cookies the size of a coin three *fen* thick. Place on the **leakage**".

③ IS of long-term festering sores. *QJYF* 21: 灸刺，則於瘡上**漏**膿水不歇，遂至癰疽羸瘦而死, "If this is cauterized or pierced, there will be unending **leakage** of pus and water from the top of the sores. This will result in obstruction-illness and impediment-illness, emaciation, and eventually death".

***Lou* 瘻, fistula** [p] AN *lou ji* 瘻疾, fistula ailment; *lou chuang* 瘻瘡, fistula sores; *lou chuang* 漏瘡, leaking sores.

PC of tubular structures releasing pus and water from openings failing to close over a long period of time. They develop in the skin or in deep-lying regions of the body from festering scrofula or ulcers that have broken open. *ZBYHL* 33: 若膿汁不盡，多變成**瘻**也, "If the flow of a purulent liquid fails to end, this often develops into **fistula**".

***Lou chou* 漏臭, leakage stench** [1]

PC of a → *hu chou* 胡臭, barbarian stench, with moisture in one's armpit, soles of the feet, palms of the hands, and intimate regions releasing a distinct odor as major sign. *BCGM* Bai bing zhu zhi yao 百病主治藥：胡臭：有體臭，腋臭，**漏臭**, "Barbarian stench includes body stench, armpit stench, and **leakage stench**". *ZBYHL* and other works call this *lou ye* 漏腋, leaking armpit.

***Lou chuang* 瘻瘡, fistula sores** [26] AN *chuang lou* 瘡瘻, fistula.

PC identical with → *lou* 瘻, fistula. *MYBL* SE *kun bu* 昆布：主十二種水腫，癭瘤聚結氣，**瘻瘡**, "It controls the twelve types of edematose swelling, goiter tumor with collected bound qi, and **fistula sores**".

***Lou chuang* 漏瘡, leaking sores** [23] AN *chuang lou* 瘡漏, sores with leakage; *lou* 漏, leakage.

PC identical with → *chuang* 瘻, sores. *QJYF* 5: 牛膝末酒服方寸匕，**漏瘡**多年不瘥，搗末敷之, "Ingest one square inch spoon of *niu xi* powder with wine. For **leaking sores** that have not healed for many years, grind to powder and apply externally".

***Lou dai* 漏帶, leakage [from below the] belt** [3]

PC CD of → *lou xia* 漏下 leaking discharge, and → *dai xia* 帶下②, discharge from below the belt. *BCGM* SE *bai zhi* 白芷：如**漏帶**癰疽諸病，三經之濕

熱也, "All diseases such as **leakage [from below the] belt**, as well as obstruction-illnesses and impediment-illnesses are conditions of moisture and heat in three conduits".

Lou er **漏耳, leaking ear** [1]

PC of → *lou chuang* 漏瘡, leaking sores, with pus flowing out of the ear(s). *PJF* 310: **漏耳**，鼻內生瘡，牙疼等疾, "Ailments such as **leaking ear**, sores growing in the nose, and toothache".

Lou gu lou **螻蛄漏, mole-cricket leakage** [2]

PC of mole-cricket-shaped sores that constitute one of the → *jiu lou* 九漏, nine types of leakage. *QJYF* 23: 荏子桔梗丸，治**螻蛄漏**，始發於頸項，狀如腫, "Pills with *ren zi* and *jie geng*. They cure **mole cricket leakage**. In the beginning it effuses on the front and back of the neck where it looks like a swelling".

Lou ji **瘺疾, fistula ailment** [4]

PC identical with → *lou* 瘺, fistula. *PJF* 292: 琥珀膏，治頸項瘰癧，初起如梅子，腫結硬強，漸若連珠，或穿穴膿潰，流汁不絕，經久難瘥，漸成**瘺疾**，並治之, "Ointment with *hu po*: It cures scrofula pervasion-illness at the neck. In their beginning they rise like a plum kernel. The swelling is unyielding and stiff. Gradually it assumes the appearance of a string of pearls. In some cases holes develop, releasing pus. The flow of liquid is continuous. This lasts long and is difficult to heal. Eventually this develops into a **fistula ailment**. It serves to cure all [these conditions] alike".

Lou ji **漏疾, leakage ailment** [5]

PC identical with → *lou* 漏①. *BCGM* SE *wang gua* 王瓜 quoting *QJYF* 50: 治一切漏, "To cure all types of leakage", writes: 一切**漏疾**, "All **leakage ailments**".

Lou jing **漏精, leaking essence/semen** [8]

PC identical with → *yi jing* 遺精, involuntary loss of essence/semen. *MYBL* SE *an shi liu* 安石榴：酸實殼，療下痢，止**漏精**, "Its sour fruit shells serve to cure discharge with free-flux illness and stop **leaking essence/semen**".

Lou lan **瘺爛, fistula festering** [3]

PC identical with → *lou shi* 瘺蝕, fistula erosion. *RHZ* SE *song zhi* 松脂：煎膏治**瘺爛**，排膿, "Boiled to a paste it cures **fistula festering**, and discharges the pus".

Lou liu **漏瘤, leaking tumor** [1]

PC identical with → *lou chuang* 漏瘡, leaking sores. *BCGM* SE *yang ti* 羊蹄 quoting *ZLBC*: 治**漏瘤**瘡，濕癬癢, 浸淫日廣，癢不可忍, "It cures leaking tumor sores, and moisture *xuan*-illness with itching. The immersion widens day by day. The itching is unbearable", writes: **漏瘤**濕癬，浸淫日廣，癢不可忍, "**Leaking tumors** with moisture xuan-illness. The immersion widens day by day. The itching is unbearable".

Lou nong **漏膿, leaking pus** [2]

IS of festering eyes. *BCGM* SE *long dan* 龍膽 quotes *HFJ*: 眼中**漏膿**：龍膽草、當歸等分，為末。每服二錢，溫水下, "For **leaking pus** in the eyes: a dose of 2 *qian* of powder made from equal amounts of *long dan cao* and *dang gui* is to be ingested with warm water".

Lou ru **瘺乳, fistula breast** [1]

PC of → *lou* 瘺, fistula, developing on a female's breast. *MYBL* SE *wang bu liu xing* 王不留行：止心煩，鼻衄，癰疽惡瘡**瘺乳**，婦人難產, "It ends heart vexation, nosebleed, obstruction-illnesses and impediment-illnesses, malign sores, **fistula breast**, as well as difficult birthing among women".

Lou shi **瘺蝕, fistula erosion** [6] AN *lou lan* 瘺爛, fistula festering.

PC of festering → *lou chuang* 瘺瘡, fistula sores. *MYBL* SE *yan shu* 鼹鼠：主癰疽，諸**瘺蝕**惡瘡, "It controls obstruction-illnesses, impediment-illnesses, and all types of **fistula erosion** and malign sores".

Lou tai **漏胎, leaking fetus** [15] AN *tai lou* 胎漏, fetal leakage; *bao lou* 胞漏, uterine leaking.

PC of vaginal bleeding during pregnancy. *ZBYHL* 43: 產難者，或先因**漏胎**，去血臟燥, "A difficult birth may be caused by **leaking fetus** resulting in a loss of blood and desiccation of the depots".

Lou xia **漏下, leaking discharge** [64] AD *lou* 漏, leakage; AN *lin lou* 淋漏, dripping leakage; *lou xue* 漏血, leaking blood.

PC with a trickling of small quantities of blood from the vaginal tract that cannot be cured over an extended period of time. Sometimes the blood comes mixed with liquids of other colors. *JGYL* Fj: 婦人則半產、**漏下**，男子則亡血、失精, "For women this results in miscarriage and **leaking discharge**. For males this results in blood loss and loss of essence/semen".

Lou xue **漏血, leaking blood** [17]

① IS of a trickling of small quantities of blood from the vaginal tract that every now and then has a turbid appearance. This term may also refer to such type of bleeding from other body parts. *YXL* SE *sang ji sheng* 桑寄生：主懷妊**漏血**不止, "It controls incessantly **leaking blood** during pregnancy".

② PC identical with → *lou xia* 漏下, leaking discharge. *ZBYHL* 38: **漏血**脈浮，不可治也, "Cases of **leaking blood** with a surface [movement in the] vessels cannot be cured".

Lou zhi **瘺痔, fistula piles** [3]

PC identical with → *zhi lou* 痔瘺, piles fistula. *BJ* SE *kong gong nie* 孔公孽：主傷食不化，邪結氣惡，瘡疽**瘺痔**, "It controls harm caused by food that fails to transform, evil [qi] nodes, qi malignity, sores and impediment-illnesses, and **fistula piles**".

Lu chuang **虜瘡, P.O.W. sores** [3]

PC identical with → *dou chuang* 痘瘡, smallpox sores. *ZHF* 2: 建武中，於南陽擊虜所得，仍呼為**虜瘡**, "In the reign period *jian wu* they got it when they came into contact with prisoners of war. Hence it is called '**P.O.W. sores**'".

Lu feng **露風, exposure wind** [2] AN *feng* 風wind.

PM explaining why wind evil was able to intrude into a human organism. *SW* 3: 因於**露風**，乃生寒熱, "If subsequently one **exposes [oneself and is affected**

by] wind, this generates cold and heat". *BCGM* refers to items suddenly **exposed and struck by wind** and therefore changing their quality.

***Lu jie* 顱解, open skull** [2]

PC identical with → *jie lu* 解顱. *BCGM* SE *zhu* 豕quoting *QJYF*: 小兒解顱 writes: 小兒**顱解**, "**Open skull** of children".

***Lu zhang* 臚脹, the abdominal wall is distended** [13]

IS identical with → *fu zhang* 腹脹①, abdominal distension. *SW* 71: 民病腠理熱，血暴溢瘧，心腹滿熱，**臚脹**, "People suffer from heat in the interstitial structures, sudden blood overflow, and malaria. The heart and abdomen are full and hot. **The abdominal wall is distended**".

***Lü zui feng* 驢觜風, donkey-mouth wind** [1]

PC of the lower lip being swollen and aching, and developing sores. *BCGM* Bai bing zhu zhi yao 百病主治藥：井華水，下唇腫痛，或生瘡，名**驢觜風**，以水常潤之，乃可擦藥, "Early morning well-water: when the lower lip is swollen and aches, and sometimes develops sores, this is called **donkey-mouth wind**. Use the [morning well-]water to moisten it and then apply a medication".

***Luan bi* 攣痹, cramps and blockage** [5]

① IS of cramped sinews and fixed bones with blocked conduit vessels. *SW* 12: 其病**攣痹**，其治宜微針, "Their diseases are **cramps and blockage**. For their treatment, fine needles are appropriate".

② PC of → *bi* 痹①a), blockage disease, with cramps and blockages. *SYCZYS* 3: 兼患水腫、消渴、**攣痹**, "A suffering jointly of edemas, melting with thirst, and **cramps and blockage**".

***Luan ji* 攣急, contraction with tension** [36]

IS of a twisted body that is difficult to stretch, accompanied by an uncomfortable contraction that in some cases may generate a feeling of pain. *LS 10*: 手心熱，臂肘**攣急**，腋腫, "The centers of the palms are hot; upper arms and elbows are **contracted with tension**, the armpits are swollen".

***Luan qu* 攣曲, cramps; crooked** [2]

① IS identical with → *luan quan* 攣拳. *QXLF* 64: 治…小腹痛引腰脊**攣曲**，身不能直, "It cures pain in the lower abdomen that pulls on lower back and spine causing a **cramp** that does not allow a person to straighten the body".

② An appearance in the growth of plants when twigs and branches assume a crooked instead of straight appearance. *BCGM* SE *rui xiang* 瑞香：攣枝者，其節**攣曲**，如斷折之狀也, "Bent twigs have joints where they are **crooked**, as if they had been broken".

***Luan quan* 攣拳, cramps** [1] AN *luan qu* 攣曲.

IS of body parts being cramped and unable to be stretched. *SYDXF* 2: 兼寒，則**攣拳**掣痛, "A double affection by cold results in **cramps** and a tugging pain".

***Luan suo* 攣縮, contraction** [16] AD *suo* 縮.

IS of the body being crooked at its joints, making it impossible to straighten it and, instead, causing it to curl up. One is unable to stretch. *BJ* SE *kuo yu* 蛞蝓：主賊風喎僻，軼筋及脫肛，驚癇**攣縮**, "It controls [facial] wryness caused by robber wind, twisted sinews and prolapse of the rectum, as well as fright epilepsy, with [body] **contraction**".

Luan suo **卵縮, egg shrinkage** [5] AN *nang suo* 囊縮scrotal shrinkage; *wai shen chu suo* 外腎搐縮, external kidneys being pulled in and shrinking.

IS of a shrinkage of the scrotum with the testicles being pulled upwards. *LS* 10: 唇青、舌卷、**卵縮**，則筋先死, "If the lips are greenish-blue, the tongue is coiled and the **eggs shrink**, the sinews have died first".

Luan tong **攣痛, contraction with pain** [15] AN *tong luan* 痛攣, pain with contraction; *ju tong* 拘痛, cramps with pain.

IS of pain affecting the extremities accompanied by a spasm making it difficult to stretch them. *ZBYHL* 48: 夫風邪中於肢節，經於筋脈，若風挾寒氣者，即拘急**攣痛**, "Now, when wind evil strikes the joints of the limbs and passes through the sinews and vessels, if the wind is accompanied by cold, it results in cramps with tension, and **contraction with pain**".

Luan tui **卵㿗, eggs affected by prominence-illness** [7]

PC of → *tui* 㿗, prominence-illness, affecting the testicles of males. *ZHF* 5: **卵㿗**，熟搗桃仁，敷之，亦療婦人陰腫，燥即易之, "**Eggs affected by prominence-illness**: Pound ripe *tao ren* to a pulp and smear them [on the afflicted region. This treatment] is also suitable for curing swelling in a woman's genital parts. When it has dried, one must replace [the pulp]".

Luan tui **卵癩, eggs affected by breakdown-illness** [2]

PC identical with → *luan tui* 卵㿗, eggs affected by prominence-illness. *WTMY* 26: 癩有四種，有腸癩、**卵癩**、氣癩、水癩, "There are four types of breakdown-illness: breakdown-illness affecting the intestines; **breakdown-illness affecting the eggs (i.e. testicles)**; qi breakdown-illness; and water breakdown-illness".

Luo li **瘰癧, scrofula pervasion-illness** [200] AN *li* 癧, pervasion-illness; *li zi* 癧子, pervasion-illness seeds; *li chuang* 癧瘡, pervasion-illness sores; *feng li* 風癧, wind pervasion-illness.

PC whereby two or three connected swellings of the size of plum or date kernels appear either on the neck or in the armpits, or somewhere else in the body. In some cases this is accompanied by fever and an aversion to cold, as well as a headache and vexation. As long as the swelling has not opened to fester it is quite hard. This stage is called *jie he* 結核, "nodular kernel". After an extended period of time it generates pus and festers, eventually developing into a fistula. The openings do not heal for a long time. This stage is also called → *shu lou* 鼠瘺, mouse fistula. *LS* 70: "寒熱**瘰癧**在於頸腋," "[Alternating sensations of] cold and heat and **scrofula pervasion-illness** on the neck and in the armpits".

Luo li jie he **瘰癧結核, nodular kernels of scrofula pervasion-illness** [18]

PC of → *lou li* 瘰癧, scrofula pervasion-illness, which have not yet opened to fester. *WTMY* 23: **瘰癧結核**令消散方, "Recipe to dissolve and disperse **nodular kernels of scrofula pervasion-illness**".

***Luo li lou* 瘰癧瘺, scrofula pervasion-illness and fistula** [4]
PC of what originally appeared to be a → *lou li* 瘰癧, scrofula pervasion-illness, but after opening to fester developed into → *lou* 瘺, fistula, in some cases with several heads developing into holes. *ZBYHL* 34: 此由風邪毒氣客於肌肉，隨虛處而停，結為**瘰癧瘺**, "This is because wind evil poison qi has settled in the muscles and the flesh. It avails itself of depleted locations, and forms nodes to become **scrofula pervasion-illness and fistula**".

***Luo li lou* 瘰癧漏, scrofula with pervasion-illness and leakage** [2]
PC identical with → *lou li lou* 瘰癧瘺, scrofula with fistula. *QJYF* 23: 雌黃芍藥丸，治**瘰癧漏**，始發於頸有根，初苦痛，令人寒熱, "Pills with *ci huang* and *shao yao*. They cure **scrofula with pervasion-illness and leakage**. [This condition] first develops at the neck and has a root. From the beginning [patients] suffer pain. It makes them experience alternating sensations of cold and heat".

- M -

***Ma* 麻, hemp[-like numbness]; numbness; tingling; numbing** [p]

① PC identical with → *ma bi* 麻痹, hemp[-like numbness] blockage. *SWXJYBS* Liu qi wei bing 六氣為病：氣行通而**麻**愈也, "Once the qi penetrates [the region again, its] **numbness** will be cured".

② IS with a feeling as if bugs/worms were moving in the skin. *YTBW* 10 SE *qi cao kou ye* 蠐螬口液:擦抹在瘡口上，覺**麻**，身上汗出，無有不活者, "If smeared on the openings of sores it causes a **tingling** feeling, and makes the body sweat, and there is no example that would not have been brought back to life again".

③ A flavor capable of generating numbness of the tip of the tongue. *BCGM* SE *hu zhang tian nan xing* 虎掌天南星：味辛而**麻**，故能治風散血, "Its flavor is acrid and generates **numbness**. Hence it is capable of treating wind and dispersing blood".

***Ma an chuang* 馬鞍瘡, horse-saddle sores** [4]

PC of → *chuang* 瘡, sores, conditions developing below the buttocks. *ZHF* 8: **馬鞍瘡**等，洗即瘥，牛領亦然, "**Horse-saddle sores** etc. heal when washed. The same applies to [sores on a] buffalo's neck".

***Ma bi* 麻痹, hemp[-like numbness] blockage** [42]

① AN *bi* 痹, blockage; numbness. IS of numbness affecting either the limbs and body as a whole, or only sections of it, with a feeling as if insects were crawling, or as if a rope tied around one body part had just been released. *WTMY* 18: 治脚氣，**麻痹**不仁，兩脚緩弱，脚腫無力, "It cures leg qi, **hemp[-like numbness] blockage** with insensitivity, both legs slacken and are weak, the legs are swollen and have no strength".

② PC with hemp[-like numbness] blockage as a major sign *HJJF* 3: 治吐瀉轉筋、癥癖疼痛、風水毒腫、冷風**麻痹**, "It cures vomiting and outflow with twisted sinews, concretion-illness and aggregation-illness, swelling resulting from wind and water poison, and **hemp[-like numbness] blockage** brought forth by cold wind".

***Ma bing* 麻病, hemp[-like numbness] disease** [1]

PC identical with → *ma bi* 麻痹, hemp[-like numbness] blockage. *SWXJYBS* Liu qi wei bing 六氣為病:俗方治**麻病**，多用烏、附, "Popular recipes to cure **hemp[-like numbness] disease** often make use of *wu* [*tou*] and *fu* [*zi*]".

***Ma dao* 馬刀, saber** [7] AN *ma dao jia yin* 馬刀挾癭, saber clinching the goiter.

PC of saber-shaped, hard → *luo li* 瘰癧, scrofula with pervasion-illness, developing in the armpits. According to Li Dongyuan 李東垣, the location where this type of scrofula develops is not decisive for its identification. He called 'saber' all types of scrofula that are hard and do not fester. LSZ adopted this view. *ZNYHL* 32: 堅而不潰者，為**馬刀**也, "Those that are hard and do not fester, they are '**saber**'".

Ma dao jia ying 馬刀挾癭, saber clinching the goiter [1]
PC identical with → *ma dao* 馬刀, saber. *LS* 81: 其癰堅而不潰者，為**馬刀挾癭**，急治之, "Obstruction-illnesses that are hard and do not fester are '**saber clinching the goiter**'. They are to be treated right away".

Ma ding 馬疔, horse pin-illness [1] AN *ma ding* 馬丁.
PC of triangular → *ding chuang* 丁瘡, pin sores, with their peaks bearing black dots while the bottom is of red color. *BCGM* SE *ling li* 鯪鯉 quotes *BaSF*: **馬疔**腫毒：穿山甲燒存性、貝母等分為末, "**Horse pin-illness** with swelling and poison: Equal parts of *chuan shan jia*, burned while retaining its nature, and *bei mu*".

Ma ding 馬丁, horse pin [1]
PC identical with → *ma ding* 馬疔, horse pin-illness. *BCGM* Bai bing zhu zhi yao 百病主治藥：穿山甲，燒研，同貝母末，傅**馬丁**, "*Chuan shan jia*, burned and ground, is externally applied together with *bei mu* powder to **horse pin**".

Ma dou 麻豆, sesame beans [8]
IS of papules resembling pockmarks in size. *MYBL* SE *lou lu* 漏蘆：熱氣瘡癢，如**麻豆**，可作浴湯, "In the case of sores with itching, resembling **sesame beans**, brought forth by heat qi, one can prepare a decoction for washing".

Ma hou bi 馬喉痹, throat blockage [as fast as a galloping] horse [2]
PC identical with → *ji hou bi* 急喉痹, acute throat blockage. *ZBYHL* 30: 熱毒之氣結於喉間，腫連頰而微壯熱，煩滿而數吐氣，呼之為**馬喉痹**, "When the qi of heat poison forms nodes in the throat, with swelling of the adjoining cheeks and a slight to strong fever, vexation, a feeling of fullness, and frequent spitting of qi, this is commonly called '**throat blockage [as fast as a galloping] horse**'".

Ma hou bi feng 馬喉痹風, throat blockage wind [as fast as a running] horse [1]
PC identical with → *zou ma hou bi* 走馬喉痹, running horse throat blockage. *BCGM* SE *ma bian cao* 馬鞭草 quoting *QJYF* 6: 馬喉痹, "Throat blockage [as fast as a running] horse", writes: **馬喉痹風**, "**Throat blockage wind [as fast as a running] horse**".

Ma jie 馬疥, horse _jie_-illness [9]
① PC of → *jie chuang* 疥瘡, *jie*-illness sores, whereby the skin forms scales and scraps, while its base is rough and thick. It itches and if scratched one does not feel any pain. *BJ* SE *liu hua* 柳華：葉，主**馬疥**痂瘡, "The leaves: they control **horse _jie_-illness**, and crust sores".
② VPC of *jie*-illness affecting horses. *BCGM* SE *ma bian cao* 馬鞭草 quotes *JiYF*: 人疥**馬疥**：馬鞭草不犯鐵器，搗自然汁半盞，飲盡，十日內愈, "For human *jie*-illness and **horse _jie_-illness**: Pound *ma bian cao* – without offending it by an iron tool – until half a cup of its natural juice is obtained. Drink this entirely. A cure will be achieved within ten days".

***Ma mu* 麻木, [numbness of] hemp and logs** [24] AN *bi mu* 痹木, blockage [with numbness like a] log.

IS. *Ma* 麻 is "hemp" and refers to an absence of sensations such as pain and itching. There is a feeling as if insects were crawling in one's flesh. The body experiences a tingling sensation as if a tightly wound rope had just been loosened. *Mu* 木 is "log" and refers to an absence of feelings such pain and itching. If pressed or pinched one fails to feel a sensation, as if one were a board of wood. Both terms are often used in combination. *QJYF* 30: 天井，主肩痛，痿痹不仁，不可屈伸，肩肉**麻木**, "[To pierce] the *tian jing* [hole] controls pain in the shoulders, dysfunction and blockage with insensitivity, an inability to bend or stretch, with the shoulder flesh experiencing **[numbness of] hemp and log**".

***Ma pi feng* 馬脾風, horse-spleen wind** [4]

PC of qi rising with rapid panting brought about by an overabundance of heat in the lung. *YKFH* 2: **馬脾風**者，肺脹也，上氣喘急，兩脅扇動，鼻張悶亂，喘喝聲嗄，痰涎壅塞，其證危惡, "**Horse-spleen wind** is a dilatation of the lung. [Patients suffer from] rising qi and rapid panting. Both flanks make a flapping movement. The nose is dilated accompanied by heart-pressure and a feeling of disorder. [Patients] pant with much noise; their voice is exclamatory. A dangerous condition".

***Ma xian* 馬癇, horse epilepsy** [3]

PC of a → *dian xian* 癲癇, peak-illness with epilepsy, which, at the time of its outbreaks, makes the patient's four limbs twitch, his mouth open wide and his head shake and make horse sounds, as well as tend to arch backwards. *QJYF* 5: **馬癇**之為病，張口搖頭，馬鳴欲反折, "The disease of **horse epilepsy**: The mouth is wide open and the head shakes. [Patients] make whickering sounds like horses and tend to arch backwards".

***Mai yi* 脈溢, vessel overflow** [5]

PC identical with → *xue han* 血汗, blood sweat. *TBC* SE *qin hua* 芹花：味苦。主**脈溢**, "Its flavor is bitter. It controls **vessel overflow**".

***Man* 滿, fullness** [ca. 142]

① IS of an uncomfortable feeling of extraordinary fullness. *SW* 5: 中**滿**者，瀉之於內, "In case of central **fullness**, drain it inside". *BCGM* refers to *xiong man* 胸滿, a feeling of fullness in the chest; *xie man* 脅滿, a feeling of fullness in the flanks; *zhong man* 中滿, a feeling of fullness in the center; *fu man* 腹滿, a feeling of fullness in the abdomen; *xin xia man* 心下滿, a feeling of fullness below the heart; *zu jing man* 足脛滿, a feeling of fullness in the feet and shin; *zhi man* 肢滿, a feeling of fullness in the extremities; *nao man* 腦滿, a feeling of fullness in the brain; etc.

② PC with an uncomfortable feeling of fullness. *SW* 12: 其民樂野處而乳食，臟寒生**滿**病，其治宜灸, "Its people find joy in living in the wilderness and in consuming milk. Their depots are cold and generate diseases of **fullness**. For their treatment, cauterization is appropriate".

***Man gan feng* 慢肝風, slow liver wind** [4]

PC of eyes of children less than one month old that do not open, or are swollen and rough, or bleed. *YYXS* 7: 慢肝風，羞日，目腫出血, "**Slow liver wind**: [children] cannot bear sunlight. Their eyes are swollen and bleed".

***Man ji* 滿急, fullness and tightness** [11] AN *ji man* 急滿, tightness and fullness.

IS of an uncomfortable feeling of fullness and pressing [qi]. *ZHF* 3: 治腫入腹，苦**滿急**害飲食方, "Recipe to cure swelling that enters the abdomen. One suffers from **fullness and tightness**, and a loss of appetite".

***Man jing* 慢驚, slow fright** [30]

PC identical with → *man jing feng* 慢驚風, slow fright wind. *XEYZZJ*, Fj: **慢驚**，因病後，或吐瀉脾胃虛損，遍身冷，口鼻氣出亦冷，手足時瘛瘲，昏睡，睡露睛。此無陽也, "**Slow fright**. This condition emerges after a disease episode or if vomiting and diarrhea result in a depletion detriment of the spleen and stomach. The entire body is cold. The qi emitted by the mouth and nose is cold too. The hands and feet are sometimes hit by clonic spasms. Patients fall into a lethargic sleep, with their eyes open. The reason is an absence of yang".

***Man jing feng* 慢驚風, slow fright wind** [2] AD *man jing* 慢驚, slow fright. AN *man pi feng* 慢脾風, slow spleen wind; *man pi jing feng* 慢脾驚風, slow spleen fright wind.

PC of a → *jing feng* 驚風, fright wind, characterized by recurrent cramps in the presence or absence of fever. The cramps are slow and not very forceful. *TPSHF* 85 RE *bai jiang can san* 白僵蠶散, powder with *bai jiang can*: 治小兒**慢驚風**，壯熱，四肢拘急，痰涎壅滯，發歇不定, "It cures **slow fright wind** in children. [Patients experience] strong heat. The four limbs cramp and are tense. Phlegm-drool is sluggish and its flow is obstructed. The periods when this condition is active and when it is dormant are not fixed".

***Man men* 滿悶, fullness and heart-pressure** [6] AN *men man* 悶滿, heart-pressure and fullness.

IS of an uncomfortable feeling of fullness and heart-pressure. *ZBYHL* 7: 頭痛，胸中**滿悶**，當吐之則愈, "In the case of headache, as well as a feeling of **fullness and heart-pressure** in the chest a cure will be achieved by making the [patient] vomit".

***Man pi* 滿痞, fullness with an obstacle-illness** [1]

IS identical with → *pi man* 痞滿①, obstacle-illness and fullness. *QJYF* 13: 胸痹之病，令人心中堅，**滿痞**急痛, "The disease of chest blockage causes hardness in a person's center, with a feeling of **fullness with an obstacle-illness**, as well as acute pain".

***Man pi feng* 慢脾風, slow spleen wind** [3]

PC identical with → *man jing feng* 慢驚風, slow fright wind. *YYXS* 10: RE *xing pi san* 醒脾散, powder to arouse the spleen: 治小兒**慢脾風**, "It cures **slow spleen wind** in children".

***Man pi jing feng* 慢脾驚風, slow spleen fright wind** [1]
PC identical with → *man jing feng* 慢驚風，slow fright wind. *YYXS* 10 RE *huo pi san* 活脾散, powder to qicken the spleen: 治小兒**慢脾驚風**, "It cures **slow spleen fright wind** in children".

***Man sai* 滿塞, fullness and blockage** [1]
IS identical with → *sai man* 塞滿①, blockage with fullness. *QJYF* 7: 風緩湯，治脚弱，舉體痹不仁，熱毒氣入臟，胸中**滿塞**不通，食即嘔吐方， "The decoction for wind that brings forth sluggishness: a recipe to cure weakness of the legs, blockage and numbness of the entire body, qi of heat poison entering the depots, **fullness and blockage** in the chest and center. The food one eats is thrown up again".

***Man shi* 滿實, fullness with repletion** [1]
PC of abdominal → *man* 滿, fullness, and → *bian mi* 便秘, constipation, brought forth by a repletion with evil qi. *ZJSHL* 5: 大滿大實，自可除下之。大承氣湯，下其**滿實**, "Massive fullness and massive repletion can be brought down. The decoction to massively support qi drains **fullness with repletion**".

***Man tong* 滿痛, fullness and pain** [14] AN *tong man* 痛滿, pain with fullness.
IS of pain associated with a feeling of extraordinary fullness. *SW* 32: 熱爭則狂言及驚，脅**滿痛**，手足躁，不得安臥, "When the heat is fought [by the proper qi, the patient] talks crazily and is frightened. The flanks experience a feeling of **fullness and pain**. The hands and the feet move restlessly. [The patient] cannot sleep peacefully".

***Mang* 盲, blindness** [p]
PC identical with → *mu mang* 目盲. *SW* 52: 刺面中溜脈，不幸為**盲**, "If one, when piercing the face, hits the stream vessel, in unfortunate [cases this] causes **blindness**".

***Mang chang qi* 盲腸氣, blind intestine qi** [4]
PC identical with → *shan qi* 疝氣, elevation-illness qi. *TPSHF* 7: 腎氣虛微，為邪冷之氣所侵，傳注於小腸，則令小腸連陰疼痛，故號**盲腸氣**也, "When the qi of the kidneys is decreased or depleted, and then [the kidneys] are intruded by the qi of evil cold which is then transferred to the small intestine, then, as a result, the small intestine and, joined to it, the yin [i.e. genital member] are painful. Hence this is called the **blind intestine qi**".

***Mao ba* 毛拔, hair plucked out** [1]
IS of loss of hair. *SW* 10: 多食苦，則皮槁而**毛拔**, "If one consumes large quantities of bitter [food], the skin will desiccate and the body **hair is plucked out**".

***Mao chi* 瞀瘛, pressure and spasms** [3]
IS of a comatose clouding with jerking [hands and feet]. *SW* 74: 諸熱**瞀瘛**，皆屬於火, "All [diseases with] heat [causing] **pressure and spasms** are associated with fire".

***Mao gui ye dao* 貓鬼野道, cat-demon-on-a-road-in-the-wilderness [disease]** [4]
PC According to the *ZBYHL* this term is to be divided into *mao gui* 貓鬼 and *ye dao* 野道. *Mao gui* 貓鬼 refers to harm inflicted on humans by the spirits of

cats they raise. *Ye dao* 野道 refers to diseases caused by *gu* 蠱 spirits roaming without a host on roads in the wilderness. Ever since the *QJYF*, the two terms have been used in combination to refer to mental states characterized by photism, phonism, singing and wailing. *QJYF* 25 lists a 治**貓鬼野道**病歌哭不自由方, "Recipe to cure the disease **cat-demon-on-a-road-in-the-wilderness** with involuntary singing and wailing".

***Mao jing chuang* 貓睛瘡, cat-eye sores** [1]

PC identical with → *han chuang* 寒瘡, cold sores. *BCGM* Bai bing zhu zhi yao 百病主治藥: 雞肉主**貓睛瘡**, "Chicken meat controls **cat-eye sores**".

***Mao shu* 冒暑, malicious summerheat** [1]

EA identical with → 傷暑②, harm caused by summerheat. *SJZL* 115: 失飢**冒暑**及風熱憂愁，使耳暴聾, "Hunger, **malicious summerheat**, wind heat, and sadness may cause the ears to become suddenly deaf".

***Mao yan jing chuang* 貓眼睛瘡, cat-eye sores** [1]

PC identical with → *han chuang* 寒瘡, cold sores. *BCGM* SE *ji* 雞 quoting *QJF*: 烏雄雞肉治**貓眼睛瘡**, "The meat of black roosters cures **cat-eye sores**".

***Mei chuang* 眉瘡, eyebrow sores** [4] AN *lian mei chuang* 煉眉瘡, tempered eyebrows sores; *mian yan chuang* 面湮瘡, facial clog-up sores; *lian yin xian* 煉銀癬, tempered silver *xuan*-illness; *lian yin chuang* 煉銀瘡, tempered silver sores.

PC of → *chuang* 瘡, sores, conditions, which develop on the eyebrows of children. They fester with seeping liquid, itch, and peel, and cannot be cured over an extended period of time. *BCGM* SE *lu* 驢 quotes *TPSHF*: 小兒**眉瘡**：黑驢屎燒研，油調塗，立效, "**Eyebrow sores** in children: Roast black donkey feces and grind to a powder, mix with oil and apply externally. Immediately effective".

***Mei he ge qi* 梅核膈氣, plum-pit occlusion qi** [1] AN *qi ye* 氣噎, qi-induced gullet occlusion.

PC of an uncomfortable feeling of a blockage caused by an alien object in the gullet which one is unable to remove by vomiting and swallowing. The *CSXZ*, published only five years prior to the *BCGM*, offers the earliest known reference to a term *mei he qi* 梅核氣, plum-pit qi [occluding the throat]. LSZ may have coined the new term 梅核膈氣 by combining the two very different disease concepts of 梅核氣 and → 膈氣, *ge qi*, occlusion qi, with a new term. *BCGM* SE *mei* 梅 quotes *GSJYF*: **梅核膈氣**，取半青半黃梅子，每個用鹽一兩淹一日夜，曬乾又浸又曬，至水盡乃止。用青錢三個，夾二梅，麻綫縛定，通裝磁罐內，封埋地下，百日取出。每用一枚，含之嚥汁，入喉即消, "For **plum-pit occlusion qi**: Take plums half-green half-yellow and cover each with 1 *liang* of salt for 1 day and 1 night. Next dry them under the sun, then immerse them [in salt] again, and then dry them again. Stop when all the water has gone. Then take 3 copper coins to enclose 2 plums, bind them together firmly with a hemp thread. This is then placed into an earthen jar, which is to be sealed and buried in the earth. Take them out after 100 days. For each [treatment] use one piece, hold it in the mouth and swallow the juice. When it enters the throat it will dissolve [the blockage]".

***Mei he qi* 梅核氣, plum-pit qi** [1]
PC identical with → *ge qi* 膈氣, occlusion qi. *BCGM* Bai bing zhu zhi yao 百病主治藥 quoting *GZQF*: 膈氣梗噎, "Occlusion qi and gullet occlusion", writes: **梅核氣, "Plum-pit qi** [occlusion]". This may have been a copying error committed by LSZ or a member of his team. The term *mei he qi* 梅核氣, plum-pit qi, is used in pre-modern literature to indicate a feeling of an alien object in the gullet which one is unable to remove by vomiting or swallowing. When this is called *ye qi* 噎氣, gullet occlusion qi, in *BCGM* Bai bing zhu zhi yao 百病主治藥, this is not the same as → *ge qi* 膈氣, occlusion qi.

***Mei hua tu xuan* 梅花禿癬, plum blossom baldness and *xuan*-illness** [1]
PC identical with → *bai tu* 白禿, white baldness. *BCGM* SE *hu ma* 胡麻quotes *PJF*: **梅花禿癬**：用清油一碗，以小竹子燒火入內煎沸，瀝豬膽汁一個和勻，剃頭擦之，二三日即愈, "For **plum blossom baldness and *xuan*-illness**: take one bowl of clear oil and pour into a [vessel] that is then to be heated with young bamboo until it boils. Then pour the juice of a hog's bile into [the oil] and mix. Shave [the patient's] head and rub [the liquid] onto it".

***Mei leng gu tong* 眉棱骨痛, painful bones behind the eyebrows** [5]
IS of pain affecting the bones above the eyes. *DXXF* 4: 又有**眉棱骨痛**，眼不可開，晝靜夜劇，宜導痰湯, "For [patients] who also suffer from **painful bones behind the eyebrows**, who do not open their eyes; with [the ailment] being dormant during daytime and serious at night, it is appropriate to use the 'decoction that guides phlegm'".

***Mei lian xuan* 眉煉癬, eyebrow tempered with *xuan*-illness** [2]
PC identical with → *lian mei chuang* 煉眉瘡, tempered eyebrows sores. *BCGM* SE *tu si zi* 菟絲子 quoting *SJSY* 3: 小兒眉練瘡, "eyebrows of children tempered with sores", writes **眉煉癬**瘡, "**Tempered eyebrows with *xuan*-illness** sores". The phrasing 小兒眉練瘡 is an erroneous version of the older term 小兒眉煉, tempered eyebrows of children, discussed in the *RMSQ* 5 for the first time.

***Mei xuan* 眉癬, eyebrow *xuan*-illness** [2]
PC of → *xuan* 癬, *xuan*-illness, developing on the eyebrows. When cured the eyebrows do not grow again. *BCGM* SE *xuan fu hua* 旋覆花 quoting *XEWSZWLF* 2: 赤芝散，治小兒眉毛眼睫，因癬退不生，名乳頰癬, "Powder with *chi zhi*: to cure the failure of eyebrows and eyelashes to grow again once a *xuan*-illness has receded. This is called 'milk-cheeks *xuan*-illness'", writes: 小兒**眉癬**：小兒眉毛眼睫，因癬退不生, "**Eyebrow *xuan*-illness** in children: When eyebrows and eyelashes fail to grow once a *xuan*-illness has receded".

***Men e* 悶惡, heart-pressure malignity** [1]
IS of an uncomfortable feeling of irritation and heart-pressure. *BCGM* SE *da dou chi* 大豆豉 quotes *MSF*: 傷寒汗出不解，已三四日，胸中**悶惡**, "Harm caused by cold, with sweating unresolved. This has already lasted for three to four days. Patients experience **heart-pressure malignity**".

***Men jue* 悶絕, heart-pressure with expiry** [20]

IS of vexation ending in a loss of consciousness. *ZBYHL* 14: 心腹絞痛脹滿，氣衝心胸，或即**悶絕**，不復識人, "Heart and abdomen experience twisting pain, with feelings of distension and fullness. The qi surges to the heart and chest. In some cases this results in **heart-pressure with expiry**. Patients no longer recognize persons".

***Men luan* 悶亂, heart-pressure with confusion** [20] AN *fan luan* 煩亂, vexation with confusion.

IS of an extreme state of vexation with heart-pressure accompanied by clouding and confusion marking one's language and behavior. *ZHF* 3: 卒中急風，**悶亂**欲死, "If someone is suddenly struck by violent wind, he will experience **heart-pressure with confusion** and be at the brink of death".

***Men man* 悶滿, heart-pressure and fullness** [3]

IS identical with → *man men* 滿悶, fullness and heart-pressure. *ZBYHL* 12: 煩心**悶滿**，不能下食, "A vexed heart, **heart-pressure and fullness**, and an inability to eat".

***Men tong* 悶痛, heart-pressure with pain** [3] AN *tong men* 痛悶, pain with heart-pressure; *teng men* 疼悶.

IS of pain accompanied by a feeling of depression or gloom. *QJYF* 13: 心**悶痛**，上氣牽引小腸，灸巨闕二七壯, "For **heart-pressure with pain** affecting the heart, with ascending qi pulling on the small intestine, cauterize the Great Tower [point] two times seven times".

***Meng ji* 夢悸, dream palpitation** [1]

IS identical with → *jing meng* 驚夢, fright dream. *BCGM* Bai bing zhu zhi yao 百病主治藥, *xie sui* 邪祟, evil curse: 古櫬板，鬼氣疰忤，中惡心腹痛，**夢悸**，常為鬼神祟撓，和桃枝煎酒服，取吐下, "Old coffin boards: Demon-qi attachment-illness and hostility, being struck by the malign with heartache and abdominal pain, and **dream palpitation**, this is often the impact of a demon-spirit's curse. Boil [old coffin boards] with the twigs of a peach tree and ingest this with wine to remove [the ailment] by vomiting and purging".

***Meng lou* 夢漏, dream leakage** [2]

PC identical with → *meng yi* 夢遺, dream emission. *PJF* 217: 清心丸，治經絡熱**夢漏**，心忪恍惚，膈熱, "Pills that clear the heart. They cure heat in conduits and network [vessels] with **dream leakage**, as well as heart agitation with absent-mindedness, and diaphragm heat".

***Meng xie* 夢泄, dream outflow** [13]

PC of wet dreams, identical with → *meng yi* 夢遺，dream emission. *MYBL* 185: 主益精，補陰氣，止虛損**夢泄**, "It controls augmentation of seminal fluid, supplements yin qi, and stops depletion injury with **dream outflow**".

***Meng yan* 夢魘, nightmare** [2]

PC identical with → *yan mei* 魘寐. *MYBL* SE *su he xiang* 蘇合香：去三蟲，除邪，令人無**夢魘**, "It removes the three types of bugs/worms, eliminates evil, and makes people have no **nightmares**".

***Meng yi* 夢遺, dream emission** [27] AN *meng xie* 夢泄, dream outflow.
PC of wet dreams, with an → *yi jing* 遺精, involuntary emission of seminal fluid, in the course of erotic dreams as a major sign. *SJZL* 185: 因邪氣乘虛客於陰為**夢遺**, "**Dream emissions** resulting from evil qi availing itself of a depletion and residing in the yin [region]".

***Mi huo* 迷惑, perplexity** [6]
IS of slowed thinking and a reduced ability to differentiate. *BJ* SE *chang pu* 菖蒲：久服輕身，不忘，不**迷惑**, "If consumed over an extended period of time, it will make the body light, prevent a person from forgetting things, and protect against **perplexity**".

***Mi jia* 米瘕, rice conglomeration-illness** [4]
PC writing error of → *mi zheng* 米癥, rice concretion-illness. *BCSY* SE *jing* 粳 quoting *QJYF* 11: 米癥常欲食米, "[Patients with] rice concretion-illness permanently wish to eat rice", writes: **米瘕**嗜米, "[Patients with] **rice conglomeration-illness** love to consume rice".

***Mi jie* 秘結, closed and bound** [6]
IS, PC identical with → *da bian mi* 大便秘, constipation. *WTMY* 27: 飲食將息過熱，熱氣蘊積**秘結**, "After one has consumed beverages and food that are too hot, heat qi will accumulate and [the passageways of stools will be] **closed and bound**".

***Mi luan* 迷亂, confusion** [4]
IS of a loss of the ability of normal thinking and differentiation. *QJYF* 1: 草石相反，**使人迷亂**, "If herbs and minerals oppose each other, this will cause **confusion** in the human mind".

***Mi men* 迷悶, perplexity with heart-pressure** [13]
IS of slowed-down thinking accompanied by an uncomfortable feeling of vexation with heart-pressure. *QJYF* 20: 手足熱，口乾燥欲得水，嘔逆**迷悶**, "The hands and feet are hot. The mouth is dry and one longs for water. [Patients] vomit with [qi] counterflow, and experience **perplexity with heart-pressure**".

***Mi mu* 眯目, dust in the eyes** [23]
PC of some small foreign objects having entered the eyes and remaining there, causing pain and making opening one's eyes difficult. *TBC* SE *chuan bao yu sheng* 穿鮑魚繩：亦主**眯目**、去刺，煮汁洗之大良也, "It also controls **dust in the eyes**, and removes stings. Boil [in water] and use the liquid to rinse the [afflicted region]. Very good".

***Mi se* 秘塞, closure** [14]
IS, PC identical with → *da bian mi* 大便秘, constipation. *WTMY* 1: 又療傷寒或始得至七八日不大便，或四五日後不大便，或下後**秘塞**者，承氣湯方, "Also, to cure cases where there has been no defecation for seven or eight days following the onset of harm caused by cold, or where there has been no defecation for four to five days after [the onset of the disease], or where following a [therapy of] discharge there is **closure**, the recipe for the 'decoction to uphold the qi' [is appropriate]".

***Mi se* 秘澀, closed and rough** [4]

IS, PC identical with → *da bian mi* 大便秘, constipation. *ZBYHL* 4: 食即欲嘔，小便如血，大便**秘澀**, "After eating one has an urge to vomit. Urine takes the appearance of blood. Defecation is **closed and rough**".

***Mi yan* 眯眼, dust in the eyes** [1]

PC identical with → *mi mu* 眯目. *PJF* 82: 治雜物**眯眼**不出方, "Recipe to cure **dust in the eyes** with the presence of various objects that fail to come out again".

***Mi zheng* 米癥, rice concretion-illness** [1]

PC of → *zheng* 癥, concretion-illness, which form when one consumes raw rice that accumulates without being digested. *ZBYHL* 19: **米癥**候, 人有好啞米，轉久彌嗜啞之…米不消化，遂生癥結, "The signs of **rice concretion-illness**: When someone likes to eat rice, and when he has eaten long enough he eats it again ... The rice is undigested and forms concretion-illness nodes over time".

***Mian gan* 面䵟, facial gloom** [32] AN *mian gan* 面皯; *hei gan* 黑䵟, gloom; *mian shang hei qi* 面上黑氣, dark qi covering the face; AD *gan* 䵟, gloom.

PC with a haggard, gloomy, and dark facial complexion as a major sign. *BJ* SE *tu si zi* 菟絲子:汁去**面䵟**, "Its juice removes **facial gloom**".

***Mian gan* 面皯, facial gloom** [3]

PC identical with → *mian gan* 面䵟. *BJ* SE *xuan hua* 旋花:主益氣，去**面皯**黑色，媚好, "It controls augmentation of qi, removes the dark complexion of **facial gloom**, and returns a charming appearance".

***Mian ji* 麵積, accumulation of flour** [1]

PC of → *shi ji* 食積②, food accumulation, brought forth by an inadequate consumption of food prepared from flour. *BCGM* Bai bing zhu zhi yao 百病主治藥：蘿卜，化**麵積**, "*Luo bo* transforms **accumulations of flour**".

***Mian pao* 面皰, facial blister** [21] AN *chi pao* 赤皰, red blister; *gu zui* 穀嘴, grain mouth.

PC of small → *chuang* 瘡, sores, developing in the face. *MYBL* SE *shan zhu yu* 山茱萸：鼻塞，目黃，耳聾，**面皰**, "Stuffed nose, yellow eyes, deafness, **facial blisters**". LSZ assumes that this is brought forth by wind and heat, and mostly affects young people.

***Mian shang fei lei* 面上痱磊, facial seething-rash pebbles** [1]

PC identical with → *fen ci* 粉刺, flour thorns". *BCGM* SE *wang gua* 王瓜 quoting *ZHBJF* 6: 土瓜根治面上疿壘，礧㔣 "*Tu gua* roots cure facial seething-rash pebbles", writes: **面上痱磊**，土瓜根搗末，漿水和勻。入夜別以漿水洗面塗藥，旦復洗之。百日光彩射人，夫妻不相識也。曾用有效, "[To cure] **facial seething-rash pebbles**, grind *tu gua* root to a powder and mix with *jiang shui*. In the evening, in addition, use [pure] *jiang shui* to wash the face and externally apply the medication. Wash again in the early morning. After 100 days glossiness will hit that person. Husband and wife will not recognize each other. [I have] used it; it is effective".

Mian shang hei an 面上黑黯, facial darkness [1]
PC identical with → *mian gan* 面皯, facial gloom. *BCGM* SE *can* 蠶 quotes *TPSHF*: **面上黑黯**：白殭蠶末，水和搽之, "For **facial darkness**: Mix a powder prepared from [dead] white, stiff silkworms with water and apply to it".

Mian shang hei qi 面上黑氣, dark qi covering the face [2]
PC identical with → *mian gan* 面皯, facial gloom. *BCGM* SE *ban xia* 半夏 quotes *ZXF*: **面上黑氣**：半夏焙研，米醋調敷, "[To cure] **dark qi covering the face**: heat *ban xia* over a slow fire and grind, mix with rice vinegar and apply externally".

Mian yan chuang 面湮瘡, facial clog-up sores [1]
PC identical with → *mei chuang* 眉瘡, eyebrow sores. *WKJY* Lj: 治小兒**面湮瘡**，俗云煉銀瘡者，是母受胎之日，食酸辣及邪味過度，多生此瘡， "To cure **facial clog-up sores** in children. This is commonly called ‚sores of tempered silver'. When a mother, on the day she conceives the child, eats too much sour and peppery food or bad substances, [the child] is likely to develop such sores".

Mian yun 面䵳, facial speckles [2]
PC identical with → *gan zeng* 皯䵳, dermal dark spots. *MYBL* SE *she xiang* 麝香：去**面䵳**、目中膚翳, "It serves to remove **facial speckles**, and a skin shade in the eyes".

Mian zha 面皶, facial sediments [2]
PC identical with → *bi zha* 鼻皶, nose sediments. *MYBL* SE *zi cao* 紫草：以合膏，療小兒瘡及**面皶**, "Prepared as an ointment it cures children's sores and **facial sediments**".

Ming long 鳴聾, ringing and deafness [3]
PC CD of → *er ming* 耳鳴②, ringing in the ears, and → *er long* 耳聾②, deafness. *QJYF* 6: 治耳**鳴聾**方，當歸、細辛、川芎、防風、附子、白芷（各六銖）, "Recipe to cure **ringing** in the ears **and deafness**: *dang gui*, *xi xin*, *chuan xiong*, *fang feng*, *fu zi*, *bai zhi*, six *zhu* each".

Ming xuan 瞑眩, dizziness with eyes closed [7]
IS of a severe version of vertigo forcing a person to close his eyes. *SSSM*: 藥弗**瞑眩**，厥疾弗瘳, "If a medication does not cause **dizziness with eyes closed**, the respective ailment will not be cured".

Mo meng 魔夢, nightmare [1]
IS of demonic illusions in one's dreams resulting in fear and horror. *BCSY* SE *pi li zhen* 霹靂針：作枕，除**魔夢**, "Prepare a headrest [made of it] to remove **nightmares**".

Mo yi 膜翳, membrane shade [3]
PC identical with → *yi mo* 翳膜, shade membrane. *YXGM* 37: 目疾**膜翳**，瘡癤癧瘤, "Eye afflictions with **membrane shade**, sores, pimples, obstruction-illnesses, and tumors.

Mu an **目暗, dim vision** [44] AN *an mu* 暗目; *yan an* 眼暗.

PC with an inability to see things clearly as major sign. *MYBL tu tou gu* 兔頭骨：肝，主**目暗**, "The liver, it controls **dim vision**".

Mu bi **木痹, log[-like numbness with] blockage** [1]

IS identical with *bi mu* 痹木, blockage [with numbness like a] log. *BCGM* SE *huang ming jiao* 黄明膠 quotes *ZXF*: 面上**木痹**：牛皮膠化，和桂末，厚塗一二分，良, "For facial **log[-like numbness with] blockage**: glue made from buffalo hide mixed with powderized *gui*, smeared [on the face] as a thick layer of one or two *fen*, is good".

Mu bing **目病, eye disease** [19]

PC identical with → *mu ji* 目疾, ailments of the eyes. *ZBYHL* 28: 凡**目病**，若肝氣不足，兼胸膈風痰勞熱，則目不能遠視, "For all **eye diseases** [the following applies]. If the liver qi is insufficient, and if at the same time the chest and diaphragm have wind and phlegm, associated with exhaustion heat, the eyes cannot see into the distance".

Mu chi **目赤, eye redness** [64] AN *yan chi* 眼赤.

① IS of eyeballs and surrounding tissue assuming a red color. *SW* 10: 凡相五色之奇脈，面黄目青，面黄**目赤**，面黄目白，面黄目黑者，皆不死也, "Whenever one observes strange [movements in the] vessels [associated with] the five complexions, when the face is yellow and the eyes are green-blue, when the face is yellow and the **eyes are red**, when the face is yellow and the eyes are white, when the face is yellow and the eyes are black, [the patient] will not die".

② PC with red eyes as major sign. *BJ* SE *rui he* 蕤核：主心腹邪結氣，明目，**目赤**, "It controls evil with bound qi in the heart and abdomen, clears the eyes, and [cures] **eye redness**".

Mu chi lan **目赤爛, eye redness and festering** [3]

PC with red and festering eyes. *TBC* SE *luan hua* 欒華：取合黄連作煎，療**目赤爛**, "Prepare a decoction together with *huang lian*. It will cure **eye redness and festering**".

Mu chi tong **目赤痛, eye redness with pain** [4]

① IS of the pupil and its surrounding tissue developing redness associated with pain. *YXL che qian zi* 車前子：毒風衝眼，**目赤痛**, "When poison wind strikes the eyes, the **eyes develop redness with pain**".

② PC with eye redness and pain. *BJ* SE *mu meng* 木虻：主**目赤痛**："It controls **eye redness with pain**".

Mu chi zhong **目赤腫, eye redness with swelling** [6]

① IS of the pupil and its surrounding tissue developing redness associated with swelling. *YXL* SE *qin bai pi* 秦白皮：去肝中久熱，兩**目赤腫**疼痛，風淚不止, "It relieves one of chronic heat in the liver, with **eye redness associated with swelling** and pain, and unending tearflow".

② PC with eye redness and swelling. *YXL* SE *shan zhi zi* 山梔子：除熱及消渴口乾，**目赤腫**病, "It eliminates diseases such as heat and melting thirst with dry mouth, as well as **eye redness with swelling**".

***Mu cuan* 目竄, scurrying eyes** [1]

IS identical with → *cuan shi* 竄視. *BCGM* Bai bing zhu zhi yao 百病主治藥：阿膠，肺風喘促，涎潮**目竄**，同紫蘇、烏梅煎服, "Take *a jiao* boiled with *zi su* and *wu mei* for lung wind with panting and urgent breathing, floods of saliva, and **scurrying eyes**".

***Mu fu* 目膚, eye skin** [2]

PC identical with *fu yi* 膚翳, dermal shade. *BCSY* SE *mi* 蜜：主牙齒疳䘌，唇口瘡，**目膚**赤障, "It controls *gan*–illness and hidden worms affecting the teeth, sores on the lips and mouth, and **eye skin** with red screen".

***Mu hei* 目黑, darkened eyes** [6] AN *yan hei* 眼黑.

IS of a feeling as if a dark screen had developed in front of the eyes, causing unclear vision. *ZBYHL* 28: 肝虛不能榮於目，致精彩不分明，故**目黑**, "The liver is depleted and unable to provide nourishment to the eyes. This leads to an inability to clearly distinguish among bright colors. Hence [one speaks of] **darkened eyes**".

***Mu hun* 目昏, dim vision** [26] AN *hun'an* 昏暗; *yan hun* 眼昏.

IS of unclear vision. *QJYF* 7, RE *ce zi jiu* 側子酒，wine with *ce zi*：患**目昏**頭眩者，彌精, "For those who suffer from **dim vision** and dizziness in their head, it will be even more effective".

***Mu ji* 目疾, ailments of the eyes** [24] AN *mu zhong ji* 目中疾, ailments in the eyes; *mu bing* 目病, eye disease; *bing mu* 病目, diseased eye; *yan ji* 眼疾, ailments of the eyes; *yan mu zhu bing* 眼目諸病, all types of eye diseases.

PC CD of diseases affecting the eyes. *WTMY* 21: 又凡**目疾**，不問少長男女等，所忌有五, "Also, there are five restrictions to be observed in the case of **ailments of the eyes**, regardless of whether young or old people, males or females are concerned".

***Mu lei* 目淚, tears** [15]

① Identical with → *yan lei* 眼淚. *MYBL* SE *zhu* 术：風眩頭痛，**目淚**出, "Wind dizziness with headache; **tears** flow".

② IS of a continuous flow of tears not stimulated by emotions. *BCGM* SE *dai mao* 瑇瑁 quotes *HFJ*: 迎風**目淚**：乃心腎虛熱也, "If one faces wind and develops **tears**, this is because of depletion heat in the heart and kidneys".

③ PC with a flow of tears as major sign. *SLBC* SE *wu xiong ji* 烏雄雞：**目淚**出不止者，以三年冠血傅目睛上，日三度, "When **tears** flow without end, smear the blood from the comb of a three-year old [black cock] on the eyeballs. Three times a day".

***Mu mang* 目盲, blindness** [19] AD *mang* 盲.

PC identical with → *shi ming* 失明, loss of vision. *SW* 3: **目盲**不可以視，耳閉不可以聽, "The **eyes are blind** and cannot be used to see. The ears are closed and cannot be used to hear".

Mu mi 目眯, dust in the eyes [1]

PC identical with → *mi mu* 眯目. *BCGM* SE *yi yu* 衣魚 quoting *QJYF* 6: 砂石草木入目中不出, "When sand or herbs or wood enter the eyes and do not come out again", writes: **目眯**, "**Dust in the eyes**".

Mu nüe 牡瘧, male malaria [3]

PC of → *nüe ji* 瘧疾, malaria ailment, with a predominance of heat over cold sensations. *BCGM* SE *chang shan shu qi* 常山蜀漆 quoting *WTMY*: 牝瘧多寒者, "Cases of female malaria are those with much cold sensation", writes: **牡瘧**獨熱不冷者, "Cases of **male malaria** are those with only heat sensation and no cold".

Mu pi 目辟, squint [1] AW 目僻.

IS identical with → *xie shi* 斜視. *LGPZL* Xu 序：**目辟**眼雕，有五花而自正。五加皮，其葉有雄雌，三葉為雄，五葉為雌，須使五葉者，作末酒浸飲之，其目喎者正, "For **squint**, there is *wu hua*. [Its application] will straighten [the eyes]. [*Wu hua*] is *wu jia pi*. The leaves of this [plant] show it to be male or female. Those with three leaves are male; those with five leaves are female. One must make use of those with five leaves, prepare a powder, steep in wine, and drink this. Wry eyes will straighten themselves again".

Mu pi 目僻, squint [1]

IS identical with → *mu pi* 目辟. *BCGM* SE *wu jia* 五加 quoting *LGPZL* Xu 序：目辟眼雕, "squint", writes: 作末浸酒飲，治**目僻**眼雕, "Prepare a powder, steep in wine, and drink to cure **squint**".

Mu re 目熱, hot eyes [9] AN → *yan re* 眼熱.

IS of an uncomfortable feeling of heat in the eyes or of feeling hot to the touch. *BJ* SE *li yü dan* 鯉魚膽：主**目熱**赤痛, "It controls **hot eyes** that are red and ache".

Mu se 目澀, the eyes are rough [10]

① IS of a dried eyeball with a rough surface. In severe cases patients develop a feeling as if they were unable to open their closed eye. *ZBYHL* 5: 大便勿強努，令人腰疼**目澀**, "One must not forcibly defecate or his lower back will ache and **the eyes become rough**".

② PC with roughness of the eyes as a major sign. *ZBYHL* 28: 液竭者，則**目澀**, "When the liquid is exhausted, **the eyes are rough**".

Mu she 木舌, wooden tongue [21]

PC with the body of the tongue massively swollen to an extent that it fills the oral cavity and at the same time is as hard as wood. *TPSHF* 36: 治**木舌**熱腫，漸大滿口，宜含馬牙硝丸方, "To cure **wooden tongue** with heat swelling that has increased until it fills the mouth, it is advisable to use the recipe to hold the pills with *ma ya xiao* in the mouth".

Mu shen 木腎, wooden [external] kidneys [3]

PC with a significantly swollen scrotum which, if pressed; appears harder than usual but is only mildly painful. One of various types of → *shan qi* 疝氣, elevation-illness qi. LSZ: this is often seen in children. *PJF* 250: 治**木腎**，乳香、沒

藥、地膽、芫菁（去翅足）, "To cure **wooden [external] kidneys**, [take] *ru xiang*, *mo yao*, *di dan*, and *yuan jing* (remove wings and feet)".

***Mu sheng chi mai* 目生赤脈, the eyes grow red vessels** [2]
PC identical with → *mu zhong chi mai* 目中赤脈, red vessels in the eye. *SJZL* 102: 治肝實，**目生赤脈**，息肉磣痛，決明子丸方, "Recipe for pills with *jue ming zi* to cure liver repletion, with the **eyes growing red vessels**, and tumorous flesh-growth with grit and pain".

***Mu shi zhao tu* 暮食朝吐, eating at dusk, vomiting at dawn** [1]
IS of vomiting undigested food in the early morning that was consumed in the evening. *JGYL* Mj: 脾傷則不磨，朝食暮吐，**暮食朝吐**，宿穀不化，名曰胃反, "When the spleen is harmed it cannot rub [the stomach]. Eating at dawn will result in vomiting at dusk. **Eating at dusk will result in vomiting at dawn.** Grains stay overnight without being digested. This is called 'stomach turnover'".

***Mu sui* 目瞧, squint** [1]
IS identical with → *yan sui* 眼瞧. *BCGM* Xu li 序例 quoting *LGPZL*: 其目喎者正, "Eye wryness will be corrected", writes: 其**目瞧**者正, "**Squint** is corrected".

***Mu wei wu shang* 目為物傷, the eye is injured by a [foreign] object** [2]
PC brought forth by injury caused to the eye from outside by a foreign object. *BCGM* SE *yang* 羊 quoting *TPSHF* 33: 眼為他物所傷"The eye is injured by a foreign object", writes: **目為物傷**, "**The eye is injured by a [foreign] object**",

***Mu xie* 目斜, slanting of an eye; squinting** [2] AN *yan xie* 眼斜.
IS of a) eyes being slanted to one side. *QJYF* 13: 治頭風眩，口喎**目斜**耳聾，大三五七散方, "To cure head wind with dizziness, wryness of the mouth, **slanting of an eye**, and deafness, [use the] recipe for 'the massive powder with [dosages of ingredients varying from] three to five and to seven [*qian*]'". b) Eyes squinting. *YXZC* 6: 口噤**目斜**，身體強直，如角弓反張之狀, "Lockjaw, **squinting**, and a stiff and straight body, resembling arched reverse strain".

***Mu xuan* 目眩, visual dizziness** [29] AW *yan xuan* 眼眩.
IS of dim vision, with darkness in front of the eyes. *SW* 40: 四肢清，**目眩**，時時前後血，病名為何, "Their four limbs are cool. Their **eyes are dizzy**. They often pass blood in front and behind. What is the name of [this] disease?"

***Mu yi* 目翳, eye shade** [54] AD *yi* 翳; AN *yan yi* 眼翳, eye shade; *fu yi* 膚翳, skin shade; *yi mo* 翳膜, shade membrane; *yi zhong* 翳腫, shade swelling; *yi miao* 翳眇 shade blindness.
PC with a speckled membrane covering the pupils, impairing vision and making a person see threads. Turbidity and scars associated with injuries to the cornea and festering sores are the major reasons for the development of such 'eye shades'. *BJ* SE *bei zi* 貝子：主**目翳**，鬼疰，蠱毒, "It controls **eye shade**, demon attachment-illness, and *gu* poison".

***Mu yu* 木郁, pent-up wood [qi]** [4]
PC of → *yu jie* 鬱結, pent-up [qi] nodes, in the liver and gallbladder. *SW* 71: **木郁**達之, "In the case of **pent-up wood [qi]**, open its way".

***Mu yun* 目運, visual movements** [1]

IS of a perception of rotating or fluttering scenery in front of the eyes. LS 10: 五陰氣俱絕則目系轉，轉則**目運**, "When all the five yin qi are cut off, then the eye[-brain] connection is twisted. When it is twisted [the patient] experiences **visual movements**".

***Mu zhang* 目障, eye screen** [3] AD *zhang* 障, screen; AN *yan zhang* 眼障.

PC of eyes with impaired vision. *YHJW* Lj: 石決明，入肝經。去**目障**，明目, "*Shi jue ming* enters the liver conduit. It removes **eye screens** and clears the eyes".

***Mu zhi* 牡痔, male piles** [p]

PC of → *zhi* 痔瘡, piles, with tumorous flesh-growths to the side of the anus that are exposed outside the anus and frequently release pus and blood. *ZBY-HL* 34: **牡痔**候：肛邊生鼠乳，出在外者，時時出膿血者是也, "The signs of **male piles**: Mouse teats develop to the side of the anus. When they appear outside [of the anus] they often release pus and blood".

***Mu zhi chuang* 木蛭瘡, wood-leech sores** [1]

PC of → *chuang* 瘡, sores, conditions resulting from bodily contact with so-called 'wood-leech' insects found in the forests in South China. *BCGM* SE *dan sha* 丹砂 quoting *YS*: 南方多雨，有物曰木癡，其大概類鼻涕，積陰而生於古木之上，聞人氣則閃閃而動。人過其下，有墮於人體間者，即立成瘡，久則遍其肌體。有客患其木癡之瘡，遇一道士謂曰：以硃砂、麝香塗之即愈, "In the South it often rains, and there is a thing called 'wood simple'. It is as small as [a drop of] nasal snivel. It is an accumulation of yin, and lives up in old trees. When it smells human qi it flickers and begins to move. When that person passes by underneath it, it may drop on that person, and this immediately generates sores. After a long time, they will cover the entire body, and one suffers from 'wooden simple sores'. I once met a Daoist who told me that smearing [a medication with the ingredients] *zhu sha* and *she xian* will cure it", writes: **木蛭瘡**毒：南方多雨，有物曰木蛭，大類鼻涕，生於古木之上，聞人氣則閃閃而動。人過其下，墮人體間，即立成瘡，久則遍體。惟以硃砂、麝香塗之，即愈, "The poison of **wood-leech sores**. In the South it often rains, and there is a thing called 'wood leech'. It is as small as [a drop of] nasal snivel. It lives up in old trees. When it smells human qi it flickers and begins to move. When that person passes by underneath it, it may drop on that person, and this immediately generates sores. After a long time, they will cover the entire body. One only needs to smear [a medication with the ingredients] *zhu sha* and *she xian* on them, and this will bring the cure".

***Mu zhong chi mai* 目中赤脈, red vessels in the eye** [4] AN *yan zhong chi mai* 眼中赤脈; *mu sheng chi mai* 目生赤脈, the eyes grow red vessels.

PC identical with → *fei xue* 飛血, flying blood. *KBBC* SE *mi meng hua* 蜜蒙花：主青盲膚翳，赤澀多眵淚，消**目中赤脈**, "It controls green blindness and skin shade, with redness, roughness and profuse tearflow, and it dissolves **red vessels in the eye**".

***Mu zhong ji* 目中疾, ailments in the eyes** [2]
PC identical with → *mu ji* 目疾, ailments of the eyes. *MYBL* SE *zi bai pi* 梓白皮：療**目中疾**, "It cures **ailments in the eyes**".

***Mu zhong re mo* 目中熱膜, heat membrane in the eyes** [3]
PC identical with → *re yi* 熱翳, heat screen. *SLBC* SE *shi mi* 石蜜：點**目中熱膜**，家養白蜜為上, "To be dropped onto **heat membrane in the eyes**. Home-made white honey is best".

***Mu zhong zhu bing* 目中諸病, all types of diseases in the eyes** [3]
PC identical with → *mu ji* 目疾, ailments of the eyes. *BCGM* SE *lu gan shi* 爐甘石 quotes *ZSF*: **目中諸病**：石連光明散, "For **all types of diseases in the eyes**, [use] the powder with [*lu gan*] *shi* and [*huang*] *lian* to brighten vision".

- N -

***Nai tou hua* 奶頭花, breast nipple blossoms** [1]

PC identical with → *ru tou lie* 乳頭裂, cracked breast nipples. *HYBC* SE *ding xiang* 丁香：治**奶頭花**，止五色毒痢, "It cures **breast nipples blossoms**, and ends multi-colored poison free-flux illness".

***Nai tou hua lie* 奶頭花裂, breast nipples blossoms cracked open** [1]

PC identical with → *ru tou lie* 乳頭裂, cracked breast nipples. *BCGM* Bai bing zhu zhi yao 百病主治藥 quoting *HYBC*: 奶頭花, "Breast nipples opened like blossoms", writes: **奶頭花裂**，**breast nipple blossoms cracked open**".

***Nai yong* 奶癰, breast obstruction-illness** [2]

PC identical with → *ru yong* 乳癰, breast obstruction-illness. *HJJF* 8: 神效托裏散，治癰疽發背、腸癰、**奶癰**, "The 'wondrously effective powder to support the interior' cures obstruction-illnesses and impediment-illnesses and effusion of the back, intestinal abscesses, as well as **breast obstruction-illness**".

***Nan chan* 難產, difficult birth** [91] AN *chan nan* 產難; *ru nan* 乳難; *sheng zi bu xia* 生子不下, a child to be born fails to descend; *tai chan bu xia* 胎產不下, a fetus to be born fails to descend.

PC of difficulties to give birth to a child on its due date. *ZBYHL* 43 lists 婦人**難產**病諸候, "All signs of the disease **difficult birth** of females".

***Nan zi bai ji* 男子敗積, destructive accumulation in males** [2]

PC of a → *ji* 積, accumulation, which in males has developed into a very serious condition. *BCGM* SE *qiao mai* 蕎麥 quotes *DNBS*: 通仙散，治**男子敗積**, "Powder to communicate with the hermits: It cures **destructive accumulations in males**".

***Nang suo* 囊縮, scrotal shrinkage** [1]

IS identical with → *luan suo* 卵縮, egg shrinkage. *SW* 31: 六日厥陰受之，厥陰脈循陰器而絡於肝，故煩滿而**囊縮**, "On the sixth day, the ceasing yin [conduits] receive it. The ceasing yin vessels move along the yin (i.e. sexual) organ and enclose the liver. Hence, there is vexation and fullness, and **the scrotum shrinks**".

***Nao beng* 腦崩, brain collapse** [3]

PC identical with → *bi yuan* 鼻淵, nasal deep-source [outflow]. *BCGM* SE *si gua* 絲瓜 quoting *YXZC* 5: 鼻中時時流臭黃水, "Malodorous yellow water constantly flows from inside the nose", writes: **腦崩**流汁：鼻中時時流臭黃水, "**Brain collapse** with liquid flow: Malodorous yellow water constantly flows from inside the nose".

***Nao bi* 腦痹, brain [pit] and blockage [pit]** [1]

PC of a → *tan he* 痰核, phlegm pit, located in the posterior section of the brain. *BCGM* SE *fu shi* 浮石 quotes *RZZZF*: 頭核**腦痹**：頭枕後生痰核，正者為腦，側者為痹, "A pit at the head [may be a] **brain [pit] or blockage [pit]**: When the back of one's head has developed a phlegm pit, if it is in the center, this is called 'brain [pit]'. If it is to the sides this is called 'blockage [pit]'".

***Nao chong* 蟯蟲, pinworm** [8]

① EA of a small parasite in the intestinal tract of humans, often causing itching in the anal region. *ZBYHL* 18: **蟯蟲**，猶是九蟲內之一蟲也，形甚細小, "**Pinworm**: one of the nine types of worms. Its physical appearance is very small".

② PC brought forth by pinworm parasites in the intestinal tract. *ZBYHL* 18: **蟯蟲**候…蟯蟲是人體虛極重者，故蟯蟲因之動作，無所不為也, "The signs of **pinworm: …** pinworms become active as a result of an extreme depletion of the human body. They can generate all types [of ailments]".

***Nao feng* 腦風, brain wind** [5]

PC of → *tou feng* 頭風, head wind, characterized by a simultaneous presence of cold evil, with headache, a feeling of cold in the neck and back, as well as running nose and tearflow. *QJYF* 13: 芎酒 治**腦風**，頭重，頸項強，淚出，"Wine with [*chuan*] *xiong* cures **brain wind** with heavy-headedness, stiffness of the neck, and tearflow".

***Nao gan* 腦疳, brain *gan*-illness** [9]

PC of → *gan chuang* 疳瘡, *gan*-illness sores, with withering hair, ulcers on the head, loss of hair, nasal itching, and body heat as major signs. *LXJ* Fj: 蓋腦散，治孩子**腦疳**鼻癢，毛髮作穗，"Now, the 'powder to press down the brain', it cures children' **brain *gan*-illness**, with nasal itching and hair turning into grain spikes".

***Nao gu teng tong* 腦骨疼痛, brain-bone pain** [1]

IS identical with → *tou tong* 頭痛①, headache. *YXL* SE *gan ju hua* 甘菊花：能治熱頭風旋倒地，**腦骨疼痛**, "It is able to cure heat and head wind spin making a person fall on the ground, as well as **brain-bone pain**".

***Nao gu tong* 腦骨痛, brain-bone pain** [2]

IS identical with → *tou tong* 頭痛①, headache. *YXL* SE *shan zhu yu* 山茱萸：治**腦骨痛**，止月水不定, "It cures **brain-bone pain**, and it ends irregular menstruation".

***Nao ju* 腦疽, brain impediment-illness** [2]

PC identical with → *dui kou* 對口, counter-orifice. *JYBJF* Yong jie bu ke yong gao yao tie he lun 癰癤不可用膏藥貼合論, "On the inadequacy of applying ointment medications to obstruction-illnesses and pimples", **腦疽**不可灸，引其氣一上，痰涎膿血並起上攻，傾人性命急於反掌，"**Brain impediment-illnesses** must not be cauterized. Once the qi is stimulated to rise, phlegm, saliva, pus and blood will rise with it and attack above. Within the shortest moment the life of that person will be jeopardized".

***Nao lou* 腦漏, brain leakage** [2]

PC of a → *bi yuan* 鼻淵, nasal deep-source [outflow], with a secretion of foul yellow purulent snivel. *BCGM* SE *bai piao* 敗瓢 quotes *JiXF*: **腦漏**流膿：破瓢、白雞冠花、白螺螄殼各燒存性，等分，血竭、麝香各五分，為末。以好酒灑濕，熟艾連藥揉成餅，貼在頂門上，以熨斗熨之，以愈為度，"For **brain leakage** with running pus: Burn a broken gourd ladle, white cockscomb, and white spiral snail shells maintaining their nature. Take equal amounts. *Xue jie* and *she xiang*, five *fen* each. Grind to a powder. Use good wine to sprinkle processed *ai*. All these drugs are to be kneaded into cookies which are to be attached to the opening in the crown of the head. Exert hot pressure with a flat iron. Stop when the cure is achieved".

***Nao ming* 腦鳴, brain sounds** [5] AN *tou nao ming xiang* 頭腦鳴響; *tou zhong ming xiang* 頭中鳴響, sounds in the head.

IS of a perception of voices and sounds in the head. *MYBL* SE *man jing shi* 蔓荊實：主風頭痛，**腦鳴**，目淚出, "It controls wind head-ache, **brain sounds**, and tearflow".

***Nao nü* 腦衄, brainbleed** [1]

PC of massive spontaneous bleeding from mouth and nose. *SJZL* 193: 凡口鼻出血不止，名**腦衄**, "All incessant bleeding from the mouth and nose is called '**brainbleed**'". The *BCGM* has this term only once in the paragraph Bai bing zhu zhi yao 百病主治藥. Elsewhere in the main text it always speaks of *kou bi da nü* 口鼻大衄, "massive bleeding from the mouth and nose".

***Nao re* 腦熱, brain heat** [8]

① PC of brain heat affecting the nose and the eyes. *SWBC* SE *ran she dan* 蚺蛇膽：小兒**腦熱**，水漬注鼻中, "For **brain heat** in children, soak it in water and pour it into the [child's] nose".

② IS identical with → *tou re* 頭熱, head heat. *RHZ* SE *yang rou* 羊肉:頭，涼。治骨蒸，**腦熱**頭眩, "Its head is of a cool nature and cures bone steaming and **brain heat** with a dizzy head".

***Nao suan* 腦酸, brain pain** [2]

IS of an uncomfortable feeling of pain and distension reaching from the upper part of the nose to the forehead. *YJQW* Lj: 嗃鼻碧雲散，治腫脹紅赤，昏暗羞明…頭痛**腦酸**, "'Bluish powder to be blown into the nose' cures swelling with distension and redness; dim vision and fear of light; headache and **brain pain**".

***Nao tong* 腦痛, brain pain** [14]

IS identical with → *tou tong* 頭痛①, headache. *LS* 5: 熱病，面青**腦痛**，手足躁, "Heat disease: the face is greenish, and the **brain is painful**; hands and feet are restless".

***Nao xie* 腦瀉, brain outflow** [2]

PC identical with → *bi yuan* 鼻淵, nasal deep-source [outflow]. *PJF* 卷 57: 川芎防風散，治積年**腦瀉**秘方, "Powder with *chuan xiong* and *fang feng*: a secret recipe to cure **brain outflow** that has lasted for several years". It was believed that the brain is the "sea of marrow", *sui hai* 髓海. It stores and there must be no efflux. Only if evil heat rises to attack the brain, and when subsequently the yang qi is no longer stable, the liquid marrow flows down into the nose resulting in turbid snivel that does not end. Hence the brain is like a deep source of water, with "brain outflow" as alternative designations of "nasal deep source [outflow]".

***Nao xie* 腦泄, brain outflow** [3]

PC identical with → *bi yuan* 鼻淵, nasal deep-source [outflow]. *BCGM* SE *fu zi* 附子 quoting *PJF* 57: 鼻淵腦瀉 writes: 鼻淵**腦泄**, "Nasal deep-source **brain outflow**".

***Nao xuan* 腦宣, brain spread** [1]

PC identical with → *bi yuan* 鼻淵, nasal deep-source [outflow]. *BCGM* SE *zao jia* 皂莢 quoting *RMSQ* 15 RE *nao xuan fang* 腦宣方, "Recipe for brain spread", writes: **腦宣**不止, "Unending **brain spread**". This may be a misinterpreted disease term. *PJF* 53 quoting this recipe writes: 腦宣方，治耳聾, "Brain spread recipe cures deafness". *RMSQ* RE *nao xuan fang* 腦宣方, "Brain spread recipe", does not mention an ailment as a therapeutic indication. However, the preceding recipe entry lists a "recipe to cure deafness", and the following entry lists "a recipe to cure ear diminution". Hence it may well be that the author of *PJF* mistook the desired effect of "causing the brain to spread (and thereby to cure deafness, etc.)" as the ailment to be cured by this recipe.

***Nao yong* 腦癰, brain obstruction-illness** [2]

PC identical with → *dui kou* 對口, counter-orifice. *TPSHF* 62: 治**腦癰**及熱毒瘡腫，宜貼黃連餅方, "To cure **brain obstruction-illnesses** and heat-poison sores with swelling, it is advisable to resort to the recipe for a paste with *huang lian* for external application.

***Nei beng* 內崩, inner collapse** [6]

PC of spitting blood and blood loss through the lower orifices following harm caused by exhaustion and internal organ bleeding. *ZBYHL* 4: 勞傷於臟腑，**內崩**之病也, "When the depots and palaces are harmed by exhaustion, this is the disease of '**inner collapse**'".

***Nei bi* 內痹, internal blockage** [2]

PC of → *bi* 痹① c), blockage, brought forth by stagnant blood in the chest and abdominal cavity. *BJ* SE *wang gua* 王瓜: 主消渴，**內痹**，瘀血，月閉, "It controls melting with thirst, **internal blockage**, stagnant blood, and blocked menses".

***Nei bing* 內病, inner disease** [1]

CD of all PC that have their onset in the inner depots and palaces. *SYDXF* 1: 外病自經絡入，**內病**自五臟郁發, "Outer diseases enter through conduits and network vessels. **Inner diseases** effuse from pent-up [qi] in the five depots".

***Nei diao* 內釣, internally pulled up by a hook** [11] AN *nei diao* 內吊, internal haul.

PC mostly among children with violent abdominal pain accompanied by a feeling of being dragged and tightness. It easily develops into → *jing feng* 驚風, fright wind. *YYXS* 10: 治嬰孩、小兒驚風**內釣**，桃符丸, "To cure children with fright wind and being **internally pulled up by a hook**, [ingest] the 'pills as effective as peach-wood charms'".

***Nei diao* 內吊, internal haul** [2]

PC identical with → *nei diao* 內釣, internally pulled up by a hook. *XEWSZWLF* 14: 腹中撮痛，乾啼無淚，腰曲背弓，上唇乾，額上有汗，此名盤腸**內吊**之痛, "An abdominal pain as if being dragged, dry weeping without tears, the lumbar region and spine bent, the upper lip dry, sweat on the forehead, this is called 'twisted intestines **hauled internally**'".

Nei han **內寒, inner cold** [7]
PC of an abundance of yin cold in the body's depots and palaces, in contrast to → *wai han* 外寒, external cold. *SW* 62: 陰盛則**內寒**, "Yin abundance results in **inner cold**".

Nei jing **內痙, internal spasms** [2]
PC of → *jing bing* 痙病, spasms disease, brought forth either by harm incurred during delivery or by an injury caused from outside. *MYBL* SE *fang feng* 防風: 主四肢攣急，字乳金瘡**內痙**, "It controls cramps affecting the four limbs, as well as **internal spasms** brought about by parturition or wounds inflicted by metal objects".

Nei ju **內疽, internal impediment-illness** [4]
PC identical with → *nei yong* 內癰, internal obstruction-illness. *MYBL* SE *long gu* 龍骨：療腸癰**內疽**陰蝕, "It cures intestinal obstruction-illness, **internal impediment-illness**, and erosion in the yin (i.e. genital) region".

Nei jue **內絕, internal severance** [3]
PC identical with → *jue yang* 絕陽, severed yang. *WPBC* SE *bian qing* 扁青：治丈夫**內絕**，令人有子, "It cures males with **internal severance**, and lets people have children".

Nei lou **內漏, internal leakage** [20]
PC of blood emitted from an external wound or from internal sores into a body cavity. *SW* 52: 刺客主人內陷中脈，為**內漏**, "If one, when piercing the visitor-host-person [hole], sinks [the needle] into the interior and hits the vessel, this causes **internal leakage**".

Nei re **內熱, internal heat** [31]
PC of internal heat, as opposed to → *wai re* 外熱 heat from outside. *SW* 45: 熱盛於中，故熱遍於身，**內熱**而溺赤也, "Heat abounds in the center. The fact is, [in this case] heat is everywhere in the body. The **internal heat** causes the urine to assume a red color".

Nei shang **內傷, internal harm** [40]
① EA PM a) of etiological agents such as extremes of any of the seven emotions, harm caused by exhaustion and overexertion, as well as unbalanced food causing qi disturbances resulting in harm to the depots and palaces that leads to further disease. *LS* 66: 若**內傷**於憂怒，則氣上逆, "If worries and anger cause **internal harm**, qi rises flowing contrary to its regular direction". b) Of an occasional intrusion of external evil qi into the internal organs. *QJYF* 5: 治腎腑臟温病，身面如刺，腰中欲折，熱毒**內傷**方, "Recipe for heat poison causing **internal harm** to cure a kidney palace and depot warmth disease, with the body and face feeling as if pierced, and a sensation in the lumbar region as if it were to break".
② CD of PCs brought forth by internal harm. *QJYF* 12: 堅中湯，治虛勞**內傷**, "The decoction to strengthen the center cures depletion exhaustion and **internal harm**".

***Nei shang zhi shi* 內傷之濕, moisture resulting from inner harm** [1]
EA of moisture generated internally following harm caused by beverages and food that manifests itself as inhibiting the functions of the organs of transporting and transforming water and other liquids. The moisture is retained in the body and may generate further disease. *BCGM* Shi ji 十劑, *zao ji* 燥劑, preparations to achieve desiccation: **內傷之濕**，生於水飲酒食及脾弱腎強, "**Moisture resulting from inner harm** originates internally from water, wine, and food, in conjunction with spleen weakness and kidney strength".

***Nei shi* 內濕, internal moisture** [1]
EA identical with → *nei shang zhi shi* 內傷之濕, moisture resulting from internal harm. *DXXF* 1: 外濕宜表散，**內濕**宜淡滲, "External moisture is to be dispersed outside. **Internal moisture** is to be drained internally by means of substances without any specific flavor".

***Nei sun* 內損, internal injury** [2]
PC of → *shang sun* 傷損, injury, inflicted by blunt force that does not break the skin but injures organs in the body's interior. *ZBYHL* 36: 壓迮墜墮**內損**候：此為人卒被重物壓迮，或從高墜下，致吐、下血，此傷五內故也, "The signs of **internal injury** resulting from pressure and falls: This results when a person is suddenly exposed to heavy pressure, or when he falls from somewhere high, and leads to blood spitting and blood downpour. These are the reasons for injuries to the five internal [organs]".

***Nei tui* 內癀, internal prominence-illness** [1]
PC identical with → *yin tui* 陰癀, yin (i.e. scrotal) prominence-illness. *BCGM* SE *ju* 橘：和劑局方治諸疝痛及**內癀**，卵腫偏墜，或硬如石，或腫至潰，有橘核丸，用之有效, "To cure all types of elevation-illness with pain and **internal prominence-illness**, with unilateral swelling and collapse of the testicles, or hardening like a stone, or swelling until they burst, the *HJJF* recipes list the pills with *ju*-pits. Their application is effective". This is the only known appearance of the term 內癀 in medical literature. Print versions of the *HJJF* available today do not list "pills with *ju*-pits". Such a recipe is listed only in *PJF* and *YFLJ*, both citing *ZSJYF* as the source. LSZ's quoting of *HJJF* may be an error. Also, neither *PJF* nor *YFLJ* refer to 內癀, internal prominence-illness, but recommend the pills with *ju*-pits: 治四種癩病, "to cure the four types of breakdown disease". 癩病 is identical with the condition 陰癀. Therefore one may assume that *nei tui* 內癀, internal prominence-illness, is identical with *yin tui* 陰癀，yin (i.e. scrotal) prominence-illness.

***Nei wai zhang* 內外障, internal and external screen** [2] AN *nei wai zhang yi* 內外障翳, internal and external obstructive shade; *nei wai zhang yan* 內外障眼, internally and externally obstructed eye.
IS CD of → *nei zhang* 內障, internal screen, and → *wai zhang* 外障, external screen. *SJZL* 102: 頭風、**內外障**、青盲、攀睛翳膜悉治，填睛育嬰丸方, "Recipe for 'pills to fill the eyeballs and raise an infant' that cure head wind, **internal and external screen**, green blindness and shade membranes covering the eyeballs alike".

***Nei wai zhang yan* 內外障眼, internally and externally obstructed eye** [1]
IS identical with → *nai wai zhang* 內外障, internal and external screen. *ZLBC* SE *long nao xiang* 龍腦香 quotes *HYBC*: 主**內外障眼**，三蟲，治五痔，明目，鎮心，秘精, "It controls **internally and externally obstructed eyes**, and the three bugs/worms, and it cures the five types of piles, clears the eyes, eases an [excited] heart, and prevents spontaneous emission of essence".

***Nei wai zhang yi* 內外障翳, internal and external obstructive shade** [7]
IS identical with → *nai wai zhang* 內外障, internal and external screen. *SJZL* 109: 治肝腎虛風上攻，眼生黑花，頭目不利及**內外障翳**, "To cure depletion wind of the liver and kidneys attacking the upper regions, with the eyes growing black flowers, impairing the functions of the head and eyes, and generating **internal and external obstructive shade**".

***Nei xu* 內虛, internal depletion; hollow; name of a pharmaceutical drug** [12]
① PC identical with → *li xu* 裏虛, interior depletion. *NJ* 48: 外痛內快，為外實**內虛**, "If the patient feels pain externally and is comfortable internally, that indicates external repletion and **internal depletion**".
② Designates the texture of pharmaceutical substances, identical with → *xu* 虛 ④, hollow. *BCSY* SE *tian men dong* 天門冬：天門冬根有十餘莖，百部多者五六十莖，根長尖，**內虛**，味苦, "The root of *tian men dong* has more than ten stems. Most of *bai bu* [roots] have 50 to 60 stems. The roots are long and pointed, **hollow**, and have a bitter flavor.
③ Alternative name of the pharmaceutical drug *huang qin* 黃芩. *BCGM* SE *huang qin* 黃芩, Shi ming 釋名, Explication of names: **內虛** 別錄, "[Called] *nei xu* in the [*MY*]*BL*".

***Nei yong* 內癰, internal obstruction-illness** [3]
PC of → *yong* 癰, obstruction-illness, developing in the body's cavities. *ZBYHL* 33: **內癰**者，由飲食不節，冷熱不調，寒氣客於內，或在胸膈，或在腸胃, "**Internal obstruction-illnesses** result from immoderate drinking and eating, when cold and heat are not balanced. Cold qi settles internally, either in the region of the chest and diaphragm, or in the intestines and the stomach".

***Nei zhang* 內障, internal screen** [18]
PC of → *mu zhang* 目障, eye screen, resulting from diseases affecting the pupil or any other tissue inside the eyes. *HYBC* SE *shi jue ming* 石决明：主青盲、**內障**, "It controls green blindness and **internal screen**".

***Nei zhi* 內痔, internal piles** [10]
PC of → *zhi chuang* 痔瘡, piles sores, located inside the anus, sometimes apparent outside the anus, with much bleeding, especially following defecation, and an unspecific pain. *WTMY* 26: **內痔**每便即有血下，下血甚者，下血擊地成孔，出血過多，身體無復血色。有痛者，有不痛者, "**Internal piles** bleed following each defecation. When the bleeding is serious, holes form where the blood hits the ground. The bleeding is excessive to a degree that the body assumes a color showing that it is unable to regenerate the blood. In some cases there is pain, in some cases there is no pain".

***Ni* 𧓍, hidden worms** [p] AN *chong ni* 蟲𧓍，hidden worm infestation.
PC of worm infestation, with various illness signs resulting from worms gnawing on different body parts. *MYBL* SE *ku shen* 苦參：療惡瘡、下部**𧓍**, "It cures malign sores, and **hidden worms** in the lower body parts".

***Ni bu li* 溺不利, urine does not flow freely** [2]
IS, PC identical with → *xiao bian bu li* 小便不利. *BCJJZ* SE *xiong qiao shi* 雄雀屎：療目痛，決癰瘺，女子帶下，**溺不利**, "It cures painful eyes, ends obstruction-illnesses and pimples, female [diseases of] discharge from below the belt, and [stimulates the passage of] **urine that does not flow freely**".

***Ni chan* 逆產, delivery of [a child in] an unnormal position** [8] AN *ni sheng* 逆生, birth of [a child in] a position contrary to normal; *dao chan* 倒產, delivery of [a child in] an inverted position; *dao sheng* 倒生, birth of [a child in] inverted position.
PC of a → *nan chan* 難產, difficult birth, with the child entering the birth canal with its feet first. *ZBYHL* 43: **逆產**者，初覺腹痛，產時未至，驚動傷早，兒轉未竟，便用力產之，則令逆也, "In the case of a **delivery of [a child in] an unnormal position**, [the woman feels abdominal pain first. Before the delivery has begun, frightful excitement causes early damage, and the turning of the child will remain incomplete. If she then applies force to deliver it, this will cause it to move [in a position] contrary to normal".

***Ni chi* 𧓍齒, hidden-worms teeth** [8]
PC identical with → *chi ni* 齒𧓍. *SLBC* SE *hu cong* 胡葱：患胡臭、**𧓍齒**人不可食，轉極甚, "If someone suffers from barbarian stench and **hidden-worms teeth,** he must not eat [*hu cong*] lest [his disease] should become extremely serious".

***Ni chong* 𧓍蟲, hidden-worms infestation** [1]
PC identical with → *chong ni* 蟲𧓍. *JGYL* Lj: 白苣不可共酪同食，作**蟲𧓍**, "*Bai ju* must not be consumed together with cheese, lest a **hidden-worms infestation** should result".

***Ni chuang* 𧓍瘡, hidden-worms sores** [18] AN *chuang ni* 瘡𧓍.
PC of → *ni* 𧓍, hidden-worms, disease with ulcers, festering and stench. *MYBL* SE *qing xiang zi* 青葙子：惡瘡疥虱，痔蝕，下部**𧓍瘡**, "For malign sores, *jie*-illness, and lice, pile erosion, and **hidden-worms sores** affecting the lower body parts.

***Ni leng* 逆冷, counterflow cold** [2]
IS identical with → *shen leng* 身冷, body cold. *JGYL* Fj: 寒疝腹中痛，**逆冷**，手足不仁, "Cold, elevation-illness, with pain in the abdomen, **counterflow cold**, and numbness of the hands and feet".

***Ni lu* 逆臚, inverted skin** [3]
PC of skin at the margins of the toes and fingernails breaking up and peeling off. *ZBYHL* 30: 手足爪甲際皮剝起，謂之**逆臚**, "When the skin at the borders of the toe and fingernails peels off and breaks up, this is called '**inverted skin**'".

Ni man **逆滿, counterflow and fullness** [2]

IS of an uncomfortable feeling of distension and fullness brought forth by a qi movement upwards, contrary to its proper direction, and often accompanied by vomiting. *JGYL* Fj: 腹中寒氣，雷鳴切痛，胸脅**逆滿**，嘔吐，附子粳米湯主之, “[If patients suffer from] cold qi in the abdomen with thunderous sounds and cutting pain, **counterflow and fullness** in the chest and flanks, as well as vomiting, the decoction with *fu zi* and *jing mi* controls this”.

Ni qi **逆氣, counterflow qi** [43]

① IS of panting, vomiting, belching and hiccough as manifestations of qi moving upward, contrary to its regular direction. *SW* 22: 肺病者，喘咳**逆氣**，肩背痛, “In the case of a lung disease, one pants and coughs from **counterflow qi**. There is pain in the shoulders and the back”.

② PC with qi moving contrary to its regular direction as a major sign. *MYBL* SE *mu he* 木核：根，療心腹**逆氣**，止渴, “The root. It cures **counterflow qi** in the heart and abdomen; it quenches thirst”.

Ni qi qiang xin **逆氣搶心, counterflow qi knocking at the heart** [3]

IS of an uncomfortable feeling of qi moving upward from below and striking at the heart depot. *WTMY* 12: 范汪療胸痹，心中痞堅，留氣結於胸中，胸滿，脅下**逆氣搶心**，枳實湯方, “Fan Wang cures chest blockage, obstacle-illness hardening in the heart, resident qi forming nodes in the chest, a feeling of fullness in the chest below the flanks and **counterflow qi knocking at the heart** with the recipe for a decoction with *zhi shi*”.

Ni se **溺澀, urine is rough** [4]

IS identical with → *xiao bian bu li* 小便不利①, urine does not flow freely. *SJZL* 179: 小腹滿，**溺澀**，有餘瀝者，為氣淋, “If the lower abdomen has a feeling of fullness and the **urine is rough**, and if there is a dribbling of remaining [urine], this is ‘qi dripping’”.

Ni sheng **逆生, birth of [a child in] an unnormal position** [6]

PC identical with → *ni chan* 逆產, delivery of [a child in] an unnormal position. *QJYF* 卷 2: 治**逆生**胎不出方, “Recipe to cure **birth of [a child in] an unnormal position** with the fetus failing to leave [the birth canal]”.

Ni shui **溺水, submersion in water; drowning** [10] AN *shui ni* 水溺.

PC of diseases resulting from submersion in water. *QJYF* 25: 夫五絕者：一曰自縊，二曰牆壁壓迮，三曰**溺水**，四曰魘寐，五曰產乳絕, “Now, the five cut-offs include, first, [appearance of death following] suicide by hanging; second, [appearance of death following] being crushed by a wall; third, [appearance of death because of] **drowning**; fourth, [appearance of death because of] nightmare demons; fifth, [appearance of death in the course of giving] birth”.

Ni shui si **溺水死, [appearance of] death from drowning in water** [5]

PC identical with → *ni si* 溺死, [appearance of] death from drowning. *PJF* 255: 治**溺水死**者，上臥倒瀝却水,便於肚上多著灰掩之，仍以皂莢末吹鼻中，即活, “To cure cases of **[appearance of] death from drowning in water**, let that person lie with his upper body inclined downwards to have the water flow off.

Then have his abdomen covered with ashes. In addition blow a *zao jia* powder into his nose. This will bring him back to life".

***Ni si* 溺死, [appearance of] death from drowning** [6] AN *ni shui si* 溺水死, [appearance of] death from drowing in water.

PC of → *cu si* 卒死, sudden [appearance of] death, resulting from drowning in water. *ZBYHL* 23: **溺死**候：人為水所沒溺，水從孔竅入，灌注腑臟，其氣壅閉，故死, "The signs of **[appearance of] death from drowning**: When someone is submerged in water, water will enter his body through the orifices. It pours into the depots and palaces, and blocks the path of qi. Hence he will die".

***Ni tong* 䘌痛, hidden-worms pain** [5]

PC CD of all → *ni* 䘌, hidden worms, diseases manifesting themselves with pain. *MYBL* SE *ran she dan* 蚺蛇膽：主心腹**䘌痛**，下部䘌瘡, "It controls **hidden-worms pain** in heart and abdomen, and hidden-worms sores in the lower body parts".

***Ni xia* 䘌下, hidden-worms discharge** [2]

PC CD of all → *ni* 䘌, hidden worms, diseases manifesting themselves with diarrhea. *ZHF* 2: 又有病**䘌下**不止者，烏頭二兩，女葳、雲實各一兩，桂二分，蜜丸如桐子，水服五丸，一日三服, "Also, in the case of the disease of incessant **hidden-worms discharge**: *wu tou* 2 *liang*; *nü wei* and *yun shi* 1 *liang* each; *gui* 2 *fen*. Prepare pills with honey, the size of *tong* seeds. Ingest five pills with water. Three doses every day".

***Ni xue* 溺血, urine with blood** [24]

① IS identical with → *niao xue* 尿血①. *SW* 37: 胞移熱於膀胱，則癃、**溺血**, "When the uterus moves heat to the urinary bladder, [this results in] protuberance-illness and **urine with blood**".

② PC identical with → *niao xue* 尿血②. *MYBL* SE *cong zhi* 葱汁：平，温，主**溺血**, "Balanced, warm. It controls **urine with blood**".

***Niao bi* 尿閉, blocked urination** [8]

IS, PC identical with → *xiao bian bu tong* 小便不通. *BCGM* SE *ju* 橘 quotes *FRDQLF*: 產後**尿閉**不通者，陳皮一兩去白為末，每空心温酒服二錢，一服即通, "In the case of **blocked urination** following delivery, take 1 *liang* of *chen pi*, discard the white parts and grind to a powder. Ingest 2 *qian* with warm wine on an empty stomach. One dose will make [the urine] flow".

***Niao bu tong* 尿不通, blocked urination** [1]

IS, PC identical with → *xiao bian bu tong* 小便不通. *PJF* 182: 神仙一塊氣，治男子婦人病**尿不通**, 氣血流滯，下元虛寒，四肢腫滿, "[The recipe called] 'lump of qi from the spirit hermits' cures males and females suffering from **blocked urination**, sluggish flow of qi and blood, depletion cold of the original [qi] in the lower parts, and swelling and a feeling of fullness in the four limbs".

***Niao chuang* 尿床, bedwetting** [11]

IS of nocturnal spontaneous enuresis while asleep. *QJYF* 5: 燒鵲巢灰井花水服之，亦治夜**尿床**, "Consuming the ashes of burned magpie nests with early morning well water also cures nocturnal **bedwetting**".

***Niao duan* 尿短, scant urination** [4]

IS identical with → *xiao bian duan* 小便短. *BCGM* SE *yang* 羊 quoting *QJYF* 水氣腫，鼓脹，小便不利, "Water qi swelling with drum distension; the urine does not flow freely", writes: 水腫**尿短**, "Water swelling with **scant urination**".

***Niao hui chuang* 尿灰瘡, urinary sand-sores** [1]

PC of → *chuang* 瘡, sores, conditions covering the inside of a child's two thighs as a result of wearing urine-soaked garments for too long. *BCGM* SE *da dou* 大豆：嚼爛，傅小兒**尿灰瘡**, "Chew until mashed and apply to **urinary sand-sores** in children".

***Niao nan* 尿難, difficult urination** [2]

IS identical with → *xiao bian bu li* 小便不利①, urine does not flow freely. *QJYF* 30: 中封、行間，主振寒溲白，**尿難**而痛, "[Piercing the needle insertion holes] *zhong feng* and *xing jian* controls shaking with cold and white urine, as well as painful and **difficult urination**".

***Niao se* 尿澀, urine roughness** [15]

IS identical with → *xiao bian bu li* 小便不利①, urine does not flow freely. *ZBY-HL* 14: 其狀：膀胱小腹皆滿，**尿澀**，常有餘瀝是也, "Its signs: the urinary bladder and lower abdomen have a feeling of fullness with **urine roughness**. A dribbling of remaining [urine] is common".

***Niao shuo* 尿數, frequent urination** [8]

IS identical with → *xiao bian shuo* 小便數. *PJF* 216 lists 治**尿數**而多者方, "Recipes to cure **urination that is frequent** and copious".

***Niao xue* 尿血, urine with blood** [75] AN *ni xue* 溺血.

① AN *xiao bian xue* 小便血. IS of bleeding through the frontal yin opening. *JGYL* Mj: 熱在下焦者，則**尿血**, "When there is heat in the lower burner, this leads to **urine with blood**".

② PC with hematuria and no pain. *SYJYBZFL* 9: 與淋不同，以其不痛，故屬**尿血**, "It differs from dribbling because there is no pain. Hence it belongs to [the conditions of] **urine with blood**".

***Nie chuang* 嚙瘡, bite wound** [4]

PC identical with → *yao chuang* 咬瘡. *MYBL* SE *hu gu* 虎骨：膏，主狗**嚙瘡**, "The ointment controls dog **bite wounds**".

***Nie shang* 嚙傷, injury from a bite** [1]

PC identical with → *yao shang* 咬傷. *BCGM* SE *huang han she* 黃頷蛇 quoting *QJYF* 25: 狂犬嚙人, "Rabid dog bites a human", writes: 猘狗**嚙傷**, "**Injury from a bite** of a rabid dog".

***Ning xue* 凝血, coagulated blood** [7]

EA PI of extravascular, hardened blood. Chinese medicine assumes that such an item, when staying in the body, may cause further diseases. *YXL lu jiang* 鹿醬：主破多年**凝血**, 能化膿為水及產後諸病, "It controls breaking through **coagulated blood** of many years. It is able to transform pus into water and [cures] all types of disease following delivery".

***Niu ma jie* 牛馬疥, *jie*-illness of oxen and horses** [1] V
PC of → *jie chuang* 疥瘡, *jie*-illness sores, affecting oxen and horses. *BCGM* SE *bai* 柏 quotes *BCBS*: 亦治**牛馬疥**, "It also cures ***jie*-illness of oxen and horses**".

***Niu pi e xuan* 牛皮惡癬, malign ox-hide *xuan*-illness** [1]
PC identical with → *niu pi xuan* 牛皮癬, ox-hide *xuan*-illness. *BCGM* SE *shui yin fen* 水銀粉 quotes *ZNF*: **牛皮惡癬**：五更食炙牛肉一片，少刻以輕粉半錢，温酒調下, "For **malign ox-hide *xuan*-illness**: 1 piece of roasted beef is to be eaten at the fifth watch. A little later half a *qian* of *qing fen* is to be ingested mixed with warm wine".

***Niu pi feng xuan* 牛皮風癬, ox-hide wind-*xuan*-illness** [6]
PC identical with → *niu pi xuan* 牛皮癬, ox-hide *xuan*-illness. *BCGM* SE *niu* 牛 quotes *GZQF*: **牛皮風癬**：生驢皮一塊，以朴消腌過，燒灰，油調搽之，名一掃光, "**Ox-hide wind-*xuan*-illness**: a piece of raw donkey hide is pickled with *pu xiao*, burned to ashes, mixed with oil and applied externally. This is called 'sweeping to have the luster return immediately'".

***Niu pi wan xuan* 牛皮頑癬, stubborn ox-hide *xuan*-illness** [2]
PC identical with → *niu pi xuan* 牛皮癬, ox-hide *xuan*-illness. *SYDXF* 19 lists 遍身牛皮癬方, ...雌黃末入輕粉，豬脂調抹, "Recipes for ox-hide *xuan*-illness affecting the entire body: "Mix *ci huang* powder with *qing fen* and lard and apply externally". *PJF* 281 quotes this and writes 遍身皮癬, "*Xuan*-illness affecting the skin of the entire body". *BCGM* SE *ci huang* 雌黃 quotes the latter version and writes **牛皮頑癬**, "**Stubborn ox-hide *xuan*-illness**".

***Niu pi xuan* 牛皮癬, ox-hide *xuan*-illness** [4] AN *niu pi feng xuan* 牛皮風癬, ox-hide wind *xuan*-illness; *niu pi wan xuan* 牛皮頑癬, stubborn ox-hide *xuan*-illness; *niu pi xue xuan* 牛皮血癬, ox-hide blood *xuan*-illness; *niu pi e xuan* 牛皮惡癬, malign ox-hide *xuan*-illness.
PC of → *xuan* 癬, *xuan*-illness a), with a stubborn, thick and hard lesion, reminiscent of an ox's neck skin. *SJZL* 137: 牛犬所飲、刀刃磨淬之餘水，取以盥濯，毒氣傳人，亦能生癬，故得於牛毒者，狀似牛皮。於諸癬中最為痹厚邪毒之甚者，俗謂之**牛皮癬**, "If for washing one uses the water given oxen and dogs to drink, or the water running from a stone used for grinding knives, poisonous qi may enter [one's organism] and cause *xuan*-illness. Those resulting from the poison of oxen will appear as ox-hide. Among all types of *xuan*-illness, those with a very numb and thick skin and with the most evil poison, they are commonly called '**ox-hide *xuan*-illness**'".

***Niu pi xue xuan* 牛皮血癬, ox-hide blood *xuan*-illness** [1]
PC identical with → *niu pi xuan* 牛皮癬, ox-hide *xuan*-illness. *BCGM* SE *yan jiao* 烟膠 quotes *JDTF*: **牛皮血癬**：烟膠三錢，寒水石三錢，白礬二錢，花椒一錢半，為末，臘豬脂調搽, "For **ox-hide blood *xuan*-illness**: *yan jiao*, 3 *qian*; *han shui shi*, 3 *qian*; *bai fan*, 2 *qian*; *hua jiao*, 1 1/2 *qian*. Prepare a powder. Mix with cured lard and apply externally".

***Niu xian* 牛癇, buffalo epilepsy** [4]
PC of a → *dian xian* 癲癇, peak-illness with epilepsy, which, at the time of its outbreaks, makes the patient's four limbs twitch and his eyes be fixed to look straight ahead, together with abdominal distension, to make him resemble a buffalo. *QJYF* 5: **牛癇**之為病，目正直視，腹脹, "The disease of **buffalo epilepsy**: the eyes stare straight ahead, and the abdomen is distended".

***Nong chuang* 膿瘡, festering sores** [4] AN *chuang nong* 瘡膿.
PC CD of open → *chuang* 瘡, sores, conditions with pus emitted as a major sign. *SJZL* 1: 民病熱中、聾瞑、血溢、**膿瘡**, "The people suffer from heated center, deafness and blindness, blood overflow, and **festering sores**".

***Nong lou* 膿瘺, putrescent fistula** [1]
PC of → *lou* 瘺, fistula, with an opening that fails to close for a long time and releases large quantities of pus and other liquids. *ZBYHL* 34: 重為熱毒氣停積生膿，常不絕，故謂之**膿瘺**也, "In serious cases heat poison stagnates and collects to develop pus. This often cannot be stopped. Hence one calls it '**putrescent fistula**'".

***Nong she* 弄舌, playing tongue** [7]
IS of a tongue, mostly among children, that is repeatedly stretched out of the mouth and immediately retracted again. It may be stretched upward or downward, to the left and to the right without ceasing to move, and it may lick the lips all around the mouth. *BJ* SE *zao xiu* 蚤休: 驚癇，搖頭**弄舌**, "Fright epilepsy, swaying head, and **playing tongue**".

***Nong shui* 膿水, pus and water** [25]
PI, a mixture of pus with watery secretions. *QJYF* 21: 凡消渴病經百日以上，不得灸刺，灸刺則於瘡上漏**膿水**不歇, "Patients who have had melting-with-thirst disease for more than one hundred days cannot be cauterized or treated with needling. If they are subjected to cauterization or piercing, this will result in unending flow of **pus and water** from above the sores". When the *BCGM* speaks of "pus and water" it mostly refers to matter discharged from local lesions.

***Nong xue* 膿血, pus and blood** [154]
PI, a mixture of pus and blood that can be discharged through cough, spitting, vomiting, diarrhea, or through local lesions resulting from pathological changes. *SW* 40: " 岐伯曰：裹大**膿血**，居腸胃之外，不可治，治之每切按之致死, "Qi Bo: [The lower abdomen] holds massive **pus and blood**, located outside of the intestines and the stomach. This must not be treated. If one treats it, each time one presses the [lower abdomen] this brings [the patient] closer to death".

***Nong xue li* 膿血痢, free-flux illness with pus and blood** [1]
PC of → *li ji* 痢疾, ailment of free-flux illness, with thin stool carrying pus and blood. *ZBYHL* 17: 夏月多苦**膿血痢**, "During summer one often suffers from **free-flux illness with pus and blood**".

***Nong zhong* 膿腫, swelling with pus** [2]
PC CD of → *chuang yang* 瘡瘍, sores, with an obvious swelling that includes pus but has not opened to fester yet. *QJYF* 30: 憂思損傷，氣積聚，腹中甚

痛，作**膿腫**, "Harm caused by grief and pondering results in qi accumulation and collection with heavy pain in the abdomen that eventually transforms into **swelling with pus**".

Nü **衄, nosebleed; spontaneous external bleeding** [p]
① IS identical with → *nü xue* 衄血①. *SW* 45: 太陽厥逆，僵仆嘔血善**衄**, "Recession with counterflow in the major yang [conduit results in the following: patients] fall, vomit blood, and tend to have **nosebleed**".
② PC identical with → *nü xue* 衄血②. *SW* 4: 春善病鼽**衄**, "In spring one tends to suffer from stuffy nose and **nosebleed**".

Nu **胬, tumorous [flesh-growth]** [p]
PC AD of → *nu rou* 胬肉. *BCGM* SE *xing* 杏 quotes *SJZL* 112: 目為物所傷，睛陷胬肉, "When the eye is harmed by an object, the eyeball sinks in and develops a tumorous flesh-growth", writes: 傷目生**胬**, "Harmed eye develops **a tumorous [flesh-growth]**".

Nü dan **女疸, *dan*-illness [caused by exhaustion with] women** [1]
PC identical with → *nü lao dan* 女勞疸, *dan*-illness resulting from exhaustion with women. *ZHF* 4: 疸病有五種，謂黃疸，穀疸，酒疸，**女疸**，勞疸也, "There are five types of the disease of *dan*-illness. They are called yellow bile, *dan*-illness [caused by] grain, *dan*-illness [caused by] wine, ***dan*-illness [caused by exhaustion with] women**, and *dan*-illness [caused by] exhaustion in general".

Nü jing bu li **女經不利, menstruation not flowing freely** [1]
PC identical with → *jing shui bu li* 經水不利. *BCTJ* SE *ma fen* 麻蕡：古方亦有用麻花者，云味苦，主諸風及**女經不利**, "Some ancient recipes also made use of *ma hua*. It is said to have a bitter flavor and to master all types of wind and **menstruation not flowing freely**".

Nü jing bu xing **女經不行, menstrual blockage** [1]
PC identical with → *yue shui bu tong* 月水不通. *BCGM* SE *zi wei* 紫葳 quotes *XSTCF*: **女經不行**：凌霄花為末，每服二錢, "**Menstrual blockage**: Grind *ling xiao hua* to a powder; the dose to be ingested is 2 *qian*".

Nü jing ji nian bu tong **女經積年不通, chronic menstrual blockage** [1]
PC of → *jing bi* 經閉, menstrual blockage, which has not been cured for an extended period of time. *BCTJ* SE *long gu* 龍骨：**女經積年不通**，必治之，用龍胎、瓦松、景天三物各少許, "**Chronic menstrual blockage** requires treatment. Use small amounts of the three items *long tai*, *wa song*, and *jing tian*".

Nu kuang **怒狂, anger with madness** [1]
IS of a tendency to easily become angry as if one were insane. LSZ speaks of this condition as *yi nu ru kuang* 易怒如狂, "to easily become angry as if one were insane". *SW* 46: 有病**怒狂**者，此病安生, "Someone suffers from **anger with madness**; how does this disease emerge?"

Nü lao **女勞, exhaustion with women** [1]
EA identical with → *fang lao* 房勞, bedchamber exhaustion. *JGYL* Mj: 黃家，日晡所發熱，而反惡寒，此為**女勞**得之, "A jaundice patient effused heat in

the late afternoon but nevertheless had an aversion to cold. He got this as a result of an **exhaustion with women.**

***Nü lao dan* 女勞疸, *dan*-illness resulting from exhaustion with women** [3] AN *nü dan* 女疸, female *dan*-illness; *nü lao huang dan* 女勞黃疸, yellow *dan*-illness resulting from exhaustion with women; *nü lao hei dan* 女勞黑疸, black *dan*-illness resulting from exhaustion with women.

PC of → *huang dan* 黃疸, yellow *dan*-illness, resulting from excessive sexual intercourse. *JGYL* Mj: 額上黑，微汗出，手足中熱，薄暮即發，膀胱急，小便自利，名曰**女勞疸**, "The forehead is dark. Some sweat appears. There is heat in hands and feet. It breaks out at dusk. The bladder is tight, and urine flows spontaneously. This is called '***dan*-illness resulting from exhaustion with women**'".

***Nü lao fu* 女勞復, recurrence because of exhaustion from [intercourse with] women** [5]

PC of a recurrence of a serious disease because of immoderate sexual activity immediately after recovery. A type of → *lao fu* 勞復, recurrence because of exhaustion. *MYBL* SE *huan hui zhi* 浣褌汁：解毒箭，並**女勞復**亦善, "Dissolves arrow poison. It is also good for treating **recurrence because of exhaustion from [intercourse with] women**".

***Nü lao hei dan* 女勞黑疸, black *dan*-illness following exhaustion with women** [2]

PC identical with → *nü lao dan* 女勞疸, *dan*-illness following exhaustion with women. *BCGM* SE *xiao shi* 消石 quoting *JGYL* 女勞疸, "*Dan*-illness following exhaustion with women", writes: **女勞黑疸**, "**Black *dan*-illness following exhaustion with women**".

***Nü lao huang dan* 女勞黃疸, yellow *dan*-illness following exhaustion with women** [8]

PC identical with → *nü lao dan* 女勞疸, *dan*-illness following exhaustion with women. *BCGM* SE *fan shi* 礬石 quoting *JGYL* 女勞疸, "*Dan*-illness following exhaustion with women", writes: **女勞黃疸**, "**Yellow *dan*-illness following exhaustion with women**".

***Nü ren san shi liu ji* 女人三十六疾, 36 types of women's ailments** [1]

PC identical with → *fu ren san shi liu ji* 婦人三十六疾. *BCGM* Bai bing zhu zhi yao 百病主治藥 quoting *QJYF* 2: 承澤丸，治婦人下焦三十六疾, "The 'pills upholding moisture' cure 36 types of ailments affecting the lower burner in women", writes: 澤蘭子，**女人三十六疾**, "*Ze lan zi*: **36 types of women's ailments**".

***Nü ren yi ji* 女人異疾, unusual ailment in women** [1]

PC of an unusual disease of menstruating women who discharge clots shaped like birds and animals. *BCGM* SE *ze xie* 澤瀉 quotes *QJF*: **女人異疾**：女人月事退出，皆作禽獸之形，欲來傷人。先將綿塞陰戶，乃頓服沒藥末一兩，白湯調下，即愈, "**Unusual ailment in women**: when women discharge their monthly affair entirely shaped like birds and animals that intend to harm humans, first use a piece of cloth to close the yin-gate, and then ingest 1 *liang* of *mo yao* powder mixed with clear hot water. This will bring the cure".

***Nu rou* 努肉, tumorous flesh-growth** [1]

PC identical with → *nu rou* 胬肉. *TPSHF* 32: 眼赤腫痛，生**努肉**侵睛，宜服前胡散方, "When the eyes are red with swelling and pain and develop **a tumorous flesh-growth** encroaching upon the eyeball, the recipe to ingest the powder with *qian hu* is advisable".

***Nu rou* 胬肉, tumorous flesh-growth** [47] AD *nu* 胬; AW *nu rou* 努肉.

① PC with the growth of a redundant fleshy object reminiscent of an insect wing developing from the canthi towards the dark part of the eye as a major sign. *TBC* SE *que shi* 雀屎：和男首子乳如薄泥，點目中，**胬肉**、赤脈貫瞳子上者即消, "Mix with the milk for a first male child to prepare a thin paste and swab into the eye. **Tumorous flesh-growth** and red vessels pervading the surface of the pupil will then dissolve".

② PI of flesh tissue protruding from sores and ulcers. *TPSHF* 61: 治諸瘡瘥後，瘡瘢**胬肉**未消, "It cures, in the scars following the healing of any type of sore, **tumorous flesh-growth** failing to dissolve".

***Nü xue* 衄血, nosebleed; spontaneous external bleeding; blood lost through spontaneous external bleeding** [148] AD *nü* 衄.

① IS of bleeding from any of the orifices in the head or from the skin, without any externally inflicted harm. The term is mostly used to signify nosebleed. *LS* 66: 陽絡傷則血外溢，血外溢則**衄血**, "When the yang network [vessel] is harmed, blood will flow out. When blood flows out, this is '**spontaneous external bleeding**'".

② PC a) with spontaneous bleeding from any orifice or through the skin. *ZBYHL* 29: 診其寸口微芤者，**衄血**, "When one examines the [patient's] inch opening and the [movement in the] vessels there is weak and hollow, this is **spontaneous external bleeding**". b) Of → *bi nü* 鼻衄, nosebleed, in particular. *DXXF* 2: **衄血**者，鼻中出血也, "As for *nü xue*, this is **loss of blood through the nose**".

③ PI of blood lost in the course of spontaneous external bleeding. *ZBYHL* 27: 或如豆汁，或如**衄血**，凝停胃裏，因即滿悶便吐, "It may resemble bean juice, and it may resemble **blood lost through spontaneous bleeding**. It coagulates and stays in the stomach. Hence [patients] experience a feeling of fullness, heart-pressure, and they defecate and vomit".

***Nü zi jing chan yu xue* 女子經產余血, surplus blood among women following delivery** [1]

PC CD of all types of diseases caused by stagnant blood following delivery. *MYBL* SE *wu zhu yu* 吳茱萸：根白皮，殺蟯蟲，治喉痹咳逆，止泄注，食不消，**女子經產余血**, "The white bark of the root kills pinworms and cures throat blockage and coughing with counterflow. It stops diarrhea and failure to digest food, and ends **surplus blood among women following delivery**".

***Nü zi yu chang* 女子育腸, birth intestine [qi] in females** [1]
PC of → *yu chang qi* 育腸氣, birth intestine qi. *BCGM* Bai bing zhu zhi bing 百病主治病, *shan qi* 疝氣, elevation-illness qi: **女子育腸**，小兒木腎, "**Birth intestine [qi] in females**; testicles [as hard as] wood in children". *BCGM* Bai bing zhu zhi bing 百病主治病, *shan tui* 疝㿉 elevation-illness and prominence-illness: 腹病曰疝，丸病曰㿉。有寒氣，濕熱，痰積，血滯，虛冷。男子奔豚、**女子育腸**、小兒木腎, "When the illness affects the abdomen, it is called 'elevation-illness'. When it effects the testicles, it is called 'prominence-illness'. [Its different manifestations] include 'cold qi', 'moisture heat', 'phlegm accumulation', 'blood sluggishness', 'depletion cold', 'running piglets' in males, '**birth intestine [qi] in females**', and testicles as hard as wood in children".

***Nüe* 瘧, malaria** [p]
PC identical with → *nüe ji* 瘧疾, malaria ailment. *SW* 35: **瘧**之始發也，先起於毫毛, "When **malaria** begins to break out, it first emerges from the finest body hair".

***Nüe bing* 瘧病, malaria disease** [4]
PC identical with → *nüe ji* 瘧疾, malaria ailment. *ZHF* 3: 治**瘧病**方，鼠婦、豆豉二七枚，合擣令相和。未發時服二丸，欲發時服一丸, "Recipe to cure **malaria disease**: Pound 27 pieces of *shu fu* and *dou chi* together until they are thoroughly mixed. Ingest two pills before an outbreak; when an outbreak is immanent ingest one pill".

***Nüe ji* 瘧疾, malaria ailment** [94] AD *nüe* 瘧; AN *nüe bing* 瘧病, malaria disease; *kai nüe* 痎瘧, *shan* 痁.
PC of recurring alternating sensations of cold and heat. *QJYF* 24: 温疫**瘧疾**，年年常患, "Warmth epidemics and **malaria ailments** make a person suffer constantly for many years".

***Nüe lao* 瘧勞, malaria exhaustion** [1]
PC identical with → *lao nue* 勞瘧, exhaustion malaria. *BCGM* SE *bie jia* 鱉甲:鱉色青入肝，故所主者，**瘧勞**寒熱，痃瘕驚癇, "Turtles have a greenish-blue color and enter the liver. Hence [*bie jia*] controls **malaria exhaustion** with alternating sensations of cold and heat, string-illness with conglomeration-illness, as well as fright epilepsy".

***Nüe li* 瘧痢, malaria-related free-flux illness** [13]
PC of → *li ji* 痢疾, ailment of free-flux illness, associated with → *nüe* 瘧, malaria. *JYBC* SE *bo lao* 伯勞：繼病，母有娠乳兒，兒有病如**瘧痢**，他日相繼腹大，或瘥或發。他人有娠，相近亦能相繼也。北人未識此病, "Transmission disease: when a pregnant mother breast-feeds an earlier child, and this child has a disease that resembles **malaria-related free-flux illness**, then the next day this will be transmitted and [the mother's] abdomen enlarged. This may recede and then break out again. If another woman is pregnant and comes close, this may also be transmitted to her. The people in the North do not know this disease".

***Nüe mu* 瘧母, malaria-mother [of lumps]** [5]

PC of a long-lasting sequence of malaria outbreaks where over time hard lumps develop below the flanks. *JGYL* Fj: 此結為癥瘕，名曰**瘧母**，急治之，宜鱉甲煎丸, "This forms nodes generating concretion-illness and conglomeration-illness; it is called '**malaria-mother [of lumps]**'. It must be treated immediately. The pills with boiled *bie jia* are appropriate".

***Nüe hou guai zheng* 瘧後怪症, queer conditions following malaria** [1]

PC of an unusual disease in the aftermath of a malaria episode with the skin of the shoulders and chest hardening and assuming a dark color, and impaired eating and drinking. *BCGM* SE *ze xie* 澤瀉 quotes *QJF*: **瘧後怪症**，口鼻中氣出，盤旋不散，凝如黑蓋色，過十日漸至肩胸，與肉相連，堅勝金石，無由飲食, "**Queer condition following malaria**: Qi is released from the mouth and nose, but it coils and fails to disperse. It congeals and assumes the appearance of a black cover. After ten days it gradually reaches the shoulders and the chest, where it connects with the flesh. Its hardness exceeds that of metal and stones. There is no space left for drinking and eating".

***Nuo chu* 搦搐, grabbing and jerking** [1]

IS identical with → *chu nuo* 搐搦, convulsions. *BCGM* Bai bing zhu zhi yao 百病主治藥: 井泉石，產後**搦搐**, "*Jing quan shi* [cures] **grabbing and jerking** following delivery". This is the only occurrence of *nuo chu* 搦搐 in the *BCGM*. It may be an early scribal error for in the paragraph on *jing quan shi* 井泉石 itself the *BCGM* has the common wording 產後搐搦.

***Nuo mi ji* 糯米積, accumulation of glutinous rice** [1]

PC of → *shi ji* 食積②, food accumulation, brought forth by an excessive consumption of food prepared from glutinous rice. *BCGM* SE *qu* 麴: 消食積、酒積、**糯米積**, "It dissolves food accumulations, wine accumulations, and **accumulations of glutinous rice**".

- O -

***Ou* 嘔, vomiting** [p]

① IS of a reflux of the stomach's contents being thrown up, accompanied by a retching sound. *SW* 38: 胃咳之狀，咳而**嘔**，**嘔**甚則長蟲出, "The appearance of stomach cough: [Patients] cough and **vomit**. When the **vomiting** is severe, long worms come out".

② PC with retching and vomiting as its main illness signs. *SW* 74: 諸痿喘**嘔**，皆屬於上, "All [cases of] dysfunction [with] panting and **vomiting**, without exception they are associated with the upper [parts of the body]".

***Ou e* 嘔噁, vomiting with nausea** [7]

IS CD of → *e xin* 噁心, malign center/nausea, and *ou tu* 嘔吐, vomiting. *HJJF* 2 RE *huo xiang zheng qi san* 藿香正氣散, powder with *huo xiang* to correct the qi: It cures 心腹冷痛，反胃**嘔噁**, "Cold pain in the heart and abdomen, turned over stomach with **vomiting and nausea".**

***Ou ku zhi* 嘔苦汁, vomiting of bitter liquid** [1]

IS of vomiting a liquid with bitter flavor. *SJZL* 193: 咳而**嘔苦汁**者，陽陵泉主之, "If someone coughs and **vomits bitter liquid**, this is controlled by [piercing the] yang-mound-fountain [hole]".

***Ou ni* 嘔逆, vomiting with countermovement [of qi]** [104]

① IS identical with → *ou* 嘔①, vomiting. *SW* 74: **嘔逆**躁煩，腹滿痛，溏泄，傳為赤沃, "[People suffer from] **vomiting with countermovement [of qi]**, overexcitement, vexation, abdominal fullness, pain, and semiliquid stools. Transmission turns this into a red downpour".

② PC identical with → *ou* 嘔②, vomiting. *SW* 74: 為丹熛瘡瘍，**嘔逆**喉痹, "It also causes vermilion flaming-heat sores and ulcers. [Patients suffer from] **vomiting with countermovement [of qi]** and throat blockage".

***Ou ni suan shui* 嘔逆酸水, vomiting with counterflow of sour water** [1]

IS identical with → *ou tu suan shui* 嘔吐酸水, vomiting of sour water. *ZLBC* SE *yang shi* 羊屎 quotes *BBSJ*: 療無故**嘔逆酸水**不止，或吐三五口，食後如此方, "Use this recipe after meals for treating unending **vomiting with counterflow of sour water** that cannot be explained, or if someone vomits three to five times".

***Ou qing shui* 嘔清水, vomiting of clear water** [3]

IS identical with → *ou tu qing shui* 嘔吐清水. *BCGM* SE *gao liang jiang* 高良姜 quoting *BCTJ* 忽心中惡，口吐清水, "There is a sudden feeling of malignity/nausea in the heart/center, and they spit clear water", writes: 忽然噁心，**嘔清水**, "[Patients] have a sudden feeling of malignity/nausea in the heart/center, and **vomit clear water**".

***Ou shang* 毆傷, injury from a blow** [1]

PC identical with → *da pu shang sun* 打撲傷損. *BCGM* SE *da dou chi* 大豆豉 quoting *QJYF* 25: 治被毆擊損傷聚血，腹滿煩惱悶方, "Recipe for injuries from an assault with blood collecting, and also a feeling of fullness in the abdomen, vexation and annoyance as well as heart-pressure", writes: **毆傷**瘀聚，腹中悶滿, "**Injuries from a blow**, with collection of stagnant [blood], and in the abdomen a feeling of heart-pressure and fullness".

Ou shi **嘔食, vomiting [when one sees] food** [1]
IS of dry vomiting or retching stimulated by looking at food. *BCGM* SE *yang* 羊 quoting *TPSHF*: 反胃，見食即嘔噦, "Turned over stomach. When [the patient] sees food he immediately vomits", writes: 反胃**嘔食**, "Turned over stomach. [The patient] **vomits when [he sees] food**". The *SYDXF* uses *ou shi* 嘔食 in the sense of → *ou tu* 嘔吐, to vomit. However, as the *BCGM* took its quote from the *TPSHF*, it may well have continued the meaning documented in that source text.

Ou shui **嘔水, vomiting of water** [1]
IS identical with → *tu shui* 吐水, vomiting of water. *BCGM* SE *jiu* 韭 quotes *ZXF* 摘玄方：用韭汁治產後**嘔水**, "Use *jiu*-juice to cure **vomiting of water** following delivery".

Ou suan shui **嘔酸水, vomiting of sour water** [1]
IS identical with → *ou tu suan shui* 嘔吐酸水. *PJF* 184: 治一切冷氣不和，面色深黃，吃食減少，腹中時痛，**嘔酸水**，大腹滑泄, "To cure all types of unbalanced cold qi, deeply yellow facial complexion, diminished intake of food, recurrent pain in the abdomen, and **vomiting of sour water**".

Ou tu **嘔吐, vomiting** [100] AD *tu* 吐.
① IS of a reverse passage of the stomach's contents as well as of bile and intestinal liquid, followed by a discharge through vomiting. This may or may not be accompanied by a retching sound. *SW* 36: 足少陰之瘧，令人**嘔吐**甚, "Malaria of the foot minor yin [conduit]: it makes a person **vomit** severely".
② PC with vomiting as its major illness sign. *JGYL* Mj: **嘔吐**而病在膈上，後思水者，解，急與之, "In the case of **vomiting** with the disease being situated above the diaphragm, when after [vomiting patients] wish to drink water, the disease has ended and one should quickly provide them with [water to drink]".

Ou tu qing shui **嘔吐清水, vomiting of clear water** [2] AN *ou qing shui* 嘔清水.
IS of spitting of clear and thin liquid. *TPSHF* 78: 治產後心腹疼痛，**嘔吐清水**，不下飲食，肉豆蔻散方, "To cure pain in the region of the heart and abdomen following delivery, **vomiting of clear water**, and an inability to eat and drink: [use the] recipe for a powder with *rou dou kou*".

Ou tu suan shui **嘔吐酸水, vomiting of sour water**[4] AN *ou suan shui* 嘔酸水, vomiting of sour water; *ou ni suan shui* 嘔逆酸水, vomiting of sour water; *ou tu ben zhi* 嘔吐酸汁, vomiting of sour juice.
IS identical with → *tu suan shui* 吐酸水. *WTMY* 6: 療**嘔吐酸水**，結氣築心，白术散方, "Recipe with *bai zhu* for curing **vomiting of sour water**, and bound qi pounding at the heart".

Ou tu suan zhi **嘔吐酸汁, vomiting of sour juice** [1]
IS identical with → *ou tu suan shui* 嘔吐酸水. *BCGM* SE *wu zhu yu* 吳茱萸 quotes *ZSJYF*: 十日一發，頭痛背寒，**嘔吐酸汁**, "It is active once every ten

days. [Patients suffer from] headache, cold in their back, and **vomiting of sour juice**".

Ou tu tan shui **嘔吐痰水, vomiting of phlegm and water**[2]

IS identical with → *tu tan shui* 吐痰水, spitting of phlegm and water. *SJZL* 54: 治上焦虛寒…不能飲食，**嘔吐痰水**，胡椒理中丸方, "To cure depletion cold in the upper burner…inability to eat and drink, **vomiting of phlegm and water**, [use the] recipe for pills with *hu jiao* to regulate the center".

Ou tu tan xian **嘔吐痰涎, vomiting of phlegmy sputum** [2]

IS of vomiting of sticky phlegm and phlegm-like sputum. *TPSHF* 48: 右脅下結聚成塊，喘咳胸痛，**嘔吐痰涎**，面黃體瘦，宜服三棱丸方, "Lumps of nodular collections form below the right flank. [Patients] cough and have chest pain. They **vomit phlegmy sputum**. Their face is yellow, and their body is emaciated. [In such cases] the recipe to ingest the pills with *san leng* is advisable".

Ou xie **嘔泄, vomiting and outflow** [1] AN *yue xie* 噦泄, retching vomiting and outflow.

PC identical with → *tu li* 吐利②, vomiting and free flow. *XEYZZJ* Qian Zhongyang zhuan 錢仲陽傳, Biography of Qian Zhongyang: 宗室王子病**嘔泄**, "A prince of the royal clan suffered from **vomiting and outflow**".

Ou xue **嘔血, vomiting of blood** [19]

① IS of vomiting that also produces blood. *SW* 38: 怒則氣逆，甚則**嘔血**, "When one is angry, the qi moves contrary [to its regular course]. In severe cases, [patients] **vomit blood**".

② PC with vomiting of blood. *LS* 4: 澀甚為**嘔血**；微澀為鼠瘻, "If it is very rough, [patients] **vomit blood**. If it is mildly rough, they have mouse fistula".

Ou yue **嘔哕, retching** [5]

IS identical with → *yue* 哕, retching. *MYBL* SE *zhu* 竹：皮茹，微寒。主**嘔哕**, "The peel, [its nature is] slightly cold. It controls **retching**".

Ou ye **嘔噎, vomiting [resulting from] gullet occlusion** [1]

IS of vomiting resulting from gullet occlusion. *QXLF* 18: 大抵翻胃未嘗不由膈噎而起…治翻胃**嘔噎**，上用大田螺, "Generally speaking, an upset stomach always results from a gullet blockage…To cure an upset stomach and **vomiting [resulting from gullet] occlusion**, [for the indications listed] above use large river snails".

Ou yue **嘔噦, vomiting** [35]

① IS identical with → *yue* 噦, retching. *QJYF* 10: 治傷寒後**嘔噦**方, "Recipe to cure **vomiting** in the aftermath of harm caused by cold".

② PC identical with → *yue ni* 噦逆②, retching with countermovement [of qi]. *ZBYHL* 18: **嘔噦**之病者，由脾胃有邪，穀氣不治所為也, "The disease of **vomiting** is caused by evil [qi] in the spleen and stomach with the result that the qi of the grain cannot be managed properly [by the spleen and stomach]".

- P -

***Pan chang* 盤腸, twisted intestine** [14] AN *pan chang qi* 盤腸氣, twisted intestine qi; *pan chang tong* 盤腸痛, twisted intestine pain.

PC of children experiencing an excruciating abdominal pain causing them to bend their back, cry and emit cold sweat. *XEWSZWLF* 14: 更有一證，發則腹中撮痛，乾啼無淚，腰曲背弓，上唇乾額上有汗，此名**盤腸**內吊之痛, "There is one more condition. When it appears there is a pinching pain in the abdomen, with dry crying without tears. The lower back is bent. The upper lip is dry, and sweat leaves from the forehead. This is called 'the pain of **twisted intestine** hauled internally'".

***Pan chang chan* 盤腸產, birth with a twisted intestine** [2] AN *pan chang sheng chan* 盤腸生產; *zi chang xian chu* 子腸先出, prior appearance of the infant's intestine; *zi chang xian xia* 子腸先下, prior descent of the infant's intestine.

PC at the time of birth with the vaginal wall or rectum appearing first and, after the child was born, being unable to retreat by themselves. *FRDQLF* 17: 趙都運恭人，每臨產則子腸先出，然後產子。產子之後，其腸不收，甚以為苦，名曰**盤腸產**。醫不能療。偶在建昌，得一坐婆施之一法而收之。其法遇產後子腸不收之時，以醋半盞，新汲冷水七分，碗調停，噀產婦面，每噀一縮，三噀收盡。此良法也，後學不可不知, "Whenever the wife of the official Zhao Duyun approached the moment of delivery, the 'infant's intestine' (i.e. uterus) appeared first, and only then did she give birth to a child. After the child was born, her intestine failed to recede. This caused her extreme suffering. It is called '**birth with a twisted intestine**'. The physicians were unable to cure this. It so happened that in Jianchang eventually she was treated by a midwife with a therapeutic approach that caused [the intestine] to recede. This approach is as follows. When she encounters a woman whose 'infant's intestine', following delivery, fails to recede, she mixes in a bowl half a cup of vinegar with 7 parts of cold water freshly drawn from a well, and spits it out of her mouth into the face of the delivering woman. After each spitting [the intestine] withdraws a bit. After three spirtings it has completely receded. This is a good approach. It must be known by students in the future".

***Pan chang sheng chan* 盤腸生產, to give birth with a twisted intestine** [3]

PC identical with → *pan chang chan* 盤腸產. *BCGM* SE *ban xia* 半夏 quoting *FRDQLF*: 盤腸產, "Delivery with a twisted intestine", writes: **盤腸生產, "To give birth with a twisted intestine"**.

***Pang guang huo* 膀胱火, bladder fire** [5]

PC and EA identical with → *pang guang re* 膀胱熱, bladder heat. *ZZN* 1: 黃柏瀉膀胱火, "*Huang bo* drains **bladder fire**".

Pang guang re **膀胱熱, heat in the bladder; bladder heat** [7] *pang guang huo* 膀胱火, bladder fire.

① PC of heat-type diseases affecting the bladder. *QJYF* 6 RE *sheng ma jian* 升麻煎, decoction with *sheng ma*: 治**膀胱熱**不已, "It cures **bladder heat** that does not end".

② EA bringing forth heat-type disease in the bladder. *ZBYHL* 14: 小便難者，此是腎與**膀胱熱**故也, "Difficulties in passing urine result from heat in the kidneys and **heat in the bladder**".

Pao **皰, blister** [p]

PC a) identical with → *mian pao* 面皰, facial blister. *ZBYHL* 27: 面皰者，謂面上有風熱氣生**皰**, "Facial blister is to say: **blisters** developing in the face following exposure to wind and heat qi". b) Of → *chuang* 瘡, sores developing in the shape of water blisters on the skin following some injury. The external skin is rather thin. Its contents mostly resemble water or pus. *BCSY* SE *bo pi* 檗皮: 主熱瘡**皰**起，蟲瘡, "It controls heat sores with the rise of **blisters**, and bug sores".

Pao chuang **皰瘡, blister sores** [5] AN *chuang pao* 瘡皰, sores with blisters.

PC CD of → *chuang* 瘡, sores, conditions with a clearly marked eruption of skin and a thick or thin wall surrounding the sores that are filled with a clear or turbid liquid. *ZBYHL* 7: 傷寒勢毒氣盛，多發**皰瘡**, "When as a result of harm caused by cold poison qi abounds, this often leads to a development of **blister sores**".

Pei lei **痞癗, clustered [seeds]-illness** [3] AN *lei zi* 癗子; *wu lei* 痦癗.

PC with small pimples or knots on the skin as its major sign. *QJYF* 5: 遍身**痞癗**如麻豆粒，年年喜發, "**Clustered [seeds]-illness** covering the entire body resemble sesame beans. They develop year after year".

Pen xue **噴血, spouting of blood** [2]

IS of rapidly spitting large quantities of blood. *BCGM* SE *hua ru shi* 花乳石 quoting *SYSS*: 涌噴血出成升斗, "Gushing and spouting of blood, emitting as much as a *sheng* or *dou*", writes: **噴血**出斗升, "[Patients] **spouting blood** emitting as much as a *dou* or a *sheng*".

Peng zhang **膨脹, swelling and distension** [9]

① IS identical with → *zhang* 脹①, distension. *QJYF* 26: 若貪味多餐，臨盤大飽，食訖覺腹中**膨脹**短氣，或至暴疾 "If one has an insatiable appetite, and eats to massive repletion, after having dined he will have a feeling of abdominal **swelling and distension**, as well as shortness of qi. In some instances this may develop into a violent ailment".

② PC with an uncomfortable feeling of swelling and distension. *BCGM* SE *ren gui* 人傀 quotes *XQYJ*: 明嘉靖乙酉，橫涇佣農孔方，忽患**膨脹**, "In the year *yi you* of the *jia qing* reign period of the Ming dynasty, a rural worker named Kong Fang from Hengjing all of a sudden suffered from **swelling and distension**".

Pi **澼, flush** [p]

PC of → *shui xie* 水瀉, watery outflow, or → *li ji* 痢疾, free-flux illness, caused by phlegm rheum stagnating in thes intestines. *MYBL* SE bai shi zhi 白石脂:

小腸**澼**，熱溏，便膿血，“Small intestinal **flush**, which is hot and viscous. Defecation is with pus and blood”.

Pi **癖 aggregation-illness** [p] AN *pi qi* 癖氣, aggregation-illness qi.
PC of painful lumps emerging from time to time in both flanks. *ZBYHL* 20: **癖**者，謂僻側在於兩脅之間，有時而痛是也，“**Aggregation-illness** is to say: something strange/out of the way (*pi* 僻) is located sideways in the costal regions. From time to time it hurts”.

Pi **痞, obstacle-illness** [p]
① IS of a feeling of uncomfortable fullness and distension. *SW* 74: 胸膈不利，心痛**痞**滿，“The chest and diaphragm are not freely passable. [Patients suffer from] heartache with **obstacle-illness** and a feeling of fullness”.
② PC of an uncomfortable distension and fullness in the chest and abdominal region. When pressed there is no pain. *SW* 70: 其色黃，其養肉，其病**痞**，其味甘，“Its color is yellow. It nourishes the flesh. Its disease is **an obstacle-illness**. Its flavor is sweet”.

Pi bi **脾痹, spleen blockage** [2] AN *wei bi* 胃痹, stomach blockage.
PC resulting from a depletion of spleen qi and a loss of its ability to move [qi to the other depots], with the four limbs slackening, and vomiting. *SW* 43: **脾痹**者，四肢解惰，發咳嘔汁，“In the case of a **spleen blockage**, the four limbs are sluggish. [Patients] cough and vomit liquid”.

Pi dan **脾疸, spleen *dan*-illness** [2]
PC of → *huang dan* 黄疸, yellow *dan*-illness, accompanied by illness signs such as heart vexation, a desire to sleep, and retching. *MYBL tong cao* 通草：療**脾疸**，常欲眠，心煩，噦出音聲，“It cures **spleen *dan*-illness**, with a permanent desire to sleep, heart vexation and noisy retching”.

Pi feng **皮風, skin wind** [1]
PC AD of → *pi fu feng* 皮膚風. *YXL* SE *xi xin* 細辛: 去**皮風**濕癢，能止眼風淚下，明目，“It removes **skin wind** with moisture and itching, and it is capable of ending eye wind with tearflow. It clears the eyes”.

Pi feng **脾風, spleen wind** [1]
PC of a spleen affection by wind evil. *SW* 42: **脾風**之狀，多汗惡風，身體怠惰，四肢不欲動，色薄微黃，不嗜食，“The appearance of **spleen wind** [is such: patients] sweat profusely and have an aversion to wind. Their body is tired and [they are] lazy; their four limbs do not wish to move. Their [facial] color is slightly yellow. They do not wish to eat”.

Pi fu feng **皮膚風, skin wind** [9] AN *pi feng* 皮風, *fu feng* 膚風，*pi jian feng* 皮間風.
PC CD of → *pi zhen* 皮疹, skin papules; → *chuan zhong* 瘡腫, sores and swelling; *tuo xie* 脫屑, desquamation, and *sao yang* 瘙癢, itching. *WTMY* 19 RE *cang er jiu* 蒼耳酒, wine with *cang er*: 大去**皮膚風**, “[Capable of] massively eliminating **skin wind**”.

Pi fu gan bi **皮膚乾閉, the skin is desiccated and blocked** [1]
IS of a skin that contains depressed fire heat and cannot sweat. *BCGM* Shi ji 十劑, LSZ: 裏閉者，火熱鬱抑，津液不行，**皮膚乾閉**，“In the case of internal

obstruction, fire heat is pent-up, the bodily liquids cannot pass, **the skin is desiccated and blocked**".

***Pi gan* 脾疳, spleen *gan*-illness** [2]
PC of → *gan* 疳, *gan*-illness, with abdominal bloating resulting from too little food, with yellow complexion, emaciation, a desire to eat strange things, and a free-flux illness with a sour stench. *XEYZZJ* 173: **脾疳**，體黃腹大，食泥土，當補脾, "**Spleen *gan*-illness**: The body is yellow, the abdomen is enlarged, [patients] consume mud. It is essential to supplement the spleen".

***Pi han* 脾寒, spleen cold** [5]
PC of a type of cold disease with spleen qi depletion brought forth by yang qi depletion or weakness. *QJYF* 8: 檳榔散，治**脾寒**，飲食不消，勞倦氣脹, "Powder with *bing lang* cures **spleen cold**, with an inability to digest beverages and food, as well as exhaustion-fatigue and qi distension".

***Pi huo* 脾火, spleen fire** [2]
PC and EA identical with → *pi re* 脾熱, spleen heat. *ZZN* 1: 白芍瀉**脾火**, "*Bai shao* drains **spleen fire**".

***Pi ji* 脾積, spleen accumulation** [10]
PC identical with → *pi qi* 痞氣, obstacle-illness qi. *ZBYHL* 卷 19: "診得**脾積**脈，浮大而長，"If an examination reveals a [movement in the] vessels associated with **spleen accumulation**, this is at the surface, massive and extended".

***Pi ji* 痞積, obstacle-illness accumulation** [10] AN *pi jie* 痞結, obstacle-illness node.
PC of an impeded flow of qi in the abdomen, resulting from immoderate eating and drinking, or from an intrusion of an external cold or heat evil. The resulting qi accumulation causes abdominal pain and abdominal swelling as major conditions. *WTMY* 12: 古今錄驗氣痞丸，療寒氣**痞積**，聚結不通，繞臍切痛，腹中脹滿，"*GJLY*: Pills for qi obstacle-illness. They cure cold qi **obstacle-illness accumulation**. [The qi] does not pass but collects and forms nodes resulting in a cutting pain around the navel. The abdomen experiences swelling and a feeling of fullness".

***Pi ji* 癖積, aggregation-illness accumulation** [2]
PC identical with → *ji pi* 積癖, accumulation aggregation-illness. *BCYY* SE *pi shuang* 砒霜：磨研酒飲，治**癖積**氣有功, "If ground to be ingested with wine it is effective in the treatment of **aggregation-illness accumulation**".

***Pi jian feng* 皮間風, wind in the skin** [1]
PC identical with → *feng shui* 風水, wind water. *TYBC* SE *bai zhu* 白朮：近多用白朮治**皮間風**，止汗消痞，補胃和中, "Nowadays one often uses *bai zhu* to cure **wind in the skin**, to end sweating and dissolve an obstacle-illness, supplement the stomach and harmonize the center".

***Pi jie* 痞結, obstacle-illness node** [4]
① EA PM *ZBYHL* 7: 熱氣乘虛而**痞結**不散, "Heat qi avails itself of a depletion and forms an **obstacle-illness node** that fails to dissipate".

② PC identical with → *pi ji* 痞積, obstacle-illness accumulation. *BJ* SE *shu qi* 蜀漆：主瘧及咳逆寒熱、腹中癥堅**痞結**, "It controls malaria as well as cough with counterflow and alternating sensations of cold and heat; abdominal concretion-illness hardnesss, and **obstacle-illness nodes**".

Pi jing **辟驚, to break up fright** [2]
TA identical with → *zhi jing* 止驚, to stop fright. *TPSHF* 98: 治風鎮心，**辟驚**除邪, "To cure wind and ease an [excited] heart; **to break up fright** and eliminate evil".

Pi lao **脾勞, spleen exhaustion** [5]
PC of a depletion exhaustion brought forth by exhaustion detriment affecting the spleen. *ZBYHL* 3: **脾勞**者，舌本苦直，不得嚥唾, "In the case of **spleen exhaustion**, the base of the tongue is plagued by stiffness. [Patients are] unable to swallow or spit".

Pi leng **脾冷, spleen cold** [3]
PC identical with → *pi han* 脾寒, spleen cold. *KBBC* SE *ru gan zi* 乳柑子：多食令人**脾冷**，發痼癖，大腸泄, "Consumed in large quantities it causes **spleen cold** resulting in obstinacy-illness with aggregation-illness and outflow from the large intestine".

Pi man **痞滿, obstacle-illness and fullness** [71] AN *man pi* 滿痞, fullness with an obstacle-illness; *sai man* 塞滿, blockage and fullness; *man sai* 滿塞, fullness and blockage.
① IS of an uncomfortable feeling of fullness and blockage. *SW* 74: 病生胠脅，氣歸於左，善太息，甚則心痛**痞滿**，腹脹而泄, "The disease develops in the subaxillary region and in the flanks; the qi turns to the left. [Patients] tend to breathe deeply. In severe cases, they [suffer from] heartache with **obstacle-illness and fullness**, from abdominal distension and outflow".
② PC with an uncomfortable feeling of fullness and and blockage. *QJYiF* 2 SE *shi long chu* 石龍芻：補內虛不足，療**痞滿**, "It supplements internal depletion and insufficiency; it cures **obstacle-illness and fullness**".

Pi miu **僻謬, eccentric and delirious [language]** [3] AN *yan yu pi yue* 言語僻越, eccentric language; *yu yan cuo miu* 語言錯謬, muddled and delirious language; *yu yan cuo wang* 語言錯妄, muddled and absurd language.
IS of a language that has no logic and fails to correctly respond to a question. *MYBL* SE *ling yang jiao* 羚羊角：除邪氣驚夢，狂越**僻謬**, "It eliminates evil qi, and fright dreams; crazy jumping and **eccentric as well as delirious [language]**".

Pi nüe **脾瘧, spleen malaria** [1]
PC of → *nüe ji* 瘧疾, malaria ailment, associated with illness signs of the spleen and stomach, such as abdominal pain and intestinal noises. *SW* 36: **脾瘧**者，令人寒，腹中痛，熱則腸中鳴, "**Spleen malaria**: it causes a person to be cold. [Patients] have a painful abdomen. When they are hot, sounds occur in their intestines".

***Pi qi* 痞氣, obstacle-illness qi** [9]
PC identical with → *pi ji* 脾積, spleen accumulation. *ZBYHL* 19: 脾之積，名曰**痞氣**, "Accumulations in the spleen are called **obstacle-illness qi**".

***Pi qi* 癖氣, aggregation-illness qi** [10]
PC identical with *pi* 癖, aggregation-illness. *SJZL* 73: **癖氣**者，聚於兩脅間，有時而痛是也, "**Aggregation-illness qi** collects in the costal regions. From time to time it hurts".

***Pi re* 脾熱, heat in the spleen; spleen heat** [11]
① PC of heat-type diseases affecting the spleen. *SW* 32: **脾熱**病者鼻先赤, "In the case of the disease **heat in the spleen**, the nose becomes red first".
② EA bringing forth heat-type disease in the spleen. *ZBYHL* 74: 小兒重舌者，心**脾熱**故也, "When children have a heavy tongue, this is because of heat in the heart and heat in **the spleen**".

***Pi re* 痞熱, obstacle-illness heat** [2]
PC identical with → *re pi* 熱痞, heat obstacle-illness. *MYBL* SE *mu li* 牡蠣：療泄精，喉痹咳嗽，心脅下**痞熱**, "Cures discharge of essence/semen; throat blockage and cough, and **obstacle-illness heat** below heart and flanks".

***Pi shi* 脾濕, spleen moisture** [18]
EC of water/moisture stagnation resulting from spleen depletion or from moisture evil having offended the spleen, impairing the spleen's potential of transporting/transforming liquid. *SJZL* 84: 治脚氣之疾，先起嶺南，稍來江東，皆由**脾濕**得之, "To cure the ailment of leg qi. It originated in Lingnan and has reached the region east of the Yangzi river. The reason for getting it is always **spleen moisture**".

***Pi shi du* 砒石毒, arsenic mineral poison** [9]
EA of the poison of arsenic. *BCGM* SE *bai zhi* 白芷 quotes *SLGJ*: 解**砒石毒**：白芷末，井水服二錢, "To dissolve **arsenic mineral poison**: ingest 2 *qian* of *bai zhi* powder with well water".

***Pi shui* 皮水, skin water** [2]
PC of → *shui zhong* 水腫, water swelling, disease with water/moisture flowing into the skin and causing a swollen surface there. If pressed, the finger sinks deep. Patients do not sweat. They are thirsty and have no aversion to cold. *JGYL* Mj: 渴而不惡寒者，此為**皮水**, "If they are thirsty and have no aversion to cold, this is a case of **skin water**".

***Pi tong* 痞痛, obstacle-illness with pain** [3]
IS of pain accompanied by a feeling of distension and fullness. In some cases a massive lump can be felt. *MYBL* SE *zhi shi* 枳實：破結實，消脹滿，心下急，**痞痛**逆氣, "It breaks open nodular concretions, dissolves swelling and fullness, and tensions below the heart and **obstacle-illness with pain**, with counterflow of qi".

***Pi wei xu* 脾胃虛, spleen and stomach depletion** [5]
PC of a joint → *pi xu* 脾虛, spleen depletion, and → *wei xu* 胃虛, stomach depletion. *ZBYHL* 17: 下斷之後，**脾胃虛**，氣逆，遇冷折之，其氣不通，則

令噦也, "Once the discharge has ended, **spleen and stomach are in a state of depletion**. The qi rises in counterflow. When it meets with cold, [the cold] will make it turn around. The qi cannot pass, and this causes retching".

***Pi xie* 脾泄, spleen outflow** [18]
PC of → *xie xie* 泄瀉, outflow, caused by spleen qi depletion and weakness, manifesting itself as abdominal distension and formless stools accompanied by vomiting. *NJ* 57: **脾泄**者，腹脹滿，泄注，食即嘔吐逆, "In the case of **spleen outflow**, the abdomen is distended with a feeling of fullness; outflow; consumed food is immediately vomited with counterflow".

***Pi xie* 積泄, [food] accumulation outflow** [2] AN *shi xie* 食泄, food outflow.
PC of → *xie xie* 泄瀉，outflow, brought forth by harm caused by food accumulations. *BCGM* Bai bing zhu zhi yao 百病主治藥：黃丹、百草霜，並治**積泄**, "*Huang dan* and *bai cao shuang* both cure [food] **accumulation outflow**".

***Pi xie* 澼泄, flushing outflow** [1]
PC identical with → *xia li* 下痢, discharge with free-flux illness. *BCTJ* SE *wu xin cao* 無心草：療**澼泄**腹痛, "It heals **flushing outflow** with abdominal pain".

***Pi xu* 脾虛, spleen depletion** [45]
PC of a depletion of the spleen with an impediment of spleen functions. *SW* 76: 肝虛、腎虛、**脾虛**，皆令人體重煩冤, "Liver depletion, kidney depletion, **spleen depletion**, all [these conditions] make a person's body become heavy, [associated with] vexation and grievance".

***Pi yin* 澼飲, flushing rheum** [2]
PC identical with → *pi yin* 癖飲, aggregation-illness rheum. *BCTJ* SE *yuan hua* 芫花 quoting Hu Qia 胡洽：胡洽治水腫及支飲、**澼飲**，加大黃、甘草並煎，五物各一兩，棗十枚，同煮如法, "Hu Qia's treatment of water swelling and propping rheum, as well as **flushing rheum**. Add *da huang* and *gan cao*, and fry together. All five items in the amount of 1 *liang*. Boil together with ten pieces of *zao*. Proceed according to the established pattern".

***Pi yin* 癖飲, aggregation-illness rheum** [3]
PC identical with → *yin pi* 飲癖, rheum aggregation-illness. *ZBYHL* 20: 此由飲水多，水氣停聚兩脅之間，遇寒氣相搏，則結聚而成塊，謂之**癖飲**, "This results from excessive rheum liquid. The liquid qi collects in the region of the two flanks. There it clashes with cold qi. As a result it forms nodular amassments that generate lumps. One calls this '**aggregation-illness rheum**'".

***Pi yu* 脾郁, pent-up spleen [qi]** [1]
EA of liver accumulation overcoming the spleen. When spleen qi fails to move, transmission and transformation end. *SYJYBZFL* 11: 肝氣不平，勝克於脾，**脾郁**不行，結聚涎沫，閉於臟氣，腑氣不舒，胃則脹滿，其脈弦遲, "When the liver qi is not balanced and manages to overpower the spleen, [this brings forth] **pent-up spleen [qi]** and [this qi] fails to move. This results in nodular collections with saliva turning into foam. The qi of the depots is locked in, and the qi of the palaces cannot move freely. As a result, the stomach is distended with a feeling of fullness, and the [movement in the] vessels is string-like and retarded".

***Pi yue* 脾約, spleen restraint** [3]

PC of constipation brought forth by harm caused to the body liquids by flaming stomach heat. *SHL* 179: 太陽陽明者，**脾約**是也, "When it affects the major yang and yang brilliance [sections], this is **spleen restraint**".

***Pi zhai* 疲瘵, weariness consumption** [2]

PC identical with → *lao zhai* 勞瘵, exhaustion consumption. *PJF* 337: 瘡瘍癰腫，聾盲喑啞，瘦瘠**疲瘵**，氣形之病有如此者, "Sores, ulcers, obstruction-illnesses, swelling, deafness, blindness, muteness, emaciation and leanness, as well as **weariness consumption**, these are diseases affecting a person's qi and physical appearance".

***Pi zhu* 癖疰, aggregation-illness attachment-illness** [1]

PC erroneous writing of *leng pi zhu* 冷痹疰, cold blockage attachment-illness, identical with → *pian feng* 偏風, unilateral wind. See *WTMY*, *ZLBC* SE *fu zi* 附子 where *leng pi zhu* 冷痹疰 is erroneously recorded as *leng pi zhu* 冷**癖疰**, "Cold **aggregation-illness attachment-illness**". *BCGM* SE *fu zi* 附子 again changes *leng pi zhu* 冷癖疰 to *ling pi zhu* 令**癖疰**, "Causes **aggregation-illness attachment-illness**".

***Pian bi* 偏痹, hemilateral blockage** [3]

PC of a → *bi* 痹① a), blockage disease, affecting only one side of the body, while the other side remains completely unaffected. *BJ* SE tian men dong 天門冬：主諸暴風濕**偏痹**，強骨髓, "It controls all types of sudden **hemilateral blockage** [induced by] moisture and wind, and strengthens bones and their marrow".

***Pian fei* 偏廢, hemilateral disablement** [2]

IS identical with → *pian ku* 偏枯, unilateral withering. *SYDXF* 13: 趁風膏，治中風，手足**偏廢**不舉, "The 'ointment that avails itself of wind' cures wind stroke, with hands and feet being **hemilaterally disabled** so that they cannot be raised".

***Pian feng* 偏風, hemilateral wind** [29] AN → *pian ku* 偏枯, hemilateral withering; → *feng pi* 風僻, wind wryness.

PC of unilateral loss of function and inability to move at one's will. Often an aftereffect of wind stroke. *SW* 42: 各入其門戶，所中則為**偏風**, "In each case it enters through the respective door. Where it strikes **hemilateral wind** results".

***Pian ku* 偏枯, hemilateral withering** [6] AN *pianfei* 偏廢, hemilateral disablement; *ban sheng kusi* 半身枯死, unilateral withering and necrosis

PC identical with → *pian feng* 偏風, hemilateral wind. *LS* 23: **偏枯**，身偏不用而痛, "In the case of **hemilateral wind**, one side of the body cannot function and is painful".

***Pian pi* 偏僻, hemilateral wryness** [1]

IS identical with → *kou wuo* 口喎, wryness of the mouth. *QJYiF* 16: 中風面目相引，**偏僻**，牙車急, "In the case of wind stroke the face and eyes pull on each other, with **hemilateral wryness** and lockjaw".

Pian qi 偏氣, hemilateral qi [2]

PC of → elevation-illness qi, *shan qi* 疝氣, with a unilateral swelling-distension. *BCGM* Bai bing zhu zhi yao 百病主治藥：甘遂，疝瘕**偏氣**，同茴香末酒服, "*Gan sui*: for elevation-illness and conglomeration-illness with **hemilateral qi**, add *hui xiang* powder and ingest with wine".

Pian shan 偏疝, hemilaterial elevation-illness [1]

PC identical with → *pian zhui* 偏墜, unilateral drop. *BCMQ* SE *gua lou shi* 栝蔞實：仍治**偏疝**，酒浸微煎，如法服之，住痛如劫, "To cure **hemilateral elevation-illness** it is to be soaked in wine and slightly boiled. If ingested according to the pattern, the pain will be eased as if [the entire problem] had been eliminated". *BCGM* SE *gua lou* 栝蔞, *gen* 根, the root: **偏疝**痛極：劫之立住。用綿袋包暖陰囊。取天花粉五錢，以醇酒一碗浸之，自卯至午，微煎滾，露一夜。次早低凳坐定，兩手按膝，飲下即愈，未下再一服, "In the case of **hemilateral elevation-illness** with pain reaching an extreme, it brings immediate relief. Take a soft bag and wrap warmly around the testicles. Then take 5 *qian* of *tian hua fen* and soak in a bowl with concentrated wine from the hour *mao* in the morning to the hour *wu* at noon. Add mild heat and let it stand open, uncovered, overnight. The next morning let [the patient] sit on a bench with his testicles hanging, and have his two hands hold his knees. When he drinks this and [the elevation] comes down, this is the cure. If it fails to descend, ingest once more".

Pian teng 偏疼, hemilateral pain [1]

IS identical with → *pian tong* 偏痛. *TPSHF* 33: 見紅白黑花，頭額**偏疼**，漸漸昏暗，不見物者，宜服羚羊角丸, "If [a patient] sees red, white and black flowers, with **hemilateral pain** affecting his forehead, and with gradual development of dim vision, or if he cannot recognize anything at all, it is advisable to ingest the pills with *ling yang jiao*".

Pian tong 偏痛, hemilateral pain [2] AN *pian teng* 偏疼.

IS of a pain affecting only one of two symmetrical body or organ structures. *ZBYHL* 39: 左脅**偏痛**者，由經絡偏虛，受風邪故也, "A **hemilateral pain** in the left flank results from hemilateral depletion of conduits and network [vessels] which then received wind evil".

Pian tou feng 偏頭風, hemilateral head wind [10]

PC of → *tou feng* 頭風, head wind, characterized by hemilateral headache. *RMSQ* 7: **偏頭風**者，少陽相火也, "In the case of **hemilateral head wind** the minor yang's minister fire is involved".

Pian tou tong 偏頭痛, hemilateral headache [1]

IS of pain affecting only one half of the head. *QJYF* 30: 前頂、後頂、頷厭, 主風眩**偏頭痛**, "[Piercing the holes] *qian ding*, *hou ding*, and *han yan* controls wind dizziness and **hemilateral headache**".

Pian xie **偏斜, hemilateral wryness** [1]

IS identical with → *wai xie* 喎斜. *JYBC* SE *huai jiao* 槐膠：破傷風，口眼**偏斜**，腰脊強硬, "Wound wind, with **hemilateral wryness** of the mouth and eyes, and stiffness of the lumbar region and lower back".

Pian zheng tou feng **偏正頭風, hemilateral and ordinary head wind** [14]

PC CD of → *pian tou feng* 偏頭風, hemilateral head wind, and → *zheng tou feng* 正頭風, ordinary head wind [affecting the entire head], i.e. variants of → *tou feng* 頭風, head wind, characterized by headache. *HJJF* 1 RE *bai long wan* 白龍丸, white dragon pills, cure **偏正頭風**, "**hemilateral and ordinary head wind**".

Pian zheng tou tong **偏正頭痛, hemilateral and ordinary headache** [11]

① IS CD of headache affecting only one half of the head, and of headache reaching from the eyes, the eybrows and the forehead to the top of the head. *SJZL* 12: **偏正頭痛**, 眉骨痛, 肢體倦怠, "**Hemilateral and ordinary headache**, pain in the eyebrow bones, and fatigue of the limbs and body".

② PC CD of pathological conditions with either hemilateral or ordinary headache as their major signs. *SJZL* 15: 療**偏正頭痛**, 解身體拘倦, 清爽神志, 通利關竅, 大川芎丸方, "For healing **hemilateral and ordinary headache**, to resolve cramps affecting the body, to clear the mind, and to make passes and orifices passable, [use] the recipe for major pills with *chuan xiong*".

Pian zhong **偏腫, hemilateral swelling** [3]

IS of a unilateral swelling of organs or of only one side of a symmetrical structure. *ZBYHL* 50: 其**偏腫**者，氣偏乘虛而行，故偏結腫也, "As for **hemilateral swelling**, in such cases the qi has availed itself of a depletion on one side only. Hence it forms nodes and swelling on only one side".

Pian zhui **偏墜, hemilaterial drop** [28] AN *pian shan* 偏疝, hemilateral elevation-illness.

PC of a → *yin shan* 陰疝, yin elevation-disease, characterized by a unilateral swelling of the scrotum. *TPSHF* 92: 治小兒**偏墜**，或氣攻小腹疼痛, "To cure **hemilateral drop** in children, with the qi sometimes attacking the lower abdomen and generating pain".

Piao she zhang **朴蛇瘴, cobra snake miasma** [1]

PC identical with → *suo hou zhang* 鎖喉瘴, throat-locking miasma. *PJF* 61: 治鎖喉瘴，又名**朴蛇瘴**，項大腫痛連喉, "To cure throat-locking miasma, which is also called '**cobra snake miasma**'. The [patient's] nape is massively swollen and painful, and this also affects the throat".

Pin guan duo tai **頻慣墮胎, repeated miscarriage** [1]

PC identical with → *shu duo tai* 數墮胎, frequent miscarriage. *BCGM* SE *du zhong* 杜仲 quotes *JBF*: **頻慣墮胎**：或三四月即墜者, "**Repeated miscarriage**: [Patients experience] a spontaneous abortion in the third or fourth month [of pregnancy]".

***Pin nüe* 牝瘧, female malaria** [3]
PC of → *nüe ji* 瘧疾, malaria ailment, with a predominance of cold over heat sensations. *GYL* Fj: 瘧多寒者，名曰**牝瘧**, "Those cases of malaria that are associated with much cold sensation, they are called '**female malaria**'".

***Po shang* 破傷, open injury; wound** [9] AW *shang po* 傷破.
PC of a → *shang sun* 傷損, injury, with opened skin. *SJZL* 21: 牛膝散方…**破傷**骨不折，以童子小便和酒調服, "The powder with *niu xi* ...For an **open injury** without bone fracture, ingest it mixed with boy's urine and wine".

***Po shang feng* 破傷風, wound wind** [59] AN *jin chuang zhong feng* 金瘡中風 wind stroke via wounds inflicted by metal objects; *po shang zhong feng* 破傷中風, wind stroke via wounds.
PC of lockjaw, arched back rigidity, and convulsions. *XSLSXDMF*: 若水與風入腦，成**破傷風**, "When water and wind enter the brain, the result will be **wound wind**".

***Po shang feng shui du* 破傷風水毒, wound wind with water poisoning** [1]
PC identical with → *zhu chuang zhong feng* 諸瘡中風, wind stroke via all possible sores. *PJF* 113: 治一切**破傷風水毒**，腫痛不可勝忍，用麝香末, "To cure all types of **wound wind with water poisoning**, and swelling with unbearable pain, use *she xiang* powder".

***Po shang feng zhong* 破傷風腫, wound wind with swelling** [2]
PC identical with → *zhu chuang zhong feng* 諸瘡中風, wind stroke via all possible sores. *QJYF* 25: 治**破傷風腫**方, "Recipe to cure **wound wind with swelling**".

***Po shang shi* 破傷濕, wounds harmed by moisture** [4] *BCGM* AD *shang shi* 傷濕.
PC of lockjaw and rigidity brought forth by the impact of water/moisture on an open wound. Similar to → *po shang feng* 破傷風, wound wind. *SYJYBZFL* 7: 瘡瘍未合，風入，為破傷風；濕入，為**破傷濕**。二者害人最急, "If wind enters sores and ulcers that have not closed yet, this results in wound wind. If moisture enters, the result is **wounds harmed by moisture**. Both types of harm are extremely serious for a person".

***Po shang zhong feng* 破傷中風, wind stroke via wounds** [38]
PC identical with → *po shang feng* 破傷風, wound wind. *SJZL* 6: **破傷中風**，牙關緊急，四肢強硬, "In the case of **wind stroke via wounds** [patients suffer from] lockjaw, and the four limbs are stiff".

***Pu sun* 撲損, injury from a blow** [31]
PC identical with → *da pu shang sun* 打撲傷損. *XSLSXDMF* RE *da huo xue dan* 大活血丹, massive pills to quicken the blood: 治**撲損**傷折，骨碎筋傷，疼痛浮腫, "To cure **injuries from blows**, with bone fracture and harmed sinews, pain and surface swelling".

-Q-

Qi ben **氣奔, qi run** [6]

① EA PM identical with → *qi ni* 氣逆, qi counterflow. *ZBYHL* 14: 邪動則**氣奔**逆上，氣上則五臟傷動, "Excited by evil [qi], the [regular] **qi runs** and ascends contrary to its regular direction. When the qi ascends, the five depots are harmed".

② PC with an unbearable itch, which does not end despite scratching that draws blood. *CXSYF* Lj quoting *QJF*: 遍身忽皮底混混如波浪聲，癢不可忍，抓之肉血出，亦不能解，為之**氣奔**, "Suddenly there is a movement, like a wave in the sea, at the base of the skin all over the body. The itch is unbearable. If scratched, blood leaves the flesh, but this fails to resolve [the itch]. This is '**qi run**'".

Qi bi **氣閉, qi closure** [14]

① PC a) identical with → *qi mi* 氣秘. *YXQY* Mj: 橘杏丸：治**氣閉**，老人、虛弱〔人〕皆可服, "The pills with *ju* and *xing* cure **qi closure**. Old people and those in a state of depletion and weakness can ingest them". b) Identical with → *qi long* 氣癃, qi protuberance-illness. *YXQY* Lj: 車前子，氣寒味甘，陰癃、**氣閉**，利水道，通小便, "*Che qian zi*: cold qi, sweet flavor. [It controls] yin protuberance-illness with **qi closure**, opens the waterways, stimulates the passage of urine". c) Deafness brought forth by a blocked passage of lung qi. *PJF* 53: 川芎湯，治耳聾**氣閉**, "The decoction with *chuan xiong* cures deafness resulting from **qi closure**".

② IS of difficult breathing, with heart-pressure and a feeling of suffocation. *PJF* 60: 忽然咽喉腫痛，手足厥，**氣閉**不通, "Suddenly the throat is swollen and painful. Hands and legs experience recession [of yang qi]. This is **qi closure**, with no passage possible".

③ PM of all types of pathological processes involving a blockage of the passage of qi. *SJZL* 12: 治風虛**氣閉**，口眼瞤動，偏正頭痛，乳香丸方, "To cure wind [intruding into a state of] depletion with **qi closure**, twitching movements of the mouth and eyes, hemilateral or ordinary headache, [use] the recipe for the pills with *ru xiang*".

Qi bi **氣閟, qi closure** [2]

PC identical with → *qi mi* 氣秘. *BCGM* SE *ju* 橘 quoting *YSJSF* Da bian men 大便門: 治**氣秘**, 老人虛弱人皆可服, "It cures qi closure. Old people and those in a state of depletion and weakness can ingest them", writes: 老人氣閟, "Old people with **qi closure**".

Qi bi **氣痹, qi blockage** [2]

PC of → *bi bing* 痹病, blockage disease, brought forth by emotional factors. *ZZJ* Mj: **氣痹**者，愁憂思喜怒過多…壅而不散，則痛；流而不聚，則麻, "In the case of **qi blockage**, one has excessively given oneself to emotions such as sorrow, grief, pondering, joy and anger…[the qi] is obstructed and fails to dissipate, and this results in pain. When it flows off and does not collect, this results in hemp[-like numbness]".

Qi bie **氣鱉, qi turtle** [6]
PC identical with → *bie jia* 鱉瘕, turtle[-shaped] conglomeration-illness. *BCGM* SE *wu yi* 蕪荑 quotes *RZZZF*: 腹中鱉瘕：平時嗜酒，血入於酒則為酒鱉；平時多氣，血凝於氣則為**氣鱉**, "Abdominal turtle conglomeration-illness: When someone regularly indulges in drinking wine, when his blood enters the wine this will result in 'wine turtle'. When someone regularly has much qi, the blood congeals with the qi, and this will result in '**qi turtle**'".

Qi bing **奇病, strange disease** [1]
PC identical with → *guai bing* 怪病, queer disease. *WTMY* 39: 邪…溢於大絡，而生**奇病**焉, "Evil…flows into the large network [vessels] where it generates a **strange disease**".

Qi bing **氣病, qi disease** [10] AN *qi ji* 氣疾, qi ailment.
PC brought forth by an unbalanced qi dynamic in depots and palaces, conduits and network vessels. There are two types, with → *qi xu* 氣虛, qi depletion; *qi hao* 氣耗, qi consumption; and → *qi tuo* 氣脫, qi loss, constituting the depletion type, and → *qi zhi* 氣滯, qi sluggishness; → *qi ni* 氣逆, qi counterflow; and → *qi jie* 氣結, qi nodes, constituting the repletion type. *SW* 23: 辛走氣，**氣病**無多食辛, "The acrid [flavor] moves to the qi; in the case of **qi diseases** one must not consume acrid [flavor] in large quantities".

Qi chong guai bing **臍蟲怪病, queer disease of navel worms** [1]
PC of an unusual disease with abdominal distension and hardening, and the release of liquid from the navel that turns into bugs/worms that cause itching. *BCGM* SE *hua shi* 滑石 quotes *QJF*: **臍蟲怪病**：腹中如鐵石，臍中水出，旋變作蟲，行繞身匝，癢難忍，撥掃不盡, "**Queer disease of navel worms**: There is a feeling in the abdomen as if there were a piece of iron or a stone. Water is released from the navel. It transforms into a movement of bugs/worms winding around the body and causing unbearable itching. If one tries to remove them with the hands, one fails".

Qi chuan **氣喘, panting** [38]
① IS identical with → *chuan* 喘①. *SW* 74: 太陰司天，客勝則首面胕腫，呼吸**氣喘**, "When the major yin [qi] controls heaven, in case the visitor [qi] dominates, then [people suffer from] *fu*-swellings on the head and in the face. They **pant** while exhaling and inhaling".
② PC identical with → *chuan* 喘②. *TBC* SE *zi wan* 紫菀：治**氣喘**，陰痿, "It cures **panting** and dysfunction of the yin [member, i.e. penis]".

Qi chuang **臍瘡, umbilical sores** [14]
PC of festering → *chuang* 瘡, sores, conditions developing in the naval region of children after the umbilical cord was cut. They cannot be healed for a long time. *ZBYHL* 50: **臍瘡**，由初生斷臍，洗浴不即拭燥，濕氣在臍中, "**Umbilical sores**: when the umbilicus of a newborn child was cut and washed, and if this was not dried immediately, the moisture qi will collect in the navel".

Qi chuang **漆瘡, lacquer sores** [42]
PC of → *chuang* 瘡, sores, conditions developing as an allergic reaction to having been affected by the qi of lacquer. After the naked skin has come into contact with lacquer qi it suddenly turns red, is inflamed and itches. Small streaks or blisters emerge. If scratched they open to fester and emit liquid. *MYBL* SE *ku ao* 苦芙: 主面目通身**漆瘡**，"It controls **lacquer sores** on the face, eyes, and the entire body".

Qi cu **氣促, panting** [10]
IS identical with → *chuan* 喘①. *YXL* SE *jie geng* 桔梗：消積聚痰涎，主肺氣，**氣促**嗽逆, "It dissolves accumulation and collection of phlegm and saliva. It controls lung qi, **panting** and cough with [qi] counterflow".

Qi duan **氣短, shortness of qi** [24]
IS of hectic breathing, with a feeling as if one were unable to continue breathing. Usually this goes along with all types of depletion conditions. *ZBYHL* 13: 虛極之人，榮衛減耗，腑臟虛弱，氣行不足，所以呼吸**氣短**也, "Persons with an extreme condition of depletion, their camp and guard [qi] are diminished. Palaces and depots are depleted and weak. The passage of qi is inadequate. Hence their breathing is characterized by a **shortness of qi**".

Qi e **氣惡, qi malignity; foul qi** [7]
① IS of foul mouth odor. *BJ* SE *kong gong nie* 孔公孽：主傷食不化，邪結**氣惡**, "It controls failure to digest food, with evil [qi] nodes and **qi malignity**".
② CD of all strong and bad odors. *BCGM* SE *tao fu* 桃符 quotes *DS*: 味辛**氣惡**，故能厭伏邪氣，制百鬼, "Flavor: acrid; **qi: foul**. Hence it is able to suppress evil qi and check all demons".

Qi fang **氣妨, qi impediment** [6]
EA PM identical with → *qi zhi* 氣滯, qi sluggishness. *BCTJ* SE *suo cao gen* 莎草根：心中客熱，膀胱間連脅下**氣妨**，常日憂愁不樂, "There is visitor heat in the heart, and there is a **qi impediment** in the bladder connecting with the region below the flanks. [Patients] are worried all the time and cannot be happy".

Qi feng **臍風, navel wind** [27] AN *xiao er zhong feng* 小兒中風, children struck by wind; *qiang bao zhong feng* 襁褓中風, struck by wind in the swaddling cloth; *rao qi feng* 繞臍風, wind encircling the navel.
PC of → *po shang feng* 破傷風， wound wind, brought forth by wind evil affecting the navel region of newborn children. *QJYF* 8: 小兒**臍風**、大人涼濕，得痓風者皆死, "If small children with **navel wind** or adults with cold moisture are, in addition, affected by spasms wind, they all die".

Qi ge **氣膈, occlusion by qi** [1]
PC. One of five types of gullet occlusion. *ZBYHL* 13: **氣膈**之為病，胸脅逆滿，咽塞，胸膈不通，噫聞食臭, "The disease of **occlusion by qi** is as follows: the chest and flanks have a [qi] counterflow and a feeling of fullness. The throat is blocked. The chest is occluded and not passable. One smells the stench of food [blocked in the patient's chest].

Qi gu **氣蠱, qi** ***gu*** [2]
PC of abdominal drum-like distension, and a feeling of heart-pressure and fullness, brought forth by qi stagnation. *PJF* 168, comment added to RE *wu ji san fang* 五積散方, recipe for the powder for five types of accumulation: 五積散，治五積六聚，並酒積蠱氣所傷…傷酒葛根湯下，傷食鹽湯下，**氣蠱**木香湯下，水蠱樟柳根湯下, "The 'powder for the five accumulations' cures the five accumulations [in the five depots] and six collections [in the six palaces], and also wine accumulation as well as damage caused by *gu* qi ... For damage caused by wine, ingest it with a decoction of *ge gen*; for damage caused by food, ingest it with brine; for **qi *gu*** ingest it with a decoction of *mu xiang*; for water *gu* ingest it with a decoction of *zhang liu* roots"

Qi ji **氣急, qi urgency** [31]
① AN *qi cu* 氣促, panting. IS identical with → *chuan* 喘①, panting. *ZHF* 2: 治胸脅痞滿，心塞，**氣急**喘急方, "A recipe for panting to cure an obstacle-illness and fullness in the chest and flanks, heart congestion and **qi urgency**".
② PC identical with → *chuan* 喘②. *QJYF* 21: 有人患**氣急**，積久不瘥，遂成水腫, "A person suffered from **qi urgency** for an extended period of time without cure. Eventually this developed into water swelling".

Qi ji **氣疾, qi ailment** [8]
PC identical with → *qi bing* 氣病, qi disease. *QJYF* 27: 病有四種，一冷痹，二**氣疾**，三邪風，四熱毒, "There are four types of disease: one, cold blockages; two, **qi ailments**; three, evil wind; four, heat poison".

Qi ji **氣積, qi accumulation** [7]
EA PM of qi halting and accumulating at any place in the body, which in turn may cause disease. *TPSHF* 71: 五臟之**氣積**，名曰積；六腑之氣聚，名曰聚也, "**Qi accumulation** in any of the five depots is called 'accumulation'. Qi collection in any of the six palaces is called 'collection'".

Qi ji **氣結, qi nodes** [10]
EA PM of a depressed qi dynamic, with the flow of qi blocked at any place in the body, which may in turn generate disease. *SW* 39: 勞則氣耗，思則**氣結**, "Exhaustion results in qi consumption. Pensiveness results in **qi nodes**".

Qi jie **氣竭, qi exhaustion** [3]
PC of a rather serious variant of depletion. *SW* 40: 病名血枯，此得之年少時，有所大脫血，若醉入房中，**氣竭**肝傷，故月事衰少不來也, "The disease is named blood withering. It is acquired in younger years either [because of] a massive loss of blood or [because] one has entered the chambers [for sexual intercourse] in a state of drunkenness [with the result that] the **qi is exhausted** and the liver is harmed. Hence, the monthly affair is weak and diminished and fails to arrive".

Qi jue **氣厥, qi recession** [9]
① EA PM identical with → *qi ni* 氣逆, qi counterflow. SW 37: 鼻淵者，濁涕下不止也，傳為衄衊瞑目，故得之**氣厥**也, "As for nasal deep-source [outflow], that is turbid snivel flowing down without end. Further transmission caus-

es nosebleed and blurred vision. The fact is, one acquires these [states] from **qi recession**".

② PC of → zu *jue* 卒厥, sudden fainting, caused by qi weakness or qi blockage. *SJZL* 1: 民病**氣厥**心痛，寒熱更作, "The people suffer from **qi recession** and heartache, with alternatingly active sensations of cold and heat".

Qi jue **氣蹶, qi recession** [1]

IS identical with → *qi ni* 氣逆, qi counterflow. *BCGM* SE *yi zhi zi* 益智子 quotes *YJZ*: 忽得吐血不止，**氣蹶**驚顫，狂躁直視, "Suddenly afflicted by unending blood spitting, with **qi recession**, shock and shivering, crazy restlessness and staring straight ahead".

Qi kuai **氣塊, qi lump** [37]

PC of swelling and lumps generated by qi stagnation in the abdomen or anywhere else in the body. In general, these lumps are pliable and form and disperse spontaneously. *QJYiF* 14: 火煉白石英、紫石英，療結滯**氣塊**, "Fire-refined *bai shi ying* and *zi shi ying* cure nodular and sluggish [qi] as well as **qi lumps**".

Qi lao **氣勞, qi exhaustion; qi is fatigued** [1]

PC identical with → *xu lao* 虛勞, depletion exhaustion. *SW* 3: 味過於咸，大骨**氣勞**，短肌，心氣抑, "When the flavors [consumed] are excessively salty, the major bones have **qi exhaustion**, the muscle[-flesh] is shortened and the qi of the heart is repressed".

Qi li **瘼癧, scrofula with pervasion-illness** [1]

PC of → *luo li* 瘰癧, scrofula with pervasion-illness, developing in the armpits or groin. *BCGM* SE *wu ming yi* 無名異 quotes *DNBS*: 股陰**瘼癧**：無名異二錢，麝香一字，研。酒半碗，午後空腹服，立效, "For **scrofula with pervasion-illness** in the groin: *wu ming yi*, 2 *qian*; *she xiang*, the amount covering 1 character [on a copper coin]. Grind and mix with half a bowl of wine. Ingest after noon on an empty abdomen. Immediately effective".

Qi li **氣痢, qi free-flux illness** [25]

PC of → *li ji* 痢疾, free-flux illness, with a qi depletion in the spleen and stomach, when cold and heat are out of balance. This is apparent as intestinal sounds and a feeling of abdominal fullness, red and white free-flux illness, lack of appetite and loss of vigor. This situation continues for long and is difficult to cure. *WTMY* 37 Shi xian ji hui fa 食鮮鯽鱠法, Pattern of consuming minced meat of fresh crucian carp: 亦療**氣痢**、赤痢, "It also cures **qi free-flux illness** and red free-flux illness".

Qi lin **氣淋, qi dripping** [15]

PC of → *lin bing* 淋病, dripping disease, with a feeling of distension and fullness in the lower abdomen, difficult, rough and painful urination, and a remnant of urine that fails to flow off entirely. *ZBYHL* 14: **氣淋**者，腎虛膀胱熱，氣脹所為也, "As for **qi dripping**, it is caused by kidney depletion and urinary bladder heat with qi distension".

***Qi long* 氣癃, qi protuberance-illness** [5]

PC of → *long* 癃, protuberance-illness, with an inability to pass urine and a feeling of distension and fullness in the lower abdomen and urinary bladder. *BJ* SE *shu fu* 鼠婦：主**氣癃**，不得小便, "It controls **qi protuberance-illness** with an inability to pass urine".

***Qi long* 氣聾, qi deafness** [1]

PC of → *er long* 耳聾②, deafness, caused by a bursting out of qi following physical overexertion. *BCGM* SE *zha er cao* 札耳草 referring to *ZJZSJ* 6: 耳聾有用氣得者, "A deafness acquired because of qi overexertion", writes: 王執中資生經，治**氣聾**方中用之, "Wang Zhizhong in his *ZJSJ* used it among the recipes to cure **qi deafness**".

***Qi lou* 氣瘺, qi fistula** [1]

PC of → *lou* 瘺, fistula, with an opening that fails to close for a long time while releasing hardly any pus or other liquid. *WKJY* Fj: 應效散，治**氣瘺**、疳瘡多年不效者, "Powder with Certain Effect: It cures **qi fistula**, and *gan*-illness sores that have not been treated effectively for many years".

***Qi luan* 氣亂, qi disorder** [5]

EA PM of a disorderly qi dynamic, with a failure to follow the regular sequence of upward and downward movement. *SW* 39: 驚則心無所倚，神無所歸，慮無所定，故**氣亂**矣, "When one is frightened, the heart has nothing to lean on, the spirit has nowhere to return, and deliberations have nowhere to settle. Hence, the **qi is in disorder**".

***Qi man* 氣滿, qi fullness** [14]

IS of an uncomfortable feeling of fullness brought about by internal qi stagnation. *SW* 19: 大骨枯槁，大肉陷下，胸中**氣滿**，喘息不便，其氣動形，期六月死, "When the major bones have dried and when major [masses of] flesh have sunk down, when there is **qi fullness** in the chest and when the breath is panting and does not flow unimpeded, while one's physical appearance shows the movement of qi, death is to be expected within six months".

***Qi men* 氣悶, qi heart-pressure** [4]

IS of difficult breathing, with a feeling of shrinking and obstruction in the region of the heart and chest. *QJYF* 20: 四肢厥冷，心煩**氣悶**，流汗, "The four limbs experience recession cold. The heart is vexed, and the **qi** makes a person have **heart-pressure**. Sweat flows".

***Qi mi* 氣秘, qi closure** [6] AW *qi bi* 氣閉, *qi bi* 氣閟.

PC of constipation brought about by sluggish qi or qi depletion. *SJZL* 17: 治風熱**氣秘**，郁李仁散方, "To cure wind heat with **qi closure** [use] the recipe for the powder with *yu li ren*".

***Qi ni* 氣逆, qi counterflow** [32]

① EA PM of qi moving in the body contrary to its normal direction, possibly generating further disease conditions. *SW* 3: 因而大飲，則**氣逆**, "Subsequent excessive drinking [causes] **qi counterflow**".

② IS identical with → *ni qi* 逆氣①, counterflow qi. *SW* 21: "太陽臟獨至，厥，喘虛**氣逆**。When only [the qi of] the major yang depot arrives, [accompanied by] receding [qi], panting, depletion, and **qi counterflow**".

Qi pi **氣癖, qi aggregation-illness** [2]

PC of → *qi* 癖, aggregation-illness, disease brought forth by qi stagnation. *SJZL 176:* 治小兒**氣癖**，上下左右，移動不常，木香丸方, "To cure children with **qi aggregation-illness**, above and below, left and right, moving here and there spontaneously, [use] the recipe for pills with *mu xiang*".

Qi re **氣熱, qi heat; qi is hot** [13]

① CC of hot weather. SW 70: 高者氣寒，下者**氣熱**, "In the high lying [regions], the qi is cold; in the low-lying [regions], the **qi is hot**".

② PQ of pharmaceutical substances of a hot nature: *YXQY* 7: 肉桂，**氣熱**，味大辛, "*Rou gui*, its **qi is hot**, its flavor is strongly acrid".

③ PC of illnesses associated with hot bodily qi. *SW* 28: 重實者，言大熱病，**氣熱**脈滿, "As for the so-called 'doubled repletion,' that is to say: a massive heat disease. [That is,] the **qi is hot** and the vessels are filled".

Qi ruo **氣弱, qi weakness** [18]

PC identical with → *qi xu* 氣虛, qi depletion. *ZBYHL* 3: 脾胃**氣弱**，大小腸偏虛，下焦偏冷，不能制於水穀者，故令大小便數也, "The **qi** of the spleen and stomach **is weak**. The large and small intestines are partially depleted; the lower burner is partially cold. They are unable to control water and grain. Hence defecation and urination increase in frequency".

Qi sai **氣塞, qi blockage** [9]

IS of difficult breathing. *MYBL* SE *gang tie* 鋼鐵：主金瘡，煩滿熱中，胸膈**氣塞**，食不化, "It controls wounds inflicted by metal objects, vexation, a feeling of fullness, and heated center, **qi blockage** in the chest and diaphragm, and an inability to digest food".

Qi san **氣散, qi dispersion** [5]

EA PM of qi dispersion which in turn may cause disease. For example, a dispersion of the spleen and stomach qi may result in intestinal efflux and prolapse of the rectum. A dispersion of lung qi may result in lung distension and pain. *QXLF* 16: 怒則氣逆，喜則**氣散**，悲則氣消, "Anger results in qi counterflow. Joy results in **qi dispersion**. Grief results in qi dissolution".

Qi shang **七傷, seven types of harm** [87]

PC CD of depletion-detriment conditions of depots and palaces, physical appearance and spirit. *BJ* SE *ma fen* 麻蕡：主五勞**七傷**，利五藏, "It controls the five types of exhaustion and the **seven types of harm**; it benefits the five depots".

Qi shang **氣上, the qi rises** [6]

PN identical with → *shang qi* 上氣, rising qi②. *SW* 39: 怒則**氣上**，喜則氣緩, "When one is angry, the **qi rises**. When one is joyous, the qi relaxes".

Qi sheng **氣盛, qi abundance** [15]

① PN of flourishing qi dynamics. *SW* 53: 穀盛**氣盛**，穀虛氣虛，此其常也, "When the grain abounds, the **qi abounds**; when the grain is depleted, the qi is depleted. That is the regular [association]".

② EA PM of an abundance of pathological qi, or the qi dynamic being blocked or moving disorderly contrary to its regular direction. *SW* 46: 夫**氣盛**血聚者，宜石而瀉之, "Now, when the **qi abounds** and blood has collected, one must drain it with a [sharpened] stone".

Qi shui **氣水, qi [blockage induced] water** [4]

PC of blockage of the qi dynamic resulting in edema disease that alternates between remission and renewed appearance. *ZBYHL* 21: **氣水**者，乍盛乍虛，乍來乍去, "As for **qi [blockage induced] water**, it alternatingly flourishes and is depleted, comes and goes".

Qi sou **氣嗽, qi cough** [5]

PC of cough with plenty of qi resulting from evil qi availing itself of a lung depletion. *TPSHF* 46: 肺氣不足，為邪所搏，則嗽而多氣，故曰**氣嗽**, "When the lung's qi is insufficient, it will be struck by evil [qi]. As a result [patients] cough with much qi. Hence this is called '**qi cough**'".

Qi tan **氣痰, qi phlegm** [6]

PC. A variant of → *tan bing* 痰病, phlegm disease, brought forth by the presence of phlegm and moisture in the lung. *WSBJ* 12: 濕在肺經，謂之**氣痰**, "When moisture is present in the lung conduits, this is called '**qi phlegm**'".

Qi teng **氣疼, qi pain** [3]

PC identical with *qi tong* 氣痛. *SLBC* SE *tuo* 鼉：療驚恐及小腹**氣疼**, "It cures fright and fear, as well as **qi pain** in the lower abdomen".

Qi tong **氣痛, qi pain** [44] AN *qi teng* 氣疼.

A large group of PCs of pain brought forth by blockages of the qi dynamic, caused by qi sluggishness, blood stasis, qi depletion, as well as cold. *ZBYHL* 4: 疝者，**氣痛**也。眾筋會於陰器。邪客於厥陰、少陰之經，與冷氣相搏，則陰痛腫而攣縮, "Elevation-illness, this is **qi pain**. All sinews meet in the genital organ. When evil settles in the ceasing yin and minor yin conduits, and clashes there with cold qi, the yin [i.e. genital organ] will be painful and swollen, and subject to contraction".

Qi tuo **氣脫, qi loss** [9]

PC brought forth by a loss of proper qi. This is often a sequel of excessive sweating, excessive diarrhea, and massive loss of blood, with incontinence and massive sweating. *SJZL* 96: 治虛冷，大便不禁，**氣脫**神昏，石硫黃湯方, "To cure depletion cold, incontinence, **qi loss** and spirit clouding, [use] the recipe for the decoction with *shi liu huang*".

Qi xia ji **臍下悸, palpitation below the navel** [1]

IS of a feeling of a racing throbbing and restlessness below the navel. *JGYL* Fj: 發汗後，**臍下悸**者，欲作奔豚, "After one has made the patient sweat, those with **palpitation below the navel** have a tendency to develop running piglets [conditions]".

Qi xia xian **氣下陷, qi downfall** [6]

PC of qi depletion leading to a loss of strength, which in turn causes the qi dynamic and inner organs to slow down or get stuck in their activities, with diarrhea and sagging inner organs as further results. *YXZC* 1: 其或泄痢，脫肛後重，大孔痛不可忍，是為**氣下陷**也, "When outflow and free-flux illness, prolapse of the rectum and a feeling of heaviness at the behind, and unbearable pain at the anus develop, this is because of a **qi downfall**".

Qi xian **氣癇, qi epilepsy** [1]

PC named in the conclusion of the *BCGM* section Bai bing zhu zhi yao 百病主治藥 where a *GLF* statement 心熱風癇, "Heart heat wind epilepsy" is quoted as: 心熱**氣癇**, "Heart heat **qi epilepsy**".

Qi xie **氣泄, qi outflow** [3]

① PM of a loss of qi in the course of profuse sweating, massive diarrhea and excessive bleeding. *SW* 39: 炅則腠理開，榮衛通，汗大泄，故**氣泄**, "When one is hot, the interstitial structures open. The camp [qi] and guard [qi] pass through. Sweat flows out profusely. Hence, there is **qi outflow**".

② PC identical with → *pi xie* 脾泄, spleen outflow. *PJF* 21: 治久患脾胃**氣泄**不止。用蕪荑五兩擣末，以飯丸如梧桐子大，每日空心午飯前，各用陳米飲下三十丸, "To cure [patients] suffering from unending spleen and stomach **qi outflow** use *wu yi*, 5 *liang*, and pound to a powder. Take rice to prepare pills the size of *wu tong* seeds. Take 30 pills daily with the liquid obtained by boiling rice on an empty stomach prior to lunch".

Qi xu **氣虛, qi depletion** [88]

PC of depletion with insufficient original qi, a decrease of the body's functions, and a diminution of its potential for defense. *SW* 53: 氣實形實，**氣虛**形虛，此其常也, "Qi repletion goes along with a repletion of one's physical appearance; **qi depletion** goes along with a depletion of one's physical appearance. That is the normal state of things".

Qi xue bi **氣血痹, qi and blood blockage** [1]

PC CD of → *qi bi* 氣痹, qi blockage, and *xue bi* 血痹, blood blockage. *BJ* SE *hou pu* 厚朴：主中風傷寒，頭痛，寒熱，驚悸，**氣血痹**, "It controls wind stroke and harm caused by cold, headache, alternating sensations of cold and heat, fright with palpitation, as well as **qi and blood blockage**".

Qi ye **氣噎, qi[-induced] gullet occlusion** [7]

① PC a) AN *ye qi* 噎氣, gullet occlusion qi. A gullet occlusion disease brought forth by cold that has entered chest and diaphragm region, with panting, palpitation, and pain in the chest and back as characteristic signs. *ZBYHL* 20: 此由陰陽不和，臟氣不理，寒氣填於胸膈，故氣噎塞不通，而謂之**氣噎**。令人喘悸，胸背痛也, "This is caused by a yin-yang disharmony, by a disregulation of depot qi, when cold qi fills the chest and diaphragm region. As a result there is a qi gullet occlusion and blocked passage, which is called '**qi[-induced] gullet**

occlusion.' It causes a person to pant and have palpitations, as well as feel pain in the chest and back". b) Identical with → *mei he ge qi* 梅核膈氣, plum-pit occlusion qi. *BCGM* Bai bing zhu zhi yao 百病主治藥：**氣噎**，咽中如有物，吞吐不出, "**Qi[-induced] gullet occlusion**, this is as if there were an object in thes gullet that cannot be removed by swallowing or vomiting".
② IS of an inability to move food down, and of food that is thrown up as soon as it has been consumed. *BCGM* SE *ding xiang* 丁香 quotes *DSTJYF*: 反胃關格：**氣噎**不通, "Turned over stomach and blockage, that is **qi[-induced] gullet occlusion** closing the passage".

Qi ying **氣癭, qi[-induced] goiter** [8]
PC of → *ying* 癭, goiter, which begins with a widening of the neck followed by gradually increasing swelling in front of the neck which in some cases grows and wanes again in accordance with the patient's mood. *ZBYHL* 50: **氣癭**之狀，頸下皮寬，內結突起膇膇然，亦漸長大，氣結所成也, "The appearance of **qi[-induced] goiter**: The skin below the neck widens. Inside nodular protusions emerge. And the swelling gradually grows bigger forming qi nodes".

Qi yong **氣壅, qi obstruction** [18]
EA PM identical with → *qi zhi* 氣滯, qi sluggishness. *QJYF* 17: 其人勞倦則咳唾血，其脈細緊浮數皆吐血，此為躁擾嗔怒得之，肺傷**氣壅**所致也, "When such persons overexert themselves, they will cough and spit blood. Their [movements in the] vessels are fine, tight, floating, and increased in speed, and they all spit blood. This is caused by stress and anger, with harm to the lung and **qi obstruction**".

Qi yu **氣鬱, pent-up qi** [24]
① PC one of → *liu yu* 六郁, the six types of pent-up [matter in the organism]. Refers to accumulation disease brought forth by mental depression, with a feeling of fullness and pain in the chest and abdomen, and a deep and rough movement in the vessels. *SW* 71: 民病**氣鬱**中滿; "People suffer from **pent-up qi** and central fullness".
② EA of a blockage of the qi dynamics inside the organism, possibly bringing forth all types of disease. *SJZL* 1: 寒氣時至，民乃和，其病淋，目瞑目赤，**氣鬱**於上而熱, "When cold qi arrives in time, the people feel well. Their diseases include dripping, the eyes do not open, and [when open] they are red. [This is] **pent-up qi** above with heat".

Qi zhang **氣脹, qi distension** [24]
IS of an uncomfortable feeling of distention brought forth by qi stagnation. *SW* 17: 上盛則氣高，下盛則**氣脹**, "If it is abundant above, the qi is [situated] high [in the body]. If it is abundant below, this is a **qi distension**".

Qi zhi **氣滯, qi sluggishness** [31] AN *qi yong* 氣壅, qi obstruction
EA PM of qi dynamic hindered in its free flow, which in turn may cause disease. *SLBC* SE *cu* 醋：**氣滯**風壅，手臂、脚膝痛。炒醋糟裹之，三兩易，當差, "In the case of **qi sluggishness** and wind obstruction, the hands and arms, legs

and knees ache. They are to be wrapped with the dregs produced in the course of making vinegar. Change three times or twice. This should bring the cure".

Qi zhi **氣痔, qi piles** [2]
PC of → *zhi chuang* 痔瘡, piles sores, associated with difficult and bloody defecation, as well as prolapse of the rectum. *ZBYHL* 34: **氣痔**，大便難而血出，肛亦出外，良久不肯入, "In the case of **qi piles** defecation is difficult and associated with a release of blood. Also, the rectum comes out, and will not be able to enter [the body] again for a long time".

Qi zhong **臍腫, umbilical swelling** [8]
PC of children with their umbilical region being red, swollen, excreting liquid and being painful. *TPSHF* 82: 治小兒**臍腫**汁出久不瘥方, "Recipe to cure **umbilical swelling** in children with liquid excretions that have not been cured for a long time".

Qi zhong **氣腫, qi swelling** [6]
PC of → *zhong ji* 腫疾, swelling ailment, brought forth by stagnant qi. *ZBYHL* 43: 輕浮如吹者，是邪搏於氣，**氣腫**也, "Those that are light and at the surface as if blown into, these are cases of evil striking at the qi. These are cases of **qi swelling**".

Qian hou bu de sou bian **前後不得溲便, inability to discharge in front or behind** [1]
IS identical with → *da xiao bian mi* 大小便秘, stool and urine are blocked. *RMSQ* 1: **前後不得溲便**，宜木通、海金沙、大黃、琥珀、八正散之屬, "In the case of an **inability to discharge in front or behind** it is advisable to ingest [medications] such as *mu tong*, *hai jin sha*, *da huang*, *hu po*, and the 'powder with eight rectifiers'".

Qian jia **嵌甲, embedded nail** [7]
PC of → *chuang* 瘡, sores, conditions with a flaming, painful swelling developing when fingernails or toenails grow too long and enter the flesh, or when one cuts one's nails and injures the flesh. Serious cases are associated with putrescence. *PJF* 300: 治**嵌甲**生入肉，常出血疼痛, "To cure **embedded nails** that have grown into the flesh. They are often accompanied by bleeding and pain".

Qian xuan **錢癬, coin[-size] *xuan*-illness** [1]
PC of → *xuan* 癬, *xuan*-illness a), with the lesion assuming a round shape like a coin. *BCGM* SE *mu jin* 木槿 quotes *JgXF*: 頭面**錢癬**：槿樹皮為末，醋調，重湯頓如膠，內傅之, "**Coin[-size] *xuan*-illness** on the head and face: Grind the bark of *jin shu* to powder, mix with vinegar, and boil extensively with plenty of water until it turns into a glue. Use this for external application".

Qiang lang lou **蜣螂瘺, dung beetle fistula** [1]
PC of → *lou* 瘺, fistula, initially developing as severely itching swelling. Once they have opened to fester there appear numerous deep holes, and bugs/worms grow in these holes. In former times it was believed that this disease results from being affected by poisonous qi of dung beetles. Hence bugs reminiscent of dung beetles were seen to grow in the holes. *ZBYHL* 34: **蜣螂瘺**候：此由飲食居處有蜣螂毒氣，入於臟腑，流於經脈所生也, "The signs of **dung beetle fistu-**

la: This results from poisonous dung beetle qi one has encountered in beverages, food or at one's living place, and that has entered one's depots and palaces whence it has flown into the conduit vessels".

***Qiang ying* 強硬, stiff and hard** [4]
Refers to a rather abnormal state of sturdiness and hardness of any item. *BCTJ* SE *she gan* 射干：葉中抽莖，似萱草而**強硬**, "Take the stalks from inside the leaves. They resemble *xuan cao* but are **stiff and hard**".

***Qiang zhi* 強直, stiff and straight** [1]
Refers to stiffness with an inability to bend. *BCTJ* SE *wei rui* 萎蕤：莖幹**強直**，似竹箭幹, 有節, "The stalks are **stiff and straight**, resembling bamboo arrow stalks with knots".

***Qiang zhong* 強中, stiff center** [8] AN *shen lou* 腎漏, kidney leakage.
PC of male adults with an erection persisting over a long time without returning to dysfunction, and a spontaneous seminal pollution or a failure to ejaculate. *ZBYHL* 5: **強中**病者，莖長興盛不痿，精液自出是也, "The disease of '**stiff center**' is as follows: The stalk is fully erected without turning limp for an extended period of time, with spontaneous seminal emission".

***Qiao cui* 憔悴, thin and pallid** [5]
IS of an unhealthy appearance, such as a yellow face and emaciation, and failing vigor. *QJYF* 19: 悲憂**憔悴**，凡是病皆須服之方, "Being worried and sad, **thin and pallid** – all persons suffering from this disease ought to ingest this recipe".

***Qie tong* 切痛, cutting pain** [9]
IS of an incisive pain with a feeling as if one were being sliced by a knife, or bitten by an animal. *ZHF* 7: 中蠱令人心腹**切痛**，如有物嚙, "If a person is struck by *gu*, this will cause him to feel a **cutting pain** in his heart and abdominal region, as if something had bitten him".

***Qin si* 寢死, [appearance of] death while asleep** [1]
PC of → *cu si* 卒死, sudden [appearance of] death, while one is asleep. *BCGM* SE *ji* 雞 quoting *ZHF* 1: 救卒死，或先病痛，或常居寢臥，奄忽而絕，皆是中死, "For sudden [appearance of death] either following prior disease and pain, or after a normal life while asleep, with a sudden cut-off, these all are cases of a fatal strike", writes: 卒死**寢死**：治卒死，或寢臥奄忽而絕，皆是中惡, "Sudden [appearance of] death and **[appearance of] death while asleep**: When treating sudden [appearance of] death, which may be a sudden cut-off during sleep, these all are cases of being struck by the malign".

***Qing mang* 青盲, green blindness** [60]
PC of → *shi ming* 失明, loss of vision, with no externally apparent changes in the eye and a clear distinction of the dark and white parts of the eye, while patients nevertheless are unable to see. *BJ* SE *gu yang jiao* 羖羊角: 主**青盲**，明目, "It controls **green blindness** and clears the eyes".

***Qing ti* 清涕, clear snivel** [4]
IS identical with → *liu qing ti* 流清涕, clear snivel flow. *SW* 43: 胞痹者，少腹膀胱按之內痛，若沃以湯，澀於小便，上為**清涕**, "In the case of a uterus

blockage, if one presses the lower abdomen and the urinary bladder, this causes internal pain as if hot water had been poured over [the lower abdomen]. Urination is rough. Above, it causes **clear snivel**".

Qing yi **青翳, greenish shade** [5]
PC of a → *mu yi* 目翳, eye shade, with a greenish speckled membrane. *BJ* SE *qin pi* 秦皮: 除熱，目中**青翳**、白膜, "To remove heat, as well as **greenish shade** and white membrane from the eyes".

Qing zhong **青腫, greenish swelling** [21] AN *yü zhong* 瘀腫, stasis swelling.
IS of topical swelling accompanied by stagnant blood underneath the skin which in turn assumes a greenish color. *QJYF* 25: 治被打擊，頭眼**青腫**方：炙肥豬肉令熱，拓上, "Recipe to cure someone who has been struck, and whose head and eyes show a **greenish swelling**: roast fat hog meat until it is hot and rub on [the greenish swelling]".

Qiu bi **鼽鼻, congested nose** [1]
PC identical with → *bi qiu* 鼻鼽, nasal congestion. *BCGM* SE *lü qing* 綠青 quoting *MYBL*: 主益氣，療鼽，止泄痢, "It controls the increase of qi, cures congested nose, and stops diarrhea and free-flux illness", writes: 益氣，止泄痢，療**鼽鼻**, "It increases qi, stops outflow and free-flux illness, and cures **congested nose**".

Qiu bing **秋病, autumn disease** [1] CD of all
PC that primarily have their onset in autumn. *QJYF* and *PJF*: 胃而有毛曰**秋病**, "If the stomach [movement in the vessels] is hair-like, this is called '**autumn disease**'". In contrast: *BCGM* Si shi yong yao li 四時用藥例, examples of using pharmaceutical drugs in the course of the four seasons: 春得**秋病**, 夏得冬病, 神而明之, 機而行之, 變通權宜, 又不可泥一也, "If in spring one gets an **autumn disease**, if in summer one gets a winter disease, one must do everything to understand this, and act flexibly and do what is expedient. It would be wrong to cling to just one principle".

Qiu li **秋痢, autumn free-flux illness** [4]
PC of → *li ji* 痢疾, free-flux illness, affecting a person in autumn. *SLBC* SE *shi* 柿：作餅及糕與小兒食，治**秋痢**, "Prepare cakes or pudding and let children eat them to cure **autumn free-flux illness**".

Qu chi **齲齒, decayed teeth** [31] AN *chi qu* 齒齲, tooth decay; *chong ya* 蟲牙, worm teeth; *zhu ya* 蛀牙, worm-borer teeth; *chong qu* 蟲齲, worm decay of teeth.
PC with decaying teeth developing holes, turning black and emitting a bad odor. In severe cases hollow teeth may crack. Also, the decay may enter the gums resulting in swelling, pain and festering. *LS* 74: 診**齲齒**痛，按其陽之來，有過者獨熱, "To examine the origins of **decayed teeth** with pain: feel [the skin] to trace the origin of the yang [heat]. Where there is excessive yang, this is a presence of heat only".

Qu sou niao chuang **蠼螋尿瘡, earwig-urine sores** [22]
PC of → *chuang* 瘡, sores, conditions forming clusters of blisters on the chest, flanks and lower back with an excruciatingly piercing pain, accompanied by

strong heat and an aversion to cold, as a major sign. This condition is reminiscent of the neurological disease herpes zoster. Formerly it was believed that the urine of earwigs, when touched by the shadow of a human, would cause this person to suffer from this disease. *ZBYHL* 25: 其成瘡，初如豆粒黑子，或如火燒，或如**蠼螋尿瘡**, "When this develops into sores it appears first as black moles like beans. Or like a burning. Or like **earwig-urine sores**".

Qu tu 取吐, **to stimulate vomiting** [91] AN *tan tu* 探吐.

TA using pharmaceutical substances or other means to stimulate vomiting to cure accumulations of pathological matter, such as phlegmy sputum, liquids, undigested food, toxic qi, or toxic matter, in the upper part of the body. *ZHF* 2: RE *chi san* 赤散：以少許納鼻中，吸之，**取吐**, "A small amount inhaled through the nose will **stimulate vomiting**".

Qu tu li 取吐利, **to stimulate vomiting and free flow** [5]

TA identical with → *qu tu xia* 取吐下, to stimulate vomiting and discharge. *QJYF* 12: RE *qi po wan bing wan* 耆婆萬病丸, "granny's pills for a myriad of diseases": 卒病欲死，服三丸如小豆，**取吐利**即瘥, "If in the case of a violent disease [a patient] comes close to dying, have him ingest three pills of the size of small beans **to stimulate vomiting and free flow**. This will bring the cure".

Qu tu xia 取吐下, **to stimulate vomiting and discharge** [5] AN *qu tu li* 取吐利.

TA using emetic and laxative pharmaceutical substances to stimulate vomiting and defecation for therapeutic purposes. *ZBYHL* 9: 不可苟依日數，輒**取吐下**, "One must not exclusively depend on the number of days [the disease has lasted] and always **stimulate vomiting and discharge**".

Qu xue 去血, **loss of blood; removal of blood; bloodletting** [22]

① PC identical with → *shi xue* 失血, loss of blood. *JGYL* Lj: 兼取崩中**去血**，或月水來過多，及至期不來, "[This recipe] is also able to eliminate [conditions such as] collapsing center with **blood loss**, as well as excessive menstruation and [menstruation] that fails to come in due time".

② TA of a) removal of extravascular stagnant blood. *MYBL* SE *bai tu huo* 白兔藿：又**去血**，可末著痛上，立消, "It also **removes blood**. Its powder may be applied on the aching location. This brings immediate dissolution". b) Bloodletting. *TBC* SE *tong xie* 銅屑：先刺腋下脈，**去血**，封之，攻腋臭神效, "First pierce the vessel below the armpit and **let blood**. Then cover it. This is wondrously effective in attacking armpit stench".

③ PTP of the removal of blood from animals. *SLBC* SE *mu gou yin jing* 牡狗陰莖：**去血**食之，却不益人也, "If eaten with its **blood removed**, it will not be beneficial to humans".

Quan mao 拳毛, **hair inverted like a fist** [15]

① PC identical with → *dao jie* 倒睫, inverted eyelashes. *RMSQ* 15:（穿山甲）治倒睫**拳毛**, "*Chuan shan jia* .. cures inverted eyelashes, (i.e.) **hair inverted like a fist**".

② Reference to curled eyelashes. *RMSQ* 15: 如用藥時，先將**拳毛**摘盡，後用藥一字, "When one is about to use pharmaceutical drugs, the entire **hair invert-**

ed like a fist is to be plucked first. Only then may one apply the medication in an amount covering one character [on a copper coin.]"

Quan xian **犬癇, dog epilepsy** [1]

PC of a → *dian xian* 癲癇, peak-illness with epilepsy, which, at the time of its outbreaks, causes contraction of the patient's hands and feet. *QJYF* 5: **犬癇**之為病，手足攣, "The disease of **dog epilepsy**: contraction of the hands and feet".

Que ban **雀斑, sparrow speckles** [12]

PC identical with → *gan zeng* 皯黷. *PJF* 51: 七白丸，治面上黶色並**雀斑**, "Pills with the seven [ingredients with the character for] 'white' [in their names]. They cure facial moles and **sparrow speckles**".

Que lou **雀瘺, sparrow fistula** [1]

PC of → *lou* 瘺, fistula, with swellings appearing at random locations, eventually opening to develop into festering fistula. In former times it was believed that after having ingested medication to cure sparrow fistula, one would discharge with one's urine items resembling sparrow eggs, or with one's feces items resembling sparrows. *ZBYHL* 34: 此由居處飲食有雀毒氣，入於臟，流於脈，發無定處，腫，因潰成瘺，服藥，有物隨小便出，狀如雀卵，故謂之**雀瘺**, "This is because poisonous qi of sparrows encountered at one's living place, in beverages and food, has entered the depots whence it has flown into the vessels. It does not effuse at fixed locations. The swelling later begins to fester and develops into fistula. Having ingested medication, [patients] will release with their urine items resembling sparrow eggs. Hence one calls this '**sparrow fistula**'".

Que luan ban **雀卵斑, sparrow-egg speckles** [3]

PC identical with → *gan zeng* 皯黷, dermal dark spots. *BCGM* SE *da huang feng* 大黄蜂: 治**雀卵斑**，面皰, "They cure **sparrow-egg speckles** and facial blisters".

Que mang **雀盲, sparrow blindness** [4]

PC identical with → *que mu* 雀目, sparrow eye. *BCJJZ* SE *que luan* 雀卵: 人患黃昏間目無所見，為之**雀盲**, "When someone suffers from an inability to see during dusk, this is called '**sparrow blindness**'".

Que mu **雀目, sparrow eye** [33] AN *que mang* 雀盲, sparrow blindness.

PC with unimpaired vision during daylight and significantly decreased vision after nightfall. *ZBYHL* 28: 人有晝而睛明，至瞑則不見物，世謂之**雀目**, "If someone's vision is clear during daylight yet he cannot see things when darkness sets in, this is commonly called '**sparrow eye**'".

Que zheng **怯證, timidity condition** [1]

PC identical with → *xu zheng* 虛證, depletion condition. *PJF* 228: 治男子婦人**怯證**，男子用小女兒小便，日進二次，乾燒餅壓之。婦人服童子小便，依前服。月余日全效, "For **timidity conditions** of men and women, men take the urine of young girls, ingest it twice a day, and press it down with dry sesame see cakes. Women ingest the urine of boys, the intake is the same as the one just outlined. In a little longer than one month this will be completely cured".

***Qun bi* 痛痹, numbness blockage** [9]

PC of → *bi* 痹, blockage, with numbness and slackening of the limbs and body. *YXL* SE *tian ma* 天麻: 能治冷氣**痛痹**，攤緩不遂, "It is capable of curing cold qi **numbness blockage**, and paralysis".

***Qun feng chuang* 裙風瘡, skirt-wind sores** [2]

PC of → feng chuang 風瘡, wind sores, affecting the legs of adult women. *BCGM* SE *tou gou* 頭垢quotes *JBF*: 婦人足瘡經年不愈，名**裙風瘡**。用男子頭垢，桐油調作隔紙膏，貼之, "If adult women suffer from sores on their feet that do not heal over the years, this is called '**skirt-wind sores**'. Take the filth from the head of a male, mix with *tong* oil and apply as a plaster on paper".

- R -

***Rao qi feng* 繞臍風, wind encircling the navel** [1]

PC identical with → *qi feng* 臍風, navel wind. *BCGM* SE *wei ling xian* 威靈仙, quotes *HSJYF*: 此藥治丈夫婦人中風不語，手足不遂，口眼喎斜，言語謇滯，筋骨節風，**繞臍風**，胎風頭風, "This drug cures males and females struck by wind who do not speak, whose hands and feet are paralysed, with their mouth and eyes wry, and their language impaired, and whose sinews, bones, and joints have wind, [also] **wind encircling the navel**, and fetus wind as well as head wind".

***Re* 熱, heat; hot; to heat** [p] ,

① Temperature of items. *SHL* RE *gua di san*, powder with *gua di*: 用**熱**湯七合煮作稀糜, "Boil with 7 *ge* of **hot** water to prepare a thin gruel".

② AN *xie re* 邪熱, evil heat; *re qi* 熱氣, heat qi. EA able to bring forth heat-type diseases. *SW* 72: **熱**淫所勝，平以咸寒, "When **heat** excess dominates, level it with salty and cold [items]".

③ AN *re bing* 熱病, heat disease; *re ji* 熱疾, heat ailment; *re zheng* 熱證. PC of exuberant yang qi brought about by various causes. *SW* 35: 如是者，陰虛而陽盛，陽盛則**熱**矣, "In such a situation, the [qi in the] yin [section] is depleted and the [qi in the] yang [section] abounds. When [the qi in] the yang [section] abounds, [the patient] is **hot**".

④ AN heat condition; *fa re* 發熱, heat effusion; *shen re* 身熱, body heat; *ti re* 體熱, body heat. IS of higher than normal body temperature or a subjective feeling of being hot. *SW* 31: **熱**雖甚不死, "The **heat** may be extreme, but he will not die".

⑤ PQ of pharmaceutical substances. Refers to those substances that have heat qi. *BJ* Introductory section: 有寒、**熱**、温、涼四氣, "[Pharmaceutical drugs] may have one of the four qi cold, **heat**, warmth, coolness".

⑥ TA by which pharmaceutical substances with a warm or hot thermoquality are used to cure diseases. *SW* 72: 寒者**熱**之, "Cold conditions are to be **heated**".

***Re an* 熱暗, heat with dim vision** [3]

IS apparent as scorching heat in the eyes associated with unclear vision. *TBC* SE *di fu zi* 地膚子 quotes *BL*: 洗目，去**熱暗**雀盲澀痛, "To rinse the eyes. It removes **heat with dim vision**; night blindness, roughness and pain".

***Re bi* 熱痹, heat blockage** [4]

PC a) of → *bi* 痹, blockage, brought forth by heat evil. *SJZL* 20: **熱痹**…腑臟壅熱，復遇風寒濕三氣至，客搏經絡，留而不行，陽遭其陰，故㾓痹熻然而熱悶也, "**Heat blockage**…if in case of depots and palaces being obstructed with heat one encounters, in addition, the three qi of wind, cold, and moisture, they will settle in the main and network conduits without proceeding further. The yang meets with the yin. Hence there will be a numbness blockage with extreme heat, and heat with heart-pressure". b) Brought forth by evil heat blocking the qi dynamics of the depots and palaces. *QJYF* 14: 左手關前寸口陽實者，小腸實也，苦心下急，**熱痹**，小腸內熱，小便赤黃, "A repletion felt at the inch-opening in front of the pass section of the wrist indicates a repletion in the small intestine. One suffers from tensions below the heart, **heat blockage**, heat in the small intestine, as well as red-yellow urine".

***Re bi* 熱閟, heat closure** [1]

PC identical with → *re mi* 熱秘, heat constipation. *BCGM*, SE *hu ma* 胡麻, *hu ma you* 胡麻油, quotes 陳藏器 Chen Cangqi: 主天行**熱閟**，腸內結熱，服一合，取利為度, "Controls heaven-sent **heat closure**, with bound heat in the intestines. Ingest 1 *ge*. Once a free flow is reached end the treatment".

***Re bing* 熱病, heat disease** [100]

PC identical with → *re* 熱③, heat. *SW* 31: 今夫**熱病**者，皆傷寒之類也, "Now, as for **heat diseases**, they all are of the type 'harm caused by cold'". *BCGM* lists numerous types of heat disease, including *tian xing re bing* 天行熱病, heaven-sent heat disease; *shang han re bing* 傷寒熱病, heat disease resulting from harm caused by cold; *han re bing* 寒熱病, cold and heat disease, It also specifies numerous signs of heat disease, such as *re bing tou tong* 熱病頭痛, heat disease with headache; *re bing fan ge* 熱病煩渴, heat disease with vexation and thirst; *re bing fa ban* 熱病發斑, heat disease with an appearance of macules.

***Re chuan* 熱喘, heat panting** [2]

PC of → *chuan* 喘, panting, brought forth by heat evil. *BCGM* Li Dongyuan sui zheng yong yao fan li 李東垣隨證用藥凡例, Outline of the application of pharmaceutical drugs by Li Dongyuan in accordance with [a patient's] condition: **熱喘**咳嗽，桑白皮、黃芩、訶子, "In the case of **heat panting** and cough: [ingest] *sang bai pi*, *huang qin*, *he zi*".

***Re chuang* 熱瘡, heat sores** [45] AN *chuang re* 瘡熱, heat sores; *biao chuang* 熛瘡, flaming-heat sores; *re yan chuang* 熱焱瘡, heat flame sores; *huo biao re chuang* 火飆熱瘡, fire flame heat sores; *huo yan re chuang* 火焱熱瘡, fire flame heat sores.

PC of → *chuang* 瘡, sores, brought forth by heat evil. *ZBYHL* 35: 風多則癢，熱多則痛；血氣乘之，則多膿血，故名**熱瘡**, "Much wind causes itching; much heat causes pain. [If wind and heat] impact the blood and qi, this will result in plentiful purulent blood. Hence one speaks of **heat sores**". *BCGM* refers to → *tian pao chuang* 天泡瘡, celestial blister sores; → *ru chuang* 蓐瘡, childbed sores; → *huo dai chuang* 火帶瘡, fire girdle sores; → *huang lan chuang* 黃爛瘡, yellow festering sores; → *huo chuang* 火瘡, fire sores; → *kou zhong re chuang* 口中熱瘡, heat sores in the mouth; → *shi ji re chuang* 時疾熱瘡, heat sores associated with seasonal ailments; → *tian huo re chuang* 天火熱瘡, celestial fire heat sores, as variants of heat sores.

***Re dan* 熱疸, heat *dan*-illness** [2]

PC identical with → *re huang* 熱黃, heat jaundice. *RHZ* SE *chun* 蓴：絲蓴，治**熱疸**，厚腸胃, "*Si chun* cures **heat dan-illness**, and strengthens the intestines and stomach".

***Re dan* 熱丹, heat cinnabar** [2]

PC identical with → *chi dan* 赤丹, red cinnabar. *BCGM* SE *lan dian* 藍澱quoting *ZMML*: 治小兒丹，藍澱傅，熱即易, "To cure cinnabar in children, externally apply *lan dian*. The heat will change", writes: 小兒**熱丹**：藍澱傅之, "**Heat cinnabar** in children, apply *lan dian* to it externally".

Re dan du **熱丹毒, heat cinnabar poison** [1]

PC identical with → *chi dan* 赤丹, red cinnabar. *BCGM* SE *zhu ma* 苧麻 quoting *MYBL*: 根，安胎，貼熱丹毒腫有效, "The root: it pacifies the fetus, and is effective when pasted on swelling from heat cinnabar poison", writes: 安胎，貼**熱丹毒**, "It pacifies the fetus; paste on **heat cinnabar poison**".

Re du feng **熱毒風, heat poison wind** [20]

PC of heat congestion in the heart and lung brought about by wind heat evil [qi], or excessive consumption of "hot" medication, or excessive consumption of alcoholic beverages. *TPSHF* 21: 夫**熱毒風**者，皆由臟腑風虛，外邪所中，心肺壅熱，風氣在於胸心，或因吃熱藥，或飲酒過度，即頭面腫熱，心神煩悶，眼目昏昏，或時語澀，痰粘壅滯，皮膚壯熱，面赤口乾，肢節不利者，是其候也, "Now, as for **heat poison wind**, all such conditions result from wind depletion of depots and palaces struck by external evil. The heart and lung are obstructed with heat, and the wind qi is in the chest and heart. The reason may be consumption of hot medication, or excessive drinking of alcoholic beverages. As a result, the head and face are swollen and hot. The heart and spirit experience vexation with heart-pressure. Vision is dimmed. In some cases language is impaired, and sticky phlegm forms obstructions. The skin is very hot. The face is red and the mouth is dry. Limbs and joints do not move freely. These are its signs".

Re du guai bing **熱毒怪病, queer disease of heat poisoning** [1]

PC of an unusual disease with red eyes and dilated nose, massive panting, macules developing all over the body, and the hair on the body and head turning stiff. *BCGM* SE *hua shi* 滑石 quotes *QJF*: **熱毒怪病**，眼赤鼻張，大喘，渾身生斑，毛髮起如銅鐵, "**Queer disease of heat poisoning**: The eyes are red, and the nose is dilated. Massive panting. Macules develop all over the body. The hair on the body and head rises as if it were of copper or iron".

Re du li **熱毒痢, heat poison free-flux illness** [6]

PC identical with → *du li* 毒痢, poison free-flux illness. *QJYF* 20: 治下焦**熱毒痢**，魚腦雜痢赤血，臍下小腹絞痛不可忍，欲痢不出方, "Recipe to cure lower burner **heat poison free-flux illness**, free-flux illness interspersed with fish brain and red blood, with unbearable twisting pain below one's navel in the lower abdomen, and also if there is an urge to [defecate as if suffering from a] free-flux illness with eventually no discharge at all".

Re fan **熱煩, heat with vexation** [15]

IS identical with *fan re* 煩熱, vexing heat. *BJ* SE *jing tian* 景天：主大熱火瘡，身**熱煩**, "Controls massive heat fire sores; the body is **hot with vexation**".

Re fei **熱痱, heat with seething rash** [5] AW 熱疿; AD *fei* 痱.

PC of itchy millet size papules developing on the skin during summer months. *QJYF* 6 RE qiang wei wan 薔薇丸, pills with *qiang wei*: 方治口瘡，身體有**熱氣痱**瘰, "A recipe to cure mouth sores, when the body has heat qi, **seething**

rash, and scrofula", *BCGM* SE *sheng ma* 升麻: **熱痱**瘙癢，升麻煎湯飲，並洗之, "For **heat with seething rash** and itching, [have the patient] drink a decoction prepared from *sheng ma*, and also use this to wash [the afflicted body parts]". *BCGM* refers to *re fei* 熱痱 also as *sao fei* 瘙痱, itching with seething rash; *fei chuang* 痱瘡, seething rash sores; *fei zhen* 痱疹, seething rash papules; *fei yang* 痱癢, seething rash with itching; *fei zi* 痱子, seething rash seeds; *fei bao* 痱皰, seething rash blisters.

Re feng **熱風, heat wind** [25]

① EA CD of → *feng* 風, wind, and → *re* 熱, heat, with the latter dominating. *QJYiF* 21: **熱風**上沖，頭面上癢、鼻中癢, "**Heat wind** rushes upward. Head and face itch, and there is itching in the nose".

② Miscellaneous PC resulting from *re feng* 熱風，heat wind. *QJYF* 8: 竹瀝飲子，患**熱風**者，必先用此，制其熱毒, "The drink with *zhu li* is the first to be applied by patients suffering from **heat wind**. It subdues its heat poison". Such a PC belongs to the category of *feng fei* 風痱, wind disablement. *JWYS* 1:**熱風，**此症初起目脫、惡風、寒戰，鼻中常流黃濁涕，或咳吐膿血，鼻崩、眼坍、耳塞，而氣閉不通，救遲則死, "**Heat wind**. This condition begins with a feeling as if the eyes were bursting. [Patients] have an aversion to wind. They feel cold and shiver. Yellow, turbid snivel flows out of the nose continuously. Sometimes [patients] vomit pus and blood. Their nose breaks down. Their eyes collapse. The ears are blocked, and the qi is closed in and cannot pass. If help is late [the patient] will die". This PC is a heat type *ma feng* 麻風, numbness wind, i.e. leprosy. *BCGM* refers to pathological conditions associated with heat wind, such as *re feng shen yang* 熱風身癢, heat wind with body itching; *re feng shou zu bu sui* 熱風手足不遂, heat wind with hands and feet not moving according to one's will; *re feng shui zhang* 熱風水脹, heat wind with edema.

Re gan **熱疳, heat *gan*-illness** [3]

PC identical with → *gan re* 疳熱, *gan*-illness with heat. *LXJ* Fj: 胡黃連丸，治孩子**熱疳**, "Pills with *hu huang lian* cure **heat *gan*–illness** in children".

Re huang **熱黃, heat jaundice** [13] AN → *re dan* 熱疸, heat *dan*-illness; → *huo huang* 火黃, fire jaundice.

PC of → *huang dan* 黃疸, yellow *dan*-illness, brought forth by heat evil. *YXL* SE *long dan* 龍膽: 治時疾，**熱黃**, "It cures seasonal ailments and **heat jaundice**".

Re huo zhuo lan chuang **熱火灼爛瘡, festering sores following scorching by heat and fire** [1]

PC identical with → *huo chuang* 火瘡, fire sores. *BCGM* SE *ji* 雞 quotes *MYBL*: 除**熱火灼爛瘡**、癇痓, "It removes **festering sores following scorching by heat and fire**, as well as epilepsy and spasms".

Re ji **熱疾, heat ailment** [24]

PC identical with → *re* 熱, heat. *YXL* SE *sheng ma* 升麻：主治小兒風，驚癇，時氣**熱疾**, "It is able to cure children suffering from wind, fright epilepsy, seasonal qi, and **heat ailment**".

***Re ji huang* 熱急黃, acute heat jaundice** [1]
PC of → *ji huang* 急黃, acute jaundice, brought forth by heat evil. *BCGM* SE *lu ru* 驢乳, main indications: 小兒**熱急黃**，多服使利, "**Acute heat jaundice** in children. Ingesting large quantities will be beneficial".

***Re jie* 熱結, heat nodes** [26]
① EA identical with → *jie re* 結熱①, bound heat. *SHL* 136: 傷寒十餘日，**熱結**在裏，復往來寒熱者，與大柴胡湯, "If harm caused by cold continues for more than ten days, **heat nodes** will form internally. In the case of recurring alternating sensations of cold and heat, give [the patient] the 'major decoction with *chai hu*'".
② PC identical with → *jie re* 結熱②, bound heat. *BJ* SE *fang kui* 防葵：主疝瘕、腸泄、膀胱**熱結**、溺不下, "It controls elevation-illness and conglomeration-illness, intestinal free-flux, **heat nodes** in the bladder, and inability to discharge urine".

***Re jie* 熱癤, heat pimples** [4]
PC of → *jie* 癤, pimples, brought forth by heat evil. *QJYF* 19: 棗葉揩**熱癤**瘡，良, "Wipe **heat pimples** with date leaves. This is good".

***Re jing* 熱驚, heat fright** [2]
PC identical with → *jing re* 驚熱, fright heat. *RHZ* SE *qin pi* 秦皮：洗肝益精明目，小兒**熱驚**，皮膚風痹, "Cleanses the liver, adds to the essence, clears the eyes; for **heat fright** in children, and wind blockage of the skin".

***Re ju* 熱疽, heat with impediment-illness** [1]
PC of → *ju* 疽, impediment-illness, brought forth by heat evil. *MYBL* SE *lu er* 鹿茸：散石淋癰腫，骨中**熱疽**, "It disperses stone dripping, obstruction-illnesses and swelling, as well as **heat with impediment-illnesses** in the bones".

***Re jue* 熱厥, heat recession** [16] AN → *huo jue* 火厥, fire recession.
PC of a) hot hands and feet as a result of an abundance of heat and a recession of yin. *SW* 45: 陰氣衰於下，則為**熱厥**。帝曰：**熱厥**之為熱也，必起於足下, "When the yin qi weakens below, this causes **heat recession**. [Huang] Di: As for the heat of **heat recession**, it always rises from the lower side of the feet". b) Cold hands and feet because of an unbalanced interaction of yin and yang in the body due to heat abundance. *SHLZHRF* 28: **熱厥**須脈沉伏而滑，頭上有汗，其手雖冷，時復指爪温, "In the case of **heat recession**, the [movement in the] vessels should be in the depth, subdued, and smooth. There is sweating on the head. The hands are cold, but at times the fingernails turn warm". *BCGM* also refers to heat recession in connection with illness conditions of pain. This may be Li Shizhen's personal interpretation.

***Re ke* 熱咳, heat cough** [14] AN *huo ke* 火咳, fire cough; *re sou* 熱嗽, heat cough; *huo sou* 火嗽; fire cough; *huo re sou* 火熱嗽, fire heat cough.
PC of → *ke sou* 咳嗽, cough, brought forth by heat evil. *WTMY* 10 RE *tian men dong jian* 天門冬煎, decoction with *tian men dong*: 主肺間**熱咳**, "It controls **heat cough** in the lung".

Re ke **熱渴 heat with thirst** [24]
IS of a feeling of agitation and heat with thirst. *MYBL* SE *sang gen bai pi* 桑根白皮：去肺中水氣，唾血**熱渴**, "It removes water qi from within the lungs, bloodspitting, and **heat with thirst**".

Re kuang **熱狂, heat with madness** [39] AN → *kuang re* 狂熱, madness with heat.
IS apparent as a fever with mental derangement. *RHZ* SE *shi gao* 石膏：治天行**熱狂**, "It cures heaven-sent **heat with madness**".

Re lao **熱勞, heat exhaustion** [26]
PC identical with → *lao re* 勞熱, exhaustion heat. *BCGM* SE *gou qi di gu pi* 枸杞地骨皮 quotes *SJZL*: **熱勞**如燎：地骨皮二兩，柴胡一兩，為末。每服二錢，麥門冬湯下, "For **heat exhaustion** resembling burns: *di gu pi*, 2 *liang*; *chai hu*, 1 *liang*. Powderize. Each dosis is 2 *qian*. Ingest with *mai men dong* decoction".

Re lei **熱淚, hot tears** [4]
IS of a feeling of hot tears. *WTMY* 21: 硝石研末，於眼四角各點一粟許，須臾**熱淚**出, "If *xiao shi* is ground to powder and given into the four canthi in a quantity of about a millet grain, within a short time **hot tears** will appear".

Re li **熱痢, heat free-flux illness** [37]
PC of → *li* 痢, free-flux illness, brought forth by heat evil. *ZHF* 2 RE *huang lian, huang bo, long gu tang* 黃連黃柏龍骨湯, decoction with *huang lian*, *huang bo*, and *long gu*: 治大下，**熱痢**, "It cures massive discharge and **heat free-flux illness**".

Re lian **熱臁, heat shanks** [1]
PC of → *lian chuang* 臁瘡, shank sores, brought forth by heat evil. *BCGM* Bai bing zhu zhi yao 百病主治藥：百草霜，**熱臁**口厚，同輕粉、麻油，作隔紙膏貼, "For [treating] **heat shanks** with hardened openings of lesions [use] *bai cao shuang*. Mixed with *qing fen* and *ma you* and apply as a paper plaster".

Re lin **熱淋, heat dripping** [42]
PC of → *lin* 淋, dripping, brought forth by heat evil. *ZBYHL* 14: **熱淋**者，三焦有熱，氣搏於腎，流入於胞而成淋也, "As for **heat dripping**, the triple burner has heat qi which hits the kidneys. It flows into the bladder and causes dripping".

Re man **熱滿, heat with a feeling of fullness** [3] AN → *re zhang* 熱脹，heat with distension.
IS identical with *re zhang* 熱脹, heat with distension. *ZBYHL* 7: 心下有水氣，其人微嘔，**熱滿**而煩悶也, "There is water qi below the heart. The person has a slight urge to vomit, as well as **heat with a feeling of fullness** and vexation with heart pressure".

Re men **熱悶, heat with heart-pressure** [16]
IS of a feeling of heat with blocked qi stream. *ZBYHL* 25: 病發之時，腹內**熱悶**, "When the illness breaks out [patients experience] abdominal **heat with heart-pressure**".

Re mi **熱秘, heat constipation** [1] AN → *re bi* 熱閟, heat closure.
PC of → *bian mi* 便秘, constipation, brought forth by heat evil. *SJZL* 97: 大便秘澀…胃蘊客熱，口糜體黃，是謂**熱秘**, "If in the case of constipated or

rough stools, visitor heat has accumulated in the stomach, and oral putrescence is accompanied by a yellow color of the body, this is called **heat constipation**".

Re nü **熱衄, heat nosebleed** [1]

PC of nosebleed brought forth by heat evil. *BCGM* Bai bing zhu zhi yao 百病主治藥：玄明粉水服、水銀，並主**熱衄**, "*Xuan ming fen* to be ingested with water, and *shui yin*, together they control **heat nosebleed**".

Re nüe **熱瘧, heat malaria** [11]

PC identical with → *wen nüe* 温瘧, warmth malaria. *WTMY* 39: 商陽…主氣滿胸中，喘息支脅，熱病汗不出，耳中生風，耳鳴耳聾時不聞，**熱瘧**口乾. [Piercing the] *shang yang* [insertion hole] controls a feeling of fullness with qi in the chest, pant-breathing with propping [fullness in the] flanks, heat disease without sweating, wind generated in the ears, sounds ringing in the ears, and deafness to the extent that occasionally one cannot hear, as well as **heat malaria** with a dry mouth".

Re pi **熱痞, heat obstacle-illness** [2] AW → *pi re* 痞熱, obstacle-illness heat.

PC of → pi 痞, obstacle-illness, brought forth by heat evil. *KBBC* SE *ge gen* 葛根：小兒**熱痞**，以葛根浸搗汁飲之良, "For **heat obstacle-illness** in children, have them drink the juice gained from pounding soaked *ge gen*; this will be beneficial".

Re qi **熱氣, heat qi; hot vapors** [113]

① AN *huo qi* 火氣, fire qi. CC. *SW* 74: 流水不冰，**熱氣**大行, "The flowing waters do not freeze. **Heat qi** prevails everywhere".

② EA identical with → *re* 熱②, heat. SW 35: 此皆得之夏傷於暑，**熱氣**盛，藏於皮膚之內，腸胃之外, "All these [states] are acquired from harm by summerheat during summer. The **heat qi** abounds; it is stored inside the skin and outside of the intestines and the stomach".

③ A male's yang qi. *SW* 39: 按之則**熱氣**至，**熱氣**至則痛止, "If one presses them, **heat qi** arrives. When **heat qi** arrives, the pain stops"

④ The physiological effects generated by pharmaceutical drugs or other therapies. *ZHF* 5: 熨令**熱氣**下，即消, "Hot pressure will cause **heat qi** to descend. This makes [the swelling] diminish".

⑤ Heated fumes/vapors. *WTMY* 26: **熱氣**熏之即愈, "Fumigating [the patient] with the **hot vapors** will bring the cure".

Re ru xue shi **熱入血室, heat has entered the blood chamber** [6]

PC of evil heat availing itself of a depletion and entering the blood chamber in the aftermath of menstruation or a delivery, with stagnant blood and heat forming nodes. *SHL* 144: 寒熱，發作有時，經水適斷者，此為**熱入血室**，其血必結, "In the case of alternating sensations of cold and heat following the timely end of menstruation, this is because **heat has entered the blood chamber**. The blood must form nodes".

Re sai **熱塞, heat with obstruction** [5]

IS of a feeling of local scorching heat associated with obstruction. *WTMY* 35: 劉氏療小兒喉痹**熱塞**方, "Mr. Liu's recipe for healing children with throat blockage, that is, **heat with obstruction**".

Re sheng **熱盛, heat abundance** [10]

① IS of high fever. *MJ* 4: 诊伤寒，**热盛**，脉浮大者，生；沉小者，死, "If a diagnosis shows harm caused by cold, **heat abundance**, and a [movement in the] vessels that is both at the surface and massive, [the patient] will survive. If [the movement in the vessels] is in the depth and minor, he will die".

② EA identified as extreme form of evil heat. *SW* 45: **熱盛**於中，故熱遍於身, "**Heat abounds** in the center. The fact is, [in this case] heat is everywhere in the body".

Re shi **熱實, heat repletion** [2]

PC of a body filled with heat resulting in a standstill of the qi dynamics of depots and palaces. *YXLSE*: 前胡；能去**熱實**，下氣，主時氣內外俱熱, "It is able to remove **heat repletion**, to drain qi, and to control seasonal qi generating heat both in the inner and outer [sections of the body]".

Re shi jie xiong **熱實結胸; bound chest because of heat repletion** [1]

PC of → *jie xiong* 結胸, bound [evil qi in the] chest, brought forth by heat evil. Among all types of chest nodes, those resulting from heat repletion constitute the majority. *SHLZHRS* 10: 有寒熱二證：有**熱實結胸**，有寒實結胸, "One distinguishes between cold and heat conditions. There is **bound chest because of heat repletion**, and there is a bound chest because of cold repletion".

Re sou **熱嗽, heat cough** [14]

PC identical with → *re ke* 熱咳. *WTMY* 9: 將息傷熱，積熱所成，故致**熱嗽**, "If one is harmed by heat while recuperating, heat accumulations form. Hence this results in **heat cough**".

Re tan **熱痰, heat with phlegm** [25]

① EA identical with → *tan re* 痰熱①, phlegm and heat. *ZBYHL* 6: 將適失宜，飲食乖度，膈內生**痰熱**, "If the balance of nourishment is missed, and in drinking and eating one violates all reason, **heat with phlegm** will develop in the diaphragm region".

② PC identical with → *tan re* 痰熱②, phlegm and heat. *SJZL* 64: **熱痰**者，由氣道壅塞，津液不通，熱氣與痰水相搏，聚而不散也，若咽喉乾燥，或塞或壅，頭目昏重，咳唾稠濁，面目熱赤，是其證也, "As for '**heat with phlegm**', because the qi path is obstructed the body liquids cannot pass, heat qi and phlegm-water clash, collect and fail to dissipate. It feels as if the throat were dry, or blocked, or obstructed; vision is dim and the head feels heavy. [Patients] spit thick, turbid saliva. The face and eyes are hot and red. These are its signs".

Re ti **熱啼, heat weeping** [2]

IS of children who do not feel well because of → *re xian* 熱癇, heat epilepsy, and weep. *BCGM* Bai bing zhu zhi yao 百病主治藥：臘雪，止兒**熱啼**, "*La xue* ends **heat weeping** among children".

Re tong **熱痛, heat pain** [46]

IS of pain associated with heat. *MYBL* SE *shi long chu* 石龍芻：除莖中**熱痛**, "Removes **heat pain** from the penis".

Re xian **熱癇, heat epilepsy** [3] AW *xian re* 癇熱, epilepsy with heat.
PC of → *xian* 癇, epilepsy, brought forth by heat evil. *TPSHF* 85: 夫小兒**熱癇**者，由氣血不和，內有積熱之所致也, "**Heat epilepsy** among children results from an imbalance of qi and blood leading to internal heat accumulations".

Re xie **熱瀉, heat outflow** [3] AW 熱泄.
PC of → *xie xie* 泄瀉, outflow, brought forth by heat evil. *SJZL* 74, RE *ru shen san* 如神散, powder with divine effects: 如**熱瀉**，新水調下, "In the case of **heat outflow**, ingest [this powder] mixed with fresh water".

Re xie **熱泄, heat outflow** [3]
PC identical with → *re xie* 熱瀉. *MYBL* SE *long dan* 龍膽: 除胃中伏熱，時氣温熱，**熱泄**下痢，去腸中小蟲，益肝膽氣，止驚惕, "It eliminates hidden heat from within the stomach, seasonal qi of warmth and heat, **heat outflow** and discharge with free-flux illness, removes small bugs/worms from within the intestines, augments the qi of liver and gallbladder, and ends fearfulness".

Re yan **熱涎, heat with saliva** [2]
PC identical with → *re tan* 熱痰, heat with phlegm②. *JYBC* SE *jin xing shi* 金星石：下**熱涎**，解眾毒, "It drains **heat with saliva** and dissolves all types of poisons".

Re yan chuang **熱焱瘡, heat flame sores** [2]
PC identical with → *re chuang* 熱瘡, heat sores. *BCSY* SE *jing jing* 荊莖：其洗灼瘡及**熱焱瘡**，有效, "If used to rinse scolding sores and **heat flame sores**, it will be effective".

Re ye **熱暍, heat stroke** [1]
PC identical with → *zhong shu* 中暑, struck by summerheat. *ZBYHL* 23: 夫**熱暍**不可得冷，得冷便死，此謂外卒以冷觸其熱，蘊積於內，不得宣發故也, "A **heat stroke** must not be met with cold. If met with cold, [the patient] will die. This is explained as a sudden clash of the heat with cold. This will lead to an accumulation inside because [the qi] will be unable to move on and effuse".

Re yi **熱翳, heat shade** [2] AN → *mu zhong re mo* 目中熱膜, heat membrane in the eyes.
PC of → *mu yi* 目翳, eye shade, which is a heat condition. It is accompanied by red eyes that ache and feel hot. *BCSY* SE *ying yu* 蘡薁：（藤汁）滴目中，去**熱翳**赤障, "[The juice from the vine] is to be dripped into the eyes to remove **heat shades** and red screens".

Re yong **熱壅, heat obstruction** [6]
PC identical with → *yong re* 壅熱①, obstruction with heat. *SLBC* SE *ku zhu ru* 苦竹茹: 主下**熱壅**, "It is responsible for moving down **heat obstruction**".

Re yong **熱擁, heat congestion** [4]
① PC identical with → *yong re* 壅熱①, obstruction with heat. *YXL* SE *diao teng* 釣藤: 能主小兒驚啼，瘈瘲**熱擁**, "It is capable of mastering fright and the crying of children, spasms, and **heat congestion**".
② PQ identical with → *yong re* 壅熱②. *BCSY* SE *chun* 蓴: 蓴雖水草，性**熱擁**, "Although *chun* is a water plant, its nature is one of **heat congestion**".

Re you dan zhong **熱游丹腫, heat-roaming cinnabar-swelling** [1]
PC identical with → *chi you dan du* 赤游丹毒, red-roaming cinnabar-poison. *BCGM* SE *gua lou* 栝樓quoting *YSCRF*: 熱游丹赤腫, "Heat-roaming cinnabar-red-swelling", writes: **熱游丹腫, "Heat-roaming cinnabar-swelling"**.

Re you huo zhuo **熱油火灼, scorching by hot oil and fire** [1]
PC identical with → *tang huo shang* 湯火傷, harm caused by boiling water and fire. *BCGM* SE *dan shen* 丹參 quotes *ZHF*: **熱油火灼**, 除痛生肌, "For **scorching by hot oil and fire**: It removes the pain and lets muscles grow".

Re you shao tong **熱油燒痛, painful burns by hot oil** [1]
PC identical with → *tang huo shang* 湯火傷, harm caused by boiling water and fire. *BCGM* SE *feng mi* 蜂蜜 quotes *HS*: **熱油燒痛**, 以白蜜塗之, "**Painful burns by hot oil**: smear white honey on them".

Re you zhuo shang **熱油灼傷; harm following sorching by hot oil** [1]
PC identical with → *tang huo shang* 湯火傷, harm caused by boiling water and fire. *BCGM* SE *bai* 柏 quotes *ZHF*: **熱油灼傷**, 柏白皮，以臘豬脂煎油，塗瘡上, "**Harm following scorching by hot oil**: boil the white bark of *bai* with cured lard to an oil and apply externally to the sores".

Re yu **熱郁, pent-up heat** [3]
PC identical with → *huo yu* 火郁, pent-up fire. *SW* 71: 其病**熱郁**, "The illnesses [caused by] them are **pent-up heat**".

Re yue **熱噦, heat retching** [4]
PC of → *yue* 噦，retching，brought forth by heat evil. *BCGM* SE *bai mao* 白茅 quoting *Shang han zong bing lun* 傷寒總病論：温病噦, "Warmth disease with retching", writes: 温病**熱噦**, "Warmth disease with **heat retching**".

Re zao **熱燥, heat and dryness; hot and dry** [3]
① PC identical with → *zao re* 燥熱③, dryness and heat. *SJBC* SE *pu sun* 蒲筍: 去**熱燥**，利小便, "It removes **heat and dryness**, and facilitates urination".
② IS identical with → *zao re* 燥熱④. *BCYY* Xu li 序例：我但胸中**熱燥**，口鼻乾, "I only experience **heat and dryness** in the chest; the mouth and nose are dry".
③ PQ identical with → *zao re* 燥熱⑤. *BCTJ* SE *sheng jiang* 生薑 quotes *CXF*: 凡人患嗽，多進冷藥，若見此方用藥**熱燥**，即不肯服，故但出藥多效，試之信然, "Whenever people suffer from a cough, they mostly ingest cold medication. When they realize that the present recipe makes use of pharmaceutical substances that are **hot and dry**, they refuse to ingest them. Hence it is essential to prescribe only medications that have often proved effective. Once they have tried them they will believe in them".

Re zhang **熱瘴, heat miasma** [2]
PC of → *zhang nüe* 瘴瘧, miasmatic malaria, with heat spells only and no cold. *PJF* 199: 治丈夫婦人患**熱瘴**, "To cure men and women suffering from **heat miasma**".

Re zhang **熱脹, heat with distension** [4]
IS of an uncomfortable feeling of heat and fullness with distension. *SW* 71: 其病中**熱脹**，面目浮腫, "Its illnesses include central **heat and distension**. The face and the eyes have surface swelling".

Re zhang **熱障, heat screen** [1]
PC of → *zhang* 障, screen [of the eyes], brought forth by heat evil. *BCSY* SE *na qi xi* 那耆悉：取汁洗目，主赤爛**熱障**, "If the eyes are rinsed with its juice, this will master redness, festering, and **heat screen**".

Re zheng **熱證, pathological heat condition** [11]
PC identical with → *re* 熱, heat. *SHL* 141: 寒實結胸無**熱證**者，與三物小陷胸湯, "If there is a bound chest because of cold repletion but no **pathological heat condition**, treat with the 'minor decoction with three items that sink into the chest'".

Re zhong **熱中, heated center** [25] AW *zhong re* 中熱.
PC of heat in the central section of the human body. *SW* 20: 是故寒熱病者，以平旦死；**熱中**及熱病者，以日中死, "Hence, those who suffer from cold and heat disease, they die at dawn. Those who have a **heated center** and who suffer from heat disease, they die at noon". LSZ identifies the following pathological conditions as most important signs of heated center: *shan ji er sou* 善飢而瘦, emaciation despite good appetite; *jie yi zhong man* 解㑊中滿, weariness and a feeling of central fullness; *zhu zhang fu da* 諸脹腹大, all types of bloatings and abdominal extension; *shang xia bu tong* 上下不通, constipation; *huo luan tu li* 霍亂吐利, cholera with spitting and free-flux[-illness]. The alternative writing *zhong re* 中熱 is supposed to convey an identical meaning, but is used in the *BCGM* less often than *re zhong* 熱中.

Re zhong **熱腫, hot and swollen** [32]
IS apparent as a localized swelling that feels hot to the touch. *LS* 10: 氣有餘則當脈所過者**熱腫**, "When there is surplus qi the regions where the respective vessel passes will be **hot and swollen**".

Re zhong feng **熱中風, wind stroke with heat** [3]
PC of → *zhong feng* 中風, wind stroke, with a particularly hot body. *YXL* SE *tian men dong* 天門冬：去**熱中風**, "It eliminates **wind stroke with heat**".

Ren fu fu tong **妊婦腹痛, a pregnant woman's abdominal pain** [2]
PC identical with → *ren shen fu tong* 妊娠腹痛, abdominal pain during pregnancy. *BCGM* SE *ju* 櫸 quoting *QJYF*: 妊娠腹中痛, "Pain in the abdomen during pregnancy" writes: **妊婦腹痛, "A pregnant woman's abdominal pain"**.

Ren fu tou yuan **妊婦頭旋, a pregnant woman's spinning head** [2]
PC of a pregnant woman's vertigo and visual dizziness, accompanied by a swelling of the face and limbs, in severe cases even with clouding and a tendency to lose consciousness. *BCGM* SE *zhu sun* 竹筍 quoting *RHZ* SE *dan zhu bing gen* 淡竹並根：懷妊人頭旋, "Spinning head during pregnancy", writes: **妊婦頭旋, "A pregnant woman's spinning head"**.

Ren shen dong tai **妊娠動胎, fetus stirred during pregnancy** [1]
PC identical with → *shang tai* 傷胎, harmed fetus. *WTMY* 33: 療婦人**妊娠動胎**，腰腹痛及血下, "To cure women with a **fetus stirred during pregnancy**, associated with lumbar and abdominal pain as well as discharge of blood".

***Ren shen fu tong* 妊娠腹痛, abdominal pain during pregnancy** [2] AN *ren fu fu tong* 妊婦腹痛, abdominal pain of pregnant women.

PC with pain in the lower abdomen resulting from fetal injury. *WTMY* 33: 療**妊娠腹痛**，或者冷痛，或者胎動，葱白當歸湯方, "For curing **abdominal pain during pregnancy**, sometimes as cold pain, sometimes as fetal movement, [use] the recipe for the decoction with *cong bai* and *dang gui*".

***Ren shen fu zhong* 妊娠浮腫, surface swelling during pregnancy** [3]

PC identical with → *ren shen shui zhong* 妊娠水腫, edematose swelling during pregnancy. *BCGM* Bai bing zhu zhi yao 百病主治藥：天仙藤，**妊娠浮腫**，謂之子氣，乃素有風氣，勿作水治，同香附、陳皮、甘草、烏藥、紫蘇煎服, "*Tian xian teng*: **surface swelling during pregnancy**, which is also called child qi, is commonly [brought forth by] wind qi. One must not treat this as if there were water. Ingest it boiled in a decoction together with *xiang fu*, *chen pi*, *gan cao*, *wu yao*, and *zi su*".

***Ren shen shang dong* 妊娠傷動, injury inflicted during pregancy** [2]

PC identical with → *shang tai* 傷胎, harmed fetus. *TPSHF* 75: 治**妊娠傷動**，腹痛下血, "To cure **injury inflicted during pregnancy**, with abdominal pain and discharge of blood".

***Ren shen shui qi* 妊娠水氣, water qi during pregnancy** [1]

PC identical with → *ren shen shui zhong* 妊娠水腫, edematose swelling during pregnancy. *WTMY* 33 lists **妊娠水氣**方三首, "Three recipes for **water qi during pregnancy**".

***Ren shen shui zhong* 妊娠水腫, edematose swelling during pregnancy** [5] AN *tai zhong* 胎腫, fetus swelling; *ren shen shui qi* 妊娠水氣, water qi during pregnancy; *ren shen fu zhong* 妊娠浮腫, surface swelling during pregnancy; *zi qi* 子氣, child qi.

PC of → *shui zhong* 水腫, edematose swelling, in the late phase of a pregnancy. *SJZL* 157: 治**妊娠水腫**，茯苓湯方, "To cure **edematose swelling during pregnancy** [use the] recipe for the decoction with *fu ling*".

***Ren shen tai dong* 妊娠胎動, fetal movement during pregnancy** [9]

PC identical with → *tai dong bu an* 胎動不安, fetal movement and restlessness. *ZBYHL* 41: **妊娠胎動**候：胎動不安, "Signs of **fetal movement during pregnancy**: the fetus moves and is restless".

***Ren shen tai si* 妊娠胎死, fetal death during pregnancy** [2]

PC identical with → *zi si fu zhong* 子死腹中, a fetus' death in the abdomen. *TPSHF* 77: 治**妊娠胎死**腹中，衣不出, "To cure **fetal death during pregnancy** in the abdomen, with the placenta failing to come out".

***Ren shen xia huang zhi* 妊娠下黃汁, discharge of yellow liquid during pregnancy** [1] AN *ren shen xia shui* 妊娠下水, discharge of water during pregnancy.

PC of vaginal discharge of yellow liquid caused by fetal injury. *BCGM* SE *shu* 秫：食鵝鴨成癥，**妊娠下黃汁**, "Consuming geese or ducks generates conglomeration-illness, and **discharge of yellow liquid during pregnancy**".

Ren shen xia shui **妊娠下水, discharge of water during pregnancy** [1]

PC identical with → *ren shen xia huang zhi* 妊娠下黄汁, discharge of yellow liquid during pregnancy. *BCGM* SE *shu* 秫 quotes *HS*: **妊娠下水**：黃色如膠，或如小豆汁, "**Discharge of water during pregnancy**: [The liquid is] yellow like glue, sometimes it resembles the juice of beans".

Ren shen xia xue **妊娠下血, discharge of blood during pregnancy** [10]

PC of vaginal bleeding caused by fetal injury. *JGYL* Lj: 婦人有漏下者，有半產後因續下血都不絕者，有**妊娠下血**者, "It may be that a woman experiences leaking discharge, or that after a miscarriage blood continues to be discharged without coming to an end, or it may be that she experiences a **discharge of blood during pregnancy**".

Ren shen yao tong **妊娠腰痛, lower back pain during pregnancy** [7]

PC of lumber pain caused by a fetal injury. *QJYF* 2: 治**妊娠腰痛**及妊娠熱病, "To cure **lower back pain during pregnancy** and heat disease during pregnancy".

Rou ci **肉刺, flesh thorn; corn** [11] AN *ji yan* 雞眼, chicken eye, corn; *rou ci* 肉杸, flesh spade, corn.

PC of skin sections developing into thick, unyielding nodes that reach deep into the flesh and are painful to the touch. Often they grow on the feet because a shoe is too tight or has an inner uneven part rubbing the feet. *ZBYHL* 30: 脚趾間生肉如刺，謂之**肉刺**, "When flesh resembling a thorn grows on the toes, this is called '**flesh thorn**'".

Rou ci **肉杸, flesh spade; corn** [2]

PC identical with → *rou ci* 肉刺, flesh thorn, corn. *ZLBC* Xu li shang 序例上 quotes *LGPZL*: 脚有**肉杸**者，取莨菪根，於褌帶上系之, "When legs develop a **flesh spade**, take the root of *lang dang* and attach it to the belt of the underpants".

Rou gan fu qi **肉乾麸起, the flesh is desiccated and bran emerges** [1]

IS of a rising of desiccated skin. *BCGM* SE *ren xue* 人血 quoting *BCSY*: 皮肉乾枯，身上麸片起, "The skin and flesh are desiccated and wither. Bran flakes emerge from the body", writes: **肉乾麸起, "The flesh is desiccated and bran emerges"**.

Rou huai **肉壞, flesh decay** [2]

PC of an unusual disease with a malodorous liquid flowing from the mouth and nose, mixed with dead items of iron color and the size of polished rice. *JFP-JF* 26: 口鼻中腥臭水流，以碗盛之，有鐵色蝦魚粳米大，走躍不住，以手捉之，即化為水，此**肉壞**矣, "From mouth and nose a stinking liquid flows. If one fills it into a bowl it contains items of an iron color as big as shrimps or polished rice. They move and jump continuously. If touched by one's hand they transform into water. This is '**flesh decay**'".

Rou ji **肉積, meat accumulation** [5]

PC of → *shi ji* 食積, food accumulation, brought forth by a consumption of meat that fails to be digested. *DXXF* 3: 阿魏丸，治**肉積**, "Pills with *a wei* cure **meat accumulation**".

***Rou jing* 柔痓, soft spasms** [3]

PC of a) → *jing bing* 痓病, spasms disease, with the special characteristic of feverish sweating without an aversion to cold. *JGYL* Fj: 太陽病，發熱汗出，而不惡寒，名曰**柔痓**, "If someone suffers from major yang disease, with effusion of heat and sweating and no aversion to cold, this is called **soft spasms**". b) Spasms disease of heat in the lung and kidneys, with muscles being soft, flaccid, and without strength. *SW* 37: 肺移熱於腎，傳為**柔痓**, "When the lung moves heat to the kidneys, [further] transmission causes **soft spasms**".

***Rou ren* 肉人, flesh man** [2]

PC of an unusual disease with sores of the size of a cherry or peach developing on the nape, displaying various colors. When these sores open the patient will lose his skin from nape to the feet. *JFPJF* 26: 項上生瘡如櫻桃大, 有五色。如瘡破, 即項皮遂斷, 上連髮捲去, 下至足脫之, 乃為**肉人**, "On the nape sores develop of the size of a cherry or peach. They display various colors. When they open, the skin of the nape will be cut. Above it rolls up and vanishes up to the hairline; downwards it is lost to the feet. This ends in a '**flesh man**'".

***Rou zheng* 肉癥, meat concretion-illness** [4]

PC of → *zheng* 癥, concretions, which form when someone continuously consumes meat and never seems to be satisfied. *QJYF* 11: 治**肉癥**，思肉不已，食訖復思者方, "Recipe to cure meat **concretion-illness**, when someone continuously longs for meat. Once he has eaten, he longs for it again".

***Rou zhui* 肉錐, flesh awl** [1]

PC identical with → *qian jia* 嵌甲, embedded nail. *BCGM* SE *kui* 葵 quoting *CXSYF* Lj: 手足甲忽然長，倒生刺肉如錐，痛不可忍, "The nails of the hands and feet suddenly grow long. They turn around and pierce the flesh like an awl. The pain is unbearable", writes: **肉錐**怪疾, "Queer ailment of **flesh awl**".

***Ru ai* 乳癌, breast tumor** [1]

PC identical with → *ru yan* 乳岩, breast rock. *BCGM* SE *ling li* 鯪鯉 quotes *DXF*: **乳癌**乳癰, 方同上, "For **breast tumor** and breast obstruction-illness: the recipe is identical with that above".

***Ru chuang* 乳瘡, breast sores** [3]

PC of → *chuang* 瘡, sores, conditions developing on the female breast. *ZHF* 5: 槲樹皮切三升，以水一斗，煮取五升，春夏冷用，秋冬溫用，洗**乳瘡**及諸敗瘡, "Cut *hu shu pi*, 3 *sheng*, and boil with 1 *dou* of water down to five *sheng*. Use cold in spring and summer and use warm in autumn and winter to wash **breast sores** and all types of decay sores".

***Ru chuang* 蓐瘡, childbed sores** [4]

PC of → *chuang* 瘡, sores, conditions of newborn children developing within their first seven days of life. *XEWSZWLF* 1: 兒自初生，至七日內外，因胎毒攻發，身生瘡者，名曰**蓐瘡**，謂在產草上生瘡也, "When in newborn children, within around the first seven days, fetal poison breaks out and causes the body to develop sores, these are called **childbed sores**. They are named so because [newborn children] develop these sores while [the children] still lie on the straw where they were delivered".

Ru du **乳毒, breast poison** [1]

PC of an infectious disease brought forth by an accumulation of milk in the breasts of nursing women. *TPSHF* 71: 婦人乳汁不下，內結成腫，名為**乳毒**，乃急於癰也, "When a female's milk is not let, it forms internal nodes and generates swelling. This is called '**breast poison**'. It is more critical than an obstruction-illness".

Ru e **乳蛾, nipple moth; acute tonsillitis** [16]

PC with red swelling and pain on both sides of the throat, in severe cases including the generation of pus forming white dots, as a major sign. *PJF* 60: 熱氣上行，結纏於喉之兩旁近外腫作，以其形似，是謂**乳蛾**, "Heat qi ascends. It forms nodes on both sides of the throat towards the outside and causes swelling there. Because of their appearance these [swellings] are called '**nipple moth**'".

Ru fa **乳發, breast effusion** [3]

PC identical with → *fa ru* 發乳, effusion of the breast. *XCWKJYF* 4: 多口者為**乳發**, 乳房堅硬者為乳石，正在乳嘴處腫者為吹乳, "If it has many openings, this is '**breast effusion**'. If the breasts are hard, this is 'breast stone'. If there is a swelling right at the mouth of the breast, this is 'inflated breast'".

Ru he **乳核, breast kernel** [2]

PC of a swelling in the region of the breast resembling a fruit kernel. It is hard and does not fester. *PJF* 325: 治**乳核**，結硬不消, "To cure **breast kernels**, with nodular hardness that fails to dissolve".

Ru jie **乳結, breast nodes** [3]

PC with a woman's milk, following delivery, not flowing freely, and stagnating in the breast instead, causing painful swelling and hardening. *MYBL* SE *xi xin* 細辛：除喉痹齆鼻，風癇癲疾，下**乳結**, "It removes throat blockage and nasal congestion, wind epilepsy with peak ailment, and discharges **breast nodes**".

Ru jing **乳痙, childbirth spasms** [1]

PC of → *jing bing* 痙病, spasms disease, contracted by women in the course of delivery. *BJ* SE *gou wu* 鉤吻：主金瘡**乳痙**，中惡風，咳逆上氣，水腫, "It controls wounds inflicted by metal objects as well as **childbirth spasms**, being struck by malign wind, coughing with qi rising in counterflow, water swelling".

Ru lao **蓐勞, childbed exhaustion** [8] AN *chan lao* 產勞, childbirth exhaustion.

PC of depletion exhaustion developed by women after childbirth. *QJYF* 3: 產後虛羸，喘乏，乍寒乍熱，如瘧狀，名**蓐勞**, "If after delivery she is emaciated, pants, and has alternating sensations of cold and heat as if she were suffering from malaria, this is called **childbed exhaustion**".

Ru lie **乳裂, breast[-nipple] cracks** [3]

PC AD of → *ru tou lie* 乳頭裂. *TPSHF* 71: 上件藥，研細塗**乳裂**處，神效, "The above-mentioned pharmaceutical substances: grind them to a fine powder and apply to the **breast[-nipple] cracks**. Wondrously effective".

***Ru nan* 乳難, difficult birth; breast disorder** [13]

PC identical with a) → *nan chan* 難產, difficult birth. *BJ* SE *hua shi* 滑石: 主身熱泄澼，女子**乳難**, "It controls body heat with outflow and flush, and [cures] women who experience a **difficult birth;** b) → *ru yong* 乳癰, breast obstruction-illness. *BJ* SE *xu duan* 續斷: 補不足，金瘡，癰，傷折跌，續筋骨，婦人**乳難**, "It supplements insufficiencies, [cures] wounds inflicted by metal [objects, cures] obstruction-illnesses, and injuries from fractures and falls, links sinews and bones, [and cures] women with **breast disorder**".

***Ru shi du* 乳石毒, stalactite mineral poison** [3]

EA identical with → *shi yao du* 石藥毒, mineral drug poison. *YXL* SE *gan cao* 甘草: 治七十二種**乳石毒**, "To cure 72 types of **stalactite mineral poison**".

***Ru shi fa* 乳石發, outbreak of stalactite mineral [poisoning]** [12] AN *ru shi fa dong* 乳石發動; *yao shi fa* 藥石發, outbreak of [stalactite] mineral drug [poisoning]; *yao shi fa dong* 藥石發動; *fu shi du fa* 服石毒發, outbreak of poisoning after ingesting [stalactite] mineral; *shi qi fa dong* 石氣發動, outbreak of [stalactite] mineral [poison] qi.

PC CD of all types of poisoning following an ingestion of medication based on *ru shi*, often accompanied by restlessness, heat, thirst, obstruction- as well as impediment-illnesses, and red eyes. *QJYiF* 15: **乳石發**, 頭痛寒熱, 胸中塞, 日晡手足煩疼方, "Recipe for [treating] **outbreak of stalactite mineral [poisoning]**, with headache, alternating sensations of cold and heat, and chest congestion, as well as vexing pain of the hands and feet in the late afternoon".

***Ru shi fa dong* 乳石發動, outbreak of stalactite mineral [poisoning]** [5]

PC identical with → *ru shi fa* 乳石發. *WTMY* 38: 療諸**乳石發動**, 口乾寒熱, 似鬼神為病方, "Recipe to cure all types of **outbreaks of stalactite mineral [poisoning]**, with dry mouth and alternating sensations of cold and heat as if this were a disease inflicted by demon-spirits".

***Ru tou lie* 乳頭裂, breast nipple cracks** [2] AD *ru lie* 乳裂; AN *ru tou lie po* 乳頭裂破, cracked open breast nipples; *ru tou po lie* 乳頭破裂; *nai tou hua* 奶頭花, breast nipple blossoms; *nai tou hua lie* 奶頭花裂，breast nipples blossoms cracked open.

PC with the female breast nipples cracking and being painful during the period of breast-feeding. *TPSHF* 71: 治婦人**乳頭裂**，痛，欲成瘡方, "Recipe to cure women with **cracked breast nipples** that are painful and may develop into sores".

***Ru tou lie po* 乳頭裂破, cracked open breast nipples** [2]

PC identical with → *ru tou lie* 乳頭裂, breast nipple cracks. *DXZFXY* 6: **乳頭裂破**，丁香末敷, "For **cracked open breast nipples**, apply *ding xiang* powder".

***Ru tou po lie* 乳頭破裂, cracked open breast nipple** [1]

PC identical with → *ru tou lie* 乳頭裂, breast nipple cracks. *PJF* 346: 亦治**乳頭破裂**, "It also cures **cracked open breast nipples**".

***Ru xia* 乳瘕, breast conglomeration-illness** [1]

PC with nodes conglomerating in the female breast without dissolving again. Their sizes differ. When they form they are painful. *BJ* SE *huai shi* 槐實：婦人**乳瘕**，子藏急痛, "[To cure] **breast conglomeration-illness** in women, as well as uterine tightness and pain".

***Ru xuan* 乳懸, hanging breast** [2]

PC of a woman's breasts that, following delivery, suddenly grow long and thin, and are unbearably painful. *SYDXF* 10: 婦人產後忽然兩乳伸長，細小如腸，垂下直過小肚，痛不可忍，危亡須臾，名曰**乳懸**, "When a woman's two breasts following delivery suddenly grow long and thin like an intestine, and hang down deeper than the lower abdomen, accompanied by unbearable pain and impending danger of life, this is called '**hanging breast**'".

***Ru yan* 乳岩, breast rock** [1] AN *ru ai* 乳癌, breast tumor.

PC with a lump in a female breast. At the beginning there is neither pain nor itching. After several years it breaks open like a rock cave. Prognosis is inauspicious. *DXXF* 5: 若不得於夫，不得於舅姑，憂怒鬱悶，昕夕累積，脾氣消阻，肝氣橫逆，遂成隱核，如大棋子，不痛不癢。數十年後，方為瘡陷，名曰奶岩，以其瘡形嵌凹似岩穴也。不可治矣。若於始生之際，便能消釋病根，使心清神安，然後施之治法，亦有可安之理…**乳岩**小破，加柴胡、川芎。右以水煎，入酒服, "If [a woman] finds no [solace with her] husband, and if she finds [solace] neither with uncle nor with an aunt, is sad and angry with pent-up [qi] and heart-pressure, accumulating from dawn to dusk, with the spleen qi disappearing and blocked, and the liver qi moving in a transverse counterflow, then hidden kernels develop of the size of chess pieces. They do not ache and they do not itch. After several decades they form indented sores, and this condition is called 'breast rock' because they are caved in like a rock cave. At this stage there is no cure. At the very beginning, though, it is possible to eliminate the root of the disease by clearing [the woman's] heart and calming her spirit. Therapeutic patterns applied later on, they too are based on the principle of calming ... When the **breast rock** has a small crack, add *chai hu* and *chuan xiong*. Boil the [ingredients mentioned] above in water and ingest with wine".

***Ru yong* 乳癰, breast obstruction-illness** [82] AN *nai yong* 奶癰.

PC of acute putrefication of a woman's breast. Often encountered if a woman, following delivery, experiences → *chui nai* 吹奶, inflated breast, or → *du ru* 妒乳, jealousy breast. *BJ* SE *mang cao* 莽草：主風頭癰腫，**乳癰**疝瘕, "It controls wind head and obstruction-illness with swelling, **breast obstruction-illness**, and elevation-illness with conglomeration-illness".

***Ru zhi bu chu* 乳汁不出, failure to produce breast milk** [1]

PC identical with → *ru zhi bu tong* 乳汁不通, blocked breast milk passage. *MYBL* SE *ze xie* 澤瀉：主大風，**乳汁不出**, "It controls massive wind and **failure to produce breast milk**".

***Ru zhi bu tong* 乳汁不通, blocked breast milk passage** [12] AN *ru zhi bu xia* 乳汁不下, failure to discharge breast milk; *ru zhi bu xing* 乳汁不行, failure to pass breast milk; *ru zhi bu chu* 乳汁不出, failure to produce breast milk; *wu ru* 無乳, to have no breast milk.

PC with women producing too little or, in severe cases, no breast milk during the period of breast-feeding. *TPSHF* 81: 治產後**乳汁不通**神效方, "Wondrously effective recipe for treating **blocked breast milk passage** following delivery".

Ru zhi bu xia **乳汁不下, failure to discharge breast milk** [9]
PC identical with → *ru zhi bu tong* 乳汁不通, blocked breast milk passage. *WTMY* 34: 崔氏療乳汁不下方, "Mr. Cui's recipe to cure **failure to discharge breast milk**".

Ru zhi bu xing **乳汁不行, failure to pass breast milk** [3]
PC identical with → *ru zhi bu tong* 乳汁不通, blocked breast milk passage. *FRDQLF* 34: 漏蘆散，療乳婦氣脈壅塞，**乳汁不行**, "The powder with *lou hu* cures obstructed qi vessels in breast-feeding women, with **failure to pass breast milk**".

Ru zhi qing shao **乳汁清少, clear breast milk in small quantities** [1]
PC with women producing, during the breast-feeding period, only small quantities of clear, watery breast milk. *BCGM* SE *shu* 鼠 quotes *ZMML*: **乳汁清少**，死鼠一頭燒末，酒服方寸匕, "[To cure women producing only] **clear breast milk in small quantities** have them ingest one square inch spoon of a burned and powderized head of a dead rat mixed with wine".

Ruan feng **軟風, softness wind** [2]
PC of slackening and weakness in the lower back and feet, and an inability to walk. *TPSHF* 69 RE *niu xi san fang* 牛膝散方, recipe for the powder with *niu xi*: 治婦人脚氣，緩弱無力，兼**軟風**, "It cures leg qi in women, with slackening and weakness, and simultaneously **softness wind**".

Ruan jiao **軟脚, soft legs** [10] AN *gu ruan* 骨軟 bone softness.
PC with atrophying and weakness of the lower extremities to the extent that standing up and walking is impossible. *YXL* SE *gou ji* 狗脊：能治男子女人毒風**軟脚**, "It is able to cure poison wind with **soft legs** of males and females".

Ruan jie **軟癤, soft pimple** [21]
PC of → *jie* 癤, pimples, that have developed pus. They may or may not have opened to release the pus. *TPSHF* 61: 治**軟癤**，赤腫疼痛不可忍方, "Recipe to cure **soft pimples** with redness, swelling, and unbearable pain".

Ruan que **軟怯, weakness** [2]
IS identical with → *ruan ruo* 軟弱. *RHZ* SE *niu xi* 牛膝：治腰膝**軟怯**冷弱, "It cures cold and **weakness** of the lower back and knees".

Ruan ruo **軟弱, weakness** [10] AN *ruan que* 軟怯.
IS identical with → *wu li* 無力①, loss of strength. *YXL* SE *shi hu* 石斛：益氣除熱，主治男子腰肢**軟弱**，健陽，逐皮肌風痹, "Augments qi, removes heat. It is responsible for the treatment of **weakness** of the lower back of males, strengthens the yang, and eliminates wind blockage from the skin and the muscles".

Ruo fang **弱房, bedroom weakness** [3]
PC with a decreased sexual potency of adult males. *SLBC* SE *mi rou* 麋肉：多食令人**弱房**，髮脚氣, "If consumed in large quantities it causes men to experience **bedroom weakness**, and to develop leg qi [disease]".

- S -

***Sai man* 塞滿, blockage and fullness** [2]

IS identical with → *pi man* 痞滿①, obstacle-illness and fullness. *TPSHF* 61: 治胸痹連心氣悶，喉中**塞滿**，赤茯苓湯方, "To cure chest blockage associated with heart qi bringing forth heart-pressure, as well as **blockage and fullness** in the throat, [use] the recipe for the decoction with *chi fu ling*".

***San chong* 三蟲, three bugs; three worms** [80]

EA a) of all microorganisms in the body that bring forth disease. *BJ* SE *li shi* 理石：明目，破積聚，去**三蟲**, "Clears the eyes, breaks open accumulations and collections, removes the **three bugs/worms**". *BCGM chong bu* 蟲部, "section: bugs/worms", LSZ: 蟲乃生物之微者，其類甚繁，故字從**三蟲**會意, "Bugs/worms are small organisms. There are very many types. This is the meaning of '**three bugs/worms**'". b) CD of *hui chong* 蛔蟲, roundworms, *chi chong* 赤蟲, red worms, and *nao chong* 蟯蟲, pinworms. *ZBYHL* 18: **三蟲**者，長蟲、赤蟲、蟯蟲也, "The **three worms** include long worms, red worms, and pinworms".

***San jiao xiao ke* 三焦消渴, triple burner's melting with thirst** [2]

PC identical with → *san xiao* 三消, three types of melting. *BCGM* SE *xi lin zhi* 錫吝脂：又主一切風氣，及**三焦消渴**，飲水，併入丸藥用, "Furthermore it controls all types of wind qi, as well as the **triple burner's melting with thirst** [disease] with [abnormal] drinking of water. It may also be used in pills".

***San jiao yue* 三焦約, triple burner restraint** [3]

PC of constipation and anuria brought forth by evil qi affecting the triple burner. *SJZL* 54: 治三焦約，大小便不通，枳殼散方, "To cure **triple burner restraint,** with no passage of stools and urine, [use] the recipe for the powder with *zhi qiao*".

***San shi* 三屍, three corpse [bugs/worms]** [18] AN *shi chong* 屍蟲, corpse bugs/worms.

EA of microorganisms that can bring forth all types of → *shi bing* 屍病, corpse [qi] disease. *ZBYHL* 23: 人身內自有**三屍**諸蟲，與人俱生，而此蟲忌惡，能與鬼靈相通，常接引外邪，為人患害, "Inside the human body there are from the beginning all the **three corpse [bugs/worms]**. They come to life together with man, but they are most malicious. They are able to communicate with demons and the numinous, and they regularly invite evil [qi] from outside, thereby causing human suffering".

***San shi liu ban feng* 三十六般風, the 36 variants of wind** [2]

PC identical with → *san shi liu feng* 三十六風, the 36 types of wind. *RHZ* SE *ma chi xian* 馬齒莧：治**三十六般風**, "It cures **the 36 variants of wind**".

***San shi liu feng* 三十六風, thirty-six types of wind** [5] AN *san shi liu zhong feng* 三十六種風, *san shi liu ban feng* 三十六般風.

CD. One example of ancient categorizations of → *feng bing* 風病, wind diseases. *BCGM* SE *jiu* 酒：菖蒲酒治**三十六風**，一十二痹，通血脈，治骨痿，久

服耳目聰明, "Wine with *chang pu* cures the **36 types of wind**, and the 12 types of blockage. It makes the blood vessels passable and cures bone dysfunction. Ingested over an extended period of time it clears ears and eyes".

***San shi liu huang* 三十六黃, thirty-six types of jaundice** [9]
PC CD of numerous variations of → *huang dan* 黃疸, yellow *dan*-illness, with the definition of these variations differing from author to author. *SJZL* 61: 三十六黃：黃病有三十六種，所載名數雖同，而證候各異, "**Thirty-six types of jaundice**: Jaundice disease may appear in 36 variations. The number [of these variations] is identical in the literature; the conditions [listed] differ [from text to text]".

***San shi liu zhong feng* 三十六種風, the 36 types of wind** [2]
PC identical with → *san shi liu feng* 三十六風. *SLBC* SE *ma chi xian* 馬齒莧：作膏主三十六種風, "Preparing a paste will control **the 36 types of wind**".

***San xiao* 三消, three types of melting** [6]
PC of three types of the disease → *xiao ke* 渴病, melting with thirst. *TPSHF* 53: 夫三消者，一名消渴，二名消中，三名消腎, "Now, as for the **three types of melting**, the first is melting with thirst; the second is central melting; the third is kidney melting".

***San xiao ke bing* 三消渴病, three types of melting-with-thirst disease** [1]
PC identical with → *san xiao* 三消, three types of melting. *SYJYBZFL* 10: 子童桑白皮湯，治三消渴病, "The decoction with unprocessed *sang bai pi* cures the **three types of melting-with-thirst disease**".

***San xiao ke ji* 三消渴疾, three types of melting-with-thirst ailment** [2]
PC identical with → *san xiao* 三消, three types of melting. *SJZL* 58: 治三消渴疾，硝石散方, "To cure the **three types of melting-with-thirst ailment**, [use the] recipe for the powder with *xiao shi*".

***San yin jing zheng* 三陰經證, pathological condition of the three yin conduits** [1]
PC CD of *tai yin bing* 太陰病, major yin disease; *shao yin bing* 少陰病, minor yin disease; *jue yin bing* 厥陰病, ceasing yin disease. *BCGM* Bai bing zhu zhi yao 百病主治藥：附子，治三陰經證, "*Fu zi* cures **pathological conditions of the three yin conduits**".

***San yin shang han* 三陰傷寒, harm caused by cold with signs in the three yin sections** [1]
CD of → *shang han*, 傷寒, harm caused by cold with signs in the major yin, minor yin, and ceasing yin sections. *ZQZSHL* 6: 三陰傷寒，太陰為始, "**Harm caused by cold with signs in the three yin sections** begins in the major yin section".

***Sao fei* 瘙疿, itching seething rash** [1]
PC identical with *re fei* 熱疿, heat with seething rash. *BCGM* SE *ci gu* 慈姑：調蚌粉，塗瘙疿, "Mix mussel-shell powder with water and smear it onto **itching seething rash**".

***Sao jie* 瘙疥, itching *jie*-illness** [3]
PC identical with → *jie sao* 疥瘙, *jie*-illness with itching. *QJYiF* 24: 諸**瘙疥**，皆單用水銀豬膏，研令極細塗之, "For all types of **itching *jie*-illness**, one employs nothing but lard with *shui yin*. It is to be ground extremely fine and then applied externally".

***Se fan bing* 澀飯病, rough-passage-of-meals disease** [2]
PC identical with → *ye ge* 噎膈, gullet occlusion. *BCSY* SE lin shi 淋石：主噎病吐食，俗云**澀飯病**者效, "This is effective to control gullet occlusion disease with vomiting of food, which is commonly called '**rough-passage-of-meals disease**'".

***Se tong* 澀痛, roughness with pain** [33] AN *tong se* 痛澀.
IS of a) pain in the eyes and/or face accompanied by a feeling of dryness and the presence of a foreign body. *QJYF* 26: 其根主目**澀痛**, "The root controls **roughness with pain** in the eyes". b) Pain in the urinary tract accompanied by difficulties in passing urine. *QJYF* 5: 患小便不通，欲小便則**澀痛**不出, "[Patients] suffer from anuria. If they intend to pass urine, they feel **roughness with pain**, and it does not leave".

***Sha bing* 沙病, sand disease** [2] AN *shui shang han* 水傷寒, water-borne harm caused by cold; *shui sha* 水沙, water-borne sand [disease].
PC resembling harm caused by cold brought forth by an affection with an improper qi, with the skin showing small red dots. *YSLYF* Fj: 辨**沙病**論…大凡才覺寒慄似傷寒，而狀似瘧。但覺頭痛，渾身壯熱，手足厥冷, "How to distinguish **sand disease**: In general [patients] tremble with a feeling of cold as if this were harm caused by cold. The entire appearance is that of malaria. However, they also suffer from headache, and the entire body is very hot. The hands and legs experience recession with counterflow".

***Sha lin* 沙淋, sand dripping** [8]
PC identical with → *shi lin* 石淋, stone dripping. *BCSY* SE *xuan cao gen* 萱草根：治**沙淋**，下水氣, "It cures **sand dripping**, and discharges water qi".

***Sha lin* 砂淋, grit dripping** [1]
PC identical with → *shi lin* 石淋, stone dripping. *ZZJ* Mj: **砂淋**者，腹臍中隱痛，小便難，其痛不可忍，須臾，從小便中下如砂石之類, "As for **grit dripping**, there is a latent pain in the abdominal navel region. Urination is difficult. After a short while, the pain is unbearable. Grit is passed together with the urine".

***Sha shi* 沙虱, sand lice** [36] AW *sha shi* 砂虱.
① EA. A small bug, in former times assumed to live in waters or at the banks of waters and being able of penetrating the skin of people and cause disease. *ZHF* 7: 山水間多有**沙虱**，甚細略不可見, "In the region of mountains and waters there are many **sand lice**. They are so tiny that they cannot be seen".
② PC brought forth by sand lice. *ZHF* 7: 藥子一物方…蛇螫，惡毛、蠍、蜈蚣等螫，**沙虱**，射工，此六病，用暖水研，赤莧和，封之, "Recipe with one single item, (i.e.) the drug seeds [of the *chuan shu* tree], for snake bite, [stings by] malign hair [caterpillar], scorpions, centipedes, as well as **sand lice** and ar-

cher, for these six diseases, grind with warm water and add *chi xian*. Then cover [the wound with] it".

***Sha shi* 砂虱, sand lice** [2]
EA identical with → *sha shi* 沙虱①. *BCGM* SE *shu yu* 鸀鳿：**砂虱**，沙中細蟲也, "**Sand lice** are tiny bugs/worms in the sand".

***Sha shi lin* 沙石淋, sand and stone dripping** [12]
PC identical with → *shi lin* 石淋, stone dripping. *SJZL* 98: 治**沙石淋**，茅根湯方, "To cure **sand and stone dripping** [use] the recipe for a decoction with *mao gen*".

***Sha zhen* 沙疹, sand papules** [1]
PC of papules rising like sand. *SLBC* SE *hu sui* 胡荽：療**沙疹**、豌豆瘡不出, "It cures **sand papules** and pea sores that do not emerge".

***Sha zheng* 沙證, sand condition** [3]
PC of an affection by external evil with headache and high fever, cold fingers and toes, and abdominal pain. *SYDXF* 2: 艾湯，試**沙證**。江南舊無，今所在有之。原其證古方不載，所感如傷寒，頭痛嘔噁，渾身壯熱，手足指末微厥，或腹痛煩亂，須臾能殺人。先濃煎艾湯試之，如吐即是。右用五月蠶蛻紙碎剪，安碗中，以盤蓋之，以百沸湯泡艾碗許，仍以別紙封裹縫良久，乘熱飲之，就臥，以厚被蓋之，汗出愈, "Decoction with *ai* to test a **sand condition**. In former times [this condition] did not exist in the Jiangnan region. Nowadays it is present there everywhere. This condition was not listed in ancient recipes. It feels like harm caused by cold, with headache and vomiting and nausea. The entire body is very hot. The ends of the fingers and toes experience slight recession. In some cases there is abdominal pain, with vexation and confusion. After a short time it will kill the [afflicted] person. First one prepares a thick decoction of *ai* [and has the patient ingest it] as a test [whether he has a sand condition]. If he vomits, this is it. [For the indications listed] above one uses paper on which silkworm moths have laid their eggs in the fifth month, cuts it and places it into a bowl. This is to be covered with a plate. Then soak *ai* with approximately a bowl of boiling water and add it [to the paper]. Now close the seams with additional paper and wait a while. Eventually have [the patient] drink this as long as it is still hot. Then he is to lie down and to be covered with a thick quilt. When he sweats, he is cured".

***Shan* 痁, malaria** [3]
PC identical with → *nüe ji* 瘧疾, malaria ailment. *JYBC* SE xian ren zhang 仙人杖：主噦氣嘔逆，辟**痁**, "It controls retching and vomiting with counterflow, and it eliminates **malaria**".

***Shan* 疝, elevation-illness** [p] AN *shan qi* 疝氣, elevation-illness qi; *shan tong* 疝痛, elevation-illness pain.
PC CD of a group of conditions characterized by violent abdominal pain, in some cases associated with constipation and anuria. *SW* 55: 病在少腹，腹痛不得大小便，病名曰**疝**, "When the disease is in the lower abdomen, [with the patient experiencing] abdominal pain and an inability to pass stools or urine. The name of the disease is **elevation-illness**".

Shan cuo **閃挫, sprain** [13]
PC of a → *shang sun* 傷損, injury, affecting the lower back region, caused by a sudden accidental movement. *HJJF* 1: 烏藥順氣散…如**閃挫**身體疼痛，温酒調服, "The 'powder with *wu yao* to make qi flow its due course'...for **sprain** with bodily pain, ingest mixed with warm wine".

Shan du **疝毒, elevation-illness with poison** [2]
PC, presumably a writing error of → *bian du* 便毒, poison [in the region] of relief. *BCGM* SE she gan 射干 quoting *BCYYBY*: 行太陰、厥陰之積痰，使結核自消，甚捷，又治便毒, "It moves phlegm accumulations in the major yin and ceasing yin [regions], causes node kernels to dissolve by themselves, and is very fast [in its effects]. It also cures poison [in the region] of relief", writes: 利積痰**疝毒**，消結核, "It is beneficial [in curing] phlegm accumulations and **elevation-illness with poison**, and dissolves node kernels".

Shan ji **痁疾, malaria ailment** [2]
PC identical with → *nüe ji* 瘧疾. *RHZ* SE *li shu gen* 李樹根：治小兒壯熱，**痁疾**，驚癇, "It cures strong heat in children, **malaria ailment**, and fright epilepsy".

Shan jia **疝瘕, elevation-illness with conglomeration-illness** [44]
PC of a lump-like swelling in the abdomen that alternately collects and then dissolves again. When it collects, patients feel pain. If squeezed it moves. *SW* 18: 寸口脈沉而弱，曰寒熱及**疝瘕**少腹痛, "If the [movement in the] vessels at the inch opening is deep inside and weak, that is called: 'cold and heat' and '**elevation-illness with conglomeration-illness**,' with pain in the lower abdomen".

Shan jing **善驚, tendency to be frightened** [5]
IS of easily being frightened, in extreme cases of panicking without apparent reason. *SW* 36: 熱間**善驚**，如有所見, "While it is hot, [patients] **tend to be frightened** as if they had seen something [frightening]".

Shan na **閃肭, sprain** [7] AN *shan zhe* 閃折, *shan sun* 閃損, *shan niu* 閃拗等.
PC of a → *shang sun* 傷損, injury, affecting the extremities and/or the body, caused by a sudden accidental movement. *SJZL* 143: 治一切傷折及驢馬墜墮，打撲**閃肭**，疼痛不可忍者，五傷接骨丸方, "Recipe for the pills for five types of injury and bonesetting to cure all types of injury and fracture, [injuries from] falling from a donkey or horse, from a blow with a **sprain** and unbearable pain".

Shan niu **閃拗, limb sprain** [2]
PC identical with → *shan na* 閃肭, sprain. *BCGM* SE *tu dang gui* 土當歸：**閃拗**手足，同荊芥、葱白煎湯淋洗之, "For **limb sprain** of the hands and feet boil together with *jing jie* and *cong bai* and use the hot liquid to wash the [afflicted body parts].

Shan nu **善怒, tendency to be angry** [7]
IS of a person being excited and easily angered, in extreme cases without any reason. *SW* 46: 陽氣者，因暴折而難決，故**善怒**也, "As for the yang qi, because [its flow] was suddenly cut off and because [this blockage] is difficult to open, one **tends to be angry**".

Shan pi **閃癖, sprain with aggregation-illness** [11]

PC of children with swelling below the flanks, loss of appetite, no digestion, yellow complexion, emaciation and desiccation of the hair. This is often accompanied by bone steaming, scrofula, and pervasion-illness. *TPSHF* 卷31: "治骨蒸勞，兩肋下有**閃癖**，漸上攻心，食少或不消化，腹內積聚不散，黃瘦久困, "To cure bone steaming with exhaustion, and **sprain with aggregation-illness** below the two flanks gradually rising to attack the heart. [Patients] eat little or may have no digestion. Accumulations and collections that fail to dissipate form in the abdomen. A yellow [complexion] and emaciation indicate long-term distress".

Shan qi **善噫, tendency to belch** [3]

IS of frequent occurrence of belching qi. *ZBYHL* 21: 脾傷，**善噫**，欲臥，面黃, "The spleen is harmed. [As a result patients have] a **tendency to belch**, a desire to lie down/sleep, and the facial complexion is yellow".

Shan qi **疝氣, elevation-illness qi** [92]

PC a) of an item having entered the scrotum, with pain, sometimes ascending, sometimes descending. *JGYL* Mj: 陰狐**疝氣**者，偏有小大，時時上下，蜘蛛散主之, "In the case of yin-fox-type **elevation-illness qi**, with one side being small and the other being enlarged, and an alternating movement up- and downward, the powder with *zhi zhu* will control this". b) Of a condition affecting the scrotum or a testicle. *WTMY* 10: 療腎虛**疝氣**，腰膝冷疼，陰囊腫癢，狐陰丸方, "To cure kidney depletion and **elevation-illness qi**, swelling and itching of the scrotum, [use] the recipe for pills [to cure] 'fox in the yin'". c) Identical with → *shan* 疝, elevation-illness. *BJ* SE *wu jia pi* 五加皮：主心腹**疝氣**，腹痛, "It controls the heart and abdomen with **elevation-illness qi**, and abdominal pain". In the *BCGM* the first two meanings dominate. The image of a "fox" implies an item moving erratically inside the body – in this case in the scrotum. *RMSQ* explains: "The item [in the scrotum] is shaped like a tile. When [the patient] lies down to sleep, it enters the lower abdomen. When he walks and stands it leaves the lower abdomen and enters the scrotum. A fox leaves its den in the morning to urinate. It enters its den at night and will not urinate there. This elevation-illness comes out and withdraws, moves upward and downward, just like a fox".

Shan sun **閃損, sprain injury** [2]

PC identical with *shan na* 閃肭, sprain. *RHZ* SE *shi yin chen* 石茵陳：治天行時疾熱狂，頭痛頭旋，風眼疼，瘴瘧。女人癥瘕，並**閃損**乏絕, "It cures heaven-sent seasonal ailments, heat madness, headache and dizziness, wind eye pain, miasmatic malaria, concretion-illness and conglomeration-illness of females, as well as a **sprain injury** with extreme exhaustion".

Shan tai xi **善太息, tendency to breathe deeply** [1]

IS of frequent deep inhaling of breath without apparent reason. *ZBYHL* 15: 膽氣不足，其氣上溢而口苦，**善太息**, "The gallbladder qi is insufficient; its qi rises and spills above, with a bitter taste in the mouth. [Patients develop a] **tendency to breathe deeply**".

***Shan tong* 疝痛, elevation-illness with pain** [30]
PC identical with → *shan* 疝, elevation-illness. *QJYF* 28: (脈)弦緊，亦為積，為寒痹，為**疝痛**, "A string-like and tight [movement in the vessels] may be a sign of accumulation, of cold blockage, and of **elevation-illness with pain**".

***Shan wang* 善忘, forgetfulness** [10]
IS identical with → *jian wang* 健忘①, forgetfulness. *BJ* SE *ru* 藺茹：除大風熱氣，**善忘**不樂, "It eliminates massive wind and heat qi, **forgetfulness** and unhappiness".

***Shan zhang* 山瘴, mountain miasma** [2]
EA identical with → *zhang qi* 瘴氣, miasmatic qi ①. *ZHBJF* 2: 度瘴散，辟**山瘴**惡氣, "The 'powder to pass through miasmatic [qi]' repels the malign qi of **mountain miasma**".

***Shan zhe* 閃折, sprain** [1]
PC identical with → *shan na* 閃肭. *BCTJ* SE *gu sui bu* 骨碎補：蜀人治**閃折**筋骨傷損，取根搗篩，煮黃米粥，和之裹傷處，良, "When the people of Shu/Sichuan treat a **sprain** with injured sinews and bones, they take the root and pound it through a sieve. Then they boil a yellow rice congee and mix the two components to wrap the injured location. This is excellent".

***Shang chuan* 上喘, panting** [3]
IS identical with → *chuan* 喘①. *YXL* SE *ting li* 葶藶：能利小便，抽肺氣，**上喘**息急，止嗽, "It frees the passage of urine, withdraws lung qi, [cures] **panting** and rapid breathing, and ends cough".

***Shang chuang* 傷瘡, wounds** [14]
PC CD of all types of → *chuang* 瘡, sores, conditions resulting from externally inflicted injury. *MYBL* SE *xia ma* 蝦蟆：療陰蝕疽癘惡瘡，猘犬**傷瘡**, "It cures erosion in the genital region, impediment-illness epidemics, malign sores, as well as **wounds** inflicted by rabid dogs".

***Shang feng* 傷風, harm caused by wind** [15]
① PM of harm caused by wind evil qi. *ZBYHL* 11: 夫瘧皆由傷暑及**傷風**所為, "Now, all states of malaria result from harm caused by summerheat or **harm caused by wind**".
② PC of a light condition resulting from an external affection by wind. *HJJF* 1: 尋常些小**傷風**，頭痛鼻塞，項強筋急, "These are various minor types of **harm caused by wind**, with headache, a blocked nose, a stiff neck, and tense sinews".

***Shang han* 傷寒, harm caused by cold** [383] AN *si shi shang han* 四時傷寒, harm caused by cold in all seasons.
PC a) general reference to heat diseases resulting from external affection. *NJ* 58: **傷寒**有五，有中風，有**傷寒**，有濕温，有熱病，有温病，其所苦各不同, "There are five types of **harm caused by cold**, including wind stroke, **harm caused by cold**, moisture-warmth, heat disease, and warmth disease. The symptoms one suffers from are all different". b) Special reference to all heat diseases brought forth by external affection by cold evil. *SHL* Shang han li **傷寒**例, examples of **harm caused by cold**: 冬時嚴寒，萬物深藏，君子固密，則不傷

於寒，觸冒之者，乃名**傷寒**耳, "In winter, when it is very cold, all things go into deep hiding. The gentleman closes himself in tightly, and will not be harmed by cold. If someone is struck by malicious [cold] nevertheless, this is called **harm caused by cold**".

Shang han biao xu **傷寒表虛, harm caused by cold with external depletion** [1]
PC of → *shang han* 傷寒, harm caused by cold, with signs such as sweating and an aversion to wind, as well as slowed movement in the vessels. *BCYY* SE *gui* 桂：張仲景桂枝湯治**傷寒表虛**，皆須此藥，是專用辛甘之意也, "Zhang Zhongjing's decoction with *gui zhi* for the treatment of **harm caused by cold with external depletion** is required in all cases where it is meaningful to apply especially acrid and sweet [flavor qualities]".

Shang han hu huo **傷寒狐惑, harm caused by cold with fox and delusion** [3]
PC identical with → *hu huo* 狐惑, fox and delusion. *ZBYHL* 8: **傷寒狐惑**候, "Signs of **harm caused by cold with fox and delusion**:" 夫狐惑二病者，是喉、陰之為病也。初得狀如傷寒，或因傷寒而變成斯病。其狀，默默欲眠，目瞑不得眠，臥起不安。蟲食於喉咽為惑，食於陰肛為狐。惡飲食，不欲聞食臭，其人面目翕赤翕黑翕白。食於上部其聲嗄，食於下部其咽乾。此皆由濕毒氣所為也, "Now, the two diseases 'fox' and 'delusion' are affecting the throat and the genital region respectively. At first they appear to be harm caused by cold, or there is harm caused by cold which gradually changes to become the present disease. The signs are sleepiness. [Patients] close their eyes but cannot sleep. They cannot calm down, neither while lying down nor when up. When bugs/worms gnaw on their throat, this is 'delusion'; when they gnaw on the genital or anal region, this is 'fox'. [Patients] have an aversion to beverages and food, and they cannot even stand the odors of food. Their face and eyes are at times red, at times dark, at times white. When [the bugs/worms] gnaw on [the patient's] upper body parts, their voice is exclamatory. When they gnaw on the lower body parts, their throat is dry. All of this is brought forth by the qi of moisture poison".

Shang han huai zheng **傷寒壞證, harm caused by cold with worsened signs** [1]
PC resulting from a mistaken treatment of → *shang han* 傷寒, harm caused by cold, with the result of an uncontrolled intermingling of yin and yang qi that is most difficult to cure. *PJF* 140: 一法治**傷寒壞證**，時或發消渴，燥煩。用新羅參不拘多少，煎湯，浸令水冷後，盛渴之時與之，頓服，熱則隨去。大抵傷寒渴者，不可多與之水，水積胸中，便為結胸。然亦須濡沫之可也, "Another therapy pattern to cure **harm caused by cold with worsened conditions**. It may be that [patients] develop melting with thirst, restlessness and vexation. In this case take any amount of Korean ginseng and put it into boiling water to let it soak until the water is cold again. This is to be given [to the patient] at the moment when his thirst has reached a peak, to be ingested immediately. It will take away the heat. Generally speaking, patients with harm caused by cold must not be given much water when they are thirsty. The water would accumulate in their chest, resulting in a bound chest. It is quite possible, though, to [quench their thirst] by moistening [their mouth] with foam". *BCGM* SE *ren*

shen 人參：**傷寒壞證**：凡傷寒時疫，不問陰陽，老幼妊婦，誤服藥餌，因重垂死，脈沉伏，不省人事，七日以後，皆可服之，百不失一，"**Harm caused by cold with worsened conditions**: Whenever in a time of epidemic harm caused by cold [a treatment is initiated] regardless of whether yin or yang [conduits are affected], and regardless of whether [patients] are old or young, or perhaps pregnant women, and if as a result the wrong medication is ingested, [the disease] will worsen so much that [the patient] may die. The movement in the vessels is deep inside and hidden; he fails to recognize people or things. After seven days any [patient] can ingest this. There will be not a single loss in a hundred cases".

***Shang han jie xiong* 傷寒結胸, bound chest following harm caused by cold** [5]
PC identical with → *jie xiong* 結胸, bound [qi in the] chest. *ZBYHL* 7: **傷寒結胸**候：結胸者，謂熱毒結聚於心胸也。此由病發於陽，而早下之，熱氣乘虛而痞結不散也。按之痛，其脈寸口浮，關上反自沉是也, "Signs of **bound chest following harm caused by cold**: bound [qi in the] chest, that is to say: heat poison forms nodular collections in the heart and chest. The reason is that the disease originates in the yang [conduits], and is purged early on. The heat qi avails itself of the depletion, and forms obstacle-illness nodes that fail to dissipate. If pressed they ache. The accompanying [movement in the] vessels at the inch-opening is at the surface, and contrary [to normal] it is deep inside above the gate-section".

***Shang han lao fu* 傷寒勞復, recurrence, because of exhaustion, of harm caused by cold** [16]
PC of a recurrence of → *shang han* 傷寒, harm caused by cold, following exhaustion. *ZBYHL* 8: **傷寒勞復**候：傷寒病新瘥，津液未復，血氣尚虛，若勞動早，更復成病，故勞復也。若言語思慮則勞神，梳頭澡洗則勞力，勞則生熱，熱氣乘虛還入經絡，故復病也。其脈沉緊者，宜下之, "Signs of a **recurrence, because of exhaustion, of harm caused by cold**: When harm caused by cold disease has just been healed and the bodily liquids have not yet recuperated, with blood and qi still depleted, if in such a situation one moves too early, then this will result in disease once again. Hence [patients suffer from] 'recurrence because of exhaustion'. If [exhaustion is based on excessive] speaking and pondering, this will result in spirit exhaustion. If [exhaustion results from] combing and washing, this is exhaustion of physical strength. Exhaustion generates heat. This heat avails itself of the depletion and furthermore enters conduits and network [vessels]. Hence a recurrence of the disease results. If the [movement in the]vessels is deep inside and firm, it is advisable to purge with a discharge".

***Shang han li* 傷寒痢, harm caused by cold with free-flux illness** [3]
PC of free-flux illness occurring in the course of a disease of the harm-caused-by-cold type. *TPSHF* 13: 治**傷寒痢**，下膿血，宜服竹茹飲子方, "To cure **harm caused by cold with free-flux illness**, with outflow of pus and blood, the recipe to ingest a drink with *zhu ru* is appropriate".

***Shang han shao yin zheng* 傷寒少陰證, harm caused by cold with signs in the minor yin section** [2]
PC identical with → *shao yin shang han* 少陰傷寒, harm in the minor yin section caused by cold. *SJZL* 25: 治**傷寒少陰證**嘔噦者，四逆湯加生薑方, "To cure **harm caused by cold with signs in the minor yin section** with vomiting, [use] the recipe for the 'decoction for counterflow in the four [limbs] amended by raw ginger".

***Shang han shi fu* 傷寒食復, recurrence, because of food, of harm caused by cold** [2]
PC of a → *shi fu* 食復, recurrence because of food, resulting from an inadequate diet consumed immediately after recovery from harm caused by cold. *ZBYHL* 8: **傷寒**病後**食復**候:, "Signs of a recurrence, because of food, following a disease of harm caused by cold". *BCGM* SE *fan* 飯：寒食飯…傷寒食復，用此飯燒研，米飲服二三錢，效, "If one consumes cold rice…and if there is a recurrence, because of food, of harm caused by cold, use this type of rice, roast it and grind it. Ingest with two to three *qian* of the liquid obtained by boiling rice. Effective".

***Shang han tai yang zheng* 傷寒太陽證, harm caused by cold with signs in the major yang section** [1]
PC identical with → *tai yang shang han*, 太陽傷寒, harm caused by cold in the major yang section. *SHLZHRS* 9: **傷寒太陽證**，衄血者乃解，蓋陽氣重故也, "**Harm caused by cold with signs in the major yang section** is resolved by nosebleed. The reason is [nosebleed carries away] a preponderance of yang qi".

***Shang han xu xue* 傷寒畜血, harm caused by cold with accumulated blood** [1]
PC of a type of → *shang han* 傷寒, harm caused by cold, where evil heat enters the interior and clashes with the blood, with stagnant heat accumulating internally. *SHL* 237: 陽明證，其人喜忘者，必有蓄血, "In cases where a person [with harm caused by cold] shows yang brilliance signs and has a tendency to forget, this must be accumulated blood". *BCGM* SE *xi* 犀: (角）磨汁，治吐血、衄血、下血，及**傷寒畜血**, "The juice obtained by grinding the horn serves to cure blood spitting, nosebleed, discharge of blood, and **harm caused by cold with accumulated blood**".

***Shang han yang ming zheng* 傷寒陽明證, harm caused by cold with signs in the yang brilliance** section [1]
PC of → *shang han* 傷寒, harm caused by cold, with signs such as a hot body and sweating, no aversion to cold, but an aversion to heat instead, and in some cases with abdominal fullness and difficulties in defecating. *SHLZHRS* 1: 大抵**傷寒陽明證**宜下，少陰證宜温, "In general, in the case of **harm caused by cold with signs in the yang brilliance** section it is advisable to purge; with signs in the minor yin section it is advisable to add warmth".

***Shang han yang zheng* 傷寒陽證, harm caused by cold with signs in the yang section** [1]
PC of → *shang han* 傷寒, harm caused by cold, with signs such as an exuberance of yang qi and heat. *SHZZZS* 7: 温疫之治與**傷寒陽證**相同, "The treatment of

warmth epidemics is identical with that of **harm caused by cold with signs in the yang section**".

Shang han yin sheng ge yang **傷寒陰盛隔陽, harm caused by cold, whereby abundant yin forms a barrier to yang** [1]
PC of a type of → *shang han* 傷寒, harm caused by cold, whereby internally abundant yin cold forms a barrier to yang in the exterior, resulting in a cold body with restlessness, and a fine and tight movement in the vessels as its characteristics. *SJZL* 21: 治**傷寒陰盛隔陽**，身冷煩躁，脈細沉緊，黑龍散方, "To cure **harm caused by cold, whereby abundant yin forms a barrier to yang**, resulting in a cold body with restlessness, and a fine and tight movement in the vessels, [apply] the recipe for 'black dragon powder'".

Shang han yin zheng **傷寒陰證, harm caused by cold with signs in the yin section** [2] AN *yin zheng shang han* 陰證傷寒.
PC of → *shang han* 傷寒, harm caused by cold, with a weakness of yang qi and an abundance of yin qi. *SJZL* 185: 治**傷寒陰證**，脈候沉細，正元湯方, "To cure **harm caused by cold with signs in the yin section** and when the movement in the vessels is deep inside and fine: [use] the recipe for the 'decoction to rectify the original [qi]'".

Shang jiao re **上焦熱, heat in the upper burner** [6]
PC of heat-type diseases affecting the upper burner. *QJYF* 20 *mai men dong li zhong tang* 麥門冬理中湯, decoction with *mai men dong* to order the interior: 治**上焦熱**，腹滿，不欲飲食, "It cures **heat in the upper burner**, abdominal fullness, and lacking desire to drink or eat".

Shang jin **傷筋, damage to sinews** [5]
① PC with major signs including injured sinews with impaired function or damaged physical condition following either an external impact or as an effect of pharmaceutical treatment. *ZBYHL* 36 lists: 金瘡**傷筋**斷骨候, "Signs of wounds inflicted by metal objects, **damage to sinews**, and bone fractures".
② PE of pharmaceutical substances, beverages, or food resulting in damage to sinews. *SW* 5: 酸**傷筋**，辛勝酸, "[If] sour [flavor causes damage, it causes] **damage to the sinews**; acrid [flavor] dominates sour [flavor]".

Shang jin gu **傷筋骨, damage to sinews and bones** [4]
① PC with major signs including injured sinews and bones with impaired function or damaged physical condition following either an external impact or as an effect of pharmaceutical treatment. *SW* 55: 病在肌膚，肌膚盡痛，名曰肌痹，傷於寒濕，刺大分小分，多發針而深之，以熱為故，無傷筋骨，**傷筋骨**，癰發若變，諸分盡熱病已止, "When the disease is in the muscles and in the skin, [with the patient experiencing] pain all over the muscles and the skin, this is called muscle blockage. [It results from] harm caused by cold and moisture. Pierce the large partings and the small partings [of the flesh]. Deploy the needle many times and insert it deeply aiming at [generating] heat. Do not damage the sinews and the bones. If **the sinews and the bones are damaged,**

obstruction-illnesses develop as [pathological] changes. When all partings [of the flesh] are completely hot, the disease has ended. Stop [the piercing]".
② PE of pharmaceutical substances, beverages, or food resulting in damage to sinews. *MYBL* SE *xing shi* 杏實：不可多食，**傷筋骨**, "One must not each much of them lest this result in **damage to sinews and bones**".

Shang po **傷破, open injury** [2]
PC identical with → *po shang* 破傷. *QJYF* 25：治被打**傷破**，腹中有瘀血方, "Recipe to cure **open injury** from a blow, with stagnant blood [that has left the vessels and is now] in the abdomen".

Shang qi **上氣, upper qi; rising qi; panting** [174]
① PN of essence qi in the upper parts of the human body. *LS* 28: **上氣**不足，腦為之不滿，耳為之苦鳴，頭為之苦傾，目為之眩, "In the case of an insufficiency of **upper qi**, this causes the brain not to be filled, the ears to suffer from sounds, the head to suffer from being inclined, and the eyes to be dizzy".
② PC of qi dynamics that should take a downward direction but move upward instead. *ZBYHL* 13: **上氣**動於胃，胃氣逆，故嘔吐也, "When **rising qi** excites the stomach, the stomach qi will move [upward] contrary to its proper direction. As a result, [patients] vomit.
③ IS of a) → *chuan* 喘①, panting. *SW* 19: 病入舍於肺，名曰肺痹，發咳**上氣**, "The disease enters the lung and lodges there. It is [now] called 'lung blockage.' It develops a cough and **rising qi**". b) → *ou tu* 嘔吐①, vomiting. *QJYF* 12: 若**上氣**嘔逆，加橘皮二兩, "In the case of **rising qi** with vomiting and counterflow, add two *liang* of *ju pi*". c) → *fou zhong* 浮腫, surface swelling. *QJYF* 12: 又加心腹脹滿，**上氣**，身面脚等並腫，垂死者，服一丸, "If to this is added a distension and a feeling of fullness in heart and abdomen, and **rising qi** with simultaneous swelling affecting the body, face and feet, and the patient being in a state of dying, let him ingest one pill".
④ PC identical with → *chuan* 喘②. *LS* 47: 肺堅則不病咳、**上氣**, "When the lung is strong one will not suffer from cough and **rising qi**".

Shang re **傷熱, harm caused by heat** [5]
PC of harm brought forth by heat evil. *BJ* SE *niu xi* 牛膝：主**傷熱**火爛, "It controls **harm caused by heat** and festering because of fire".

Shang re **上熱, heat in the upper [sections of the body]** [9]
PC of heat in the upper sections of the human body. *SW* 71: 病**上熱**血溢, "The illnesses [caused by] them include **heat in the upper [sections of the body]** and overflowing blood". LSZ identifies the following pathological conditions as the most important signs of heat in the upper sections: → *chuan man* 喘滿, panting and fullness; → *zhu ou* 諸嘔, all types of vomiting; → *tu suan* 吐酸; sour spitting; → *xiong pi* 胸痞, obstacle-illness in the chest; *xie tong* 脅痛, pain in the flanks; → *yin shi bu xiao* 食飲不消, inability to digest liquid and solid food; → *tou shang chu han* 頭上出汗, sweating on the head.

***Shang ru* 傷乳, harm caused by breast-milk** [3]

PC of children harmed by breast-feeding with abdominal distension, vexation and heart-pressure as well as, in serious cases, diarrhea. *YYXS* 3: **傷乳**則面黃，心熱則舌重生瘡, "In case of harm caused by breast-milk the [child's] facial complexion is yellow. When the heart is affected by heat the tongue will be heavy and develop sores".

***Shang shi* 上視, vision turned upward** [4] AN *dai yan* 戴眼, eyes turned upward; *diao yan* 吊眼, hauled eyes; *yan fan bu xia* 眼翻不下, eyes turned upward without coming down.

IS of eyeballs turned upward, with patients being unable to move them. *TPSHF* 82: Zhi xiao er tai han zhu fang 治小兒胎寒諸方, All recipes to cure fetal cold: 治小兒五十日以來，胎寒腹痛，微熱而驚，聚唾弄舌，軀啼**上視**，此癇之候, "It cures children who at the age of 50 days [suffer from] fetal cold with abdominal pain, slight heat with fright, accumulation of saliva and non-directional movements of the tongue. The body is bent forward, [the child] weeps and **vision is turned upward**. These are the signs of epilepsy".

***Shang shi* 傷食, harm caused by food** [7]

① EA PM brought forth by consumption of food that proves to be harmful. *BJ* SE *kong gong nie* 孔公孽：**傷食**不化，邪結氣惡, "**Harm caused by food** that fails to transform, with evil [qi] nodes and qi malignity [leaving from the mouth]".
② PC brought forth by harmful food. *MYBL* SE *kong gong nie* 孔公孽：主男子陰瘡，女子陰蝕及**傷食**病, "It controls sores in the private region of males, erosion in the female genital region, as well as the disease **harm caused by food**".

***Shang shi* 傷濕, harm caused by moisture** [3]

① PC identical with → *po shang shi* 破傷濕, wounds harmed by moisture. *BCGM* SE *bai hua she* 白花蛇：瀕湖白花酒治中風、**傷濕**, "Binhu's wine with *bai hua* cures wind stroke and **harm caused by moisture**".
② EA of moisture that has entered wounds, causing them to fester and impeding normal healing. *BCGM* SE *gui* 桂 quoting *YHCF*: 治小兒臍腫，取桂心炙令熱，熨之, "To cure umbilical swelling of small children: take *gui xin* and roast until hot, then exert hot pressure [with it]", writes: 嬰兒臍腫，多因**傷濕**，桂心炙熱，熨之, "Umbilical swelling often results from **harm caused by moisture**. [For treatment] roast *gui xin* until hot and exert hot pressure [with it]".

***Shang shi* 傷螫, injury from a sting** [9]

PC identical with → *shi shang* 螫傷. *BCGM* SE *ma xie* 麻鞋 quoting *WTMY* 40: 蜈蚣螫人, "Centipede stings a human person", writes: 蜈蚣**傷螫**, "**Injury from a** centipede **sting**".

***Shang shu* 傷暑, harm caused by summerheat** [13]

① PC identical with → *shu* 暑④, summerheat. *MYBL* SE *gua lou gen* 栝樓根：莖、葉療中熱**傷暑**, "Stem and leaves cure heatstroke and **harm caused by summerheat**".
② EA of summerheat evil. *SW* 53: 氣虛身熱, 得之**傷暑**, "If the qi is depleted while the body is hot, this is acquired through **harm caused by summerheat**".

Shang shui **傷水, harmed by water** [8]

PC of having fallen into water or of open sores that have been affected by water which eventually brings forth a disease. *BCGM* SE *gu wen qian* 古文錢 quotes *RCF*: **傷水**喘急，因年少飲冷水驚恐所致者, "If someone is **harmed by water** and pants hastily, this is because this person consumed cold water and was terrified in his youth".

Shang shui lan **傷水爛, harmed by water with festering** [1]

PC of damaged and festering skin brought forth by excessive soaking in water. *BCGM* SE *ji chang cao* 雞腸草 quoting *YXL* 洗手足水爛, "Wash hands and feet [harmed by] water with festering", writes 洗手足**傷水爛**, "Wash hands and feet **harmed by water with festering**".

Shang sun **傷損, injury** [36] AW *sun shang* 損傷.

PC of all types of bodily injuries, including damaged tissue or functions of the skin and flesh, sinews and bones, as well as organs, inflicted by harmful external causes or pharmaceutical effects, or resulting from an improper lifestyle, with major signs including pain and functional impairment. *MYBL* SE *bai jiao* 白膠：療吐血下血，崩中不止，四肢酸疼，多汗淋露，折跌**傷損**, "It cures blood spitting and blood discharge, unending collapsing center, sour pain affecting the four limbs, profuse sweating and dripping [like] dew drops, as well as **injuries** resulting from fracturing [a bone] and falls".

Shang tai **傷胎, harmed fetus** [4] AN *sun tai* 損胎, injured fetus; *sun dong tai qi* 損動胎氣, injured fetus qi; *ren shen shang dong* 妊娠傷動, injury inflicted during pregnancy; *ren shen dong tai* 妊娠動胎, fetus stirred during pregnancy.

PC CD of harm or injuries inflicted upon a fetus because of one of the following causes: an illness or excessive exhaustion of the mother during pregnancy, or immoderate sexual intercourse. *QJYF* 2：治妊娠**傷胎**，結血心腹痛, "It cures **fetal harm** inflicted during pregnancy, with bound blood and abdominal pain".

Shang xiao **上消, upper melting; dissolve above** [2]

① AN *ge xiao* 膈消, diaphragm melting. PC of the upper burner manifesting itself in → *xiao ke* 消渴, melting with thirst, with thirst and much drinking. *SWBJQYBMJ* Xiao ke lun 消渴論，**上消**者上焦受病，又謂之膈消病也。多飲水而少食，大便如常，或小便清利，知其燥在上焦也, "In the case of '**upper melting**' the upper burner has been affected by a disease. It is also called the 'disease of diaphragm melting'. One drinks a lot of water, and eats little. Defecation is normal. In some cases urine is clear and passes freely. This indicates that the upper burner is affected by dryness".

② TA of dispelling water evil and have it leave the organism by means of sweating from the upper parts of the body. *BCGM* SE *li yu* 鯉魚 quotes *YFZY*: 水腫脹滿：赤尾鯉魚一斤，破開，不見水及鹽，以生礬五錢研末，入腹內，火紙包裹，外以黃土泥包，放灶內煨熟取出，去紙、泥，送粥。食頭者**上消**，食身、尾者下消，一日用盡。屢試經驗, "For water swelling with distension and a feeling of fullness: 1 *jin* of a red tail carp is to be opened. It must not be touched by water and salt. Grind 5 *qian* of *sheng fan* to a powder and put this into [the fish's] stomach. Then wrap it with fire-proof paper and enclose this with yellow clay. Place into an oven and heat until done. Then remove the paper and the clay, and prepare a congee. Those who eat the head will **dissolve [swellings] above**; eating the body and the tail will dissolve [swellings] below. Use up within one day. It has proven effective in numerous tests".

Shang xu **上虛, depletion above** [2]

PC of depletion affecting a person's body's upper part. *SW* 10: 徇蒙招尤，目冥耳聾，下實**上虛**，過在足少陽、厥陰，甚則入肝, "Dizziness and shaking, blurred vision and deafness, [this is] repletion below and **depletion above**. The excess is in the foot minor yang and ceasing yin [conduits]. If it is serious, it enters the liver".

Shang zhe **傷折, fracture** [14]

PC identical with → *zhe shang* 折傷. *QJYF* 25: 治從高墮下，**傷折**疾痛，煩躁啼叫不臥方, "Recipe to cure **fractures** and pain following a fall from somewhere high, with vexation, agitation and weeping and an inability to lie down to rest".

Shang zhong **傷腫, injury swelling** [1]

IS of topical swelling resulting from an injury. *SJZL* 10: 治風腰脚痛不得履地，及拗折**傷腫**，瘀血攻痛，三神散方, "To cure wind causing pain in one's lower back and feet so that one is unable to walk, as well as fractures with **injury swelling**, and stagnant blood [having left the vessels and] attacking [other body parts] causing pain, [use the] recipe for the 'powder of the three spirits'".

Shang zhong **傷中, damaged center** [43]

PC brought forth by damage inflicted upon any essential internal matter, such as essence qi and blood, not just central qi. *BJ* SE *shu yu* 署預：主**傷中**, 補虛羸, "It controls a **damaged center**, and supplements depletion and emaciation".

Shao jing **少精, shortness of seminal fluid** [5]

PC of adult males with a scantness of seminal fluid. *MYBL* SE *qin pi* 秦皮：療男子**少精**，婦人帶下, "It cures **shortness of seminal fluid** of males, and [diseases of] discharge from below the belt in women".

Shao qi **少氣, shortness of qi** [30]

① IS of weak and short breathing, and feeble speech. *SW* 19: 其不及則令人喘，呼吸**少氣**而咳, "When it is inadequate, this makes a person pant; he exhales and inhales being **short of qi** and coughs".

② PC brought forth by qi depletion, with shortness of qi/breath as a major sign. *SW* 17: 脾脈搏堅而長，其色黃，當病**少氣**, "When the beating in the vessels of the spleen is firm and extended and when the complexion is yellow, [the patient] must suffer from being **short of qi**".

Shao yang bing **少陽病, minor yang disease** [1]

PC identical with → *shao yang zheng*, 少陽證, minor yang pathological condition. *SHL* 272: **少陽病**欲解時，從寅至辰上, "The time a **minor yang disease** tends to resolve is from *yin* to *chen* (i.e. from 3 a.m. to 9 a.m.)".

***Shao yang tou tong* 少陽頭痛, minor yang headache** [1]
PC of → *tou tong* 頭痛, headache, extending along the course of the minor yang conduits resulting from an intrusion of wind cold into the minor yang conduits. That is, the pain affects mainly the two temples at the sides of the forehead. *SJZL* 24: **少陽頭痛**，脈弦細而發熱, "In the case of **minor yang headache**, the [movement in the] vessels is string-like and fine, and [patients] effuse heat".

***Shao yang zheng* 少陽證, minor yang pathological condition** [4] AN *shao yang bing* 少陽病, minor yang disease.
PC in the course of harm caused by cold where evil affects the minor yang blocking the pivotal qi dynamics and the conduit qi, with alternating sensations of cold and heat, a feeling of fullness in the chest and flanks, a bitter taste in the mouth, a dry throat, dizzy eyes, and a string-like, fine movement in the vessels as frequent signs. *SHL* 5: 傷寒二三日，陽明、**少陽證**不見者，為不傳也, "If after harm caused by cold has lasted for two to three days no yang brilliance and no **minor yang pathological conditions** are visible, then it has not been transmitted further".

***Shao yin bing* 少陰病, minor yin disease** [5] AN *shao yin zheng* 少陰證, minor yin pathological condition.
PC in a later phase of harm caused by cold disease brought forth by harm to the proper qi, a weakening of the disease qi, and an exhaustion of the entire body. *SHL* 285: **少陰病**，脈細沉數，病為在裏，不可發汗, "A **minor yin disease**: the [movement in the] vessels is fine and deep inside. The disease is in the interior. One must not cause sweating".

***Shao yin tou tong* 少陰頭痛, minor yin headache** [3]
PC of headaches resulting from insufficient kidney yang qi and an internal abundance of yin cold, accompanied by recession cold affecting the hands and feet, and a movement in the vessels that is deep and fine. *SWBJQYBMJ* Fj: 細辛，**少陰頭痛**不足, "*Xi xin* [cures] **minor yin headache** with insufficient [qi]".

***Shao yin zheng* 少陰證, minor yin pathological condition** [7]
PC identical with → *shao yin bing* 少陰病, minor yin disease. *BCGM* SE *gan cao* 甘草 quoting *SHL* 311: 少陰病二三日，咽痛者，可與甘草湯, "When a minor yin disease has lasted for two to three days with the [patient's] throat aching, one can give the decoction with *gan cao*", writes: 傷寒咽痛：**少陰證**，甘草湯主之, "**Minor yin pathological condition**: the decoction with *gan cao* controls it".

***Shao yin shang han* 少陰傷寒, harm in the minor yin section caused by cold** [1] AN *shang hang shao yin zheng* 傷寒少陰證, harm caused by cold with signs in the minor yin section.
PC of → *shang han* 傷寒, harm caused by cold, with signs such as a minute, fine movement in the vessels, and a desire to sleep. *QJYF* 8 RE *da yan mi tang* 大岩蜜湯, massive cliff honey decoction: 並主**少陰傷寒**, "It also controls **harm in the minor yin section caused by cold**".

She an 舌喑, **tongue silence**; **muteness** [2] AN *she bu neng yan* 舌不能言, the tongue cannot speak.

IS of an inability to speak because the tongue cannot move. *XMLF* 2: 內奪而厥，**舌喑**不能言，二足廢，不為用。腎脈虛弱，其氣厥不至，舌不仁。經云：喑俳，足不履用，聲音不出者, "In the case of internal deprivation with recession, the **tongue is silent** and one cannot speak. The two feet are lame and cannot be used. The [movement in the] kidney vessels is depleted and weak. Its qi has receded and fails to arrive. The tongue is numb. The Classic states: 'mute and lame, the feet cannot be used for walking, and no sound is emitted'".

She ben jiang 舌本強, **tongue base stiffness** [3]

IS identical with → *she jiang* 舌強, tongue stiffness. *ZBYHL* 1: 驚悸恍惚，少顏色，**舌本強**，善憂悲，是為心氣之虛也, "Fright with palpitation and absent-mindedness, loss of complexion, **tongue base stiffness**, a tendency to worry and mourn: these are [the signs of] heat qi depletion".

She bu neng yan 舌不能言, **the tongue cannot speak** [1]

IS identical with → *she an* 舌喑, muteness. *WTMY* 39: 大迎：一名髓孔…足陽明脈氣所發，灸三壯，主寒熱，頸瘰癧，癲疾，口病，喘…口不收，**舌不能言**，不得嚼, "The [needle insertion hole] *da ying*: an alternative name is *sui kong*...This is where the qi of the foot yang brilliance vessel effuses. When cauterized with three cones, it controls alternating sensations of cold and heat, scrofula pervasion-illness at the neck, ailments of peak-illness, wry mouth, panting...when one is unable to close the mouth, **the tongue is unable to speak**, and [patients] are unable to chew".

She che 舌坼, **tongue fissures** [3]

IS of fissures developing on the tongue surface. In severe cases the fissures may release blood. *LGPZL* Xu 序：口瘡**舌坼**，立愈黃蘇, "Mouth sores and **tongue fissures** are cured instantaneously with [*gen*] *huang* and [*zi*] *su*".

She chu 舌出, **tongue protrusion** [8]

IS of a tongue that is stretched out of the mouth and cannot be retracted. *QJYF* 10: 故督郵顧子獻得病已瘥未健，請華佗視脈。曰：雖瘥尚虛未得復，陽氣不足，慎勿勞事。余勞尚可，女勞則死，當吐舌數寸。其婦聞其夫瘥，從百餘里來省之，經宿交接，中間三日發熱口噤，臨死**舌出**數寸。病新瘥未滿百日，氣力未平復，而犯房室略無不死, "Former local inspector Gu Zixian had been cured of a disease but he did not feel healthy. He asked Hua Tuo to examine [the movements in] his vessels. [Hua Tuo] told him: Although you have been cured, there is still a depletion that has not been restored to normal yet. Your yang qi is insufficient. You must be careful not to exhaust yourself. While other types of exhaustion may be possible, exhaustion [through intercourse] with women will kill you. Your tongue will protrude several *cun*. When his wife learned that her husband had been cured, she came from a hundred miles away to have intercourse with him. They met for an entire night. Three days later he effused heat and developed a clenched jaw. Close to his death his **tongue protruded** several *cun*. If a disease has not been cured for one hundred days, and if [a person's] strength has not been restored to normal, and if contrary to a warning one enters the bedroom [for intercourse], there is hardly a chance he will not die".

She dan **舌淡, tasteless tongue** [1]

IS of a dull, tasteless sensation on the tongue. *BCGM* Bai bing zhu zhi yao 百病主治藥：**舌淡**：白术，燥脾, "For **tasteless tongue**, *bai zhu* dries the spleen. LSZ: 舌苦是膽熱，甘是脾熱，酸是濕熱，澀是風熱，辛是燥熱，咸是脾濕，淡是胃虛, "A bitter taste of the tongue results from gallbladder heat; a sweet taste [of the tongue] results from spleen heat; a sour taste results from moisture heat; a roughness results from wind heat; an acrid taste results from dryness heat; a salty taste results from spleen moisture; a **tasteless** [**tongue**] results from stomach depletion".

She duan **舌短, tongue shortening** [3]

IS of a milder form of → *she suo* 舌縮, tongue contraction. *TPSHF* 4: 心黃者，目赤，舌上生瘡，心悶喘急，多言無度，或笑或嗔，微微汗出，口乾**舌短**，起臥不安, "In the case of heart jaundice the eyes are red, and sores emerge on the tongue. Heart-pressure is associated with hectic panting. [Patients] speak a lot, without restraint. Sometimes they laugh, sometimes they are angry. They sweat a little. Their mouth is dry and the **tongue is shortened**. [Patients] rise and lie down without calming down".

She gan **舌乾, desiccated tongue** [4]

IS of either a feeling of having a dry tongue, or of an appearance of the tongue surface as if it lacked moisture. *SW* 31: 五日少陰受之，少陰脈貫腎絡於肺，系舌本，故口燥**舌乾**而渴, "On the fifth day, the minor yin [conduits] receive it. The minor yin vessels penetrate the kidneys and enclose the lung. They are attached to the base of the tongue. Hence, the mouth is dry, the **tongue is desiccated**, and one is thirsty".

She gan **舌甘, sweet taste of the tongue** [1]

IS of a sensation of a sweet taste on the surface of the tongue despite the fact that one has not ingested any beverage or food. *BCGM* Bai bing zhu zhi yao 百病主治藥：**舌甘**：生地黄、芍藥、黄連, "For **sweet taste of the tongue**: *sheng di huang*, *shao yao*, *huang lian*". LSZ: 舌苦是膽熱，甘是脾熱，酸是濕熱，澀是風熱，辛是燥熱，咸是脾濕，淡是胃虛, "A bitter taste of the tongue results from gallbladder heat; a **sweet taste** [**of the tongue**] results from spleen heat; a sour taste results from moisture heat; a roughness results from wind heat; an acrid taste results from dryness heat; a salty taste results from spleen moisture; a tasteless [tongue] results from stomach depletion".

She gan ying **舌乾硬, the tongue is desiccated and hard** [1]

IS of a tongue that is dry and cannot be moved freely. *BCGM* SE *wu jing* 蕪菁 quoting *TPSHF*: 身體腫強，舌乾燥硬, "The body is swollen and stiff. The tongue is dry and hard", writes: 身體強，**舌乾硬**, "The body is stiff. **The tongue is desiccated and hard**".

She gen jiang ying **舌根強硬, stiff and hard tongue base** [1]

IS identical with → *she jiang* 舌強, tongue stiffness. *TPSHF* 19: 治卒中風不語，**舌根強硬**，宜服此方，陳醬（五合，三年者妙），人乳汁（五合）。右件藥，相和研，以生布絞取汁，不計時候，少少與服。良久當語，“To cure sudden wind stroke with loss of speech and a **stiff and hard tongue base** it is advisable to ingest the following recipe. Seasoned bean sauce (5 *ge*, those of 3 years are best), human milk (5 *ge*). Grind these two drugs together, and wring them through a fresh piece of cloth to obtain the juice. Give [the patient] a very small amount to ingest, regardless what time it is. After a rather long time he will regain his speech”.

She gong **射工, archer** [61]

① AN *duan hu* 短狐, short[-tail] fox; *shui nu* 水弩, water crossbow; *bao qiang* 抱槍, rifle holder. EA. A small bug in ancient times believed to live in waters and be capable of “shooting” poison from its mouth at people, thereby causing disease. *ZHF* 7: 江南有**射工**毒蟲, “ In the region south of the Yangzi there is a poisonous bug, the ‘**archer**’”.

② PC caused by the poison of the archer. *ZHF* 8: 扁鵲陷水丸，療內脹病，並蠱疰中惡等，及蜂百毒、溪毒、**射工**, “Bian Que’s pills for immersion in water cure diseases of inner distension, and *gu*-attachment-illness as well as being struck by the malign. Also, [it eliminates] the hundred poisons of wasps, rivulet poison, and **archers**”.

She hei **舌黑, black tongue** [1]

IS of the tongue assuming a black color. *TPSHF* 11: 治陰毒傷寒，面青，張口出氣，心下硬，身不熱，只額上有汗，煩渴不止，**舌黑**多睡, “To cure yin-poison with harm caused by cold. [Patients have] a greenish face. Their mouth is wide open and releases qi. There is a hardening below the heart. The body is not hot. Only on the forehead is there sweat, with unending vexation and thirst. They have a **black tongue** and they sleep a lot”.

She hui du **蛇虺毒, snake venom poison; snake venom poisoning** [5] AN *she hui shang* 蛇虺傷, injury caused by snake venom; *du she shang chi* 毒蛇傷, injury caused by a poisonous snake; *e she hui shang* 惡蛇虺傷, injury caused by the venom of a malign snake; *she hui shang ren* 蛇虺傷人, a snake’s venom harms a person; *du she shang* 毒蛇傷, injury caused by a poisonous snake; *she shang du* 蛇傷毒, poisoning resulting from an injury caused by a snake; *du she shang ren* 毒蛇傷人, a poisonous snake harms a person.

PC with major signs including all types of local reactions to poisoning, or those affecting the entire body, stimulated by the bites of a poisonous snake. *BCSY* SE *cai ju ji shi* 蔡苴機屎：主**蛇虺毒**, 兩頭麋屎也, “It controls **snake venom poisoning**. These are the excrements of elks with two heads”.

She hui shang **蛇虺傷, injury caused by snake venom** [2]

PC identical with → *she hui du* 蛇虺毒, snake venom poisoning. *BCGM* SE *ban bian lian* 半邊蓮 quotes *SYSF*: **蛇虺傷**，搗汁飲，以滓圍塗之, “For **injury caused by snake venom**, pound [this] and ingest the resulting liquid. Apply the sediment externally all around [the wound]”.

She hui shang ren **蛇虺傷人, harm caused to man by snake venom** [1]
PC identical with → *she hui shang* 蛇虺傷, harm caused by snake venom. *BCGM* SE *su* 蘇 quotes *QJYF*: **蛇虺傷人**：紫蘇葉搗飲之, "For **harm caused to man by snake venom**: Pound the leaves of *zi su* and drink [the liquid]".

She jia **蛇瘕, snake conglomeration-illness** [7]
PC of → *jia* 瘕, conglomeration-illness, in the abdomen that has the shape of a snake and moves when squeezed. It was believed that the formation of such aggregations is associated with the consumption of snakes or an inadvertent ingestion of food contaminated with snake sperm. *ZBYHL* 19: 其病在腹，摸揣亦有蛇狀，謂**蛇瘕**也, "The disease is situated in the abdomen. When touched it appears to have the shape of a snake. It is called **snake conglomeration-illness**".

She jian **舌蹇, tongue sluggishness** [1]
IS of a sluggish tongue movement impairing one's speech. *BCGM* SE *shu jiao* 蜀椒 quotes *JiuJF*: 舌蹇語吃：川椒，以生麵包丸。每服十粒，醋湯送下, "For **tongue sluggishness** and stuttering: Prepare pills from *chuan jiao* with a coating of unprocessed flour. Each time ingest 10 pills. To be ingested with vinegar decoction".

She jiang **舌強, tongue stiffness** [10] AN *she ben jiang* 舌本強, tongue base stiffness; *she gen jiang ying* 舌根強硬, stiff and hard tongue base.
IS of a stiff and hard tongue that is difficult to move. *ZBYHL* 1: 風邪之氣，若先中於陰，病發於五臟者，其狀奄忽不知人，喉裏噫噫然有聲，**舌強**不能言, "The qi of wind evil, if it first strikes the yin [conduits], and when the disease [qi] effuses into the five depots: its appearance is such that [a patient] suddenly does not recognize others. In his throat he makes sounds like *yi-yi*; his **tongue is stiff** and he cannot speak".

She jiao **舌焦, parched tongue** [2]
IS of a tongue surface that is both dry and shows a parched, black color. *BJ* SE *shi gao* 石膏：主中風寒熱，心下逆氣驚喘，口乾**舌焦**, "It controls wind stroke with alternating sensations of cold and heat, counterflow of qi below the heart with fright panting, a dry mouth and **parched tongue**".

She ku **舌苦, bitter taste of the tongue** [3]
IS of a sensation of a bitter taste on the surface of the tongue despite the fact that one has not ingested any beverage or food. *PJF* 153: 熱病後脾胃氣虛，四肢乏力，骨節煩疼，口乾**舌苦**，不思飲食, "In the aftermath of a heat disease, spleen and stomach qi is depleted. The four limbs lack strength, the bone joints are distressed with pain. The mouth is dry and **the tongue has a bitter taste**. One does not wish to eat or drink". *BCGM* Bai bing zhu zhi yao 百病主治藥：**舌苦**是膽熱，甘是脾熱，酸是濕熱，澀是風熱，辛是燥熱，咸是脾濕，淡是胃虛, "A **bitter taste of the tongue** results from gallbladder heat; a sweet taste [of the tongue] results from spleen heat; a sour taste results from moisture heat; a roughness results from wind heat; an acrid taste results from dryness heat; a salty taste results from spleen moisture; a tasteless [tongue] results from stomach depletion".

***She lou* 蛇瘺, snake fistula** [2]

PC of → *lou* 瘺, fistula, associated with fever and an aversion to cold. The swelling does not emerge at any fixed location. It opens to fester and develops into fistula. In former times it was believed that snake fistula differs from sparrow fistula in that, after treatment, patients discharge items resembling snakes in their urine. *ZBYHL* 34: 由居處飲食有蛇毒氣，入於腑臟，流於經脈，寒熱結腫，出處無定，因潰成瘺。服藥，有物隨小便出，如蛇形狀，謂之**蛇瘺**, "This is because poisonous qi of snakes encountered at one's living place, in beverages and food, has entered the depots and palaces whence it has flown into the conduit vessels. [Patients] experience sensations of cold and heat, as well as nodular swelling that appears at no fixed locations. The swelling later begins to fester and develops into fistula. Having ingested medication, [patients] will release items resembling snakes with their urine. [Hence] one calls this '**snake fistula**'".

***She ma* 舌麻, tongue hemp[-like numbness]** [3]

IS of a numb tongue with a complete inability to sense a flavor. *PJF* 218: 咽乾，**舌麻**失味，不喜飲食， "The throat is dry. The **tongue is [as numb as] hemp** and has lost its ability to distinguish flavors. Patients find no pleasure in drinking or eating".

***She mi* 舌糜, tongue erosion** [1]

IS of a tongue that develops sores and festers. *YXRM* 4: 熱…在上焦，則咽乾，口燥而臭，**舌糜**唇瘡, "If there is heat in the upper burner, then the throat dries, the mouth is desiccated and malodorous, the **tongue erodes**, and the lips develop sores".

***She mo chuang* 蛇漠** (possibly erroneous for *mo* 沫) **瘡, snake spread** (for foam) **sores** [2]

PC of → *chuang* 瘡, sores, conditions developing from human contact with saliva spat by poisonous snakes onto plants during the seventh and eighth month. *BCSY* SE *fu she* 蝮蛇：吐口中涎沫於草木上，著人身腫成瘡，卒難主療，名曰**蛇漠瘡**, "They spit the saliva foam from their mouth onto plants. When humans touch this they develop a swelling and eventually sores. This is most difficult to cure. It is called '**snake spread sores**'".

***She nü* 舌衄, spontaneous bleeding of the tongue** [2]

PC of a spontaneous bleeding of the tongue. *SYDXF* 17: 舌無故出血，名**舌衄**，炒槐花為末，摻之而愈 "When the tongue bleeds without apparent cause, this is called '**spontaneous bleeding of the tongue**'. Roast *hui hua* to prepare a powder, and rub it [onto the tongue]. This brings the cure".

***She pan li* 蛇盤癧, snake-coil pervasion-illness** [1] AN *She pan luo li* 蛇盤瘰癧, snake-coil scrofula with pervasion-illness

PC of numerous → *luo li* 瘰癧, scrofula with pervasion-illness, growing around the neck. *SYDXF* 19: 海菜丸，治癧生於頭項上交接，名**蛇盤癧**者，宜早治之, "Pills with *hai cai*. They cure scrofula developing at the intersection of the head and nape. Those called '**snake-coil pervasion-illness**' are to be treated early".

***She pan luo li* 蛇盤瘰癧, snake-coil scrofula with pervasion-illness** [2]

PC identical with → *she pan li* 蛇盤癧. *BCGM* SE *hai zao* 海藻 quoting *SY-DXF* 19: 蛇盤癧, "Snake-coil pervasion-illness", writes: **蛇盤瘰癧**, "**Snake-coil scrofula with pervasion-illness**".

***She se* 舌澀, tongue roughness** [3]

IS of a sensation as if there were some roughness on the surface of the tongue despite the fact that one has not ingested any beverage or food. *HJJF* 3: 大沉香丸，治一切冷氣攻心腹刺痛，胸膈噎塞，嘔吐痰水，噫氣吞酸，口苦**舌澀**，不思飲食, "The large pills with *chen xiang*, they cure all types of conditions where cold qi attacks heart and abdomen causing a piercing pain, with blockage of the chest, diaphragm and gullet, vomiting of phlegm and water, belching and sour regurgitation, a bitter taste in the mouth and **tongue roughness**. There is no intention to drink or eat". *BCGM* Bai bing zhu zhi yao : 舌苦是膽熱，甘是脾熱，酸是濕熱，澀是風熱，辛是燥熱，咸是脾濕，淡是胃虛, "A bitter taste of the tongue results from gallbladder heat; a sweet taste [of the tongue] results from spleen heat; a sour taste results from moisture heat; a roughness results from wind heat; an acrid taste results from dryness heat; a salty taste results from spleen moisture; a tasteless [tongue] results from stomach depletion".

***She shang* 蛇傷, injury caused by snakes** [25]

PC CD of all types of harm caused by snakes, including bites of poisonous and non-poisonous snakes, as well as being squeezed by a snake winding around a person's body, or body part. *TBC* SE *huai xiang zi* 蘹香子：主諸瘺，霍亂及**蛇傷**, "It controls all types of fistula, cholera, and **injury caused by snakes**".

***She shang chu xue* 舌上出血, bleeding on the tongue** [6] AN *she shang chu xue* 舌上血出; *she shang wu gu chu xue* 舌上無故出血, spontaneous bleeding on the tongue.

PC identical with → *she nü* 舌衄, tongue bleeding. *QJYF* 6: 治**舌上出血**如泉方，燒鐵篦熟爍孔中，良, "Recipe to cure **bleeding on the tongue** as if there were a fountain: Heat one tooth of an iron comb until it is very hot and insert it into the hole [from which the blood is gushing]. Good".

***She shang du* 蛇傷毒, harm caused by snake poisoning** [3]

PC identical with → *she hui du* 蛇虺毒②, venomous snake poisoning. *YXL* SE *bai ying qiu yin* 白頸蚯蚓：乾煮熬末用之，主**蛇傷毒**, "Dried, boiled and prepared as a powder it controls **snake poisoning**".

***She shang sheng tai* 舌上生胎, fur-growth on the tongue** [2]

IS identical with → *she tai* 舌胎, tongue fur. *SHLS* 3: 傷寒，**舌上生胎**，不拘滑白黃黑，俱用井水浸青布片，於舌上洗淨後，用生薑片子時時浸水刮之，其胎自退, "In the case of harm caused by cold there is **fur-growth on the tongue**. Regardless of whether it is smooth, white, yellow, or black, in all cases use well water in which a piece of blue cloth has been soaked and wash the surface of the tongue with it. Then take a slice of raw ginger and repeatedly dip it into water and wipe the [fur]. The fur will vanish as a result" .

She shang wu gu chu xue **舌上無故出血, spontaneous bleeding on the tongue** [1]
PC identical with → *she shang chu xue* 舌上出血, bleeding on the tongue. *BCGM* SE *ba dou* 巴豆：**舌上無故出血**，以（巴豆油）熏舌之上下，自止, "For **spontaneous bleeding on the tongue**, use [*ba dou* oil] to steam the upper and the lower side of the tongue, and [the bleeding] will end".

She shang xue chu **舌上血出, bleeding on the tongue** [1]
PC identical with → *she shang chu xue* 舌上出血. *SJZL* 69: 治**舌上血出**不止，阿膠散方, "Recipe for the powder with *a jiao* cures unending **bleeding on the tongue**".

She suan **舌酸, sour taste of the tongue** [1]
IS of a sensation of a sour taste on the surface of the tongue despite the fact that one has not ingested any beverage or food. *HJJF* 3: 口苦**舌酸**，胸滿短氣，肢體怠惰, "The mouth is bitter and the **tongue has a sour taste**. A feeling of fullness in the chest and shortness of qi. The extremities and body slacken". *BCGM* Bai bing zhu zhi yao 百病主治藥：舌苦是膽熱，甘是脾熱，酸是濕熱，澀是風熱，辛是燥熱，咸是脾濕，淡是胃虛, "A bitter taste of the tongue results from gallbladder heat; a sweet taste [of the tongue] results from spleen heat; a sour taste results from moisture heat; a roughness results from wind heat; an acrid taste results from dryness heat; a salty taste results from spleen moisture; a tasteless [tongue] results from stomach depletion".

She suo **舌縮, tongue contraction** [4]
IS of a retraction of the tongue into the depth of the oral cavity, making it difficult to extend. *TPSHF* 4: 臟腑壅滯，口乾**舌縮**，神思不安, "The depots and palaces are obstructed with [qi] sluggishness. The mouth is dry and the **tongue contracted**. The spirit and thoughts are not calm".

She tai **舌胎, tongue fur** [5] AN *she shang sheng tai* 舌上生胎.
IS of the appearance on the surface of the tongue of a thick fur-like coating. The character *tai* 胎 (lit.: "fetus", "uterus", "source") in *she tai* 舌胎is a near-homophone of what may have been the original character used to designate a fur-like coating: *tai* 苔, lit. "moss". *BCGM* SE *sheng jiang* 生薑 quoting *SHLS* 3: 舌上生胎，不拘滑白黃黑, "When a coating develops on the tongue, regardless of whether it is smooth, white, yellow or black", writes: 舌上生胎，諸病**舌胎**，以布染井水抹，後用薑片時時擦之，自去, "Fur-growth on the tongue, and all [other] types of diseases of **tongue fur**: Wipe [the tongue] with a piece of cloth moistened with well water, and then rub [the tongue surface] repeatedly with a piece of ginger".

She ti **蛇體, snake body** [1]
PC identical with → *lin ti* 鱗體, scaly body. *XEWSZWLF* 20: "鱗體者，謂皮膚之上，如蛇皮鱗甲之狀，故又名**蛇體**, "A 'scaly body' is to say: an appearance of scales, like a snake, on the skin. Hence it is also called '**snake body**'".

She xian **蛇癇, snake epilepsy** [3]
PC of a → *dian xian* 癲癇, peak-illness with epilepsy, which, at the time of its outbreaks, makes the patient's four limbs twitch, accompanied by a shaking head

and a tongue moving here and there. *BJ* SE *she tui* 蛇蜕：味咸，平。主小兒百二十種驚癇，瘈瘲，癲疾，寒熱，腸痔，蟲毒，**蛇癇**, "Its flavor is salty, balanced. It controls 120 types of fright epilepsy in children, convulsion, ailments of peak-illness, alternating sensations of cold and heat, intestinal piles, poison of bugs/worms, and **snake epilepsy**".

She xian **舌咸, salty taste of the tongue** [1]

IS of a sensation of a salty taste on the surface of the tongue despite the fact that one has not ingested any beverage or food. *BCGM* Bai bing zhu zhi yao 百病主治藥：**舌咸**：知母瀉腎For **salty taste of the tongue**, *zhi mu* drains the kidneys". LSZ: 舌苦是膽熱，甘是脾熱，酸是濕熱，澀是風熱，辛是燥熱，咸是脾濕，淡是胃虛, "A bitter taste of the tongue results from gallbladder heat; a sweet taste [of the tongue] results from spleen heat; a sour taste results from moisture heat; a roughness results from wind heat; an acrid taste results from dryness heat; a salty taste results from spleen moisture; a tasteless [tongue] results from stomach depletion".

She xin **舌辛, acrid taste of the tongue** [1]

IS of a sensation of an acrid taste on the surface of the tongue despite the fact that one has not ingested any beverage or food. *BCGM* Bai bing zhu zhi yao 百病主治藥：**舌辛**：黃芩、巵子，瀉肺, "For **acrid taste of the tongue**: *huang qin* and *zhi zi* serve to drain the lung". LSZ: 舌苦是膽熱，甘是脾熱，酸是濕熱，澀是風熱，辛是燥熱，咸是脾濕，淡是胃虛, "A bitter taste of the tongue results from gallbladder heat; a sweet taste [of the tongue] results from spleen heat; a sour taste results from moisture heat; a roughness results from wind heat; an acrid taste results from dryness heat; a salty taste results from spleen moisture; a tasteless [tongue] results from stomach depletion".

She ying chu xue **舌硬出血, tongue hardness with bleeding** [2]

PC with a hardening of the tongue and bleeding from its surface as major sign. *BCGM* SE *mu zei* 木賊 quoting *PJF* 59: 舌硬忽出血不止, "The tongue is hard and suddenly develops unending bleeding", writes: **舌硬出血, "Tongue hardness with bleeding"**.

She zao **舌燥, tongue desiccation** [1]

IS of a desiccated tongue surface lacking moisture. *QJYF* 19: 病苦**舌燥**咽腫，心煩咽乾…名曰腎實熱也, "The disease of **tongue desiccation** and throat swelling, vexed heart and throat dryness is called 'kidney repletion with heat'".

She zhang **蛇瘴, snake miasma** [4]

PC identical with → *biao chuang* 瘭瘡, flaming heat sores. *WKZZ* 4: 瘭疽，一名**蛇瘴**，川、廣烟瘴地面有之 "Flaming-heat impediment-illnesses are also called '**snake miasma**'. They occur in Sichuan and Guangzhou, i.e. regions with smoky miasma".

She zhang **舌脹, tongue distension** [13]

IS, PC identical with → *she zhong* 舌腫, tongue swelling. *QJYF* 6: 治**舌脹**滿口不得語方，䗪蟲（三十枚），鹽（一升），上二味，以水三升，煮三沸，含之，稍稍嚥之，日三, "Recipe to cure **tongue distension** to a degree that it fills the mouth and one cannot speak: 30 ground beetles; salt, 1 *sheng*. Boil these two substances with 3 *sheng* of water three times until bubbling. Hold [the liquid] in the mouth, and swallow it in very small quantities".

***She zheng* 蛇癥, snake concretion-illness** [2]

PC of → *zheng* 癥, concretion-illness, that forms when someone inadvertently consumes living bugs/worms or snakes that gather in the abdomen *QJYF* 11: 治**蛇癥**方。白馬尾切長五分，以酒服方寸匕，大者自出, "Recipe to cure **snake concretion-illness**: ingest with wine one square-inch spoon of white horse tail cut in the length of five *fen*. Large ones will leave by themselves".

***She zhi* 失志, loss of mind** [10]

PC of a slight mental confusion resulting from fright and fear, from sadness and pondering, or from chronic peak-illness with epilepsy. *YXL* SE *huang jin xie* 黄金屑：主小兒驚傷五藏，風癎，**失志**, "In children it controls fright harming the five depots, wind epilepsy, and **loss of mind**".

***She zhong* 舌腫, tongue swelling** [13] AN *she zhang* 舌脹, tongue distension.

① IS of a swollen, distended tongue. In severe cases the tongue fills the entire mouth. In very severe cases the tongue may protrude from the mouth. *QJYF* 16: 胃絕不治五日死，何以知之？**舌腫**，溺血，大便赤泄, "When the stomach [qi] is interrupted and if this is not treated, death will follow within five days. How does one know? The **tongue is swollen**, the urine is bloody, and defecation is a red outflow".

② PC with a swollen tongue as its major sign. *ZBYHL* 50: **舌腫**候：心候舌，脾之絡脈出舌下。心脾俱熱，氣發於口，故**舌腫**也, "The signs of **tongue swelling**: The condition of the heart is visible in the condition of the tongue. The network vessel of the spleen leaves from underneath the tongue. When the heart and spleen both have heat, their qi effuses through the mouth. Hence the **tongue is swollen**".

***She zi* 舌紫, purple tongue** [2]

IS of the base of the tongue assuming a dark purple color. *BCGM* SE *niu* 牛 quoting *SJZL* 61: 舌上紫色，甚則舌面坼裂, "The surface of the tongue assumes a purple color. In severe cases it will develop fissures", writes: **舌紫**面裂, "**Purple tongue** with surface fissures".

***Shen bu shou she* 神不守舍, unsettled spirit** [3] AN *shen zhi bu shou* 神志不守, unruly spirit of the heart; *xin shen bu an* 心神不安, restless spirit of the heart; *xin shen bu ding* 心神不定, instable spirit of the heart.

IS of abnormal mental conditions brought forth by a harassment of the spirit with the result that it is no longer securely settled in the heart. *HJJF* 1: **神不守舍**，風涎潮作，手足抽掣, "When the **spirit is unsettled**, a tidal wave of wind drool emerges, and the hands and feet are drawn in in cramps".

***Shen bu zu* 神不足, spirit [qi] insufficiency** [2] AN *xin shen bu zu* 心神不足, heart spirit [qi] insufficiency.

PC of forgetfulness and palpitation with fear brought forth by depletion of spirit qi, and a disharmony of qi and blood. *PJF* 337: 心氣虛乏而**神不足**之屬，皆以

氣血不調之故也, "All [conditions] associated with heart qi depletion and **spirit [qi] insufficiency** result from a disharmony of qi and blood".

***Shen chan* 身顫, the body shivers** [2]
IS of the entire body displaying an uncontrolled trembling movement. *BCGM* SE lu 驢 quotes *SYXJ*: 主中風頭眩，心肺浮熱，手足無力，筋骨煩疼，言語似澀，一身動搖。烏驢頭一枚，燖洗如法，蒸令極熟，細切，更於豉汁內煮，著五味調，點少酥食，"To master wind stroke with a dizzy head: the [movement in the vessels of] the heart and lung is at the surface, associated with heat. Hands and feet lack strength. The sinews and bones are vexed and painful. Language appears rough, and the entire body sways. Wash and prepare with fire 1 head of a black donkey according to the rules. Steam it until it is very well done. Cut it into fine slices and boil them in the juice of salted, fermented beans. Regulate with the five flavors, heat until crisp, and eat", writes: 中風頭眩：心肺浮熱，肢軟骨疼，語蹇**身顫**。用烏驢頭一枚，如食法，豉汁煮食, "Wind stroke with a dizzy head: the [movement in the vessels of] heart and lung is at the surface, associated with heat. The limbs are soft and the bones ache. Speech is impaired, and **the body shivers**. Take 1 head of a black donkey and prepare as if it were for a meal. Then boil with salted, fermented beans, and eat this".

***Shen chun* 沈唇, leaking lips** [2] AN chun shen 唇沈, lip leakage.
PC identical with → *jin chun* 緊唇, tight lips. *BCGM* SE *shan yu* 鱔魚 quoting *MYBL*: 主補中，益血，療沈唇, "It controls by supplementing the center and augmenting blood, and it heals moist lips", writes: 補中益血，療**沈唇**, "It supplements the center, augments blood, and heals **leaking lips**".

***Shen diao* 腎釣, kidneys pulled upward by a hook** [4]
PC with a pulling pain felt in the scrotum and the lumbar and abdominal region. One of various types of → *shan qi* 疝氣, elevation-illness qi. *RHZ* SE *shu jiao* 蜀椒：治賁豚，伏梁氣及內外**腎釣**, "It cures running piglet, hidden-beams qi and [a feeling as if] one's internal as well as external **kidneys** [i.e. testicles] **were pulled upward by a hook**".

***Shen feng* 腎風, kidney wind** [5]
PC identified by LSZ as sores and itching developing on the scrotum and lower limbs. The concept of "kidney wind" appears first in *SW* 42: **腎風**之狀，多汗惡風，面痝然浮腫，脊痛不能正立，其色炲，隱曲不利, "The appearance of **kidney wind** [is such]: [patients] sweat profusely and have an aversion to wind. Their face develops a surface swelling of the *mang*-type. The spine aches and they cannot stand upright. Their [facial] color is [that of] soot. The passage through the hidden bend (i.e. the penis) is impeded". This definition was accepted by most authors in subsequent centuries, but is quite different from the meaning seen in the *BCGM*, SE *lu* 驢, quoted from the *QXLF*: **腎風**下注生瘡, "When **kidney wind** flows down it generates sores".

***Shen gan* 腎疳, kidney *gan*-illness** [2]
PC of → *gan* 疳, *gan-illness*, with an extreme degree of emaciation, and frequent appearance of ulcers affecting the ears, nose, teeth and lower body parts. *XE*-

YZZJ Fj: **腎疳**，極瘦，身有瘡疥，當補腎, "**Kidney *gan*-illness** is associated with extreme emaciation. The body has sores with *jie*-illness. It is essential to supplement the kidneys".

Shen gan hei shou **身乾黑瘦, the body is desiccated, black and emaciated** [2]
IS of an emaciated body of dark color and desiccated skin. *WSYJF* 5: 鼓脹，**身乾黑瘦**，多渴煩悶, "Drum distension. **The body is desiccated, black and emaciated**. One is often thirsty, with vexation and heart-pressure".

Shen han **腎寒, cold in the kidneys** [1]
PC identical with → *shen leng* 腎冷. *QJYF* 19: 虛則**腎寒**，耳聾或鳴，汗出，腰痛不得俯仰, "Depletion results in **cold in the kidneys**. The ears are deaf, and may hear a ringing. [Patients] sweat; their lower back aches, and they can neither bend nor lift their body.

Shen hua **腎滑, smooth [flow from the] kidneys** [1]
PC identical with → *jing hua* 精滑, smooth flow of essence/semen. *BCGM* SE *ge li* 蛤蜊 quotes Wang Haogu 王好古：主濕嗽**腎滑**之疾, "It controls the ailments of moist cough and **smooth [flow from the] kidneys**".

Shen huang **腎黃, kidney jaundice** [2]
PC of → *huang dan* 黃疸, yellow *dan*-illness, accompanied by illness signs of kidney depletion such as anuria and tinnitus, painful lumbar region and back, weakness of legs and knees. *WTMY* 4: **腎黃**，小便不通，氣急心悶，五色黃，瓜蒂散方, "For **kidney jaundice** with an inability to pass urine, qi urgency and heart-pressure, as well as for all [other types of] jaundice, [use] the recipe for a powder with *gua di*".

Shen hun **神昏, spirit clouding** [4]
IS identical with → *hun kui* 昏憒, muddle-headedness. *BCJJZ* SE *jiu* 酒：人飲之，使體弊**神昏**，是其有毒故也, "When one drinks it, it harms the body and causes **spirit clouding**. The reason is that it is poisonous".

Shen huo **腎火, kidney fire** [6]
PC and EA identical with → *shen re* 腎熱, kidney heat. *SWBJQYBMJ* Lj: 知母泄**腎火**助陰, "*Zhi mu* drains **kidney fire** and assists the yin".

Shen ji **腎積, kidney accumulation** [2]
PC identical with → *ben tun* 奔豚, running piglet. *ZBYHL* 19：積聚候，診得**腎積**脈，沉而急。苦脊與腰相引痛, "The signs of accumulation and collection: examination reveals a **kidney accumulation** [movement in the] vessels; it is deep inside and urgent. [Patients] complain about pain in the spine extending down to the lower back".

Shen jiang **身強, stiff body** [5]
IS of a stiff body with difficulties moving. *QJYF* 1: 虛而**身強**，腰中不利，加磁石、杜仲, "In the case of depletion with a **stiff body**, and if there is an uncomfortable feeling in the lower back, add *ci shi* and *du zhong*".

***Shen jing* 神驚, spirit fright** [3]
IS identical with → *xin jing* 心驚, heart fright. *BCGM* SE hu 虎 quoting *SLBC*: 主小兒疳痢，驚神不安, "It controls *gan*-illness with free-flux illness in children, with a frightened spirit that does not find rest", writes: **神驚**不安, "**The spirit is frightened** and restless".

***Shen ju* 深疽, deep-reaching impediment-illness** [1]
PC of a → *ju* 疽, impediment-illness, located in the depth of the tissue. *QJYF* 22: 有久癰余瘡，敗為**深疽**者，在腨脛間，喜生瘡中水惡露，寒凍不瘥，經年成骨疽, "When an obstruction-illness or any other sores last for a long time, [and the patient's condition] deteriorates with the generation of **deep-reaching impediment-illnesses**, sores filled with water and malign dew tend to develop in the region of his calves and shins. If they are exposed to freezing cold and are not healed, in the course of several years, they will form bone impediment-illnesses".

***Shen jue* 腎厥, kidney recession** [5]
PC of headache caused by kidney yang depletion. *PJBSF* 2: 腎氣不足，氣逆上行，頭痛不可忍，謂之**腎厥**, "When the kidney qi is insufficient, with an upward movement of qi counterflow, and an unbearable headache, this is called '**kidney recession** '".

***Shen kun* 神困, spirit inertia** [1]
IS of mental weakness and sleepiness with a longing to lie down. *SJZL* 96: 治膈上虛熱，喉咽噎塞，小便赤澀，**神困**多睡，酸棗仁丸方, "To cure depletion heat above the diaphragm, blockage of the throat, red and rough urine, **spirit inertia** with much sleep, [use] the recipe for the pills with *suan zao* kernels".

***Shen lao* 腎勞, kidney exhaustion** [5]
PC of a depletion exhaustion brought forth by exhaustion detriment affecting the kidneys. *ZBYHL* 3: **腎勞**者，背難以俯仰，小便不利，色赤黃而有餘瀝，莖內痛，陰濕，囊生瘡，小腹滿急, "In the case of **kidney exhaustion**, bending the back is difficult. The urine fails to flow freely; its color is red-yellow, and there is a remainder that trickles. One feels pain inside the stalk; one's private parts are moist. The scrotum develops sores. The lower abdomen has a feeling of fullness and tightness".

***Shen leng* 身冷, the body is cold** [18] AN *ti han* 體寒; *ni leng* 逆冷, counterflow cold.
IS of a feeling of cold, or of the body's exterior being exposed to low temperatures. *JGYL* Fj: 唇口青，**身冷**，為入臟即死, "The lips and mouth are green-blue, and **the body is cold**. If this enters the depots, one will die".

***Shen leng* 腎冷, kidney cold; cold of the testicles** [15]
① AN *shen han* 腎寒, cold in the kidneys. PC of internal abundance of yin and cold brought forth by a depletion and weakness of the kidneys and insufficiency of yang qi. *QJYF* 16: 脹滿、**腎冷**、瘕積、泄利，灸天樞百壯 "For distension and fullness, **kidney cold**, conglomeration-illness accumulations, and free-flux illness cauterize the *tian shu* [point] one hundred times".

② IS of cold of the testicles. *WTMY* 7: 集驗療**腎冷**及疼，疝氣滯後，灌方, "The *JiYF* has a recipe for an enema to cure **cold of the testicles** and pain, elevation-illness qi, and difficult defecation".

Shen lou **腎漏, kidney leakage** [2]

PC identical with → *qiang zhong* 強中, powerful center. *BCGM* SE *bu gu zhi* 補骨脂 quotes *QJF*: 玉莖長硬不痿，精出捏之則脆癢如刺針，名**腎漏**, "The jade stalk (i.e. the penis) is hard and fails to shrink for a long time. When pinched while seminal fluid is discharged then there is a feeling of brittleness and itching as if being pierced with a needle. This is called '**kidney leakage**'".

Shen nüe **腎瘧, kidney malaria** [3]

PC of → *nüe ji* 瘧疾, malaria ailment, associated with illness signs of the kidney conduits, such as fear of cold, difficult defecation, and pain in the back and lumbar region. *SW* 36: **腎瘧**者，令人洒洒然，腰脊痛宛轉，大便難, "**Kidney malaria**: it makes a person shiver. [Patients] writhe with pain in the lower back and spine. Defecation is difficult".

Shen qi lao **腎氣勞, kidney qi exhaustion** [1]

PC identical with → *shen lao* 腎勞, kidney exhaustion. *YXL* SE *zhi mu* 知母: 主治心煩躁悶，骨熱勞往來，生產後蓐勞，**腎氣勞**，憎寒虛損, "It is responsible for curing heart vexation, restlessness and heart-pressure, recurring bone heat and exhaustion, childbed exhaustion following delivery, **kidney qi exhaustion**, aversion to cold, and depletion detriment".

Shen qian han **身前寒, the body front is cold** [1]

IS of a feeling of cold in the frontal section of the body. *BCGM* Zang fu xu han biao ben yong yao shi 臟腑虛寒標本用藥式：發熱蒸蒸，身前熱，**身前寒**, "Effusion of heat with steaming; [sometimes] the body front is hot, [sometimes] **the body front is cold**".

Shen re **腎熱, heat in the kidneys; kidney heat** [2] AN → *shen huo* 腎火, kidney fire.

① PC of heat-type diseases affecting the kidneys. *SW* 32: **腎熱**病者頤先赤, "In the case of the disease **heat in the kidneys**, the chin becomes red first".

② EA bringing forth heat-type disease in the kidneys. *ZBYHL* 49:**腎熱**，其氣則澀，故令水道不利, "In the case of **heat in the kidneys**, the [movement in the vessels of the patient's] qi is rough. Hence it makes the passageways of water impassable".

Shen re **身熱, body heat; the body is hot** [76]

IS identical with → *fa re* 發熱, effusion of heat. *SW* 5: 陽勝則**身熱**，腠理閉, "When yang dominates, **the body is hot** and the interstitial structures close".

Shen shi **腎濕, kidney moisture** [2]

① EA of an inability of water/moisture transformation because of kidney depletion, or of moisture evil harming the kidneys, with water/moisture stagnation as a consequence. *ZBYHL* 5: 久久變為水病，**腎濕**故也, "After a long time this changes into a water disease. The reason is **kidney moisture**".

② PC of an oozing, moist scrotum. *MYBL* SE *wu hui* 烏喙：主風濕，丈夫**腎濕**陰囊癢, "It controls wind and moisture, and **kidney moisture** with scrotum itching in males".

Shen suo **腎縮, shrinkage of [external] kidneys** [5]

PC with the testicles of newborns shrinking and pulled upward into a position where they cannot be felt. *SYDXF* 11: 七日**腎縮**，乃初生受寒所致, "If on the seventh day **the [external] kidneys shrink**, then this is because a newborn has been affected by cold".

Shen ti zhong **身體重, the body feels heavy** [3]

IS identical with → *shen zhong* 身重. *SW* 1: 今五臟皆衰，筋骨解墮，天癸盡矣。故髮鬢白，**身體重**，行步不正，而無子耳, "[At this age] the five depots are all weak and the sinews and the bones have become sluggish. The heaven *gui* is used up entirely. Hence, the hair on the head and on the temples turns white and **the body feels heavy**. [A male of that age] no [longer] walks upright and no [longer] has children".

Shen tuo **神脫, spirit loss** [2]

PC of a separation of yin and yang, with life being in great danger. LSZ identifies *shen tuo* 神脫 as including → *tuo yin* 脫陰, loss of yin, and → *tuo yang* 脫陽, loss of yang. *BCGM* Ba ji 八劑：脫陽者見鬼，脫陰者目盲，此**神脫**也，非澀藥所能收也, "In the case of a loss of yang, one sees demons; In the case of a loss of yin, one turns blind. This is '**spirit loss**'. It cannot be retrieved by roughening medication".

Shen xiao **腎消, kidney melting** [8]

PC identical with → *xia xiao* 下消, lower melting. *WTMY* 11: 渴，飲水不能多，但腿腫脚先瘦小，陰痿弱，數小便者。此是腎**消病**也, "One is thirsty, but cannot drink much water. The thighs are swollen; and the legs become emaciated. Dysfunction and weakness of the yin [member, i.e. penis], with increased urination. This is the disease of **kidney melting**".

Shen xie **腎泄, kidney outflow** [4]

PC of patients experiencing semiliquid outflow once or twice at the hour of five *geng*, and continuing for years without ending. *PJBSF* 4: 五味子散，治**腎泄**，五味子（二兩，揀），吳茱萸（半兩，細粒綠色者）。上二味同炒香熟為度，細末。每服二錢，陳米飲下。頃年有一親識，每五更初欲曉時，必溏痢一次，如是數月。有人云：此名**腎泄**，腎感陰氣而然，得此方服之而愈, "The powder with *wu wei zi* cures **kidney outflow**. *Wu wei zi* (2 *liang*, choice quality), *wu zhu yu* (1 half *liang*, fine kernels of a green color). These two substances are to be roasted until a strong fragrant odor has been produced. Prepare a fine powder. Each dose consists of 2 *qian*, to be ingested with the liquid obtained by boiling old rice. A year or so ago, an acquaintance every morning at the 5th *geng* at daybreak inevitably experienced a free-flux illness of semiliquid stools. This went on for several months. Someone said: This is called '**kidney outflow**'. This is so when the kidneys are affected by yin qi. He got hold of this recipe, ingested it, and was cured".

Shen xu **腎虛, kidney depletion** [86]
PC of a kidney depletion with impeded kidney function. *SW* 49: 內奪而厥，則為喑俳，此**腎虛**也, "Internal deprivation and [subsequent] recession results in muteness and lameness. This is a **kidney depletion**".

Shen xu xiao ke **腎虛消渴, melting with thirst associated with kidney depletion** [3]
PC identical with → *xiaxiao* 下消, lower melting. *BCSY* SE *jiayu* 嘉魚：治**腎虛消渴**及勞損羸瘦，皆煮食之, "It cures **melting with thirst associated with kidney depletion**, with exhaustion detriment and emaciation. Always consume boiled".

Shen ying **腎硬, kidneys hardness** [2]
PC of kidney depletion cold of old people that is difficult to cure even by ingesting medications meant to supplement the kidneys. *BCGM* SE *yang* 羊 quotes *JFBJF*: 老人**腎硬**：治老人腎臟虛寒，內腎結硬，雖服補藥不入, "**Kidney hardness** of old people: To cure depletion cold of an old person's kidneys. When the internal kidneys are bound and have hardened, one may ingests kidney-supplementing medication - it will not be able to enter".

Shen zao **腎燥, kidney dryness** [7]
PC brought forth by a loss and depletion of kidney yin qi. *SJZL* 58: 三曰腎消，以渴而復利，**腎燥**不能制約言之 "The third type is called kidney wasting. It is named this way because [patients experience] thirst with repeated free flow [of urine resulting in] uncontrollable **kidney dryness**".

Shen zhi bu shou **神志不守, unruly spirit and mind** [2]
IS identical with → *shen bu shou she* 神不守舍, unsettled spirit. *SYJYBZFL* 12: 張真君茯苓丸，治心腎氣虛，**神志不守**，小便淋瀝，或不禁, The True Lord Zhang's pills with *fu ling* cure qi depletion of heart and kidneys, **unruly spirit and mind**, and urine dripping, sometimes with incontinence.

Shen zhi bu zu **神志不足, spirit and mind [qi] insufficiency** [2]
PC of forgetfulness and bone steaming brought forth by heart and kidney qi insufficiency. *YXRM* 2: 牡丹皮治**神志不足**，神屬心，志屬腎，故八味丸用之以補心腎也, "*Mu dan pi* cures **spirit and mind [qi] insufficiency**. The spirit is associated with the heart; the mind is associated with the kidneys. Hence one uses the pills with the eight ingredients to supplement the heart and kidneys".

Shen zhong **身重, the body feels heavy** [23] AN *ti zhong* 體重; *shen ti zhong* 身體重.
IS of a feeling of extreme heaviness in the body, together with a sensation of fatigue. *JGYL* Fj: 風濕，脈浮，**身重**，汗出, "[In the case of an affection by] wind and moisture, the [movement in the] vessels is at the surface. **The body feels heavy**. [Patients] sweat".

Shen zhu **腎疰, kidney attachment-illness** [2]
PC of a chronic pain in the lumbar region that fails to heal. *BCYY* SE *ju you* 橘柚：**腎疰**、腰痛、膀胱氣痛，微炒核，去殼為末，酒調服，愈, "For **kidney attachment-illness**, lower back pain, bladder qi pain, slightly roast the kernels, remove their shells and grind to a powder. Ingest mixed with wine. This brings the cure".

Sheng chan sun pao **生產損脬, bladder damaged during delivery** [1]

PC identical with → *chan fu pao sun* 產婦脬損, damage to a delivering woman's bladder. *BCGM* SE *juan* 絹：**生產損脬**，小便淋瀝不斷, "**Bladder damaged during delivery** [is associated] with unceasing urine dripping".

Sheng po **聲破, broken voice** [2]

IS identical with → *sheng ya* 聲啞, impaired speech; muteness. *SJZL* 193: 上氣氣閉咳逆，咽冷**聲破**，灸天突五十壯, "In the case of rising qi, qi closure, and cough with counterflow, when the throat is cold and the **voice is broken**, cauterize the *tian tu* [hole] fifty times".

Sheng shi bu chu **聲失不出, loss of voice** [1]

PC identical with → *shi yin* 失音. ① *BCGM* SE *ma bo* 馬勃 quotes *ZXF*: **聲失不出**：馬窊勃、馬牙消等分，研末，沙糖和丸芡子大。噙之, "For **loss of voice**: grind equal amounts of *ma pi bo* and *ma ya xiao* and use powderized sugar to form pills the size of *qian* seeds. They are to be held in the mouth".

Sheng ya **聲啞, impaired speech; muteness** [2] AN *sheng ya* 聲瘂, impaired speech; muteness-disease.

IS of impaired speech, with the voice being low and deep, rather than full and mellow. *SJZL* 66: 治積年咳嗽，**聲啞**，芫根丸方, "Recipe for pills with *yuan gen* to cure cough lasting for years and **impaired speech**".

Sheng ya **聲瘂, impaired speech; muteness-disease** [2]

IS identical with → *sheng ya* 聲啞, impaired speech/muteness. *BCGM* Bai bing zhu zhi yao 百病主治藥 quoting from the main entry of *renshen* 人參：肺熱聲啞, "Lung heat and impaired speech", writes: 肺熱**聲瘂**, "Lung heat and **muteness-disease**".

Sheng yin **聲喑, muteness** [1]

IS identical with → *yin* 喑①. *BCGM* Bai bing zhu zhi yao 百病主治藥：黃芩，熱病**聲喑**，同麥門冬丸服, "Ingest *huang qin* together with the pills with *mai men dong* for heat disease with **muteness**".

Sheng yin bu chu **聲音不出, loss of voice** [1]

IS identical with → *shi yin* 失音② a). *BCGM* SE *ji ti bi sheng* 屐屜鼻繩 quotes *ZHF*: 屍咽痛癢：**聲音不出**。履鼻繩燒灰，水服之, "For corpse throat with pain and itching, and **loss of voice**: burn shoe strings to ashes and ingest with water".

Sheng zi bu xia **生子不下, failure of a child to descend** [1]

PC identical with → *nan chan* 難產, difficult delivery. *BCGM* SE *zha chan* 蚱蟬：小兒驚癇，婦人生子不下, "[It cures] children with fright epilepsy, and women with a **failure of a child [that is to be born] to descend**".

Shi **濕, moisture; to moisten** [p]

① AN *shi bing* 濕病, moisture disease; *shi qi* 濕氣, moisture qi. PC that is difficult to cure and hence lasts for an extended period of time. The disease has its seat in the lower parts of the body; it manifests itself through turbid secretions and is often accompanied by a failure of the spleen's and stomach's functions of transportation and transformation. *SW* 71: 其病**濕**，下重, "The illnesses [caused by] them include **moisture** with pressure below".

② AN *shi qi* 濕氣, moisture qi. EA of the evil qi that is capable of bringing forth moisture disease. It includes moisture causing harm from inside, and moisture affecting the body from outside. *SW* 3: 因於**濕**，首如裹, "As a result of **moisture**, the head [feels] as if it were wrapped up".

③ IS of local liquid seeping or sweat. *SW* 3: 汗出見**濕**，乃生痤疿, "When sweat flows and meets with **moisture** [from outside the body], this generates acne and seething rashes.

④ TA of moistening. *BCSY* Xu li 序例：**濕**可去枯, "**Moistening** is able to eliminate dryness".

⑤ PQ. Ancient criterion of categorizing pharmaceutical substances, referring to drugs with a moistening function. *BCSY* Xu li 序例：藥有宣、通、補、泄、輕、重、澀、滑、燥、**濕**十種，是藥之大體, "There are ten types of pharmaceutical drugs, including those that spread, penetrate, supplement, and drain, and those that are able to lift, press down, roughen, smoothen, dry and **moisten**. These [ten types of functions] include the entire *materia medica*"..

Shi **螫, sting** [p]

EA identical with → *shi ren* 螫人, to sting a person. *QJYF* 25: 治蜂**螫**方，豬脂、蜜（各半升），蠟（二兩）。上三味，和煎如膏，候冷以塗之, "Recipe to cure bee/wasp **sting**: lard, honey (one half *sheng* of each), wax (2 *liang*). Boil these three ingredients together to form a paste. Wait until it has cooled and use for external application".

Shi bi **濕閟, moisture closure** [1]

PC of constipation with intestines and stomach being affected by moisture. *BCGM* SE *bing lang* 檳榔 quoting *PJF* RE *bing lang san* 檳榔散, powder with *bing lang*: 亦治腸胃有濕，大便秘澀, "It also cures the intestines and stomach when they are affected by moisture, with defecation blocked and rough", writes: 大腸**濕閟**：腸胃有濕，大便秘塞, "**Moisture closure** of the large intestine: intestines and stomach are affected by moisture. Defecation is blocked".

Shi bi **濕痹, moisture blockage** [68] AN ***bi shi*** 痹濕.

PC of → *bi bing* 痹病, blockage disease, brought forth by moisture evil. *BJ* SE *che qian zi* 車前子：利水道小便，除**濕痹**, "It eases the flow of urine through the waterways, and eliminates **moisture blockage**".

Shi bi qi **濕痹氣, qi blockage caused by moisture** [2]

PC identical with → *shi bi* 濕痹, moisture blockage. *MYBL* SE *qin gui* 秦龜：主除**濕痹氣**，身重，四肢關節不可動搖, "It controls elimination of **qi blockages caused by moisture**. The body feels heavy, and the joints of the four limbs cannot be moved".

Shi bing **時病, seasonal disease** [3]

PC identical with → *tian xing* 天行, heaven-sent [disease]. *ZBYHL* 9: **時病**始得，一日在皮，二日在膚，三日在肌，四日在胸，五日入胃，入胃乃可下也, "When one has just been affected by a **seasonal disease**, on the first day it is in the skin. On the second day it is in a deeper layer of the skin. On the third day it is in the muscles. On the fourth day it is in the chest. On the fifth day it enters the stomach. Once it has entered the stomach it can be discharged".

***Shi bing* 濕病, moisture disease** [6]

PC identical with → *shi* 濕②. *QJYiF* 9: 傷寒與痓病、**濕病**及熱暍相濫，故敘而論之, "Harm caused by cold is interrelated with spasms, **moisture disease**, as well as heat and sunstroke. Hence they are discussed [here]".

***Shi bing* 屍病, corpse [qi] disease** [3]

PC CD of all diseases associated with *shi* 屍, corpse [qi], such as → *shi zhu* 屍注, corpse [qi] influx, → *fei shi* 飛屍, flying corpse [qi], → *dun shi* 遁屍, run-away corpse [qi]. *ZBYHL* 23: 以其**屍病**注易傍人，故為屍注, "Because the corpse [qi] disease flows into a person nearby it causes a 'corpse [qi] influx'". Under the heading Shi bing zhu hou 屍病諸候, "All signs of **corpse [qi] diseases**", it lists *shi zhu* 屍注, corpse [qi] influx, *fei shi* 飛屍, flying corpse [qi], *dun shi* 遁屍, run-away corpse [qi], and states that all these diseases 變狀多端，其病大體略同，而有小異，但以一方治之, "May assume many forms. Basically they are identical, but in the details of their appearance they may differ. Still, they can be cured with one and the same recipe".

***Shi bing* 虱病, lice disease** [2]

PC resembling an abdominal accumulation caused by living lice. *BCSY* SE *shu bi* 梳篦：**虱病**是活虱入腹為病如癥瘕者, "The **lice disease** is a disease resembling concretion-illness and conglomeration-illness; it is caused by living lice having entered the abdomen".

***Shi chong* 屍蟲, corpse bugs/worms** [9]

EA identical with → *san shi* 三屍, three corpse [evils]. *ZBYHL* 47: **屍蟲**為性忌惡，多接引外邪，共為患害, "The nature of **corpse bugs/worms** is most malign. They often invite evil [qi] from outside, and together they cause suffering".

***Shi chou* 濕臭, moisture with stench** [1]

IS of topical emission of liquid and stench. *ZBYHL* 31: 氣血不和，為風邪所搏，津液蘊瘀，故令**濕臭**, "If qi and blood are not in harmony, they are attacked by wind evil. The body liquids are blocked in their flow. **Moisture with stench** is the result".

***Shi chu guai bing* 虱出怪病, queer disease of lice appearance** [1]

PC with the appearance of lice all over the body after one has gone to bed, and with itching and pain. *BCGM* SE *shi yan* 食鹽 quotes *QJF*: **虱出怪病**：每至臨臥, 渾身虱出約及五升, 隨手血肉俱壞, 每宿漸多, 癢痛不可名狀, 惟吃水臥坐床上, 晝夜號哭, 舌尖血出不止, 牙齒俱黑, 唇動鼻開, "**Queer disease of lice appearance**. Each time one goes to bed lice appear, all over the body, as many as would fill 5 *sheng*. Blood and flesh decay immediately. This increases every night. The itching and pain are undescribable. All one consumes is water, and one sleeps sitting on the bed, wailing day and night. The tip of the tongue bleeds unendingly. The teeth are all black. The lips move and the nose opens".

Shi chuang **蝕瘡, erosion sores** [8] AN *chuang shi* 瘡蝕, sores erosion.
PC CD of open → *chuang* 瘡, sores, conditions reaching deeper than usual. *BJ* SE *yu shi* 礜石：主寒熱，鼠瘺，**蝕瘡**，死肌, "It controls alternating sensations of cold and heat, mouse fistula, **erosion sores**, and dead muscles".

Shi chuang **濕瘡, moist sores** [24]
PC of all → *chuang* 瘡, sores, that are moist or emit liquid. *QJYF* 5: 治**濕瘡**方：濃煎地榆汁，洗浴，每日二度, "Recipe for **moist sores**: Prepare a concentrated decoction of *di yu* juice. Rinse. Twice each day".

Shi dan **濕疸, moisture *dan*-illness** [2] AN *shi huang* 濕黃, moisture jaundice
PC of → *huang dan* 黃疸, yellow *dan*-illness, caused mainly by moisture evil. *ZBYHL* 12: **濕疸**病者，脾胃有熱，與濕氣相搏, "As for **moisture *dan*-illness**, this is a disease where heat in the spleen and stomach clashes with moisture qi".

Shi du **食毒, food poison; food poisoning** [19]
① EA of the poison in a victual. *QJYF* 2 has 解**食毒**第一, "To resolve **food poison**, nr. 1".
② PC of poisoning brought forth by inadequate food and beverages. *WTMY* 31: 古今錄驗療諸**食毒**方, "A recipe from the *GJLY* to cure all types of **food poisoning**". Food poisoning documented in the *BCGM* include *jun du* 菌毒, mushroom poisoning; *mian du* 麵毒, flour poisoning; *cai du* 菜毒, vegetable poisoning; *rou du* 肉毒, meat poisoning, and *yu xie du* 魚蟹毒, fish and crab poisoning.

Shi du **時毒, seasonal poison** [1]
PC identical with → *yi du* 疫毒, epidemic poison. *QXLF* 11: 普濟消毒飲子，**時毒**治驗, "The 'drink for all-encompassing help to dissolve poison'. It has proved to be effective in the cure of **seasonal poison**".

Shi du **石毒, mineral poison; mineral poisoning** [2]
① EA identical with → *shi yao du* 石藥毒, mineral drug poison. *WTMY* 38: 去**石毒**, 麻黄湯方, "Recipe for a decoction with *ma huang* to remove **mineral poison**".
② PC identical with → *ru shi fa* 乳石發, outbreak of stalactite mineral [poisoning]. *QJYiF* 22: 治**石毒**, 或十年、二十年、三十年而發者, "To cure **mineral poisoning** which may break out within ten years, twenty years, or thirty years".

Shi du **螫毒, poisonous bite; poisonous sting** [9]
① PC identical with → *yao du* 咬毒, bite poisoning. *BJ* SE *guan jun* 雚菌：去長蟲，白癬，蟯蟲，蛇**螫毒**, "It serves to remove long worms, white *xuan*-illness, pinworms, and snake **bite poisoning**".
② EA of a poisonous hair or poisonous sting by insects and reptiles. *BCGM* SE *que weng* 雀甕：俗呼毛蟲，又名楊瘌子，因有**螫毒**也, "It is commonly called hairy bug, and also *yang la zi*, because it has a **poisonous sting**".

Shi er xian **十二癇, twelve types of epilepsy** [3]
PC of → *xian ji* 癇疾, epilepsy ailment, classified into twelve categories. *MYBL* SE *long chi* 龍齒：主…小兒五驚**十二癇**，身熱不可近, "It controls the five types of fright and **twelve types of epilepsy** in children".

Shi feng **濕風, moisture and wind** [5]

PC brought about by moisture and wind with pain in hands and feet, as well as painful and itching skin. *YXL* SE *han fang ji* 漢防己：能治**濕風**，口面喎斜，手足疼, "It is able to cure **moisture wind** with wryness of the mouth and face, and painful hands and feet".

Shi fu **食復, recurrence because of food** [19] AN 食勞, food exhaustion.

PC of a recurrence caused by an inadequate diet consumed immediately after a serious disease was cured. See also → *lao fu* 勞復, recurrence because of exhaustion. *ZBYHL* 9: 病新瘥者，脾胃尚虛，穀氣未復，若即食肥肉、魚鱠、餅餌、棗、栗之屬，則未能消化，停積在於腸胃，使脹滿結實，因更發熱，復為病者，名曰**食復**也, "When a disease has just been cured, the spleen and stomach are still depleted, and the qi of grain has not returned yet. If in such a situation one consumes food such as fat meat, herring, pastry, dates, or chestnuts, he will be unable to digest this. The food will remain in the stomach and the intestines, and cause bloating, a feeling of fullness, as well as nodes and repletion. If as a result, there is a renewed effusion of heat, and the disease recurs, this is called **recurrence because of food**".

Shi guo **濕瘑, moist lair-illness** [3]

PC of moist and festering → *guo chuang* 瘑瘡, lair-illness sores. *ZBYHL* 35: **濕瘑**瘡候，其瘡痛癢，搔之汁出，常濡濕者, "The signs of **moist lair-illness** sores: These sores are painful and itch. If scratched, liquid comes out. They are always moist".

Shi han **濕汗, moisture with sweating** [1]

IS of profuse topical moisture and sweating. *SJZL* 101: 治腋下**濕汗**不止，及足心、手掌、陰下、股裏，常如汗濕臭者方, "Recipes to cure unending **moisture with sweating** under the armpits, as well as constant conditions resembling sweating with moisture stench on the soles of the feet, on the palms of the hands, below the private parts, and on the insides of the thighs.

Shi hui **石蛔, stone[-like] roundworm** [4]

PC of intractable and difficult to cure → *hui chong* 蛔蟲②, roundworm, disease. *BCSY* SE *si ren chen ji xi* 死人枕及席：**石蛔**者，醫療既癖，蛔蟲轉堅，世間藥不能遣, 所以須鬼物馳之，然後乃散，故令煮死人枕服"As for **stone[-like] roundworm**, when medically treated it forms an aggregation-illness. The roundworms turn hard, and no medication on earth is able to eliminate them. This is why one must resort to demonic items to get it moving and then to have it dispersed. Hence [the patient] is ordered to prepare and ingest a decoction from a dead person's headrest".

Shi huo luan **濕霍亂, moist cholera** [2]

PC of → *huo luan* 霍亂, cholera, including vomiting and diarrhea. *WTMY* 6: 上吐下痢者，名為**濕霍亂**, "If someone suffers from vomiting above and free-flux illness below, this is called **moist cholera**".

Shi ji **時疾, seasonal ailment** [51]

PC identical with → *tian xing* 天行, heaven-sent [disease]. *WTMY* 13: 五疰丸：一名神仙丸, 一名千金丸, 一名轉疰丸, 一名司命丸, 一名殺鬼丸。療萬病, 邪鬼疰忤, 心痛上氣, 厭夢蠱毒, 傷寒**時疾**疫癘方, "The pills for the five types of attachment-illness: Another name: 'pills of spirits and hermits'. Another name: 'pills worth thousands in gold'. Another name: 'pills transforming attachment-illness'. Another name: 'pills guarding life'. Another name: 'pills that kill demons'. They are a recipe to cure a myriad of diseases, attachment-illness and hostilities by evil demons, heart pain with rising qi, nightmares and *gu* poisoning, harm caused by cold, **seasonal ailments**, and epidemics".

Shi ji **食積, food accumulation** [50]

① EA PM identical with → *su shi* 宿食①, food remaining in the body over night. *JYBC* SE *meng shi* 礞石：**食積**不消，留滯在臟腑, "[It controls] **food accumulations** failing to dissolve and stagnating sluggishly in the depots and palaces". *BCGM* Bai bing zhu zhi yao 百病主治藥 traces pathological conditions such as distension and fullness, jaundice, leg qi, pain in the heart and abdominal region, as well as pain in the lower flanks to food accumulation.

② PC identical with *su shi* 宿食②, food remaining in the body overnight. *SJZL* 71: 治**食積**，隱見時作, "To cure **food accumulation** that is alternatingly dormant and then active again".

Shi ji re chuang **時疾熱瘡, heat sores associated with seasonal ailments** [1]
AN → *shi ji re biao chuang* 時疾熱熛瘡, flaming-heat sores associated with seasonal ailments.

PC of → *re chuang* 熱瘡, heat sores, developing in the aftermath of → *shi ji* 時疾, seasonal ailments. *RHZ* SE *xiao mai* 小麥：麩，涼。治**時疾熱瘡**，湯火瘡爛，撲損傷折瘀血，醋炒貼罯, "Cold bran cures **heat sores associated with seasonal ailments**; festering sores resulting from boiling water and fire; bruises, injuries, fractures, and stagnant blood [that has left the vessels]. Stir-fry in vinegar and apply locally".

Shi jiao **屍脚, corpse leg** [5]

PC of an inclination of one's leg to break regardless of whether it is winter or summer. *ZBYHL* 30: **屍脚**者，脚跟坼破之名也, 亦是冬時觸犯寒氣所以然。又言脚踏死屍所臥地，亦令脚坼破, "As for **corpse leg**, this is the designation of a fractured leg or heel. It may also be that [a leg] was struck by cold qi in winter. It is also said that stepping on the ground where a corpse had been lying causes a leg to fracture".

Shi jiao qi **濕脚氣, moist leg qi** [1]

PC of edema affecting the leg and knee in the course of a → *jiao qi* 脚氣, leg qi, disease. *TPSHF* 45: 其候：脚膝浮腫, 故名**濕脚氣**也, "The signs are: the legs and knees are swollen. Hence it is called **moist leg qi**".

Shi jie **濕疥, moisture *jie*-illness** [1]

PC of → *jie chuang* 疥瘡, *jie*-illness sores, of small size and with weak skin emitting a flow of liquid as the major sign. *ZBYHL* 35: **濕疥**者，小瘡，皮薄，常有

汁出, "**Moisture *jie*-illness**: [This condition manifests itself] as small sores. The skin is thin. There is a continuous release of liquid".

***Shi jing* 失精, involuntary loss of essence/semen** [16]

PC identical with → *yi jing* 遺精. *JGYL* Fj: 脈得諸芤動微緊，男子**失精**, "The movement felt in the vessels is hollow and slightly tense. Males experience **involuntary emission of essence**".

***Shi ju* 石疽, stone impediment-illness** [1]

PC of → *ju* 疽, impediment-illness, brought forth by cold, with the affected region being both quite thick, hard as stone, and of a relatively small circumference. *ZNYHL* 33: 其寒毒偏多，則氣結聚而皮厚，狀如痤癤，堅如石，故謂之**石疽**也, "If there is a unilateral preponderance of cold, the qi will form nodular collections and the skin thickens. The appearance is that of acne pimples. They are hard as stone. Hence they are called '**stone impediment-illness**'".

***Shi jue* 屍厥, corpse[-like condition because of qi] recession** [12]

PC of sudden unconsciousness. Patients are unable to recognize people, while the pulse remains normal. *SW* 63: 人身脈皆動，而形無知也，其狀若屍，或曰**屍厥**, "This makes all the vessels in the [affected] person's body move while his physical appearance gives no response. These people resemble a corpse. Sometimes it is called **corpse[-like condition because of qi] recession**.

***Shi lan* 濕爛, moist festering** [14]

IS of topical emission of liquid together with festering. *ZBYHL* 30: 風邪寒濕之氣搏於瘡，則微腫**濕爛**, "When the qi of wind evil, cold, and moisture affects the sores, this results in a slight swelling and **moist festering**".

***Shi lan chuang* 濕爛瘡, moist and festering sores** [1]

PC of all → *chuang* 瘡, sores, which are moist or emit liquid and simultaneously fester. *PJF* 300: 淨肌散，治一切臀腿手足**濕爛瘡**, "The 'powder to cleanse flesh' cures all types of **moist and festering sores** on the buttocks, legs, hands and feet".

***Shi lao* 食勞, food exhaustion** [2]

① PC identical with → *shi fu* 食復, recurrence because of food. *QJYF* 10: 治食勞方，麺二升煮取汁服之, "Recipe for curing **food exhaustion**: Boil two *sheng* of flour in water. Consume the liquid".

② EA of immoderate eating and drinking. *TPSHF* 49: 治食癥癖氣，**食勞**，宿食不消，痰逆，京三棱丸方, "To cure food-induced qi concretion-illness and aggregation-illness, **food exhaustion** with food that remains in the body overnight without being digested, and phlegm counterflow, [use] the recipe for pills with *jing san leng*".

***Shi lao huang* 食勞黃, food exhaustion jaundice** [2]

PC identical with *gu dan* 穀疸, grain *dan*-illness. *PJF* 195: 棗礬丸，治**食勞黃**，目黃身黃者, "Pills with *zao fan* cure **food exhaustion jaundice**. The eyes and the entire body are yellow".

***Shi leng* 濕冷, moisture and cold; moisture-cold** [2]

PC identical with → *han shi* 寒濕, cold-moisture. *QJYF* 8: 排風湯，治男子婦人風虛**濕冷**, "The 'decoction to expel wind' cures wind [intruding into a state of] depletion and **moisture-cold** of males and females".

***Shi li* 濕痢, moisture free-flux illness** [2]

PC of → *li ji* 痢疾, free-flux illness, where moisture qi troubles the spleen. It is accompanied by a feeling of heaviness in the body, abdominal distension, fatigue and lack of strength, as well as lack of appetite. *QXLF* 13 **濕痢**久不斷，體瘦多昏，坐則閉目，食不下, "**Moisture free-flux illness** that cannot be stopped for a long time. The body is emaciated and often [patients are] mentally disturbed. When they sit down, they close their eyes. They cannot eat".

***Shi lin* 石淋, stone dripping** [66] AN *sha lin* 沙淋, sand dripping; *sha shi lin* 沙石淋, sand and stone dripping.

PC of difficult urination, or sudden interruption of urine flow, with an uncomfortable feeling and pain in the urinary tract, an unbearable twisting pain in the lower back and abdomen, and the excreted urine appearing as small stones. *BJ* SE *shi dan* 石膽：主明目，目痛，金瘡，諸癇痙，女子陰蝕痛，**石淋**，寒熱, "It is responsible for clearing eyesight, [and cures] aching eyes, wounds inflicted by metal objects, all types of epilepsy and spasms, erosion in the female genital region, **stone dripping**, and alternating sensations of cold and heat".

***Shi liu* 虱瘤, lice tumor** [3]

PC of tumors generated by lice or parasitic microorganisms resembling lice, with localized itching. When the tumors open lice appear. *BCGM* SE *ren shi* 人虱 quotes *JSL*: 浮梁李生背起如盂，惟癢不可忍，人皆不識。醫士秦德立云：此**虱瘤**也。以藥傅之，一夕瘤破，出虱斗余, "Mr. Li from Fuliang had a growth like a jar on his back. The itching was unbearable. Nobody knew what this was. Qin Deli, a physician, said: This is a **lice tumor**. He applied a medication to it. After one night had passed the tumor broke open and more than a bushel of lice left it".

***Shi lou* 濕漏, moist leakage** [1]

PC of → *yong* 癰, obstruction-illness, and → *jie* 癤, pimples, releasing pus and water. *QJYF* 22：治石癰堅如石，不作膿者方…又治**濕漏**諸癰癤, "The recipe to cure non-festering stone obstruction-illnesses that are hard as a stone…It also cures obstruction-illnesses and pimples with **moist leakage**".

***Shi ming* 失明, loss of vision, blindness** [22] AN *mu mang* 目盲; *gu* 瞽; *xia* 瞎.

PC with loss of vision. *ZBYHL* 28: 生白障者，是疾重極，遍覆黑睛，滿眼悉白，則**失明**也, "When a white screen develops, a severe peak of the ailment is reached. It covers the entire black part of the eyeball and makes the entire eye appear white. **Loss of vision** is the result".

***Shi ni* 失溺, loss of urine** [5]

IS identical with → *yi niao* 遺尿. *MYBL* SE *gou ji* 狗脊：療**失溺**不節，男子脚弱腰痛, "It cures uncontrolled **loss of urine**; weak legs in males and pain in the lower back".

Shi ni **濕䘌, moisture hidden-worms infestation** [5]

PC of worms infestation whereby moisture has entered the spleen and stomach in a situation of depletion and weakness resulting from incessant diarrhea. The illness signs are frequent panting, ulcers on the upper lip, mental vexation, and depression, or ulcers on the lower lip, and anal decay. In severe cases the lips, mouth, and gums all develop ulcers. The teeth blacken and decay; blood and watery liquid flow freely. *ZBYHL* 18: **濕䘌**病，由脾胃虛弱，為水濕所乘，腹內蟲動，侵食成䘌也, "The disease of **moisture hidden-worms infestation** results from an intrusion of moisture into a depleted and weak spleen and stomach. This causes worms to move in the abdomen. They enter and feed [on the organs], and this causes hidden-worms infestation".

Shi nüe **食瘧, food malaria** [5] AN *ji nüe* 積瘧, accumulation malaria.

PC of → *nüe ji* 瘧疾, malaria ailment, associated with food accumulation. The clinical appearance, in addition to regularly recurring alternating sensations of cold and heat, includes a feeling of distension and pain in the stomach tract and abdomen, sometimes with a tendency to avoid eating. *WTMY* 5: 服藥忌飽飯，**食瘧**斷後食如常，萬不失一, "When ingesting this medication one must not eat to repletion. After the **food malaria** has been ended, one may eat as usual. Not one treatment in a myriad of cases will fail".

Shi qi **時氣, seasonal qi** [77]

① PC identical with → *tian xing* 天行, heaven-sent [disease]. *ZHBJF* 2 lists a *zhi shang han shi qi wen bing fang* 治傷寒**時氣**温病方, "Recipe to cure harm caused by cold, **seasonal qi**, and warmth disease".

② EA *ZBYHL* 42: 此時普行此氣，故云**時氣**也 "In this season this qi is universally active. Hence it is called **seasonal qi**.

③ The normal climatic qi associated with any of the four seasons. *QJYF* 27: 衣食寢處皆適，能順**時氣**者，始盡養生之道, "If clothing, food, rest, and work are all appropriate, and if one is able to live in accordance with the **seasonal qi**, then this is all there is to the Dao of nourishing life".

Shi qi **濕氣, moisture qi** [63]

① EA identical with → *shi* 濕①, moisture. *SW* 5: 地之**濕氣**，感則害皮肉筋脈, "When one is affected by the **moisture qi** of the earth, this harms the skin, the flesh, the sinews, and the vessels".

② PC identical with → *shi* 濕②, moisture. *DXZFXY* Yi'an shi yi 醫案拾遺, Medical case histories to supplement omissions: 一人年三十患**濕氣**，四肢疼痛，兩足難移, "A man at the age of 30 suffered from **moisture qi**. His four extremities were painful, and he had difficulties moving his legs".

③ The qi of rain and moisture in nature. *SW* 71: 三之氣，天政布，**濕氣**降，地氣騰, "The third qi: The policy of heaven is widespread. **Moisture qi** descends; the qi of the earth surges".

Shi qi **屍氣, corpse qi** [3]

① EA bringing forth exhaustion-consumption. *ZBYHL* 23: 人有觸值死屍，或臨屍，其**屍氣**入腹內，與屍蟲相接成病, "When someone touches a corpse, or is near a corpse, the **corpse qi** enters his abdomen where it encounters corpse bugs/worms to generate disease".

② PC resulting from inhaling corpse qi, with the corpse qi reaching heart and abdomen where it generates a piercing pain as well as distension and a feeling of fullness, accompanied by qi urgency. *ZBYHL* 23:其發亦心腹刺痛，脹滿氣急。但聞**屍氣**則發，故謂之**屍氣**, "When it breaks out, [patients] feel a piercing pain in the heart and abdomen, with distension, a feeling of fullness and qi urgency. One only needs to inhale **corpse qi** and it will break out. Hence it is called '**corpse qi**'".

③ The stench emitted by a rotting corpse. *BCGM* SE *bao yu* 鮑魚 quoting *TBC*: 鮑似屍臭, "*Bao*-fish stinks like a corpse", writes: 彌臭似**屍氣**, "Its stench resembles that of **corpse qi**".

Shi qi fa dong 石氣發動, **outbreak of [stalactite] mineral [poison] qi** [1]

PC identical with → *ru shi fa* 乳石發, outbreak of stalactite mineral [poisoning]. *BCSY* SE *long zhu* 龍珠：主諸熱毒, **石氣發動**, 調中, 解煩, "It controls all types of heat poisoning and **outbreaks of [stalactite] mineral [poison] qi**; it regulates the center, and resolves vexation".

Shi re 實熱, **repletion heat** [23]

PC of a) an overabundance of yang heat without a weakening yet of proper qi. *ZBYHL* 35: 凡疽發於脛，名曰兔嚙瘡。一名血實瘡。又隨月生死。蓋月食之類，非脛瘡也。尋此瘡，亦風濕搏於血氣，血氣**實熱**所生，故一名血實, "All impediment-illnesses effusing at the shins are called 'hare teeth sores'. Another name is 'blood repletion sores'. They wax and wane with the moon. Now, sores of the 'lunar eclipse' type do not emerge on the shins. If one looks for these sores [discussed here], they emerge when wind and moisture clash with blood and qi, and blood and qi develop **repletion heat**. Hence another name is 'blood repletion'". b) An overabundance of internal heat with blocked passage of stools and urine. *WTMY* 6: 中焦**實熱**閉塞，上下不通, "The central burner has **repletion heat** and is blocked. The passages above and below are closed".

Shi re 濕熱, **moisture and heat** [253] CD of *shi* 濕, moisture, and *re* 熱, heat.

① EA identified as simultaneous appearance of moisture and heat. *SW* 3: **濕熱**不攘，大筋緛短，小筋弛長, "If **moisture and heat** are not driven out, the large sinews will shrink and shorten; the small sinews will slacken and extend".

② PC brought about by moisture and heat. *TYBC* SE *yin chen hao* 茵陳蒿：仲景茵陳梔子大黃湯治**濕熱**也, "[Zhang] Zhongjing used the decoction with *yin chen hao* seeds and decoction with *da huang* to cure **moisture and heat**". *BCGM* lists many diseases associated with moisture and heat, such as *pi wei shi re* 脾胃濕熱, moisture and heat affecting spleen and stomach; *xia jiao shi re* 下焦濕熱, the lower burner affected by moisture and heat.

③ CC of late summer when moisture and heat interact. *SW* 71: 四之氣，溽暑**濕熱**相薄, "The fourth qi: Humidity and summerheat; **moisture and heat** strike each other".

Shi re bu tong **實熱不通, repletion heat blocking the passage [of stools]** [2]

PC of → *da bian mi* 大便秘①, constipation, brought forth by body repletion with heat. *YXQY* Lj: 瀉諸**實熱不通**，下大便，蕩滌腸胃中熱, "It drains all **heat repletion blocking the passage [of stools]**. It stimulates defecation. It purges the heat in the intestines and stomach".

Shi ren **螫人, to sting a person** [41] AD *shi* 螫, sting; AN *shi nie* 螫嚙, [injury from] sting and bite; *ding shi* 叮螫，[injury from a] sting.

EA of a sting or bite with poisonous teeth by a venomous bug/worm or snake that may generate a poisoning injury affecting either a body region or the entire human body. *BCJJZ* SE *shi long zi* 石龍子：一種喜緣籬壁，名蝘蜓，形小而黑，乃言**螫人**必死, "An animal that prefers to live in hedges and walls, named *yan ting*. It is small and black. It is said that when it **stings a person**, [this person] will have to die". *BCGM* lists the following animals that may sting a person: *wu song* 蜈蚣, centipede; *xie chai* 蠍蠆, scorpion; *du she* 毒蛇, poisonous snake; *du feng* 毒蜂, poisonous wasp; *she xie* 蛇蠍, snakes and scorpions; *she feng* 蛇蜂, snakes and bees/wasps; *fu she* 蝮蛇, pallas pit viper; zhu she 諸蛇, all types of snakes; *mao chong* 毛蟲, hairy bugs/worms; *feng chai* 蜂蠆, bees/wasps and scorpions; *sang xie* 桑蠍, mulberry scorpion; *shou gong* 守宮, palace guardian; *chong yi* 蟲蟻, bugs/worms and ants. It also mentions the animals' organs causing a sting, such as *chong ci* 蟲刺, a worm's/bug's sting; *xie ci* 蠍刺, a scorpion's sting, and *ran si bei mao* 蛅蟖背毛, hair on the back of *ran-si* caterpillars.

Shi ru fan chu **食入反出, regurgitation of food** [2]

IS of food being thrown up again from the stomach. This may be in the evening after having eaten in the morning, or in the morning after having eaten in the evening, and also vomiting immediately after having eaten. *QXLF* 18: 食不得入，是有火也，**食入反出**，是無火也, "An inability to consume food shows a presence of fire; a **regurgitation of food** shows an absence of fire".

Shi ru ji tu **食入即吐, vomiting after having eaten** [5]

IS identical with *shi yi ji tu* 食已即吐, vomiting after having eaten. *QJYiF* 10: 少陰病，食入即吐, "When the minor yin has a disease, [patients] **vomit after having eaten**".

Shi shang **螫傷, injury from a sting** [38] AW *shang shi* 傷螫; *shi ren* 螫人, to sting a person; *shi nie* 螫嚙, [injury from] sting and bite; *ding shi* 叮螫，[injury from a] sting.

PC of a → *shang sun* 傷損, injury, that is a → *zhong du* 中毒, poisoning, caused by poisonous sting or teeth of a venomous bug/worm or snake. *PJF* 307: 治蠍**螫傷**，詩曰：曾聞蠍螫徹心田，休候雞兒叫曉天。耳塞調來疼處抹，除毒減痛却依元, "To cure an **injury from a** scorpion **sting**, a poem says: I have heard, an **injury from a** scorpion **sting** goes right into the heart. But it is not necessary to wait for the rooster to crow at dawn. Just prepare some earwax and smear it on where the pain is located. This will remove the poison, diminish the pain, and restore [the patient's] original condition". *BCGM* lists the following animals as potential causers of an injury from a sting: *she hui* 蛇虺, venomous viper; *du she* 毒蛇, poisonous snake; *du feng* 毒蜂, poisonous wasp; *she chong* 蛇蟲, snakes and bugs/worms; *zhu she* 諸蛇, all types of snakes; *she xie* 蛇蠍, snakes and scorpions; *fu she* 蝮蛇, pallas pit viper; *xie chai* 蠍蠆, scorpion; *feng xie* 蜂蠍, wasps/bees and scorpions; *feng chai* 蜂蠆, scorpion.

Shi sheng **失聲, loss of voice** [7]
PC and IS identical with → *shi yin* 失音. *ZHF* 3: 治卒**失聲**，聲噎不出方, "Recipe to cure sudden **loss of voice** when no sound can be released".

Shi shui **石水, stone water** [8]
PC of → *shui zhong* 水腫, water swelling, disease with abdominal distension and hardening, and an emaciation of the four limbs. *SW* 7: 陰陽結斜，多陰少陽曰**石水**，少腹腫, "In the case of nodes where yin and yang [vessels branch out] diagonally, with more on the yin and less on the yang [part], this is called '**stone water**'. The lower abdomen is swollen".

Shi sou **濕嗽, moisture cough** [2]
PC of → *ke sou* 咳嗽, cough, brought forth by moisture evil. *RMSQ* 6: **濕嗽, moisture cough**: 趙君玉妻病嗽，時已十月矣。戴人處方六味；陳皮、當歸、甘草、白术、枳殼、桔梗。君玉疑其不類嗽藥。戴人笑曰：君怪無烏梅、罌粟殼乎？夫冬嗽，乃秋之濕也。濕土逆而為嗽，此方皆散氣除濕，解急和經。三服帖然效矣, "The wife of Zhao Junyu had already suffered from a cough for ten months. Dairen devised a recipe with six ingredients: *chen pi*, *dang gui*, *gan cao*, *bai zhu*, *zhi ke*, and *jie geng*. Junyu voiced her doubts that these are not drugs related to cough. Dairen laughed and told her: You wonder why [this recipe] does not include *wu mei* and *ying su ke*? Now, coughing in winter, this is the moisture of autumn. Moisture and soil move towards each other, and this results in a cough. All ingredients of this recipe serve to disperse qi and to eliminate moisture. They resolve tightness and harmonize the conduits. Ingesting three doses will show the desired effect".

Shi tan **食痰, food [and] phlegm** [1]
PC. A variant of → *tan bing* 痰病, phlegm disease, brought forth by a simultaneous presence of undigested food and phlegm. *RYJY* RE *er chen tang* 二陳湯, decoction with two matured ingredients: 夫二陳湯，內有半夏，其煨熱，若風痰、寒痰與**食痰**則相宜, "Now, as for the 'decoction with the two matured ingredients', among its ingredients is *ban xia*. If heated over a slow fire it is suitable for [treating] wind phlegm, cold phlegm, and **food phlegm**".

Shi tan **濕痰, moisture and phlegm** [38] AW *tan shi* 痰濕, phlegm and moisture.
① EA of → *shi* 濕①, moisture, and *tan* 痰, phlegm, jointly bringing forth disease. *DXXF* 2: 熱痰能降，**濕痰**能燥, "Heat and phlegm can be brought down; **moisture and phlegm** can be dried up".
② PC brought forth by moisture and phlegm. *DXXF* 2: 風痰多見奇證，**濕痰**多見倦怠軟弱, "Wind and phlegm is often associated with strange pathological signs. **Moisture and phlegm** is often accompanied by ennui and weakness".

Shi ting **食停, food halt** [1]
PC identical with → *shi zhi* 食滯, food stagnation. *BCGM* SE *xing* 杏 quotes *YSJCF*: 一切**食停**，氣滿膨脹, 用紅杏仁三百粒，巴豆二十粒同炒，色變去豆不用，研杏為末，橘皮湯調下"In all cases of **food halt** with qi fullness, swell-

ing and distension, take 200 red pieces of *xing ren* and 20 pieces of *ba dou*, to be roasted together. When the color changes, discard the [*ba*] *dou*, they must not be used. Grind the *xing* [*ren*] to a powder, and ingest mixed with a *ju pi* decoction".

Shi tong **時痛, intermittent pain** [3]
IS of a pain that is felt sporadically. Sometimes it appears to be gone; sometimes it is present again. *LS* 6: 寒痹之為病也，留而不去，**時痛**而皮不仁, "The disease of cold blockage stays and does not go away. There is **intermittent pain**, and the skin is numb".

Shi wen **濕温, moisture and warmth** [1]
PC brought forth by a simultaneous affection with moisture evil and heat evil. *NJ* 58: 傷寒有五，有中風，有傷寒，有**濕温**，有熱病，有温病，其所苦各不同, "There are five types of harm caused by cold: wind stroke, harm caused by cold, **moisture and warmth**, heat disease, and warmth disease. Each of them causes a different ailment".

Shi xian **食癇, food epilepsy** [3]
PC of → *xian bing* 癇病, epilepsy disease, among children improperly fed with milk. *ZBYHL* 45: **食癇**者，因乳哺不節所成, "**Food epilepsy** is caused by immoderate breast-feeding".

Shi xie **食泄, food outflow** [1]
PC identical with *ji xie* 積泄, accumulation outflow. *BCGM* SE *huang lian* 黄連 quotes *HRXT*: 脾積**食泄**：川黄連二兩，為末，大蒜搗和丸梧子大，每服五十丸，白湯下, "Spleen accumulation with **food outflow**: *chuan huang lian*, 2 *liang*, powderize; *da suan*; pound and prepare to pills the size of *wu* seeds. Each time ingest 50 pills with clear hot water".

Shi xie **濕瀉, moisture outflow** [4]
PC of diarrhea brought forth by moisture harming the spleen and stomach. *DXXF* Lj: **濕瀉**由坐臥濕處，以致濕氣傷脾，土不克水, "**Moisture outflow** results from sitting or lying at a moist place with the result that moisture qi harms the spleen. Soil does not overcome water".

Shi xie **濕泄, moisture outflow** [5]
PC identical with → *shi xie* 濕瀉, moisture outflow. *BCGM* Bai bing zhu zhi yao 百病主治藥：山藥，**濕泄**，同蒼朮丸服, "*Shan yao*: In case of **moisture outflow**, ingest together with *cang zhu* pills".

Shi xin feng **失心風, loss-of-heart wind** [4]
PC identical with → *dian feng* 癲病, peak-illness. *ZBZZZS* Shen zhi men, 神志門, Section spirit and mind: 癲病，俗謂之**失心風**，多因抑鬱不遂，傺無聊而成。精神恍惚，言語錯亂，喜怒不常，有狂之意，不如狂之甚。狂者暴病，癲則久病也, "Peak-illness is commonly called '**loss-of-heart wind**'. This is often caused by a depression, when [a person] is hindered in his activities, and his life has no meaning. He is absent-minded, and his language is chaotic. Happiness and anger are irregular. He seems to be mad, but it is not a serious condition of madness. Madness is a sudden, violent disease. Peak-illness is a chronic disease".

Shi xing 時行, seasonally active [disease] [49]
PC identical with → *tian xing* 天行, heaven-sent [disease]. *ZBYHL* 9: **時行**病者，是春時應暖而反寒，夏時應熱而反冷，秋時應涼而反熱，冬時應寒而反温，此非其時而有其氣，是以一歲之中，病無長少，率相似者，此則**時行**之氣也, "**Seasonally active diseases** emerge when in spring when it should be warm, it is cold instead, when in summer when it should be hot it is cold instead, when in autumn when it should be cool it is hot instead, and when in winter when it should be cold it is warm instead. This is the presence of a qi whose time has not come. If in the course of a year the severity or lengths of diseases [affecting various people] are very similar, then this is a **seasonally active** [disease] qi".

Shi xing re biao chuang 時行熱熛瘡, seasonally active flaming-heat sores [1]
PC identical with → *shi ji re chuang* 時疾熱瘡, heat sores associated with seasonal ailments. *BCGM* Bai bing zhu zhi yao 百病主治藥：羊膽，**時行熱熛瘡**，和酢服, "The gallbladder of sheep: ingest with vinegar for **seasonally active flaming-heat sores**".

Shi xuan 濕癬, moisture _xuan_-illness [12]
PC of → *xuan* 癬, *xuan*-illness, local red and moist lesions brough forth jointly by wind and moisture, with a larger proportion of moisture than wind. *ZBYHL* 35: **濕癬**者，亦有匡郭，如蟲行，浸淫，赤，濕癢，搔之多汁成瘡, "**Moisture *xuan*-illness** also has an outer wall. [Patients feel] as if there were bugs/worms moving. There are [skin lesions] soaked [with pus and/or liquid], redness, moisture, and itching. Scratching it will release much liquid and generate sores".

Shi xue 失血, loss of blood [27] AN *qu xue* 去血.
PC of a loss, through bleeding, of a large quantity of blood. *ZBYHL* 36: 夫金瘡**失血**，則經絡空竭，津液不足, "Now, if there is a **loss of blood** because of wounds inflicted by metal objects, then the conduits and network [vessels] are empty and [the body] does not have enough liquids". *BCGM* has *lao zhai shi xue* 勞瘵失血, loss of blood because of exhaustion; *chang feng shi xue* 腸風失血, loss of blood because of intestinal wind; *shang zhong shi xue* 傷中失血, loss of blood because of harm in the center.

Shi yan 屍咽, corpse [bugs/worms] throat [14]
PC of a disease affecting the throat with pain and itching and loss of voice. *ZBYHL* 30: **屍咽**者，謂腹內屍蟲，上食人喉咽生瘡。其狀或癢或痛, "**Corpse [bugs/worms] throat** is to say: corpse bugs/worms in the abdomen rise to gnaw on the throat and thereby cause sores. The [disease] manifests itself sometimes as itching and sometimes as pain.

Shi yang 濕癢, moisture itching [37]
IS of topical emission of liquid together with itching. *BJ* SE *she chuang zi* 蛇床子：主婦人陰中腫痛，男子陰痿**濕癢**, "It controls swelling and pain in the female private parts. In males dysfunction of the yin [member, i.e. penis], with **moisture itching**".

Shi yao du 石藥毒, **mineral drug poison** [4] AN *ru shi du* 乳石毒, stalactite mineral poison; *shi du* 石毒, mineral poison; *wu shi du* 五石毒, the five mineral poisons.
EA CD of the poison of medication based on finest stalactite powder ingested to strengthen the body. *QJYF* 24: **石藥毒**：用白鴨屎、人參汁, "For **mineral drug poison**: use the feces of white ducks and *ren shen* juice".

Shi ye 食噎, **gullet occlusion by food** [2]
PC identical with → *ye bing* 噎病, gullet occlusion disease. *MYBL* SE *ling yang jiao* 羚羊角：除邪氣驚夢，狂越僻謬及**食噎**不通, "To eliminate evil qi with fright and dreams, crazy jumping with absurd behavior, as well as **gullet occlusion by food** failing to pass".

Shi yi 時疫, **seasonal epidemic** [6]
PC identical with → *wen yi* 瘟疫, warmth-illness epidemic. *QJYF* 9 RE *xiong huang wan* 雄黃丸, pills with *xiong huang*: 卒中惡病及**時疫**，吞如梧子一丸，燒彈大一丸戶內, "In the case of the disease of suddenly being struck by the malign and **seasonal epidemics**, swallow one pill the size of a *wu* seed and burn one pill the size of a bullet inside the house".

Shi yi ji tu 食已即吐, **vomiting after having eaten** [2]
IS of vomiting soon after one has had a meal. *JGYL* Mj: **食已即吐**者，大黃甘草湯主之, "When [patients] **vomit after having eaten**, this will be controlled by a decoction with *da huang* and *gan cao*".

Shi yin 失音, **loss of voice** [81] AN *shi sheng* 失聲.
① PC with a loss of voice resulting from a local throat disease as the major sign. *ZBYHL* 48: 暴寒氣客於喉厭，喉厭得寒，即不能發聲，故卒然**失音**也。不能語者，語聲不出，非牙關噤也, "Suddenly cold qi settles at the throat lid. When the throat lid is affected by cold, [the patient] suddenly experiences a **loss of voice**. That he cannot speak, this is because no sound is released. It is not because of clenched jaw".
② IS of a) an inability to produce voice sounds because of a local throat disease. *QJYF* 8: 喑不能言及喉痹**失音**，皆風邪所為也, "Muteness with an inability to speak, and throat blockage with a **loss of voice**, all these are caused by wind evil". b) Being struck by wind and a resulting tongue lameness making it impossible to speak. *QJYF* 8: 猝倒悶絕，即不能語便**失音**，半身不隨, "Sudden fall, with heart-pressure and unconsciousness. [Patients] cannot speak; they have **lost their voice**. Half their body is paralyzed".

Shi yong 石癰, **stone obstruction-illness** [12]
PC of → *yong* 癰, obstruction-illness, which feels hard, has a root reaching deep into the skin, with the skin not being overly hot, and which begins to fester only after an extended period of time. *ZBYHL* 32: 此寒多熱少，堅如石，故謂之**石癰**也, "This is mostly cold and rarely hot, and it is hard as a stone. Hence it is called '**stone obstruction-illness**'".

Shi yu 食郁, **pent-up food** [3]
PC of one of → *liu yu* 六郁, the six types of pent-up [matter in the organism]. Refers to accumulation disease brought forth by stagnant food and beverages,

with sour regurgitation and a feeling of fullness such that one cannot eat. *DXXF* 3: **食郁**者，噯酸，腹飽不能食, "In the case of **pent-up food**, sour regurgitation, and a feeling of fullness, with [patients] being unable to eat".

***Shi yu* 濕郁, pent-up moisture** [5]

① EA of moisture blocking the qi dynamics. It clogs and cannot be overcome. *DXSJ* Lj: 清濁相混，**濕郁**為熱, "When the clear and the turbid mix, this results in **pent-up moisture** causing heat".

② PC of congestion brought forth by moisture evil that does not dissipate. One of the six types of pent-up [qi], yu 郁. *DXXF* 3: **濕郁**者，周身走痛，或關節痛，遇陰寒則發，脈沉細, "In the case of **pent-up moisture**, the entire body feels pain, or at least the joints ache. This develops if one encounters cold. The [movement in the] vessels is deep inside and fine".

***Shi zheng* 食癥, food concretion-illness** [2]

PC of → *zheng* 癥, concretion-illness, associated with a sudden craving for food as its characteristic sign. *ZBYHL* 19: **食癥**候：有人卒大能食，乖其常分, "The signs of **food concretion-illness**: When someone suddenly consumes massive quantities of food, vastly exceeding normal portions".

***Shi zheng* 虱癥, lice concretion-illness** [3]

PC of → *zheng* 癥, concretions-illness, which forms when lice crushed with one's teeth and swallowed in excessive quantities collect in the organs without being digested. *ZBYHL* 19: **虱癥**候：人有多虱而性好嚙之，所嚙既多，腑臟虛弱，不能消之，不幸變化生癥，而患者亦少, "The signs of **lice concretion-illness**: When someone has many lice and prefers to chew them, and if those chewed are too many, in case the depots and palaces are depleted and weak and are unable to dissolve them, it may be that they are transformed into concretion-illness. However, not many suffer from this".

***Shi zhi* 食滯, sluggish food** [3] AN *shi ting* 食停, food halt; *ting shi* 停食, halting food.

PC of beverages and food in the stomach and intestines not being digested in due time. *SJZL* 172：消肌疳煩熱，化腸胃**食滯**, "It dissolves muscle *gan*-illness and vexing heat; it transforms **sluggish food** in the intestines and the stomach".

***Shi zhi* 食痔, food piles** [2]

PC of → *zhi* 痔, piles, resulting from an ingestion of inadequate food and beverages. *TBC* SE *xiao mai qu* 小麥麴：主小兒痢，消**食痔**, "It controls free-flux illness in children, and dissolves **food piles**".

***Shi zhi* 濕滯, sluggish moisture** [1]

EA identical with → *liu shi* 留濕, abiding moisture. *PJF* 154: 風淫、**濕滯**、血刺、痰攻，皆能作痛, "Wind excess, **sluggish moisture**, blood [clot] piercing, and phlegm attack – they all have the potential to cause pain".

***Shi zhong* 濕腫, moisture swelling** [13]

① AN *zhong shi* 腫濕, swelling with moisture. IS of topical swelling and emission of liquid. *TPSHF* 82: 治小兒臍風，**濕腫**久不瘥方, "Recipes for navel wind among children, and **moisture swelling** that does not heal over an extended period of time".

② PC of → *shui zhong* 水腫, edema, brought forth by moisture evil. *QJYF* 7 RE *tai fu bai gao* 太傅白膏, the Grand Instructor's white paste: 治百病。傷寒咽喉不利，頭項強痛，腰脊兩脚疼。有風痹、**濕腫**，難屈伸，不能行步, "It cures the one hundred diseases: Harm caused by cold with throat blockage. Stiffness and pain affecting head and neck. Pain in the lower back, the spine and the two legs. When there is a wind blockage, **moisture swelling**, difficulties of bending and stretching, and inability to walk".

Shi zhu **溼注, moisture influx** [2]

EA of moisture entering various regions of the body. *ZZN* SE *wei rui* 萎蕤：男子**濕注**腰痛, "It is used [to cure] males with **moisture influx** resulting in pain in the lower back".

Shi zhu **屍注, corpse [qi] influx** [13]

PC identical with → *shi zhu* 屍疰, corpse [qi] attachment-illness. *ZHF* 1: **屍注**、鬼注病者…不的知其所苦，而無處不惡，累年積月，漸就頓滯，以至於死，死後復傳之旁人，乃至滅門, "Patients suffering from **corpse [qi] influx**, and demon influx…have no idea why they suffer but they feel bad all over. This may continue for months or years…eventually they die. After they have died [the disease] is transmitted to a bystander until the entire family has perished".

Shi zhu **屍疰, corpse [qi] attachment-illness** [14] AN *shi zhu* 屍注, corpse [qi] influx. PC identical with → *gui zhu* 鬼疰, demon attachment-illness. *SYJYBZFL* 10: 夫骨蒸、殗殜、復連、**屍疰**、勞疰、蟲疰、毒疰、熱疰、冷疰、食疰、鬼疰等，皆曰傳屍者，以疰者、注也，病自上注下，與前人相似，故曰疰, "Bone steaming, an early mild stage of corpse transmission, repeated connection, **corpse [qi] attachment-illness**, exhaustion attachment-illness, bug attachment-illness, poison attachment-illness, heat attachment-illness, cold attachment-illness, food attachment-illness, and demon attachment-illness, they all are variants of corpse [qi] transmission. The character *zhu* 疰 is to say *zhu* 注, 'to flow'. The disease flows from one generation to the next. Its appearance is similar to that of the previous [afflicted] person. Hence it is called *zhu* 疰, 'influx-illness'". With the character *zhu* 疰 identified here as a combination of the radical *ni* 疒 signifying "illness" with the component *zhu* 主 of *zhu* 注, the term *shi zhu* 屍疰 may also be interpreted/translated as "corpse [qi] influx-illness".

Shou bing **瘦病, emaciation disease** [10]

PC identical with → *xu lao* 虛勞, depletion exhaustion. *WTMY* 13: 廣濟療**瘦病**，每日西即赤色，脚手酸疼，口乾壯熱，獺肝丸方, "The *GJF* [has] the recipe for pills with otter liver to cure **emaciation disease**. Each time when the sun is in the West [the patient] has a red color, the legs and hands are in sour pain. The mouth is dry and very hot".

Shou chan **手顫, the hands shiver** [1]

IS of uncontrolled shivering movements of the hands. *BCGM* Zhu shui you du 諸水有毒，All poisonous waters: 酒中飲冷水，成**手顫**, "If one drinks cold water after having consumed wine, the **hands** will **shiver**".

Shou cui **瘦悴, emaciation and distress** [6]

① IS of an emaciated body and a distressed facial complexion. *WTMY* 6: 素有冷病，年衰力弱，膚肉**瘦悴**，此則積冷在胃, "If someone has a cold disease for his entire life, if over the years he becomes weaker and weaker, if skin and flesh are **emaciated and distressed**, then this is a case of cold accumulating in the stomach".

② PC of diseases whose main sign is emaciation and distress. *RHZ* SE *ren ru* 人乳：治**瘦悴**，悅皮膚，潤毛髮, "It cures **emaciation and distress.** It returns luster to the skin, and makes the hair shine glossy again".

Shou feng **首風, head wind** [3]

PC of → *tou feng* 頭風, head wind, characterized by headache accompanied by profuse sweating, an aversion to wind, and a hot body. *SW* 42: **首風**之狀，頭面多汗惡風…頭痛不可以出內, "The appearance of **head wind** [is as follows: patients] sweat profusely on the head and in the face and have an aversion to wind…They have headaches and cannot leave the indoors".

Shou ji **瘦瘠, emaciation to leanness** [1]

IS identical with → *ji shou* 肌瘦, muscle-flesh emaciation. *BCSY* SE *dong hai fu ren* 東海夫人：主虛羸勞損，因產**瘦瘠**, "It controls depletion and thinness, exhaustion detriment, as well as **emaciation to leanness** following delivery".

Shou ji **瘦疾, emaciation ailment** [4]

PC identical with → *shou bing* 瘦病, emaciation disease. *WTMY* 13 quotes *Jiu-JF*: 療**瘦疾**方，甘草三兩，炙, "A recipe to cure **emaciation ailment**: *gan cao*, 3 *liang*, roasted".

Shou quan **手拳, cramped hand** [1]

IS of hands cramped like a clenched fist. *WTMY* 13: 其病口噤**手拳**，氣不出, "The disease manifests itself as a clenched jaw and **cramped hands**; the qi is not released".

Shou sun **瘦損, emaciation detriment** [4]

PC identical with → *xu lei* 虛羸, depletion and thinness. *WTMY* 39: 膏肓俞：主無所不療，諸羸弱、**瘦損**、虛勞、夢中失精、上氣咳逆、狂惑妄誤, "[To pierce] the *gao huang* transporter serves to cure every [ailment]: all types of thinness and weakness, **emaciation detriment**, depletion exhaustion, loss of semen while dreaming, cough with qi rising contrary to it normal course, madness and delusion, and deliberate lying ".

Shou tai **瘦胎, to thin a fetus** [3]

TA causing a fetus to emaciate to ease birth. LSZ considers this to be a method to ease delivery by making sluggish qi pass in a woman who experiences qi stagnation prior to delivery. *FRDQLF* 16: **瘦胎**易產，胡陽公主每產累日不下，南山道士進此方, "**To thin a fetus** and ease delivery: each time when the princess of Huyang gave birth and [the child] failed to descend for several days, the Daoist of Nanshan gave this recipe".

Shou xue **瘦削, emaciated to thinness** [5]
IS identical with → *ji shou* 肌瘦, muscle-flesh emaciation. *ZHF* 4: 久者積年，輕者才百日，漸至**瘦削**，五臟氣竭，則難可復振，治之湯方， "Chronic ones accumulate for a year; light cases last just one hundred days. [Patients] are gradually **emaciated to thinness**. The qi of their five depots is exhausted, and it is difficult to recover".

Shou yang ming tou tong **手陽明頭痛, hand yang brilliance headache** [1]
PC identical with → *yang ming tou tong* 陽明頭痛, yang brilliance headache. *YXQY* Lj: 香白芷，氣温，味大辛，治**手陽明頭痛**, "*Xiang bai zhi*, qi: warm, flavor: very acrid. It cures **hand yang brilliance headache**".

Shou zu dong yao **手足動搖, shaking movements of hands and feet** [1]
IS of uncontrolled shaking of hands and feet. *HYXS* Lj: 氣促喘悶，**手足動搖**，似搐非搐, "The qi is hurried, with panting and heart-pressure. **Hands and feet display a shaking movement** as if they had been pulled, when in fact they were not".

Shou zu duo ye **手足嚲曳, drooping hands and feet** [3] AW 手足軃曳.
IS of feeble hands and feet that hang down and cannot be raised. *PJF* 93: 烏龍丹，治癱瘓風，**手足嚲曳**，口眼喎斜，言語謇澀，步履不正, "The 'black dragon elixir' cures paralysis wind, **drooping hands and feet**, slanted mouth and eyes, difficulties speaking, and inability to walk upright".

Shou zu duo ye **手足軃曳, drooping hands and feet** [1]
IS identical with → *shou zu duo ye* 手足嚲曳. *YSJCF* 1: 中風不省人事，涎潮口噤，語言不出，**手足軃曳**, "Struck by wind with an inability to recognize people or items. A flood of saliva and clenched jaw. Inability to speak. **Drooping hands and feet**".

Shou zu duan han **手足端寒, cold in the tips of hands and legs** [1]
IS of cold in the tips of the feet and legs. *MYBL* SE *qiang lang* 蜣螂：主**手足端寒**，肢滿賁豚, "It controls **cold in the tips of hands and legs**, fullness in the extremities and running piglet syndrome".

Shou zu han **手足寒, hands and legs are cold** [3]
IS identical with → *shou zu jue ni* 手足厥逆, recession with counterflow in the hands and legs. *SHL* 305: 少陰病，身體痛，**手足寒**, "When the minor yin has a disease, the entire body is in pain; the **hands and legs are cold**".

Shou zu jue han **手足厥寒, recession with cold in the hands and legs** [1]
IS identical with → *shou zu jue ni* 手足厥逆, recession with counterflow in the hands and legs. *SHL* 351: **手足厥寒**，脈細欲絕者，當歸四逆湯主之, "In the case of **recession with cold in the hands and legs**, when the movement in the vessels is fine and tends to stop, the decoction with *dang gui* for counterflow in the four [limbs] controls it".

***Shou zu jue leng* 手足厥冷, recession with cold in the hands and legs** [6]

IS identical with → *shou zu jue ni* 手足厥逆, recession with counterflow in the hands and legs. *SHL* 340: 病者**手足厥冷**, "The disease is **recession with cold in the hands and legs**".

***Shou zu jue ni* 手足厥逆, recession with counterflow in the hands and legs** [8]
AN *shou zu jue leng* 手足厥冷, recession with cold in the hands and legs; 手足冷 *shou zu leng* , the hands and legs are cold; *shou zu ni leng* 手足逆冷, counterflow with cold in the hands and legs; *shou zu han* 手足寒, the hands and feet are cold; *shou zu jue han* 手足厥寒, recession with cold in the hands and legs.

IS of hands and legs that feel as cold as ice when touched. *SHL* 317: **手足厥逆**，脈微欲絕, "**Recession with counterflow in the hands and legs**. The [movement in the] vessels is weak and at the brink of interruption".

***Shou zu leng* 手足冷, hands and legs are cold** [5]

IS identical with → *shou zu jue ni* 手足厥逆, recession with counterflow in hands and legs. *SHL* 148: 頭汗出，微惡寒，**手足冷**, "The head sweats. [The patient] has a slight aversion to cold. The **hands and legs are cold**".

***Shou zu ni leng* 手足逆冷, counterflow with cold in the hands and legs** [5]

IS identical with → *shou zu jue ni* 手足厥逆, recession with counterflow in the hands and legs. *SHL* 337: 厥者，**手足逆冷**者是也, "As for recession, this is when there is **counterflow with cold in the hands and legs**".

***Shou zu quan* 手足拳, hands and feet cramped** [2]

IS of hands and feet cramped and unable to be stretched. *ZBYHL* 8: 四肢拘急，小腹㽲痛，**手足拳**, "The four extremities cramp and are tense. The lower abdomen is affected by flatulent pain. The **hands and feet are cramped**".

***Shou zu zhi mo wei jue* 手足指末微厥, slight recession in the tips of the fingers and toes** [2]

IS of a feeling of slight cold in the tips of hands and feet. *SHZG* Mj: **手足指末微厥**，脈浮數而緊者，邪熱在表, "**Slight recession in the tips of the fingers and toes**. The [movement in the] vessels is at the surface, frequent, and tight. Evil heat is in the body's outer sections".

***Shu* 癙, mouse-illness** [1]

PC identical with → *shu lou* 鼠瘺, mouse fistula. *BCGM* SE *mao* 貓：狸頭治**癙**及鼠嚙人瘡, "The head of a racoon dog cures **mouse-illness** and sores resulting from mice biting humans".

***Shu* 暑, summer; summerheat** [p]

① The season of summer. *ZBYHL* 23: 人盛**暑**之時，觸冒大熱，熱毒氣入臟腑, "When during mid**summer** a person is affected by the malicious in the form of massive heat, and the poison qi of heat enters the depots and palaces".

② AN *shu qi* 暑氣, qi of summerheat. Summerheat. CC of burning heat. *SW* 5: 喜怒不節, 寒**暑**過度, 生乃不固, "If joy and anger are unrestrained, if cold and **summerheat** exceed the norms, life no longer exists on a solid [foundation].

③ AN *shu qi* 暑氣, qi of summerheat; *shu re* 暑熱, summerheat; *shu ye* 暑暍, summerheat. EA of heat qi during summer causing harm to man. *SW* 3: 因於

暑, 汗, 煩則喘喝, 靜則多言, 體若燔炭, 汗出而散, "As a result of **summerheat** and sweat, if [the patient suffers from] uneasiness, he will pant with much noise; if he is at peace, he [nevertheless] speaks a lot. The body resembles burning coal. Flowing sweat makes [the internal heat] disperse".

④ AN *shu bing* 暑病, summerheat disease. PC brought forth either by the qi of summerheat, or a cold affliction in winter caused by summerheat. *SW* 31: "後夏至日者為病**暑**, "Those cases following summer solstice day, they constitute a suffering from **summerheat**". *BCGM* 百病主治藥 distinguishes between 受暑中暍, "Affection by heat during summer", and 受涼中暑, "Affection by summerheat during a cool period". However, in its main text, there is no strict division between 中暍, struck by heat, and 中暑, struck by summerheat. *BCGM* lists the following as *shu bing* 暑病, "summerheat disease": *zhong shu* 中暑, struck by summerheat; *fu shu* 伏暑, hidden summerheat; *shang shu* 傷暑, harm caused by summerheat; *mao shu* 冒暑, malicious summerheat; *shu shi* 暑濕, summerheat with moisture; *shu feng* 暑風, summerheat with wind; *shu xie* 暑瀉, summerheat outflow; *shu du* 暑毒, summerheat poison.

***Shu bing* 暑病, summerheat disease** [1]

PC identical with → *shu* 暑④, summerheat. *SHL* Shang han li 傷寒例：**暑病**者, 熱極重於溫也, "As for **summerheat disease**, the heat is extreme and stronger than in the case of a warmth [disease]".

***Shu du* 暑毒, summerheat poison** [16]

EA of a rather violent version of → *shu* 暑, summerheat, evil. *SJZL* 34: 心藏神而惡熱, 若冒觸**暑毒**, 蘊蓄於五臟, 則陰陽不能升降, 經絡不得宣通, 故奄然悶絕, "The heart stores the spirits and has an aversion to heat. If it encounters the malicious in the form of **summerheat poison**, which collects in the five depots, then yin and yang [qi] are unable to rise and descend, and the conduits and network vessels are no longer passable. Hence there is sudden heart-pressure and cut-off".

***Shu duo tai* 數墮胎, frequent miscarriage** [1] AN *pin guan duo tai* 頻慣墮胎.

PC of repeated spontaneous terminations of pregnancies. *ZBYHL* 41: 妊娠**數墮胎**候…血氣不足，故不能養胎，所以致胎數墮, "The signs of a pregnant woman's **frequent miscarriage**...blood and qi are insufficient. Hence she is unable to nourish a fetus. As a result she experiences frequent spontaneous abortions".

***Shu feng* 暑風, summerheat wind** [1]

PC brought about by → *shu* 暑 summerheat, evil [qi] with mental confusion and convulsions. *QYXJ* 2: **暑風**，暑毒入心，痰塞心孔，昏迷搐搦, "In the case of **summerheat wind**, summerheat poison has entered the heart. Phlegm blocks the heart holes, and [the patient] is comatose with convulsions".

***Shu li* 暑痢, summerheat free-flux illness** [1]

PC of → *li ji* 痢疾, free-flux illness, which appears in summer and is brought about by summerheat and moisture. *SYDXF* 6: 柏皮湯，治**暑痢**, "Decoction with *bo pi* cures **summerheat free-flux illness**".

***Shu li* 鼠瀝, mouse pervasion-illness** [1]

PC identical with → *shu lou* 鼠瘺, mouse fistula. *BCGM* Bai bing zhu zhi yao 百病主治藥 quoting the main text: 鼠瘺, "Mouse fistula", writes: **鼠瀝, "Mouse pervasion-illness"**.

***Shu lou* 鼠漏, mouse leakage** [5]

PC identical with → *shou lou* 鼠瘺, mouse fistula. *QJYF* 23: 治**鼠漏**，瘡瘥復發及不愈，出膿血不止方, "Recipe to cure **mouse leakage**, whereby the sores if healed reappear and cannot be cured, associated with unending festering and bleeding".

***Shu lou* 鼠瘺, mouse fistula** [72] AN *shu lou* 癙瘺, mouse-illness fistula; *shu* 癙, mouse-illness.

PC identical with → *luo li* 瘰瀝, scrofula with pervasion-illness. *LS* 70: **鼠瘺**之本，皆在於臟，其末上出於頸腋之間, "The root of **mouse fistula** always lies in the depots. The tip emerges from between the neck and armpits".

***Shu lou* 癙瘺, mouse-illness fistula** [1]

PC identical with → *shu lou* 鼠瘺, mouse fistula. *BCGM* SE *mao* 貓：殺蟲治疳及痘瘡變黑，瘰瀝**癙瘺**惡瘡, "It kills bugs/worms and cures *gan*-illness as well as smallpox sores that have turned black, scrofula with pervasion-illness, **mouse-illness fistula**, and malign sores".

***Shu nai zhi* 鼠奶痔, mouse-nipple piles** [1]

PC identical with → *shu zhi* 鼠痔, mouse piles. *ZLBC* SE *pu huang* 蒲黃：治**鼠奶痔**：蒲黃末，空心温酒下方寸匕，日三, "To cure **mouse-nipple piles**: Ingest one square-inch-size spoon full of *pu huang* powder with warm wine on an empty stomach three times a day".

***Shu nue* 暑瘧, summerheat malaria** [2]

PC of → *nue ji* 瘧疾, malaria ailment, during summer with only minor sensations of cold and strong sensations of heat, or only of heat with no cold. *SYDXF* 115: 先寒後熱名寒瘧, 先熱後寒名温瘧, 但熱不寒名**暑瘧**, "If a cold sensation comes first and a heat sensation follows, this is called 'cold malaria'. If a heat sensation comes first and a cold sensation follows, this is called 'warmth malaria'. If there is only a heat sensation with no cold sensation, this is called '**summerheat malaria**'".

***Shu qi* 暑氣, summerheat qi** [3]

① CC identical with → *shu* 暑②, summerheat. *HNHLJ* 4: **暑氣**多夭, 寒氣多壽, "Much **summerheat qi** entails early death; much cold qi entails long life".

② EA identical with → *shu* 暑③, summerheat. *HJJF* 2 RE *si ni tang* 四逆湯, decoction for counterflow in the four [limbs]: 常服消**暑氣**, 分水穀, "If regularly ingested it will dissolve **summerheat qi**, and divide liquid [lit. "water"] and solid [lit. "grain"] food".

***Shu re* 暑熱, summerheat** [7]

EA identical with → *shu* 暑. *ZBYHL* 39: 宿經傷**暑熱**，今因產虛…故發作成瘧也, "The conduits have long been harmed by **summerheat**. Now, because of a depletion following delivery...[the patient] develops malaria".

***Shu ru zhi* 鼠乳痔, mouse-breast piles** [1]
PC identical with → *shu nai zhi* 鼠奶痔, mouse-nipple piles. *BCGM* SE *niu* 牛 quoting *ZLBC*: 鼠奶痔 writes: **鼠乳痔**, "**Mouse-breast piles**".

***Shu shi* 暑濕, summerheat with moisture** [6]
EA of an interaction of → *shu* 暑, summerheat, and → *shi* 濕, moisture, evil. *QJYiF* 24: 遇**暑濕**涼氣者, 多生此病, "If one encounters **summerheat with moisture** and cool qi, this will often give rise to this disease". This is not to be confused with a reference to 暑濕 in *ZBYHL*: 其風**寒暑**濕, 魅魃魍魎, 皆謂為邪也: "Wind, cold, **summerheat and moisture**, and various types of demons, they all are called 'evils'".

***Shu xie* 暑瀉, summerheat outflow** [1]
PC of → *xie xie* 泄瀉, outflow, during summer caused by summerheat evil. *PJF* 38: 黃龍丸, 治腸風臟毒及**暑瀉**熱瀉, "The 'Yellow Dragon Pills' cure intestinal wind, depot poisoning, as well as **summerheat outflow**, and heat outflow".

***Shu xie* 暑泄, summerheat outflow** [1]
PC identical with → *shu xie* 暑瀉. *BCGM* SE *shen qu* 神麴 quotes *ZHBYF*: 壯脾進食：療痞滿**暑泄**, 麴朮丸, "They strengthen the spleen and allow food to enter: To cure an obstacle-illness with a feeling of fullness and **summerheat outflow**, [use the] pills with *qu* and *zhu*".

***Shu ye* 暑暍, summerheat** [1]
EA identical with → *shu* 暑③. *BCGM* SE *ren niao* 人尿：蓋臍乃命蒂, **暑暍**傷氣, 温臍所以接其元氣之意, "Now, the umbilicus is the base of one's life. When **summerheat** has harmed the qi, then the meaning of warming the umbilicus is to hold the [patient's] original qi".

***Shu zhi* 鼠痔, mouse piles** [4] AN *ju zhi* 舉痔, raised piles; *shu nai zhi* 鼠奶痔, mouse-nipple piles; *shu ru zhi* 鼠乳痔, mouse-breast piles.
PC of → *zhi chuang* 痔瘡, piles sores, which develop inside the anus with many tumorous flesh-growths resembling breast nipples. *PJF* 297: 穀道四面肉如奶，名鼠痔, "Flesh-growths on all four sides of the path of grain resembling breast nipples are called '**mouse piles**'".

***Shui* 水, water; liquid** [p]
① PS *BCGM* has *shui bu* 水部, water section, as heading of 43 types of water, such as *yu shui* 雨水, rain water, used as pharmaceutical substances: 今集**水**之關於藥食者，凡四十三種，分為二類：曰天，曰地, "Here are gathered 43 types of **water** used in pharmacy and dietetics. They fall into two groups, i.e. celestial and earth [waters]".
② PN of those yin body liquids that are supposed to have a nourishing and moistening function. They are juxtaposed with fire in a relationship of mutual control. *SW* 34: 少**水**不能滅盛火, "Diminished **water** cannot extinguish intensely burning fire".
③ PC of all types of swelling of the facial region or four limbs brought forth by water/liquids retained in the human body, in extreme cases including edematous swelling of the entire body or gatherings of water/liquid in the chest and

abdominal cavities. *SW* 20: 病水者，以夜半死, "This who suffer from **water** disease die at midnight".
④ AN *shui qi* 水氣, water qi; *shui shi* 水濕, moisture of water.
EA capable of bringing forth water disease. Its nature is similar to that of moisture, but it lends itself more easily to unchecked spreading. *SW* 33: 水在腹者，必使目下腫也, "When there is **water** in the abdomen, it must cause swelling below the eyes".

Shui bing **水病, water disease** [42]
PC identical with a) → *shui* 水③, water. *SW* 61: **水病**下為胕腫大腹，上為喘呼，不得臥, "**Water diseases**: below they cause *fu*-swellings in the upper abdomen, above they cause panting exhalation". b) → *shui du* 水毒, water poisoning. *ZHF* 7: 水毒中人，一名中溪，一名中灑，一名**水病**, "When water poison strikes a person, this is also named 'struck by a rivulet'; 'struck by sprinkling water'; '**water disease**'".

Shui chuan **水喘, water panting** [1]
PC of → *chuan* 喘, panting, brought forth by internal stagnation of water rheum. *YS* 4: **水喘**，有人先因咳嗽發喘，胸膈痞悶，難於倒頭，氣上湊者，宜早利水道，化痰下氣, "**Water panting**. In cases where people develop panting in connection with a cough, with their chest and diaphragm [region] feeling as if they had an attachment-illness or heart-pressure, and if they find it difficult to lie down with qi pressing upwards, then it is advisable to free the passageways of water as soon as possible, and to transform phlegm and discharge qi".

Shui ding **水疔, water pin-illness** [3]
PC of → *ding chuang* 疔瘡, pin-illness sores, with the sores being numb without pain, and assuming a yellow-black color. *RZZZF* 22: 此疾雖自風毒而來，其諸觸犯不可不信。如石疔之忌，瓦礫磚石；麻子疔之忌，麻衣麻仁；火疔之忌，火光炙煿；**水疔**之忌，飲水渡河, "This ailment is caused by wind poison. Nevertheless, there are all types of contact offenses that must be taken into regard. Such as [patients with] stone pin-illness, they must not come into contact with broken tiles, bricks or stones. [Patients with] hemp-seed pin-illness, they must not come into contact with garments made from hemp or hemp seeds. [Patients with] fire pin-illness, they must not come into contact with the light of fire and roasting and frying. [Patients with] **water pin-illness**, they must not drink water or wade through a river".

Shui du **水毒, water poison** [14]
① EA identical with → *xi du* 溪毒①, rivulet poison. *ZHF* 7: **水毒**中人，一名中溪，一名中灑，一名水病, "When **water poison** strikes humans, this may also be called 'struck by a rivulet', 'struck by sprinkling water', 'water disease'".
② AN *zhong xi* 中溪, struck by a rivulet; *zhong shui* 中水, struck by water; *shui bing* 水病, water disease. PC identical with → *xi du* 溪毒②. *ZBYHL* 25: 自三吳已東及南，諸山郡山縣，有山谷溪源處，有**水毒**病，春秋輒得, "From Sanwu both eastward and southward, in all mountain prefectures and mountain counties, where there are springs of small rivers of mountain valleys, there is **water poison** disease. One often acquires it during spring and autumn".

Shui fu zhang man **水腹脹滿, abdominal water distension and a feeling of fullness** [1]

PC identical with → *shui zhang* 水脹, water distension. *TBC* SE *shu jiao* 蜀椒: 主**水腹脹滿**，利小便, "It controls **abdominal water distension and a feeling of fullness**, and frees urination".

Shui gu **水穀, water and grain; liquid and solid food; water grain** [53]

① Liquid and solid food. *SW* 43: 榮者，**水穀**之精氣也, "The camp [qi], that is the essence qi of **water and grain**".

② PN of a type of grain. *SWBJQYBMJ* Fj: 麻，木穀而治風；豆，**水穀**而治水 "Sesame is a wood grain and cures wind [disease]. Beans are a **water grain** and cure water [disease]".

Shui gu **水蠱, water *gu*[-distension]** [25]

PC identical with → *gu zhang* 鼓脹①, drum[-like] distension. *ZHF* 4: 治卒大腹水病方，鬼扇，細擣絞汁，服如雞子，即下水，更復取**水蠱**， "Recipes to cure water disease with sudden abdominal enlargement: *Gui fan*, pound to a fine pulp and wring to obtain its juice. If consumed in the amount of an egg, this will drain water. It also eliminates **water *gu*[-distension]**".

Shui gu **水鼓, water drum** [4]

PC identical with → *shui gu* 水蠱, water *gu* [-distension]. *SKLBC* SE *da dou* 大豆：和桑柴灰汁煮之，下**水鼓**腹脹, "Boil it in water in which the ashes of mulberry firewood have been dispersed. It purges abdominal distension of **water drum**".

Shui gu bu hua **水穀不化, water and grain failing to transform** [1]

IS identical with → *shui gu bu xiao* 水穀不消, water and grain failing to dissolve. *QJYF* 28: 小腹痛，癥疝，**水穀不化**，宜服大平胃丸, "For pain in the lower abdomen, concretion-illness and elevation-illness, and when **water and grain fail to transform**, it is advisable to ingest the 'pills that massively pacify the stomach'".

Shui gu bu xia **水穀不下, water and grain failing to move down** [2]

IS of an inability to swallow beverages or food. *WSBJ* 11: 備急如聖散，治時氣纏喉，風漸入咽喉，閉塞，**水穀不下**，牙關緊急，不省人事, "The 'powder that prepares people for urgencies like a sage' cures seasonal qi constricting the throat, wind gradually entering the throat, and closing it with the result that **water and grain fail to move down**. The mandibular joints are firmly clenched. Patients do not recognize other people or things".

Shui gu bu xiao **水穀不消, water and grain failing to dissolve** [4] AN *shui gu bu hua* 水谷不化, water and grain failing to transform.

IS of aqueous stools mixed with undigested food. *QJYF* 13: 瀉心湯，治老小下痢，**水穀不消**，腸中雷鳴, "The 'decoction to drain the heart' cures discharge with free-flux illness of old and young patients, **water and grain failing to dissolve**, thunder-like sounds in the intestines".

Shui gu li **水穀利, water and grain free-flux [illness]** [1]

PC of a diarrhea where a depletion of stomach and intestines has eliminated the ability of these organs to digest solid food with the result that they are discharged together with water/liquid. *ZBYHL* 40: 腸虛則泄，故變為利也，此下利是**水穀利**也, "Intestinal depletion leads to outflow. Hence this changes to free-flux [illness]. This type of discharge with free-flux is **water and grain free-flux [illness]**". *BCGM* also has *shui gu xia li* 水谷下利, "Water and grain discharge with free-flux".

Shui gu li **水穀痢, water and grain free-flux-illness** [6]

PC of → *li ji* 痢疾, free-flux illness, of a mucous bloody stool interspersed with undigested solid food. This is often the result of evil qi availing itself of a regular depletion. *ZBYHL* 17: 脾胃大腸虛弱，而邪氣乘之，故為**水穀痢**也, "The spleen, stomach and large intestine are depleted and weak so that evil qi can enter. This then results in **water and grain free-flux-illness**".

Shui gu xia li **水穀下利, water and grain discharge with free-flux** [1]

PC identical with → *shui gu li* 水穀利, water and grain free-flux [illness]. *BCGM* SE *chun chu* 椿樗：**水穀下利**及每至立秋前後即患痢，兼腰痛, "**Water and grain discharge with free-flux** as well the free-flux-illness suffers from prior to and after the date 'spring begins' are both accompanied by lower back pain".

Shui ji **水疾, water ailment** [4]

PC identical with → *shui* 水, water③. *ZBYHL* 5: 診其脈，心脈滑甚為善渴。其久病變，或發癰疽，或成**水疾**, "If upon examination of the [movements in the] vessels one finds a very smooth [movement] in the heart vessels, and [patients] long for something to drink. After an extended period of time the disease undergoes a change. It may bring forth obstruction- and impediment-illnesses, or it may develop into a **water ailment**".

Shui jiang bu xia **水漿不下, water and broth failing to move down** [2] AN *yan shui bu xia* 嚥水不下, water drunk fails to move down.

IS of a closed throat permitting neither liquid nor solid food to pass. *BJ* SE *luo shi* 絡石：主 …口乾舌焦，癰腫不消，喉舌腫，**水漿不下**, "It controls…dry mouth and parched tongue, obstruction-illnesses and swellings that fail to dissolve, swelling of the throat and tongue, **water and broth failing to move down**".

Shui lan shang **水爛傷, harmed by water with festering** [1]

PC identical with → *shang shui lan* 傷水爛. *BCGM* SE *zhan si* 占斯 quoting *YXL* 洗手足水爛瘡, "To wash hands and feet with festering sores [harmed by] water" writes: 洗手足**水爛傷**, "To wash hands and feet **harmed by water with festering**".

Shui li **水利, watery free-flux [illness]** [1]

PC identical with → *shui xie* 水泄, water diarrhea. *TPSHF* 47: 治霍亂，**水利**不止，吐不下食，兼煩渴，草豆蔻散方, "To cure cholera, and unending **watery free-flux [illness]**, with vomiting and an inability to eat, as well as vexation and thirst, [use the] recipe for the powder with *cao dou kou*".

Shui li 水痢, **watery free-flux-illness** [33]

PC of → *li ji* 痢疾, free-flux illness with water-thin feces discharged with urgency. *QJYiF* 3 SE *lü cao* 葎草：主五淋，利小便，止**水痢**, "It controls the five types of dripping, stimulates the free flow of urine, and stops **watery free-flux-illness**".

Shui ni 水逆, **water counterflow** [2]

PC of → *tai yang zhong feng* 太陽中風, wind stroke in the major yang [conduits], with fever, irritation and thirst, and if one drinks water/liquid it is immediately thrown up again. *SHL* 74: 中風，發熱六七日不解而煩，有表裏證，渴欲飲水，水入則吐者，名曰**水逆**，五苓散主之, "If one is struck by wind and has had unending effusion of heat for six, seven days, as well as vexation, with pathological signs internally and externally, and if he is thirsty and wishes to drink water, with the water consumed being thrown up again, then this is called **water counterflow**. The powder with *wu ling* controls it".

Shui nu 水弩, **water crossbow** [5]

EA identical with → *she gong* 射工①, archer. *ZHF* 7: 治卒中射工**水弩**毒方第六十五, "Recipe for **water crossbow** poison nr. 65 to cure a sudden strike by the archer".

Shui ni 水溺, **submersion in water** [1]

PC identical with → *ni shui* 溺水. *BCGM* SE *zao jiao* 皂角 quoting *WTMY* 溺死一宿者, "Those having been dead following submersion for one night" writes: **水溺**卒死一宿者, "Those who died following **submersion in water** and have been dead for one night".

Shui pi 水癖, **water aggregation-illness** [4]

PC identical with → *zhi yin* 支飲, propping rheum. *ZBYHL* 21: **水癖**，由飲水漿不消，水氣結聚而成癖，在於兩脅之側，轉動便痛，不耐風寒，不欲食而短氣是也, "**Water aggregation-illness**: When one has drunk water or thick liquid that fail to dissolve, the water qi forms nodular collections and generates aggregation-illness in the two upper flanks. Physical movement generates pain, and one cannot stand wind or cold. Patients have no appetite and are short of qi".

Shui pi 水痞, **water obstacle-illness** [2]

PC of a feeling of blockage and fullness below the heart brought forth by stagnant water/moisture accumulating there. *BCGM* SE *ze xie* 澤瀉：去脬中留垢，心下**水痞**, "It eliminates filth residues from the bladder, and **water obstacle-illness** from below the heart".

Shui qi 水氣, **water qi** [174]

① PC identical with → *shui* 水③, water. *JGYL* Mj lists **水氣**病脈證並治, "**Water qi** disease – its [movements in the] vessels, signs, and cures".

② EA identical with → *shui* 水④. *SW* 34: 夫不得臥，臥則喘者，是**水氣**之客也, "Now, when someone cannot lie down and when, if he lies down, he pants, this is a case of **water qi** settling".

③ PN of kidney qi. *BCYY* Zong xu 總序, General Introduction: 蓋愁憂思慮則傷心，心傷則血逆竭，血逆竭，故神色先散，而月水先閉也。火既受

病，不能榮養其子，故不嗜食。脾既虛，則金氣虧，故發嗽。嗽既作，**水氣**絕，故四肢乾。木氣不充，故多怒。鬢髮焦，筋痿。俟五臟傳遍，故卒不能死，然終死矣, "Now, worrying and contemplation harm the heart. When the heart is harmed the blood flows contrary to its normal direction and is used up. Hence the spirit [of the heart and its associated] complexion disperse first, and menstruation is blocked. When the fire has received this disease, it cannot nourish its child [i.e. the spleen]. Hence [patients] do not wish to eat. Once the spleen has been depleted, the metal qi is insufficient, resulting in a cough. When the patient coughs the [movement of] **water qi** is cut off. Hence the four limbs dry out, and the wood qi is not complete. As a result [patients] are often angry. Their hair is scorched and their sinews turn limp. The entire transmission involves all the five depots. Hence [patients] do not die immediately, but in the end they must die".

***Shui sha* 水沙, water-borne sand [disease]** [1]

PC of → *sha bing* 沙病, sand disease. *SYDXF* 2: 沙證…兩足墜痛，亦名**水沙**, "The signs of sand [disease]…Both legs feel like they are sagging and painful. Another name is '**water-borne sand [disease]**'".

***Shui shang han* 水傷寒, water-borne harm caused by cold** [1]

PC identical with → *sha bing* 沙病, sand disease. *SYDXF* 2: 艾湯，試沙證。江南舊無，今所在有之。原其證古方不載，所感如傷寒，頭痛嘔噁，渾身壯熱，手足指末微厥，或腹痛煩亂，須臾能殺人。先濃煎艾湯試之，如吐即是。右用五月蠶蛻紙碎剪，安碗中，以盤蓋之，以百沸湯泡艾碗許，仍以別紙封裹縫良久，乘熱飲之，就臥，以厚被蓋之，汗出愈,…又名**水傷寒**, "Decoction with *ai* to test a sand condition. In former times [this condition] did not exist in the Jiangnan region. Nowadays it is present there everywhere. This condition was not listed in ancient recipes. It feels like harm caused by cold, with headache and vomiting and nausea. The entire body is very hot. The ends of the fingers and toes experience slight recession. In some cases there is abdominal pain, with vexation and confusion. After a short time it will kill the [afflicted] person. First one prepares a thick decoction of *ai* [and has the patient ingest it] as a test [whether he has a sand condition]. If he vomits, this is it. [For the indications listed] above one cuts paper prepared from silkwom sloths of the 5th month and places it into a bowl. This is to be covered with a plate. Then soak the *ai* bowl a little while in boiling hot water, and close the seams with additional paper for a long time. Have [the patient] avail himself of the heat and drink this. Then he is to lie down and to be covered with a thick quilt. When he sweats, he is cured…Another name is '**water-borne harm caused by cold**'".

***Shui shi* 水濕, the moisture of water** [18]

① EA identical with → *shui* 水④, water *ZBYHL* 18: 若脾胃和，則土氣強盛，**水濕**不能侵之, "When the spleen and stomach are in harmony, the qi of soil is strong and flourishes, and **the moisture of water** is unable to intrude".
② PC identical with → *shui* 水③. *XMLF* 8: 濕病本不自生，因於大熱怫鬱，水液不能宣通，即停滯而生**水濕**也, "A moisture disease cannot come about by itself. As a result of massive heat there is anger with pent-up [qi], and the wa-

ter/liquids cannot be transported further. Hence they are sluggish and stagnate and bring forth **the moisture of water**[disease]".

③ Natural water. *BCYY* SE *liu hua* 柳華：小黑子因風而起，得**水濕**處便生, "The small black seeds open because of wind. Where they receive the **moisture of water** they grow easily".

Shui sou **水嗽, water cough** [1]

PC of → *ke sou* 咳嗽 brought forth by internal stagnation of water rheum. *PJF* 139: 傷寒咳嗽：肺主氣，氣逆而不下，則嗽…其間**水嗽**三症不可無辨, "The signs of harm caused by cold with cough. The lung rules the qi. When the qi flows contrary to its normal direction and fails to move down, then [patients] cough…It is essential to distinguish among three variants of **water cough**".

Shui tui **水㿉, water prominence-illness** [1]

PC of swollen, enlarged testicles associated with an edematose swelling of the entire body. *BCGM* Bai bing zhu zhi yao 百病主治藥 quoting from recipes attached to SE *mu li* 牡蠣：水病囊腫, "Water disease with testicle swelling", writes: **水㿉, "Water prominence-illness"**.

Shui xie **水泄, watery outflow** [27] AN *shui xie* 水瀉, *shui* li 水利, water free-flux [illness].

PC of watery diarrhea. *QJYF* 2: 治婦人**水泄**、痢方：灸氣海百壯三報, "Recipe to cure **watery outflow** and free-flux illness in women: cauterize the *qi hai* with 100 cones, three times".

Shui xie **水瀉, watery outflow** [27]

PC identical with → *shui xie* 水泄. *TPSHF* 59: 治**水瀉**不止，茱萸丸方, "To cure unending **watery outflow**, [use the] recipe for pills with *zhu yu*".

Shui xu **水蓄, water amassment** [1]

PC identical with → *xu shui* 畜水, amassed water. *BCYY* SE *ze xie* 澤瀉：**水蓄**渴煩，小便不利，或吐或瀉，五苓散主之, "In the case of **water amassment** with thirst and vexation, blocked urination and at times vomiting, at times outflow, the powder with *wu ling* will master it".

Shui xu huo ji **水虛火極, water depletion with extreme fire** [1]

EA, PM of a → *yin xu huo dong* 陰虛火動, yin depletion with excited fire, resulting from a unilateral insufficiency of yin body liquid. *BCGM* SE *qiu shi* 秋石：病淋者**水虛火極**，則煎熬成沙成石, 小便之煉成秋石，與此一理也, "When [patients] suffer from dripping, with **water depletion with extreme fire**, the boiling will generate sands or stones. When tempering of urine with fire generates *qiu shi*, then this is the same principle".

Shui ye cheng che qing leng **水液澄徹清冷, watery fluids being extremely clear and cold** [2]

IS of diarrhea that is as liquid and clear as water. *SW* 74: 諸病**水液澄徹清冷**，皆屬於寒, "Without exception, all diseases of **watery fluids being extremely clear and cold** are associated with cold".

Shui ye hun zhuo **水液渾濁, turbidity of watery fluids** [1]
IS of turbid urine. *SW* 74: 諸轉反戾，**水液渾濁**，皆屬於熱, "Without exception, all types of contortions and **turbidity of watery fluids** are associated with heat".

Shui yi **水溢, water spill** [1]
IS identical with → *chu zhi* 出汁, discharge of liquid. *BCGM* SE *qian niu zi* 牽牛子 quotes *RZZZF*: 漏瘡**水溢**，乃腎虛也, "In the case of leaking sores and **water spill**, [the underlying condition] is kidney depletion".

Shui yin **水飲, watery rheum** [17]
① EA identical with → *shui* 水④, water. *SW* 70: 濕氣變物，**水飲**內蓄，中滿不食, "Moisture qi changes beings. **Watery rheum** accumulates inside [the body]. There is a feeling of central fullness and [people] do not eat".
② PC identical with → *shui* 水③. *WTMY* 8 RE *da gan sui wan* 大甘遂丸, massive pills with *gan sui*: 療大**水飲**病, "They cure massive **water rheum** disease".

Shui yin **水癮, water hidden-illness** [10]
PC identical with → *shui zhong* 水腫, edema. *BCSY* SE *zi teng* 紫藤：主**水癮**病, "It controls the disease of **water hidden-illness**".

Shui yin feng **水銀風, mercury wind** [1]
PC mentioned only once in the *BCGM*, and nowhere else in earlier or contemporary medical texts. Hence its etiology and signs remain unclear. *RHZ* SE *zhu* 豬：肉療水銀風, "The meat cures mercury wind".

Shui ying **水癭, water goiter** [1]
PC of unspecified types of → *ying liu* 癭瘤, goiter tumor. The term *shui ying* **水癭**, **water goiter**, is rarely seen in ancient medical texts; the illness signs of this condition are not described anywhere. The term itself suggests a pliable bag-like swelling filled with liquid. *WTMY* 23: 崔氏云凡**水癭**、氣癭可瘥，石癭不可治, "Mr. Cui states: All cases of **water goiter** and qi goiter can be cured. Stone goiter is incurable".

Shui yu **水郁, pent-up water [qi]** [2]
PC of water and moisture qi accumulation forming nodes and blockages. *SW* 71: 水郁折之, "In the case of **pent-up water [qi]**, break it".

Shui zhang **水脹, water distension** [19] AN *shui fu zhang* 水腹脹, abdominal water distension.
PC identical with → *gu zhang* 鼓脹①, drum[-like] distension. *LS* 36: 邪氣內逆，則氣為之閉塞而不行，不行則為**水脹**, "When evil qi counterflows internally, then the [proper] qi is blocked and barred from further movement. When it no longer moves this will result in **water distension**".

Shui zheng **水癥, water concretion-illness** [3]
PC of nodes and hardenings in the abdomen brought forth by accumulations of stagnant water. *ZBYHL* 21: **水癥**者，由經絡痞澀，水氣停聚，在於腹內，大小腸不利所為也。其病腹內有結塊堅強, "As for **water concretion-illness**, the reason is that water qi has stagnated and collected in the abdomen because of an obstacle-illness and roughness in the conduits and network vessels. As a

result, the large and small intestines are no longer freely passable. The disease manifests itself as abdominal nodes and hardenings".

Shui zhong **水腫, water swelling; edema** [241]

PC identical with → *shui* 水③, water. *SW* 61: 水病下為胕腫大腹，上為喘呼，不得臥者，標本俱病，故肺為喘呼，腎為**水腫**, "Water diseases: below they cause *fu*-swelling in the upper abdomen, above they cause panting exhalation. If [the patient] cannot lie down, tip and root both have the disease. As a fact, the lung causes panting exhalation and the kidneys cause **water swelling**".

Si hun **死昏, death[-like] clouding** [1]

IS of a mental clouding that includes a complete lack of response to any stimulus, as if the patient were dead. *BCGM* SE *ji* 雞 quoting from the *QJYF* the passage 魘死不自覺, "Nightmare with death[-like] unconsciousness", writes: 卒魘**死昏**, "Sudden nightmares with **death[-like] clouding**".

Si ji **死肌, dead muscle** [37]

① IS of festering, dead flesh and muscles that may have lost sensitivity and function. *BJ* SE *bai xian* 白鮮：濕痹，**死肌**不可屈伸起止行步, "Moisture blockage [results in] **dead muscles** that cause a person to be unable to bend or stretch, to rise or stop, or to walk".

② PC of atopical existence of dead muscles. *BJ* SE *luo shi* 絡石：主風熱**死肌**，癰傷, "It controls wind heat and **dead muscles**, obstruction-illnesses and wounds".

③ PI of muscle tissue that has decayed and as a consequence has lost sensitivity and moving function. *BJ* SE *luo shi* 絡石：逐骨節皮膚**死肌**, "It eliminates **dead muscles** from the joints and skin".

Si lü **思慮, pondering** [17]

EA of harmful long-term intense pondering. *NJ* 49: 憂愁**思慮**則傷心，形寒飲冷則傷肺, "Worrying and **pondering** harm the heart. A cold body and cold beverages harm the lung".

Si shi shang han **四時傷寒, harm caused by cold in all four seasons** [3]

PC identical with → *shang han* 傷寒, harm caused by cold. *SJZL* 21: 治**四時傷寒**初覺，桂心湯方, "For treating a first awareness of **harm caused by cold in all four seasons**: the recipe for the decoction with *gui xin*".

Si shui **嗜睡, somnolence** [2]

IS of a continuous urge to sleep, regardless of whether it is day or night. If called, such patients wake up. Woken up they immediately fall asleep again. *ZBYHL* 18: 手足心熱，腰痛**嗜睡**, "The palms of the hands and the soles of the feet are hot. The lower back aches and [patients] are **somnolent**".

Si tai bu xia **死胎不下, a dead fetus fails to be discharged** [9]

PC identical with → *zi si fu zhong* 子死腹中, a fetus' death in the abdomen. *PJF* 357, Chan nun zi si fu zhong 產難子死腹中, Difficult delivery and a fetus has died in the abdomen: 治**死胎不下**,其證指甲青,舌青,脹悶甚者,口中作屎臭…其胎即化血水而下, "To cure [a condition] where a **dead fetus fails to be discharged**. The signs are greenish-blue fingernails, and a greenish-blue tongue, with extreme distension and heart-pressure. From within the mouth a stench like feces is emitted...The fetus will eventually be transformed to blood liquid and be discharged".

Si tai zai fu **死胎在腹, a dead fetus in the abdomen** [1]
PC identical with → *zi si fu zhong* 子死腹中, a fetus' death in the abdomen. *PJF* 328, RE *chen xiang wan ying wan* 沉香萬應丸, pills with *chen xiang* that generate a myriad responses: **死胎在腹**，不過二丸, "For **a dead fetus in the abdomen,** not more than two pills".

Si wo **嗜臥, a desire to lie down** [11]
IS of extreme fatigue of the body and limbs, mental inertia, and a frequent desire to lie down on a bed. *SW* 16: 病不已，令人益**嗜臥**, "The disease [that was to be healed] does not end. [This] increasingly makes a person **desire to sleep**".

Si zhi bing leng **四肢冰冷, the four limbs are as cold as ice** [2]
IS identical with → *si zhi ni leng* 四肢逆冷, counterflow with cold in the four limbs. *BCGM* SE *huang yao zi* 黃藥子, quoting *YJSJYF*: **四肢冰冷**，唇青腹脹, "**The four limbs are as cold as ice.** The lips are greenish-blue and the abdomen is distended".

Si zhi fan leng **四肢煩冷, vexation and cold in the four limbs** [?]
IS of cold in the upper and lower extremities accompanied by a feeling of agitation. *BCTJ* SE *xiang ru* 香薷：霍亂轉筋，煮飲服之，無不差者。若**四肢煩冷**，汗出而渴者，加蓼子同切，煮飲, "For cholera with twisted sinews, ingest it as a decoction, and not a single case will remain uncured. In the case of **vexation and cold in the four limbs**; and when [the patient] sweats and is thirsty, cut it together with *liao zi* and boil a decoction".

Si zhi han **四肢寒, the four limbs are cold** [1]
IS identical with → *si zhi ni leng* 四肢逆冷, counterflow with cold in the four limbs. *QJYF* 28: 脈澀，**四肢寒**者死, "Those whose [movement in the] vessels is rough, and whose **four limbs are cold**, will die".

Si zhi han jue **四肢寒厥, cold with recession in the four limbs** [1]
IS identical with → *si zhi ni leng* 四肢逆冷, counterflow with cold in the four limbs. *BJ* SE *chang shi* 長石：主身熱，**四肢寒厥**, "It controls body heat, and **cold with recession in the four limbs**".

Si zhi han nüe **四肢寒瘧, cold malaria affecting the four limbs** [1]
IS identical with → *si zhi ni leng* 四肢逆冷, counterflow with cold in the four limbs. *BCTJ* SE *ta gan* 獺肝：主傳屍勞極，**四肢寒瘧**，虛汗客熱, "It controls corpse [evil] transmission with extreme exhaustion, **cold malaria affecting the four limbs**, and depletion sweating with visitor heat".

Si zhi jue **四肢厥, recession in the four limbs** [1]
IS identical with → *si zhi ni leng* 四肢逆冷, counterflow with cold in the four limbs. *QJYF* 30: 列缺，主**四肢厥**，喜笑, "[The needle insertion hole] *lie jue*: it controls **recession in the four limbs**, and a tendency to laugh".

Si zhi jue ji **四肢厥急, recession with tension in the four limbs** [1]
IS identical with *si zhi ju ji* 四肢拘急, cramps and tension of the four limbs. Possibly a writing error in the *BCGM* SE *zhu dan* 豕膽 quoting from the *ZJSHL* 7：吐已下斷，汗出而厥，四肢拘急不解，脈微欲絕者，通脈四逆加豬膽汁湯主之, "When the vomiting has ended and the discharge has been halted, while [the patient continues] to sweat [in a manner] associated with recession, so that the four limbs are cramped with tension, and the [movement in the] vessels is so weak that it is at the brink of being cut off, then the 'decoction to penetrate the vessels in the case of counterflow in the four [limbs]' with added hog bile will control this", writes: 霍亂病吐下已斷，汗出而厥，**四肢厥急**，脈微欲絶者，通脈四逆湯加豬膽汁主之, "When in the treatment of cholera, the vomiting and the discharge have been halted, while [the patient continues] to sweat [in a manner] associated with recession, so that **the four limbs have recession with tension**, and the [movement in the] vessels is so weak that it is at the brink of being cut off, then the 'decoction to penetrate the vessels in the case of counterflow in the four [limbs] with added hog bile' will master this".

Si zhi jue leng **四肢厥冷, recession with cold in the four limbs** [4]
IS identical with → *si zhi ni leng* 四肢逆冷, counterflow with cold in the four limbs. *QJYF* 9: 唇青面黑，**四肢厥冷**，其脈沉細緊數, "The lips are greenish-blue, the face is black. There is **recession with cold in the four limbs**. The [movement in the] vessels is in the depth, fine, tight, and frequent".

Si zhi jue ni **四肢厥逆, recession with counterflow in the four limbs** [3]
IS identical with → *si zhi ni leng* 四肢逆冷, counterflow with cold in the four limbs. *ZBYHL* 18: 陰陽毒病無常也，或初得病便有毒，或服湯藥，經五六日以上，或十餘日後不瘥，變成毒者。其候身重背強，喉咽痛，糜粥不下，毒氣攻心，心腹煩痛，短氣，**四肢厥逆**，嘔吐，體如被打，發斑，此皆其候, "The disease of yin-yang poisoning takes no regular course. It may be that an initial disease has been associated with poison from its beginning. It may also be that [a patient] has ingested decoction medication for more than five, six days, or even longer than ten days without being cured, at which point he develops a poison. The signs are a heavy body and stiff back, pain in the throat, even gruel cannot be passed down. The poison qi attacks the heart, resulting in vexation and pain in the heart and abdomen, shortness of qi, **recession with counterflow in the four limbs** and vomiting. The body looks as if beaten, and develops macules. All these are its signs".

Si zhi jue qi **四肢厥氣, qi recession in the four limbs** [1]
IS identical with → *si zhi ni leng* 四肢逆冷, counterflow with cold in the four limbs. *BJ* SE *wan jiao* 蔓椒：除**四肢厥氣**，膝痛, "It eliminates **qi recession in the four limbs**, and pain in the knees".

Si zhi leng **四肢冷, the four limbs are cold** [2]
IS identical with → *si zhi ni leng* 四肢逆冷, counterflow with cold in the four limbs. *ZHBJF* 2: 唇青面黑，**四肢冷**，脈沉細而緊數, "The lips are greenish-blue, the face is black. **The four limbs are cold**. The [movement in the] vessels is deep inside, fine, tight, and frequent".

***Si zhi ni leng* 四肢逆冷, counterflow with cold in the four limbs** [7] AN *si zhi jue leng* 四肢厥冷, recession with cold in the four limbs; *si zhi jue ni* 四肢厥逆, recession with counterflow in the four limbs; *si zhi leng* 四肢冷, the four limbs are cold; *si zhi bing leng* 四肢冰冷; the four limbs are as cold as ice; *si zhi han* 四肢寒; the four limbs are cold; *si zhi han nüe* 四肢寒瘧; cold malaria in the four limbs; *si zhi han jue* 四肢寒厥; cold recession in the four limbs; *si zhi jue* 四肢厥, recession in the four limbs; *si zhi jue qi* 四肢厥氣; receding qi in the four limbs.

IS of cold upper and lower extremities, which feel as cold as ice when touched. *ZHBJF* 3: 若**四肢逆冷**，吐清汁，宛轉啼呼者。取桂一兩，㕮咀，以水三升，煮取二升，去滓，適寒温，盡服, "In the case of **counterflow with cold in the four limbs**, with [patients] spitting greenish liquid and winding and crying, take *gui*, 1 *liang*, chew and boil in 3 *sheng* of water down to two *sheng*. Discard the dregs, adjust the temperature and ingest completely".

***Si zhi qing* 四肢清, the four limbs are cool** [2]

IS identical with → *si zhi ni leng* 四肢逆冷, counterflow with cold in the four limbs. *SW* 40: 先唾血，**四肢清**，目眩，時時前後血, "In the beginning, [patients] spit blood and their **four limbs are cool**. Their eyes are dizzy. They often pass blood in front and behind".

***Si zhi quan leng* 四肢拳冷, the four limbs are [twisted into] fists and are cold** [1]

IS of the four limbs being twisted with a feeling of cold. *BCGM* SE *hui dang* 褌襠 quotes *JJF*: 中鬼昏厥：**四肢拳冷**，口鼻出血。用久污溺衣燒灰，每服二錢，沸湯下。男用女，女用男, "Demon stroke with clouding and recession: **The four limbs are [twisted into] fists and are cold**. The mouth and nose bleed. Take a diaper soiled with urine over a long time and burn to ashes. For each dose ingest 2 *qian*, and swallow with hot water. Males use [the diaper] of females; females use those of males".

***Si zhi wei jue* 四肢微厥, slight recession in the four limbs** [1]

IS of a slight cold in the upper and lower extremities. *BYCY* 19: 竊謂前症若熱毒方出，忽被風寒閉塞，肌竅血脈不行，身體作痛，或**四肢微厥**, "I venture to say that when in the case of the above-mentioned conditions heat poison is emitted, and in this situation [the body] is suddenly closed by wind cold so that the sinews, the orifices and the blood vessels can no longer operate, the entire body aches, and in some cases there is **slight recession in the four limbs**".

***Si zhi zhong* 四肢重, the four limbs feel heavy** [1] AN *si zhi zhong ruo* 四肢重弱.

IS of a feeling of unbearable heaviness in the four extremities, and a sensation of fatigue when one starts moving. *BJ* SE da zao 大棗：身中不足，大驚，**四肢重**, "An inadequacy [of qi] in the body. Massive fright. **The four limbs feel heavy**".

***Si zhi zhong ruo* 四肢重弱, the four limbs feel heavy and weak** [1]

IS identical with → *si zhi zhong* 四肢重, the four limbs feel heavy. *BJ* SE *gui jia* 龜甲：濕痹，**四肢重弱**，小兒囟不合, "Moisture blockage. **The four limbs feel heavy and weak.** In children, the fontanelles fails to close".

Song ji **忪悸, agitated palpitation** [2]
IS identical with → *xin ji* 心悸①, heart palpitation. *QJYF* Fj: 棗仁湯，治大虛勞，夢泄精，莖核微弱，血氣枯竭，或醉飽傷於房室，驚惕**忪悸**，小腹裏急方, "The decoction with *zao ren* is a recipe to cure massive depletion exhaustion, wet dreams, weakness of the stalk and kernels (i.e. penis and testicles], as well as harm caused by entering the bedroom [for intercourse] intoxicated with wine and heaving eaten to repletion, fearfulness and **agitated palpitation**, and tensions in the lower abdomen".

Sou **嗽, cough** [p]
① IS identical with → *ke sou* 咳嗽①. *ZHF* 2: 若**嗽**，加栝蔞二兩, "If [the patient] **coughs**, add two *liang* of *gua lou*".
② PC identical with → *ke sou* 咳嗽②. *ZBYHL* 10: 水停心下，則上乘於肺，故令**嗽**, "If water stagnates below the heart, it will then ascend and avail itself of the lung. As a result [the patient] will **cough**".

Sou ni **嗽逆, cough with [qi] counterflow** [2]
PC identical with → *ke sou* 咳嗽②, cough. *YXL* SE *bai shi ying* 白石英：治**嗽逆**上氣, "It cures **cough with [qi] counterflow**, [that is,] ascending qi".

Sou shuo **溲數, frequent urination** [4]
IS identical with → *xiao bian shuo* 小便數, frequent urination. *JGYL* Mj: 氣盛則**溲數**，**溲數**即堅, "If qi is present plentiful this will result in **frequent urination**. **Frequent urination** leads to a hardening [of stools]".

Sou xue **嗽血, blood cough; to cough up blood** [16]
① IS identical with → *ke xue* 咳血①. *SJZL* 68: 治肺損，吐血**嗽血**, "To cure harm to the lung, with blood spitting and **coughing up blood**".
② PC identical with → ke xue 咳血②. *ZZYJ* 4: **嗽血**，熱壅於肺能**嗽血**，久嗽損肺亦能**嗽血**, "**Blood cough**: Heat that is obstructed in the lung can result in **coughing up blood**. If any cough continues for an extended period of time it too can lead to **coughing up blood**".

Su bing **宿病, abiding disease** [2]
PC identical with → *su ji* 宿疾, abiding ailment. *BCJJZ* SE *shu mi* 黍米：又有穄米與黍米相似, 而粒殊大, 食不宜人, 言發**宿病**, "Also, *ji mi* looks very much like *shu mi*, but the seeds are rather big. Eating this is not good for humans. It is said it will cause **abiding disease**".

Su chuang **粟瘡, millet sores** [2]
PC of millet-size → *chuang* 瘡, sores, conditions developing in the genital region. *WTMY* 26 lists 陰邊**粟瘡**方五首, "Five recipes for **millet sores** adjacent to the yin region".

Su gou **宿垢, overnight filth** [6] AN *liu gou* 留垢.
PP of pathological matter remaining in the intestines and in the bladder, accumulating there as feces or urine, or as pus and blood. *YXQY* Lj: 治熱淫於內一也；去腸內**宿垢**二也；破堅積熱塊三也, "The first is: to cure internal heat excess. The second is to remove **overnight filth** from within the intestines. The third is to break hardened accumulations and heat lumps".

Su ji **宿疾, abiding ailment** [7] AN *su bing* 宿病, abiding disease; *gu ji* 故疾, chronic ailment; *gu bing* 故病, chronic disease.

CD of PCs showing a slow development. *QJYF* 13: 治久寒**宿疾**, 胸腹中痛, "To cure **abiding ailments** of long-lasting cold with pain in the chest and abdomen".

Su leng **宿冷, abiding cold** [5]

PC of abiding → *leng bing* 冷病, cold disease. *ZBYHL* 2: 除臟腑內**宿冷**, "Eliminates **abiding cold** in the depots and palaces".

Su shi **宿食, food remaining in the body overnight** [61]

① EA PM of food and beverages remaining undigested in the stomach and intestines for an extended period of time. *SHL* 241: 大下後，六七日不大便，煩不解，腹滿痛者，此有燥屎也。所以然者，本有**宿食**故也, "If after a massive discharge there is no defecation for six or seven days, with a vexation that fails to be resolved, and a feeling of fullness and pain in the abdomen, this is because of the presence of dried feces. The reason is that in the beginning this was a case of **food remaining in the body overnight**".

② AN *shi ji* 食積, food accumulation. PC brought forth by abiding food. *JGYL* Fj: 腹滿、寒疝、**宿食**病脈證治, "[Movements in the] vessels, pathological conditions, and cure of abdominal fullness, cold elevation-illness, and **food remaining in the body overnight**".

Su shui **宿水, abiding water** [8]

EA of water evil stagnating in the human body. *WTMY* 7: 又療心腹脹滿，腹中有**宿水**，連兩肋滿悶，氣急衝心坐不得。郁李仁丸方, "Furthermore, to cure distension and a feeling of fullness in the heart and abdomen, **abiding water** in the abdomen, and a feeling of fullness in the two flanks as well as heart-pressure, with qi urgently moving against the heart and making it impossible to sit, [use] the recipe for pills with *yu li ren*".

Su tong **宿痛, abiding pain** [1]

PC of a pain that is constantly present. *BCGM* SE *jiu* 酒：蠶沙酒，治風緩頑痹，諸節不隨，腹內**宿痛**, "Wine made from silkworm excrements cures wind sluggishness and stubborn blockage, when all joints fail to function as one would like them to, with **abiding pain** in the abdomen".

Su xu **素虛, habitual depletion** [1]

A chronically depleted and weak constitution. *YXRM* 1: **素虛**者得之，為骨蒸怯症, "If one feels such [a movement in the vessels when examining] persons with a **habitual depletion**, then this indicates a condition of bone steaming and timidity".

Su xue **宿血, residual blood** [48] AN *lao xue* 老血, old blood;

① AN *liu xue* 留血, residual blood; *chen xue* 陳血, aged blood. EA of → *yu xue* 瘀血②, stagnant blood, forming long-term accumulations in the body that are difficult to dissolve and may in turn cause further diseases. *ZBYHL* 42: 過年不產，由挾寒冷**宿血**在胞而有胎，則冷血相搏，令胎不長，產不以時, "She [was pregnant and] did not give birth for more than a year. The reason is that she had cold and **residual blood** in her womb together with the fetus. As a result,

the cold and the blood struck each other. This prevented the growth of the fetus, and delayed delivery beyond the appropriate time".
② PC brought forth by residual blood. *TBC* SE *shan hu* 珊瑚：主**宿血**，去目中翳, "It controls **residual blood** and removes shades from within the eyes".

Su yin **宿飲, abiding rheum** [5]
EA of → *yin* 飲①, rheum, collecting in the body. *ZLBC* SE *jiu* 韭：黃帝云：霜韭凍，不可生食，動**宿飲**, "Huang Di: *Jiu* exposed to frost cannot be consumed in a raw state. It activates **abiding rheum**".

Su zheng **宿癥, abiding concretion-illness** [6]
PC of long-lasting → *zheng* 癥, concretion-illness. *YXL* SE wa na qi 膃肭臍：主治男子**宿癥**氣塊, "It controls **abiding concretion-illness** and qi lumps in males".

Su zhi **宿滯, abiding [qi] with sluggishness** [8]
① EA PM identical with → *ji zhi* 積滯①, accumulation and sluggishness. *TPSHF* 49: 食飲**宿滯**，積聚成病, "**Abiding [qi] with sluggishness** of food and beverages [resulting in] accumulation and collection generates disease".
② PC identical with → *ji zhi* 積滯②, accumulation and blockage. *YXL* SE *xuan ming fen* 玄明粉：治心熱煩躁並五藏**宿滯**, "It cures heart heat with vexation and restlessness, and also **abiding [qi] with sluggishness** in the five depots".

Suan bi **痠痹, feeling of soreness [caused by a] blockage** [2]
IS of an uncomfortable sensation of soreness. *BCGM* SE xuan ming fen 玄明粉 quoting *XJ*: 手脚痠, "The hands and legs experience a feeling of soreness", writes: 手脚**痠痹**, "Hands and legs experience a **feeling of soreness [caused by a] blockage**".

Suan fa **蒜髮, garlic hair** [5]
IS of gray hair. *BCJJZ* SE fa pi 髮髲：人今呼斑髮為**蒜髮**, "Nowadays people speak of gray hair as '**garlic hair**'".

Suan shui **痠水, sour water** [16]
IS identical with *tun suan* 吞酸, acid swallowing. *BJSY* SE *kuai* 鱠：除膀胱水，喉中氣結，心下**痠水**, "It eliminates water from the bladder, qi nodes in the throat, and **sour water** below the heart".

Suan si **痠嘶, distress** [1]
IS identical with → *suan xi* 痠㪷. *BCGM* SE *rang he* 蘘荷 quotes *MYBL*: 温瘧寒熱，**痠嘶**邪氣, "[It cures] warmth malaria with alternating sensations of cold and heat; **distress** and evil qi".

Suan teng **痠疼, soreness** [13]
IS identical with → *suan tong* 痠痛. *BJ* SE *fei lian* 飛廉：主骨節熱，脛重**痠疼**, "It controls heat in the bones and joints, and a feeling of heaviness and **soreness** in the shins".

Suan tong **痠痛, soreness** [17] AN *suan teng* 痠疼; *teng suan* 疼痠.
IS of pain together with a feeling of feebleness. *SW* 36: 先足脛**痠痛**者，先刺足陽明十指間出血, "If it [appeared] initially as **soreness** in the feet and shins, first pierce the foot yang brilliance [conduit] between the ten toes to let blood".

***Suan xi* 酸嘶, distress** [1] AN *suan si* 酸嘶.
IS of an uncomfortable, distressed feeling. *BJ* SE mu meng 木虻：瘀血，血閉，寒熱**酸嘶**, "Stagnant blood, blood closure, alternating sensations of cold and heat with **distress**".

***Suan xin* 酸心, sour center** [3]
IS identical with → *cu xin* 醋心, vinegar center. *HJJF* 9: 小地黄丸，治妊娠**酸心**，吐清水，腹痛，不能飲食, "Pills with *di huang* and only a small number [of further ingredients] cure **sour center** (i.e. stomach) during pregnancy, vomiting of clear water, abdominal pain, and an inability to drink or eat".

***Suan zhong* 酸重, a feeling of soreness and heaviness** [1]
IS of a feeling of soreness or deep-seated heaviness affecting the entire body or parts of it. *RHZ nao sha* 硇砂：丈夫腰胯**酸重**，四肢不任, "In males, the lower back and the hips experience **a feeling of soreness and heaviness**. The four extremities fail to function".

***Sui gu ju* 髓骨疽, marrow and bone impediment-illness** [1]
PC identical with → *gu ju* 骨疽, bone impediment-illness. *MYBL* SE *shi hui* 石灰：療**髓骨疽**, "It cures **marrow and bone impediment-illness**".

***Sui yi* 髓溢, marrow spill** [2]
PC of one's teeth gradually growing to the extent that eventually they push the mouth wide open and make it difficult to eat. *BCGM* SE *zhu* 术 quoting *JFPJF* 22: 牙齒逐日微長，漸漸脹開口，難為飲食，蓋**髓溢**所致, "The teeth grow a bit longer day by day, gradually widening and opening the mouth and making it difficult to drink and eat. Now, this is brought forth by **marrow spill**", writes: 牙齒日長，漸至難食，名**髓溢**病, "The teeth grow longer day by day until eventually one finds it difficult to eat. This is called '**marrow spill**' disease".

***Sun chuang zhong feng* 損瘡中風, wind stroke via wounds and sores** [1]
PC identical with → *zhu chuang zhong feng* 諸瘡中風, wind stroke via all possible sores. *SLBC* SE *qin jiao* 秦椒, for external treatment of **損瘡中風, "wind stroke via wounds and sores"**.

***Sun dong tai qi* 損動胎氣, fetus qi excited by an injury** [2]
PC identical with → *shang tai* 傷胎, harmed fetus. *PJF* 344: 治妊娠**損動胎氣**，腹內結痛, "To cure **fetus qi excited by an injury** during pregnancy, with intraabdominal nodes and pain".

***Sun shang* 損傷, injury; injured** [33]
① PC identical with → *shang sun* 傷損. *QJYF* 1: **損傷**之病，亦以眾矣, "There are many diseases of **injury**".
② PM of physically harming or impairing functions of the organs of the human body. *ZBYHL* 4: 腎肝**損傷**，故因嘔逆唾血也, "**Injured** kidneys and liver cause vomiting with counterflow, and blood spitting".

***Sun tai* 損胎, injured fetus** [4] AN *tai sun* 胎損, fetal injury.
PC identical with → *shang tai* 傷胎, harmed fetus. *TPSHF* 77: 治妊娠**損胎**，下血不止, "It cures **injured fetus** during pregnancy, and unceasing discharge of blood".

***Sun xie* 飧泄, outflow of [undigested] food** [4] AW *sun xie* 飧瀉.

PC of water-like diarrhea with food being discharged undigested. SW 17: 久風為**飧泄**, "Wind staying for a long time causes **outflow of [undigested] food**".

***Sun xie* 飧瀉, outflow of [undigested] food** [2]

PC identical with → *sun xie* 飧泄. *BCGM* SE *zhu* 朮 quoting *SWBJQYBMJ* Mj: 不飲水而穀完出，名曰飧泄…泄止後服椒朮丸, "[Patients] have not drunk water and yet their food [lit. grain] is released undigested. This is called 'outflow of [undigested] food'...Once the outflow has been stopped, [patients] ingest the pills with [*shu*] *jiao* and [*cang*] *zhu*", writes: **飧瀉**久痢：椒朮丸, "For **outflow of [undigested] food** and long-lasting free-flux illness, [ingest] the pills with [*shu*] *jiao* and [*cang*] *zhu*",

***Sun xue* 損血, bleeding from an injury; to harm the blood; blood resulting from an injury** [4]

① PC of a → *shang sun* 傷損, injury, with blood spitting and blood discharge. *QJYiF* 7: 大補益當歸丸，治產後虛羸不足…或**損血**吐下及金瘡等方, "The pills with *dang gui* for massive supplementation, they are a recipe to cure depletion following delivery, with emaciation and insufficiency…and also **bleeding resulting from injury**, as well as wounds inflicted by metal objects".

② PM of pathological changes undergone by the blood inside the body resulting from various causes. *TPSHF* 30: 虛勞**損血**，則不能榮養於筋, "When depletion exhaustion **harms the blood**, it will no longer be able to nourish the sinews".

③ PP identical with → *sun yu* 損瘀, blood that has left the vessels following an injury. *WTMY* 17: 卒然損傷於腰而致痛也，此由**損血**搏於背脊所為, "If a person has been suddenly injured in the lower back and feels pain there, the reason is that the **blood resulting from the injury** is striking against the spine and back".

***Sun yu* 損瘀, blood that has left the vessels following an injury** [1]

PP of blood that has left the vessels (hematoma) following a bodily injury. *YXL* SE *bai pu xi* 敗蒲席：從高墜下，**損瘀**在腹刺痛，此蒲合臥破敗者良, "For [treating persons who] having fallen from somewhere high and [now] have **blood that has left the vessels following an injury** with piercing pain. Those mats that have been worn out by [people] sleeping on them are best".

***Suo du* 鎖肚, locked belly** [1]

PC of newborns within the first three days following delivery with the anus closed and allowing no passage of stools. *YKLC* 3:**鎖肚**者，由胎中受熱，熱毒壅盛結於肛門，閉而不通, "**Locked belly**: this is because they were affected by heat while still in the womb. The heat poison caused obstruction with nodes of abundance at the anus which got blocked and became impassable".

***Suo hou zhang* 锁喉瘴, throat-locking miasma** [1] AN *po she zhang* 朴蛇瘴.

PC with a massive swelling and pain of the nape affecting the throat. *PJF* 61: 治**鎖喉瘴**，又名朴蛇瘴，項大腫痛連喉, "To cure **throat-locking miasma**, which is also called 'pure snake miasma'. The nape is massively swollen and painful, and this also affects the throat".

- T -

Tai bing **胎病, fetal diseases** [1]

PC related to pregnancy. *PJF* 337: 古今療**胎病**方有類十首，不問虛實冷熱，殆死者活。此方（茯苓丸）緣妊娠忌桂，所以熬, "There are dozens of recipes, throughout the ages, to cure **fetal diseases**, regardless of whether it is a depletion or repletion, a cold or heat, whether the fetus has died, or is still alive. Because *gui* must not be ingested during pregnancy, the present recipe requires it to be boiled".

Tai chan bu xia **胎產不下, failure of a fetus in birth to descend** [1]

PC identical with → *nan chan* 難產, difficult delivery. *BCGM* SE *jiu* 酒：婦人崩中下血，**胎產不下**, "[It cures] women experiencing a collapsing center with discharge of blood, and a **failure of a fetus in birth to descend**".

Tai chan zhu bing **胎產諸病, all diseases related to fetus and delivery** [3]

PC CD of women's diseases related to pregnancy and delivery. *BCGM* SE *chong wei* 茺蔚：若治腫毒瘡瘍，消水行血，婦人**胎產諸病**，則宜並用為良, "When treating swelling from poison, sores and ulcers, to dissolve water and make blood flow, and for **all diseases** in women **related to a fetus and delivery**, it is advisable to use them together as a good approach".

Tai chi **胎赤, fetal red** [2]

PC identical with → *tai chi yan* 胎赤眼, fetal red eyes. *ZBYHL* 28: **胎赤**者，是人初生，洗目不淨，令穢汁浸漬於眥，使瞼赤爛，至大不瘥，故云**胎赤**, "As for 'fetal red', this is when the liquid to rinse a newborn's eyes is not clean, and lets dirty liquid enter the corners of the eyes, this causes the eyelids to turn red and fester. This cannot be healed until adulthood. Hence it is called '**fetal red**'".

Tai chi feng yan **胎赤風眼, fetal red wind eyes** [1]

PC identical with → *tai chi yan* 胎赤眼, fetal red eyes. *BCGM* SE *huai* 槐 quoting *QHYF* 6: 治胎赤眼方, "Recipe to cure fetal red eyes", writes: **胎赤風眼**, "**Fetal red wind eyes**".

Tai chi lan yan **胎赤爛眼, fetal red festering eyes** [1]

PC identical with → *tai chi yan* 胎赤眼, fetal red eyes. *BCGM* SE *shou gong* 守宮 quoting *SJZL*: 胎赤眼連睫赤爛, "Fetal red eyes and eyelashes red and festering", writes: **胎赤爛眼**, "**Fetal red festering eyes**".

Tai chi yan **胎赤眼, fetal red eyes** [6] AD *tai chi* 胎赤, fetal red; AN *tai chi feng yan* 胎赤風眼, fetal red wind eyes; *tai chi lan yan* 胎赤爛眼, fetal red festering eyes.

PC of red festering eyes of children from birth on that remain uncured for a long time. *SJZL* 102: 治**胎赤眼**久不瘥，昏暗漠漠，瞳仁脹痛，羚羊角湯方, "To cure **fetal red eyes** that have not been cured for an extended period of time, with [patients having] dim vision, and the pupil being distended and painful, [use] the recipe for the decoction with *ling yang jiao*".

***Tai dong* 胎動, fetal movement** [p]
PC identical with → *tai dong bu an* 胎動不安, fetal movement and restlessness. *MYBL* SE *sheng di huang* 生地黄：傷身**胎動**下血，胎不落, "[It serves to cure] an injured body with **fetal movement** and a discharge of blood, [and initiates birth when] the fetus does not descend".

***Tai dong bu an* 胎動不安, fetal movement and restlessness** [9] AN *tai zang bu an* 胎臟不安, fetal restlessness; *tai qi bu an* 胎氣不安, fetal restlessness; *ren zhen tai dong* 妊娠胎動, fetal movement during pregnancy; AD *tai dong* 胎動, fetal movement.
PC of a painful lumbar region and abdomen during pregnancy, with an excited fetus that appears to descend, sometimes associated with small quantities of water or blood leaving from the vagina. *ZBYHL* 41: **胎動不安**者，多因勞役氣力，或觸冒冷熱，或飲食不適，或居處失宜。輕者止轉動不安，重者便致傷墮, "**Fetal movement and restlessness** often result from [a woman's] exhaustion and excessive exertion of strength, or from being affected by the malicious in the form of cold and heat, or from inadequate beverages and food, or from failing to balance her times of resting and activity. In light cases, [the fetus] simply moves and is restless. Serious cases may end in a premature descent".

***Tai dong po xin* 胎動迫心, fetal movement pressing against the heart** [1]
PC identical with → *zi shang chong xin* 子上衝心, a child rises and clashes with the heart. *BCGM* SE *ai* 艾 quotes *ZMML*: **胎動迫心**, 作痛, "**Fetal movement pressing against the heart**: it causes pain".

***Tai dong shang bi* 胎動上逼, fetal movement pressing upward** [1]
PC identical with → *zi shang chong xin* 子上衝心, a child rises and clashes with the heart. *BCGM* SE *gong nu xian* 弓弩弦 quotes *YLJY*: **胎動上逼**, 弩弦系帶之立下, "**Fetal movement pressing upward**: Wear a bowstring of a bow or crossbow as a girdle and [the fetus] will come down immediately".

***Tai dong shang ge* 胎動上膈, fetal movement rising towards the diaphragm** [1]
PC identical with → *zi shang chong xin* 子上衝心, a child rises and clashes with the heart. *BCGM* Bai bing zhu zhi yao 百病主治藥 quoting *YLJY*: 胎動上逼, "Fetal movement pressing upward", writes: **胎動上膈**, "**Fetal movement rising towards the diaphragm**".

***Tai du* 胎毒, fetal poison** [21]
EA of heat poison transferred from a mother's body to a fetus during pregnancy, resulting in a child's predisposition for developing smallpox and other diseases. *XEWSZWFL* 1: 因**胎毒**攻發，身生瘡者，名曰蓐瘡, "If [a child] was struck by **fetal poison**, and if it then develops sores, they are called 'childbed sores'".

***Tai feng* 胎風, fetal wind** [9]
PC of a) → *jing feng* 驚風, fright wind, developed by children within 100 days following delivery. *YYXS* 11 RE *bian jin dan* 扁金丹, gold leaf elixir: 治小兒**胎風**諸癇, "It cures **fetal wind** and all types of epilepsy in children". b) Dermal sores of newborn children. *BYCY* 3: **胎風**：小兒初生，其身有如湯潑火傷者，此皆乳母過食膏粱所致也, "**Fetal wind**: when in newborn children the body ap-

pears as if scorched by boiling water, this is always because the feeding mother has consumed too much rich food".

***Tai gou* 胎垢, fetal filth** [1]

PC identical with → *lin ti* 鱗體, scaly body. *XEWSZWLF* 20: **胎垢**，謂生下體皮黑垢若鱗者也, " '**Fetal filth**' is to say: immediately following delivery the [child's] skin has black filth as if [covered with] scales".

***Tai han* 胎寒, fetal cold** [7]

PC of depletion cold and abdominal pain of newborns because of harm caused to the mother's yang qi by her excessive affection with cold during pregnancy. *ZBYHL* 47: 兒在胎之時，母取冷過度，冷氣入胞，令兒著冷，至兒生出，則喜腹痛，不肯飲乳，此則**胎寒**, "When during the child's presence in the womb the mother consumes excessive cold, this cold will enter the womb where it attaches itself to the child. When the child is born, it is likely to have abdominal pain and it will not be willing to drink milk. This is **fetal cold**".

***Tai jing* 胎驚, fetal fright** [6]

PC of → *jing feng* 驚風, fright wind, occurring in children within the first month following delivery. *BCGM* Bai bing zhu zhi yao 百病主治藥 quotes *RZZZF*: 小兒**胎驚**，琥珀、防風各一錢，硃砂半錢，為末。豬乳調一字，入口中，最妙, "For children with **fetal fright** [use] *hu po* and *fang feng*, 1 *qian* each, *zhu sha* 1 half *qian*, and prepare a powder to be mixed with as much hog milk as fits on a character of a coin. Insert this into the [child's] mouth. Extremely wondrously [effective]".

***Tai jing tian diao* 胎驚天吊, fetus with fright hauled-by-heaven** [1]

PC identical with → *tian diao jing feng* 天吊驚風, hauled-by-heaven fright wind. *BCGM* Bai bing zhu zhi yao 百病主治藥 quoting recipes attached to SE *xie* 蠍：天釣驚風, "Hooked-up-by-heaven fright wind", writes: **胎驚天吊**, "**Fetus with fright hauled-by-heaven**".

***Tai lei* 胎羸, fetal thinness** [1]

PC of an emaciation and weakness of newborn children because of insufficient nourishment during pregnancy. *HSYT* Fj: 予之**胎羸**，賴此再造，願與人人共之, "I administered them in a case of **fetal thinness**, and based on their [effect] have prepared them again. I should like to share them with everyone".

***Tai li* 胎痢, fetal free-flux illness** [1]

PC identical with → *tai qian li* 胎前痢, free-flux illness preceding delivery. *BCGM* Bai bing zhu zhi yao 百病主治藥, SE *ji luan huang* 雞卵黃：**胎痢**，同黃丹燒服, "For **fetal free-flux illness**, consume roasted together with *huang dan*".

***Tai lou* 胎漏, fetal leaking** [8]

PC identical with → *lou tai* 漏胎, leaking fetus. *TPSHF* 75: 治妊娠**胎漏**，下血不止, "It cures **fetal leaking** during pregnancy, with an unending discharge of blood".

***Tai qi bu an* 胎氣不安, fetal restlessness** [4]
PC identical with → *tai dong bu an* 胎動不安, fetal movement and restlessness. *TPSHF* 74: 治妊娠傷寒，煩熱頭痛，**胎氣不安**，或時吐逆，不下食，白术散方, "For curing harm caused by cold during pregnancy, vexation with heat and headache, **fetal restlessness**, sometimes accompanied by vomiting with counterflow and an inability to ingest food, [use] the recipe for the powder with *bai zhu*".

***Tai qi bu zhang* 胎氣不長, fetal qi failing to grow** [1]
PC with the uterus being too small for the present stage of pregnancy, and the fetus being alive but showing only a retarded growth. *BCGM* SE *li yu* 鯉魚 quoting *WTMY* 33: 懷胎不長, "The fetus fails to grow", writes: **胎氣不長**, "The **fetal qi fails to grow**".

***Tai qi shang chong* 胎氣上沖, fetal qi that rises and clashes [with the heart]** [1]
PC identical with → *zi shang chong xin* 子上衝心, a child rises and clashes with the heart. *BCGM* Bai bing zhu zhi yao 百病主治藥：竹瀝，**胎氣上沖**，煩躁，日頻飲之, "Dried bamboo sap: drink several times daily [to cure] **fetal qi that rises and clashes [with the heart]**, and vexation with restlessness.

***Tai qian li* 胎前痢, free-flux illness preceding delivery** [1]
PC identical with → *yun li* 孕痢, pregnancy-related free-flux illness. *BCGM* Bai bing zhu zhi yao 百病主治藥 quoting *QJYF* SE *yi dai* 衣帶：治妊娠痢下, "It cures pregnancy-related free-flux illness", writes: 故衣帛主**胎前痢**, "Old clothes' silk controls **free-flux illness preceding delivery**".

***Tai re* 胎熱, fetal heat** [8]
PC referring to a) a situation where a pregnant woman has been affected by heat that was able to enter the womb. *SJZL* 54: 下焦腸胃伏熱，婦人**胎熱**產難, "In the case of heat hidden in the lower burner, the intestines and the stomach, and when pregnant women have **fetal heat** and have difficulties giving birth". b) a disease brought forth in children by wind evil that has entered their mother's womb during her pregnancy, with the heat poison abiding in the child's depots and palaces after delivery. *TPSHF* 82 lists a 治小兒**胎熱**撮口方, "recipe for oral intake to cure children with **fetal heat** and pursed mouth".

***Tai shang chong xin* 胎上衝心, a fetus rises and clashes with the heart** [1]
PC identical with → *zi shang chong xin* 子上衝心, a child rises and clashes with the heart. *FRDQLF* 77: 療妊娠忽下血，**胎上衝心**，手足逆冷, "To cure sudden discharge of blood during pregnancy, with the **fetus rising and clashing with the heart**, and the hands and feet affected by counterflow cold".

***Tai shang qiang xin* 胎上搶心, a fetus rises and knocks at the heart** [1]
PC identical with → *zi shang chong xin* 子上衝心, a child rises and clashes with the heart. *FRDQLF* 12: **胎上搶心**，則悶絕欲死，冷汗自出，喘滿不食, "When **a fetus rises and knocks at the heart**, then this results in heart-pressure and an interruption [of qi flow] bringing a person close to death. Cold sweat leaves the body spontaneously. [Patients] pant, have a feeling of fullness, and do not eat".

Tai si bu xia 胎死不下, **a fetus has died and fails to descend** [2]

PC identical with → *zi si fu zhong* 子死腹中, a fetus' death in the abdomen. *FRDQLF* 17：如胎死不下，煎紅花，温酒調下, "If a **fetus has died and fails to descend**, boil *hong hua* and ingest mixed with warm wine".

Tai si fu zhong 胎死腹中, **a fetus' death in the abdomen** [12]

PC identical with → *zi si fu zhong* 子死腹中. *QJYF* 2：真珠湯，治胎死腹中方, "Decoction with *zhen zhu*, a recipe to cure **a fetus' death in the abdomen**".

Tai sun 胎損, [1] fetal injury

PC identical with → *shang tai* 傷胎, harmed fetus. *BCTJ* SE *zhu gen* 苧根：孕婦胎損方所須, "A required ingredient of recipes for pregnant women with **fetal injury**".

Tai ti 胎啼, **fetal cry** [3] AN *fu zhong er ku* 腹中兒哭, a child crying in the abdomen; *fu nei zhong ming* 腹內鐘鳴, a bell ringing in the abdomen.

PC of sounds heard out of a pregnant woman's abdomen. *BCGM* Bai bing zhu zhi yao 百病主治藥：胎前，子煩，胎啼, "[During] pregnancy: child[-bearing] vexation; **fetal cry**".

Tai xian 胎癇, **fetal epilepsy** [2]

PC of a → *dian xian* 癲癇, peak-illness with epilepsy, breaking out in infants at an age of less than 100 days. It was assumed that this is caused if a fetus in the mother's abdomen is frightened prior to delivery. *TPSHF* 100: 小兒胎癇、奶癇、驚癇，一依此灸一壯, "Infantile **fetal epilepsy**, breastmilk epilepsy, and fright epilepsy, they are to be cauterized once in accordance with this".

Tai xuan 胎癬, **fetal *xuan*-illness** [3]

PC of → *tou xuan* 頭瘡, head *xuan*-illness, growing on the head of a small child. It itches and releases water, and when scratched with the fingers it spreads and multiplies. *PJF* 363: 小兒頭生瘡，手爬處即延，謂之胎癬, "When children grow sores on their head which spread when scratched, this is called '**fetal *xuan*-illness**'".

Tai yang bing 太陽病, **major yang disease** [4]

PC of an intrusion, during a disease of harm caused by cold, into the body of wind cold resulting in a fight between proper and evil qi, and a loss of balance between camp and guardian qi, with an aversion to cold, fever, pain and stiffness in the head and neck, as well as a surface movement in the vessels. *SHL* 3: 太陽病，或已發熱，或未發熱，必惡寒、體痛、嘔逆、脈陰陽俱緊者，名為傷寒, "A **major yang disease**, in some cases with an effusion of heat, in some cases without an effusion of heat, definitely with an aversion to cold, a feeling of body heaviness, vomiting with counterflow, and a hard [movement] in both the yin and yang vessels, this is called harm caused by cold".

Tai yang shang han 太陽傷寒, **harm in the major yang section caused by cold** [1] AN *shang han tai yang zheng* 傷寒太陽證, harm caused by cold with signs in the major yang section.

PC of a type of → *shang han* 傷寒, harm caused by cold, with signs such as a movement in the vessels at the surface, stiff and aching head and neck, as well as an aversion to cold. *SHL* 119: **太陽傷寒**者，加温針必驚也, “If in the case of **harm in the major yang section caused by cold** one applies a warmed needle, this will shock [the patient]”.

Tai yang tou tong **太陽頭痛, major yang headache** [5]
PC of → *tou tong* 頭痛, headache, extending along the course of the major yang conduits resulting from an intrusion of wind cold into the major yang conduits. That is, the pain affects the region from the top to the back of the head, in severe cases it reaches the nape. *SJZL* 24: **太陽頭痛**，必發熱惡寒, “In the case of **major yang headache** [patients] will effuse heat and have an aversion to cold”.

Tai yang xue tong **太陽穴痛, major yang holes pain** [2]
IS of → *tou tong* 頭痛①, headache, mainly affecting the major yang needle insertion holes on both sides of the head. *WSBJ* 9: 救苦神白散，治男子婦人偏正頭疼，眉骨、兩**太陽穴痛**, “The 'wondrously effective powder with [*cong*] *bai* to rescue from suffering' cures hemilateral and ordinary headache in males and females, as well as **pain** affecting the eyebrow bones and the two **major yang holes**”.

Tai yang zhong feng **太陽中風, wind stroke in the major yang [conduits]** [2]
PC identical with → *zhong feng* 中風② b) wind stroke, struck by wind. *SHL* 38: **太陽中風**，脈浮緊、發熱、惡寒、身疼痛、不汗出而煩躁者，大青龍湯主之, “**Wind stroke in the major yang [conduits]**: the [movement in the] vessels is at the surface and tight. [Patients] effuse heat and develop an aversion to cold; their body is in pain. They do not sweat and are mentally irritated. The Large Greenish Dragon Decoction controls it”.

Tai yi bu xia **胎衣不下, the placenta fails to descend** [20]
PC identical with → *bao yi bu xia* 胞衣不下. *BCSY* SE *ou shi* 藕實：葉及房，主血脹腹痛，產後**胎衣不下**, “Leaves and capsules: they master blood distension and abdominal pain, and when **the placenta fails to descend** following birth”.

Tai zang bu an **胎臓不安, fetal depot restlessness** [1]
PC identical with → *tai dong bu an* 胎動不安, fetal movement and restlessness. *PJF* 340：白术散，治妊娠霍亂，吐瀉過多，傷冷，**胎臓不安**, “The powder with *bai zhu* cures pregnancy-related cholera, excessive vomiting and outflow, harm caused by cold, and **fetal depot restlessness**”.

Tai zheng **胎蒸, fetal steam** [2]
PC with a pregnant woman's red and swollen face, a bitter taste in her mouth and a dry throat, as well as fever and emaciation. *TBC* SE hu huang lian 胡黃連：治婦人**胎蒸**，虛驚, “It cures women with **fetal steam** and depletion fright”.

Tai zhong **胎腫, fetal swelling** [4]
PC identical with → *ren shen shui zhong* 妊娠水腫, edematose swelling during pregnancy. *BCGM* SE *zhu ling* 豬苓：治淋腫脚氣，白濁帶下，妊娠子淋**胎腫**，小便不利, “Cures dripping with swelling and leg qi, white-turbid discharge from below the belt, dripping during pregnancy and **fetal swelling**, as well as blocked urination”.

***Tan* 痰, phlegm** [p]

① PI of a) a fluid secreted from the respiratory tract that can be thrown out by means of coughing. *WTMY* 39: 寒熱喉痹，咳逆**痰**沫，胸中滿，不得喘息，胸痛, "Alternating sensations of cold and heat, with throat blockage, cough and counterflow with **phlegm** and foam, a feeling of fullness in the chest, and an inability to breathe with panting, as well as chest pain". b) A sticky fluid secreted from the upper digestive tract that can be eliminated by means of vomiting. *QJYF* 19: 食飲苦吐酸**痰**，嘔逆，泄下少氣, "When eating and drinking they suffer from vomiting sour **phlegm**, cough with counterflow, diarrhea and shortness of qi". c) Sticky matter collecting at the site of pathological change. *ZHF* 4: 治胸中多**痰**，頭痛不欲食, "To cure the presence of much **phlegm** in the chest, with headache and lack of appetite".

② EA of phlegm that may bring forth further ailments. *ZHF* 4: **痰**厥氣上衝所致，名為厥頭痛，吐之即瘥, "It it is brought forth by **phlegm** and recessive qi rushing upward. This is called recesssion headache. Once it has been thrown up the cure is achieved".

③ PC brought forth by phlegm. *JGYL* Mj: 膈上病**痰**，滿喘咳吐, "Above the diaphragm one suffers from **phlegm**. There are feelings of fullness, panting, cough, and vomiting". *BCGM* Bai bing zhu zhi yao 百病主治藥 distinguishes among six phlegm PCs: **痰**有六：濕、熱、風、寒、食、氣也, "There are six types of **phlegm** [condition]: moisture[-type], heat[-type], wind[-type], cold[-type], food[-type], and qi[-type phlegm]".

***Tan* 癱, paralysis; left side paralysis** [p]

① IS of an inability to raise the four limbs, with the muscles and joints having no strength so that they are unable to support the body in standing or walking. *SJZL* 7: 其證四肢不舉，筋脈關節無力，不可枝梧者，謂之**攤**（**癱**）"If the signs are such that one cannot raise his four limbs, and if sinews and joints have no strength and cannot give support, then this is called '**paralysis**'".

② PC If a → *tan huan* 癱瘓, paralysis, affects the left side, the abbreviation is *tan* 癱. *HJJF* 1: 乳香應痛丸，治一切風氣，左**癱**右瘓，口眼喎斜，半身不遂，語言謇澀, "Pills with *ru xiang* that respond to pain cure all types of wind qi, **left side paralysis**, right side paralysis, with the mouth and eyes becoming slanted, and one half of the body not following one's will. The [patient's] language is impeded".

***Tan bing* 痰病, phlegm disease** [5]

PC brought forth by the presence of phlegm. *DXZFXY* 2: **痰病**久得澀脈，卒難得開，必費調理, "If a **phlegm disease** persists over an extended period of time, the [movement in the] vessels will be rough. This is difficult to resolve in a short time; one must make great efforts to restore health!"

***Tan chuan* 痰喘, phlegm panting** [35] AN *xian chuan* 涎喘, saliva panting.

PC of → *chuan* 喘②, panting, caused by phlegm, often accompanied by cough emitting phlegm. *TPSHF* 31: 治骨蒸勞、咳嗽上氣、**痰喘**，寒熱，四肢瘦弱，宜服獺肝丸方, "To cure bone steaming with exhaustion, cough with rising qi, **phlegm panting**, alternating sensations of cold and heat, and weakness affecting the four limbs, the recipe to ingest the pills with otter liver is advisable".

***Tan du* 痰毒, phlegm poison** [3]

EA of → *tan* 痰, phlegm, that may cause disease. *TPSHF* 6: 令目眩頭旋，心腹痞滿，常欲嘔吐，不思飲食，皆由**痰毒**壅滯也, "The reason for dizziness and a spinning head, an obstacle-illness and a feeling of fullness in the heart and abdomen, a permanent urge to vomit, and a lack of appetite and thirst, is always **phlegm poison** obstruction and [qi] sluggishness".

***Tan ge* 痰膈, phlegm occlusion** [4]

PC of → *ge qi* 膈氣, occlusion qi, resulting from congestion brought forth by a mutual interference of phlegm and qi. *TPSHF* 51: 治肺脾風壅，**痰膈**，不下食飲，頭目昏悶，四肢煩疼，旋覆花散方, "To cure lung and spleen wind congestion, **phlegm occlusion**, when food and beverages fail to descend, with clouding affecting the head and eyes, as well as heart-pressure and vexation pain affecting the four limbs, [ingest] the recipe for the powder with *xuan fu hua*".

***Tan he* 痰核, phlegm kernel** [6]

PC identical with → *luo li jie he* 瘰癧結核, scrofula with pervasion-illness with nodular kernels. *SZYS* 9：**痰核**，即瘰癧也，少陽經鬱火所結, "**Phlegm kernel** is identical with scrofula with pervasion-illness. These are nodes resulting from pent-up fire in the minor yang conduits".

***Tan hou* 痰齁, phlegm roaring** [5] AN *tan xiao* 痰哮.

PC of → *xiao chuan* 哮喘, roaring panting, brought forth by phlegm and saliva congestion. *BCGM* SE *mao* 貓 quotes *YXZC*: **痰齁**發喘：貓頭骨燒灰，酒服三錢，便止, "**Phlegm roaring** with panting: Burn the skull bones of a cat to ashes, and ingest 3 *qian* with wine. It will end immediately".

***Tan huan* 癱瘓, paralysis** [24] AW 癱緩，攤緩.

① IS of an inability to move hands and legs autonomously. *SJZL* 5: 治中風，積涎在膈下，四肢**癱瘓**, "To cure wind stroke, with saliva collecting below the diaphragm and **paralysis** of the four limbs".

② AD *tan* 癱, *huan* 瘓; AN *tan huan feng* 癱瘓風, paralysis wind; *tan huan feng* 攤緩風, *tan huan feng* 癱緩風, *feng huan* 風癱. PC with paralysis as the major disease sign. *WTMY* 14: 療熱風**癱瘓**常發者方, "Recipes to cure frequent outbreaks of **paralysis** resulting from heat and wind".

***Tan huan* 癱緩, paralysis** [22]

IS PC identical with → *tan huan* 癱瘓, paralysis. *QJYF* 7: **癱緩**頑痹方, "Recipes [to cure] **paralysis** and stubborn blockage".

***Tan huan* 攤緩, paralysis** [3]

IS PC identical with → *tan huan* 癱瘓, paralysis. *WTMY* 7: **攤緩**頑痹方, "Recipes [to cure] **paralysis** and stubborn blockage".

***Tan huan feng* 癱瘓風, paralysis wind** [2]

PC identical with → *tan huan* 癱瘓②, *WTMY* 3 quotes *GJF*: **癱瘓風**及諸風，手足不隨，腰脚無力, "In the case of **paralysis wind**, and all types of wind, the hands and feet do not follow one's will; the lower back and legs have no strength".

***Tan huan feng* 癱緩風, paralysis wind** [1] AN *tan huan pian feng* 攤瘓偏風
PC identical with → *tan huan* 癱瘓②, paralysis. *QJYF* 12 RE *yuan hua san* 芫花散, powder with yuan hua: **癱緩風**，十二兩和酒三斗, "[To cure] **paralysis wind** [ingest] 12 *liang* together with 3 *dou* of wine".

***Tan huan feng* 攤緩風, paralysis wind** [2]
PC identical with → *tan huan* 癱瘓②, paralysis. *ZLBC* SE *a jiao* 阿膠 quotes *GJF*: 療**攤緩風**及諸風，手脚不遂，腰脚無力者, "It cures **paralysis wind** and all other types of wind; with the hands and legs not following [one's command], and the lower back and the legs lacking strength".

***Tan huan pian feng* 攤緩偏風, partial paralysis wind** [1]
PC identical with → *tan huan feng* 癱瘓風, paralysis wind. *ZLBC* SE *a jiao* 阿膠 quotes *GJF*: 療攤緩風及諸風，手脚不遂，腰脚無力者, "It cures paralysis wind and all other types of wind; with the hands and legs not following [one's command], and the lower back and the legs lacking strength". This is quoted again in *BCGM* SE *a jiao* 阿膠 where the term given is **攤緩偏風**, "**Partial paralysis wind**".

***Tan huo* 痰火, phlegm fire** [13] AN → *huo tan* 火痰, fire phlegm.
EA or PC identical with → *tan re* 痰熱, phlegm heat. *DXSJ* Fj: 諸病尋**痰火**，**痰火**生異證, "In all disease episodes look for **phlegm fire**. **Phlegm fire** generates abnormal pathological signs".

***Tan ji* 痰積, phlegm accumulation** [10]
① AN *ji tan* 積痰, accumulated phlegm. EA of → *tan* 痰②, phlegm, which has accumulated somewhere in the body. *DXXF* 4: **痰積**作痛者，二陳加南星、半夏, "In the case of pain resulting from **phlegm accumulation**, [take the 'decoction with] the two matured ingredients' and add *nan xing* and *ban xia*".
② PC brought forth by accumulated phlegm. *QJYF* 18: 松蘿湯，治胸中**痰積**、熱，皆除方, "The decoction with *song luo* is a recipe to cure **phlegm accumulation** and heat in the chest by eliminating them all".

***Tan jie* 痰結, phlegm nodes** [17]
PC brought forth by a non-transformation of phlegm, desiccation of body liquids, and the formation of sticky phlegm nodes. *BJ* SE chang shan 常山：主傷寒寒熱，熱發，温瘧鬼毒，胸中**痰結**，吐逆, "It controls harm caused by cold with alternating sensations of cold and heat, heat effusion, warmth malaria and demon poison, as well as **phlegm nodes** in the chest and vomiting with counterflow".

***Tan jing* 痰驚, phlegm fright** [1]
PC of chronic fright wind brought forth by phlegm resulting from spleen depletion. *BCGM* SE *hou pu* 厚朴 quoting *XEYZZJ*: 小兒吐瀉或誤服冷藥，脾虛生風，因成慢驚, "When children vomit and have outflow, or if they mistakenly ingest medication of a cold nature, their spleen will be depleted and generate wind. Hence this generates slow fright", writes: 小兒吐瀉，胃虛及有痰

驚, "When children vomit and have diarrhea, their stomach is depleted and they have **phlegm fright**".

Tan jue **痰厥, phlegm recession** [30]

① EA of blocked phlegm and closed-in qi causing headaches. *ZHF* 4: 其病是胸中膈上，**痰厥**氣上衝所致，名為厥頭痛, "This disease is in the chest above the diaphragm. It was brought forth by **phlegm recession** and qi rushing upward. It is called recession headache.

② PC of recession cold affecting the four limbs, brought forth by an abundance of phlegm and closed-in qi. In severe cases this may include the pathological condition of black-out with loss of consciousness, and an inability to recognize things and persons. *SYDXF* 2: 順元散，治暴患**痰厥**，氣虛，身微冷，面淡白，昏悶不知人事, "The 'powder favorable for the original [qi]' cures violent affection by **phlegm recession**, qi depletion, a slightly cold body, a pale facial complexion, clouding with heart-pressure and an inability to recognize persons or things".

Tan ke **痰咳, phlegm cough** [6]

PC identical with → *tan sou* 痰嗽. *SYDXF* 1: 白术散，治傷寒氣脈不和，憎寒壯熱，鼻塞腦悶, 涕唾稠粘，**痰咳**壅滯, "The powder with *bai zhu* cures harm caused by cold with an imbalance in the qi [movement in the] vessels, an aversion to cold and strong heat, a blocked nose and cerebral heart-pressure, thick and sticky snivel and saliva, as well as **phlegm cough** with obstruction and [qi] sluggishness".

Tan liu **痰瘤, phlegm tumor** [2]

PC identical with → *luo li* 瘰癧, scrofula with pervasion-illness. *BCGM* SE *tian nan xing* 天南星：**痰瘤**結核：南星膏治人皮肌頭面上生瘤及結核，大者如拳，小者如栗，或軟或硬，不疼不癢，宜用此藥, "**Phlegm tumor** and nodular kernel: Ointment with *nan xing* cures tumors and nodular kernels growing in the skin of a person's head and face. Large ones are like a fist; small ones are like a chestnut. They may be soft or unyielding. They neither ache nor itch. This medication is suitable for these [ailments]".

Tan luan **癱攣, paralytic contraction** [1]

PC identical with → *tan* 癱①, paralysis. *BCGM* SE *qian fen* 鉛粉 quotes *YDXL*: 長幼為毒熏蒸，多痿黄**癱攣**而斃, "If the old or young are exposed to toxic fumes, this will often result in dysfunction with jaundice, **paralytic contraction**, and death".

Tan man **痰滿, phlegm fullness** [4]

PC of → *man* 滿, fullness, brought forth by phlegm rheum. *ZHF* 4: 若患**痰滿**及溏泄，可除飴耳, "If the patient suffers from **phlegm fullness** and semi-liquid outflow, the maltose can be omitted".

Tan mi **痰迷, phlegm confusion** [13]

PC of mental disturbance with forgetfulness, loss of consciousness, and aphasia brought forth by an abundance of phlegm saliva diminishing the patient's mental capacities. *SYDXF* 9: 加味茯苓湯，治**痰迷**心胞，健忘失事，言語如痴,

"The decoction with *fu ling* and additional substances cures **phlegm confusion** affecting the heart enclosure, forgetfulness, and silly talking".

Tan ni **痰逆, phlegm counterflow** [5]

① PC of a qi dynamic ascending contrary to its regular direction with nausea, vomiting and an inability to ingest beverages and food, resulting from blockages of regular qi dynamics caused by phlegm abundance. *TPSHF* 51: 夫**痰逆**不下食者，由胸膈壅滯，津液不通，痰水結聚，不能消散，流行於脾，脾性惡濕，得水則脹滿，心胸不利，多痰而逆，故令不下食也, "Now, **phlegm counterflow** and an inability to ingest food results from obstruction and [qi] sluggishness in the region of the chest and diaphragm, with body liquids being unable to pass. Phlegm and liquid form nodular collections that are unable to dissolve and disperse and flow into the spleen. The spleen hates moisture, and if it takes in liquid it distends and has a feeling of fullness. The heart and chest are no longer open for passage. There is much phlegm moving contrary to its regular direction. Hence this makesa person incapable of ingesting food.

② IS CD of throwing up phlegm saliva. *TPSHF* 11: 治傷寒邪熱傷心，恍惚狂言，時有**痰逆**，不欲飲食，宜服人參散方, "To cure harm caused by cold, and evil heat harming the heart, with absent-mindedness and crazy talking, as well as occasional **phlegm counterflow** and loss of appetite, the recipe to ingest the powder with *ren shen* is advisable".

Tan nüe **痰瘧, phlegm malaria** [16]

PC of → *nüe ji* 瘧疾, malaria ailment, associated with phlegm. The clinical appearance, in addition to regularly recurring alternating sensations of cold and heat, includes a feeling of distension and fullness in chest and abdomen, and vomiting with counterflow of phlegm-like saliva. *WTMY* 5: 烏梅丸，瘵瘧，無問温瘴**痰瘧**，悉皆主之方, "Pills with *wu mei* cure malaria. Regardless of whether it is a warmth miasma or **phlegm malaria**, this is a recipe that controls them all".

Tan ou **痰嘔, phlegm vomiting** [2]

PC of vomiting, with or without retching sound, brought forth by phlegm rheum. *SJZL* 44: 每至秋夏，臟腑不調，氣逆**痰嘔**, "Always by the time of autumn and summer, when the depots and palaces have lost their balance, qi moves contrary to its normal direction, and [patients suffer from] **phlegm vomit**".

Tan pi **痰澼, phlegm flush** [20]

PC identical with → *tan pi* 痰癖, phlegm aggregation-illness. *QJYF* 18: 斷膈湯，治胸中**痰澼**方, "Decoction to break through barriers: a recipe to cure **phlegm flush** in the chest".

Tan pi **痰痞, phlegm obstacle-illness** [4]

PC of → *pi* 痞, obstacle-illness, brought forth by congealed phlegm qi. *BCSY* SE *ci mu* 慈母：取枝、葉炙黃香，作飯，下氣止渴，令人不睡主小兒**痰痞**, "Take the twigs and the leafs, and roast them until they turn yellow and develop a fragrant scent. Then prepare a meal with them. It causes the discharge of qi and quenches thirst. It lets a person not asleep and controls **phlegm obstacle-illness** in children".

***Tan pi* 痰癖, phlegm aggregation-illness** [18] AW *tan pi* 痰澼, phlegm flush.
PC of → *pi* 癖, aggregation-illness, disease brought forth by stagnant phlegm rheum. *BJ* SE *ba dou* 巴豆：破癥瘕結聚，堅積，留飲，**痰癖**, "It breaks through concretion-illness and conglomeration-illness, nodular collections, hard accumulations, abiding rheum, and **phlegm aggregation-illness**".

***Tan qi* 痰氣, phlegm [and] qi** [51]
① EA of collecting phlegm and stagnant qi, with phlegm and qi striking at each other and blocking passageways. This in turn brings forth all types of pathological conditions. *ZBYHL* 14: 胸膈痰飲多者，嗽則氣動於痰，上搏喉咽之間，**痰氣**相擊，隨嗽動息，呼呷有聲，謂之呷嗽, "If large quantities of phlegm rheum collect in the region of the chest and diaphragm, coughing will make qi move against the phlegm, with the latter rising and striking the region of the throat and gullet. **Phlegm and qi** strike at each other in accordance with the cough's being active or dormant. Exhalation has a creaking sound. This is called creaking cough". *BCGM* Bai bing zhu zhi yao 百病主治藥 lists the following conditions as brought forth by 'phlegm qi': 諸風證, all types of wind conditions; 諸氣證, all types of qi conditions; 咳嗽, cough; 喘逆, panting with [qi] counterflow; 積聚癥瘕, accumulation and collection, concretion-illness and conglomeration-illness; 脅痛, painful flanks; 腰痛, painful lower back.
② PC brought forth by a mutual blockage of phlegm and qi. *TBC* SE *sheng jiang* 生薑：薑，久服通神明，主風邪，主**痰氣**, "*Jiang*, if ingested over an extended period of time will brighten the mind. It controls wind evil, and **phlegm qi**".

***Tan qi jie xiong* 痰氣結胸, bound chest because of phlegm qi** [2]
PC identical with → *xiao jie xiong* 小結胸, minor bound chest. *BCGM* SE *yin zhu* 銀硃 quoting *HYXS*: 平常小兒，多有小結胸證 然陷胸湯內有黄連極苦，難以施之。嬰孩如發表後，但用鶴頂丹為治, "Children often have conditions of 'minor bound chest'. Now, the 'decoction sinking into the chest' has *huang lian* as one of its ingredients. This is a very bitter [substance] and must not be administered. When a child manifests [minor bound chest], the only way to cure this is by means of the 'crane's neck elixir'", writes: **痰氣結胸**：鶴頂丹：不問陰陽虛實，"For **bound chest because of phlegm qi** [use] the 'crane's neck elixir'. Regardless of whether [the disease] is of a yin or yang type, a depletion or repletion".

***Tan re* 痰熱, phlegm and heat, phlegm heat** [58] AW → *re tan* 熱痰, AN → *tan huo* 痰火, phlegm and fire.
① EA referring to → *tan* 痰, phlegm, and → *re* 熱, heat, simultaneously causing illness. *ZBYHL* 6: **痰熱**之氣熏肝，肝候目，故目無所見而疼痛, "The qi of **phlegm and heat** smokes the liver. The eyes are the external indicators of the liver's [condition]. Hence the eyes cannot see and are painful". *BCGM* considers phlegm and heat to be a serious etiological agent and identifies conditions such as vomiting, dry retching, forgetfulness, headache, dizziness, cough, panting, epilepsy, and fright wind as related to phlegm and heat.

② PC brought forth by phlegm and heat. *MYBL* SE *huang qin* 黃芩：療**痰熱**, "It heals **phlegm heat**".

Tan shi **痰食, phlegm and food** [5]

EA of a simultaneous presence of phlegm rheum and undigested food. *PJF* 165: 白朮丸，治**痰食**咳嗽，脈緩面黃，肢體沉重, "Pills with *bai zhu* cure [the presence of] **phlegm and food** associated with coughing. The [movement in the] vessels is slow and the facial complexion is yellow. The limbs and body feel very heavy. *BCGM* Bai bing zhu zhi yao 百病主治藥，嘈雜吞酸、瘧疾、心下痞滿均有由**痰食**所致一類, "Clamoring [stomach] with acid swallowing; malaria ailment; an obstacle-illness and a feeling of fullness below the heart: all these conditions are brought forth by [a simultaneous presence of] **phlegm and food**".

Tan shi **痰實, phlegm repletion** [8]

PC of a → *tan* 痰③, phlegm, disease with blockage resulting from phlegm abundance and no qi depletion. *MYBL* SE *qian hu* 前胡：主療痰滿，胸脅中痞，心腹結氣，風頭痛，去**痰實**，下氣, "It controls phlegm fullness, an obstacle-illness in the chest and flanks, bound qi nodes in the heart and abdomen, and wind headache. It removes **phlegm repletion** and causes qi to descend".

Tan shi **痰濕, phlegm and moisture** [7]

EA of a) → *shi tan* 濕痰①, moisture and phlegm. *PJF* 167: 白朮散治…**痰濕**不止，膈不利, "The powder with *bai zhu* cures…unending presence of **phlegm and moisture** with blocked diaphragm". b) General reference to all sorts of → *tan* 痰, phlegm. *BCGM* Bai bing zhu zhi yao 百病主治藥: lists **痰濕**, "**phlegm and moisture**", as causes of cough, and distinguishes among *qi tan* 氣痰, qi phlegm; *feng tan* 風痰, wind phlegm; *tan re* 痰熱, phlegm with heat; *tan han* 寒痰, cold phlegm.

Tan shui **痰水, phlegm and water; rheumy liquid** [40]

① EA of → *tan* 痰, phlegm, and → *shui* 水, water, jointly bringing forth disease. *MYBL* SE *zhu* 朮：消**痰水**，逐皮間風水結腫, "It dissolves **phlegm and water**, and it dispels wind and water from the skin, forming nodes and swelling".
② IS of vomiting and defecation of matter that resembles phlegm and water. *BCGM* Shen nong ben jing ming li 神農本經名例：以十棗湯一服，下**痰水**數升, "With one dosage of the 'decoction with ten jujubes', one can discharge several *sheng* of **rheumy liquid**".

Tan sou **痰嗽, phlegm cough** [53] AN *tan ke* 痰咳.

PC of cough resulting from the presence of phlegm, with much phlegm emitted together with the cough. Once the phlegm is emitted the cough stops. Or, the cough is associated with heart-pressure and sticky phlegm that is not easily eliminated. *TPSHF* 14: **痰嗽**，多唾稠粘，胸膈不利, "In the case of **phlegm cough**, [patients] emit thick, sticky saliva. The chest and diaphragm are blocked".

Tan tu **痰吐, phlegm vomiting** [3]

PC of vomiting brought forth by phlegm rheum. *HYKY* 10: **痰吐**者，其兒胃氣本虛，復感寒邪，生痰作熱，留滯胸膈，故吐, "In the case of **phlegm vom-**

iting, the respective child's stomach qi is habitually depleted, and was repeatedly affected by cold evil. This has produced phlegm and heat, which has become residually sluggish in the region of the chest and diaphragm. Hence [patients] vomit".

***Tan tu* 探吐, to stimulate vomiting** [12]
TA identical with → *qu tu* 取吐. *RMSQ* 11: 凡傷寒疫癘一法：若無藥之處，可用酸齏汁一大碗，煎三五沸，去菜葉，飲訖；候少時，用釵子咽喉中**探吐**，如此三次；再煎葱醋湯投之；衣被蓋覆，汗出而瘥, "A method to be applied for all cases of epidemic harm caused by cold. If this is a place where no medication is at hand, one can use a large bowl of sour spices juice. This [is obtained by] boiling three times, and having the liquid bubble five times. Then the vegetable leaves are discarded and all [the liquid] is to be ingested. After a little while **vomiting is stimulated** by bringing a hairpin into the throat. This is to be repeated three times. Next an onion vinegar decoction is to be administered, and [the patient] is to be covered with clothes or a quilt. When he sweats he is cured".

***Tan tuo* 痰唾, phlegm spittle** [4]
EA identical with → *tan* 痰②, phlegm. *BCSY* SE xuan gou gen 懸鉤根：子如梅，酸美，人食之醒酒，止渴，除**痰唾**，去酒毒, "The seeds are plums, sour and delicious. A person who eats them will be sobered up, and any thirst will be quenched. They remove **phlegm spittle** and they eliminate wine poison".

***Tan xian* 痰癇, phlegm epilepsy** [1]
PC of a → *dian xian* 癲癇, peak-illness with epilepsy, brought forth by phlegm, with patients awakening from dreams with fright and jerking as if they were crazy. *QXLF* 64: **痰癇**為病，此患似張狂, "The disease of **phlegm epilepsy**: patients appear to be in a state of madness".

***Tan xian* 痰涎, phlegm saliva** [94]
① PI identical with → *tan* 痰①, phlegm. *TPSHF* 20: 治風痰心昏，恍惚不能言語，**痰涎**流溢，宜服秦艽散方, "To cure wind phlegm with mental clouding, absent-mindedness with an inability to speak, as well as **phlegm saliva** flow and spillage, the recipe to ingest the powder with *qin jiao* is advisable".
② EA identical with → *tan* 痰②, phlegm. *TPSHF* 85: 夫小兒天吊者，由臟腑風熱，脾胃生涎，**痰涎**既生，心膈壅滯，邪熱蘊積，不得宣通之所致, "Now, as for the condition of 'children hauled by heaven', this is brought forth by the following: Wind heat affects the depots and palaces. This makes the spleen and stomach generate saliva. Once **phlegm saliva** has been generated, the region of the heart and diaphragm will be obstructed with [qi] sluggishness. Evil heat accumulates and blocks free passage".

***Tan xiao* 痰哮, phlegm roaring** [1]
PC identical with → *tan hou* 痰齁. *BCGM* SE *zhu ma* 苧麻 quotes *YXZC*: 痰哮咳嗽，苧根煅存性，為末，生豆腐蘸三五錢食，即效, "**Phlegm roaring**: Roast *zhu gen* in such a way that its nature is maintained and grind to a powder. Ingestion of 3 *qian* dipped in fresh bean curd brings an immediate effect".

***Tan xue* 痰血, phlegm and blood** [6]

① EA. A combination of → *tan* 痰②, phlegm and → *yu xue* 瘀血, stagnant blood. *SYDXF* 14: 產後**痰血**結滯，發為潮熱，心胸如火，煩躁口乾，諸藥不效, "When following delivery **phlegm and blood** form nodes and are sluggish, this causes a heat wave. The heart and chest feel as if there were a fire. [Patients experience] vexation, restlessness and a dry mouth. No medication whatsoever is effective".

② IS of blood found in thrown-up phlegm, and phlegm mixed with blood. *SW* 38: 肺虛壅，咳嗽喘滿，咯**痰血**, "The lung is depleted and obstructed. [Patients] cough, pant, and have a feeling of fullness. They cough up **phlegm mixed with blood**".

***Tan yin* 痰飲, phlegm rheum** [108]

① EA CD of → *tan* 痰, phlegm, and → *yin* 飲, rheum, as pathological products that have accumulated in the body and that are excreted in the process of pathological changes affecting the depots and palaces. They may block the passage of qi and blood and thereby become pathogenic factors. *JGYL* Mj: 心下有**痰飲**，胸脅支滿，目眩，苓桂术甘湯主之, "There is **phlegm rheum** below the heart. The chest and the flanks experience propping fullness. Vision is dim. The decoction with [*fu*] *ling*, *gui* [*zhi*], [*bai*] *zhu*, and *gan* [*cao*] will master this".

② PC of a) pathological conditions brought forth by phlegm and rheum, including all conditions related to phlegm and rheum. *JGYL* Mj: 病**痰飲**者，當以温藥和之, "If someone suffers from **phlegm rheum**, this should be harmonized with a warmth medication". b) A specific type of phlegm disease. If someone was well-fed some time ago and is emaciated now, and liquid drips into his intestinal region with sounds, this is its major sign. *JGYL* Mj: 其人素盛今瘦，水走腸間，瀝瀝有聲，謂之**痰飲**, "This person was well-fed some time ago and is emaciated now, liquid drips into his intestinal region with sounds. This is called '**phlegm rheum**'".

***Tan yong* 痰壅, phlegm obstruction** [16]

IS of large quantities of phlegm thrown up through cough or vomiting. In some cases the sound of breathing indicates the presence of large quantities of phlegm in the respiratory tract. *YXL* SE fu ling 茯苓：主肺痿**痰壅**，治小兒驚癇，療心腹脹滿, "It controls lung dysfunction with **phlegm obstruction**. It cures fright epilepsy in children. It cures distension and a feeling of fullness in the region of the heart and abdomen".

***Tan yu* 痰郁, pent-up phlegm** [1]

PC of one of → *liu yu* 六郁, the six types of pent-up [matter in the organism]. Refers to accumulation disease brought forth by phlegm stagnation in the lung, with excitement leading to panting. The movement in the vessels at the inch opening is deep inside and smooth. *DXXF* 3: **痰郁**者，動則喘，寸口脈沉滑, "In the case of **pent-up phlegm**, excitement results in panting; the [movement in the] vessels at the inch opening is deep inside and smooth".

***Tan zhi* 痰滯, phlegm sluggishness** [7]
EA identical with → *ting tan* 停痰, halting phlegm. *TPSHF* 5: 治腎臟虛損，上焦**痰滯**，多唾稠濁，腹脅脹滿，吃食微少，宜服赤茯苓丸方, "To cure depletion harm in the kidney depot, **phlegm sluggishness** in the upper burner, with large quantities of thick and turbid saliva, distension and a feeling of fullness in the abdomen and flanks, as well as minimal ingestion of food, the recipe to ingest the pills with *chi fu ling* is advisable".

***Tan zhu* 痰注, phlegm influx** [3]
PC of extremities that are painful and difficult to move, brought forth by an intrusion of phlegm and humidity into the conduits and network vessels, and bone joints. *PJF* 164: 天仙飲治**痰注**臂痛, "The decoction with *tian xian* [*teng*] cures **phlegm influx** with pain in the arms".

***Tang dang huo shao* 湯盪火燒, scorching by boiling water, burns by fire** [1]
PC identical with → *tang huo shang* 湯火傷, harm caused by boiling water and fire. *BCGM* SE *zhi zi* 梔子：**湯盪火燒**，梔子末和雞子清，濃掃之, "For **scorching by boiling water and burns by fire**, prepare a thick paste by mixing *zhi zi* powder with the clear parts of chicken eggs, and use this to wipe [the burns]".

***Tang huo chuang* 湯火瘡, boiling water and fire sores** [14]
PC identical with → *huo chuang* 火瘡, fire sores. *ZBYHL* 35: **湯火瘡**候，凡被湯火燒者, "Signs of **boiling water and fire sores**: this includes all burns caused by boiling water and fire".

***Tang huo shang* 湯火傷, harm caused by boiling water and fire** [30]
PC of injuries caused by contact with very hot items such as boiling water and oil or fire. *BCSY* SE *wu gu wa* 烏古瓦：主**湯火傷**, "It controls **harm caused by boiling water and fire**". *BCGM* uses terms such as → *tang huo shang zhuo* 湯火傷灼, harm following burns by boiling water and fire; → *tang huo zhuo shang* 湯火灼傷; → *tang huo shao zhuo* 湯火燒灼, burns by boiling water and fire; → *tang tang huo shao* 湯盪火燒, scorching by boiling water, burns by fire; → *you shang huo zhuo* 油傷火灼, harm following burns by oil and fire; → *re you huo zhuo* 熱油火灼, scorching by hot oil and fire; → *re you zhuo shang* 熱油灼傷; harm following sorching by hot oil; → *re you shao tong* 熱油燒痛, painful burns by hot oil.

***Tang huo shang chuang* 湯火傷瘡, wounds caused by boiling water and fire** [16]
PC identical with → *huo chuang* 火瘡, fire sores. *BCGM* SE *ying zi tong* 罌子桐：塗脛瘡、**湯火傷瘡**, "Apply on shin sores, and **wounds caused by boiling water and fire**".

***Tang huo shang zhuo chuang* 湯火傷灼瘡, sores following harm from scorching by boiling water and fire** [1]
PC identical with → *huo chuang* 火瘡, fire sores. *BCGM* SE jing zhong tai ji ping 井中苔及萍 quotes *ZLBC* : 陶隱居云：廢井中多生苔、萍，及磚土間生雜草、萊藍，既解毒，在井中者彌佳…亦療**湯火灼瘡**, "Tao Yinju says: Moss and duckweed, as they often grow in discarded wells, and all sorts of herbs and *lai lan* growing between bricks and stones, dissolve poison. Those from wells

are the best…They also cure **sores following harm from scorching by boiling water and fire**".

Tang huo shao chuang **湯火燒瘡, sores following burning by boiling water and fire** [1]

PC identical with → *huo chuang* 火瘡, fire sores. *BCGM* SE *fen xi* 粉錫 quoting an unknown work allegedly compiled by Sun Zhenren: **湯火燒瘡**：胡粉，羊髓和，塗之, "**Sores following burning by boiling water and fire**: Mix *hu fen* with bone marrow of sheep, and apply externally".

Tang huo shao zhuo **湯火燒灼, burns by boiling water and fire** [3]

PC identical with → *tang huo shang* 湯火傷, harm caused by boiling water and fire. *BCGM* SE *bai ye* 柏葉 quoting *BCTJ*: 其方采葉入臼中，濕搗，令極爛如泥，冷水調作膏，以治大人及小兒湯湯火燒，塗傅於傷處，用帛子系定，三二日瘡當斂，仍滅瘢, "The recipe: pluck its leaves and pound them wet in a mortar until they are extremely sodden, like mud. Add cold water to prepare a paste. This serves to cure adults and children alike who have been scalded by boiling water or burnt by fire. It is to be applied on the damaged location, and fixated with a textile bandage. After two or three days, the sores will be closed, and the scars will vanish", writes: **湯火燒灼**：柏葉生搗塗之，系定二三日，止痛滅瘢, "For **burns by boiling water and fire**: Fresh *bai* leaves are to be pounded and applied externally. [The paste] is to be bandaged and fixated for two to three days. This will end the pain and make the scars vanish".

Tang huo zhuo chuang **湯火灼瘡, sores following scorching by boiling water and fire** [9]

PC identical with → *huo chuang* 火瘡, fire sores. *WTMY* 29: 備急療**湯火灼瘡**方，柳皮燒灰如粉敷之, "Recipe for emergency treatment of **sores following scorching by boiling water and fire**: apply willow bark burned to ashes like a powder".

Tang huo zhuo shang **湯火灼傷, harm following burns by boiling water and fire** [8]

PC identical with → *tang huo shang* 湯火傷, harm caused by boiling water and fire. *BCGM* SE *bai lian* 白斂: **湯火灼傷**：白斂末傅之, "For **harm following burns by boiling water and fire**: a powder made of *bai lian* is to be applied externally".

Tang xie **溏泄, semiliquid outflow** [10]

① AN *bian tang* 便溏, viscous defecation. IS of thin, viscous, formless stool. SW 69: 病反腹滿，腸鳴，**溏泄**，食不化，渴而妄冒, "Illnesses contrary [to what is normal are:] abdominal fullness, intestinal sounds, **semiliquid outflow**, failure to digest food, thirst and confusion by the malicious".

② PC with semiliquid stools as major sign. *ZHF* 4: 若患痰滿及**溏泄**，可除飴, "If [the patient] suffers from phlegm, fullness, and **semiliquid outflow**, one may omit the sugar [from the recipe]".

Teng bi **疼痹, painful blockage** [4]
PC identical with → *tong bi* 痛痹. *BJ* SE fang feng 防風：風行周身，骨節**疼痹**，煩滿, "Wind moves through the entire body. The bones and joints experience a **painful blockage**, with vexation and a feeling of fullness".

Teng ji **疼急, sudden violent pain** [1]
IS identical with *ji tong* 急痛. *BCJJZ* SE *zhi shi* 枳實：枳樹莖及皮，療水脹，暴風骨節**疼急**, "Stems and bark of the *zhi* tree serve to cure water distension, and **sudden violent pain** in the bones and joints brought forth by fierce wind".

Teng leng **疼冷, cold pain; to be painful and cold** [9]
IS identical with → *leng tong* 冷痛, cold and pain. *MYBL* SE *ce zi* 側子：主癰腫，風痹歷節，腰脚**疼冷**, "It controls obstruction-illness swelling, wind blockage with penetration of joints, **cold pain** in the lower back and legs".

Teng men **疼悶, pain with heart-pressure** [3]
IS identical with → *men tong* 悶痛. *QJYF* 24: 冷氣入陰囊，腫滿恐死，日夜**疼悶**，不得眠, "When cold qi enters the scrotum, this results in swelling and a feeling of fullness and fear of death. Day and night one has **pain with heart-pressure**, and cannot sleep".

Teng ruo **疼弱, pain with weakness** [3] AN *tong ruo* 痛弱.
IS of pain affecting the body and extremities accompanied by a feeling of weakness. *MYBL* SE *shi liu huang* 石硫黃：咳逆上氣，脚冷，**疼弱**無力, "Cough with rising qi counterflow. The legs are cold, and patients feel **pain with weakness**; they lack strength".

Teng suan **疼酸, soreness** [5]
IS identical with → *suan tong* 酸痛. *SW* 74: 諸病胕腫，**疼酸**驚駭，皆屬於火, "All diseases [such as] *fu*-swelling, **soreness**, and shock, are associated without exception with fire".

Ti chou **體臭, body odor** [1]
PC of → *hu chou* 胡臭, barbarian stench, released as a distinct stench from the body. *SJZL* 101: 狐臭者指其腋間，**體臭**者舉其大概, "Fox odor refers to [an odor from] the armpits. **Body odor** refers to the entire [body's odor]".

Ti han **體寒, body cold** [5]
IS identical with → *shen leng* 身冷. *WTMY* 38: 若**體寒**者，倍人參，減黃芩, "In the case of **body cold**, add *ren shen*, omit *huang qin*".

Ti jin **體噤, goose pimples** [1]
IS of goose pimple swellings on the skin. *RHZ* SE *xin yi* 辛荑：治頭痛憎寒，**體噤**瘙癢, "They cure headaches with an aversion to cold, **goose pimples** and itching".

Ti re **體熱, body heat; the body is hot** [5]
IS identical with → *fa re* 發熱, effusion of heat. *ZBYHL* 4: **體熱**如火，煩躁無汗, "**The body is hot** as fire; [patients experience] vexation and agitation. No sweating".

Ti xiao ma li 啼笑罵詈, **crying, laughing, insulting, cursing** [1]
IS of a mental derangement with irregular crying and laughing, as well as insulting and cursing both persons close to oneself and strangers. *QJYF* 13: 心病其色赤，心痛短氣，手掌煩熱，或**啼笑罵詈**，悲思愁慮, "In the case of a heart disease, the complexion is red. The heart aches and [the patient] is short of qi. The palms are affected by vexing heat. In some cases [patients] **cry, laugh, insult, and curse**. They may be sad, or thinking, or worrying, or pondering".

Ti xu 體虛, **body depletion; hollow body** [15]
① PC identical with → *xu* 虛①, depletion. *ZBYHL* 1: 血痹者，由**體虛**，邪入於陰經故也, "Blood blockage is brought forth by evil entering the yin conduits following **body depletion**".
② identical with → *xu* 虛③, hollow [substance]: *BCGM* SE *ren shen* 人參：薺苨**體虛**無心，桔梗體堅有心而味苦, "*Ji ni* has a **hollow body** without a center; *jie geng* has a solid body with a center. Its flavor is bitter".

Ti xue 涕血, **bleeding through nasal mucus** [2]
IS of blood emitted with the mucus from the nose. *BCTJ* SE *ti hu* 醍醐 quoting *WTMY* 唾涕血出, "Bleeding through saliva and nasal mucus", writes: 鼻中**涕血**, "**Bleeding through the nasal mucus** from within the nose".

Ti zhong 體重, **the body feels heavy; the body is heavy** [22]
① IS identical with → *shen zhong* 身重. *SW* 5: 年五十，**體重**，耳目不聰明矣, "At the age of fifty, **the body feels heavy**; the ears and the eyes are no longer clear".
② Physical feature of pharmaceutical substances, referring to drugs with a compact and large mass. *BCTJ* SE *tao hua shi* 桃花石：其色似桃花，光潤而**體重**，以舐之不著舌者為佳, "Its color is reminiscent of that of peach blossoms; it has luster and **the body is heavy**. Those that do not stick to one's tongue when licked are best".

Tian chuang 甜瘡, **sweet sores** [5]
PC of → *chuang* 瘡, sores, conditions, mostly affecting children, that emerge on the head, face and ears, with seeping liquid and itching that cannot be cured for an extended period of time. *PJF* 272: 治**甜瘡**，以大棗去核，實以綠礬，火燒微存性，研細貼之, "To cure **sweet sores**, take a large jujube, remove the kernel and fill with *lü fan*. Roast slightly over a fire to maintain its nature. Then grind to a fine powder and apply this to the [sores]".

Tian diao jing feng 天吊驚風, **hauled-by-heaven fright wind** [2] AW *tian diao jing feng* 天釣驚風. AN *jing feng tian diao* 驚風天吊, fright wind hauled-by-heaven; → *xiao er tian diao* 小兒天吊, children hauled-by-heaven; *tian diao jing xian* 天吊驚癇, hauled-by-heaven fright epilepsy; *ke wu tian diao* 客忤天吊, hauled-by-heaven following visitor's hostility; *xiao er tian diao* 小兒天釣, children hooked-up by heaven.
PC of a type of → *jing feng* 驚風, fright wind, where the patient's eyes are turned upwards, as if "hauled-by-heaven". *XEYZZJ* 5: 琥珀散…治**天吊驚風**發搐, "Powder with *hu po*…cures **hauled-by-heaven fright wind** with convulsions".

***Tian diao jing feng* 天釣驚風, hooked-up-by-heaven fright wind** [1]
PC identical with → *tian diao jing feng* 天吊驚風, hauled-by-heaven fright wind. *BCGM* SE *xie* 蠍 quotes *TPSHF*: **天釣驚風**：翻眼向上, "In the case of **hooked-up-by-heaven fright wind**, the eyes are turned upwards".

***Tian diao jing xian* 天吊驚癇, hauled-by-heaven fright epilepsy** [3] AN *jing xian tian diao* 驚癇天吊.
PC identical with → *tian diao jing feng* 天吊驚風, hauled-by-heaven fright wind. *RHZ* SE *sang gen bai pi* 桑根白皮：研汁治小兒**天吊驚癇**, "Crushed to a juice it cures **hauled-by-heaven fright epilepsy** in children".

***Tian huo dan du* 天火丹毒, celestial fire cinnabar poison** [1]
PC identical with → *dan du* 丹毒, cinnabar poison. *QJYF* 22: 丹毒，一名天火, "Cinnabar poison, alternative name: celestial fire". *BCGM* SE *zhi* 雉：燒灰和麻油，傅**天火丹毒**, "Burn to ashes and mix with *ma you*. Smear [this] on **celestial fire cinnabar poison**".

***Tian huo re chuang* 天火熱瘡, celestial fire heat sores** [1]
PC of heat sores that appear as prickly heat in their early stages, then gradually change into blisters with liquid and acquire a red color resembling fire sores. *BCGM* SE *yun tai* 芸薹quoting *WTMY* 29: 近效療火油及天火瘡，初出似沸子，漸漸大如水泡，似火燒瘡赤色, "The *Jin xiao* [states]: to heal fire oil [sores] and celestial fire sores. When they first appear they resemble bubbles of boiling water. They gradually grow larger until they resemble water blisters. They look like sores resulting from fire burns", writes: **天火熱瘡**：初起似痱，漸如水泡，似火燒瘡，赤色，急速能殺人, "**Celestial fire heat sores**: When they first emerge they resemble a seething rash. Gradually they assume the appearance of water blisters. Their color is red, and they may quickly kill a person".

***Tian kui bu tong* 天癸不通, menstrual blockage** [2]
PC identical with → *yue shui bu tong* 月水不通. *BCGM* SE *ma* 馬 quotes *JiXF*: 婦人**天癸不通**，煅存性為末，每服三錢, "[To cure] women with **menstrual blockage**, process over heat while retaining its nature, and grind to a powder. Each dose should be 3 *qian*".

***Tian pao chuang* 天泡瘡, celestial blister sores** [3]
PC of sores with the appearance of blisters filled with water or pus, especially in children. *WKLL* 7: 一兒十餘歲，背側患水泡數顆，發熱，脈數, 此肺胃風熱所致，名曰**天泡瘡**, "A child in its teens suffered from numerous water blisters to the side of the spine, associated with heat effusion and a [movement in the] vessels with increased frequency. This was brought forth by wind and heat affecting the lung and stomach. It is called **celestial blister sores**".

***Tian pao shi chuang* 天泡濕瘡, celestial blister moisture sores** [11]
PC identical with → *tian pao chuang* 天皰瘡, celestial blister sores. *BCGM* SE *wu ming yi* 無名異 quoting *PJF*: 天皰瘡, "Celestial blister sores", writes: **天泡濕瘡**, "**Celestial blister moisture sores**".

***Tian pao shui chuang* 天泡水瘡, celestial blister water sores** [2]
PC of → *tian pao chuang* 天泡瘡, celestial blister sores, with the liquid in the blisters assuming the appearance of water. *BCGM* SE *huang yao zi* 黃藥子 quotes *BHJJF*: **天泡水瘡**，黃藥子末，搽之, "**Celestial blister water sores**: Apply *huang yao zi* powder to it".

***Tian she du* 天蛇毒, celestial snake poison** [9]
PC a) identical with → *tian she tou* 天蛇頭, celestial snake head. *BCGM* Bai bing zhu zhi yao 百病主治藥：瘭疽喜著十指，狀如代指，根深至肌…俗名**天蛇毒**, "Flaming-heat impediment-illnesses tend to develop on the ten fingers. They look like 'deputy fingers'. Their root reaches into the depth to the muscles…They are commonly called '**celestial snake poison**'". b) Of → *chuang* 瘡, sores, conditions developing all over the body when a person was bitten by a poisonous insect called *tian she* 天蛇, 'celestial snake'. *MXBT* 25: 嘗有一田家忽病癩，通身潰爛，號呼欲絶，西溪寺僧識之，曰：此**天蛇毒**耳，非癩也, "Once there was someone named Tian who suddenly developed repudiation-illness. His entire body festered. He screamed and was at the brink of ending [his life]. A priest of the Western Creek Temple learned of this. He said: This is **celestial snake poison**. It is not repudiation-illness".

***Tian she tou* 天蛇頭, celestial snake head** [3]
PC of → *chuang* 瘡, sores, conditions developing at the fingertips, with the finger tips burning and turning red and swollen and painful as the major characteristic. *BCGM* SE *wu song* 蜈蚣 quotes *QXLF*: **天蛇頭**瘡：生手指頭上。用蜈蚣一條，燒烟熏一二次即愈, "**Celestial snake head** sores: They develop at the fingertip. Use 1 centipede, roast and fumigate [the sores] with its smoke once or twice and it will be healed".

***Tian xing* 天行, heaven-sent [disease]; widely active [disease]** [122] AN *shi qi* 時氣, seasonal qi; *shi xing* 時行 seasonally active [disease]; *shi ji* 時疾, seasonal ailment; *shi bing* 時病, seasonal disease.
PC of epidemic diseases brought forth by qi that is not associated with the annual season during which it causes the disease. *ZBYHL* 46: 四時之間，忽有非節之氣傷人，謂之**天行**, "If in any of the four seasons humans are suddenly harmed by a qi that is not associated with that particular annual period, this is called **heaven-sent [disease]**".

***Tian zao dan du* 天灶丹毒, celestial stove cinnabar poisoning** [1]
PC of → *dan du* 丹毒, cinnabar poisoning, starting from the back. *BCGM* SE *liu* 柳：**天灶丹毒**：赤從背起。柳木灰，水調塗之, For **celestial stove cinnabar poisoning**, with red [sores] developing from the back, burn willow wood to ashes, mix with water and apply this externally".

***Tian zhu du chuang* 天柱毒瘡, celestial pillar poisoning sores** [2]
PC of → *chuang* 瘡, sores, conditions the size of a coin developing at the location of the Great Hammer needle insertion hole in the neck, with yellow liquid seeping incessantly. *BCGM* SE *lu* 驢 quoting *SJZL*: 天柱瘡生脊大椎上, "The celestial pillar sores develop in the back on the Great Hammer". writes: **天柱毒**

瘡生脊大椎上, "The **celestial pillar poisoning sores** develop in the back on the Great Hammer".

***Tian zhu gu dao* 天柱骨倒, celestial pillar bone inversion** [5] AN *xiang ruan* 項軟, soft nape.

PC of children having a weak neck after having been sick, their head falling to one side, and an inability to keep it upright. *YYXS* 26：漢東王先生《家寶》治小兒久患疳疾，體虛，久不進飲食，患來日久，諸候退，只是**天柱骨倒**, "Mr. Wang from Handong in his *Jia bao* cured a child suffering from the ailment of *gan*-illness. Its body was weak and it could not ingest beverages and food for a long time. After the suffering had continued for an extended period of time, all [disease] signs vanished, except for a **celestial pillar bone inversion**".

***Tiao sheng* 挑生, poke life [technique]** [6]

Ancient method of poisoning people. Fish, meat, or rice are processed in a certain way to poison visitors. *LNWSF* Mj: 廣南**挑生**殺人，以魚肉延客，對之行厭勝法，魚肉能反生於人腹中，而人以死, "When they use the **poke life [technique]** to kill people by poison in the Guang nan region they attract visitors with fish or meat and apply a magic method. The fish or meat will come to life again in the victim's abdomen, eventually causing that person's death".

***Tiao zhen* 挑針, poking needle; sty** [2]

PC identical with → *tou zhen* 偷針, sty. *BCGM* SE *chang pu* 菖蒲 quotes *SYSF*: 眼瞼**挑針**：獨生菖蒲根，同鹽研傅, "**Poking needle** in the eyelid: grind the root of an individually grown *chang pu* together with salt, and apply externally".

***Ting er* 聤耳, shedding ear; purulent ear** [59]

PC with pus and water emitted through the ear duct as the major sign. *ZBYHL* 29: **聤耳**者，宗脈之所聚，腎氣之所通。足少陰，腎之經也。勞傷血氣，熱乘虛也，入於其經，邪隨血氣至耳，熱氣聚則生膿汁，故謂之**聤耳**, "A **shedding ear** is where the basic vessels collect, and where the kidney qi passes through. The foot minor yin [vessel] is the vessel of the kidneys. When blood and qi are harmed because of exhaustion, heat will avail itself of the depletion and enter this particular conduit. There the evil [heat] follows the blood and qi and reaches the ears. When the heat qi collects then this generates purulent liquid. Hence this is called **shedding ear**". LSZ regards moisture heat as the cause of purulent ears.

***Ting han* 停寒, stagnant cold** [1]

EA identical with → *ji leng* 積冷, accumulated cold. *HJJF* 3: SE *mu xiang bing zi* 木香餅子：常服寬胸膈，散滯氣，消**停寒**, "Regularly consumed it widens the chest and diaphragm, disperses sluggish qi, and dissolves **stagnant cold**".

***Ting shi* 停屍, uninterred corpse, uninterred corpse [qi]** [3]

① An uninterred corpse. *HYBC* SE *yu* 玉：時七月中旬，長安毒熱，預**停屍**四宿，而體色不變, "During the middle ten days period of the 7th month, there was a toxic heat in Chang'an. **Corpses not interred** for four nights did not change color".

② PC of sudden clenched jaw and heartache, in serious cases resulting in death, brought forth by an affection with the qi emitted by an uninterred corpse. *QJYF* 12 RE *san wu bei ji wan* 三物備急丸, pills with three items to be prepared for urgencies: 若中惡客忤，心腹脹滿、刺痛，口噤氣急，**停屍**卒死者，以暖水若酒服大豆許三枚，老小量與, "In the case of having been struck by the malign, and a visitor's hostility, with a feeling of distension and pain in the heart and abdominal region, piercing pain, clenched jaw and qi urgency, and if one has suddenly died/fallen unconscious because of **uninterred corpse** [**qi**, have the patient] consume three portions of large beans with warm water and wine. The dosage varies with the patient's age".

Ting shi **停食, stagnant food** [1]

PC identical with → *shi zhi* 食滯, food stagnation. *PJF* 206: 嘔吐門：當辨其脈證，施以治法。中寒，則脈沉緊，四肢厥冷，飲食不下，當以温暖之藥調之。挾暑，則脈弦數，煩躁而渴，又當清涼之。**停食**，則消化之, "Section of vomiting: It is essential to distinguish the movements in the vessels and pathological conditions, and devise the therapeutic method. In the case of harm caused by cold, the [movement in the] vessels is deep inside and tight. When beverages and food do not descend, they are to be blended with warming medications. If summerheat is involved, the [movement in the] vessels is string-like and increased in frequency. When [the patient] is vexed, restless and thirsty, he should be cooled. When there is **stagnant food**, dissolve and transform it".

Ting shui **停水, stagnant water/liquid** [10]

① EA of water evil having accumulated in the human body. *ZBYHL* 41: 胎間水氣，子滿體腫者，此由脾胃虛弱，臟腑之間有**停水**，而挾以妊娠故也, "If during pregnancy water qi fills the child and causes the body to swell, this is because of a depletion and weakness of the spleen and stomach. **Stagnant water** has accumulated in the region of the depots and palaces and is held there because of the pregnancy".

② Reference to stagnant water in the natural environment. *BCSY* SE *yin shui liu quan* 陰水流泉：五月六月勿飲澤中**停水**, "During the 5th and the 6th months do not drink **stagnant water** from the swamps".

Ting tan **停痰, stagnant phlegm** [18] AN *liu tan* 留痰, abiding phlegm; *tan zhi* 痰滯, phlegm sluggishness.

EA of → *tan* 痰②, phlegm, stagnating and accumulating in the body. *ZHF* 4: 治腹中冷癖，水穀癥結，心下**停痰**，兩脅痞滿，按之鳴轉，逆害飲食， "To cure cold aggregation-illness in the abdomen, with water and grain forming hidden-illness nodes, and **stagnant phlegm** below the heart. In both flanks there is an obstacle-illness and a feeling of fullness. If one presses [the phlegm], it will make sounds and change its position. It will move [upward] to harm beverages and food".

Tong bi **痛痹, painful blockage** [6]

① PC of → *bi* 痹① a), blockage disease, which manifests itself mainly as pain and is often brought forth by cold evil. SW 43: 寒氣勝者為**痛痹**, "When cold qi dominates, this results in **painful blockage**".

② IS identical with → bi tong 痹痛. *ZBYHL* 38：令人支滿，裏急**痛痹**，引小腹重，腰背如刺狀，四肢不舉, "It causes people to have propping fullness, with internal tightness and **painful blockage**. It pulls on the lower abdomen and generates a feeling of heaviness there. The lower back and the spine feel as if pierced. The four limbs cannot be raised".

***Tong chu* 痛楚, severe pain** [7]

IS identical with → *tong teng* 痛疼. *PJBSF* 10：其内人患砂石淋者，十三年矣，每漩**痛楚**不可忍，溺器中小便下砂石，剝剝有聲, "His wife suffered from sand and stone dripping for 13 years. Whenever she turned, she felt unbearably **severe pain**. When she passed urine into a chamber pot, the stones fell down with a clack-clack sound".

***Tong ci* 痛刺, piercing pain** [9]

IS identical with → *ci tong* 刺痛. *PJF* 187：枳實桔梗湯治胸痹心下氣堅，**痛刺**不可俯仰, "Decoction with *zhi shi* and *jie geng*: to cure chest blockage and qi hardenings below the heart; with **piercing pain** making it impossible to bend the body up or down".

***Tong er* 通耳, open passage ear; to open the passage of the ears** [2]

① PC with pus flowing from inside the ears as a major sign. *WTMY* 22: 療**通耳**膿水出方, "Recipe to cure pus and water released by an **open passage ear**".

② TA of opening the ears to free passage of qi and blood. *ZBYHL* 41: 其食宜稻，其羹宜魚雁，是謂盛榮，以**通耳**目而行經絡, "The appropriate food is rice, and the appropriate soup is made of wild geese. This is called 'rich diet' and serves **to open the passage of ears** and eyes, and to make the conduits and network [vessels] passable".

***Tong feng* 痛風, pain wind** [15]

PC of → *bi* 痹, blockage, with rheumatic pain in the limb joints following an intrusion of evil qi such as wind, cold, moisture, and/or heat. *QJYF* 17: 氣盛有餘，則肩背**痛風**汗出，"An overabundance of qi. As a result, the shoulders and back experience **pain wind** with sweating". *BCGM* 4 Bai bing zhu zhi yao 百病主治藥：**痛風**，屬風、寒、濕、熱，挾痰及血虛、污血，"**Pain wind** is associated with wind, cold, moisture, and heat, accompanied by phlegm and blood depletion, or foul blood". It includes → *li jie feng* 歷節風, pervading joints wind, and → *bai hu feng* 白虎風, white tiger wind.

***Tong jiang* 痛強, pain with stiffness** [2]

IS identical with *jiang tong* 強痛, stiffness with pain. *BJ* SE bi jie 萆薢：主腰背**痛強**，骨節風寒濕周痹, "It controls **pain with stiffness** affecting the lower back and the back; as well as a blockage in the bones and joints brought forth by wind, cold, and moisture".

***Tong jing* 通睛, open eyeball** [2]

PC with → *tong ren bu zheng* 瞳人不正, incorrect pupil position, as the major sign. *SYDXF* 16:小兒**通睛**六十八：小兒雙眼睛通者，欲觀東邊，則見西畔, "**Open eyeball** in children, 68: When a child has open eyeballs in both eyes, then it will look westward when it wishes to see eastward".

Tong luan **痛攣, pain with contraction** [1]

IS identical with → *luan tong* 攣痛. *QJYF* 19: 腰背痛者，皆是腎氣虛弱，臥冷濕當風得之。不時速治，喜流入脚膝，或為偏枯冷痹緩弱疼重。 若有腰**痛攣**，脚重痹急，宜服之, "Pain in the lumbar region and back is always brought forth by kidney qi depletion and weakness, and results from lying [with such a condition] at a cold and moist place where one is affected by wind. If this is not cured quickly in time, [the wind] will flow into the legs and knees, or it will generate unilateral withering, cold blockage, slackening, pain and a feeling of heaviness. If the lower back region is affected by **pain with contraction**, if the legs are heavy, with blockage and tension, it is advisable to ingest this".

Tong man **痛滿, pain and fullness** [8]

IS identical with → *man tong* 滿痛, fullness and pain. *ZHF* 3: 心煩恍惚，腹中**痛滿**，或時絕而復甦者。取釜下土五升，搗篩，以冷水八升和之。取汁盡服之。口已噤者，強開，以竹筒灌之，使得下，入便愈，甚妙, "The heart is vexed and [patients are] absent-minded. In the abdomen they feel **pain and fullness**. If it happens that [a patient appears] to have died and then regains consciousness, take 5 *sheng* of soil from underneath a cauldron, pound through a sieve, and mix this with 8 *sheng* of cold water. Ingest the entire liquid. Those with lockjaw, their mouth is to be opened [by force], and [the liquid] is to be administered through a bamboo tube. When it is sent down this way, the [afflicted] person will be cured. This is quite wondrous".

Tong men **痛悶, pain with heart-pressure** [4]

IS identical with → *men tong* 悶痛, heart-pressure with pain. *QJYF* 18: 若齒齗無色，舌上盡白, ...唇內如粟瘡者，心內懊惱**痛悶**, 此蟲在上蝕其五臟, "When the gums have lost their color, and the surface of the tongue is completely white...and if inside the lips there are sores resembling millet grains, with a feeling of annoyance in their heart, and **pain with heart-pressure**, then this indicates the presence of bugs/worms gnawing on the five depots".

Tong ren bu zheng **瞳人不正, incorrect pupil position** [5] AN *tong xie* 瞳斜, slanted pupil.

IS where one eye is capable of seeing straight ahead while the pupil of the second eye is directed sideward. *PJF* 364: 夫目偏視者，皆由心肝臟風邪所攻，**瞳人不正**，顧視常偏, "When the eyes look sideward, this is always caused by wind evil affecting the heart and liver depots. [As a result] the **pupil assumes an incorrect position** and [patients] continuously look towards one side".

Tong ruo **痛弱, pain with weakness** [2]

IS identical with → *teng ruo* 疼弱. *TPSHF* 72: 治婦人月水不通，心腹煩悶，四肢**痛弱**，金花散方, "Recipe for a powder with *jin hua* to cure blocked menstruation, vexation with heart-pressure affecting the heart and abdomen, and **pain with weakness** in the four extremities".

Tong se **痛澀, pain with roughness** [5]

IS identical with a) → *se tong* 澀痛 a), roughness with pain, affecting the eyes. *TPSHF* 32: 治眼暴赤，熱腫**痛澀**方, "Recipe to cure sudden redness of the eyes, heat swelling, and **pain with roughness**". b) → *se tong* 澀痛 b), roughness with pain, affecting the urinary tract. *TPSHF* 58: 治卒淋瀝，小便**痛澀**，當歸散方, "Recipe for a powder with *dang gui* to cure sudden urinary dripping, and **pain with roughness** during urination".

Tong xie **瞳斜, slanted pupil** [1]
IS identical with → *tong ren bu zheng* 瞳人不正, incorrect pupil position. *BCGM* SE *ren shen* 人參 quotes *RZZZF*: 驚後**瞳斜**：小兒驚後瞳人不正者, "'**Slanted pupil** resulting from fright', this is an incorrect pupil position resulting in children following an exposure to fright".

Tong zhang **痛脹, painful distension** [8]
IS identical with → *zhang tong* 脹痛, distension with pain. *SW* 60: 次絡季脅引少腹而**痛脹**，刺譩譆, "When the network in the lateral abdomen and free ribs pulls on the lower abdomen, resulting in **painful distension**, pierce the *yi-xi* [hole]".

Tong zhu **痛注, painful influx** [1]
IS identical with → *zhu tong* 注痛, influx pain. *QJYF* 15: 猝中風，口噤不能言，四肢緩縱，偏攣急**痛注**, "Sudden wind stroke with clenched jaws and an inability to speak, the four limbs slacken, there are unilateral cramps and **painful influx**".

Tou chan **頭顫, the head shivers** [1]
IS of uncontrolled shivering movements of the head. *BCGM* Bai bing zhu zhi yao 百病主治藥：沒藥、血竭、乳香，並消腫止痛生肌，癰疽**頭顫**，熟水研服, "*Mo yao*, *xue jie*, and *ru xiang*, they all dissolve swelling, stop pain, and generate muscles, [also, for] obstruction- and impediment-illnesses, and when the **head shivers**, grind [these substances] with boiled water and ingest this".

Tou chuang **頭瘡, head sores** [107]
PC of → *chuang* 瘡, sores, conditions forming on the head. *BJ* SE *xia ku cao* 夏枯草：主寒熱，瘰癧，鼠瘺，**頭瘡**, "It controls alternating sensations of cold and heat, scrofula with pervasion-illness, mouse fistula, and **head sores**".

Tou e tong **頭額痛, forehead pain** [1]
IS of → *tou tong* 頭痛①, headache, mainly affecting the forehead. *YXRM* 2: SE *ge gen* 葛根：甘，平。善解肌，陽明**頭額痛**乃宜, "Sweet, balanced, good for relaxing the muscles, and suitable for yang brilliance [conduit] **forehead pain**".

Tou feng **頭風, head wind** [162] AN *feng tou* 風頭, wind head; *tou nao feng* 頭腦風, head and brain wind; *tou mu feng* 頭目風, head and eye wind; *pian zheng tou feng* 偏正頭風, hemilateral and proper head wind; *nao feng* 腦風, brain wind; *shou feng* 首風, head wind; *lei tou feng* 雷頭風, thundering head wind.
PC of wind evil attacking the head followed by pain, or dizziness, or itching. *JGYL*: **頭風**摩散方，大附子（一枚，炮），鹽（等分）。右二味為散，沐了，以方寸匕，已摩疢上，令藥力行, "Recipe for a powder to be rubbed [on the head for curing] **head wind**. 1 large piece of *fu zi*, boiled; equal amount of salt. Prepare a powder of these two substances. Wash [the patient's] hair and rub the amount of a spoon of the size of a square inch [into the head] above the lo-

cation of the ailment. This will activate the strength of the medication". *BCGM* refers to numerous pathological conditions of head wind, such as *tou feng tou tong* 頭風頭痛, head wind with headache; *tou feng xuan yun* 頭風眩運, head wind with dizziness; *tou feng bai xie* 頭風白屑, head wind with a white scaling.

***Tou feng* 頭瘋, head wind-illness** [1]
PC identical with → *tou feng* 頭風, head wind. *BCGM* SE *mi feng* 蜜蜂 quoting *BJ*: 主風頭，除蠱毒，補虛羸傷中。久服令人光澤好顏色，不老, "It controls wind-head, eliminates *gu* poison, supplements depletion with emaciation with harm to the center. Ingested over a long time it provides luster and a good complexion", writes: **頭瘋**, 除蠱毒, 補虛羸傷中。久服令人光澤, 好顏色, 不老, "[It cures] **head wind-illness,** eliminates *gu* poison, supplements depletion with emaciation, and [cures] harm to one's center. Ingested over a long time it provides luster and a good complexion".

***Tou gan* 頭乾, desiccated head** [1]
IS of desiccated, withered hair. *WTMY* 13: **頭乾**瘰癧，頭髮黃聳分去，或乍痢乍瘥，諸狀既多，不可備說，大黃煎丸方, "For **desiccated head** and scrofula with pervasion-illness, when the hair turns yellow and is partially lost, in some cases with sudden free-flux illness and sudden remission, and so many signs, it is impossible to name them all, [use] the recipe for the pills with boiled *da huang*".

***Tou he* 頭核, head kernel** [1]
PC of → *tan he* 痰核, phlegm kernel, developing on the back of the head. *BCGM* SE *fu shi* 浮石：**頭核**腦痹：頭枕後生痰核, "**Head kernel** with brain blockage is a phlegm kernel developing on the back of the head".

***Tou hun* 頭昏, clouded head** [2]
IS of a dazed and unwell feeling in the head, with a lack of mental alertness. In severe cases this is associated with unstable walking. *TPSHF* 30: 治虛勞乏弱, 四肢無力, **頭昏**目暗, 身體疼痛, 不欲吃食, 宜服羚羊角丸方, "To cure depletion with exhaustion to fatigue and weakness, with the four extremities lacking strength, **clouded head** with dim vision, with the body feeling pain all over, and a lack of appetite, the recipe to ingest the pills with *ling yang jiao* is advisable".

***Tou mian feng tong* 頭面風, head and face wind** [12]
PC of wind evil attacking the head and face, with → *tou feng* 頭風, head wind, and → *tou mian you feng* 頭面游風, wind roaming in the head and face. *ZBYHL* 2: **頭面風**者，是體虛，諸陽經脈為風所乘也。諸陽經脈，上走於頭面, "As for **head and face wind,** as the body is depleted all yang conduit vessels are occupied by wind. It moves upward through all yang conduit vessels to the head and face".

***Tou mian you feng* 頭面游風, wind roaming in the head and face** [7]
PC brought about by wind moisture and wind dryness, with a red, swollen, and itching face. In severe cases patients scratch their face to an extent that the skin opens and liquid flows out. *QJYF* 13: 菊花散，治**頭面游風**方，"Powder with *ju hua*: a recipe to cure **wind roaming in the head and face**".

Tou mu bu qing **頭目不清, clouded head and eyes** [3]
IS of a perception of one's brain lacking clarity. This is a mild sign of → *tou hun* 頭昏, clouded head. *SJZL* 14: 治心神驚悸，**頭目不清**，金箔十珍丸方, "To cure mental fright with palpitation, and **clouded head and eyes**, [use] the recipe for the 'pills with gold foils and ten treasures'".

Tou mu feng **頭目風, head and eyes wind** [2]
PC identical with → *tou feng* 頭風, head wind. *BCYY* 11, SE xuan fu hua 旋覆花：葉如大菊…去**頭目風**。其味甘苦辛，亦走散之藥也, "Its leaves resemble those of a large chrysanthemum...It eliminates **head and eyes wind**. Its flavor is sweet, bitter, and acrid, and it belongs to the pharmaceutical substances exerting a dispersing effect".

Tou nao da feng **頭腦大風, massive head and brain wind** [1]
PC identical with → *tou nao feng* 頭腦風, head and brain wind. *MYBL* 2, SE yang rou 羊肉：味甘，大熱，無毒。主緩中，字乳余疾，及**頭腦大風**，汗出，虛勞寒冷，補中益氣，安止驚, "Its flavor is sweet, and it is very hot. It has no poison. It controls slowing down of the center, all ailments following delivery, as well as **massive head and brain wind**, sweating, depletion exhaustion, and sensations of cold. It supplements the center and augments qi, and it calms and ends fright".

Tou nao feng **頭腦風, head and brain wind** [1]
PC identical with → *tou feng* 頭風, head wind. *BCTJ* SE *bo he* 薄荷：舊不著所出州土，而今處處有之。莖、葉似荏而尖長，經冬根不死，夏秋采莖葉，暴乾。古方稀用，或與薤作虀食。近世醫家治傷風，**頭腦風**，通關格與小兒風涎，為要切之藥，故人家園庭間多蒔之, "In former times the place of origin [of *bo he*] was not known; nowadays it is available everywhere...In recent times medical experts have used it to cure harm caused by wind, **head and brain wind**, and it is considered an indispensable medication to open passages and [to cure] wind drool in children. Hence people cultivate it in their gardens".

Tou nao ming xiang **頭腦鳴響, sounds in the brain** [1]
IS identical with → *nao ming* 腦鳴. *BCGM* SE *ming* 茗 quotes *YFZY*: **頭腦鳴響**，狀如蟲蛀，名大白蟻, "**Sounds in the brain** resembling moths are called 'big termites'".

Tou re **頭熱, the head is hot** [6] AN → *nao re* 腦熱, the brain is hot.
IS of a patient's feeling of dryness and heat in his head, or of a third person feeling heat when touching the patient's head with his hand. *SW* 28: 脈實滿，手足寒，**頭熱**, "When the vessels are replete and full, while the feet and the hands are cold, and **the head is hot**, [how is that]?"

Tou teng **頭疼, headache** [5]
IS, PC identical with → *tou tong* 頭痛. *QJYF* 3: 產後余疾，胸中少氣，腹痛，**頭疼**, "Additional ailments following delivery: diminished qi in the chest, abdominal pain, **headache**".

Tou tong **頭痛, headache** [345] AW *tou teng* 頭疼; AN *nao tong* 腦痛, brain pain; *nao gu teng tong* 腦骨疼痛, brain bone pain; *ding tong* 頂痛, vertex pain.

① IS of pain affecting the entire head or parts of it. *SW* 31: 兩感於寒者, 病一日則巨陽與少陰俱病, 則**頭痛**口乾而煩滿, "In case of double affection by cold, when the disease is in its first day, then the great yang [conduit] and the minor yin [conduit] both have the disease. As a result, **the head aches**, the mouth is dry, and there is vexation and fullness".

② PC with headache as its main illness sign. *SW* 10: **頭痛**巔疾, 下虛上實, "Hence, **headache** and peak-illness, [this is] depletion below and repletion above".

Tou xuan **頭眩, the head is dizzy** [22]

IS identical with → *xuan yun* 眩運①, vertigo. *SW* 74: 厥陰之勝，耳鳴**頭眩**, "When the ceasing yin dominates, [patients hear] ringing [sounds] in the ears and **the head is dizzy**.

Tou xuan **頭旋, head spin** [34] AN *tou yun* 頭運, head movement.

IS of a feeling of vertigo as if one's own body and the scenery around were revolving. *ZHF* 4: 治穀疸者，食畢**頭旋**，心怫鬱不安而發黃, "To cure grain *dan*-illness, this is, when following a meal [patients] develop **head spin**, their heart experiences anger and pent-up [qi] and restlessness, and they develop a yellow [complexion]".

Tou yang **頭瘍, head ulcer** [5]

PC CD of all → *chuang yang* 瘡瘍, sores and ulcers, developing on the head. *BJ* SE *li lu* 藜蘆：主蠱毒，咳逆，泄痢腸澼，**頭瘍**，疥瘙，惡瘡, "It controls *gu* poison, cough with [qi] counterflow, outflow and free-flux illness and intestinal flush, **head ulcers**, *jie*-illness with itching, and malign sores".

Tou yun **頭運, head movement** [17]

IS of vertigo identical with → *tou xuan* 頭旋, head spin. *SJZL* 151, 治婦人月水不調，手足煩熱，**頭運**心煩，大黃丸方, "To cure women with irregular menstruation, whose hands and feet are affected by vexing heat, who experience **head movement** and heart vexation, [use] the recipe for the pills with *da huang*".

Tou zhen **偷針, stealthy needle; sty** [1] AN tiao zhen 挑針, poking needle.

PC with a small red node turning into a festering swelling developing in the eyelid as a major sign. *ZBYHL* 28: 人有眼內眥頭忽結成皰，三五日間便生膿汁，世呼為**偷針**, "If, at the end of the inner canthi of a person, a blister suddenly grows and develops pus within the next three to five days, then this is commonly called '**stealthy needle**'".

Tou zhong **頭重, heavy head** [4]

IS of a feeling of the head being extremely heavy and indisposed. *SHL* 392: **頭重**不欲舉, 眼中生花, 膝脛拘急, "The **head is so heavy** one does not wish to raise it. The vision of the eyes is blurred. The knees and shins cramp and are tense".

Tou zhong ming xiang **頭中鳴響, sounds in the head** [1]

IS identical with → *nao ming* 腦鳴, sounds in the brain. *ZSYT* 5: 戴復庵云：**頭中鳴響**，有虛有實, "Dai Fu'an states: **sounds in the head** may indicate depletion or repletion".

Tu **吐, [silent] vomiting ; spitting; difficult exhalation; emetic therapy** [p]

① IS a) of a reflex of the stomach's contents being thrown up, with no retching sound as its main characteristic. This term is often used as an abbreviation of → *ou tu* 嘔吐①, vomiting. *SW* 69: 脅痛而**吐**甚, "Pain in the flanks and severe **vomiting**". b) Of spitting phlegm and other matter from the mouth. *JGYL* Fj: 風舍於肺…蓄結癰膿，**吐**如米粥, "Wind settles in the lung…It collects with nodes forming obstruction-illnesses and pus. [Patients] **spit** [matter] resembling rice congee". c) Of an impeded exhalation. *BJ* SE *mu gui* 牡桂：主上氣咳逆，結氣，喉痹**吐**吸, "It controls rising qi and cough, with [qi] moving contrary to its normal direction, bound qi, throat blockage resulting in **difficult** in- and **exhalation**".

② PC AD of → *ou tu* 嘔吐②, vomiting. *SYDXF* 12: 硫黄散，治**吐**並驚**吐**, "Powder with *liu huang* cures **vomiting** and fright with **vomiting**.

③ TA AD of → *tu fa* 吐法, application of emetics to stimulate therapeutic vomiting. *SW* 70: **吐**之下之，補之瀉之，久新同法, "[Laws exist to emit it through] **vomiting**, to discharge it, to supplement it, and to drain it. Chronic and newly acquired [illnesses are treated] following the same laws".

④ Purposely spitting matter from the mouth. *QJYiF* 15: 絞取汁，熱含冷**吐**, "Wring to obtain the juice. Heat it and [have the patient] hold it in his mouth. When it has turned cold he **spits** it out".

Tu bai mo **吐白沫, spitting of white foam** [2]

IS of spitting a foam-like white secretion. *ZHF* 7: 蜀椒閉口者有毒，戟人咽，氣便欲絕，又令人**吐白沫**, "The *shu jiao* that closes the mouth is poisonous. It pierces the throat, and breathing comes close to being interrupted. Also, it makes a person **spit white foam**".

Tu chu qing bi xian **吐出青碧涎, spitting of jade-green saliva** [1]

IS of vomiting phlegm-like sputum of a jade-green color. *BCGM* SE *tong qing* 銅青 quotes *JYF*: 碧琳丹治痰涎潮盛，卒中不語…**吐出青碧涎**, 瀉下惡物, 大效, "The virid-jade-elixir serves to treat a profuse emergence of phlegm and saliva, sudden stroke and an inability to speak…when [patients] **spit jade-green saliva**, and if through outflow they discharge malign stuff, it is greatly effective".

Tu chuang **秃瘡, baldness sores** [27]

PC of → *tou chuang* 頭瘡, head sores, with itching on the head at first, that destroy the skin later and eventually cause the loss of one's hair. *ZHF* 5：又一方，加黄連二兩，亦療得**秃瘡**, "And a further recipe: add 2 *liang* of *huang lian*. It also cures **baldness sores**".

Tu fa **吐法, method to stimulate vomiting** [8]

TA using pharmaceutical substances or other means to stimulate vomiting, including stimulation of saliva and tear flow, as well as sneezing to cure accumulations of pathological matter, such as phlegm sputum, undigested food, or toxic matter, in the upper part of the body. *SJZL* 4: **吐法**之用，不可妄施, "The application of **the method to stimulate vomiting** must not be haphazard".

Tu li **吐利, vomiting and free flow** [83] AN *tu xie* 吐瀉, vomiting and outflow; *tu xie* 吐泄, vomiting and outflow.

① AN *tu xia* 吐下, vomiting and discharge. IS of → *xie xie* 泄瀉, outflow, accompanied by → *ou tu* 嘔吐, vomiting. *SHL* 383: 病發熱、頭痛、身疼、惡寒、**吐利**者，此屬何病? "If someone suffers from an effusion of heat, headaches, pain in the entire body, an aversion to cold, with **vomiting and free flow**, with what disease are these [illness signs] associated?"

② AN *ou xie* 嘔泄, vomiting and outflow. PC with vomiting and outflow. SW 70：其氣逆，其病**吐利**, "Its qi moves contrary [to its regular course]. Its illnesses are **vomiting and free flow**".

③ PE causing vomiting and outflow. *JGYL* Lj: 食諸菌中毒，悶亂欲死…服諸**吐利**藥，並解, "If one were poisoned by eating mushrooms, with heart-pressure and chaotic [qi] as if one were about to die…ingest any medication causing **vomiting and free flow**, and all this will be resolved".

Tu na **吐納, controlled breathing** [1]

A technique aiming at health maintenance by means of controlling the frequency, spacing and force of in- and exhalation by eliminating distracting thoughts, calming one's mental activities, and harmonizing one's sentiments. *MYBL* Preface by Tao Yinju 陶隱居序：**吐納**餘暇，頗游意方技, "During leisure time when I did not practice **controlled breathing** I let my thoughts roam to the techniques of the prescription [controls]".

Tu ni **吐逆, vomiting with [qi] counterflow** [75]

① IS identical with *tu* 吐①, vomiting. *SHL* 29: 厥, 咽中乾, 煩躁**吐逆**者，作甘草乾薑湯與之, "In the case of recession, dryness in the throat, vexation and restlessness, and **vomiting with [qi] counterflow**, prepare a decoction with *gan cao* and *gan jiang* and give it [to the patient]".

② PC identical with → *tu* 吐②, vomiting. *ZBYHL* 74: 愈腸胃不能受食，**吐逆**, "To heal an inability of intestines and stomach to accept food, and **vomiting with [qi] counterflow**".

Tu nü **吐衄, [blood] spitting and spontaneous external bleeding** [34]

IS and PC CD of → *tu xue* 吐血, to spit blood, and → *nü xue* 衄血, spontaneous external bleeding. *ZBYHL* 27: "思慮傷心，心傷則**吐衄**, "Pondering harms the heart. When the heart is harmed, [patients suffer from **blood**] **spitting and spontaneous external bleeding**".

Tu ou **吐嘔, vomiting** [1]

PC identical with → *ou tu* 嘔吐②, vomiting. *MYBL* SE *bai zhi* 白芷：療風邪，久渴，**吐嘔**, "It cures wind evil, chronic thirst, and **vomiting**".

Tu qing shui **吐清水, vomiting clear water**[8]

IS of vomiting a clear and thin liquid, or of producing clear and thin liquid without vomiting. The former variant is also called *ou tu qing shui* 嘔吐清水; the latter is also called *kou tu qing shui* 口吐清水. *ZBYHL* 18: 長蟲，蛔蟲也，長一尺，動則**吐清水**, "Longworms are identical with roundworms. They are 1 *chi* long. When they move [patients will] **vomit clear water**".

***Tu ru* 吐乳, vomiting breastfed milk** [20]

IS of newborns vomiting the milk they have been breastfed. *QJYF* 26: niu ru zhi 牛乳汁：牛乳汁，味甘微寒無毒，補虛羸，止渴，入生薑、葱白，止小兒**吐乳**, 補勞, "Cow milk, flavor: sweet, slightly cold, no poison. It supplements depletion with emaciation, and stops thirst. With *sheng jiang* and *cong bai* it stops **vomiting of breastfed milk** in children, and supplements exhaustion".

***Tu she* 吐舌, tongue poking** [6]

IS of patients frequently sticking their tongue out of their mouth without immediately retracting it. *BJ* SE wei xian 薇銜：主風濕痹歷節痛，驚癇**吐舌**, "It controls wind moisture blockage and pain pervading the joints, fright epilepsy and **tongue poking**".

***Tu shi* 吐食, vomiting of food** [70]

IS of throwing up undigested food from the stomach. *ZBYHL 7:* 太陰之為病，腹滿**吐食**，不可下, "When the major yin [section] is affected by disease, the abdomen will have a feeling of fullness with **vomiting of food**. In this case one must not purge".

***Tu shui* 吐水, vomiting of water** [29] AN *ou shui* 嘔水.

IS of vomiting liquid phlegm. *QJYF* 26: 胡桃，味甘冷滑無毒，不可多食，動痰飲。令人噁心，**吐水**，吐食, "*Hu tao*, sweet flavor, cold, smooth, no poison. One must not eat much of it. It excites phlegm rheum. It makes people feel nauseous (lit. have a feeling of a malign center), and leads to **vomiting of water**, and vomiting of food". In view of different appearances of the liquid vomited, specialists distinguish among → *tu qing shui* 吐清水, vomiting of clear water; *tu tan shui* 吐痰水, vomiting of phlegm-water; *tu bai mo* 吐白沫, vomiting of white foam; *tu suan shui* 吐酸水, vomiting of sour water.

***Tu suan chou shui* 吐酸臭水, vomiting of sour and foul water** [2]

IS of vomiting of liquids that have a sour flavor and a foul odor. *BCSY* SE *zhang cai* 樟材：味辛，温，無毒。主惡氣，中惡心腹痛，鬼注，霍亂，腹脹，宿食不消，常**吐酸臭水**。酒煮服之。無藥處用之, "Acrid flavor, warm, no poison. It controls malign qi, being struck by the malign with heart and abdominal pain, demon influx, cholera, abdominal distension, food that remains in the body overnight without being digested, and frequent **vomiting of sour and foul water**".

***Tu suan shui* 吐酸水, vomiting of sour water** [5] AN *ou tu suan shui* 嘔吐酸水, vomiting of sour water.

IS of vomiting a liquid of sour flavor. *QJYF* 16: 治中散，食後**吐酸水**方, "Powder to regulate the center, a recipe for **vomiting of sour water** after one has eaten".

***Tu tan shui* 吐痰水, vomiting of phlegm and water** [4] AN *ou tu tan shui* 嘔吐痰水.

IS of vomiting of thin phlegm. *WTMY* 8: 茯苓湯，主風痰氣發，即嘔吐欠呿，煩悶不安，或**吐痰水**者方, "Decoction with *fu ling*. It controls wind phlegm qi effusion, that is, a recipe for vomiting and yawning, vexation, heart-pressure, and restlessness. In some cases there is **vomiting of phlegm and water**".

Tu xia **吐下, vomiting and discharge** [76]

① IS a) identical with → *tu li* 吐利①, vomiting and free flow. *SHL* 76: 若更發汗，必吐下不止, "If sweating is induced one more time, this will result in unending **vomiting and discharge**". b) Blood, turbid liquid, and parasites discharged from the oral cavity, anus, or genital tract. *JGYL* Lj: 吐下白沫，身體痹冷, "**Vomiting and discharge** of white foam; the entire body experiences blockage and cold".

② TA combining emetics and purgatives. *SHL* 264: 兩耳無所聞、目赤、胸中滿而煩者，不可吐下, "When both ears are deaf, when the eyes are red, and when there is a feeling of fullness in the chest associated with vexation, one must not use [therapies] causing **vomiting and discharge**".

Tu xie **吐瀉, vomiting and outflow; to stimulate vomiting and outflow** [70]

① IS identical with → *tu li* 吐利①, vomiting and free flow. *TPSHF* 9: 治傷寒六日，**吐瀉**，百骨疼痛，脚冷腹熱，宜服人參散方, "To cure harm caused by cold lasting for six days, **vomiting and outflow**, pain affecting all the bones, cold legs and abdominal heat, the recipe for ingesting the powder with *ren shen* is advisable.

② PC identical with → *tu li* 吐利②, vomiting and free flow. *XEYZZJ* Fj：小兒傷於風冷，病**吐瀉**, "When children are harmed by wind and cold, their disease is **vomiting and outflow**".

③ PE identical with → *tu li* 吐利③, to stimulate vomiting and free flow. *RHZ* SE ban mao 斑貓：生即**吐瀉**人, "[Ingested] without prior pharmaceutical processing it will **stimulate** people to develop **vomiting and outflow**.

Tu xie **吐泄, vomiting and outflow; to stimulate vomiting and outflow** [11]

① IS identical with → *tu li* 吐利①, vomiting and free flow. *BCGM* SE huang qi 黃耆 quoting *BCMQ*: 如患內傷，脾胃衰弱，飲食怕進，怠惰嗜眠，發熱惡寒，嘔吐泄瀉，及夫脹滿痞塞，力乏形羸，脈息虛微，精神短少, "If one suffers from internal harm, with the spleen and stomach weakened, and an aversion to beverages and food, a feeling of being tired and a desire to sleep, an effusion of heat and an aversion to cold, with vomiting and outflow, abdominal distension with a feeling of fullness, obstacle-illness with blockage, weakness and emaciation, a depletion [movement in the] vessels, and faint breathing, with a diminished spirit", writes: 凡內傷脾胃，發熱惡寒，**吐泄**怠臥，脹滿痞塞，神短脈微, "When there is internal harm to spleen and stomach, [this will result in] an effusion of heat and an aversion to cold, **vomiting and outflow** and a desire to lie down, distension with a feeling of fullness, obstacle-illness and blockage. The spirit is deficient, and the [movement] in the vessels is faint".

② PC identical with *tu xie* 吐瀉②, vomiting and outflow. *BCGM* SE hua shi 滑石 quoting *PJF*: 藿香吐液散，治大人小兒，諸嘔逆吐瀉，或霍亂不安, "The powder with *huo xian* for vomiting liquid cures adults and children alike with all types of vomiting with counterflow and vomiting with outflow, or cholera with restlessness", modifies the indications to:伏暑**吐泄**，或吐，或泄，或瘧，小便赤，煩渴, "**Vomiting and outflow** brought forth by latent summerheat, with either vomiting, or outflow, or malaria, red urine, and vexation with thirst".

③ PE identical with → tu xie 吐瀉, to stimulate vomiting and outflow. *BCGM* SE zao xiu 蚤休 quoting *RHZ*: 吐瀉瘰癧 writes: 吐泄瘰癧, "[Apply medication] **stimulating vomiting and outflow** [to cure] scrofula with pervasion-illness".

Tu xu huo wang **土虛火旺, soil depletion with strong fire** [1]
EA, PM of a → *yin xu huo dong* 陰虛火動, yin depletion with excited fire, resulting from an insufficiency of spleen, i.e. soil, yin. *BCGM* SE *ren shen* 人參 quoting LYW: 如土虛火旺之病，則宜生參, "For diseases such as **soil depletion with strong fire** it is advisable to use fresh [*ren*] *shen*".

Tu xue **吐血, to spit blood** [342]
① IS CD of blood being spat from one's oral cavity, mostly with an origin in the stomach it may also originate in the lung or nose. *LS* 13: 甚成息賁，脅急吐血, "In severe cases this generates rapid breathing, tightness of flanks and **blood spitting**".
② PC with blood spitting. *JGYL* Mj: 夫吐血，咳逆上氣，其脈數而有熱，不得臥者，死, "Now, if [patients] **spit blood** and cough with qi rising in counterflow, their [movements in the] vessels being accelerated, and if they have heat and cannot sleep, they will die".

Tu yao **吐藥, emetics** [13]
A category of pharmaceuticsl substances used to stimulate therapeutic vomiting. *ZBYHL* 10: 瘴氣候，三日以上，氣浮於上，填塞心胸，使頭痛胸滿而悶，宜以吐藥，吐之必愈, "The signs of miasmatic qi. After more than three days, the qi rises to the surface and fills the heart and chest causing headaches, a feeling of fullness in the chest and heart-pressure. [In this situation] it is suitable to take **emetics**. Once it has been vomited [the patient] will be cured".

Tu yu **土郁, pent-up soil [qi]** [2]
PC of spleen and stomach qi accumulation forming nodes. *SW* 71: 土郁奪之, "In the case of **pent-up soil [qi]**, take it away".

Tu zhong **凸腫, bulging swelling** [1]
IS of an area that is normally slightly sunken in but now protrudes because of a swelling. *BCGM* SE *fu zi* 附子 quotes *QJF*: 足釘怪疾，兩足心凸腫，上生黑豆瘡, "The strange ailment of foot pin-illness sores: the soles of both feet have a **bulging swelling** with black bean sores developing on top of them".

Tui **癀, prominence-illness** [p]
PC identical with → *yin tui* 陰癀, yin (i.e. scrotal) prominence-illness. *ZBYHL* 34: **癀**病之狀，陰核腫大，有時小歇，歇時終大於常, "The appearance of **prominence-illness**: The testicles are swollen. At some time [the swelling] may end for a short while. When this time ends, it is still larger than normal".

Tui **瘣, breakdown-illness** [p]
PC identical with → *yin tui* 陰癀, yin (i.e. scrotal) prominence-illness. *QJYF* 24: 男**瘣**，灸手季指端七壯, "[To cure] **breakdown-illness** in males cauterize the fingertip of the smallest finger seven times".

***Tui ji* 癩疾, ailment of breakdown-illness** [1]
PC identical with → *yin tui* 陰㿉, yin (i.e. scrotal) prominence-illness. *YXL* SE *di fu zi* 地膚子：與陽起石同服，主丈夫陰痿不起，補氣益力，治陰卵**癩疾**, "Ingested together with *yang qi shi* it controls dysfunction of the yin [member, i.e. penis] in males unable to achieve erection, supplements qi and increases strength, and cures testicles affected by the **ailment of breakdown-illness**".

***Tui ji* 㿉疾, ailment of prominence-illness** [1]
PC identical with → *yin tui* 陰㿉, yin (i.e. scrotal) prominence-illness. *BCGM* SE *hai zao* 海藻 quoting *YXL*: 消男子癩疾, "It dissolves the ailment of breakdown-illness in males", writes: 消男子**㿉疾**, "It dissolves the **ailment of prominence-illness** in males".

***Tui shan* 㿉疝, breakdown-illness with elevation-illness** [12]
PC identical with → *yin tui* 陰㿉, yin (i.e. scrotal) prominence-illness. *SW* 49: 厥陰者辰也，三月陽中之陰，邪在中，故曰**㿉疝**少腹腫也, "Ceasing yin is *chen*; the third month is the yin in the yang. The evil is in the center. Hence, [the text] states: **breakdown-illness with elevation-illness**, the lower abdomen is swollen".

***Tui shan* 癩疝, breakdown-illness with elevation-illness** [10]
PC identical with → *yin tui* 陰㿉, (i.e. scrotal) prominence-illness. *QJYF* 24: 治**癩疝**，卵偏大，氣上，不能動方, "Recipe to cure **breakdown-illness with elevation-illness**, when one testical is enlarged with rising qi, and [the patient] cannot move".

***Tui zhong* 癩腫, breakdown-illness with swelling** [4]
PC identical with → *yin tui* 陰㿉, yin (i.e. scrotal) prominence-illness. *BCGM* SE *gan lan* 橄欖：陰腎**癩腫**：橄欖核、荔枝核、山楂核等分，燒存性，研末，每服二錢, "[To cure] yin[-member, i.e. penis, and] kidneys [i.e. testicles] affected by **breakdown-illness with swelling**: burn equal amounts of *gan lan he*, *li zhi he*, *shan zha he* while maintaining their nature, and grind to a powder. The dosage to be ingested is 2 *qian*".

***Tun suan* 吞酸, sour swallowing** [15]
IS of acidic liquid moving upward from the stomach into the throat, and being swallowed again after it fails to leave the mouth. The patient feels irritated by the sour flavor. *ZBYHL* 20: 痰水結聚，停於胸膈之間，時令人**吞酸**氣逆, "Phlegm and water form nodular collections that stagnate in the region of chest and diaphragm. At times this causes **sour swallowing** with qi counterflow".

***Tuo* 唾, spittle; to spit phlegm; to spit** [203]
① PN of spittle and saliva, i.e. liquids secreted in the oral cavity. *SW* 23: 心為汗，肺為涕，肝為淚，脾為涎，腎為**唾**，是謂五液, "The heart generates sweat. The lung generates snivel. The liver generates tears. The spleen generates saliva. The kidneys generate **spittle**. These are the so-called 'five fluids'".
② IS of spitting phlegm. *SW* 19: 上見欬**唾**，下為氣泄, "Above there appears coughing and **spitting**; below it is qi outflow".

③ Identical with *tu* 吐, spitting from the mouth. Commonly used in combination with additional terms to denote IS, such as *tuo xue* 唾血, to spit blood; *tuo xian* 唾涎, to spit saliva; *tuo nong* 唾膿, to spit pus. *SW* 17: 肺脈搏堅而長，當病**唾**血, "When the beating in the vessels of the lung is firm and extended, [the patient] must suffer from **spitting** blood".

Tuo gang **脫肛, prolapsed rectum** [129] AN *da chang tuo* 大腸脫; prolapsed large intestine; *dong chang ting chu* 洞腸挺出, prolapse of the cavernous intestine; *chang tou ting chu* 腸頭挺出, prolapse of the intestinal ending; *jie chang* 截腸, severed intestine.

PC of a prolapse of the mucous membrane or an entire section of the rectum to outside of the anus. *BJ* SE *kuo yu* 蛞蝓：主賊風喎僻，軼筋及**脫肛**, "It controls [facial] wryness caused by robber wind, twisted sinews, and **prolapsed rectum**".

Tuo jing **脫精, involuntary tossing of seminal fluid** [4] AN *jing tuo* 精脫.

PC identical with a rather extreme → *yi jing* 遺精, involuntary loss of seminal fluid. *RHZ* SE *dai zhe* 代赭：止瀉痢，**脫精**，尿血，遺溺, "It stops outflow and free-flux illness, **involuntary tossing of seminal fluid**, urine with blood, and enuresis".

Tuo jiu **脫臼, dislocation** [4]

PC of a dislocation of joints, with the ends of the bones abnormally separated. This harms the body structures upholding the joints so that they no longer function properly. *SJZL* 143: 治一切打撲，驢傷馬墜，**脫臼**損折，兼定痛疼，接骨膏方, "A recipe for an ointment to cure all [injuries resulting from] hits or falls, traumata inflicted by donkeys and falls from horses, **dislocations** and fractures. At the same time it serves to stop pain and set bones".

Tuo xue **唾血, to spit blood** [33]

① IS of coughed up phlegm with blood, or spittle with blood. *SW* 38: 肺咳之狀，咳而喘息有音，甚則**唾血**, "The appearance of lung cough: [Patients] cough and their breath is panting with noises. In severe cases, they **spit blood**".

② PC with spitting of blood. *SW* 17: 肺脈搏堅而長，當病**唾血**, "When the beating in the vessels of the lung is firm and extended, [the patient] must have the disease **spitting blood**".

Tuo xue **脫血, loss of blood** [2]

PC identical with → *wang xue* 亡血. *SW* 40: 年少時，有所大**脫血**, "It is acquired in younger years because of a massive **loss of blood**".

Tuo yang **脫陽, loss of yang [qi]** [8]

PC of a weakening and eventual exhaustion of yang qi, resulting in a severe imbalance of yin and yang qi, and a departing of the human spirit. A very serious condition often following massive vomiting, diarrhea, and sweating, as well as excessive sexual intercourse. *NJ* 20: **脫陽**者見鬼，脫陰者目盲, "Those with a **loss of yang [qi]** will see demons; those with a loss of yin [qi] will turn blind".

***Tuo yang* 脫陰, loss of yin [qi]** [1]

PC of a weakening and eventual exhaustion of yin body liquids and blood, resulting in a severe imbalance of yin and yang qi, and a departing of the human spirit. A very serious condition often following massive vomiting, diarrhea, sweating, and bleeding, as well as continuing high fever. *NJ* 20: 脫陽者見鬼，脫陰者目盲, "Those with a loss of yang [qi] will see demons; those with a **loss of yin [qi]** will turn blind".

- W -

Wai **咼, slanted mouth; wryness** [p]
IS identical with → *kou wai* 口咼, wryness of the mouth. *BCGM* SE *kuo yu* 蛞蝓：**咼**，苦乖切，口戾也, "[The term] 咼, [pronounced *kuai* out of] *k*[*u*] and [*g*]*uai*, has the meaning of '**slanted mouth**'".

Wai gan **外感, external affection** [11]
① EA PM of evil agents such as the "six excesses" or epidemics that cause disease in the human body having intruded into it from its environment. *WTMY* 5: **外感**惡氣，亦生此疾, "**External affection** with malign qi will also generate this ailment".
② CD of PCs resulting from an external affection. *YXZC* 1: 適遇風雨外襲，遂成內傷挾**外感**之證, "If one happens to be struck externally by wind and rain, this will subsequently generate a condition of internal harm associated with an **external affection**".

Wai gan zhi shi **外感之濕, moisture affecting the body from outside** [1] AD *wai shi* 外濕, external moisture.
EA of moisture evil entering the human body from outside. *BCGM* Shi ji 十劑, *zao ji* 燥劑, drying preparations: **外感之濕**，雨露嵐霧地氣水濕，襲於皮肉筋骨經絡之間, "[In the case of] **moisture affecting the body from outside**, rain, dew, mountain haze and fog, qi of the earth, as well as water and moisture have attacked and entered skin, flesh, sinews, bones, conduits and network vessels".

Wai han **外寒, outer cold** [4]
① PC of an extreme aversion to cold, or of shivering indicating cold in the body's outer spheres, in contrast to → *nei han* 內寒, inner cold. *SW* 62: 陽虛則**外寒**，陰虛則內熱, "Yang [qi] depletion results in **outer cold**; yin [qi] depletion results in inner heat".
② EA referring to a cold evil that affects the human body from outside. *TPSHF* 84: 內中冷氣及傷於**外寒**, "Internally struck by cold qi, and harmed by **outer cold**".

Wai pi **咼僻, wryness** [8]
IS of the mouth only, or of both the mouth and eyes being slanted to one side. Identical with → *kou wai* 口咼 and *wai xie* 咼斜. *QJYF* 8: 中風，手臂不仁，口面**咼僻**, "As a result of wind stroke, the hands and arms are numb, with **wryness** of the mouth and face".

Wai re **外熱, external heat** [3]
PC of heat in the external sections of the body, the opposite to → *nei re* 內熱, internal heat. *SW* 62: 腠理閉塞，玄府不通，衛氣不得泄越，故**外熱**, "The interstitial structures are blocked. The dark palaces are impassable. [As a result] the guard qi cannot flow out transgressing [the skin]. Hence, [there is] **external heat**".

Wai shang **外傷, external damage** [6] CD of all
PC of damage to the human body through its exterior skin. *SJZL* 6: 如**外傷**，用此藥（銀花散）貼瘡口, "In the case of **external damage** use this medication (the powder with *yin hua*) and apply it to the wound".

Wai shen chu suo **外腎搐縮, the external kidneys are pulled in and shrink** [1]
IS identical with → *luan suo* 卵縮, egg shrinkage, i.e. shrinkage of the testicles. *SYDXF* 8: 小腹緊痛，**外腎搐縮**, "The lower abdomen is tight and aches. **The external kidneys are pulled in and shrink**".

Wai shi **外濕, external moisture** [1]
EA identical with → *wai gan zhi shi* 外感之濕, moisture affecting the body from outside. *DXXF* 1: **外濕**宜表散，內濕宜淡滲, "**External moisture** is to be dispersed to the outside. Internal moisture is to be drained internally using substances with a blant flavor".

Wai xie **喎斜, wryness** [37] AN *wai pi* 喎僻, *pian xie* 偏斜, *wai xie* 喎邪, wryness evil.
IS of eyes and mouth being slanted to one side. *QJYiF* 16: 偏枯拘屈，口面**喎斜**, "Unilateral withering with cramps, with **wryness** of the mouth and face". *BCGM* has *kou mian wai xie* 口面喎斜, wryness of the mouth and face; *kou yan wai xie* 口眼喎斜, wryness of the mouth and eyes; *kou mu wai xie* 口目喎斜.

Wai xie **喎邪, wryness evil** [1]
IS identical with → *wai xie* 喎斜, wryness. *QJYF* 8: 緩弱不收，便利無度，口面**喎邪**, "[The limbs are] slack and weak and unable to contract. Urine flows freely without restriction. The mouth and face show **wryness evil**".

Wai zhang **外障, external screen** [1] AN *wai zhang yi* 外障翳, external obstructive shade.
PC of → *mu zhang* 目障, eye screen, resulting from diseases affecting the external tissues of the eyes, such as eyelids, the two canthi, as well as the white and black sections of the eye. *SJZL* 109, 治眼生胬肉侵睛、**外障**，雖已鉤割熨烙，亦宜服此，除風湯方, "Recipe for a decoction to remove wind to cure eyes developing a tumorous flesh-growth entering the eyeball, and generating an **external screen** despite having been opened with a sickle and cauterized".

Wai zhang yi **外障翳, external obstructive shade** [1]
PC identical with → *wai zhang* 外障, external screen. *SJZL* 111, 治眼**外障翳**，水照丸方, "Recipe for the 'water illumination pills' to cure eyes with an **external obstructive shade**".

Wai zhi **外痔, external piles** [8]
PC of → *zhi chuang* 痔瘡, piles sores, forming holes releasing blood that are visible outside the anus, and with distinct swelling and pain. *QJYF* 23 lists 治**外痔**方, "Recipes to cure **external piles**".

Wan bi **頑痹, stubborn blockage** [36]
PC of chronic and difficult to cure → *bi bing* 痹病, blockage diseases. *ZBYHL* 2: 久而不治，令人**頑痹**, "If it is not cured over an extended period of time, it will make a person develop a **stubborn blockage**".

Wan bing **丸病, disease of the balls (i.e. testicles)** [1]
PC affecting the testicles, identical with → *yin kui* 陰癀, yin (i.e. scrotal) prominence-illness. *BCGM* Bai bing zhu zhi yao 百病主治藥：腹病曰疝，**丸病**曰癀, "When the disease is in the abdomen it is called 'elevation-illness'. When the **disease is in the balls (i.e. testicles)** it is called '*yin* [i.e. scrotal] prominence-illness'".

Wan bing **萬病, the myriad of diseases; all diseases** [8]
PC of "all diseases", identical with → *bai bing* 百病, the one hundred diseases. *ZBYHL* 1: 惟須向曉清靜時行氣, 大佳, 能愈**萬病**, "All that is necessary is to move the qi at dawn at a clear and calm time. This is very good, and can cure **the myriad of diseases**".

Wan chuang **頑瘡, stubborn sores** [11]
PC CD of → *chuang* 瘡, sores, conditions lasting long without being cured. *WKJYao* Fj: 若**頑瘡**痼疾，脾胃虛弱，營氣不能滋養患處，以致寒邪內襲而不愈，宜用小艾炷頻灸瘡口, "In the case of an obstinacy-illness ailment of **stubborn sores**, when the spleen and stomach are depleted and weak, and when the camp qi is no longer able to provide nourishment to the ailing location, with the result that cold evil attacks the interior and this cannot be cured, it is advisable to use a small mugwort-lamp wick to repeatedly cauterize the opening of the sores".

Wan die **踠跌, [injury from] fracturing and falling** [6]
PC CD of → *wan zhe* 踠折, fracture, and → *die pu shang sheng* 跌扑傷損, injury from falls. *MYBL* SE *wo niu* 蝸牛：主賊風喎僻，**踠跌**, 大腸下脫肛，筋急及驚癇, "It cures [facial] wryness caused by robber wind, **[injuries] from fracturing and falling**, descent of the large intestine with prolapse of the rectum, as well as sinew tension and fright epilepsy".

Wan dou ban chuang **豌豆斑瘡, pea[-size] macules sores** [3]
PC identical with → *wan dou chuang* 豌豆瘡, pea sores. *BCGM* SE *yun tai* 芸薹 quoting *WTMY*: 豌豆瘡, writes: **豌豆斑瘡, pea[-size] macules sores**.

Wan dou chuang **豌豆瘡, pea sores** [12] AN *wan dou ban chuang* 豌豆斑瘡, pea[-size] macules sores.
PC identical with → *dou chuang* 痘瘡, smallpox sores. *ZBYHL* 9: 夫熱病皰瘡者，此由表虛裏實，熱氣盛則發瘡，重者周匝遍身。若瘡色赤、頭白、則毒輕，色紫黑則毒重。其形如豌豆，故名**豌豆瘡**, "Now, as far as heat diseases with blister sores are concerned, they result from outer depletion and inner repletion. When heat qi abounds it will effuse as sores. In severe cases they cover the entire body. When the color of the sores is red with a white head, then the poisoning is minor. When the color is crimson-red and black, then the poisoning is severe. Their shape is that of beans. Hence they are called '**pea sores**'".

Wan feng **頑風, stubborn wind** [3] AW *feng wan* 風頑. AN *jiu feng* 久風, long-lasting wind; *lao feng* 老風, old wind.
PC of stubborn, difficult-to-cure wind diseases. *HYBC* SE *qin gui* 秦龜：治婦人赤白漏下，破積癥，**頑風**冷痹，關節氣壅。或經卜者更妙, "They cure

red and white leaking discharge of women, break open accumulations and concretion-illness, **stubborn wind** and cold blockage, as well as qi obstruction in the joints. Those that were used for divination are particularly effective".

Wan ma **頑麻, stubborn hemp[-like numbness]** [3]

IS of a chronic → *ma bi* 麻痹, hemp[-like numbness] blockage. *TPSHF* 19: 治風痹，關節不利，手足**頑麻**，宜服白花蛇散方, "To cure wind blockage, when the joints do not move freely, and when hands and feet are affected by **stubborn hemp[-like numbness]**, the recipe to ingest the powder with *bai hua she* is advisable".

Wan shang **踠傷, fracture harm** [1]

PC identical with → *wan zhe* 踠折, fracture. *MYBL* SE *xu duan* 續斷：止痛生肌肉，及**踠傷**，惡血腰痛，關節緩急, "It ends pain and generates muscle, and [it cures] **fracture harm**, malign blood with lower back pain, and alternating sensations of sluggishness and tightness of the joints".

Wan sun **踠損, fracture injury** [1]

PC identical with → *wan zhe* 踠折, fracture. *KBBC* SE *ye tuo zhi* 野駝脂：主頑痹風瘙，惡瘡毒腫死肌，筋皮攣縮，**踠損**筋骨, "It controls stubborn blockage and wind itching, malign sores, poison swelling, and dead muscles, as well as sinew and skin contractions, and **fracture injury** of the sinews and bones".

Wan tan **頑痰, stubborn phlegm** [7]

① EA identical with → *jie tan* 結痰, bound phlegm. *ZYMZ* 2: 老痰，即結痰，**頑痰**，堅結膠固，吐咯難出, "Chronic phlegm that is identical with bound phlegm and **stubborn phlegm**. It forms hard nodes like glue. It is difficult to emit by vomiting or coughing".

② PC brought forth by stubborn phlegm, with this disease persisting over extended periods of time and being difficult to cure and the gluey phlegm being difficult to emit. *DXZFXY* 2: 五倍子佐他藥，大治**頑痰**, "When *wu pei zi* is combined with further pharmaceutical drugs it serves effectively to cure **stubborn phlegm**".

③ IS of an emission of gluey phlegm pieces. *GZYL* Chi ni lun 吃逆論：大吐**頑痰**數碗，大汗昏睡，一日而安, "When [the patient] massively throws up several bowls of **stubborn phlegm**, with profuse sweating, and a deep sleep, he will be fine after one day".

Wan xuan **頑癬, stubborn *xuan*-illness** [4]

PC of → *xuan* 癬, *xuan*-illness, that cannot be cured for a long time. *HJJF* 指南總論：疥疽**頑癬**，與摩風膏、白龍丸、滑肌散、清心丸, "For *jie*-illness, impediment-illness, and **stubborn *xuan*-illness** apply the 'ointment to rub off wind', 'white dragon pills', the 'powder to smoothen the muscles', and the 'pills to clear the heart'".

Wan yi **頑翳, stubborn shade** [4]

PC of → *mu yi* 目翳, eye shade, that is difficult to cure and continues for an extended period of time. *TPSHF* 33: 治眼久積**頑翳**蓋覆瞳仁，宜點朴硝散方, "To cure eyes with a **stubborn shade** that has collected over an extended period of time to cover the pupil, it is advisable [to use] the recipe to swab them with the powder containing *pu xiao*".

Wan zhe **踠折, fracture** [5] AN *wan shang* 踠傷, fracture harm; *wan sun* 踠損; *wei zhe* 踒折.

PC of a → *shang sun* 傷損, injury, resulting from an improper bending of an extremity either because of an accident or because of pressure exerted. *MYBL* SE *di huang* 地黃：墮墜**踠折**，瘀血，留血，衄鼻，吐血，皆搗飲之, "For falls with **fracture**, stagnant blood [that has left the vessels], bleeding, nosebleed, blood spitting, always pound [it to obtain a liquid] and drink this".

Wang jian **妄見, illusionary visions** [5]

IS of a feeling of illusionary visions, that is, to believe to see things that in fact do not exist. *MYBL* SE *gui jiu* 鬼臼：療咳嗽喉結，風邪煩惑，失魄**妄見**, "It cures cough and throat nodes, wind evil, vexation, and delusions, loss of *po*-soul and **illusionary visions**".

Wang jin **亡津, loss of body liquids** [1]

PC AD of → *wang jin ye* 亡津液. *BCGM* Shi ji 十劑：脫者，氣脫也，血脫也，精脫也，神脫也。脫則散而不收，故用酸澀溫平之藥，以斂其耗散。汗出亡陽，精滑不禁，泄痢不止，大便不固，小便自遺，久嗽**亡津**，皆氣脫也, "A 'release' may be a release of qi, a release of blood, a release of seminal fluid, and a release of spirit. In the case of a release, [the qi, blood, etc.] disperses and is not collected again. Hence one resorts to sour, astringent, warming and neutral medications to gather what is dispersed. When sweat leaves [the body], this is a loss of yang. In case of spontaneous emission of seminal fluid, incessant outflow and free-flux illness, instability of defecation, spontaneous urination, and a long-lasting cough, with a **loss of body liquids**, all these are losses of qi".

Wang jin ye **亡津液, loss of body liquids** [3] AD *wang jin* 亡津, loss of body liquids.

PC brought forth by an excessive wastage of body liquids, often resulting from malpractice such as having patients undergo erroneous treatments of sweating, purging, or vomiting, or seen in the aftermath of long-lasting cough and massive diarrhea. *SHL* 59: 大下之後，復發汗，小便不利者，**亡津液**也, "If after a massive discharge and repeated sweating urine does not flow freely, this is because of a **loss of body liquids**".

Wang xue **亡血, loss of blood** [9] AN *xue tuo* 血脫, blood release; *tuo xue* 脫血, release of blood.

PC CD of massive blood loss brought forth by whatever reason. *JGYL* Fj: 男子面色薄者，主渴及**亡血**，卒喘悸，脈浮者，裏虛也, "When males have a pale complexion, this is because of thirst associated with a **loss of blood**. In the case of sudden panting and palpitation, when the [movement in the] vessels is floating at the surface, this is an internal depletion".

Wang yan **妄言, absurd language; false statement** [9]

① IS identical with → *kuang yan* 狂言, crazy language. *SW* 16: 口目動作，善驚**妄言**, "When the [qi of the] yang brilliance [vessel] is finished, mouth and eyes move in [senseless] activity. [The patient] tends to be fearful and [utters] **absurd language**".

② Refers to speaking in a grandiloquent style, with many errors. *BCSY* SE *qian sui lei* 千歲虆：云千歲虆，謂蘡薁者，深是**妄言**, "To speak of *qian sui lei* and say that it is *ying yu* is certainly a **false statement**".

Wang yang **亡陽, lost yang** [6]

Serious PC of an exhaustion and possibly total loss of yang qi. *SHL* 283: 病患脈陰陽俱緊, 反汗出者, **亡陽**也, "If the patient suffers with yin and yang [movements in the] vessels being both tight, and contrary [to what one might expect] releases sweat, this is [a condition of] **lost yang**".

Wang you suo jian **妄有所見, illusory visions** [1]

IS identical with → *wang jian* 妄見, illusionary visions. *ZBYHL* 23: 病苦恍惚，屍厥不知人，**妄有所見**, "The patient suffers from absent-mindedness; corpse[-like condition because of qi] recession with failure to recognize people; **illusory visions**".

Wang yu 妄語, absurd language [9]

IS identical with → *kuang yan* 狂言, crazy language. *JGYL* Lj: 心急發熱，**妄語**如狂, "The heart is hectic and [patients] effuse heat. They use **absurd language** as if they were crazy".

Wei **痿, dysfunction, to cause dysfunction** [p]

① PC a) of an atrophy and feebleness of the four extremities. In particular, this affects the legs, which may no longer be able to let a person walk or stand. In severe cases the muscle tissue will shrink. *SW* 44: 治**痿**者獨取陽明, "To cure **dysfunction**, select only the yang brilliance". b) Identical with → *yin wei* 陰痿 ②, dysfunction of the yin [member, i.e. penis]. *MYBL* SE *mi zhi* 麋脂：不可近陰，令**痿**, "One must not let it come close to one's yin (i.e. penis), lest it cause **dysfunction**.

② Side effects of pharmaceutical substances, causing a male's genital organ to become dysfunctional. *BCJJZ* SE *mi zhi* 麋脂：尋麋性乃爾淫快，不應**痿**人陰, "It lies in the nature of elks to enjoy sex; hence it cannot be able **to cause dysfunction** in a man's yin [member]".

Wei bi **胃痹, stomach blockage** [1]

PC identical with → *pi bi* 脾痹, spleen blockage. *BJ* SE *ku cai* 苦菜：主五藏邪氣，厭穀**胃痹**, "It controls evil qi affecting the five depots, lack of appetite and **stomach blockage**".

Wei bi **痿躄, dysfunction with an inability to walk** [8] AD *bi* 躄, inability to walk.

PC of atrophy and weakness of the lower legs with an inability to stand or walk. In severe cases the muscle tissue will shrink. *SW* 44: 五臟因肺熱葉焦，發為**痿躄**, "Because the lung is hot and the lobes burn, the five depots develop **dysfunction with an inability to walk**".

Wei bi **痿痹, dysfunction and blockage** [32]

PC CD of → *bi* 痹① a), blockage, and → *wei* 痿① a), dysfunction. *BJ* SE *niu xi* 牛膝：主寒濕**痿痹**，四肢拘攣，膝痛不可屈伸, "It controls cold and moisture **dysfunction and blockage**, with the four limbs being cramped and contracted, and the knees aching and unable to be stretched and bent".

Wei fan **胃反, stomach turnover** [4]

PC identical with → *fan wei* 反胃, turned over stomach. *BJ* SE *qian dan* 鉛丹：主吐逆**胃反**，驚癇癲疾, "It controls vomiting with counterflow [of qi] and **stomach turnover**; fright epilepsy and peak ailment".

Wei han **胃寒, stomach cold** [1]

PC of a cold-type disease with stomach qi depletion brought forth by an inadequate presence of spleen yang qi. *QJYF* 15: 脾病虛則**胃寒**，寒則腹中鼓脹, "When the spleen suffers from depletion, then **stomach cold** results. The cold brings forth a drum-like distension of the abdomen".

Wei han **畏寒, fear of cold** [8]

① IS identical with → *wu han* 惡寒, aversion to cold. *XMLF* 12: 或熱極悶塞，不得宣通，陽極似陰，中外喜熱而反**畏寒**者, "In some cases the heat reaches an extreme with heart-pressure and blockage making any further passage impossible. When yang has reached an extreme it resembles yin. In the center and in the outer sections there is a tendency to feel hot and contrary [to what is normal the patient] has a **fear of cold**".

② A characteristic of animals and plants which cannot stand cold weather. *BCGM* SE *mo li* 茉莉：其性**畏寒**，不宜中土, "Its nature is a **fear of cold**. The central regions [of China] are not suitable for it".

Wei huang **萎黃, wilting with jaundice; wilting and yellow** [9]

① IS identical with → *wei huang* 痿黃①, dysfunction with jaundice *ZBYHL* 48: 凡瘀血在內，顏色**萎黃**，氣息微喘, "In all cases of stagnant blood [that has left the vessels and is now] in the interior the facial complexion will be **wilting and jaundiced**; breathing will be slightly panting".

② Description of yellow color assumed by green plants when drying. *BCGM* SE *cong* 蔥 erroneously quoting *QJYF* 22: 取薑黃、蔥葉，煮沸漬之, "Take *jiang huang* and *cong* leaves, and steep in boiling liquid", writes: 代指毒痛，取**萎黃**蔥葉煮汁，熱漬之, "[To treat] an index finger that is poisoned and aches, take **wilting and yellowed** onion leaves and boil them to prepare a juice, and steep the [finger] in the hot liquid".

Wei huo **胃火, stomach fire** [18]

PC EA identical with → *wei re* 胃熱, stomach heat, heat in the stomach. *JFFH*: 謂之舍利別者，皆取時果之液，煎熬如餳而飲之，稠之甚者，調以沸湯，南人因名之曰煎。味雖甘美，性非中和，且如金櫻煎之縮小便，杏煎、楊梅煎、蒲桃煎、櫻桃煎之發**胃火**，積而至久，濕熱之禍，有不可勝言者, "For the so-called sherbet the liquid of fruit in season is boiled until it is like malt-sugar, and then it is drunk. When it is too thick, it is mixed with hot water. Hence the people in the South call it a 'decoction'. The flavor may be sweet and delicious, but its nature is definitely not neutral or harmonious. Also, when boiled with golden cherries, it withholds urination. When boiled with almonds, red bayberries, rose-apples, or cherries, it will cause **stomach fire**. When this accumulates over a long time, it ends in the undescribable disaster of moisture heat".

***Wei jian re* 胃間熱, heat in the stomach** [23]
PC EA identical with → *wei re* 胃熱, stomach heat, heat in the stomach. *MYBL* SE *shi* 柿：止口乾，**壓胃間熱**，"It ends dryness in the mouth and suppresses **heat in the stomach**".

***Wei jue* 痿蹶, dysfunction with loss of mobility** [8] AN *wei jue* 痿厥, dysfunction with recession.
PC of atrophy and weakness of the lower legs with an inability to stand or walk, in severe cases with a shrinkage of muscle tissue and a sensation of ice cold when touched (hence the notion of warm, yang qi having receded from the region). *BJ* SE *zi wan* 紫菀：去蠱毒，**痿蹶**，安五藏，"It removes *gu* poison, [cures] **dysfunction with loss of mobility**, and it pacifies the five depots".

***Wei jue* 痿厥, dysfunction with recession** [2]
PC identical with → *wei jue* 痿蹶, dysfunction with loss of mobility. *SW* 2: 逆之則傷腎，春為**痿厥**，奉生者少，"Opposing it harms the kidneys. In spring this causes **dysfunction with recession**. There is little to support generation".

***Wei jue* 踒蹶, sprain with loss of mobility** [1]
PC identical with pfeilpfeil*wei jue* 痿蹶, dysfunction with loss of mobility. *BCGM* SE *fu zi* 附子 quoting *BJ*: 主風寒，咳逆邪氣，溫中，金瘡，破癥堅積聚血瘕，寒濕踒躄，拘攣膝痛，脚疼冷弱，不能行步，"It controls wind cold and cough with counterflow of evil qi; warms the center, [cures] wounds inflicted by metal objects; breaks open concretion-illness hardness, accumulation and collection, with blood comglomeration-illness; [cures] cold moisture with sprain and limping; cramps with contraction and aching knees; legs that ache, are cold and weak, so that one cannot walk", writes: 風寒咳逆邪氣，寒濕**踒蹶**，拘攣膝痛，不能行步，破癥堅積聚血瘕，金瘡，"Wind cold and cough with counterflow of evil qi, cold moisture with **sprain with loss of mobility**, cramps with contraction and aching knees so that one cannot walk, breaks open concretion-illness hardness, accumulation and collection, with blood conglomeration-illness, [cures] wounds inflicted by metal objects".

***Wei kou re* 胃口熱, stomach mouth heat** [2]
EA referring to heat stasis in the stomach mouth blocking the downward passage of food. *DXXF* 2: 噤口痢者，**胃口熱**甚故也，"Where [patients suffer simultaneously from] lockjaw and free-flux illness, this is because of extreme **stomach mouth heat**".

***Wei ku* 痿枯, dysfunction with withering** [1]
IS of weakness of the four extremities, in particular of the feet, combined with an appearance of emaciation following the shrinking of muscles and flesh. *MYBL* SE *long gu* 龍骨：療心腹煩滿，四肢**痿枯**，"To heal vexation and a feeling of fullness in the heart and abdominal region, as well as **dysfunction with withering** of the four extremities".

Wei leng **畏冷, fear of cold** [2]
IS identical with → *wu han* 惡寒, aversion to cold. *ZHBJF* 22: 食猶不消，惡食**畏冷**, "As if food remained undigested. They have an aversion to food and they **fear cold**".

Wei ni **胃逆, stomach counterflow** [1]
PC identical with → *fan wei* 反胃, turned over stomach. *SLBC* SE *wei* 蝟：皮燒灰酒服治**胃逆**, "Its skin burned to ashes ingested with wine cures **stomach counterflow**".

Wei pi **痿癖, dysfunction with aggregation illness** [1]
PC identical with → *wei pi* 痿躄, dysfunction with limping. *BCGM dang gui* 當歸 quotes [Wang] Haogu 好古：主**痿癖**嗜臥，足下熱而痛, "It controls **dysfunction with aggregation illness** and a desire to lie down. The soles of the feet are hot and painful". In surviving texts written by Wang Haogu this term cannot be found. *SWXJYBS* Liu qi wei bing 六氣為病 and *RMSQ* 10 have: 痿厥嗜臥，足下熱而痛. *BCGM* SEs *di huang* 地黃 and *tian men dong* 天門冬 both have 痿蹶嗜臥，足下熱而痛. Hence 痿癖 may be a copying error.

Wei qiang **胃強, stomach strength** [1]
PC identical with → *wei re* 胃熱①, stomach heat. *ZJSHL* 5: 腸燥**胃強**，以苦泄之, "In the case of intestinal dryness and **stomach strength**, use bitter [flavor] to drain them".

Wei re **胃熱, heat in the stomach; stomach heat** [14]
① PC of heat-type diseases affecting the stomach. *QJYF* 25: 主脾生病，實則**胃熱**，熱則腹中切痛，痛則陽病，陽脈反大於寸口三倍，病則舌強筋轉，卵縮牽陰股，引髀痛，腹脹身重, "[This conduit] rules the spleen and is responsible for its diseases. In the case of repletion this will be **stomach heat.** Such heat results in a cutting pain in the abdomen. When such pain exists then this is a yang disease. The [movement in the] yang vessels at the inch opening is three times as massive as normal. [Patients] suffer from a stiff tongue and twisted sinews. Their testicles shrink and are drawn in, with pain extending into the thighs. The abdomen is enlarged and the body feels heavy".
② AN *wei huo* 胃火, stomach fire; *wei zhong re* 胃中熱, heat in the stomach; *wei kou re* 胃口熱, stomach mouth heat; *wei jian re* 胃間熱, heat in the stomach. EA bringing forth heat-type disease in the stomach. *LS* 80: **胃熱**則消穀，穀消故善飢, "**Stomach heat** dissolves grain. When the grain is dissolved one tends to be hungry".

Wei re xiao ke **胃熱消渴, melting with thirst associated with stomach heat** [2]
PC of → *xiao ke* 消渴, melting with thirst, brought forth by heat in the stomach. The basic pathological mechanism of 'melting with thirst' comprises a yin depletion with dryness and heat in the triple burner. Hence a 'melting with thirst' associated mainly with stomach heat is a → *zhong xiao* 中消, central melting. *ZLBC* SE *su mi* 粟米：陳者味苦，主**胃熱消渴**，利小便, "Old ones have a bitter flavor. They control **melting with thirst associated with stomach heat**, and they free the passage of urine".

***Wei ruan* 痿軟, dysfunction with softening** [5]
IS of a weakness of the four limbs, especially of the lower extremities with an inability to walk or stand. *YXQY* Lj: 使兩足膝中氣力湧出，**痿軟**實時去矣, "It causes the strength of qi to gush forth from the two feet and the knees. The **dysfunction with softening** will end immediately".

***Wei ruo* 痿弱, dysfunction with weakness** [13]
① IS identical with → *wei ruan* 痿軟, dysfunction with softening. *BCGM* Bai bing zhu zhi yao 百病主治藥 quoting *YXQY*: 痿軟實時去, "The dysfunction with softening will be ended immediately", writes: 去**痿弱**, "It eliminates **dysfunction with weakness**".
② PC a) AW 萎弱, wilting with weakness. Identical with → *yin wei* 陰痿, dysfunction of the yin [member, i.e. penis]. *HYBC* SE *wu ming mu pi* 無名木皮：主陰腎**痿弱**，囊下濕癢, "It controls yin[-member, i.e. penis, and] kidney [i.e. testicles] **dysfunction with weakness**, and moisture itching below the scrotum". b) Identical with → *xu ruo* 虛弱, depletion weakness. *SWBJQYBMJ* Fj: 五臟**痿弱**，榮衛涸流, "The five depots have **dysfunction with weakness**; camp and guardian [qi] dry up and flow off".

***Wei ruo* 萎弱, wilting with weakness** [1]
PC identical with → *wei ruo* 痿弱. *BCGM* SE *a yue hun zi* 阿月渾子 quoting *HYBC wu ming mu pi* 無名木皮：主陰腎痿弱，囊下濕癢, "It controls dysfunction and weakness of the yin[-member, i.e. penis, and] kidneys", writes: 陰腎**萎弱**，囊下濕癢, "**Wilting with weakness** of the yin[-member, i.e. penis, and] kidneys [i.e. testicles], and moisture itching below the scrotum".

***Wei xie* 微泄, mild outflow** [6]
IS of a mild form of → *xie xie* 泄瀉①, outflow, mentioned in the *BCGM* as a side effect following the intake of some pharmaceutical drugs. *BCSY* SE *zhu rou* 豬肉：肝，主脚氣，空心，切作生，以薑、醋進之，當**微泄**, "The liver. It controls leg qi. To be consumed on an empty stomach. Cut and prepare raw. Ingest with ginger and vinegar. [Its intake may be] associated with **mild outflow**".

***Wei xu* 胃虛, stomach depletion** [26]
PC of a depletion of the stomach with an impediment of stomach functions. *MJ* 2: **胃虛**，右手關上脈陽虛者，足陽明經也，病苦脛寒，不得臥，惡寒洒洒，目急，腹中痛, "**Stomach depletion**: When the [movement in the] vessels at the gate section of the right hand shows a yang depletion, this is the leg yang brilliance conduit. Patients suffer from shin cold and cannot lie down to sleep. They have an aversion to cold and shiver. Their eyes are tense, and they feel pain in their abdomen".

***Wei xu xiao ke* 胃虛消渴, melting with thirst associated with stomach depletion** [2]
PC of the depletion variant of → *zhong xiao* 中消, central melting. *BCGM* SE *yang* 羊 quotes *GJLY*: **胃虛消渴**：羊肚爛煮，空腹食之, "**Melting with thirst associated with stomach depletion**: thoroughly boil a lamb stomach, and consume on an empty abdomen".

Wei yue **胃噦, stomach retching** [2]
PC of dry heaving brought forth by cold evil entering the stomach after it has been affected by a warmth disease. *BCGM* SE *zi* 梓：治溫病復感寒邪，變為**胃噦**，煮汁飲之, "To cure a repeated affection with cold evil in the course of a warmth disease resulting in **stomach retching**, consume its boiled juice".

Wei zhe **踒折, fracture** [11]
PC identical with → *wan zhe* 踠折, fracture. *MYBL* SE *tang yi* 唐夷：主療**踒折**, "It controls the healing of **fractures**".

Wei zheng **危證, critical condition** [4] AW *wei zheng* 危症; AN *xian zheng* 險證.
CD of all PC that are very serious and may lead to an unfortunate outcome within a short time. By adding a prefix, they may be associated with a specific group of serious medical problems, such as 婦人胎前產後諸疾危證, "critical conditions of all types of perinatal ailments in women". *QXLF* 41: 久病而脹, 脾土已敗, 最為**危證**, 治難取效, "With distension in the course of an old disease, when the spleen, i.e. soil, is already destroyed, this is a most **critical condition**; in treating it one hardly achieves a good result".

Wei zheng **危症, critical condition** [2]
PC identical with → *wei zheng* 危證. *YXGM* 22: 言胃弱者陰弱也, 虛之甚也。病患見此, 似為**危症**, "When it says 'the stomach is weak', this is a yin weakness. It is an extreme depletion. If one sees a patient suffering from this, it appears as a **critical condition**".

Wei zhong **微腫, slight swelling** [9]
IS of a light → *fu zhong* 浮腫, surface swelling. *SW* 18: 目裹**微腫**如臥蠶起之狀，曰水, "When the eyelids are **slightly swollen**, resembling a silkworm rising from sleep, that is called: 'water'".

Wei zhong ni leng **胃中逆冷, counterflow with cold in the stomach** [1]
IS of a feeling of cold in the stomach accompanied by nausea and an urge to vomit. *BCTJ SE shan jiang* 山薑：主暴冷及**胃中逆冷**，霍亂腹痛, "It controls sudden cold and **counterflow with cold in the stomach**, cholera and abdominal pain".

Wei zhong re **胃中熱, heat in the stomach** [23]
PC EA identical with → *wei re* 胃熱, stomach heat, heat in the stomach. *MYBL* SE *huang qin* 黃芩：療痰熱，**胃中熱**, "It cures phlegm heat and **heat in the stomach**".

Wei zu **足痿, foot dysfunction** [1]
IS of atrophy and weakness of the lower legs with an inability to stand or walk. *SW* 44: 宗筋縱，帶脈不引，故**足痿**不用也, "The basic sinew slackens and the belt vessel fails to pull [tight]. Hence, the **feet suffer from dysfunction** and cannot be used".

Wen **瘟, warmth-illness** [7]
PC AD of → *wen yi* 瘟疫, warmth-illness epidemic. *SJZL* 33: 水調塗五心及額上、鼻中、耳門，辟**瘟**甚驗, "Mix with water and apply to the chest, the

palms and the soles, as well as to the forehead, in the nose and on the ears to ward off **warmth-illness**. Very effective".

***Wen bing* 瘟病, warmth-illness disease** [2]

PC identical with → *wen yi* 瘟疫, warmth-illness epidemic. *SYJYBZFL* 6: 以此論之，則知**瘟病**、飧泄、咳嗽，不可拘也, "Having seen this one knows: **warmth-illness disease**, outflow of undigested food, and cough cannot be restrained".

***Wen bing* 溫病, warmth disease** [27] AN *bing wen* 病溫, warmth disease; *wen ji* 溫疾; warmth disease; *wen qi* 溫氣, warmth qi.

DC of heat diseases brought forth by external warmth evil. *SW* 3: 冬傷於寒，春必**溫病**, "If one was harmed in winter by cold, in spring one will develop a **warmth disease**".

***Wen chuang* 吻瘡, lip sores** [11] AN *yan kou chuang* 燕口瘡, swallow's mouth sores.

PC of → *chuang* 瘡, sores, conditions with swelling, pain and festering of the lips that cannot be cured for an extended period of time. *BCSY* SE *jia jian* 甲煎：小兒頭瘡，**吻瘡**，耳後月蝕瘡，並傅之, "Apply to [ailments] such as children's head sores, **lip sores**, and moon eclipse sores behind the ears".

***Wen du* 溫毒, warmth poison** [10]

DC of diseases brought forth by the evil qi of heat poison. *ZHBJF* 2 lists a *hei gao fang* 黑膏方, black paste recipe: 治**溫毒**發斑，大疫難救, "It cures **warmth poison** with an effusion of macules, and massive epidemics that are difficult to control".

***Wen feng* 溫風, warmth wind** [1]

EA of an unexpected, unseasonable climatic warmth. *MYBL* SE *ling yang jiao* 羚羊角：療傷寒，時氣寒熱，熱在肌膚，**溫風**注毒伏在骨間, "It cures harm caused by cold, [alternating sensations] of cold and heat because of seasonal qi, heat in the muscles and the skin, **warmth wind** influx with poison abiding in the bones". *QJYF* 4: 遇冬天時行**溫風**, 至春夏病熱頭痛, "If in winter one encounters a **warmth wind** as seasonal [qi], this will lead to a disease of heat with headache in spring and summer".

***Wen gui* 溫鬼, warmth demon** [4]

EA of → *wen bing*, 溫病, warmth disease. *BJ* SE *mu xiang* 木香：主邪氣，辟毒疫**溫鬼**, "It controls evil qi, and eliminates poison, epidemics, and **warmth demons**".

***Wen ji* 溫疾, warmth ailment** [10]

PC identical with → *wen bing*, 溫病, warmth disease. *BJ* SE *lian shi* 楝實：主**溫疾**傷寒，大熱煩狂, "Controls **warmth ailment** and harm caused by cold, [associated with] massive heat, vexation, and madness".

***Wen li* 瘟癘, warmth-illness epidemic** [1]

PC identical with → *wen yi* 瘟疫, warmth-illness epidemic. *SYJYBZFL* 5: 民病**瘟癘**，治法宜用辛涼平其上，咸寒調其下, "The people suffer from **warmth-illness epidemic**. The appropriate treatment strategy is to apply acrid cooling and neutral [medications] to their upper [body parts], and salty and cold [medications] to harmonize their lower [body parts]".

Wen li **溫癘, warmth epidemic** [3]

PC identical with → *wen yi* 瘟疫, warmth-illness epidemic. *QJYiF* 13: 止穀瘵病，辟**溫癘**惡鬼，久久可度世, "It serves to end [the intake of] grain and to heal disease; it wards off **warmth epidemics** and malign demons. Taken over a long time it can deliver the world from suffering".

Wen nüe **瘟瘧, warmth disease malaria** [1]

PC identical with → *wen nüe* 溫瘧, warmth malaria. *SJZL* 37 RE *mu xiang bing lang wan* 木香檳榔丸, pills with *mu xiang* and *bing lang*: 治嵐瘴及**瘟瘧**大效, "They cure hazy miasma and **warmth malaria**. Very effective".

Wen nüe **溫瘧, warmth malaria** [49] AN *wen nüe* 瘟瘧, warm disease malaria; *re nüe* 熱瘧, heat malaria; *dan nüe* 癉瘧, solitary [heat] malaria, *wen re nüe ji* 溫熱瘧疾, warmth and heat malaria disease.

PC of malaria where many alternating sensations of fever are accompanied by only a few alternating sensations of cold, or where patients suffer from fever only with no cold spells at all. *JGYL* Fj: **溫瘧**者，其脈如平，身無寒但熱，骨節疼煩，時嘔, "In the case of **warmth malaria**, the [movement in the] vessels is as normal. The body never feels cold, only hot. Bones joints experience discomforting pain. At times [patients] vomit".

Wen qi **溫氣, warmth qi** [8]

① Refers to the warmth of the human body's yang qi or any other physical item. *SW* 62: 寒氣積於胸中而不瀉，不瀉則**溫氣**去, "When receding qi rises contrary [to its regular course], cold qi accumulates inside the chest and does not flow away. When it does not flow away, then the **warmth qi** leaves".

② PC identical with → *wen bing*, 溫病, warmth disease. *MYBL* SE *ren ni* 人溺：療寒熱頭疼、**溫氣**, "Cures cold and heat spells with headache, **warmth qi**.

Wen qi **瘟氣, warmth-illness qi** [2]

EA identical with → *yi qi* 疫氣, epidemic qi. *SJZL* 33, RE *liu jin san* 流金散, liquid gold powder: 每月初一，以兩許當庭燒之，能辟**瘟氣**, "On the first day of each month burn a small amount in the front courtyard. This is able to ward off **warmth-illness qi**".

Wen re **溫熱, warmth (and) heat; warm-heated** [19]

① PC identical with → *wen bing* 溫病, warmth disease. *ZBYHL* 10: 因**溫熱**病，發汗、吐、下之後，熱邪雖退，而血氣損傷，腑臟皆虛，故因玆而生諸病, "Following a **warmth and heat** disease, and after the application of sudorific, emetic, and laxative therapies, the heat evil may have retreated, but the blood and qi have been harmed nevertheless, and the depots and palaces are all depleted. Because of this all types of diseases may emerge".

② EA identical with → *re* 熱, heat. *ZBYHL* 46: 其下利者，是腸胃宿虛，而感於**溫熱**之病，熱氣入於腸胃，與水穀相搏，腸虛則泄，故下利也, "Those who suffer from free-flux discharge, their intestines and stomach have

been depleted for some time and were then affected by the disease of **warmth and heat**. Heat qi has entered their intestines and stomach, where it clashed with liquid and solid food. As the intestines are depleted this results in outflow. Hence there is free-flux discharge".
③ PQ *SW* 70: 氣溫氣熱，治以**溫熱**，強其內守, "Warm qi and hot qi, treat [them] with **warmth and heat**; strengthen their being guarded internally".
④ Temperature quality of objects: *QJYF* 25: 納酒及小便各一合，**溫熱**頓服, "Mix one *ge* of wine and urine, and swallow **warm-heated**".

***Wen re nüe ji* 溫熱瘧疾, warmth and heat malaria ailment** [1]
PC identical with → *wen nüe* 溫瘧, warmth malaria. *RHZ* SE *bai lian* 白蘞: 止驚邪，發背，瘰癧，腸風痔瘺，刀箭瘡，撲損，**溫熱瘧疾**, "Ends fright evil, effusion of the back, scrofula with pervasion-illness, intestinal [bleeding as swift as] wind; hemorrhoidal fistula; wounds inflicted by a knife and arrow, **warmth and heat malaria disease**".

***Wen yi* 瘟疫, warmth-illness epidemic** [32] AD *wen* 瘟; *yi* 疫; *li* 癘; AN *wen yi* 溫疫; warmth epidemic; *yi wen* 疫瘟, epidemic warmth-illness; *wen bing* 瘟病, warmth-illness disease; *wen li* 瘟癘, warmth epidemic; *wen li* 溫癘, warmth epidemic; *yi bing* 疫病, epidemic disease; *yi ji* 疫疾, epidemic ailment; *shi yi* 時疫, seasonal epidemic; *li yi* 癘疫, epidemic; *wen li* 溫癘, warmth epidemic; *du li* 毒癘; poison epidemic; *yi li* 疫癧, epidemic pervasion-illness; *yi li* 疫癘, epidemic.
PC DC of acute communicable diseases brought forth by an epidemic qi. *ZHBJF* 2 RE *bi wen yi yao gan san* 避**瘟疫**藥乾散, "Dried powder of pharmaceutical drugs to ward off **warmth-illness epidemics**".

***Wen yi* 溫疫, warmth epidemic** [28]
PC identical with → *wen yi* 瘟疫, warmth-illness epidemic. *ZHBJF* 8 RE *Pei shi wu du shen gao* 裴氏五毒神膏, Mr. Pei's wondrous paste with the five poisons: 並療時行**溫疫**, "It also cures seasonally active **warmth epidemics**".

***Wen yi qi* 瘟疫氣, warmth-illness epidemic qi** [3]
EA identical with → *yi qi* 疫氣, epidemic qi. *BCGM* SE *bao yu* 鮑魚 quoting *ZHF* 3: 鮑魚頭燒三指撮, 小豆七枚, 合末服之, 女用豆二七枚, "Burn the head of *bao yu* [to ashes to obtain as much as] can be picked up with three fingers. Seven *xiao dou*. Mix the powders and ingest this. Women use two times seven beans", writes: 鮑魚頭燒灰方寸匕，合小豆末七枚，米飲服之，令**瘟疫氣**不相染也, "Burn the head of *bao yu* to ashes. Mix the amount filling a square inch size spoon with powder prepared from seven *xiao dou*. Ingest with the liquid obtained by boiling rice decoction. This will prevent one from being infected with **warmth-illness epidemic** qi".

***Wen yi qi* 溫疫氣, warmth epidemic qi** [1]
EA identical with → *yi qi* 疫氣, epidemic qi. *SLBC* SE *ran she dan* 蚺蛇膽: 肉，主**溫疫氣**。可作膾食之, "The meat controls **warmth epidemic qi**; it can be consumed as chopped meat".

Wen zhang **瘟瘴, warmth-illness miasma** [3]

PC identical with → *zhang li* 瘴癘, miasmatic epidemic. *RHZ* SE *ba qia* 菝葜：治時疾**瘟瘴**, "It cures seasonal ailments and **warmth-illness miasma**".

Wen zhang **溫瘴, warmth miasma** [4]

PC identical with → *zhang li* 瘴癘, miasmatic epidemic. *ZBYHL* 10: 假令本有冷，今得**溫瘴**，雖暴壯熱煩滿，視寒正須溫藥汗之, "If [the patient] originally was affected by cold, and now [in addition] is affected by **warmth miasma**, even if the heat is violent with vexation and a feeling of fullness, one must [nevertheless] keep the cold in mind and it is appropriate to apply warming medication to cause sweating".

Wen zhu **溫疰, warmth attachment-illness** [2]

PC of a → *zhu bing* 疰病, attachment-illness disease, with an aversion to cold associated with fever. *MYBL* SE *bei zi* 貝子：除寒熱**溫疰**，解肌，散結熱, "It eliminates cold and heat spells, and **warmth attachment-illness**, relaxes muscles, and disperses bound heat".

Weng bi **齆鼻, stuffed nose** [7]

PC with a blocked nose unable to distinguish odors as major sign. *MYBL* SE *xi xin* 細辛：除喉痹、**齆鼻**、風癇、癲疾, "It removes throat blockage, **stuffed nose**, wind epilepsy, and the ailment of peak-illness".

Wo jie **窩疥, lair[-illness] and *jie*-illness** [1]

PC modified writing of → *guo jie* 瘑疥, lair-illness and *jie*-illness. *BCGM* Bai bing zhu zhi yao 百病主治藥, quoting the paragraph on *shui yin* 水銀, instead of *guo jie* 瘑疥 writes: **窩疥, lair[-illness] and *jie*-illness**.

Wu dan **五疸, five types of *dan*-illness** [4]

PC referring to five different types of → *huang dan* 黃疸, yellow *dan*-illness. *BJ* SE *zi cao* 紫草：主心腹邪氣，**五疸**, "It controls evil qi in the heart and abdomen, and the **five types of *dan*-illness**". The "five types of *dan*-illness" have been defined differently by medical authorities. The most widely accepted definition originates from *JGYL*: *gu dan* 穀疸, grain *dan*-illness; *jiu dan* 酒疸, wine *dan*-illness; *hei dan* 黑疸, dark *dan*-illness; *nü lao dan* 女勞疸, *dan*-illness resulting from exhaustion with women; *huang dan* 黃疸, yellow *dan*-illness. This definition is repeated in *BCGM*, *zhu* 豕, Zhi gao fu 脂膏附方 with only a modification from *nü lao dan* 女勞疸 to *nü dan* 女疸. "female *dan*-illness". In contrast, *BCGM* Bai bing zhu zhi yao 百病主治藥: *yu re huang dan* 瘀熱黃疸, stagnant heat yellow *dan*-illness; *pi xu huang dan* 脾虛黃疸, spleen depletion yellow *dan*-illness; *shi ji huang dan* 食積黃疸, food accumulation yellow *dan*-illness; *yu xue huang dan* 瘀血黃疸, stagnant blood yellow *dan*-illness, and *yin huang* 陰黃, yin jaundice.

Wu dian **五癲, five types of peak-illness** [1]

PC of five types of peak-illness. *ZBYHL* 37: **五癲**：一曰陽癲，二曰陰癲，三曰風癲，四曰濕癲，五曰勞癲，此蓋隨其感處之由。又有牛、馬、豬、雞、狗之癲，皆以其癲發之時，聲形狀似於牛、馬等，故以為名也, "The **five types of peak-illness** are the following. The first is yang peak-illness. The second is yin peak-illness. The third is wind peak-illness. The fourth is moisture peak-illness. The fifth is exhaustion peak-illness. These [designations] are based on the respective point of departure. Also, there is buffalo, horse, hog, chicken, and dog peak-illness. These names are based on the sounds emitted and shapes assumed by patients at the time of the outbreak of the disease when they resemble a buffalo, or a horse, etc". *BCGM* fails to give these details.

Wu du **五毒, the five poisons** [8]

EA of a) the five poisonous pharmaceutical substances: *dan sha* 丹砂, *shi dan* 石膽, *xiong huang* 雄黃, *yu shi* 礜石, *ci shi* 磁石. *BCTJ* SE *dan sha* 丹砂：鄭康成注《周禮》，以丹砂、石膽、雄黃、礜石、磁石為**五毒**，古人惟以攻創瘍, "In his comment on the *Zhou li*, Zheng Kangcheng regards *dan sha*, *shi dan*, *xiong huang*, *yu shi*, and *ci shi* as the **five poisons**. In ancient times people relied on nothing else to cope with sores and ulcers". b) The five types of → *gu du* 蠱毒, *gu* poison, i. e., *she gu* 蛇蠱, snake *gu*; *qiang lang gu* 蜣螂蠱, dung beetle *gu*; *ha ma gu* 蝦蟆蠱, toad *gu*; *ke dou gu* 蝌蚪蠱; *cao gu* 草蠱, herbal *gu*. *MYBL* SE *tao xiao* 桃梟：殺精魅**五毒**不祥, "It serves to kill what is inauspicious, such as spirit seduction-specters and the **five poisons**. c) CD of all types of → *du qi* 毒氣, poison qi, that bring forth sores and ulcers, including *dong fang qing du* 東方青毒, greenish poison of the East; *nan fang chi du* 南方赤毒, red poison of the South; *xi fang bai du* 西方白毒, white poison of the West; *bei fang hei du* 北方黑毒, black poison of the North; *zhong yang huang du* 中央黃毒, yellow poison of the center. *QJYiF* 29: 禁**五毒**法：吸東方青毒，南方赤毒，西方白毒，北方黑毒，中央黃毒。天毒、地毒、水毒、火毒、霧毒、塵毒、死生毒，百毒之精，知汝姓名，天毒上升，地毒下藏，百毒止息，五毒滅亡。惡毒須出，毒腦破，毒腹出，毒腸止。不止不已，拘汝牙、折汝齒。吸吸叱叱。急急如律令, "Method to banish the **five poisons**: 'I inhale greenish poison of the East, red poison of the South, white poison of the West, black poison of the North, yellow poison of the center. Heaven's poison, earth's poison, poison of water, poison of fire, poison of fog, poison of dirt, poison of death and life, spirits of all poisons: I know your names! Heaven's poison rise! Earth's poison descend and be stored! The hundred poisons stop; the five poisons vanish. Malign poisons must come out. Poison in the brain will be broken. Poison in the abdomen will come out. Poison in the intestine will stop. If you do not halt, if you do not end, I will grasp your teeth, I will break your teeth.' Inhale, inhale, shout, shout: 'Quick, quick, this is like a command!'"

Wu e **忤惡, the hostile and malign** [6]

EA, originally referring to demonic beings, causing sudden loss of consciousness, with an inability to recognize people. The hands and legs are cold, and in some cases blood flows from the mouth and nose. LSZ listed this EA together with → *xie mei* 邪魅, evil seduction-specters, and → *gui qi* 鬼氣, demon qi. *BCGM* SE *re tang* 熱湯, hot water, quoting *BCSY*: 忤死, "[Appearance of] death because of the hostile", writes: **忤惡**卒死, "Sudden [appearance of] death because of the **hostile and malign**".

Wu feng **惡風, aversion to wind** [16]

PC brought about by an encounter with wind, in severe cases leading to shivering. *SW* 33: 惡風而振寒, "[The patient] has an **aversion to wind** and shakes from cold".

Wu gan **五疳, five types of *gan*-illness** [20]

PC CD of five types of → *gan* 疳, *gan*-illness. *ZBYHL* 18: **五疳**，一是白疳，令人皮膚枯燥，面失顏色, "**Five types of *gan*-illness**: one is white *gan*-illness. It makes a person's skin wither and desiccate. The face loses its complexion". The five types of *gan*-illness referred to in the *ZBYHL* are *bai gan* 白疳, white *gan*-illness; *chi gan* 赤疳, red *gan*-illness; *nao gan* 蟯疳, pinworm *gan*-illness; *gan ni* 疳䘌, *gan*-illness with hidden-worms; *hei gan* 黑疳, black *gan*-illness. *BCGM* mentions only the term 'five types of *gan*-illness', but fails to delineate these five types in detail. Different authors have identified the 'five types of *gan*-illness' with different meanings. Beginning with the Song, most authors have spoken of the five types as heart, liver, spleen, lung, and kidney *gan*-illness.

Wu ge **五膈, five [types of] occlusion** [4] AN *wu ge qi* 五膈氣, five types of occlusion qi.

PC referring to five types of occlusion, each resulting from different causes: *you ge* 憂膈, occlusion by grief; *hui ge* 恚膈, occlusion by rage; *qi ge* 氣膈, occlusion by qi; *han ge* 寒膈, occlusion by cold; *re ge* 熱膈, occlusion by heat. *ZBYHL* 13: 眾方說**五膈**，互有不同，但傷動之由有五，故云五膈氣, "All recipes speak of '**five types of occlusion**'. They resemble each other, but they have five different causes. Hence one speaks of the 'five occlusion qi'".

Wu ge qi **五膈氣, five [types of] occlusion qi** [4]

PC identical with → *wu ge* 五膈, five [types of] occlusion. *ZBYHL* 13: 眾方說五膈，互有不同，但傷動之由有五，故云**五膈氣**, "All recipes speak of 'five types of occlusion'. They resemble each other, but they have five different causes. Hence one speaks of the '**five [types of] occlusion qi**'".

Wu gu **無辜, *wu gu*; [lit: "innocent"]** [11] AN *wu gu gan* 無辜疳, *wu gu* with *gan-illness.*

PC of → *gan* 疳, *gan*-illness, accompanied by scrofula affecting the head and neck. This is often associated with emaciation of the body, desiccation of the hair, with the head and neck affected by nodes that are glossy and pliable in their early stages and fester and bleed incessantly at a later stage. Authors in pre-modern literature have traced this disease to children's clothing left to dry under a clear sky overnight. When a bird crying '*wugu*, *wugu*' flew over these garments and a child was given them to wear the next day, it would develop this disease. Beginning with the Song era, this explanation lost its appeal. *ZBYHL* 48：小兒面黃髮直，時壯熱，飲食不生肌膚，積經日月，遂致死者，謂之**無辜**, "Now, when children have a yellow facial complexion, when their hair stands up straight, when they repeatedly develop strong heat, when beverages and food fail to generate muscles and flesh, and if this continues for days and months, and eventually ends in death, then this is called ***wu gu***".

Wu gu gan **無辜疳, *wu gu* with *gan*-illness; [lit: "innocent" with *gan*-illness]** [6]
PC identical with → *wu gu* 無辜 , *wu gu*. *TPSHF* 86: 夫小兒**無辜疳**者，其候：面黃髮直，時時壯熱，飲食不生肌膚，積經日月，遂致死者， "Now, when children have ***wu gu* with *gan*-illness** the signs are as follows: the facial complexion is yellow, the hair stands up straight, they repeatedly develop strong heat, beverages and food fail to generate muscles and flesh. Eventually this will end in death".

Wu han **惡寒, aversion to cold** [53] AN *wei han* 畏寒, fear of cold; *wei leng* 畏冷; *zeng han* 憎寒, hate of cold.
IS of a feeling of the body's fear of cold. *SW* 60: 汗出頭痛，身重**惡寒**, "[One suffers from] sweating and headache; the body feels heavy and has an **aversion to cold**".

Wu huan **五緩, the five types of slackening** [8]
① IS identical with → *huan* 緩①， slackening. *QJYF* 8: 石南湯，治六十四種風，注走入皮膚中如蟲行，腰脊強直，**五緩**六急，手足拘攣， "Decoction with *shi nan* [leaves]: It cures the 64 types of wind flowing into the skin and creating a sensation of crawling insects there. The lumbar region and back are stiff and straight. The **five types of slackening** and the six types of tension [will result]. The hands and feet cramp and contract".
② PC with slackening. *BJ* SE *gan qi* 乾漆：安五藏，**五緩**六急，風寒濕痹, "It serves to pacify the five depots, the **five types of slackening** and the six types of tension, as well as wind cold moisture blockage".

Wu ji **五積, five types of accumulation** [5]
PC CD of five types of → *ji* 積, accumulation, associated with one of the five depots, i.e. *fei qi* 肥氣, lung qi; *fu liang* 伏梁, hidden beam; 痞氣, obstacle-illness qi; *xi ben* 息賁, rapid breathing; *ben tun* 賁豚, running piglets. *WTMY* 39： **五積**：肥氣、伏梁、痞氣、息賁、賁豚, "The **five types of accumulation**: lung qi, hidden beam, obstacle-illness qi, rapid breathing, and running piglets".

Wu jue **五絕 the five cut-offs** [1]
PC identical with → *wu jue si* 五絕死, the five cut-offs with [an appearance of] death. *QJYF* 25: 夫**五絕**者：一曰自縊, 二曰牆壁壓迮, 三曰溺水, 四曰魘寐, 五曰產乳絕, "Now, **the five cut-offs** include, first, [appearance of death following] suicide by hanging; second, [appearance of death following] being crushed by a wall; third, [appearance of death because of] drowning; fourth, [appearance of death because of] nightmare demons; fifth, [appearance of death in the course of giving] birth".

Wu jue ji bing **五絕急病, the five cut-offs with acute disease** [1]
PC identical with → *wu jue si* 五絕死, the five cut-offs with [an appearance of] death. *ZLBC* SE *ban xia* 半夏 quotes *ZMML*: 治五絕：一曰自縊, 二曰牆壁壓, 三曰溺水, 四曰魘魅, 五曰產乳, "To cure the five cut-offs: First, [appearance of death following] suicide by hanging; second, [appearance of death following] being crushed by a wall; third, [appearance of death because of] drowning; fourth, [appearance of death because of] nightmare seduction-spec-

ters; fifth, [appearance of death in the course of] birth. *BCGM* SE *ban xia* 半夏 quotes *ZMML* from *ZLBC*: **五絕急病**：一曰自縊, 二曰牆壓, 三曰溺水, 四曰魘魅, 五曰產乳, "**The five cut-offs with acute disease**: first, [appearance of death following] suicide by hanging; second, [appearance of death following] being crushed by a wall; third, [appearance of death because of] drowning; fourth, [appearance of death because of] nightmare seduction-specters; fifth, [appearance of death in the course of giving] birth.

Wu jue si **五絕死 the five cut-offs with [an appearance of] death** [4] AN *wu jue* 五絕, the five cut-offs; *wu jue ji bing* 五絕急病, the five cut-offs with acute disease. PC of a → *cu si* 卒死, appearance of death, resulting from five different types of accidents. *WTMY* 28: 删繁療**五絕死**方：一曰自縊, 二曰牆壁所迮, 三曰溺水, 四曰魘魅, 五曰產乳, "The *SF*'s recipe for curing **the five cut-offs with [an appearance of] death**, including, first, [appearance of death following] suicide by hanging; second, [appearance of death following being] crushed by a wall; third, [appearance of death because of] drowing; fourth, [appearance of death because of] nightmare seduction-specters; fifth, [appearance of death in the course of giving] birth. LSZ in *BCGM* 百病主治藥 Bai bing zhu zhi yao: 五絕：縊死、溺死、壓死、凍死、驚死, "The five cut-offs include [appearance of] death following suicide by hanging, [appearance of] death by drowing, [appearance of] death by being crushed, [appearance of] death from freezing, [appearance of] death from fright/shock".

Wu lai **烏癩, black repudiation-illness** [3] AN *chi lai* 赤癩, red repudiation-illness. PC of → *lai* 癩, repudiation-illness where the skin itches as if bugs/worms were crawling in it. Also, lumps the size of peach or plum kernels rise from the skin, with red and black papules. In front of their eyes patients perceive items as if there were drooping silk threads. The heart is shocked and fearful. The hands and feet are numb and feel no pain if pierced with a needle. The elbows are as if tied with a string. Patients are unable to walk. *ZBYHL* 2: 凡癩病，皆是惡風及犯觸忌害所得。初覺皮毛變異，或淫淫苦癢如蟲行，或眼前見物如垂絲，言語無定，心常驚恐。皮肉中或如桃李子，隱疹赤黑，手足頑痹，針刺不痛，脚下不得踏地。凡食之時，開口而鳴，語亦如是，身體瘡痛，兩肘如繩縛，此名**黑癩**, "All types of repudiation-illness are brought forth by malign wind and the encounter with something forbidden and harmful. In the beginning [patients] notice changes in the skin and hair. In some cases they feel an extreme itch as if there were insects crawling. Or in front of their eyes they see items like silk threads. Their language is not stable, their heart if repeatedly affected by fright and fear. In their skin and flesh there is something like peaches and plums, with minute red and black pimples. Hands and feet are affected by a stubborn blockage. When pierced with a needle, they do not feel pain. With their legs they cannot walk. When it is time to eat they open the mouth and make the cries of birds. Their language is of the same type. The body has sores and is painful. The two elbows feel as if tied with a rope. This is called **black repudiation-illness**".

Wu lai feng chuang **烏癩風瘡, black repudiation-illness wind sores** [2]

PC of → *da feng* 大風②, massive wind, disease with red and black papules on the skin. *BCGM* SE *lü cao* 葎草 quotes *SJZL*: **烏癩風瘡**，葛葎草三秤切洗。益母草一秤切，以水二石五斗，煮取一石五斗，去滓入瓮中，浸浴一時方出，坐密室中。又暖湯浴一時，乃出，暖臥取汗，勿令見風。明日又浴。如浴時瘙癢不可忍，切勿搔動，少頃漸定。後隔三日一作，以愈為度, "**Black repudiation-illness wind sores**: *Ge* and *lü cao*: 3 *cheng* each, cut and wash. *Yi mu cao*, 1 *cheng*, cut. Add water, 2 stones and 5 *dou*, and boil down to 1 stone and five *dou*. Discard the dregs and [fill the liquid] into an earthen jar. Soak [the afflicted body part in the liquid] for a while and then take it out again. [Have the patient] sit in a closely sealed room, and again have him bathe in the warm liquid for a while, and then get out again. Have him lie down, warmly covered, until he sweats. He must not be touched by wind. The next day have him bathe again. When [the skin] itches while he his bathing, he must not scratch even if it is unbearable. Slowly [the disease] will be checked. Later the therapy is to be applied every third day. It ends when a cure is achieved".

Wu lao **五勞, five types of exhaustion** [103] AW 五癆, five types of exhaustion-illness; AN *wu zang lao* 五臟勞, exhaustion affecting the five depots.

PC of depletion detriment affecting the five depots. *BJ* SE *rou cong rong* 肉蓯蓉：主**五勞**七傷，補中，除莖中寒熱痛，養五藏, "It controls the **five types of exhaustion** and seven types of harm. It supplements the center, eliminates cold and heat pain from the penis, and nourishes the five depots". *BCGM* SE *chai hu* 茈胡：時珍曰：勞有**五勞**，病在五臟, "There are **five types of exhaustion**; [in each case,] the disease affects [one of] the five depots".

Wu lao **五癆, five types of exhaustion-illness** [1]

PC identical with → *wu lao* 五勞, five types of exhaustion. *BCGM* SE *huang qin* 黄芩 quoting *QJYF*: 巴郡太守奏三黄丸治男子五勞七傷, 消渴, "The *tai shou* official from the prefecture Ba submitted the 'pills with three [ingredients with the character] *huang* [in their names]' to cure the five types of exhaustion and seven types of harm of males, and melting with thirst", writes: 巴郡太守奏加減三黄丸：療男子**五癆**七傷，消渴, "The *tai shou* official from the prefecture Ba submitted the 'pills with three [ingredients with the character] *huang* [in their names] that are to be amended or diminished [in accordance with individual requirements]' to cure **the five types of exhaustion-illness** and seven types of harm of males, and melting with thirst,

Wu lei **瘔瘰, clustered [seeds]-illness** [4]

PC identical with → *pei lei* 瘔瘰. *BCGM* SE *ban mao* 斑蝥 quoting *SJZL*: 面上如有瘔瘰未消者，用乾斑貓末，以生油調成膏，傅患上, "When cluster-illness seeds appear on the face and fail to dissolve, use dry *ban mao* powder, mix with fresh oil to prepare a paste and apply this externally to the affected area", writes: 面上**瘔瘰**：大風，面上有紫瘔瘰未消。用乾斑蝥末，以生油調傅, "**Clustered [seeds]-illness** on the face: when in the case of massive wind, on the face appear crimson-colored clustered seeds that fail to dissolve, use dry *ban mao* powder, mix with fresh oil to prepare a paste and apply this externally".

Wu li **無力, loss of strength** [54]

① AN *ruan ruo* 軟弱, weakness. IS of a depletion and weakness of the entire body or any of its parts, with an inability to continue to function normally. *ZBYHL* 7: 其初患之狀，手足煩疼，腰脊**無力**，夜臥煩躁, "The early signs of this ailment include feelings of vexing pain in the hands and feet, **loss of strength** in the spine and lumbar region, and a feeling of vexation and restlessness when going to bed at night".

② Pulse condition. A weaker than usual movement in the vessels. *ZZJ* Mj: 其右關脈舉按皆**無力**，而往來澀, "All vessel [movements] at the gate on the right have **no strength**; their passage is rough".

③ PQ of an insufficient effect of a pharmaceutical substance. *ZHF* 7: 當作數升湯，以小蒜五寸，㕮咀投湯中，莫令大熱，熱即**無力**，捩去滓，適寒溫以浴, "One must prepare a decoction of several *sheng*. Take small pieces of garlic with a length of five *cun*. Chew them and place them into the hot water. Do not let the liquid become too hot. When it is [too] hot this results in a **loss of [the drug's] strength**. [Put the wet drugs into a cloth and] twist it to remove the dregs [from the liquid]. Adjust the temperature until it is suitable for bathing".

Wu li **五痢, the five types of free-flux illness** [2]

PC CD of numerous types of → *li ji* 痢疾, the ailment of free-flux illness. *QJYF* 15: 泄注，**五痢**，便膿血，重下腹痛，灸小腸俞百壯, "For outflow, **the five types of free-flux illness**, defecation with pus and blood, a feeling of heavy pressure in the lower section of the body with abdominal pain, cauterize the small intestine transportation point one hundred times".

Wu lin **五淋, the five types of dripping** [64]

PC CD of the five types of dripping, i.e. → *shi lin* 石淋, stone dripping; → *qi lin* 氣淋, qi dripping; → *gao lin* 膏淋, pasty dripping; → *lao lin* 勞淋, exhaustion dripping; → *re lin* 熱淋, heat dripping. *BJ* SE *sang piao xiao* 桑螵蛸：通**五淋**，利小便水道, "It opens the passage in the case of **the five types of dripping**; it stimulates the flow of urine and clears the passageways of water".

Wu long **五癃, the five types of protuberance-illness** [14]

PC CD of various types of → *long* 癃, protuberance-illness, disease, without distinctions as clear-cut as the → 五種淋, five types of dripping. *BJ* SE *hua shi* 滑石：主勞熱邪氣，**五癃**閉不通，利小便水道, "It controls exhaustion heat with evil qi, and the **five types of protuberance-illness** with impenetrability. It stimulates the passage of urine and opens the water tracts".

Wu nei beng sun **五内崩損, the five internal collapse injuries** [1]

PC of serious injuries inflicted upon the five depots, with → *tu xue* 吐血, blood spitting, assuming an appearance of blood gushing from the victim's mouth. *BCGM* SE *hua rui shi* 花蕊石 quoting *SYSS*: 五臟崩損, 涌噴血出成升斗, "Collapse injuries of the five depots, with the quantity of blood gushing filling *sheng*- and *dou*-measures", writes: **五内崩損**, 噴血出斗升, "**The five internal collapse injuries**, with the quantity of blood gushing filling *dou*- and *sheng*-measures".

***Wu nüe* 五瘧, five types of malaria** [2]

PC CD of five types of → *nüe ji* 瘧疾, malaria ailment. A concrete identification of what these five types were meant to be has not been recorded in known medical literature. *ZLBC* SE *tian shu shi* 天鼠屎 quotes *JYJZ*: 治五瘧方, "Recipe to cure five types of **malaria**".

***Wu pi* 無皮, absence of skin** [5]

PC of children with their body having no skin and assuming a faint red complexion. *XEWSZWLF* 1: 兒生，身如凝血，若**無皮**者，死, "When a child is born with its body appearing like coagulated blood, and if **it has no skin**, it will die".

***Wu re* 惡熱, an aversion to heat** [8]

IS of an aversion to heat, or a refusal to touch hot objects. *SHL* 182: 身熱，汗自出，不惡寒反**惡熱**也, "The body is hot. Spontaneous sweating. No aversion to cold, on the contrary: **an aversion to heat**".

***Wu ru* 無乳, to have no breast milk** [5]

PC identical with → *ru zhi bu tong* 乳汁不通, blocked breast milk passage. *SLBC* SE *ye zhu* 野豬：脂，主婦人**無乳**者，服之即乳下, "The lard cures women who **have no breast milk**. Once this is ingested, breast milk will be discharged".

***Wu ruan* 五軟, the five types of softness** [1]

PC of children with congenital deficiencies, as are soft hands, soft nape, soft legs, soft lower back, and soft back, as their major signs. *YYXS* 3：小兒**五軟**，不治。手軟、項軟、脚軟、腰軟、背軟, "**The five types of softness** among children that cannot be cured: soft hands, soft nape, soft legs, soft lower back, soft back".

***Wu se dai xia* 五色帶下, multi-color discharge from below the belt** [5]

PC of → *dai xia bing* 帶下病, diseases of discharge from below the belt, with a discharge of turbid matter of mixed colors from the vagina, sometimes green as pus, sometimes dark red as rotten blood, sometimes watery and turbid like the slop from rinsing rice. *QJYF* 26: 治**五色帶下**方：服大豆紫湯，日三服, "Recipe to cure **multi-color discharge from below the belt**: Ingest the 'purple decoction with *da dou*' three times daily".

***Wu se dan du* 五色丹毒, multi-color cinnabar poison** [10]

PC of → *dan du* 丹毒, cinnabar poison, with rashes of varying color. *BCGM* Bai bing zhu zhi yao 百病主治藥, *dan du* 丹毒, cinnabar poison, quoting *QJYF* 22: 治小兒五色丹方, "Recipe to cure children [suffering from] multi-color cinnabar", writes: 犀角、羚羊角、豬屎汁、黃龍湯，**五色丹毒**，飲二合，並塗, "*Xi jiao*, *ling yang jiao*, hog feces juice, and the decoction with *huang long*, in the case of **multi-color cinnabar poison**, drink 2 *ge* and also apply externally".

***Wu se li* 五色痢, multi-color free-flux illness** [1]

PC of → *li ji* 痢疾, free-flux illness, assuming various colors. *QJYF* 3: 膠蠟湯，治產後三日內，下諸雜**五色痢**方, "Decoction with [*a*] *jiao* and [*mi*] *la* is a recipe to cure discharge of **five-color free-flux illness** occurring on the third day after delivery".

Wu sha jing feng **烏沙驚風, black sand fright wind** [1]

PC of → *jing feng* 驚風, fright wind, characterised by a virid-black color covering the entire body. *BCGM* SE *huang tu* 黄土: quotes *XEMJ*: **烏沙驚風**，小兒驚風遍身都烏者。急推向下，將黄土一碗，搗末，入久醋一鍾，炒熱包定熨之，引下至足，刺破為妙, "**Black sand fright wind:** When children are black all over the body because of fright wind, this should quickly be pushed down. Take 1 bowl of yellow soil and grind to a powder. Add 1 cup of old vinegar, heat this and apply as compresses. This will pull it down into the feet. Pricking there to open is best".

Wu shang jing tu **物傷睛突, the eyeball is injured by a foreign object and protrudes** [1]

PC of an injury of an eye caused from outside by a foreign object with the eyeball protruding as major sign. *BCGM* SE *di huang* 地黄 quoting *SJZL* 112: 目為外所傷，輕者因物撞擊，胞瞼腫痛，重者或致目睛突出，但眼帶未斷, "When the eyes are injured by an impact from outside, in light cases the eyelids are swollen and ache as a result of a blow from a foreign object. In severe cases this may cause the eyeballs to protrude without severence of the eyeribbon", writes: **物傷睛突**：輕者瞼胞腫痛，重者目睛突出，但目系未斷, "When **the eyeball is injured by a foreign object and protrudes**, in light cases the eyelids are swollen and ache. In severe cases the eyeballs protrude without the eye connection [with the brain] being severed".

Wu shang jing xian **物傷睛陷, the eyeball is injured by a foreign object and sinks in** [2]

PC of an injury of an eyes caused from outside by a foreign object with the eyeballs sinking in as the major sign. *BCGM* SE *di fu* 地膚 quoting *SJZL* 112: 目為物所傷睛陷, "The eye is injured by a foreign object and the eyeball sinks in", writes: **物傷睛陷, "The eyeball is injured by a foreign object and sinks in"**.

Wu shi **五屍, five types of corpse [qi]** [19]

PC CD of the five diseases attributed to corpse evil. *ZHF* 1: 五屍者，飛屍、遁屍、風屍、沉屍、屍疰也，其狀皆腹痛脹急，不得氣息。右搗蒺藜子，蜜丸如胡豆，服二丸，日三, "The **five types of corpse [qi]** include 'flying corpse [qi], run-away corpse [qi], wind[-type] corpse [qi], sunken corpse [qi], and corpse [qi] attachment-illness. Their signs are abdominal pain, distension, and tightness; [patients] cannot breathe. It is best to pound *ji li zi* and form pills with honey the size of *hu dou*. [For each dosage] ingest two pills, three times a day".

Wu shi du **五石毒, five types of mineral poison** [1]

EA identical with → *shi yao du* 石藥毒, mineral drug poison. *QJYF* 24 lists: 解五石毒第三, "[Recipes] to dissolve the **five types of mineral poison**, section 3".

Wu si **忤死, [appearance of] death from hostility** [1]

PC identical with → *ke wu si* 客忤死, [appearance of] death from a visitor's hostility. *JYBC* SE *re tang* 熱湯：主**忤死**。先以衣三重, 藉**忤死**人腹上, 乃取銅器若瓦器盛湯著衣上, 湯冷者去衣, 大冷者換湯, 即愈, "To master **[the appearance of] death from hostility**: First lay three pieces of garment on the abdomen of the person with **[the appearance of] death from hostility**. Then take a bronze or earth vessel, fill with hot water, and place on the garments. Once the hot water has cooled down, remove the garments. When it has become very cold, exchange it for hot water again. This brings the cure".

Wu sou **五嗽, five types of cough** [1]

PC CD of five types of cough, including *shang qi sou* 上氣嗽, cough with ascending qi; *yin sou* 飲嗽, rheum cough; *zao sou* 燥嗽, dry cough; *leng sou* 冷嗽, cold cough; *xie sou* 邪嗽, evil [qi] cough. *WTMY* 9: 深師療**五嗽**，一曰上氣嗽，二曰飲嗽，三曰燥嗽，四曰冷嗽，五曰邪嗽, "Master Shen cures the **five types of cough**. The first is called 'qi cough', the second is called 'rheum cough', the third is called 'dry cough', the fourth is called 'cold cough', the fifth is called 'evil [qi] cough'".

Wu tun **誤吞, having mistakenly swallowed [something unsound]** [70]

PC of a poisoning or injury brought forth by inadvertently or consciously swallowing something that is poisonous or otherwise harmful. *ZHF* 6: **誤吞**釘及箭、金針、錢鐵等物方。多食肥羊脂，諸般肥肉等。自裹之，必得出, "Recipe for having **mistakenly swallowed** a nail, an arrow, a metal needle, a coin or a piece of iron: Eat much lamb fat, and all kinds of fat meat. This will bind it and it will come out".

Wu wei **五痿, five types of dysfunction** [1]

IS CD of five types of → *wei* **痿**, dysfunction, disease. *SYJYBZFL* 9: 麋角丸，治五痿, "Pills with elk horn cure the **five types of dysfunction**".

Wu xian **五癇, five types of epilepsy** [5]

PC of → *xian ji* 癇疾, epilepsy ailment, classified into five categories based on their roots in one of the five depots and specifics of their appearance. *WTMY* 35: 廣濟療小兒驚癇，體羸不堪，療子母**五癇**煎方, "The *GJ* [*F* lists] a 'decoction recipe to cure the **five types of epilepsy** in children and mothers'. It cures fright epilepsy in children and extreme physical emaciation". *SYJYBZFL* 9: 夫**五癇**合屬五臟, "Now, the **five types of epilepsy** are associated with the five depots".

Wu xie **五邪, the five evils** [7]

CD of all PC that are caused by an evil curse, with an altered psychic state as major sign. *MYBL* SE *ling li jia* 鯪鯉甲：主**五邪**, 驚啼悲傷, "It controls **the five evils**, with fearful weeping and sorrow". *ZBYHL* 3: 故病有五邪：一曰中風, 二曰傷暑, 三曰飲食勞倦, 四曰中寒, 五曰中濕, "Now, diseases may result from five evils: first, wind stroke; second, harm caused by summerheat; third, exhaustion from beverages and food; fourth, being struck by cold; fifth, being struck by moisture", that is, it uses 五邪 as reference to the common "five evil [qi]". In contrast, *QJYF* 14: 茯神湯，治五邪氣入人體中，見鬼妄語，有所見聞，心悸跳動，恍惚不定方, "The decoction with *fu shen* is a recipe to cure the intrusion of the five evil qi into the human body, when as a result [patients] see demons and use absurd language, they claim to see and hear something, they experience severe heart palpitation, with absent-mindedness and mental instability", uses 五邪 as a reference to all sorts of evil spirits. "Five" is here simply an imaginary number. *BCGM* follows the usage of the latter.

Wu xin fa re **五心發熱, heat effusion in the five centers** [1]

IS identical with → *wu xin fan re* 五心煩熱, vexation with heat in the five centers. *BCGM* SE *shui xian* 水仙：作香澤，塗身理髮，去風氣。又療婦人五**心發熱**，同干荷葉、赤芍藥等分，為末，白湯每服二錢，熱自退也, "[The blossoms to] generate fragrance and luster. Smeared on the body and used to dress the hair on the head, they remove wind qi. Also, they serve to cure women with **heat effusion in the five centers**. Prepare a powder with equal amounts of dried *he ye* and *chi shao yao*. Each dosis is to ingest 2 *qian* with clear hot water. This will cause the heat to retreat".

Wu xin fan re **五心煩熱, vexing heat in the five centers** [5] AN *Wu xin fa re* 五心發熱, heat effusion in the five centers; *Wu xin fan zao* 五心煩躁, vexing agitation in the five centers

IS of a feeling of vexation-agitation with fever at the five "*xin* 心, center" locations, namely: *xin kou* 心口, heart opening/upper stomach opening; the two palm centers of the hands, and the centers of the two soles of the feet. *ZBYHL* 31: 熱腫者，四肢熱如火炙之狀，移無常處，或如手，或如盤，著背腹是；劇則皆熱如火，遍身熠熠然，**五心煩熱**，唇口乾燥，如注之狀。此皆風邪搏血氣所生。以其移無常處，故謂流腫, "Heat swelling: …In severe cases all [limbs] are hot as fire. The entire body glows. There is **vexing heat in the five centers**; the lips and mouth are dry, as if [their liquid] had been poured out. All such cases result from wind evil striking the blood. The places it turns to are not determined. Hence one speaks of a 'flowing swelling'". *BCGM* occasionally calls this → *wu xin fan zao* 五心煩躁, vexing agitation in the five centers, and → *wu xin fa re* 五心發熱, heat effusion in the five centers.

Wu xin fan zao **五心煩躁, vexing agitation in the five centers** [1]

IS identical with → *wu xin fan re* 五心煩熱, vexing heat in the five centers. *BCGM* SE *bie* 鱉 quotes *QYXJ*: 小兒疳勞：治潮熱往來，**五心煩躁**，盜汗咳嗽，用鱉血丸主之, "Children with gan-illness exhaustion: To cure tidal heat waves that come and go, **vexing agitation in the five centers**, and robber sweat with cough, use the pills with soft turtle blood to control this".

Wu xun xing jing **五旬行經, menstruation beyond age 50** [1]

PC of → *jing bing* 經病, menstrual disease, in which a woman older than 50 years continues to menstruate, with the duration of each menstruation exceeding normal periods. *BCGM* SE *qian cao* 茜草 quotes *JYF*: **五旬行經**：婦人五十後，經水不止者，作敗血論, "**Menstruation beyond age 50**: When a woman who is older than 50 years continues to menstruate, one must take into account that [an internal disease may] have made her blood rot".

Wu ye **五噎, five types of gullet occlusion** [8]

PC referring to five types of → *ye bing* 噎病, gullet occlusion disease, resulting from different causes: *qi ye* 氣噎, gullet occlusion by qi; *you ye* 憂噎, gullet occlusion by anxiety; *shi ye* 食噎, gullet occlusion by food; *lao ye* 勞噎, gullet occlusion by exhaustion; *si ye* 思噎, gullet occlusion by pondering. *ZBYHL* 20: 夫五噎，謂一曰氣噎，二曰憂噎，三曰食噎，四曰勞噎，五曰思噎, "Now, as for the **five types of gullet occlusion**, the first is called gullet occlusion by qi, the second is called gullet occlusion by anxiety, the third is called gullet occlusion by food, the fourth is called gullet occlusion by exhaustion, the fifth is called gullet occlusion by pondering".

***Wu yin* 五飲, five types of rheum** [2]
PC CD of five types of → *yin* 飲, rheum, disease. *SJZL* 47 lists a *xin fa ban xia san fang* 新法半夏散方, recipe for a powder with *ban xia* based on a new approach: 治五飲酒癖, "It cures the **five types of rheum** and wine aggregation-illness". *BCGM* lists three different versions of 'five types of rheum': First, in Bai bing zhu zhi yao 百病主治藥, paragraph on → *tan yin* 痰飲, phlegm rheum: 支、留、伏、溢、懸, "propping [rheum], abiding [rheum], deep-lying [rheum], spillage [rheum], and suspended [rheum]". Second, SE *zhu* 朮：留、癖、痰、溢、流, "abiding [rheum], aggregation-illness [rheum], phlegm [rheum], spillage [rheum], and flowing [rheum]". Third, SE *yuan hua* 芫花：支、懸、伏、痰、溢, "propping [rheum], suspended [rheum], deep-lying [rheum], phlegm [rheum], and spillage [rheum]".

***Wu ying* 五癭, five types of goiter** [1]
PC CD of five types of → *ying* 癭, goiter. *QJYF* 24: **五癭**丸方，取鹿靨以佳酒浸令沒，炙乾，納酒中，更炙令香，含，咽汁，味盡更易，盡十具愈, "Recipe for the pills for **five types of goiter**. Roast a deer's thyroid gland soaked in good wine until it is dry. Place in wine again and roast again and again until a fragrant smell emerges. Place in the mouth and swallow the juice. Change for a new one once the flavor has ended. After ten times [the disease] will be healed".

***Wu yu* 五郁, the five types of pent-up [qi]** [1]
PC of five types of accumulation disease brought forth by five types of abnormal weather conditions that affect the heart, liver, spleen, lung, and kidneys. *YXQY* Fj lists 五郁之病, "Diseases of **the five types of pent-up [qi]**".

***Wu zang feng* 五臟風, wind affecting the five depots** [2]
PC of wind intrusion into the five depots. CD of → *xin feng* 心風, heart wind; → *fei feng* 肺風, lung wind; → *pi feng* 脾風, spleen wind; → *gan feng* 肝風, liver wind; and → *shen feng* 腎風, kidney wind. *SW* 42: 風中五臟六腑之俞，亦為臟腑之風…**五臟風**之形狀不同，願聞其診及其病能, "[Qi Bo:] When the wind strikes the transporters of the five depots and six palaces, this, too, causes wind of the depots and palaces. [Huang Di:] In what way do the physical manifestations of **wind [affecting] the five depots** differ? I should like to hear about their diagnosis and about the manifestations of the [respective] diseases".

***Wu zang lao* 五臟勞, five types of depot exhaustion** [1]
PC identical with → *wu lao* 五勞, five types of exhaustion. *SLBC* SE *luo su* 落蘇：主寒熱，**五臟勞**, "It controls alternating sensations of cold and heat, and the **five types of depot exhaustion**".

Wu zang nüe **五臟瘧, five types of depot malaria** [2] AN *zang nüe* 臟瘧, depot malaria.

PC CD of *xin nüe* 心瘧, "heart malaria", *gan nüe* 肝瘧, liver malaria; *pi nüe* 脾瘧, spleen malaria; *fei nüe* 肺瘧, lung malaria; *shen nüe* 腎瘧, kidney malaria. *WTMY* 5: 療**五臟瘧**及一切諸瘧法，灸尺澤七壯, "Method to cure the **five types of depot malaria** and all other types of malaria: cauterize the *chi ze* [insertion point] severn times".

Wu zang re **五臟熱, heat in the five depots** [3]

PC CD of → *xin re* 心熱, heart heat, → *gan re* 肝熱, liver heat, → *pi re* 脾熱, spleen heat, → *fei re* 肺熱, lung heat, and → *shen re* 腎熱, kidney heat. *ZBYHL* 8 lists 傷寒**五臟熱**候, "Signs of harm caused by cold, with **heat in the five depots**".

Wu zhi **五痔, five types of piles** [74]

PC a) CD of various types of → *zhi bing* 痔病, piles disease. *BJ* SE *huai shi* 槐實：止涎唾，補絕傷，**五痔**，火瘡, "It ends the flow of saliva, supplements in the case of extreme harm, [and cures] the **five types of piles**, and fire sores". b) CD of → *mu zhi* 牡痔, male piles; → *jiu zhi* 酒痔, wine piles; → *chang zhi* 腸痔, intestinal piles; → *xue zhi* 血痔, blood piles; → *qi zhi* 氣痔, qi piles. *SBC* SE *mi tuo seng* 蜜陀僧：**五痔**：謂牡痔、酒痔、腸痔、血痔、氣痔, "The **five types of piles** are called male piles, wine piles, intestinal piles, blood piles, and qi piles".

Wu zhu **五疰, the five types of attachment-illness** [2]

PC referring to a limited variety of → *zhu bing* 疰病, attachment-illness disease. *QJYF* 8: 金牙酒，療積年八風**五疰**, "Wine with *jin ya* serves to cure the eight types of wind and **the five types of attachment-illness** that have lasted for years".

Wu zi **無子, to have no child; childlessness** [53]

PC with an inability, in the course of a marriage, to become pregnant over an extended period of time. *LS* 71: 地有四時不生草，人有**無子**，此人與天地相應者也, "If throughout the four seasons the earth does not grow herbs, this is like man **having no children**. This is how man and heaven correspond".

- X -

***Xi ben* 息賁, running breath** [4] AN *fei ji* 肺積, lung accumulation.
PC of → *ji* 積, accumulation, associated with the lung. It has the shape of a cup turned upside down. It is located below the ribs on the right. It cannot be cured for a long time. It is accompanied by an aversion to cold and fever, as well as by coughing and panting respiration. *NJ* 56: 肺之積，名曰**息賁**，在右脅下，覆大如杯。久不已，令人洒淅寒熱，喘咳，發肺壅, "Accumulations in the lung are called '**running breath**'. They are located below the ribs on the right side and have the size of a cup turned upside down. They last a long time without healing. They make the [afflicted] person shiver with alternating sensations of cold and heat, and they make him pant and cough, and develop obstructions in his lung".

***Xi bi* 膝痹, knee blockage** [2]
PC of → *bi* 痹① a), blockage, affecting the knees. *YXL* SE *kong gong nie* 孔公孽：主治腰冷，**膝痹**，毒風，男女陰蝕瘡, "It is responsible for curing lower back cold, **knee blockage**, poison wind, and erosion sores affecting the genital regions of males and females".

***Xi du* 溪毒, rivulet poison** [41] AN *shui du* 水毒, water poison.
① EA. A tiny bug assumed to live in bodies of water and supposedly capable of striking humans when they enter the water, thereby causing disease. *ZHF* 7: 治卒中**溪毒**方, "Recipe to cure sudden strike by **rivulet poison**".
② PC resulting from being struck by rivulet poison. *ZHF* 7: 今東間諸山縣，無不病**溪毒**，春月皆得, "Nowadays in all the mountain counties of Dongxian, there is no one who has not fallen ill with **rivulet poison**. Everybody was affected during the spring months".

***Xi fu* 膝浮, knee floating** [1]
IS of a feeling, resulting from weakness and softness of the feet and knees, as if, when walking, one were not stepping on solid ground, but floating. *BCGM* SE *gan song xiang* 甘松香：脚氣**膝浮**，煎湯淋洗, "For leg qi and **knee floating**, prepare a decoction and use for bathing".

***Xi mian* 喜眠, a tendency to sleep** [1]
IS identical with → *duo shui* 多睡, profuse sleeping. *MYBL* SE *ma* 馬：頭骨，主**喜眠**, "Its skull bones control **a tendency to sleep**".

***Xi ou* 喜嘔, tendency to vomit** [3] AN *hao ou* 好嘔.
IS of a frequent urge to vomit. *SHL* 96: 心煩**喜嘔**，或胸中煩而不嘔, "Heart vexation and a **tendency to vomit**. In some cases [patients feel] vexation in their chest but do not vomit".

***Xi rou* 瘜肉, tumorous flesh-growth** [39] AW 息肉.
PC CD of redundant growths anywhere on the human body. In general they have a glossy appearance, are soft, and do not ache. Often they emerge in the nasal cavity, and in the throat. *BCSY* SE *bo luo hui* 博落回：主惡瘡癭根，瘤

贅，**瘜肉**，白癜風, "It controls malign sores and [eliminates] goiter to its root, tumor redundancy, **tumorous flesh-growths**, and white patches wind".

***Xi rou* 息肉, tumorous flesh-growth** [28]

PC identical with → *xi rou* 瘜肉. *BJ* SE *shi hui* 石灰：殺痔蟲，去黑子**息肉**, "It kills piles bugs/worms, and removes black spots as well as **tumorous flesh-growths**".

***Xi wang* 喜忘, forgetfulness** [3]

IS identical with → *jian wang* 健忘①, forgetfulness. *MYBL* SE *bai ma jing* 白馬莖：白馬蹄，味甘，平，熱，無毒。療婦人下白崩。赤馬蹄，療婦人赤崩。齒，主小兒驚癇。頭膏，平，主生髮。毛，主女子崩中赤白。心，主**喜忘**, "The hoofs of white horses have a sweet balanced flavor, are hot, and have no poison. They serve to heal women with a discharge of white [liquid because of] collapsing [center]. The hoofs of red horses serve to heal women with a discharge of red [liquid because of] collapsing [center]. The teeth control fright epilepsy in children. A paste made from the head is balanced [in flavor] and controls generation of [new] hair. The hair [of a horse] controls collapsing center in women with red and white [discharge]. The heart [of a horse] controls **forgetfulness**".

***Xi xuan* 細癬, minute *xuan*-illness** [1]

PC of → *xuan* 癬, *xuan*-illness a), with a comparatively small lesion. *QJYF* 23 lists 治**細癬**方, "Recipes to cure **minute *xuan*-illness**".

***Xi yue* 喜噦, tendency to retch** [1]

IS of a frequent occurrence of dry retching. *ZBYHL* 18: 胃蟲，令人嘔吐，胃逆**喜噦**, "A stomach bug causes vomiting. The stomach [qi] flows contrary [to its normal direction] and one has a **tendency to retch**.

***Xia* 下, discharge; let-down; to ingest [medication]** [p]

① IS a) of pus, blood, water or watery stool discharged through the anus. *SW* 28: 帝曰：腸澼下白沫何如？岐伯曰：脈沉則生，脈浮則死, "[Huang] Di: 'In the case of intestinal flush **discharging** pus and blood, how is that?' Qi Bo: 'When the [movement in the] vessels is suspended and interrupted, then [the patient] will die'". b) Of water, stones, and water discharged through the urinary tract. *QJYF* 21: 當下石子如豆卵，以石盡止, "This will cause **discharge of** stones of a size ranging from beans to eggs. Stop once all stones have left". c.) Of blood, water, leucorrhea, or any turbid matter, as well as fetus or placenta discharged from a female's genital tract. *JGYL* Lj: 婦人經水閉不利，臟堅癖不止，中有乾血，下白物，礬石丸主之, "When a woman's period fails to flow, and when her uterus continuously develops hardenings of aggregation-illness, and if this includes dried blood and the **discharge** of white matter, pills with *fan shi* will master this".

② TA a) of applying medication to stimulate defecation, discharge of liquids, or the smoothening of intestinal passage to cure accumulations in the stomach and intestines, hardening of stools, stagnating liquids, as well as repletion heat accumulation. *SHL* 36: 太陽與陽明合病，喘而胸滿者，不可下，宜麻

黃湯, "When the major yang [conduit] and yang brilliant [conduit] are both affected by a disease, and when [patients] pant and have a feeling of fullness in their chest, and are unable to **discharge** [urine and stools], the decoction with *ma huang* is appropriate". b) Of all therapies meant to pass down something, including hastening delivery, stimulating lactation, transforming accumulations, stimulating the outflow of liquids, mildly removing extravascular blood, stimulating the passage of qi, etc. *RMSQ* 2: 催生下乳、磨積逐水、破經泄氣，凡下行者，皆下法也, "To hasten delivery and stimulate the **let-down** of lactation, to grind accumulations and to discharge water, to break through conduits and cause the outflow of qi, all these [methods of] stimulating a **discharge** are 'methods of **discharging [matter]**'". c) Of all aggressive therapies meant to stimulate the discharge of pathological body products, such as to remove phlegm, pus, extravascular blood, *gu* poison, etc. *BJ* SE *jia su* 假蘇：破結聚氣，下瘀血，除濕痹, "It breaks through nodular collections of qi, **discharges** stagnant blood, and eliminates moisture blockages".

③ The intake of medication. *JGYL* Lj: 煉蜜和丸梧子大，酒下十五丸, "Smelt with honey and prepare pills of the size of *wu* seeds. **Ingest** 15 pills with wine".

***Xia* 瞎, injured eye, blindness** [2]

PC AD of → *shi ming* 失明, loss of vision. *SJZL* 194: 兩目大眥二穴，只可背睛斜飛，不得直針，直即傷睛致**瞎**，不可治也, "The two holes in the inner canthi of the two eyes can only receive a needling in a slanting approach aiming at the back of the eyeball. They must not receive a straight needling. A straight [needling] will harm the eyeball and lead to **blindness** that is incurable".

***Xia gan* 下疳, lower-region *gan*-illness** [19] AN *yin gan* 陰疳, yin-region *gan*-illness.

PC of festering ulcers developing in the external genital region of adult males and females, often developing into chronic, difficult to cure ailments. By some authors traced to unhygienic practice of sexual intercourse. *WKJYF* Lj: **下疳**者，乃男子玉莖生瘡，此病皆由所欲不遂，或交接不潔，以致邪毒浸漬，發成瘡毒, "In the case of **lower-region *gan*-illness**, males develop sores on their jade-stalk. This disease originates from unfulfilled longing, or from unclean intercourse resulting in being soaked with evil poison which then develops into sores poison".

***Xia huang shui* 下黃水, discharge of yellow water** [3]

① IS of a discharge of yellow liquid by women from their urinary tract. *BCGM* SE *dao* 稻 quotes *JXCB*: 胎動不安：**下黃水**。用糯米一合，黃芪、芎藭各五錢，水一升，煎八合，分服, "When the fetus moves and [patients] **discharge yellow water**, use polished glutinous rice, 1 *ge*, *huang qi*, *xiong qiong*, 5 *qian* each, boil in 1 *sheng* of water down to 8 *ge*. Ingest in several portions".

② Discharge of yellow liquid from a lesion. *BCSY* SE *she rui cao* 蛇芮草：主蛇虺及毒蟲等螫。取根、葉擣傅咬處，當**下黃水**, "It controls the effects of poisonous snake bites. Take the root and the leaves, pound them and apply the pulp to the bitten area. This will **discharge yellow water**".

Xia li **下痢, discharge with free-flux illness** [273] AN *li xia* 痢下, free-flux illness discharge; *xie li* 泄痢, outflow with free-flux illness; *xie li* 瀉痢.

PC a) identical with → *li ji* 痢疾, free-flux illness ailment. *BJ* SE *mi la* 蜜蠟：主**下痢**膿血, "It controls **discharge with free-flux illness** with pus and blood". b) Identical with *xia li* 下利②, discharge with free-flux. *ZHF* 7: 若藥中有巴豆，**下痢**不止, "If the medication includes *ba dou*, [its intake will cause] unending **discharge with free-flux illness**".

Xia li **下利, discharge with free flow, to cause discharge with free flow** [52]

① IS a) identical with → *xie xie* 泄瀉①, outflow. *SHL* 123: 飲食如故，時時**下利**，寸脈浮、關脈小細沉緊，名曰臟結, "When drinking and eating are normal, with recurrent **discharge with free flow**, and the [movement in the] vessels in the inch section is floating, while at the pass section it is minor, fine, deep inside, and tied, then this is called 'depot bind'".

② PC identical with → *xie xie* 泄瀉②, outflow. *SHL* 366: **下利**，脈沉而遲，其人面少赤、身有微熱、**下利**清穀者，必郁冒汗出而解, "The [movement in the] vessels of [patients suffering from] **discharge with free flow** is deep inside and retarded. If their face is slightly red, and if their body is mildly hot, and if the **discharge with free flow** consists of clear [liquid and undigested] food, then this must be pent-up malicious [qi] that can be resolved once they have been stimulated to sweat".

③ TA of stimulating defecation and urination. *BCGM* Shi ji 十劑 LSZ: 食郁微則山查、神麴以消之，甚則上涌**下利**以去之，皆宣劑也, "For a mild case of pent-up food, use *shan cha* and *shen qu* to dissolve it. In severe cases it is to be removed by having it gush upward or by **causing discharge with free flow**. These are all remedies applied for draining".

Xia li qing gu **下利清穀, discharge with free flow of clear liquid and food** [2]

IS of thin, watery excrements with the passage of undigested food. *SHL* 317: **下利清穀**，裏寒外熱，手足厥逆，脈微欲絕, "**Discharge with free flow of clear liquid and food**. There is inner cold and outer heat. The hands and feet experience recession with counterflow. The [movement in the] vessels is subtle, and on the verge of complete interruption".

Xia nong **下膿, discharge of pus; to discharge pus** [3]

① IS of feces carrying pus. *QJYF* 10: 赤白**下膿**，小兒得之三日皆死, "If children happen to have red and white [free-flux illness] with a **discharge of pus**, they will die within three days".

② TA of stimulating the discharge of pus. *YJJYF* Yong jiu chuang kou bu he lun 癰久瘡口不合論, "On obstruction-illnesses where the opening of the sores fails to close for a long time": 退毒**下膿**，漏蘆湯, "To push back poison and **discharge pus**, [use] the decoction with *lou lu*".

Xia nong xue **下膿血, discharge of pus and blood** [6]

IS identical with → *bian nong xue* 便膿血, defecation with pus and blood. *MYBL* SE *huang shi zhi* 黃石脂：泄痢腸澼，**下膿血**, "Outflow, free-flux illness with intestinal flush and **discharge of pus and blood**".

Xia re 下熱, heat in the lower [sections of the body] [1]

PC of heat in the lower sections of the human body. *ZBYHL* 6: 陰囊臭爛，坐席厚，下熱故也, "When the scrotum has a bad stench with putrefaction, this is because one has sat on a thick mat with **heat in the lower [sections of the body]"**. LSZ identifies the following major pathological conditions as signs of heat in the lower sections of the body: → *bao zhu xia po* 暴注下迫, sudden outpour with downward pressing; → *shui ye hun zhuo* 水液渾濁, turbidity of watery fluids; *xia bu zhong man* 下部腫滿, distension and fullness in the lower body; *xiao bian lin li huo bu tong* 小便淋瀝或不通, dripping urine or anuria; *da bian bi jie xia li* 大便閉結下痢, constipation and discharge with free-flux illness.

Xia shui 下水, discharge of water [41]

① TA to remove liquids retained in the body by means of stimulating urine flow. *BJ* SE *qin jiao* 秦艽：主寒熱邪氣，寒濕風痹，肢節痛，**下水**，利小便, "It controls cold and hot evil qi; blockage resulting from cold, moisture, and wind, pain in the limbs and joints. It **discharges water**, and stimulates urination".

② IS a) identical with → *shui xie* 水泄, watery outflow. *MYBL* SE *bai shi zhi* 白石脂：療五藏驚悸不足，心下煩，止腹痛**下水**, "Cures palpitation with fear brought forth by insufficiency in the five depots, and vexation felt below the heart, and stops abdominal pain and **discharge of water**". b) Of a discharge of liquid by women from their urinary tract. *BCGM* SE *shu* 秫 quotes *MSF*: 妊娠下水，黃色如膠，或如小豆汁。秫米、黃芪各一兩, "When pregnant women **discharge water** with a yellow color like glue, or like red bean juice, [ingest] 1 *liang* each of husked sorghum and *huang qi*".

③ Discharge of liquid from the anus as a reaction to the ingestion of certain medications. *ZHF* 4: 真蘇合香，水銀，白粉等分。蜜丸服，如大豆二丸，日三，當下水, "Genuine *su he xiang*, *shui yin*, and cosmetic powder, equal portions, ingest as honey pills. Ingest two pills of the size of soy beans over a period of three days. This will cause a **discharge of water**".

Xia shui gu 下水穀, discharge of water and grain [1]

IS identical with → *shu gu bu xiao* 水穀不消, water and grain fail to dissolve. *PJF* 211: 治赤白痢，**下水穀**，食不消，用麵熬粟米粥, "To cure red-white free-flux illness, and **discharge of water and grain**, when food fails to dissolve, use flour to boil a millet congee".

Xia si 嚇死, [appearance of] death from intimidation [1]

PC identical with → *jing si* 驚死. *BCGM* Bai bing zhu zhi yao 百病主治藥：醇酒, 驚怖死, 俗名**嚇死**, 灌之, "For [appearance of] death from fright/shock, commonly called '**[appearance of] death from intimidation**', use unmixed wine and forcibly instill it [into the patient]".

Xia xian xue 下鮮血, discharge of fresh blood [2]

IS of blood of a fresh, red color leaving with the stools. *BCGM* SE *mu lian* 木蓮 quoting *HJJF* 6: 大便鮮血, 臍腹疼痛, "Stools with fresh blood. Navel and abdomen are in pain", writes: 大便鮮血, 疼痛肛出, "Stools with fresh blood. A painful prolapse of the rectum". Bai bing zhu zhi yao 百病主治藥 writes: **下鮮血, "Discharge of fresh blood"**.

Xia xiao **下消, lower melting, to dispel below** [2]

① AN *shen xiao* 腎消, kidney melting; *shen xu xiao ke* 腎虛消渴, melting with thirst associated with kidney depletion; *xia xu xiao ke* 下虛消渴, melting with thirst associated with depletion below. PC of → *xiao ke* 消渴, melting with thirst, associated with a diseased lower burner. Major signs: thirst and frequent passage of an ointment-like urine. *LSMC* Fj: **下消**者，煩躁引飲，耳葉焦乾，小便如膏, "In the case of **lower melting**, vexation and restlessness with thirst, the ear lobes are burned to desiccation. The urine is viscous like a paste".

② TA of dispelling water evil and have it leave the organism from the lower orifices of the body by means of urination. *BCGM* SE *li yu* 鯉魚, quotes *YFZY*: 食頭者上消，食身、尾者**下消**, "If one consumes its head, this will dispel above; if one consumes the body and the tail this will **dispel below**".

Xia xie **下泄, discharge with outflow; to drain** [13]

① IS identical with → *xie xie* 泄瀉①, outflow. *SW* 45: 少陰厥逆，虛滿嘔變，**下泄**清，治主病者, "Recession with counterflow in the minor yin [conduit results in the following]: depletion with a change to fullness, vomiting, and a **discharge with clear outflow**. Treat the [conduit] ruling the disease".

② PC identical with → *xie xie* 泄瀉, outflow②, *YD* SE *hou pu* 厚朴：大溫。主**下泄**，腹痛, "Very warm. Controls **discharge with outflow** with abdominal pain".

③ PM of a disease-caused downward movement of qi that normally moves upward. *LS* 22: 氣**下泄**，不治, "**Discharge with outflow** of qi. Do not treat".

④ TA CD of numerous different therapies aiming at stimulating excretion, draining liquids, facilitating intestinal passage, precipating qi, and removing extravascular blood. *SWBJQYBMJ* Fj 上涌**下泄**，奪其病之大勢, "Causing upward gushing and **discharge with outflow** will remove the major strength from any disease".

Xia xu **下虛, depletion below** [25]

PC of depletion of a person's body's lower part. *SW* 10: 頭痛巔疾，**下虛**上實，過在足少陰、巨陽，甚則入腎, "Headache and peak-illness, [this is] **depletion below** and repletion above. The excess is in the foot minor yin and great yang [conduits]. If it is serious, it enters the kidneys".

Xia xu chuang **蝦須瘡, shrimp-feelers sores** [1]

PC of an extremely serious type of → *xi du* 溪毒, rivulet poison, conditions. The skin develops deep-reaching sores. When the root of the sores is pulled out it resembles the feelers of shrimps. The prognosis of such sores is inauspicious. *BCSY* SE *shu yu niao* 鸀瑦鳥：須臾即根入至骨，其根拔出如蝦須，瘡號**蝦須瘡**, "Immediately the root enters and reaches the bones. When this root is pulled out it looks like the feelers of a shrimp. Such sores are called '**shrimp-feelers sores**'".

Xia xu xiao ke **下虛消渴, melting with thirst associated with depletion below** [4]

PC identical with → *xia xiao* 下消, lower melting. *BCGM* SE niu 牛 quoting *ZYJYGLF*: 消渴，心脾中熱，下焦虛冷，小便多, "Melting with thirst, heat in the heart and spleen. The lower burner is depleted and cold. Urination is increased", writes: **下虛消渴**：心脾中熱，下焦虛冷，小便多, "**Melting with**

thirst associated with depletion below: heat in the heart and spleen. The lower burner is depleted and cold. Urination is increased".

Xia xue 下血, **discharge of blood** [492]

① IS CD of all types of blood loss through the anterior or posterior yin opening, including blood stools (seen most often), vaginal bleeding, and hematuria (encountered least often). *SW* 48: 腎脈小搏沉，為腸澼**下血**, "When the kidney vessel is small and beats deep inside, this is intestinal flush with **discharge of blood**".

② PC with a loss of blood through the lower orifices as major sign. *JGYL* Mj: **下血**，先便後血，此遠血也，黃土湯主之, "For **discharge of blood**, if one first defecates and then bleeds, this is remote bleeding. The decoction with loess controls this".

③ TA of quickening blood and removing stagnancies. *BJ* SE *tian ming jing* 天名精：主瘀血，血瘕欲死，**下血**止血, "It controls stagnant blood, and blood conglomeration-illness to the extent that one comes close to death. It causes a **discharge of [the stagnant] blood**, and it thereby stops [uterine] bleeding".

Xia zhong 下重, **pressure below** [2]

IS identical with → *hou zhong* 後重, a feeling of heavy pressure at one's behind. *JGYL* Mj: 熱利**下重**者，白頭翁湯主之, "If one experiences heat free-flux[-illness] with **pressure below**, this is controlled by the decoction with *bai tou weng*".

Xia zhu 下注, **downward influx** [7] AN *Xia zhu* 下疰, downward attachment-illness

PM of a disease's movement from above into the lower regions of the human body. *SJZL* 8: 治風冷**下注**，腰脚痿弱，步履無力，萆薢丸方, "To cure a wind cold **downward influx**, when the lumbar region and the legs are limp and weak, and if walking lacks strength, [resort to] the recipe for pills with *bi jie*".

Xia zhu 下疰, **downward attachment-illness** [1]

PM identical with → *xia zhu* 下注, downward influx. *SJZL* 10: 治風腰脚疼痛，**下疰**脚膝，行步不得，或腫癢，或在兩膝腫痛，久療不瘥，漸至足脛細小少力，虎骨散方, "To cure wind with painful lower back and legs, **downward attachment-illness** in the legs and knees, with an inability to walk, sometimes accompanied by swelling and itching, sometimes with the two knees swelling and aching, which cannot be healed for a long time and gradually results in an emaciation and loss of strength of the feet and shins, [use] the recipe for the powder with tiger bones".

Xian 癇, **epilepsy** [p] AN *dian xian* 癲癇, peak-illness with epilepsy; *xian ji* 癇疾, epilepsy ailment; *xian bing* 癇病, epilepsy disease.

PC of a seizure-type blockage of consciousness, with cataplexy and twitching. *SW* 48: 二陰急為**癇**厥，二陽急為驚, "When the second yin [vessel] is tense, this is epilepsy and recession. When the second yang [vessel] is tense, this is fright".

Xian bing 癇病, **epilepsy disease** [6]

PC identical with → *xian* 癇, epilepsy. *QJYF* 5: 少小所以有**癇病**及痙病者，皆由臟氣不平故也, "When young people suffer from **epilepsy disease** and spasms disease it is always because the qi in their depots is unbalanced".

Xian chao **涎潮, saliva upsurge** [11] AN *xian yong* 涎壅, saliva obstruction.
IS of large quantities of phlegm present in the respiratory tracts evidenced by sounds produced during in- and exhalation. *SJZL* 6: 治卒中風，**涎潮**發搐, 金虎丹方, "To cure sudden wind stroke, **saliva upsurge** and convulsions, [use] the recipe for the Golden Tiger Elixir".

Xian chi **癎瘛, epilepsy with spasms** [1]
PC CD of → *xian bing* 癎病 and → *chi bing* 瘛病, convulsion disease. *SHZG* Mj RE *yi yuan san* 益元散, powder to augment the original [qi]: 主**癎瘛**驚悸健忘, "It controls **epilepsy with spasms**, fear with palpitation, and forgetfulness".

Xian chu **癎搐, epileptic convulsions** [1]
IS of convulsions displayed by patients suffering from → *dian xian* 癲癎, peak-illness with epilepsy. This is an abbreviation of *dian xian chu nuo* 癲癎搐搦. *BCGM* Bai bing zhu zhi yao 百病主治藥：白花蛇、烏蛇，定**癎搐**, "*Bai hua she* and *wu she* fix **epileptic convulsions**".

Xian chuan **涎喘, saliva panting** [3]
PC identical with → *tan chuan* 痰喘, phlegm panting. *PJF* 162: 無憂丸，治年深日遠，咳嗽**涎喘**，夜臥不安, "The 'pills to remove all worries' cure long-lasting cough with **saliva panting**, and restlessness when one goes to bed at night".

Xian hou **咸齁, salty roaring** [1]
PC identical with → *yan hou* 鹽齁, salt roaring. *BCGM* Bai bing zhu zhi yao 百病主治藥：木鱉子，小兒**咸齁**，磨水飲，即吐出痰，重者三服即效, "*Mu bie zi*: For **salty roaring** in children, grind with water and have them drink this. They will immediately vomit and throw out phlegm. In severe cases three dosages will be effective".

Xian huang **癎黃, epilepsy jaundice** [2]
PC of a → *huang dan* 黃疸, yellow *dan*-illness, with the entire body assuming a deep yellow color, accompanied by a desire to sleep and an inability to speak, weakness of the four extremities, and spitting of sticky saliva. *SJZL* 61: **癎黃**，病患身如金色，不多言語，四肢無力，好眠臥，口吐粘涎者，宜服茵陳湯方, "**Epilepsy jaundice**: patients have a body the color of gold. They do not speak much. Their four limbs have no strength. They love to lie down and sleep. From their mouth they spit a sticky saliva. In such cases the recipe to ingest the decoction with *yin chen* is advisable".

Xian ji **癎疾, epilepsy ailment** [40]
PC identical with → *xian* 癎, epilepsy. *MYBL* SE *chi tou* 鴟頭：主頭風眩顛倒，**癎疾**, "It controls head wind with dizziness and peak inversion, as well as **epilepsy ailment**".

Xian ji **涎積, saliva accumulation** [3]
PC of → *ji* 積, accumulation, of phlegm-like saliva. *SJZL* 72: 治積聚癥塊及**涎積**等，續隨子丸方, "To cure accumulation and collection, concretion-illness with lumps, as well as **saliva accumulation**, [use] the recipe for pills with *xu sui zi*".

Xian jing **癇痙, epilepsy and spasms** [12]
PC CD of → *xian bing* 癇病, epilepsy, and *jing bing* 痙病, spasms disease. *BJ* SE *shi dan* 石膽：主明目、目痛，金瘡，諸**癇痙**, "It controls clarification of the eyes, painful eyes, wounds inflicted by metal objects, and all types of **epilepsy and spasms**".

Xian re **癇熱, epilepsy with heat** [4]
PC identical with → *re xian* 熱癇, heat epilepsy. *MYBL* SE *niu huang* 牛黃：療小兒百病，諸**癇熱**, "It heals all types of children's diseases, and all types of **epilepsy with heat**" .

Xian ru **哯乳, to regorge breast-milk** [4]
IS of breast-fed children vomiting the breast-milk. *BCSY* SE *lu zhong chong* 蘆中蟲：**哯乳**，乳飽後哯出者是, "**To regorge breast-milk**: This is when [a child] after having been breast-fed emits [the milk again]".

Xian sou **涎嗽, saliva cough** [1]
IS of cough with an emittence of much phlegm and saliva. *PJF* 64: 發聲散，治語聲不出, 胸滿短氣，**涎嗽**喘悶, "The powder to [help a person to] emit sounds: It cures an inability to speak, a feeling of fullness in the chest, with shortness of qi, and **saliva cough**, panting and heart-pressure".

Xian xiao **咸齁, salt roaring** [1]
PC identical with → *yan hou* 鹽齁. *BCGM* SE *mu bie zi* 木鱉子 quotes *ZXF*: 小兒**咸齁**：大木鱉子三四個，磨水飲，以雪糕壓下，即吐出痰, "**Salt roaring** in children: Grind three or four large pieces *mu bie zi* in water and prepare a [cold] drink [decoction]. This it to be forced down [into the body] with ice cream. This will immediately cause vomiting and eliminate the phlegm".

Xian yong **涎壅, saliva obstruction** [1]
IS identical with → *xian chao* 涎潮, saliva upsurge. *SJZL* 6: 治卒中風暗風，旋暈，痰厥頭痛，胸膈**涎壅**，言語謇澀等疾，牛黃丸方, "To cure ailments such as sudden wind stroke, dimness wind, and vertigo, phlegm recession with headache, **saliva obstruction** in the region of the chest and diaphragm, as well as impeded speech, [use] the recipe for pills with *niu huang*".

Xian zheng **險證, perilous condition** [2]
PC identical with → *wei zheng* 危證, dangerous condition. *BCGM* SE *ren shen* 人參：痘疹**險證**：保元湯, "For the **perilous condition** of smallpox papules: the 'decoction that preserves the original [qi]'".

Xiang ban chuang **香瓣瘡, fragrant clove sores** [3]
PC of chronic → *chuang* 瘡, sores, conditions developing in the face to the side of the ears with gradual immersion by filthy liquid. *PJF* 276: 其瘡多生於男子、婦人面上，常言**香瓣瘡**, "This type of sore frequently develops on the faces of men and women. It is commonly called '**fragrant clove sores**'".

Xiang bo zhong feng **襁褓中風, wind stroke [in the age] of swaddling clothes** [1]
PC identical with → *qi feng* 臍風, navel wind. *BCGM* SE *lu mao* 驢毛 allegedly quoting *QJYF*: **襁褓中風**取驢背前交脊中毛一拇指大，入麝香豆許，以乳汁和，銅器中慢炒為末。乳汁和，灌之, "For **wind stroke [in the age] of**

swaddling clothes take hair of an amount equalling the size of a thumb from the back of a donkey where in the front it intersects with the spine, add a little bean of *she xiang*, mix with breast milk, and gently roast in a copper vessel to eventually prepare a powder. This is again mixed with breast-milk to be instilled [into the child].

Xiang he **項核, nape kernel** [2]
PC of a swelling in the nape resembling a fruit kernel. It is hard and does not fester. *BCGM* Bai bing zhu zhi yao 百病主治藥：山藥，同蓖麻，生塗**項核**, "Fresh *shan yao* and *bi ma* are to be externally applied to **nape kernels**".

Xiang huo **相火, minister fire** [60]
① AN *yin huo* 陰火, yin fire. PN of a potential of liver and kidneys to provide the organism with warmth, to support its physiological functions, and to maintain the sexual abilities of men and women. *SWBJQYBMJ* Fj: 心為君火，腎為**相火**, "The heart is [the location of] the ruler fire; the kidneys are [the location of] the **minister fire**".
② EA of a tendency towards excess eventually causing harm with the generation of depletion fire, which in turn consume the true yin. Hence this causes pathological conditions of yin depletion with fire excess. *PWL* Mj: **相火**，下焦胞絡之火，元氣之賊也, 火與元氣不兩立，一勝則一負, "**Minister fire** is the fire of the network enclosing the bladder in the lower burner; it is the robber of original qi. Fire and the original qi occupy the same position. If one dominates, the other must suffer".
③ PC of yin depletion with fire excess caused by uncontrolled activity of the minister fire. *BCGM* SE huang qin 黃芩：用黃芩以治手足少陽**相火**，黃芩亦少陽本經藥也, "Use huang qin to cure **minister fire** in the minor yang [conduits] of hands and feet. *Huang qin* serves also as a drug for the minor yang conduit itself".

Xiang ji **項急, nape tension** [3]
IS of difficulties in the region of the nape in raising or lowering the head accompanied by uncomfortable contraction. *QJYF* 9: 治患霧氣者，心內煩悶少氣，頭痛**項急**，起則眼眩欲倒，身微熱，戰掉不安，時復憎寒，心中欲吐，吐時無物方, "Recipe to cure patients suffering from fog qi, with vexation, heart-pressure and diminished qi, headaches and **nape tension**. When one rises, the eyes turn dizzy and one is likely to fall to the ground. The body is mildly hot and restless. Time and again it has an aversion to cold. In the center there is an urge to vomit, but the vomiting has no matter to be thrown up".

Xiang jiang **項強, stiff nape** [18]
IS of a stiff nape with difficulties turning the head. *SW* 74: 頭痛，喉痹，**項強**, "[People suffer from] headache, throat blockage, and **stiff nape**".

Xiang ruan **項軟, soft nape** [5]
PC identical with → *tian zhu gu dao* 天柱骨倒, celestial pillar-bone inversion. *HYXS* Mj: 筋骨俱弱，則**項軟**，垂下無力，又名天柱倒, "When the sinews and bones are all weak, this results in a **soft nape**. [The head] falls and [the nape]

has no strength [to hold it upright]. Another name is 'celestial pillar-bone inversion'".

Xiang zui **項贅, nape redundancy** [1]

IS CD of all types of redundancy growths in the nape. *YS* 6: 華亭有一老僧，昔行脚河南管下，寺僧僮僕無一不病癭。時有洛僧共寮，每食取攜行苔脯同餐。經數月，僧**項贅**盡消，若未嘗病。寺僧訝嘆，乃知海岸咸物，能愈是疾, "In Hua ting there was an old monk. Once he travelled in the jurisdiction of Henan. The monks in the monasteries, and all their servants – not a single one of them did not have a goiter. At one time he shared the hut with the monks from Luo. For meals he took them to consume dried meat prepared from algae. After several months had passed, the monks' **nape redundancy** had completely disappeared, as if they had never had a disease. The monks sighed with astonishment. Now they knew that salty items from the coast were able to cure this ailment".

Xiao bian bi **小便閉, minor relief blocked; blocked urination** [5]

IS, PC identical with → *xiao bian bu tong* 小便不通. *QJYF* 19: 病先發於腎，少腹腰脊痛, 胻酸。一日之膀胱，背膂筋痛，**小便閉**。二日上之心，心痛。三日之小腸，脹。四日不已，死, "The disease develops first in the kidneys. The lower abdomen, the lower back, the spine all ache, and the shins feel sore. On the first day it moves into the urinary bladder. The spine and the sinews ache, and **urination is blocked**. On the second day it moves into the heart, and the heart aches. On the third day it moves into the small intestine and causes distension there. If on the fourth day it is not healed, [the patient] will die".

Xiao bian bi se **小便閉塞, minor relief blocked; blocked urination** [1]

IS identical with → *xiao bian bu tong* 小便不通①. *LSMC* Lj 治**小便閉塞**不通，乃血澀致氣不通而竅澀也, "To cure **blocked urination**, this is roughness of the blood leading to a roughness of the aperture that blocks the flow of qi".

Xiao bian bi zhang **小便閉脹, minor relief blockedblocked urination with distension** [1]

IS identical with → *xiao bian bu tong* 小便不通①, blocked urination. *BCGM* SE *cong* 葱 quoting *PJBSF* 3: 治小便難，小腸脹, "It cures difficult urination and small intestine distension", writes: **小便閉脹, "Blocked urination with distension"**.

Xiao bian bu jin **小便不禁, minor relief uncontrolled; urinary incontinence** [21]

AW *xiao bian shi jin* 小便失禁.

IS of an unnoticed and spontaneous flow of urine while the patient is fully awake. *ZBYHL* 14: 小便不禁者，腎氣虛，下焦受冷也。腎主水，其氣下通於陰。腎虛下焦冷，不能溫制其水液，故**小便不禁**也, "As for urinary incontinence, this is kidney qi depletion and an affection of the lower burner with cold. The kidneys rule the water. Their qi descends and passes through the yin (i.e. lower body and genital organs). When the kidneys are depleted and the lower burner is cold, the [latter] is unable to warm and control the bodily liquids. Hence there is **urinary incontinence**".

***Xiao bian bu kuai* 小便不快, minor relief retarded; prolonged urination** [1]
IS identical with → *xiao bian bu li* 小便不利①, urine does not flow freely. *SJZL* 98: 治氣淋，**小便不快**，大黃丸方, "The recipe for pills with *da huang* cures qi dripping with **prolonged urination**".

***Xiao bian bu li* 小便不利, minor relief impeded; urine does not flow freely** [53]
AW *niao bu li* 溺不利; AN *xiao bian mi* 小便秘, urine is blocked.
① AN *xiao bian nan* 小便難, difficult urination; *niao nan* 尿難; *niao se* 溺澀, rough urination, *niao se* 尿澀, *xiao bian se* 小便澀; *xiao bian bu kuai* 小便不快. IS of a difficult discharge of even small amounts of urine. *SW* 36: 足厥陰之瘧，令人腰痛少腹滿，**小便不利**如癃狀, "Malaria of the foot ceasing yin [conduit]: It causes a person's lower back to ache and gives the lower abdomen [a feeling of] fullness. The **urine does not flow freely**; it resembles a protuberance-illness".
② PC of diseases with inhibited urine flow as a major sign. *ZBYHL* 14: 熱搏其臟，熱氣蘊積，水行則澀，故**小便不利**也, "Heat pounds on the organs. Heat qi accumulates. As a result, the passage of water is rough. Hence **urine does not flow freely**".

***Xiao bian bu tong* 小便不通, minor relief blocked; blocked urination** [98] AW *niao bu tong* 尿不通; *niao bi* 尿閉; *xiao bian bi* 小便閉, et al.
① IS of a pressing urge to pass urine without being able to relieve oneself. *JGYL* Mj: 濁氣下流，**小便不通**, "Turbid qi flow downward, with **blocked urination**".
② PC identical with → *long* 癃 a), protuberance-illness. *ZBYHL* 14: **小便不通**，由膀胱與腎俱有熱故也, "The cause of **blocked urination**: both the urinary bladder and the kidneys have heat".

***Xiao bian duan* 小便短, minor relief shortened; scant urination** [4]
IS of a single passage of a small amount of urine. *YXRM* 4: **小便短**而黃者，補中益氣湯加麥門冬、五味子、山藥以補脾腎, "In the case of **scant** and yellow **urination**, supplement the spleen and the kidneys with the 'decoction to supplement the center and increase qi', amended with *mai men dong*, *wu wei zi*, and *shan yao*".

***Xiao bian fan li* 小便反利, minor relief, contrary [to the nature of the disease] unimpeded; free flow of urine despite [the nature of the disease]** [1]
IS identical with → *xiao bian zi li* 小便自利, spontaneous free flow of urine. *BCGM* SE *feng mi* 蜂蜜 quoting *SHL* 233: 小便自利, "Free flow of urine", writes: **小便反利, "Free flow of urine despite [the nature of the disease]**.

***Xiao bian hua shuo* 小便滑數, minor relief smooth and frequent; smooth and frequent urination** [5]
IS of frequently repeated urination associated with urinary incontinence. *KBBC* SE *wu yao* 烏藥：能補中益氣，偏止**小便滑數**, "It is able to supplement the center and increase qi. It is especially capable of stopping **smooth and frequent urination**".

***Xiao bian jie* 小便結, minor relief bound; bound urination** [2]
IS identical with → *xiao bian bu tong* 小便不通①, blocked urination. *BCGM* SE *bo mu* 檗木 quotes [Zhang] Yuan su 元素：黃檗之用有六：瀉膀胱龍

火，一也；利**小便結**，二也；除下焦濕腫，三也；痢疾先見血，四也；臍中痛，五也；補腎不足，壯骨髓，六也, "The usage of *huang bo* is sixfold: It drains dragon fire from the urinary bladder. That is the first. It opens the passage of **bound urination**. That is the second. It eliminates moisture swelling from the lower burner. That is the third. [It cures] the ailment of free-flux illness where blood appears first. That is the fourth. Pain in the navel. That is the fifth. It supplements kidney insufficiency and strengthens the bones and their marrow. That is the sixth".

Xiao bian jing chu **小便精出, minor relief with release of essence; urination with emission of essence** [2] AW *xiao bian yi jing* 小便遺精.

IS of a passage of urine mixed with semen. *BCYY* SE *chi shi zhi* 赤石脂：赤石脂，今四方皆有，以舌試之，粘著者為佳。有人病大腸寒滑，**小便精出**，諸熱藥服及一斗二升，未甚效。後有人教服赤石脂、乾薑各一兩，胡椒半兩，同為末，醋糊丸如梧桐子大，空心及飯前米飲下五七十丸，終四劑，遂愈, "Nowadays, *chi shi zhi* is available everywhere. Those that have a sweet flavor when tested with the tongue are best. There was a man who suffered from cold smoothness in his large intestine, and **urination with emission of essence**. He ingested all types of heating medications, in quantities of 1 *dou* to 2 *sheng*, but without good effect. Later someone told him to ingest pills the size of *wu tong* seeds made, with vinegar as a binder, from a powder prepared from 1 *liang* each of *chi shi zhi* and *gan jiang*, and ½ *liang* of *hu jiao*, to be ingested with a cold rice decoction on an empty stomach before meals. Each dose was 50 to 70 pills. After four doses the cure was achieved".

Xiao bian li **小便利, minor relief unimpeded; free flow of urine** [50]

① IS of excessive urination. *SHL* 127: 太陽病，**小便利**者，以飲水多，必心下悸, "If in the case of major yang disease there is **free flow of urine**, there must be palpitation below the heart as a result of drinking much water".

② TA of freeing an inhibited flow of urine. That is, the positive effects of treating conditions such as dripping, protuberance-illness, and edema. *JGYL* Mj: 日三服。不知，增至七八丸。以**小便利**，腹中溫為知, "Ingest three times daily. If this does not result in a cure increase the dosage to seven, eight pills. The cure is achieved when the **urine flow is freed**, and warmth is felt in the abdomen".

Xiao bian mi **小便秘, minor relief blocked; urine is blocked** [2]

IS, PC identical with → *xiao bian bu li* 小便不利, urine does not flow freely. *SYJYBZFL* 3 da huang zuo jing tang 大黃左經湯：喘，加桑白皮、紫蘇；**小便秘**，加澤瀉, "[If the patient] pants, add *sang bai pi* and *zi su*. [In case his] urine is blocked, add *ze xie*".

Xiao bian mi se **小便秘澀, minor relief blocked and rough; urine is blocked or rough** [1]

IS identical with → *xiao bian bu li* 小便不利①, urine does not flow freely. *ZLBC* SE *da dou chi* 大豆豉 quotes *MTKH*: 蝦蟇小者有毒, 主人**小便秘澀**, 臍下憋, 疼痛至死者。以生豉一合, 投新汲水半碗, 浸令水濃, 頓飲之, 愈, "Small toads with poison control [conditions] where a person's **urine is blocked and rough**. It is stopped up below the navel, with excruciating pain. Take 1 *ge* of fresh [*da dou*] *zhi* and allow it to macerate in a half bowl of water freshly drawn from a well until the water has become viscous. Then have [the patient] immediately drink this, and he will be cured".

Xiao bian nan **小便難, minor relief with difficulty; difficult urination** [3]

IS identical with → *xiao bian bu li* 小便不利①, urine does not flow freely. *SHL* 20: 太陽病，發汗，遂漏不止，其人惡風，**小便難**，四肢微急，難以屈伸者，桂枝加附子湯主之，"In the case of major yang disease, if one causes sweating, the subsequent flow will not end. The person has an aversion to wind, and **urination is difficult**. The four limbs are mildly tense, making it difficult to bend and stretch them. The decoction with *gui zhi* amended with *fu zi* will control this".

Xiao bian pin shuo **小便頻數, frequent minor relief; frequent urination** [27]

IS identical with → *xiao bian shuo* 小便數, frequent urination. *SJZL* 35: 治勞瘧，毛髮枯焦，寒熱不定，飲食減少，肌肉消瘦，面色青黑，兩足無力，非時足冷，**小便頻數**，大便不調，夜夢泄精。鱉甲煮散方，"To cure exhaustion malaria, with desiccation of hair on the body and head and irregular alternation of cold and heat spells, when patients drink and eat less and show emaciation of the muscles and flesh, with a greenish-dark complexion, the two feet being without strength, and the feet unexpectedly turning cold, **frequent urination**, irregular passage of stools, and ejaculation while dreaming at night, [use the] recipe for a powder with boiled turtle shell".

Xiao bian pin yi **小便頻遺, minor relief with repeated loss [of urine]; repeated loss of urine** [2]

IS of frequent → *yi niao* 遺尿, loss of urine. *BCGM* SE *ji* 雞 quotes *MYBL* SE *ji bi zhi li huang pi* 雞肶胵裏黃皮：主治泄痢，**小便頻遺**，除熱止煩，"It controls outflow with free-flux illness and **repeated loss of urine**; it eliminates heat and ends vexation".

Xiao bian se **小便澀, minor relief with roughness; urine roughness** [13]

IS identical with → *xiao bian bu li* 小便不利①, urine does not flow freely. *ZBYHL* 6: 其風濕停水而腫者，則必腫而煩熱，或**小便澀**而腫，"In case of swelling because of wind moisture and stagnating water, there must be swelling associated with vexing heat; in some cases the swelling is associated with **urine roughness**".

Xiao bian shi jin **小便失禁, uncontrolled minor relief; urinary incontinence** [3]

IS identical with → *xiao bian bu jin* 小便不禁. *KBBC* SE *zeng dai hui* 甑帶灰：主胃反，**小便失禁**、不通及淋，"It controls stomach turnover, **urinary incontinence**, [urine that] does not flow freely, and dripping".

Xiao bian shu yi **小便數遺, minor relief with frequent loss [of urine]; repeated loss of urine** [1]

IS identical with → *xiao bian pin yi* 小便頻遺. *BCGM* Bai bing zhu zhi yao 百病主治藥：雞腸草，止**小便數遺**，"*Ji chang cao* stops **repeated loss of urine**".

Xiao bian shuo **小便數, frequent minor relief; frequent urination** [42] AW *xiao bian pin shuo* 小便頻數, *niao shuo* 尿數, *sou shuo* 溲數.

IS of a frequent passage of urine. *LS* 10: 汗出中風，**小便數**而欠, "If one is struck by wind while he sweats, [this results in] **frequent urination** together with yawning".

Xiao bian xia zhuo **小便下濁, minor relief with discharge of turbid [urine]; discharge of turbid urine** [1]

IS identical with → *bai zhuo* 白濁①, white turbidity. *BCGM* SE *fu ling* 茯苓 quoting *HJJF* RE *wei xi wan* 威喜丸, pills with *wei xi* (i.e. *fu ling*): 小便白濁, "The urine is white-turbid", writes: **小便下濁, "Discharge of turbid urine"**.

Xiao bian xue **小便血, minor relief with blood; urine with blood** [6]

IS identical with → *niao xue* 尿血①. *ZBYHL* 27: 心家有熱，結於小腸，故**小便血**也, "When there is heat in the heart, nodes will form in the small intestine. Hence there is **blood in the urine**".

Xiao bian yi **小便遺, involuntary minor relief; involuntary loss of urine** [1]

IS identical with → *yi niao* 遺尿, [involuntary] loss of urine. *BCGM* Bai bing zhu zhi yao 百病主治藥：虛則欠咳**小便遺**, "Depletion brings forth yawning, cough, and an **involuntary loss of urine**".

Xiao bian yi chuang **小便遺床, minor relief with loss [of urine] in one's bed; bed-wetting** [1]

IS identical with → *niao chuang* 尿床. *BCGM* SE *ma xie* 麻鞋 quotes *JXF*: **小便遺床**：麻鞋尖頭二七枚，燒灰，歲朝井華水服之, "For **bedwetting**: burn 27 tips of hemp shoes to ashes and consume them with early morning well water drawn on the first day of the New Year".

Xiao bian yi jing **小便遺精, minor relief with loss of essence; urination with loss of semen** [1]

IS identical with → *xiao bian jing chu* 小便精出, urination with emission of essence. *BCGM* SE *lian ou* 蓮藕 quotes *YLJY*: **小便遺精**：蓮子心一撮，為末，入辰砂一分，每服一錢，白湯下，日二, "For **urination with loss of semen**: Take of *lian zi xin* the amount one can hold with three fingers and prepare a powder. Add *chen sha*, 1 *fen*. Each dose is 1 *qian*. Ingest with clear boiled water. Twice a day".

Xiao bian yi shi **小便遺失, minor relief with loss [of urine]; involuntary loss of urine** [3]

IS identical with → *yi niao* 遺尿. *DXSJ* Mj: **小便遺失**者肺虛也, "**Involuntary loss of urine** is [associated with] lung depletion".

Xiao bian yi shu **小便遺數, minor relief with frequent loss [of urine]; repeated involuntary loss of urine** [2]

IS CD of → *yi niao* 遺尿, involuntary loss of urine, and → *xiao bian shu* 小便數, frequent urination. *QJYF* 17: 寒則欠咳，**小便遺數**, "Cold brings forth yawning and cough, and **repeated involuntary loss of urine**".

Xiao bian zi li **小便自利, spontaneous, unimpeded minor relief; spontaneous free flow of urine** [5] AN *xiao bian fan li* 小便反利, free flow of urine despite [the nature of the disease].

IS of an uninhited flow of urine. Commonly used as a diagnostic category to note the absence of an inhibition of urination. *SHL* 125: 太陽病，身黃、脈沉結、少腹硬、小便不利者，為無血也；**小便自利**，其人如狂者，血證諦也, "In the case of major yang disease, when the body is yellow, the [movement in the] vessels is deep inside and bound, the lower abdomen is hardened, and urine does not flow freely, this is a lack of blood. In the case of a **spontaneous free flow of urine**, if the person behaves insane, this is definitely a blood condition".

Xiao bian zi yi **小便自遺, minor relief with spontaneous loss [of urine]; involuntary loss of urine** [1]

IS identical with → *yi niao* 遺尿. *BCGM* Shi ji 十劑; Se ji 澀劑：大便不固，**小便自遺**, "The stools are not solid; **involuntary loss of urine**".

Xiao bing **小病, minor disease** [1]

PC CD of light diseases with only minor damage to a person's body. The opposite of → *da bing* 大病, massive disease. *SW* 13: **小病**必甚, 大病必死, "**Minor diseases** will be serious; massive diseases will end in death".

Xiao bu xiu **笑不休, laughing without end** [3]

IS of mental irregularity with endless laughing. *SW* 62: 神有餘則**笑不休**，神不足則悲, "When the spirit has [assumed a state of] surplus, then one **laughs without end**; when it has [assumed a state of] insufficiency, then one is sad".

Xiao chan **小產, miscarriage** [1]

PC identical with → *ban chan* 半產. *FKCY* Lj: 大產如栗熟自脫，**小產**如生采破其皮殼, "A normal birth is like a chestnut that has ripened and falls down by itself. A **miscarriage** is as if it were harvested before it has ripened with its skin and shell being broken open".

Xiao chang re **小腸熱, heat in the small intestine** [3]

PC of heat-type diseases affecting the small intestine. *ZBYHL* 15: 小腸象火，旺於夏。手太陽其經也，心之腑也。水液之下行為溲便者，流於小腸。其氣盛為有餘，則病**小腸熱**，焦竭乾澀，小腸昔脹，是為小腸之氣實也，則宜瀉之, "The small intestine is the image of fire; it flourishes in summer. The hand major yang [conduit] is its conduit. It is the palace associated with the heart [depot]. When water-liquids are passed down to be discharged as urine, they flow into the small intestine. When it abounds, this will bring forth a surplus, and the resulting disease will be **heat in the small intestine**. Its desiccation will make passage through it rough, and the small intestine will eventually distend. The reason is a qi repletion in the small intestine which needs to be drained".

Xiao chang xu **小腸虛, small intestine depletion** [1]

PC of a depleted small intestine intruded by cold. *MJ* 2: **小腸虛**，左手寸口人迎以前脈陽虛者，手太陽經也, "**Small intestine depletion**: when the [movement in the] vessels at the inch opening of the left hand and in front of the *ren ying* [insertion hole] shows a yang depletion, this is the hand major yang conduit".

Xiao chang yong **小腸癰, obstruction-illness of the small intestine** [2]

PC identical with → *chang yong* 腸癰, intestinal obstruction-illness. *TPSHF* 61: 關元隱隱而痛者，小腸疽也；上肉微起者，**小腸癰**也, "When the *guan yuan* hole has a minute pain, this [signals] an impediment-illness in the small intestine; when the flesh above it rises slightly, this is an **obstruction-illness of the small intestine**".

Xiao chuan **哮喘, roaring panting** [7] AN *hou xiao* 齁哮, *hou chuan* 齁喘; *xiao ji* 哮疾, roaring ailment; *ga qi* 呷氣, creaking qi.

PC of panting accompanied by a roaring sound in the throat. *DXXF* 2: **哮喘**必用薄滋味，專主於痰，宜大吐, "[To cure] **roaring panting** one must employ [victuals or pharmaceutical substances with] a weak flavor that are especially suited to master the phlegm. The [patient] should vomit large quantities".

Xiao er cha tui **小兒差穨, diverging descent [of the testicles] of children** [3]

PC of children with unequal sized testicles as a major sign. *CBSY* SE *du fu yu* 杜父魚：主小兒差穨。差穨，核大小也, "It controls **diverging descent [of the testicles] of children**. 'Diverging descent' is [to say:] the pits differ in size".

Xiao er fu dou **小兒麩豆, children's bran-beans** [2] AN *fu dou chuang* 麩豆瘡, bran-beans sores.

PC CD of → *ma zhen* 麻疹, sesame papules, and → *dou zhen* 痘疹, smallpox papules. *HYBC* SE *xi jiao* 犀角：主風毒攻心，毷氉熱悶，擁毒赤痢，**小兒麩豆**，風熱驚癇，並宜用之, "It controls wind poison attacking the heart, with restlessness, heat and heart-pressure; it blocks poison and red free-flux illness, **children's bran-beans**, as well as wind heat and fright epilepsy – for all these conditions its use is appropriate".

Xiao er gua chang **小兒刮腸, brushed intestines of children** [1]

PC of serious → *li ji* 痢疾, ailment of free-flux illness, in children with lockjaw and an inability to consume food, closed eyes and abdominal pain and internal cramps with an unsuccessful urge to defecate. *HYKY* 11: 又有毒氣侵胃口亦不飲食，或痢疾因食毒物，不見腸頭，鮮血頻滴，肛門寬大深黑可畏，腹肚疞痛，裏急後重，名曰刮腸, "It may also be that poison qi enters the stomach and [the child can] not drink or eat. Or it suffers from the ailment of free-flux illness because it has eaten poisonous items. The tip of the intestine does not appear. Fresh blood repeatedly drops from the anus which is widened and so dark black that one may be frightened. The abdomen is in continuous pain. [Patients suffer from] internal cramps and a feeling of heavy pressure at their behind. This is called 'brushed intestines'". *BCGM* SE *zhu* 豖 writes: **小兒刮腸**：痢疾，禁口閉目至重者, "**Brushed intestines of children**: A very serious condition of free-flux illness with lockjaw and closed eyes".

Xiao er jing xian **小兒驚癇, fright epilepsy in children** [82]

PC AN → *jing feng* 驚風, fright wind. *YYXS* 9: **小兒驚癇**，古醫經方論但云陰陽癇，而今人乃云急慢驚, "**Fright epilepsy in children** was always called 'yin yang epilepsy' in ancient discourses on medical recipes. Nowadays people call it acute or slow fright".

Xiao er liu xian **小兒流涎, drooling in children** [6]

PC of children with a constant flow of saliva from their mouth. *BCGM* SE *yang* 羊 quoting *QJYF*: 小兒口中涎出, "Saliva released from the mouths of children", writes: **小兒流涎, "drooling in children"**.

Xiao er nai ju **小兒奶疽, children's breast-feeding impediment-illness** [1]

PC not mentioned in any other medical text. Possibly a writing error for → *nai xuan* 奶癬, breast-*xuan*-illness, as *feng xiang* 楓香 was often used for treating breast-*xuan*-illness during the Yuan and Ming era. *BCGM* SE *feng xiang zhi* 楓香脂 quotes *HYQS*: **小兒奶疽**：生面上，用楓香為膏，攤貼之, "**Children's breast-feeding impediment-illness**: when it grows on the face prepare a paste from *feng xiang* and apply externally".

Xiao er nai pi **小兒奶癖, breast-milk aggregation-illness in children** [3]

PC identical with → *xiao er ru pi* 小兒乳癖. *BCYY* SE *ying shi bai* 鷹屎白：治**小兒奶癖**，黃，鷹糞白一錢，蜜佗僧一兩，舶上硫黃一分，丁香二十一個, "To cure **children with breast-milk aggregation-illness** and yellow [complexion]: *ying shi bai*, 1 *qian*; *mi tuo seng*, 1 *liang*; *bo shang liu huang*, 1 *fen*; *ding xiang*, 21 pieces".

Xiao er pi feng **小兒脾風, children's spleen wind** [1]

PC of children producing much saliva, sleeping much, and being unable to consume breast milk. *TPSHF* 89: 治**小兒脾風**，多涎，心胸壅悶，不下乳食，昏昏多睡，鉛霜散方, "To cure **children's spleen wind** with much saliva. The heart and chest are obstructed and feel heart-pressure. The children do not consume breast-milk. They are dizzy and sleep much. [Use] the recipe for the powder with *qian shuang*".

Xiao er qi bing **小兒魃病**, children's jealousy-demon disease [3] AN *ji bing* 繼病, transmission disease.

PC of children under two years of age who, following a second pregnancy of their mother, lose weight to emaciation, are tired and have their hair wither. This was believed to result from their being cursed by the jealousy demon. *TPSHF* 88: 治**小兒魃病**諸方：小兒所有此魃病，由婦人懷妊之時，有惡神導其腹中胎妒嫉而制服他小兒令病也。…治小兒生十餘月後，母又有娠，令兒精神不爽，身體萎瘁，名為魃病, "All recipes to cure **children's jealousy-demon disease**: Children have this 'jealousy-demon disease' when their mother is pregnant [again] and a malign demon causes jealousy against the fetus in the abdomen and then causes the other child to have a disease. … [These recipes] cure children whose mother ten months or more after their birth is pregnant again which causes the child's essence-spirit to feel unwell, with the result that the entire body fails to function properly. This is called jealousy-demon disease".

Xiao er ru huo **小兒乳霍, cholera among children being breast-fed** [3]

PC of breast-fed children with abdominal pain, vomiting and diarrhea. *BCSY* SE *sang du chong* 桑蠹蟲：又主**小兒乳霍**, "It also controls **cholera among children being breast-fed**".

***Xiao er ru pi* 小兒乳癖, breast-milk aggregation-illness in children** [4] AN *xiao er nai pi* 小兒奶癖.

PC of children who fail to digest breast-milk and as a result develop lumps in their abdomen or flanks while assuming a yellow complexion and losing weight. *TPSHF* 88: **小兒乳癖**結實，或有滯惡，停積不散，令兒日漸羸瘦，面色萎黄, "**Children's breast-milk aggregation-illness** with nodular repletion, sometimes with stagnant malign [qi] that halts and accumulates without dispersing and causes children to gradually lose weight every day, with their faces assuming a wilting yellow complexion".

***Xiao er she jiang zhong* 小兒舌強腫, stiff, swollen tongue in children** [1]

PC identical with → *mu she* 木舌, wooden tongue. *BCGM* Bai bing zhu zhi yao 百病主治藥 quoting from the main text on SE *cu* 醋：木舌腫強, "Wooden tongue swollen and stiff", writes: **小兒舌強腫, "Stiff, swollen tongue in children"**.

***Xiao er she mo* 小兒舌膜, tongue membrane in children** [1]

PC with a white membrane enclosing the tongue, in some cases the entire back of the tongue, as major sign. It was believed that this membrane must be removed lest the patient will be mute. *BCGM* SE *fan shi* 礬石 quotes *ZBF*: **小兒舌膜**：初生小兒有白膜皮裹舌，或遍舌根，可以指甲刮破令血出，以燒礬末半緑豆許傅之。若不摘去，其兒必啞, "**Tongue membrane in children**: When in a newborn child a white membrane-skin encloses the tongue, in some cases the entire tongue root, one may scratch, with the fingernail, the tongue until it bleeds. Then a mixture of roasted *fan* powder with about half a green bean is smeared on it. If it is not removed, the child will be mute".

***Xiao er tian diao* 小兒天吊, children hauled-by-heaven** [6]

PC identical with → *tian diao jing feng* 天吊驚風, hauled-by-heaven fright wind. *TPSHF* 85, RE *tian ma wan* 天麻丸, pills with *tian ma*: 治**小兒天吊**，眼目翻上，手足抽掣，發歇不定, "They cure **children hauled-by-heaven**, with their eyes turned upward; experiencing hand and foot spasms. The periods when this condition is active and when it is dormant are not fixed".

***Xiao er tian diao* 小兒天釣, children hooked-up by heaven** [1]

PC identical with → *tian diao jing feng* 天吊驚風, hauled-by-heaven fright wind. *BCGM* SE *yun tai* 芸薹 quoting *SJZL* 172: 小兒天瘹, "Children with the hooked-up-by-heaven illness", writes: **小兒天釣, "Children hooked-up by heaven"**.

***Xiao er xian yin* 小兒癇喑, children's epilepsy muteness** [1]

PC of muteness in children brought forth by an outbreak of → *dian xian* 癲癇, peak-illness with epilepsy. *BCGM* SE *hu zhang tian nan xing* 虎掌天南星 quotes *QYXJ*: **小兒癇喑**，癇後喑不能言。以天南星濕紙包煨，為末，雄豬膽汁調服二字, "**Children's epilepsy muteness**: when [children] are mute and cannot speak following an epilepsy [seizure]. Wrap *tian nan xing* in moist paper and roast over a slow fire. Then grind to a powder and mix with the bile of a boar. Ingest the amount covering 2 characters on a coin".

Xiao er zheng re **小兒蒸熱, steaming heat in children** [1]

PC referring to an emaciated, feverish body brought forth by spleen depletion and too little intake of food. *WSBJ* 19: 肥兒丸，治**小兒蒸熱**, "Chubby Child Pills cure **steaming heat in children**".

Xiao er zhong feng **小兒中風, infant wind stroke** [5]

PC identical with → *qi feng* 臍風, navel wind. *QJYF* 5: 石膏湯，治**小兒中風**，惡痱不能語，口眼了戾，四肢不隨方, "Decoction with *shi gao*, a recipe to cure **infant wind stroke**, with malign disability and an inability to speak, the mouth and eyes distorted, and the four limbs not following one's intentions".

Xiao ga **哮呷, roaring and creaking** [1]

IS of hectic, difficult breathing with a creaking sound emitted from the throat. *PJF* 136: 二黃丸，治喘嗽，**哮呷**氣急, "Pills with the two *huang*[-ingredients]: to cure panting with cough, **roaring and creaking**, qi urgency".

Xiao gu **消穀, to melt grain** [33]

① PN of the function of the spleen and stomach to 'melt and transform' liquid and solid food, and of the effects of pharmaceutical substances to support this function. *MYBL* SE *zhu* 术：益津液，暖胃，**消穀**, "It augments body liquids, warms up the stomach, and **melts grain**".

② IS of an immediate return, following the intake of food, of a feeling of hunger. *LS* 80：胃熱則**消穀**，穀消則善飢, "Stomach heat will cause the **melting of grain**. Once the grain has melted one tends to feel hungry again".

Xiao ji **哮疾, roaring ailment** [1]

PC identical with → *xiao chuan* 哮喘, roaring panting. *BCGM* SE *wo luo* 蝸螺 quotes *ZXF*: 小兒**哮疾**：向南牆上年久螺螄為末，日晡時以水調成，日落時舉手合掌皈依，吞之效, "**Roaring ailment** of children: Remove snail shells from an old wall facing south and grind to a powder. Mix the powder with water in the late afternoon. At sundown have [the child] raise its hands and put both palms together as is done in Buddhist religious ceremonies. Have [the child] swallow it and it will be effective".

Xiao jie xiong **小結胸, minor bound chest** [2]

PC of → *jie xiong* 結胸, bound chest, brought forth by phlegm and heat. *SHL* 138: **小結胸**病，正在心下，按之則痛，脈浮滑者, "**Minor bound chest**: The disease is located right below the heart. If one presses there, [patients] feel pain. The movement in the vessels is at the surface and smooth".

Xiao ke **消渴, melting with thirst, diabetes** [334]

① PC a) manifesting itself as an urge to drink, eat, and urinate more than normal. This is **melting with thirst** in the broadest sense. *ZBYHL* 5: 夫**消渴**者，渴不止，小便多是也, "Now, as for melting with thirst, one is always thirsty, and urinates often". b) Diabetes in a narrow sense, with an urge to drink and urinate much, with the urine having a sweet taste. *WTMY* 11: **消渴**病有三。一渴而飲水多，小便數，無脂似麩片甜者，此是消渴病也, "There are three types of the disease **melting with thirst**. First, if one is thirsty and drinks much water, and if urination is frequent, [with the urine] being sweet and having no fat flakes, then this is melting with thirst disease”.

② IS of thirst and an urge to drink more than normal. *SHL* 71: 太陽病，發汗後…若脈浮，小便不利，微熱，**消渴**者，五苓散主之，“If in the course of a major yang disease following sweating … the movement in the vessels is at the surface, urine does not flow freely, one's temperature is slightly raised, and one experiences **melting with thirst**, then the powder with *wu ling* will control this”.

***Xiao ke bian shui* 消渴變水, melting with thirst transformed to edema** [3]
PC of → *shui zhong* 水腫, edema, brought forth in the aftermath of → *xiao ke* 消渴, melting with thirst. *BCGM* SE *su* 蘇 quotes *SJZL*: **消渴變水**，服此令水從小便出，“For **melting with thirst transformed to edema** ingest this. If one consumes it, it will expel the water via urination”.

***Xiao ke yin yin* 消渴引飲, melting with thirst leading to drinking** [14]
IS identical with → *xiao ke* 消渴②, melting with thirst. *QJYF* 19 RE *zeng sun shen li tang* 增損腎瀝湯, decoction to augment loss for dripping kidneys: 又治腎氣不足，**消渴引飲**，小便過多，腰背疼痛者，“It further cures insufficient kidney qi, **melting with thirsting leading to drinking**, excessive urination, and pain in the back and lumbar region”. Entries in the *BCGM* suggest that this is either a sign of the disease of diabetes, or of heat-related diseases.

***Xiao lao* 小勞, minor exhaustion** [5]
EA of a slight exhaustion. *ZHF* 2: 大病瘥後，**小勞**便鼻衄，“When a massive disease has been cured, and **minor exhaustion** leads to nosebleed”.

***Xiao shen* 消腎, melting kidneys** [4]
① PC identical with → *shen xiao* 腎消. *TPSHF* 53: 飲水隨飲便下，小便味甘而白濁，腰腿消瘦者，**消腎**也，“If one drinks water and it is passed as urine immediately, with the urine having a sweet flavor and being white and turbid, and the lumbar region and the legs becoming emaciated, then this is **melting kidneys**”.

② PE of toxic pharmaceutical substances on the kidneys. *BCTJ* SE *shang lu* 商陸：又一種名赤菖，苗、葉絕相類，不可用，服之傷筋**消腎**，須細辨之，“Another species is called ‘red calamus’. Its seedlings and leaves are very similar, but must not be used. If consumed they harm the sinews and they cause **kidney melting**. One must be careful to distinguish between the two”.

***Xiao sou bi* 小溲閉, blocked urination** [1]
IS, PC identical with → *xiao bian bu tong* 小便不通. *RMSQ* 3: 夫一井之水，而功用不同，豈烹煮之間，將行藥勢，獨不擇夫水哉？昔有患**小溲閉**者，眾工不能瘥，予易之長川之急流，取前藥而沸之，一飲立溲，“Now, the water of one and the same well may have different effects. How can it be that through boiling we activate the strength of a pharmaceutical substance, and yet do not choose [from among different] waters? Formerly, those suffering from **blocked urination** could not be healed by all the practitioners. I changed [the water and resorted to] that taken from a swiftly flowing stream. I used the same drugs as before and boiled them, and one ingestion immediately restored urination”.

Xiao zhong **消中, melting center** [9]

PC identical with → *zhong xiao* 中消. *WTMY* 11: 吃食多，不甚渴，小便少，似有油而數者，此是**消中**病也, "[Patients] eat much, but are not very thirsty. The amounts of urine passed are small. The urine appears to be oily, and is passed frequently. This is the disease of **melting center**".

Xie **泄, outflow; to cause an outflow** [p]

① IS a) identical with with → *xie xie* 泄瀉①, outflow. *SW* 7: 一陽發病，少氣善咳善**泄**, "When the first yang develops a disease, [patients] are short of qi and tend to cough. [There is also] a tendency toward **outflow**". b) Identical with → 遺精, seminal emission. *TPSHF* 5: 小便白濁，夢寐頻**泄**, "The urine is white and turbid, with frequent **outflow** while [patients are] asleep".

② PC identical with → *xie xie* 泄瀉②, outflow. *SW* 17: 胃脈實則脹，虛則**泄**, "If the [movement in the] vessels of the stomach is replete, then this is distension. When it is depleted, then this is **outflow**".

③ PM identical with *xia xie* 下泄③, discharge with outflow. *SW* 18: 乳之下其動應衣，宗氣**泄**也, "As for the movement reflected by the garments below the breast, [if it is interrupted and does not arrive, in this case] this is an **outflow** of the basic qi".

④ TA identical with → *xia xie* 下泄④, to discharge with outflow; to drain. *SW* 22: 肺苦氣上逆，急食苦以**泄**之, "When the lung suffers from qi rising contrary [to its regular course], quickly consume bitter [flavor] **to cause its outflow**".

Xie **瀉, outflow; to drain** [p]

① IS a) identical with with → *xie xie* 泄瀉①, outflow. *SW* 74: 清氣動下，少腹堅滿而數便**瀉**, "Cool qi moves below. The lower abdomen is firm and full and [patients suffer from] frequent **outflow** of urine and stools". b) CD of a diarrhea-type excretion of formless or liquid matter, including blood, pus, water, and watery exrements. *ZBYHL* 32: 赤疽發額，不**瀉**，十餘日死, "If a red impediment-illness develops at the forehead, without **outflow**, [the patient] will die after ten or so days".

② PC identical with → *xie xie* 泄瀉②, outflow. *ZHF* 8: 卒得吐**瀉**、霍亂、蠱毒, "If one suddenly experiences vomiting and **outflow**, as well as cholera, *gu* poisoning…".

③ TA a) of a large group of therapies opposed to *bu* 補, "supplementation", and meant to attack an evil. *SW* 20: 實則**瀉**之，虛則補之, "In case of repletion, **drain** it. In case of depletion, supplement it". b) Identical with → *xia xie* 下泄④, to discharge with outflow; to drain. *SW* 5: 中滿者，**瀉**之於內, "In case of central fullness, **drain** it inside".

Xie bi **邪痹, evil [qi] blockage** [1]

PC CD of blockages in depots and palaces, conduits and network vessels brought forth by evil qi. *MYBL* SE *suan* 蒜：理胃，溫中，除**邪痹**毒氣, "It regulates the stomach, warms the center, and eliminates **evil blockage** and poison qi".

Xie du **邪毒, evil poison** [8]

EA of evil qi capable of causing all types of disease. *ZBYHL* 31: 毒腫之候，與風腫不殊，時令人壯熱，其**邪毒**甚者，入腹殺人, "The signs of poison swelling are identical with those of wind swelling. After some time they make a person become very hot. When an **evil poison** is extreme and enters the abdomen, it will kill that person".

Xie e **邪惡, evil and malign [qi]** [22]

EA CD of pathogenic evil affecting the body from outside. *BJ* SE *mi wu* 蘼蕪：咳逆，定驚氣，辟**邪惡**，除蠱毒鬼疰，去三蟲, "It controls coughing with counterflow [of qi], stabilizes fright qi, eliminates **evil and malign [qi]**, discards *gu* poison and demon attachment-illness, and removes the thee types of bugs/worms".

Xie feng **脅風, flanks wind** [5]

PC of pain in the flanks. *MYBL* SE *du gui* 牡桂：心痛，**脅風**脅痛，溫筋通脈，止煩出汗, "[It controls] heart pain, **flanks wind**, aching flanks. Warms sinews, penetrates vessels. Ends vexation, stimulates sweating".

Xie jie **邪結, evil [qi] node** [4]

PC of rather deep-lying accumulations of pathogenic items. *BJ* SE *kong gong nie* 孔公孽：主傷食不化，**邪結**氣惡, "It controls harm caused by undigested food, with **evil [qi] nodes** and qi malignity".

Xie jing **泄精, involuntary emission of essence** [50]

PC identical with → *yi jing* 遺精. *MYBL* SE *xun cao* 熏草：主明目，止淚，療**泄精**, "It controls clearing eyesight, stops tears, and cures **involuntary emission of essence** (i.e. seminal fluid)".

Xie li **泄利, unimpeded free-flux** [12]

① IS identical with → *xie xie* 泄瀉①, outflow. *SHL* 318: 少陰病，四逆，其人或咳、或悸、或小便不利、或腹中痛、或**泄利**下重者，四逆散主之, "Minor yang diseases are associated with four counterflows. When the afflicted person coughs, or experiences palpitation, or has impeded urine flow, or feels pain in the abdomen, or has **unimpeded free-flux** with a feeling of heaviness below, then the 'powder for the four counterflows' will master this.

② PC identical with → *xie xie* 泄瀉②, outflow. *SW* 19: 脈細，皮寒，氣少，**泄利**前後，飲食不入，此謂五虛, "A fine [movement in the] vessels, cold skin, being short of qi, **unimpeded free-flux** in front and behind, beverages or food do not enter [the stomach], these are called the five depletions".

Xie li **瀉利, unimpeded free-flux** [4]

IS identical with with → *xie xie* 泄瀉①, outflow. *ZBYHL* 45: 傷寒，是寒氣客於皮膚，搏於血氣，使腠理閉密，氣不宣洩，蘊積毒氣，頭痛、體疼而壯熱也。其熱歇後而利者，是熱從表入裏故也。表熱雖得解，而裏熱猶停腸胃，與水穀相併，腸胃虛則泄利。其狀，利色黃。若壯熱不止，則變為血利。若重遇冷，則冷熱相加，則變赤白**瀉利**也, " 'Harm caused by cold' is to say: cold qi settles in the skin and strikes the blood and qi. It causes the interstitial structures to close so that the qi cannot flow off. This leads to accumulations of poison qi, with headaches, a painful body and strong heat. When the heat has ended and free flow is possible again, this is so because the heat has moved from the body's outer sections into its interior. The external heat may appear to have been resolved, but now the heat stagnates internally in the intestines and the stomach where it unites with water and grain. In the case of intestinal and stomach depletion, this leads to unimpeded outflow, as is indicated by a yellow color of the free flow. When the heat is strong and does not end, then a change occurs to bloody free flow. When [patient] is exposed to cold again, then cold and heat add to each other, and a change occurs to red-white **unimpeded free-flux**".

***Xie li* 泄痢, outflow with free-flux illness** [115]
PC identical with *xia li* 下痢, discharge with free-flux illness. *BJ* SE *fan shi* 礬石：主寒熱，**泄痢**, "It controls alternating sensations of cold and heat, as well as **outflow with free-flux illness**".

***Xie li* 瀉痢, outflow with free-flux illness** [55]
PC identical with → *xia li* 下痢, discharge with free-flux illness. *RHZ* SE *hai tong pi* 海桐皮：消痰下氣，除煩治水，調中，止**瀉痢**, "It dissolves phlegm and drains qi. It removes vexation and cures water, regulates the center, and stops **outflow with free-flux illness**".

***Xie lou* 脅漏, flank leakage** [2]
PC of → *lou chuang* 漏瘡, leaking sores, in the region of the flanks. *BCGM* SE *niu* 牛：**脅漏**，出水不止，用烏牛耳垢傅之，即瘥, "For **flank leakage** releasing water continuously: smear the dirt from the ears of a black ox on it. This will bring the cure".

***Xie lou* 蠍瘺, scorpion fistula** [1]
PC of → *lou* 瘺, fistula, with a swelling developing in the neck or in the armpits resembling a scorpion. This is associated with fever and an aversion to cold. When they open to fester they develop into fistula. This is a chronic disease that fails to heal. Within the sores small bugs/worms resembling scorpions are seen to grow. *ZBYHL* 34: **蠍瘺**候，此由飲食居處有蠍蟲毒氣，入於腑臟，流於經脈所生也。或生掖下，或生頸邊，腫起如蠍蟲之形，寒熱而潰成瘺。久則瘡裏生細蠍蟲也, "The signs of **scorpion fistula**: This is because [the patient] has encountered the poisonous qi of scorpions in beverages and food and at his domicile. It enters the palaces and depots and flows into the conduit vessels. It may effuse into the armpits or to the side of his neck. The swelling looks like a scorpion. [Patients] experience alternating sensations of cold and heat. Eventually it festers and develops into fistula. After a long time small scorpions grow in the sores".

***Xie mei* 邪魅, evil seduction-specter** [20]
EA PC identical with → *gui mei* 鬼魅, demon seduction-specter. *ZHF* 3: 若或悲泣呻吟者，此為**邪魅**，非狂，自依邪方治之, "If [a patient] is grieved and weeps silently and groans, this is an **evil seduction-specter**. If [his behavior] is not crazy, he is to be treated with recipes for [disease brought forth by the] evil".

***Xie ni* 邪逆, evil counterflow** [4]
CD of PCs brought forth by a disease evil abiding at a specific location in the body and impairing its normal functioning. *BJ* SE *she gan* 射干：主咳逆上氣,

喉痹咽痛, 不得消息, 散結氣, 腹中**邪逆**, "It controls coughing with counterflow, i.e. rising qi, throat blockage with gullet pain that cannot be dissolved. It disperses bound qi, and **evil counterflow** in the abdomen". The term also appears in later quotes, including *BCGM*, of four passages from the *BJ* and *MYBL*. There is no known definition of its meaning in any text. The definition given here is tentative; it is based on the four quotes in the *BCGM*.

Xie nue **邪瘧, evil [qi] malaria** [17]
PC identical with → *nue ji* 瘧疾, malaria. *PJF* 18: 七寶鎮心丸，治心風，狂語錯亂，似如**邪瘧**，發作有時, 'Pills with seven treasured ingredients to ease an [excited] heart' cure heart wind, crazy language and disorderly behavior. The appearance is that of **evil [qi] malaria** with its periodic outbreaks".

Xie nüe **泄瘧, outflow and malaria** [1]
PC CD of → *xie xie* 泄瀉, outflow, and → *nüe ji* 瘧疾, malaria. *BCGM* SE *shao jiu* 燒酒：通膈噎而散痰飲，治**泄瘧**而止冷痛也, "It opens food barriers and disperses phlegm rheum. It cures **outflow and malaria**, and ends cold pain".

Xie pi **泄澼, outflow and flush** [6] AN *pi xie* 澼泄, flushing outflow.
PC identical with → *li ji* 痢疾, ailment of free-flux illness. *MYBL* SE *bai la* 白蠟：療久**泄澼**，後重見白膿, "It heals prolonged **outflow and flush**, with a feeling of heavy pressure at one's behind and the appearance of white pus".

Xie qi **邪氣, evil qi** [247]
EA CD of all types of etiological agents. All etiological agents, regardless of whether they have originated outside the body or whether they have been generated inside the body, can be termed 'evil qi'. *SW* 3: 數犯此者，則**邪氣**傷人，此壽命之本也, "If this [qi of heaven] is offended repeatedly, then **evil qi** harms humanity. [Hence] this [qi of heaven] is the basis of one's lifespan".

Xie re **邪熱, evil heat** [43]
EA identical with → *re* 熱, heat. *ZBYHL* 8: 此由寒毒氣傷於太陰經也。太陰者肺也。肺主氣，肺虛，為**邪熱**所客，客則脹，脹則上氣也, "This [disease] results from cold poison qi harming the major yin conduit. The major yin is the lung. The lung rules the qi. In the case of lung depletion, **evil heat** settles there. Such a settling brings forth distension. In the case of distension the qi rises".

Xie shi **斜視, squint** [1] AN *mu pi* 目辟; *yan sui* 眼矓.
IS of a failure of both eyeballs to automatically assume parallel positions to focus on one object. *XEYZZJ* Fj: 因潮熱，申、酉、戌時不甚搐而喘，目微**斜視**，身體似熱，睡露睛，手足冷，大便淡黃水。是肺旺，當補脾治心肝, "Subsequent to tidal heat, convulsions and panting will not be excessive at *shen*, *you*, and *xu* hours. The eyes have a slight **squint**. The body appears hot. [People] sleep with open eyes. The hands and feet are cold. Defecation produces water of a bland-yellow color. As this is an excess activity of the lung, it is essential to supplement the spleen and to heal the heart and liver".

***Xie sou* 邪嗽, evil [qi] cough** [1]

PC CD of all types of cough resulting from an affection with evil qi. *WTMY* 9: 深師療五嗽，一曰上氣嗽，二曰飲嗽，三曰燥嗽，四曰冷嗽，五曰**邪嗽**，四滿丸方, "*Shen shi* cures the five types of cough. The first is named 'qi cough', the second is named 'rheum cough', the third is called 'dry cough', the fourth is called 'cold cough', the fifth is called '**evil [qi] cough**'. [It calls for] the recipe for the 'fourfold fullness pills'".

***Xie sui* 邪祟, evil curse** [8]

CD of all PC resulting from a demon's curse. *ZLBC* SE *can tui* 蠶退 quotes *BYF*: 若或悲泣呻吟者, 此為**邪祟**。以蠶紙作灰, 酒水任下, 差, "If someone weeps with grief and moans, this is an **evil curse**. Burn paper with silkworm eggs to ashes, and ingest with wine and water. This will banish [the curse]". *BCGM* SE *zhu tong qi* 諸銅器 quotes *DTQL*: 山精水魅多歷年代, 故能為**邪祟**。三代鐘鼎彝器, 歷年又過之, 所以能辟祟也, "Mountain spirits and water seduction-specters have existed for ages. Hence they are able to issue an **evil curse**. Funeral objects such as bells and vessels from the three Ancient Dynasties have an even longer history. Hence they are able to remove such curses".

***Xie xie* 泄瀉, outflow** [55] AD *xie* 泄, *xie* 瀉; AN *li* 利, free flow; *xia li* 下利, discharge with free-flux; *xia xie* 下泄, discharge with outflow.

① AN *zi li* 自利, unimpeded free flow; *xie li* 泄利, free outflow; *xie li* 瀉利. IS of frequent discharge of thin or liquid excrements. *QJYF* 3: 治產後虛冷，洞下，心腹絞痛，兼**泄瀉**不止方, "Recipes for treating postpartum depletion cold, with vacating downpour, twisting pain in the heart and abdomen, as well as unending **outflow**".

② AN *li xia* 利下, free flow discharge. PC with outflow. *SJZL* 26: 治產後**泄瀉**，日久不止，煩渴睏倦，不思飲食，地榆散方, "Recipe for the powder with *di yu* to cure postpartum **outflow** that does not end for days, with vexation, thirst, and fatigue, as well as lack of appetite".

***Xie xue* 瀉血, blood outflow** [86]

IS of a) anal bleeding. *YXL* SE *qian gen* 茜根：吐血，**瀉血**用之, "Use it for [treating] blood spitting and **blood outflow**". b) Vaginal bleeding. *ZBYHL* 42: 墮胎損經脈，損經脈，故血不止也。**瀉血**多者，便致煩悶，乃至死也, "An abortion injures the conduit vessels. When the conduit vessels are injured this results in unending bleeding. Massive **blood outflow** leads to vexation and heart-pressure, and may end in death". c) Pus and, mostly, blood in one's stools in the course of free-flux illness. *YXL* SE *niu jiao sai* 牛角鰓：止冷痢**瀉血**, "It ends cold free-flux illness with **blood outflow**".

***Xie xue nong* 泄血膿, outflow of blood and pus** [1]

IS identical with → *bian nong xue* 便膿血, defecation with pus and blood. *BCGM* SE *jiu* 韭 quoting *BCSY* 止泄白膿, "It ends outflow of white pus", writes: 止**泄血膿**, "It ends **outflow of blood and pus**".

***Xie yan* 邪魘, evil nightmare** [1]
PC identical with → *yan mei* 魘寐. *SJZL* 5: 鬼氣、**邪魘**、屍厥、暴亡不省人事等疾，至聖太一散方, "For ailments such as demon qi, **evil nightmares**, corpse[-like condition because of qi] recession, sudden loss of consciousness with an inability to recognize people, resort to the recipe for the 'powder to reach sagehood and great unity'".

***Xie yu* 邪郁, pent-up evil [qi]** [1]
EA identical with → yu 郁①, pent-up [qi]. *BCGM* SE *shui yin fen* 水銀粉：水銀乃至陰毒物，因火煅丹砂而出，加以鹽、礬煉而為輕粉，加以硫黃升而為銀硃，輕飛靈變，化純陰為燥烈。其性走而不守，善劫痰涎，消積滯。故水腫風痰、濕熱毒瘡被劫，涎從齒齦而出，**邪郁**為之暫開，而疾因之亦愈, "*Shui yin* is a poisonous substance of extreme yin-quality. It is produced by means of a fire refinement process from cinnabar, another refinement with salt and *fan* creating *qing fen*, then sublimation with *liu huang* to generate *yin zhu*, then another modification by means of sublimation to create a pure yin-substance of extreme ferocity. Its nature is to move; it cannot be guarded. It is good in removing phlegm and saliva, and in dissolving accumulations of sluggish [qi]. Hence when it removes water swelling and wind phlegm, moisture heat and poison sores, if saliva emerges from the gums and **pent-up evil** [qi] is given a temporary opening there, then the cause of the ailment is cured too".

***Xie zhu* 邪疰, evil attachment-illness** [3]
PC identical with → *gui zhu* 鬼疰, demon attachment-illness. *BJ* SE *shi yan* 食鹽：主殺鬼蠱,**邪疰**毒氣, "It controls killing of demon *gu*, **evil attachment-illness**, and poison qi".

***Xie zhu* 泄注, outpour** [2]
PC identical with → *shui xie* 水泄, watery outflow. *MYBL* SE *wu zhu yu* 吳茱萸：根白皮殺蟯蟲，治喉痹，咳逆，止**泄注**, "The white bark of its root kills pinworms, cures throat blockage and cough with qi counterflow, and stops **outpour**".

***Xin bi* 心痹, heart blockage** [3]
PC resulting from excessive pondering harming the spirit of the heart, with a feeling of heart-pressure, secret anguish in the heart, and lack of appetite. *SW* 10: 積氣在中，時害於食，名曰**心痹**。得之外疾，思慮而心虛, "Accumulated qi in the center. Occasionally this is harm caused by food. It is called **heart blockage**. If one gets it as an external disease, [the reason is that] one has been thinking and pondering [about something] and the heart is depleted".

***Xin bing* 新病, new disease; modern-day disease** [3]
PC a) CD of all diseases with a rather short duration that have been acquired only recently. The opposite of → *jiu bing* 久病, old disease. *SW* 17: 征其脈與五色俱不奪者, **新病**也, "If it is verified that the [movement in the] vessels is diminished and that the complexion is not lost, it is a **new disease**". b) CD of all modern-day diseases that are not mentioned in ancient recipes. *YXQY* Xu 序：潔古治病, 不用古方, 但云：古方**新病**, 不相宜, 反以害人, "When [Zhang] Jiegu

cured diseases, he did not use ancient recipes. He merely stated: Ancient recipes and **modern-day diseases** do not fit each other. On the contrary, their use will harm people".

Xin chong **心忡, heart anxiety** [2]

IS of a feeling of worry and misgivings in the heart without any apparent reason. *NKTY* Fj: 徹夜不寐，**心忡**不寧，此脾血尚虛, "[If the woman suffers from] a failure to sleep for the entire night, **heart anxiety** and restlessness in her heart, this is a continuing blood depletion in the spleen".

Xin fan **心煩, heart vexation** [60]

IS identical with → *fan men* 煩悶, vexation with heart-pressure. *SW* 10: **心煩**頭痛，病在膈中, "In case of **heart vexation** and headache, the disease is in the diaphragm".

Xin fei da xiao chang re **心肺大小腸熱 heat in the heart, the lung, the large and the small intestines** [1]

CD of → *xin re* 心熱, heat in the heart; → *fei re* 肺熱, heat in the lung; → *da chang re* 大腸熱, heat in the large intestine; → *xiao chang re* 小腸熱, heat in the small intestine. *BCGM* SE *sha tang* 沙糖 quotes *RHZ*: 潤**心肺大小腸熱**，解酒毒。臘月瓶封窖糞坑中，患天行熱狂者，絞汁服，甚良, "It provides moisture to **heat in the heart, the lung, the large and the small intestines**, resolves wine poison. In the *la* month store it in a sealed jar in the cesspool. When the time comes where people suffer from heaven-sent (i.e. epidemic) heat and madness, wring the juice from it and ingest it. This is very good.".

Xin fei re **心肺熱, heat in the heart and lung** [2]

CD of → *xin huo* 心火, heart fire, and → *fei huo* 肺火, lung fire. *BCGM* Bai bing zhu zhi yao 百病主治藥：麥門冬除**心肺熱**, "*Mai men dong* eliminates **heat in the heart and lung**".

Xin feng **心風, heart wind** [18]

PC of a heart affection by wind evil. *SW* 42: **心風**之狀，多汗惡風，焦絕善怒嚇，赤色, 病甚則言不可快, 診在口, 其色赤, "The appearance of **heart wind** [is such]: [patients] sweat profusely and have an aversion to wind. When the burning is extreme, they tend to be angry and cry out. Their [facial] color is red. When the disease is severe, [patients find] it impossible to speak cheerfully. This is diagnosed in the mouth. The color there is red". *BCGM* refers to heart wind in the context of a loss of the heart's function to control the spirit and mind, e.g. *xin feng fa kuang* 心風發狂, heart wind with fits of madness; *xin feng jing re* 心風驚熱, heart wind with fright and heat; *xin feng dian xian* 心風癲癇, heart wind with peak-illness epilepsy; *xin feng fan men* 心風煩悶, heart wind with vexation and heart-pressure, and *xin feng jian wang* 心風健忘, heart wind with forgetfulness.

Xin fu tong **心腹痛, heartache and abdominal pain** [113]

① IS of a feeling of pain anywhere in a region including the heart pit and navel. *ZBYHL*16: **心腹痛**者，由腑臟虛弱，風寒客於其間故也, "In the case of

heartache and abdominal pain the reason is a palace and depot depletion weakness. Wind cold has settled inside of them".

② AN *xin pi tong* 心脾痛, heartache and spleen pain.

PC with heartache and abdominal pain. *BJ* SE *bai ji* 白棘：主**心腹痛**, "It controls **heartache and abdominal pain**". LSZ identifies "heartache and abdominal pain" as a sign of a disease in the spleen itself, brought forth by a variety of EA such as → *han* 寒, cold; → *re* 熱, heat; → *tan* 痰, phlegm; → *chong* 蟲, bugs/worms; → *shiji* 食積, food accumulation, and → *xu lao* 虛勞, depletion exhaustion.

Xin gan huo **心肝火, heart and liver fire** [3]
CD of → *xin huo* 心火, heart fire, and → *gan huo* 肝火, liver fire. *BCGM* Bai bing zhu zhi yao 百病主治藥：黃連瀉**心肝火**, "*Huang lian* drains **heart and liver fire**.

Xin han **心寒, heart cold** [3] AN → *han xin* 寒心, cold heart.
IS of a feeling of cold in the heart cave. *SW* 36: 肺瘧者，令人**心寒**, "Lung malaria: it makes a person feel **heart cold**".

Xin huang **心黃, heart jaundice** [3]
PC of → *huang dan* 黃疸, yellow *dan*-illness, accompanied by psychiatric illness signs such as heart-pressure, hectic panting, an excessive talkativeness and laughing, restlessness, and absent-mindedness. *TPSHF* SE *a bo le* 阿勃勒：心膈間熱風，**心黃**, "[It cures] heat wind in the region of heart and diaphragm, as well as **heart jaundice**".

Xin huo **心火, heart fire; heart, i. e. fire** [43]
① PC and EA, identical with → *xin re* 心熱, heat in the heart; heart heat. *SWBJQYBMJ* Fj: 中風偏枯者，由**心火**暴盛, "If someone has been struck by wind with hemilateral withering, this is because of a sudden flaring up of **heart fire**".

② PN as an alternative designation for *xin* 心, heart. The heart is associated with fire. Hence the designation *xin huo* 心火, heart, i. e. fire. *SW* 69: 寒氣流行，邪害**心火**，民病身熱，煩心躁悸, "If in a year [associated with water] there is great excess [of the qi] of water, cold qi prevails everywhere. The evil harms **the heart, (i.e.) the fire**. People suffer from body heat and a vexed heart with restlessness and palpitation".

Xin ji **心悸, heart palpitation** [5]
① AN *song ji* 忪悸, agitated palpitation. IS of a feeling of the heart racing, often associated with mental restlessness. *SHL* 49: 若下之，身重**心悸**者，不可發汗，當自汗出乃解, "When purging it, if the body feels heavy and experiences **heart palpitation**, one must not induce sweating. The sweat should leave [the patient] spontaneously. This will solve it".

② PC with heart palpitation. *QJYF* 3 RE *ren shen wan* 人參丸, pills with *ren shen*: 亦治男子虛損**心悸**, "They also cure depletion injury with **heart palpitation** in males".

Xin ji **心積, heart accumulation** [3]
PC identical with → *fu liang* 伏梁, hidden beam. *ZBYHL* 19: 診得**心積**脈，沉而芤，時上下無常處。病悸，腹中熱，面赤，咽乾，心煩，掌中熱，甚

即唾血, "If upon an examination one finds a [movement in the] vessels of **heart accumulation**, it is deep inside and scallion-stalk[-like]. At times it is above, at times below, and it has no fixed location. Patients experience palpitations, abdominal heat, a red face, a dry throat, heart vexation and heat in their palms. In severe cases they spit blood".

***Xin jing* 心驚, heart fright** [3] AN *shen jing* 神驚, spirit fright.
IS of mental restlessness and fearfulness. *ZBYHL* 31: 犯疔瘡，謂疔瘡欲瘥，更犯觸之，若大嗔，及食豬、魚、麻子，並狐臭人氣熏之，皆能觸犯之，則更極，乃甚於初。更令瘡熱焮腫，先寒後熱，四肢沉重，頭痛**心驚**，嘔逆煩悶，則不可治, " 'Offended pin-illness sores' is to say: When pin-illness sores are about to heal and at this stage are offended again, as for instance by a massive emotion of anger, or by meals with pork, fish, hemp seeds, or if they are exposed to human fox-odor qi – all these may offend them – they again become serious, even more so than they were originally. These [offenses] cause the sores to be hot again and make them swell. There is a feeling of cold first and of heat afterwards. The four limbs feel sunken and heavy. Headaches come with **heart fright**. Vomiting with counterflow, vexation and heart-pressure".

***Xin lou* 心漏, heart leakage** [1]
PC of → *lou chuang* 漏瘡, leaking sores, in the region of the heart and chest. *YS* 6 quotes *YJZ* 6: 時康祖大夫患**心漏**二十年，當胸數竅，血液長流，屢訪名醫，皆云不可治, "*Dai fu* Shi Kangzu suffered from **heart leakage** for twenty years, with blood and [other] liquid flowing from several openings in his chest for a long time. He repeatedly consulted eminent physicians. They all said that it could not be cured".

***Xin men* 心悶, the heart experiences heart-pressure** [28]
IS of an uncomfortable feeling of vexation and heart-pressure in the heart region. *ZBYHL* 2: 冷折於氣血，使人面青**心悶**，嘔逆吐沫，四肢痛冷, "When cold conflicts with qi and blood, this makes a person's face turn virid and his **heart experience heart-pressure**. He will vomit with counterflow, and spit foam. The four extremities ache and are cold".

***Xin nü* 心衄, spontaneous heart bleeding** [2]
PC of spitting small amounts of blood. *QJYF* 12: 治忽吐血一二口，或者**心衄**，或者內崩方 "Recipe to cure sudden spitting of one or two mouthfuls of blood, this may by **spontaneous heart bleeding**, or internal collapse".

***Xin nüe* 心瘧, heart malaria** [2]
PC of → *nüe ji* 瘧疾, malaria ailment, associated with mental conditions such as heart vexation and, in extreme cases, mental confusion, madness, and restlessness. *SW* 36: **心瘧**者，令人煩心甚，欲得清水，反寒多，不甚熱, "**Heart malaria**: it causes a person's heart to be very vexed. [Patients] long for cool water. Contrary [to what might be expected,] they are often cold and not very hot".

Xin pi tong **心脾痛, heartache and spleen pain** [7]

PC identical with → *xin fu tong* 心腹痛②, heartache and abdominal pain. *SJZL* 55: 治**心脾痛**，霍亂吐瀉，蓬莪术丸方, "To cure **heartache and spleen pain**, cholera with vomiting and outflow, [use] the recipe for the pills with *peng e zhu*".

Xin qi tong **心氣痛, central qi pain** [19]

PC with pain in the stomach as a major sign. *SJZL* 55: 治**心氣痛**，悶亂，山杏煎方, "To cure **central qi pain**, heart-pressure with [stomach] disorder, [use] the recipe with boiled *shan xing*". When the *BCGM* speaks of 心氣痛, this is mostly a reference to pain in the stomach duct. *BCGM* also has *xin qi ci tong* 心氣刺痛, central qi piercing pain; *xin qi teng tong* 心氣疼痛, central qi pain; *xin qi leng tong* 心氣冷痛, central qi cold pain.

Xin re **心熱, heat in the heart; heart heat** [38]

① PC of heat-type diseases affecting the heart. *SW* 32: **心熱**病者顏先赤, "In the case of the disease **heat in the heart**, the forehead becomes red first".

② AN *xin huo* 心火, heart fire. EA bringing forth heat-type heart disease. *WTMY* 17: 若心煩而不得睡者，**心熱**也。若但虛煩而不得臥者，膽冷也, "If the heart is vexed, and the [patient] cannot sleep, this is [because of] **heart heat**. If there is simply depletion with vexation and [the patient] cannot lie down to rest, then this is gallbladder cold".

Xin re **焮熱, scorching heat** [4]

IS apparent as localized burning heat in the skin. *ZBYHL* 36: 云是野狐尿棘刺頭，有人犯之者，則多中於人手指、足指，腫痛**焮熱**。有端居不出而著此毒者，則不必是狐尿刺也，蓋惡毒氣耳。故方亦云惡刺毒者也, "It is said that this is because the urine of a wild fox has pierced the head. When a person encounters it, he often experiences swelling, pain and **scorching heat** at the fingers and toes. If someone lives properly and does not go out, and still is affected by this poison, then this is certainly not a fox urine piercing. Rather this is malign poison qi. Hence the recipe also speaks of poisoning from a malign sting".

Xin shan **心疝, heart elevation-illness** [2]

PC of heartache caused by cold qi, and accompanied by counterflow cold in the four extremities with the lips and mouth assuming a greenish-blue color. *ZBY-HL* 20: 由陰氣積於內，寒氣不散，上衝於心，故使心痛，謂之**心疝**也。其痛也，或如錐刀所刺，或陰陰而疼，或四肢逆冷，或唇口變青，皆其候也, "When yin qi collects internally, and cold qi fails to dissipate and rushes upward against the heart, this causes heartache. One calls this **heart elevation-illness**. This pain is sometimes as if one were pierced with an awl or a knife, sometimes it is a weak pain. Or the four limbs experience counterflow cold. Or the lips and the mouth change their complexion to greenish-blue. All these are its signs".

Xin shen bu an **心神不安, restless spirit of the heart** [1]

IS identical with → *shen bu shou she* 神不守舍, unsettled spirit. *QJYF* 3: 甘草丸，治產後心虛不足，虛悸，**心神不安**, "Pills with *gan cao* cure heart depletion with insufficient [qi] following delivery, depletion palpitation, and **restless spirit of the heart**".

Xin shen bu ding **心神不定, instable spirit of the heart** [1]
IS identical with → *shen bu shou she* 神不守舍, unsettled spirit. *QJYF* 14: 治心氣不足，虛悸恐畏，悲思恍惚，**心神不定**，惕惕然驚者方, "Recipe to cure insufficiency of heart qi, depletion palpitation with fear, sorrowful pondering, absent-mindedness, **instable spirit of the heart**, and shyness".

Xin shen bu jiao **心腎不交, failure of the heart and kidneys to communicate** [3]
PC caused by a loss of balance between the kidney yin and the heart yang, often accompanied by heart palpitation and insomnia, robber sweat and involuntary emission of essence. *PJF* 33: 降心丹，治**心腎不交**，盜汗遺精, "The elixir to tame the heart cures **failure of the heart and kidneys to communicate**, with robber sweat and involuntary emission of essence".

Xin shen bu zu **心神不足, heart spirit [qi] insufficiency** [2]
PC identical with → *shen bu zu* 神不足, spirit [qi] insufficiency. *BCGM* SE *chen xiang* 沉香 quoting *BYXF* 心神不安, "restless spirit of the heart", writes: **心神不足**, "**heart spirit [qi] insufficiency**".

Xin teng **心疼, heartache** [8]
IS and PC identical with → *xin tong* 心痛. *RHZ* SE *bei ting sha* 北庭砂：女人血氣**心疼**，丈夫腰胯酸重, "In females [it cures] **heartache** because of blood and qi [abnormalities]; in males, distress and a feeling of soreness and pressure in the lower back and hips".

Xin tong **心痛, heartache** [p] AN *xin teng* 心疼.
① IS of pain felt in the heart and in the stomach pit. *JGYL* Fj: 胸痹不得臥，**心痛**徹背者，栝蔞薤白半夏湯主之, "In the case of chest blockage one cannot sleep, with **heartache** penetrating one's back, this will be controlled by a decoction with *gua lou*, *xie bai* and *ban xia*".
② PC with heartache. *SW* 17：細則氣少，澀則**心痛**, "If it is fine, then the qi is diminished. If it is rough, then the **heart aches**". *BCGM* uses *xin tong* 心痛 for a broad range of issues, including *jiu zhong xin tong* 九種心痛, the nine types of heartache, such as pain in the heart itself, etc.; *xiong bi xin tong* 胸痹心痛, chest blockage heartache, and also pain in the stomach duct; *shi ji xin tong* 食積心痛, food accumulation heartache, and pain in the gallbladder duct; *hui chong xin tong* 蛔蟲心痛, roundworm heartache.

Xin tou yang yang yu tu **心頭瀁瀁欲吐, a floating sensation on top of the heart, and an urge to vomit** [1]
IS of an uncomfortable feeling of unrest in the stomach region with an urge to vomit. *BCSY* SE *jing li* 荊瀝：飲之，去心悶煩熱，頭風旋運目眩，**心頭瀁瀁欲吐**，卒失音, "Consumed as a drink it removes heart-pressure and vexation heat, head wind, vertigo and dizziness, and a **floating sensation on top of the heart and an urge to vomit**, as well as sudden loss of one's voice".

***Xin xia ji* 心下悸, palpitation below the heart** [3]

① IS of a feeling of a racing throbbing and restlessness below the heart. *SHL* 64: 發汗過多，其人叉手自冒心，**心下悸**欲得按, "If one makes a patient sweat excessively, he will touch his heart region with both his hands joined. He experiences **palpitation below the heart** and wishes to exert pressure there".

② PC with palpitation below the heart. *JGYL* Mj: **心下悸**者，半夏麻黄丸主之, "Cases of **palpitation below the heart** are controlled by the pills with *ban xia* and *ma huang*".

***Xin xia jian* 心下堅, hardening below the heart** [4]

IS of an uncomfortable distension and heart-pressure felt in the heart pit. If pressed there, a hardening can be felt. *JGYL* Fj: 脈緊大而遲者，必**心下堅**, ""When the [movement in the] vessels is tight, massive and slow, there must be a **hardening below the heart**".

***Xin xia pi* 心下痞, obstacle-illness below the heart** [9]

PC with a feeling of fullness and heart-pressure in the stomach duct below the heart. If pressed this region is pliable and patients do not feel pain. *SHL* 154: **心下痞**，按之濡，其脈關上浮者，大黃黃連瀉心湯主之, "An **obstacle-illness below the heart**: If pressed [one's finger] can sink into it, and if the [movement in the] vessels above the pass is at the surface, it will be controlled by the decoction with *da huang* and *huang lian* that drains the heart".

***Xin xia xuan* 心下懸, dangling below the heart** [1]

PC with a feeling of the stomach duct below the heart being empty, unsettled and "dangling", i.e. not firmly fixed. *MYBL* SE *da zao* 大棗：療**心下懸**，除腸澼, "It cures **dangling below the heart**; it eliminates intestinal flush".

***Xin xian* 囟陷, caved-in top of the head** [6]

PC of small children with a fontanelle that has not closed yet and is caved in. *ZBYHL* 48：**囟陷**候，此謂囟陷下不平也，由腸內有熱，熱氣熏臟，臟熱，即渴引飲。而小便泄痢者，即腑臟血氣虛弱，不能上充髓腦，故囟陷也, "Signs of a **caved-in top of the head**: That is to say, the top of the head is caved in and not flat. The reason is: When there is heat in the intestines, the heat qi will fumigate the depots. When the depots are hot, then [the patient] will be thirsty and seeks to drink. Now, when the urine flows freely, blood and qi in the palaces and depots will be depleted and weak, and cannot ascend to fill the brain with marrow. This results in a **caved-in top of the head**".

***Xin xian* 心癇, heart epilepsy** [2]

PC of a → *dian xian* 癲癇, peak-illness with epilepsy, which, at the time of its outbreaks, causes the patient's four limbs to twitch, with a red face, heat below the heart, shortness of qi and a breathing that is weak and fast. *QJYF* 5: **心癇**之為病，面赤，心下有熱，短氣息微數, "The disease of **heart epilepsy**: a red face, heat below the heart, shortness of qi, weak and fast breathing".

***Xin xiong jia cuo* 心胸甲錯, scaly skin on the heart and chest** [4]

IS of a dry and rough skin in the region of the heart (i.e. stomach) and chest coming off as flakes. It feels thorny when touched and looks like fish scales.

BCTJ SE *yi yi ren* 薏苡人：韋丹治肺癰，**心胸甲錯**者，淳苦酒煮薏苡人令濃，微溫頓服之, "If *wei* elixir is used to cure lung obstruction-illness and **scaly skin on the heart and chest**, one boils *yi yi ren* in pure bitter wine until a dense liquid is left and ingests it once when it is slightly warm".

Xin xu **心虛, heart depletion; hollow** [38]

① PC of a depleted heart and a blockage of heart functions. *SW* 10: 思慮而**心虛**，故邪從之, "One thinks and ponders and the result is **heart depletion**. Hence evil [qi] follows this [lead and enters]".

② Condition of pharmaceutical substances, identical with → *xu* 虛③, hollow. *LGPZL* SE *bing lang* 檳榔：半白半黑並**心虛**者，不入藥用, "Those that are half white, half black and **hollow**, do not lend themselves to pharmaceutical use".

Xin xuan **心痃, heart string-illness** [2]

PC of → *xuan* 痃, string-illness, caused by a consumption of *ren shen* 人參 in summer. *BCGM* SE *ren shen* 人參, Zheng wu 正誤, Correction of errors, quotes *LGPZL* 4: 夏中少使，發**心痃**之患也. 李時珍認為：雷斆反謂發**心痃**之患，非矣。痃乃臍旁積氣，非心病也。人參能養正破堅積，豈有發痃之理, "[Lei Xu states:] "In summer, one should consume only small amounts lest he suffers from **heart string-illness**. LSZ: When Lei Xu stated that [*ren shen*] causes ailments of stomach turnover and **heart string-illness**, he was wrong. The string-illness is a qi accumulation to the side of the navel; it is not a heart disease. *Ren shen* is capable of nourishing proper [qi] and breaking up hard accumulations. How could it be that it leads to a string-illness?"

Xin xuan **心懸, heart suspension** [1]

PC with a feeling of the stomach not being firmly fixed and dangling in a hollow space. *BJ* SE *bai hao* 白蒿：療**心懸**，少食常飢, "It cures **heart suspension**; [patients] eat small amounts, and are always hungry".

Xin xuan **心眩, heart dizziness** [2]

PC of dizziness experienced by females with extreme feelings of → *xuan yun* 眩運, vertigo, and a perception of heaven and earth revolving. *FRDQLF* 4: 治女人頭旋，即天動地轉，名曰**心眩**, "To cure females with their head revolving, that is, as if heaven and earth were moving around them. This is called '**heart dizziness**'".

Xin zhong **焮腫, scorching swelling** [3]

IS identical with → *re zhong* 熱腫, heat and swelling, a topical swelling together with a hot skin. *SJZL* 183: 發背癰疽疼痛，熱毒**焮腫**，赤硬有膿, "Effusion of the back with painful obstruction- and impediment-illnesses, and heat poison [causing] **scorching swelling**. The area is red, hard, and contains pus".

Xin zhong **囟腫, swollen top of the head** [4]

PC of small children with a fontanelle that has not closed yet and is swollen and protruding.. *XEWSZWLF* 17: 陰陽氣逆，上衝而**囟腫**也。熱則腫而軟，冷則腫而硬, "Yin and yang qi rush upward in counterflow, causing a **swollen top of the head**. If it is heat then the swelling is soft. If it is cold then the swelling is hard".

Xin zhong **心忪, heart agitation** [10]

IS of a feeling of fear and restlessness in the heart without any apparent reason. *ZBYHL* 12: 穀疸之狀，寒熱不食，食畢頭眩，**心忪**怫鬱不安而發黃, "The appearance of grain *dan*-illness: [patients] experience alternating sensations of cold and heat and do not [wish to] eat. Following a meal, they develop head spin, with **heart agitation**, anger with pent-up [qi] and restlessness, and they develop a yellow complexion".

Xing chi **行遲, retarded [beginning of] walking** [4]

PC of children with an inability, at age three, to walk. *TPSHF* 89：骨氣虛弱，筋脈無力，故**行遲**也, "The bone qi is depleted and weak. The sinew vessels have no strength. Hence [these children have] a **retarded [beginning of] walking**".

Xing han **形寒 body cold** [1]

EA indicating the affection of the body by cold. *LS* 4: **形寒**, 寒飲則傷肺, "If in the case of **body cold** one consumes cold beverages, this will harm the lung".

Xiong bi **胸痹, chest blockage** [33]

PC of → *bi* 痹① a), blockage disease, brought forth by blood stasis, cold[-induced qi] conglomeration, or phlegm nodes, with a feeling of pressure and pain in the chest and back. *JGYL* Fj: **胸痹**之病，喘息咳唾，胸背痛，短氣, "The disease of **chest blockage** [is marked by] panting, coughing and spitting, pain in the chest and back, and shortness of qi".

Xiong pi **胸痞, chest obstacle-illness** [4]

PC of an uncomfortable feeling of distension and heart-pressure in the region of the stomach, chest and flanks, accompanied by dry retching and belching. *SYJYBZFL* 4: **胸痞**證者，胃中不和，心下堅硬，乾嘔，惡寒汗出，噫氣不除, "As for the condition of '**chest obstacle-illness**', it comprises discomfort in the stomach, a hardening below the heart, dry vomiting, an aversion to cold and sweating, as well as belching that does not end".

Xiong shou shang **熊獸傷, harm caused by bears and [other] animals** [1]

PC of injuries inflicted by wild animals. *BCGM* Bai bing zhu zhi yao 百病主治藥 quoting the main entries on *su* 粟 and *li* 栗：熊虎爪傷, "Harm caused by the claws of bears and tigers", writes: **熊獸傷, "Harm caused by bears and other beasts"**.

Xiong zhong re **胸中熱, heat in the chest** [4]

① PC of heat-type diseases in the chest. *SW* 32: 熱病氣穴：三椎下間, 主**胸中熱**, "In the case of heat disease, the qi holes [to be treated are the following: Those] located below the third vertebra rule **heat in the chest**".

② IS of heat in the chest. *SW* 63: 邪客於手陽明之絡，令人氣滿胸中，喘息而支胠，**胸中熱**, "When an evil has settled in the network [vessels] of the hand yang brilliance [conduits], it makes the [affected] person experience qi fullness inside of his chest. His breath is panting and he has a [feeling of] propping [fullness] in his upper flanks. There is **heat in the chest**".

Xiu ming **羞明, shy of light** [15]

IS of a feeling of roughness and pain in the eyes accompanied by tears when looking into a source of light. *TPSHF* 87: 治小兒腦疳，鼻塞頭痛，眼目昏暗，**羞明**怕日，吹鼻龍腦散方, "Recipe for a powder with *long nao* to be blown into the nose to cure brain *gan*-illness in childen, with stuffed nose and headache, dim vision, and **shyness of light** associated with a fear of the sun".

Xiu xi li **休息痢, dormant free-flux illness** [16]

PC of → *li ji* 痢疾, free-flux illness, that at times is dormant, at times is active and cannot be healed for an extended period of time. *ZBYHL* 17: 其痢乍發乍止，謂之**休息痢**也, "When the free-flux illness at times is active and then rests again, this is called '**dormant free-flux illness** '".

Xu **虛, depleted [movement in the vessels]; depletion; hollow; false** [p]

① AN *ti xu* 體虛, body depletion. PM of a depletion of the proper qi of the human body, with a diminution of physiological functions and a decrease of the organism's defense potential. *SW* 10: 是謂五並，**虛**而相併者也, "These are the so-called 'five accumulations.' In the case of a **depletion** mutual accumulations occur".

② AN *xu bing* 虛病, depletion disease; *xu ji* 虛疾, depletion ailment; *xu zheng* 虛證, depletion condition; *xu ruo* 虛弱, depletion and weakness; *xu lei* 虛羸, depletion and thinness. PC of all types of a depleted and weak condition brought forth by → *xu* 虛①, depletion. *SW* 20: 實則瀉之，**虛**則補之, "In case of repletion, drain it. In case of **depletion**, supplement it". As the nature of the items depleted varies, there are also → *qi xu* 氣虛, qi depletion; → *xue xu* 血虛, blood depletion; → *yang xu* 陽虛 yang [qi] depletion; → *yin xu* 陰虛, yin [qi] depletion., as well as conditions of depletion associated with individual depots and palaces.

③ AN *ti xu* 體虛, hollow body;; *nei xu* 內虛, hollow interior; *xin xu* 心虛, hollow center..Pharmaceutical substances of a loose or hollow structure. *BCJJZ* preface: 以藥升分之者，謂藥有**虛**實、輕重，不得用斤兩，則以昇平之, "To measure [pharmaceutical drugs] with a 'pharmaceutical bushel' has the following rationale: some drugs are **hollow**, others not; some are light, others are heavy – they cannot be measured on the basis of their weight. They should be measured using a bushel".

④ "False". *BCGM* Shen nong ben cao ming li 神農本草名例, "On the names in Shen nong's Materia Medica": 名實既**虛**，寒溫多謬, "The associations of names and substances are **false**; [statements on] the cold and warm [nature of substances] are wrong".

Xu bai **虛敗, depletion detriment** [1]

EA identical with → *xu jie* 虛竭, depletion exhaustion. *HJJF* 7: 兼治乾濕脚氣，消中消渴，及諸風氣等疾，由腎氣**虛敗**者, "It cures both dry and moist leg qi, melting center and melting with thirst, as well as all ailments associated with wind qi that arise from the kidney qi **depletion detriment**".

***Xu bei* 虛憊, depletion and fatigue** [9]

① PC identical with → *xu* 虛②, depletion. *ZBYHL* 38: 婦人月水下，惡血未盡，其人**虛憊**, "When women discharge their monthly liquid, and the malign blood is not discharged completely, such persons have **depletion and fatigue**".

② IS identical withpfeilpfeil *xu fa* 虛乏, depletion and exhaustion. *TPSHF* 44: 腰痛不可忍，**虛憊**無力，宜服鹿角丸方, "If [a patient's] lower back is in unbearable pain, and if [that person] suffers from **depletion and fatigue** and lack of strength, the recipe to ingest the pills with deer horn is advisable".

***Xu bi* 虛閉, depletion closure** [15]

PC of constipation and anuria brought forth by depletion. *HYXS* Lj: 治大府**虛閉**，氣連日不通, "To cure **depletion closure** of the large [intestine] palace, if qi cannot pass for several consecutive days".

***Xu bing* 虛病, depletion disease** [3]

PC identical with → *xu* 虛②, depletion. *GZYL* Yang lao lun 養老論：局方用暖劑，為劫**虛病**也, "The *JF* uses warming remedies to end **depletion disease**".

***Xu chuan* 虛喘, depletion panting** [3]

PC of → *chuan* 喘, panting, resulting from an insufficiency of proper qi. *YXL* SE *huang qi* 黄耆：內補，主**虛喘**, "For internal supplementation. It controls **depletion panting**".

***Xu fa* 虛乏, depletion and exhaustion** [17]

① PC identical with → *xu* 虛②, depletion. *MYBL* SE *yi tang* 飴糖：主補**虛乏**，止渴，去血, "It controls supplementation of **depletion and exhaustion**, stops thirst, and removes blood".

② IS of decreased body functions and abilities. *ZBYHL* 5: 夫人渴病者，皆由臟腑不和，經絡虛竭所為。故病雖瘥，血氣未復，仍**虛乏**也, "Now, when someone has a thirst disease, this is always the result of a disharmony among depots and palaces with a depletion-exhaustion of conduits and network [vessels]. Hence the disease may have been healed, but as long as blood and qi have not recovered yet, the status is one of **depletion and exhaustion**".

Xu feng **虛風, depletion wind** [10]

① EA of non-seasonal climatic conditions able to cause disease in man. *LS* 50: 黃色薄皮弱肉者，不勝春之**虛風**, "[Patients] whose skin is yellow and thin, and whose flesh is weak, are unable to overcome a spring-time **depletion wind**".

② PC identical with → *man pi feng* 慢脾風, slow spleen wind. *YTBW* 2: 慢脾風一名**虛風**, "Another name for slow spleen wind is **depletion wind**".

***Xu han* 虛寒, depletion cold** [96] AN *xu leng* 虛冷.

PC brought forth by inadequate presence and lowered function of yang qi. *JGYL* Fj: 便難，兩胠疼痛，此**虛寒**從下上也, "In the case of difficult defecation, and when the two flanks are painful, this is because **depletion cold** is rising from below".

***Xu han* 虛汗, depletion sweating** [35]

PC of sweating brought forth by an insufficiency of qi and blood, i.e. of yang and yin qi. *BJ* SE *song luo* 松蘿：主嗔怒邪氣，止**虛汗**，頭風，女子陰寒腫

痛, "It controls evil qi of anger and resentment; it ends **depletion sweating**, head wind, as well as cold swelling and pain in the private parts of females".

Xu han li **虛寒痢, depletion-cold free-flux illness** [1]
PC of → *leng li* 冷痢, cold free-flux illness, with body depletion. *BCGM* Bai bing zhu zhi yao 百病主治藥：糯殼爆米花，以薑汁服，治禁口痢、**虛寒痢**, "Shells of glutinous rice and puffed rice ingested with *jiang* juice cure lock-jaw with free-flux illness, as well as **depletion-cold free-flux illness**".

Xu han nüe ji **虛寒瘧疾, depletion-cold malaria ailment** [2]
PC of → *han nüe* 寒瘧, cold malaria, affecting persons with a depletion. *BCGM* SE *yang* 羊 quotes *JYF*: **虛寒瘧疾**：羊肉作臛餅，飽食之, "For the **ailment of depletion-cold malaria** prepare a mutton meat cake and [have the patient] eat it to his fill".

Xu han xia li **虛寒下痢, depletion-cold discharge with free-flux illness** [1]
PC identical with → *xu han li* 虛寒痢, depletion-cold free-flux illness. *BCGM* SE *gang tie* 鋼鐵 quotes *RCF*: **虛寒下痢**：腸滑不禁。針砂七錢半，官桂一錢，枯礬一錢，為末，以涼水調攤臍上下，縛之。當覺大熱，以水潤之。可用三四次，名玉胞肚, "In the case of **depletion-cold discharge with free-flux illness**, the intestines experience a smooth passage that cannot be stopped. Prepare a powder of *zhen sha*, 7 ½ *qian*, *guan gui*, 1 *qian*, and *ku fan*, 1 *qian*. Mix it with cold water, smear it on the region above and below the [patient's] navel, and bandage it. When he has a sensation of massive heat, moisten it with water. This can be applied three or four times. It is called 'jade embraced abdomen'".

Xu han xie li **虛寒泄痢, depletion-cold outflow with free-flux illness** [1]
PC identical with → *xu han li* 虛寒痢, depletion-cold free-flux illness. *BCGM* SE *dao* 稻,: 稻米暖脾胃，止**虛寒泄痢**, "*Dao mi* warms the spleen and stomach, and ends **depletion-cold outflow with free-flux illness**".

Xu hou **虛吼, depletion roar** [1] AN *xu ming* 虛鳴.
IS of rattling sounds in the intestines brought forth by stagnating water in the abdomen. *YXL* SE *hou pu* 厚朴：能主療積年冷氣，腹內雷鳴**虛吼**，宿食不消，除痰飲，去結水, "It is able to cure cold qi that has accumulated over years, thunderous rumbles and **depletion roar** in the abdomen, with food that remains in the body overnight and fails to dissolve, and eliminates phlegm rheum, as well as bound water".

Xu hua **虛滑, depleted and slippery** [8]
PC of an insufficiency of proper qi that has lost its power of securing and containing, eventually resulting in diarrhea. *ZBYHL* 17: 腸間**虛滑**，所以因下痢而便腸垢也, "When the intestines are **depleted and slippery,** this will result in discharge with free-flux illness with a relief of intestinal filth".

Xu huang **虛黃, depletion jaundice** [1]
IS of a skin that turns yellow and loses its luster. *SJZL* 61: 面目**虛黃**，不能食，宜服葫蘆飲方, "Face and eyes have **depletion jaundice**. [Patients] are unable to consume food. The recipe to ingest the drink with *hu lu* is advisable".

***Xu huo* 虛火, depletion fire** [21]

PC identical with → *xu re* 虛熱, depletion heat. *DXXF* 1: 實火可瀉，黃連解毒之類；**虛火**可補，小便降火極速, "Repletion fire can be drained with substances resolving poison such as *huang lian*. **Depletion fire** can be supplemented; urine brings the fire down very fast".

***Xu ji* 虛疾, depletion ailment** [2]

PC identical with → *xu* 虛②, depletion. *QJYF* 29: 凡諸**虛疾**，水穀沉結流離者，當灸腹背宜多，不可過百壯, "For all types of **depletion ailments**, when water and grain (i.e. liquid and solid food) sink deep in the body and form nodes, or when they flow away or dissipate, it is appropriate to cauterize the abdomen and back many times, but not more than a hundred times".

***Xu jia* 虛家, person with a depletion** [1]

Patient with a depleted and weak body. *SHL* 166: 諸亡血**虛家**，不可與瓜蒂散, "The powder with *gua di* must never be given to **persons with a depletion** who have lost blood".

***Xu jie* 虛竭, depletion exhaustion** [4] AN *xu bai* 虛敗, depletion detriment.

EA of an extreme weaking of a person's physical body or capabilities that may result in various diseases. *ZBYHL* 5: 渴病者，皆由臟腑不和，經絡**虛竭**所為, "Now, when someone has a thirst disease, this is always the result of a disharmony among depots and palaces with a **depletion-exhaustion** of conduits and network [vessels]".

***Xu kun* 虛困, depletion weariness** [1]

IS of sleepiness and weariness brought forth by exhaustion. *TPSHF* 18: 治熱病鼻衄出多，面無顏色，昏悶**虛困**，熟乾地黃散方, "To cure profuse nose-bleeding associated with heat disease, when the face loses its color, with dizziness, heart-pressure, and **depletion weariness**, [use] the recipe for a powder with heat-dried *di huang*".

***Xu lao* 虛勞, depletion exhaustion** [159] AD *lao* 勞; AN *lao ji* 勞疾, exhaustion ailment; *lao bing* 勞病, exhaustion disease; *lao zheng* 勞證, exhaustion condition; *lao sun* 勞損, exhaustion detriment; *lao shang* 勞傷, exhaustion harm; *lao jian* 勞劣, exhaustion diminution; *lao qi* 勞氣, qi exhaustion.

PC of → *xu zheng* 虛證, depletion condition, brought forth by harm affecting the human body, its depots and palaces, and its qi and blood. These conditions are also called → *xu sun* 虛損, depletion detriment. Depletion exhaustion also includes pathological conditions manifesting themselves as infectious or consumptive depletion conditions, such as → *lao zhai* 勞瘵, exhaustion consumption, and → *chuan shi lao* 傳屍勞, exhaustion through corpse [evil] transmission. *JGYL* Fj: **虛勞**裏急，諸不足，黃芪建中湯主之, "Cases of **depletion exhaustion** with internal tightness and an all-around insufficiency, they are controlled by the decoction with *huang qi* that strengthens the center".

***Xu lao feng* 虛勞風, depletion-exhaustion wind** [1]

PC identical with → *lao feng* 勞風, exhaustion wind. *YSZY* SE *ye tuo* 野駝：駝峰，治**虛勞風**。有冷積者，用葡萄酒溫調峰子油，服之良, "Camel hump serves to cure **depletion-exhaustion wind**. For those with cold accumulation, mix warm grape wine and with the oil from a hump. To ingest this has good results".

***Xu lei* 虛羸, depletion and thinness** [41] AN *lei ruo* 羸弱, thinness and weakness; *shou sun* 瘦損, emaciation detriment; *xu shou* 虛瘦, depletion emaciation.

PC of → *xu* 虛, depletion, with an emaciated physical appearance, a depleted and weak proper qi, and decreased functions of the depots and palaces. *BJ* SE *shu yu* 薯蕷：補**虛羸**，除寒熱邪氣, "It supplements **depletion and thinness**, and it eliminates the evil qi of cold and heat".

***Xu leng* 虛冷, depletion cold** [76]

PC identical with → *xu han* 虛寒. *SHL* 122: 不能消穀，以胃中**虛冷**，故吐也, "If someone is unable to digest grain (i.e. solid food), this is because of **depletion cold** in his stomach. Hence he will vomit".

***Xu leng li* 虛冷痢, depletion-cold free-flux illness** [1]

PC identical with → *xu han li* 虛寒痢, depletion-cold free-flux illness. *BCGM* Bai bing zhu zhi yao 百病主治藥 quotes *SLBC* SE *niu gan* 牛肝：牛肝、牛䏶，**虛冷痢**，並醋煮食, "For **depletion-cold free-flux illness**, ox bile and ox stomach are to be consumed boiled in vinegar".

***Xu li* 虛痢, depletion free-flux illness** [14]

PC of old persons and women in childbed who have a weak body and suffer from diarrhea, or if depletion in other persons lasts for an extended period of time, eventually resulting in diarrhea. *HYBC* SE *pi pa* 蓽茇：主老冷心痛，水瀉**虛痢**, "It controls chronic cold with heartache, watery outflow and **depletion free-flux illness**".

***Xu lie* 虛劣, depletion and diminution** [3]

PC identical with → *xu* 虛②, depletion. *QJYiF* 18: 前胡建中湯, 主大勞**虛劣**，寒熱嘔逆, "The 'decoction with *qian hu* to strengthen the center' controls massive exhaustion, **depletion and diminution**, cold and heat spells, as well as vomiting and counterflow".

***Xu lin* 虛淋, depletion dripping** [1]

PC identical with → *lao lin* 勞淋, exhaustion dripping. *BCGM* Bai bing zhu zhi yao 百病主治藥：五淋者，熱淋、氣淋、**虛淋**、膏淋、沙石淋也, "The five types of dripping: heat dripping, qi dripping, **depletion dripping**, pasty dripping, and sand dripping".

***Xu lou* 虛漏, depletion leakage** [1]

PC of a loss of semen brought forth by insufficient proper qi associated with a loss of its power of securing and containing. *KBBC* SE *yi zhi zi* 益智子：主遺精**虛漏**，小便餘瀝，益氣安神, "It controls loss of essence/semen associated with **depletion leakage**; trickling of residual urine, and it increases the qi and pacifies the spirit".

***Xu man* 虛滿, depletion and fullness** [2]

IS of an uncomfortable feeling of fullness brought forth by qi depletion or stagnant qi. *SW* 45: 少陰厥逆，**虛滿**嘔變，下泄清，治主病者, "Recession with counterflow in the minor yin [conduit results in the following]: **depletion and**

fullness, changing to vomiting, and a discharge with clear outflow. Treat the [conduit] ruling the disease".

***Xu mi* 虛秘, depletion blockage** [8] AN *xu zao* 虛燥, depletion desiccation.
PC of constipation brought forth by depletion. *SJZL* 47: 氣虛津液枯乾，大便**虛秘**者，最宜服之，磨滯丸方, "In the case of qi depletion and when the body liquids have dried up, with defecation undergoing **depletion blockage**, the most appropriate medication to ingest is the recipe for 'pills that grind sluggishness'".

***Xu ming* 虛鳴, depletion rumble** [2]
IS a) of a feeling of sounds in the ears brought forth by a depletion. *RHZ* SE *ze xie* 澤瀉：主頭旋，耳**虛鳴**，筋骨攣縮, "It controls spinning head, **depletion rumble** in the ears, and contraction of the sinews and bones. b) Identical with → *xu hou* 虛吼, depletion roar. *HYBC* SE *yi zhi zi* 益智子：主水腫浮氣，結聚宿滯不消，腹中**虛鳴**, "It controls water swelling and floating qi, nodular collections that abide, are sluggish, and fail to dissolve, and **depletion rumble** in the abdomen".

***Xu nei* 虛餒, depleted and feeble** [1]
PC identical with → *xu* 虛②, depletion. *BCGM* SE *sheng ma* 升麻 LSZ: 此乃賦素弱，元氣**虛餒**，及勞役飢飽，生冷內傷，脾胃引經最要藥也, "This is a most important remedy guiding through the conduits of the spleen and stomach for treating patients with a weak constitution, whose original qi is **depleted and feeble**, and who, hungry after arduous labor, [eat] to repletion, with fresh and cold [food] leading to inner harm".

***Xu qi* 虛氣, depletion qi** [7]
PC of depletion and weakness together with sluggish qi and counterflowing qi. *ZHF* 3: 凡此滿或者**虛氣**，或者風冷氣，或者水飲氣，此方皆治之, "This recipe cures all cases of fullness associated with either **depletion qi,** or wind and cold qi, or water and rheum qi".

***Xu qie* 虛怯, depletion; hollow** [3]
① PM identical with → *xu* 虛①, depletion. *SYDXF* 2: 治**虛怯**人患瘧，未可進常山等藥, "To cure people with **depletion** who suffer from malaria, it is not appropriate to prescribe drugs such as *chang shan*".
② Identical with → *xu* 虛③, hollow. *SLBC* SE *su mi* 粟米：少**虛怯**，只爲灰中種之，又不鋤治故也, "It is very rare that they are **hollow**. They can only be grown in ashes. This is because they cannot be treated with a hoe".

***Xu re* 虛熱, depletion heat** [93] AN *xu huo* 虛火, depletion fire; *yin huo* 陰火, yin fire.
PC of a) fever brought about by a depletion of yin, *jin* 津 liquid, qi and blood. *ZBYHL* 9: 五臟有**虛熱**，脾胃不和，津液竭少, "The five depots have **depletion heat**. The spleen and stomach have lost their balance, and the body-liquids are diminished". b) Abdominal extension due to harm caused by cold, without blockage of stool and urine. *ZJSHL* 4: 心下痞，按之濡…**虛熱**也, "A obstacle-illness below the heart. It appears soggy when pressed. …This is **depletion heat**". When the *BCGM* refers to *xu re* 虛熱, depletion heat, it mostly means a).

Xu ren **虛人, to cause depletion in a person; person with a depletion** [21]
① A person caused to have a depletion condition. *QJYF* 5: 紫丸無所不療，雖下不**虛人**, "There is no [ailment] Purple Pills are unable to heal. Although they drain, they do not **deplete the patient**".
② A person with a depleted and weak body. *ZBYHL* 6: **虛人**亦治，又與此藥相宜, "**Persons with a depletion** can also be cured. This medication is perfectly suited for them".

Xu ruo **虛弱, depletion and weakness** [43] AN *lei ruo* 羸弱, thinness and weakness. PC identical with → *xu* 虛②, depletion. *SHL* 174: 附子三枚恐多也，**虛弱**家及產婦，宜減服之, "[In some cases] three pieces of *fu zi* may be too much. For persons with **depletion and weakness**, and women who have just given birth, it is appropriate to ingest less".

Xu shou **虛瘦, depletion emaciation; hollow and shriveled** [3]
① PC identical with → *xu lei* 虛羸, depletion and thinness. *PJF* 353: 黃芪飲子，治產後體**虛瘦**，四肢少力, "The drink with *huang qi* cures physical **depletion emaciation** following delivery, with the four limbs lacking strength".
② Designation of pharmaceutical substances that are hollow and shriveled. *BCGM* SE *bai bu* 百部：其根長者近尺，新時亦肥實，但乾則**虛瘦**無脂潤爾, "The root is almost one *chi* long. When it is fresh, it is fat and solid. But when dried it is **hollow and shriveled** and lacks fat and moisture".

Xu shui **畜水, amassed water** [2] AW *shui xu* 水蓄, water amassment.
PC of water that fails to pass on and collects in the realm of the lower burner instead, causing a lower bloated abdomen with blocked urination. *BCGM* SE hua shi 滑石 quoting *SHZG* Mj: 益元散…消**蓄水**，止渴利中, "The Powder to Benefit the Original [Qi]…dissolves **amassed water**, ends thirst und makes the center passable", writes: 益元散…止渴，消**畜水**, "The Powder to Benefit the Original [Qi]… ends thirst and dissolves **amassed water**".

Xu sun **虛損, depletion detriment** [121]
PC of → *xu* 虛, depletion, brought forth by various injuries. *MJ* 2: 寸口脈濡，陽氣弱，自汗出，是**虛損**病, "If the [movement in the] vessels at the inch opening is soggy, if the yang qi is weak, and if the patient sweats spontaneously, this is the disease **depletion detriment**".

Xu xie **虛邪, depletion evil** [2]
EA of evil qi originating in the mother depot. *NJ* 58: 從後來者為**虛邪**，從前來者為實邪, "Those coming from behind (in the Five Phases sequence of mutual generation) represent a **depletion evil**. Those coming from ahead represent a repletion evil".

Xu xie **虛泄, depletion outflow** [10]
PC of old people, women in childbed, or persons after an illness who have a weak body and whose depots and palaces are depleted and weak, resulting in diarrhea. *WTMY* 6: 療中焦虛寒洞泄，人參湯補**虛泄**方, "To cure depletion cold in the central burner with outflow, [use] the recipe for a decoction with *ren shen* to supplement **depletion outflow**".

***Xu xie* 虛瀉, depletion outflow** [4]

PC identical with → *xu xie* 虛泄. *HYBC* SE *ju jiang* 蒟醬：主咳逆上氣，心腹蟲痛，胃弱**虛瀉**，霍亂吐逆，解酒食味, "It controls cough with qi rising in counterflow, bug pain in the heart and abdomen, stomach weakness with **depletion outflow**, cholera with spitting counterflow. It resolves [the bad] flavor of wine and food".

***Xu xue* 畜血, amassed blood** [10]

① EA of → *yu xue* 瘀血②, stagnant blood, which has merged with internal heat. *SHL* 237: 其人喜忘者，必有**蓄血**, "When such persons have a tendency to be forgetful the reason must be **amassed blood**".

② PC brought forth by a merger of stagnant blood with heat when, during an episode of harm caused by cold, heat abounds and meets stagnant blood. The major clinical signs are a hot body, hardening of the lower abdomen, hardening of stools, free flow of urine, and a tendency to be forgetful. In severe cases patients behave as if they were mad. *SHMLL* Mj: **蓄血**之證，又有輕重焉。如狂也，喜忘也，皆蓄血之甚者，須抵當湯丸以下之, "The conditions of **amassed blood** may be light or severe. They may include states like madness and a tendency to be forgeful. In all severe cases of amassed blood one must use an appropriate decoction or pills to discharge it". *BCGM* quotes 蓄血 as **畜血**.

***Xu yi* 虛遺, depletion efflux** [1]

PC identical with → *xu lou* 虛漏, depletion dribbling. *BCGM* Bai bing zhu zhi yao: 白膠，**虛遺**，酒服, "*Bai jiao*: for **depletion efflux** ingest with wine".

***Xu zao* 虛燥, depletion desiccation; hollow and desiccated** [3]

① PC of insufficient body liquids and blood losing their moistening and nourishing functions. *PJF* 207: 痢，則津液空竭，臟腑**虛燥**, "As a result of free-flux illness the body liquids are exhausted and the depots and palaces have **depletion desiccation**".

② Hollow and desiccated pharmaceutical substances. *BCTJ* SE *huo xiang* 藿香 quotes *FYHXF*: 零藿**虛燥**。古人乃以合熏香, "*Ling huo* is **hollow and desiccated**. The ancients used it for preparing incense".

***Xu zhai* 虛瘵, depletion consumption** [1]

PC identical with → *lao zhai* 勞瘵, exhaustion consumption. *HSYT* Lj RE *lu zui wan* 鹿 峻丸, pills with *lu zui*: 用起**虛瘵**危疾尤捷, "They offer especially quick results when they are used to raise patients from as dangerous a disease as **depletion consumption**".

***Xu zhang* 虛脹, depletion with distension** [13]

IS of an uncomfortable feeling of distension in the abdomen or affecting other parts of the body, brought forth by qi depletion or qi stagnation. *JGYL* Mj: **虛脹**者為氣, "In the case of **depletion with distension**, the qi is involved".

***Xu zheng* 虛證, depletion condition** [5]

PC identical with → *xu* 虛②, depletion. *SYDXF* 8: 薑朮湯，治**虛證**停飲，怔忡, "Decoction with *jiang* and *zhu* cures **depletion condition** and stagnating rheum, as well as fearsome throbbing".

Xu zhong **虛腫, depletion swelling** [23]

① PC of → *zhong ji* 腫疾, swelling ailment, brought forth by qi depletion. *ZBY-HL* 3: 夫病後，經絡既虛，受於風濕，膚腠閉塞，榮衛不利，氣不宣洩，故致**虛腫**, "Now, when conduits and network [vessels] are depleted after a disease, and they receive wind and moisture, then the interstices are closed and neither camp nor guardian [qi] can pass. The qi is unable to flow off. Hence this leads to **depletion swelling**". In the *BCGM* the concept of 'depletion swelling' is rather broad. It sometimes refers to swelling ailments brought forth by qi stagnation or by stagnant water, e.g. Bai bing zhu zhi yao 百病主治藥：**虛腫**者屬氣, "**Depletion swelling** is associated with qi;" 水氣**虛腫**, "**depletion swelling** [because of] water qi".

② IS of massive swelling showing, when pressed, no hardness. *QJYF* 9: 五香麻黃湯，治傷寒忽發腫，或著四肢，或在胸背，**虛腫**，浮如吹狀, "The 'decoction with *ma huang* and five fragrant ingredients' cures harm caused by cold without subsequent swelling, sometimes affecting the four limbs, sometimes the chest and back, **depletion swelling** floating on the surface as if blown up".

Xuan **痃, string-illness** [p] AN → *xuan qi* 痃氣, string-illness qi.

PC of acute pain located in the abdomen to the left and right of the umbilicus. *TPSHF* 49: **痃**者，在腹內近臍左右，各有一條筋脈急痛，大者如臂，次者如指, 因氣而起，如弦之狀，名曰痃氣也. "**String-illness** is situated in the abdomen immediately to the left and right of the navel. On both sides a line of sinew vessels causes acute pain. Large ones are the size of an arm; smaller ones the size of a finger. One calls this 痃氣, 'string-illness qi', because the formation of the qi assumes the shape of a string (弦 *xian*)".

Xuan **眩, vertigo** [p]

IS identical with → *xuan yun* 眩運, vertigo. *LS* 20: 大便難，肩背頸項痛，時**眩**, "Defecation is difficult. The shoulders, back, nape and neck ache. At times [patients experience] **vertigo**".

Xuan **癬, *xuan*-illness** [p] AN *xuan chuang* 癬瘡, *xuan*-illness sores; *chuang xuan* 瘡癬.

PC a) of dermal lesions with initially erythema, papules, and itching gradually extending in all directions to form an irregular ring with clear boundaries. The skin is slightly elevated with small papules, blisters, and/or scales and scraps. The central lesion may appear to heal spontaneously, and it may reappear. *ZBY-HL* 35: **癬**病之狀，皮肉隱胗如錢文，漸漸增長，或圓或斜，癢痛，有匡郭，裏生蟲，搔之有汁, "The signs of the disease ***xuan*-illness**: the skin and flesh develop dormant papules like script on a coin. This grows gradually larger. Sometimes it is round; sometimes its circumference is irregular. There is itching and pain. The boundaries are marked by a wall. Inside it grows worms. When scratched, liquid appears". b) CD of local lesions with itching, release of liquid and shedding of scabs. *QJYiF* 13: 頭瘡禿**癬**，醋酒洗去痂, "For head sores, baldness, and ***xuan*-illness**, rinse with vinegar and wine to remove the crust".

***Xuan chuang* 癬瘡, *xuan*-illness sores** [28]

PC identical with → *xuan* 癬, *xuan*-illness. *WTMY* 30: **癬瘡**方一十一首, "Eleven recipes for ***xuan*-illness sores**".

***Xuan dao* 眩倒, dizziness with fall** [2] AW *xuan pu* 眩仆.

IS of severe vertigo with the patient being unable to stand securely, or even falling to the ground. *MYBL* SE *du ruo* 杜若：主**眩倒**，止痛，除口臭氣, "It controls **dizziness with fall**, ends pain, and eliminates malodorous qi from the mouth".

***Xuan jia* 痃瘕, string-illness with conglomeration-illness** [5]

PC identical with → *xuan pi* 痃癖, string-illness with aggregation-illness. *BCGM* SE *bie* 鱉：鱉色青入肝，故所主者，瘧勞寒熱，**痃瘕**驚癇, "Soft-shelled turtles have a greenish-blue color and enter the liver. Hence they master malaria exhaustion with alternating sensations of cold and heat, **string-illness with conglomeration-illness**, and fright epilepsy".

***Xuan jie* 癬疥, *xuan*-illness and *jie*-illness** [1]

PC identical with → *jie xuan* 疥癬, *jie*-illness and *xuan*-illness. *BCSY* SE *ren ni* 人溺：口中涎及唾，取平明未語者，塗**癬疥**良, "Take saliva and spittle from [the patient's] mouth in the morning before he has begun to speak and smear on [the skin sections affected by] ***xuan*-illness and *jie*-illness**. Good [effect]".

***Xuan lu* 宣露, [tooth] exposure** [16]

PC a) of the third stage of → *zou ma ya gan* 走馬牙疳, running horse dental *gan*-illness, with signs of the first stage → *peng sha* 崩砂, collapsing sand, and second stage → *kui cao* 潰槽, bursting trough, as well as appearance of blood. *HYKY* 18: 又盛血出，名曰**宣露**, "When even more abundant, blood appears. This is called 'drained dew'". b) Identical with → *ya xuan* 牙宣, tooth exposure. *QJYF* 6: 凡齒齦**宣露**，多是疳䘌及月蝕, "Cases of teeth and gums **exposure** are mostly *gan*-illness with hidden worms and lunar eclipse".

***Xuan mao* 眩冒, veiled eyes dizziness** [9]

IS of → *xuan yun* 眩運, vertigo, with severe cases resulting in a clouding. *SW* 19: 太過則令人善忘，忽忽**眩冒**而巔疾, "When it is greatly excessive, then this causes a person to be forgetful; he experiences **veiled eyes dizziness** and suffers from peak-illness".

***Xuan pi* 痃癖, string-illness with aggregation-illness** [11] AN *xuan pi qi* 痃癖氣, string-illness with aggregation-illness qi.

PC CD of → *xuan* 痃, string-illness, and → *pi* 癖, aggregation-illness. *QJYiF* 19: 療十年**痃癖**方, "[A recipe] to heal **string-illness with aggregation-illness** that has lasted for ten years".

***Xuan pi qi* 痃癖氣, string-illness with aggregation-illness qi** [18]

PC identical with *xuan pi* 痃癖, string-illness with aggregation-illness. *WTMY* 12: 廣濟療**痃癖氣**，兩肋妨痛方, "The *GJF* has a recipe to cure **string-illness with aggregation-illness qi**. It helps against pain in the ribs on both sides".

***Xuan pu* 眩仆, dizziness with fall** [1]

IS identical with → *xuan dao* 眩倒. *SW* 74: 民病厥心痛，嘔血，血泄，鼽衄，善悲，時**眩仆**. "People suffer from recession heartache, blood vomiting, blood outflow, stuffy nose, nosebleed, and a tendency toward sadness. Occasionally they experience **dizziness and fall** to the ground.

***Xuan qi* 痃氣, string-illness qi** [1]

PC identical with *xuan* 痃, string-illness. *WTMY* 12: 救急療腹中**痃氣**，連心以來相引痛緊急方, "The *Jiuj*[*F*] has a recipe to heal abdominal **string-illness qi** connecting with the heart and causing pain and tension".

***Xuan xuan tu* 旋旋吐, repeated vomiting** [1]

IS of slow and continuous vomiting. *BCGM* SE *gan zhe* 甘蔗 quotes *MSF*: 主胃反，朝食暮吐，暮食朝吐，**旋旋吐**者, "It controls stomach turnover with vomiting at dawn after having eaten at dusk, and vomiting at dusk after having eaten at dawn, as well as **repeated vomiting**".

***Xuan yin* 懸飲, suspended rheum** [1]

PC of → *yin* 飲②, rheum, disease brought forth by rheum flowing into the region below the flanks with cough and vomiting causing pain. *JGYL* Mj: 水流在脅下，咳吐引痛，謂之**懸飲**, "When water flows to below the flanks, and if there is cough and vomiting with a pulling pain, then this is called '**suspended rheum**'".

***Xuan yong* 懸癰, suspended obstruction-illness** [7]

① PC of → *yong* 癰, obstruction-illness, developing either in the perineum or in the bend between the jaws and pharynx. *YLQF* 7: **懸癰**，生穀道、外腎之間, "**Suspended obstruction-illnesses** develop between the anus (lit.: grain path) and the testicles (lit.: external kidneys)".

② AP: the uvula. *ZBYHL* 2: **懸癰**是音聲之關, "The **suspended obstruction-illness** is the gate for sounds".

***Xuan yun* 眩運, dizziness with movement; vertigo** [45] AW *xuan yun* 旋運; *yun xuan* 運眩; *tou xuan* 頭眩, the head is dizzy.

① IS of a perception of the body and its surroundings as revolving, together with darkness developing in front of the eyes. *SJZL* 17: 治風頭旋，眼目昏痛，**眩運**，倦怠，心忪，芎藭散方, "To cure head wind spinning; visual clouding with pain and **dizziness with movement**, exhaustion and heart agitation, [use] the recipe for the powder with *xiong qiong*". LSZ: 眩是目黑，運是頭旋, "眩 stands for darkness in front of the eyes; 運 stands for a revolving movement perceived in the head".

② PC with vertigo as its main pathological sign. *XMLF* 3: **眩運**嘔吐，謂風熱之甚也, "**Vertigo** with vomiting, that is to say: excessive wind heat".

***Xuan yun* 旋運, vertigo** [11]

IS identical with → *xuan yun* 眩運①, vertigo. *TPSHF* 79: 治產後崩中，頭目**旋運**，神志昏迷，四肢煩亂，不知人事，熟乾地黃散方, "To cure collapsing center after delivery; **vertigo** affecting head and eyes; mental confusion, vexing confusion affection the four limbs, and if one fails to recognize persons and things, [use] the recipe with prepared *gan di huang*".

Xue beng **血崩, blood collapse** [97]

PC of excessive vaginal bleeding, identical with → *beng zhong* 崩中, collapsing center. *MYBL* SE *shui su* 水蘇：主吐血、衄血、**血崩**, "It controls spitting of blood, nosebleed, and **blood collapse**".

Xue bi **血閉, [menstrual] blood blockage** [55] AN *bi xue* 閉血, blocked [menstrual] blood.

PC of a) → *jing bi* 經閉 menstrual blockage. *BJ* SE *juan bai* 卷柏：女子陰中寒熱痛，癥瘕，**血閉**，絕子, "[It cures] females experiencing cold [pain] and heat pain in their genital region, concretion-illness and conglomeration-illness, **[menstrual] blood blockage**, and childlessness". b) Rather serious cases of → *yü xue* 瘀血③, stagnant blood. *BJ* SE *huang qin* 黄芩：主諸熱黄疸，腸澼泄痢，逐水，下**血閉**, "It controls all types of heat and yellow *dan*-illness, intestinal flush and outflow with free-flux illness, eliminates water, and brings down a **[menstrual] blood blockage**".

Xue bing **血病, blood disease** [55] AN *xue ji* 血疾, blood ailment; *xue zheng* 血證, blood condition.

PC CD of all types of diseases brought forth by abnormal states of blood, such as all types of extravascular stagnant blood, etc. *SW* 23: 咸走血，**血病**無多食咸, "The salty [flavor] moves to the blood; in the case of **diseases in the blood** one must not consume salty [flavor] in large quantities".

Xue ci **血刺, blood piercing** [9]

PC of pain in the heart and abdomen caused by stagnant blood. *BCSY* RE *xun zhu tang* 焊豬湯, decoction with boiled pork: 主產後**血刺**，心痛欲死，取一盞溫服之, "It controls **blood piercing** following delivery, with heartache to the extent that one is at the verge of expiring. Take one small cup and ingest warm".

Xue fan **血煩, blood vexation** [1]

PC of females who following delivery experience heart-pressure as a result of blood stasis. *BCGM* Bai bing zhu zhi yao: 百病主治藥：蒲黄，血運、血癥、**血煩**、血痛、胞衣不下，並水服二錢, "For *pu huang* [to cure] blood[-induced brain] movements, blood concretion-illness, **blood vexation**, blood pain, and failure of the placenta to come down [following delivery], ingest 2 *qian* with water".

Xue feng **血風, blood wind** [30]

PC introduced in *ZBYHL* 15 as brought about by an intrusion of wind evil qi into an unbalanced state of qi and blood, mostly in women. *TPSHF* 69: **血風**…由體虛，氣血不調，為風冷所侵故也, "**Blood wind**…is caused by an intrusion of wind cold into a state of physical depletion and failing balance between qi and blood".

Xue feng chi yan **血風赤眼, bleeding wind-red-eye** [1]

PC identical with → *xue feng yan* 血風眼, bleeding wind-eye. *BCGM* SE *wu zei yu* 烏賊魚 quotes *YSJCF* 11: 婦人血風眼, "Bleeding wind-eye in women", writes: 血風赤眼，女人多之, "**Bleeding wind-red-eye**: women are affected by it often".

Xue feng nao yun **血風腦運, blood and wind brain-movements** [1]
PC identical with → *xue yun* 血運, blood[-induced brain] movements. *BCGM* SE *xi er* 枲耳：**血風腦運**：方見發明下, "For **blood and wind brain-movements**, see the recipes in the section 'Explanations'".

Xue feng tong **血風痛, blood-wind pain** [1]
PC of → *xue feng* 血風, blood wind, with pain as a major sign. *BCGM* Bai bing zhu zhi yao 百病主治藥：茺蔚子，治風解熱，莖葉，治**血風痛**, "*Chong wei*. The seeds cure wind and resolve heat. The stem and leaves cure **pain from blood-wind**".

Xue feng yan **血風眼**, bleeding wind-**eye** [1] AN xue feng chi yan 血風赤眼, bleeding wind-red-eye.
PC of → *feng yan* 風眼, wind eye, in women of child-bearing age. *YSJCF* 11: 通聖散，治婦人**血風眼**, "The 'recipe for communication with the sages': it cures **bleeding wind-eye** in women".

Xue hai tong **血海痛, painful sea of blood** [1]
PC of pain in the region of the uterus. *BCGM* SE *wu yao* 烏藥 quotes *QKMY*: 婦人**血海痛**，男子疝氣，茴香湯下, "For **painful sea of blood** in women and elevation-illness qi of males, ingest with a decoction with *hui xiang*".

Xue han **血汗, blood sweat** [7] AN *han xue* 汗血, sweat blood; *mai yi* 脈溢, vessel overflow; *ji nü* 肌衄, spontaneous muscle bleeding.
PC of bleeding from the muscle tissue without apparent external injury. *SJZL* 69: 治**血汗**從膚腠出，神白散方, "To cure **blood sweat** leaving through the dermal interstices, [use] the recipe for the 'wondrously effective powder with [*ren zhong*] *bai*'".

Xue huang **血黃, blood jaundice** [2]
PC of → *huang dan* 黃疸, yellow *dan*-illness, accompanied by nosebleed and dryness in the mouth, and in some cases with blood leaving with the stools and urine. *TPSHF* 55: 治**血黃**，羚羊角散方, "To cure **blood jaundice**, [use] the recipe for the powder with *ling yang jiao*".

Xue ji **血疾, blood ailment** [4]
PC identical with → *xue bing* 血病, blood disease. *RHZ* SE *di yu* 地榆：月經不止，血崩，產前後諸**血疾**, "Incessant menstruation; blood collapse; all types of **blood ailments** prior to and following delivery".

Xue ji **血積, blood accumulation** [16]
① EA PM of stagnant blood accumulating and failing to pass on. This in turn may cause further diseases. *ZBYHL* 31: 惡肉者…春冬被惡風所傷，風入肌肉，結瘀，**血積**而生也, "In the case of malign flesh…if one was harmed by malign wind in spring or winter, this wind has entered the muscles and the flesh. There it stagnates and forms nodes. This generates **blood accumulation**".
② PC identical with → *ji xue* 積血, accumulated blood. *ZHF* 8: 蛇銜膏，療癰腫，金瘡瘀血，產後**血積**，耳目諸病, "*She xian* paste cures obstruction-ill-

nesses with swelling, wounds inflicted by metal objects with stagnant blood, **blood accumulation** following delivery, as well as all diseases affecting the ears and eyes".

Xue jia **血瘕, blood conglomeration-illness** [26]

PC of → *jia* 瘕, conglomeration, which has formed from stagnant blood and fails to dissolve. Such a condition mostly develops in women with irregular menstruation or out of stagnant blood present in the body following delivery. *BJ shui zhi* 水蛭：主逐惡血，瘀血，月閉，破**血瘕**, "It controls elimination of malign blood, stagnant blood, and blocked menses, and it crushes **blood conglomeration-illness**.

Xue jie **血結, blood nodes** [33]

① EA PM identical with → *jie xue* 結血, "bound blood". *LS* 27: 視其虛實，及大絡之**血結**而不通，及虛而脈陷空著而調之, "Examine whether it is a situation of depletion or repletion. It is either **blood nodes** in the large network [vessels] causing blockage, or it is a condition of depletion with the empty vessels being caved in. Regulate this accordingly".

② PC brought forth by accumulations of stagnant blood. *WPBC* SE *shi liu huang* 石硫黃：治婦人**血結**, "It cures **blood nodes** in women".

Xue jie xiong **血結胸, bound chest because of blood [1]** [1]

PC of a → jie xiong 結胸, bound chest, resulting from an interaction of evil heat and stagnant blood in the chest. *SHQSJ* 3: 胸腹脹滿硬痛，身熱，漱水不嚥，喜忘如狂，大便黑，小便利，名**血結胸**, "[A feeling of] swelling, fullness, hardening and pain in chest and abdomen, with body heat, gargling water that cannot be swallowed, forgetfulness as in madness, black stool and blocked urine, this is called **bound chest because of blood**".

Xue jin **血噤**, blood lockjaw [7]

PC of women having lost their voice with a clenched mouth following delivery. *RHZ* SE *yuan zhi* 遠志：主婦人**血噤**失音，小兒客忤, "It controls women displaying **blood lockjaw** with loss of voice; in children: a visitor's hostility".

Xue jing bu yun **血經不勻, menstrual irregularity** [1]

PC identical with → *yue shui bu tiao* 月水不調. *RHZ* SE *wang bu liu xing* 王不留行：治發背、游風、風疹，婦人**血經不勻**及難產, "It cures effusion of the back, roaming wind, and wind macules, as well as **menstrual irregularity** and difficulties giving birth".

Xue ju **血聚, blood collection** [6]

① EA PM identical with → *xue ji* 血積①, blood accumulation. *QJYF* 3: 治子門閉，**血聚**腹中生肉癥, "To cure closure of the uterus opening, with **blood collection** and meat concretion-illness in the abdomen".

② PC identical with → *xue jie* 血結②, blood nodes. *ZLBC* SE *gan di huang* 乾地黃 quotes *MSF*: 若**血聚**，以針決之, "In the case of **blood collection**, open it with a needle".

Xue jue **血厥, blood recession** [4] AN *yu mao* 郁冒, pent-up malicious [qi].

PC of women who, without apparent reason, experience profuse sweating and sudden loss of consciousness. The body is as dead, and after a while they wake up again". *PJBSF* 7: 名曰郁冒，亦名**血厥**，婦人多有之, "It is called pent-up malicious [qi]. Another name is '**blood recession**'. Women often have it".

Xue ke **血渴, bleeding and thirst** [8]

PC of an excessive blood loss in women during delivery with thirst. *BCSY* SE *bai mang bo* 敗芒箔：主產婦血滿腹脹痛，**血渴**，惡露不盡, "It controls, in women giving birth, blood fullness with abdominal distension and pain, **bleeding and thirst**, and persistent flow of lochia".

Xue ku **血枯, blood desiccation** [15] AN *jing shui ku* 經水枯, desiccation of menstrual liquid.

PC of → *jing bi* 經閉, menstrual blockage, resulting from decay of essence and exhaustion of the blood because of an injury in early years. *SW* 40: 病名**血枯**，此得之年少時，有所大脫血，若醉入房中，氣竭肝傷，故月事衰少不來也, "The disease is named **blood desiccation**. It is acquired in younger years either [because of] a massive loss of blood or [because] one has entered the [women's] chambers in a state of drunkenness [with the result that] the qi is exhausted and the liver is harmed. Hence, the monthly affair is weak and diminished and fails to arrive".

Xue kuai **血塊, blood clot** [26]

① PI of extravascular blood forming lumps. In some cases they may remain inside the body; in other cases they may be discharged from the body. Such an item, when staying in the body, may cause further diseases. *SJZL* 161: 取下**血塊**如雞肝，是效, "It serves to discharge **blood clots** resembling chicken liver. Truly effective".

② PC of lumps swelling in the abdominal cave as a result of stagnant blood accumulating there. *WTMY* 13: 療婦人腹內冷癖**血塊**，虛脹，月經不調, "It cures, in the abdomen of females, cold aggregation-illness with **blood clots**, depletion distension, and irregularities in the monthly period".

Xue kui **血潰, blood festering** [2]

PC of an unusual disease with the whites of the eyes gradually turning black while vision remains unimpaired, the hair on the body and on the head stiffening, and even though patients can still eat and drink they are unable to speak. *JFPJF* 26: 眼白人渾黑, 見物依舊, 毛髮直如鐵條, 雖能飲食, 不語如大醉, 名曰**血潰**, "When the white parts of the eyes turn black, while one can still see things as normal, and the hair on the body and on the head rises straight as if it were iron sticks. Although [patients] are able to drink and eat, they cannot speak, as if they had drunken to intoxication. This is called '**blood festering**'".

Xue lai **血癩, blood repudiation-illness** [1]

PC identical with → *chi lai* 赤癩, red repudiation-illness. *YXL* SE *qiang huo* 羌活：能治賊風，失音不語，多癢，**血癩**, "It can be used to cure robber wind, loss of voice, frequent itching, and **blood repudiation-illness**".

***Xue lao* 血勞, blood exhaustion** [4]

PC of a depletion exhaustion with extremely weak menstruation, or in severe cases complete failure to menstruate. *YXL* SE *shui zhi* 水蛭：主破女子月候不通，欲成**血勞**、癥塊, "It controls by breaking open the blocked passage of menstruation, and a tendency to develop into **blood exhaustion** and concretion-illness with lumps".

***Xue li* 血痢, bleeding free-flux illness** [131] AN *li xue* 痢血, free-flux illness with blood.

PC of thin stool interspersed with blood, or a → *li ji* 痢疾, free-flux illness ailment, consisting of only fresh blood or dark blood. *MYBL* SE *li chang* 鱧腸：主**血痢**, "It controls **bleeding free-flux illness**".

***Xue li* 血瀝, blood trickling** [7]

EA PM identical with → *yue xue* 瘀血①, stagnant blood. *YXL* SE *xi xin* 細辛：主血閉，婦人**血瀝**腰痛, "It controls blood closure, and in women **blood trickling** with pain in the lower back region".

***Xue lin* 血淋, blood dripping** [64]

PC of → *lin bing* 淋病, dripping disease, with painful passage of bloody urine as a major sign. *ZBYHL* 14: **血淋**者，是熱淋之甚者，則尿血，謂之血淋。心主血，血之行身，通遍經絡，循環腑臟。其熱甚者，血則散失其常經，溢滲入胞，而成**血淋**也, "As for **blood dripping**, this is an extreme case of heat dripping. As a result one passes blood with the urine. Hence it is called blood dripping. The heart rules the blood. When the blood passes through the body it penetrates the conduits and network vessels and circumvents the depots and palaces. In the case of extreme heat, the blood disperses. It leaves the regular conduits and pours into the bladder. This then generates **blood dripping**". *BCGM* Bai bing zhu zhi yao 百病主治藥：小便血：不痛者為尿血，主虛；痛者為**血淋**，主熱, "If the urine contains blood: If there is no pain, this is urine with blood; it is brought forth by depletion. If it is painful, this is **blood dripping**; it is brough forth by heat".

***Xue liu* 血瘤, blood tumor** [1]

PC of soft → liu 瘤, tumors, which neither ache nor itch and that, if pressed, generate extravascular blood. *WTMY* 23: 不癢不痛，又不堅強，按之柔軟，此**血瘤**也, "If they neither itch nor ache, and if they are not hard, but are soft if pressed, then these are **blood tumors**". *BCGM* SE *shi* 豕 quoting *RYBC*: **血瘤**, **blood tumor**, erroneously writes: 血溜, blood current. In contrast, *BCGM* Bai bing zhu zhi yao 百病主治藥 correctly writes 血瘤, blood tumor.

***Xue lu* 血露, blood dew, lochia** [4]

Identical with → *e lu* 惡露①, malign dew. *ZBYHL* 43: " 或新產**血露**未盡，而取風涼，皆令風冷搏於血, "In some cases, following delivery, the **blood dew** may not have departed entirely when it is affected by wind coolness. This results in wind cold beating against the blood".

Xue men **血悶, blood heart-pressure** [14]

PC of vexation and pressure felt in the region of the heart and chest and being caused by extravascular blood or blood stagnation. *TBC* SE *zhe shang mu* 折傷木：主傷折筋骨疼痛，散血補血，產後**血悶**, "It controls pain in harmed and broken sinews and bones; it disperses blood, and it supplements blood. [It cures] **blood heart-pressure** following delivery".

Xue mi **血秘, blood blockage** [1] AN *da chang xue mi* 大腸血閟, closure of the large intestine because of blood.

PC of constipation brought forth by blood stagnation or blood depletion. *YXQY* Lj: 治大便血結、**血秘**、血燥，通潤大便, "It cures stools with blood nodes, **blood blockage**, and blood dryness; it moistens stools and stimulates defecation".

Xue ni **血逆, blood counterflow** [4]

PC of great body heat associated with headache and heart vexation . *MYBL* SE *chong wei zi* 茺蔚子：療**血逆**，大熱，頭痛，心煩, "It cures **blood counterflow**, with massive heat, headache and heart vexation".

Xue ning **血凝, blood coagulation** [10]

EA PM identical with → *yu xue* 瘀血①, stagnant blood. *ZBYHL* 1: 夏遇痹者為脈痹，則**血凝**不流，令人萎黃, "If one is affected by a blockage in summer, then this will be a vessel blockage. As a result, the **blood coagulates** and fails to flow. This causes people to have a wilting-yellow complexion".

Xue qi **血氣, blood and qi** [210]

① EA CD of stagnant blood and blocked qi, often with special emphasis on stagnant blood. *SW* 62: **血氣**以並，病形以成, "When **blood and qi** have collected, and the disease has assumed a physical manifestation". *BCGM* has *xue qi tong* 血氣痛, "blood and qi [induced] pain", *xue qi duo tai* 血氣墮胎, "blood and qi [induced] abortion", and *xue qi fu zhang* 血氣腹脹, "blood and qi [induced] abdominal distension".

② PC brought forth by stagnant blood together with blocked qi – a condition often seen in women. *BJ* SE *tian shu shi* 天鼠屎：主面癰腫，皮膚洗洗時痛，腹中**血氣**, "It controls obstruction-illnesses with swelling in the face. Skin that has pain when it is washed. [Stagnant] **blood and** [blocked] **qi** in the abdomen". *BCGM* has *fu ren xue qi* 婦人血氣, "[stagnant] blood and [blocked] qi in females;" *nü ren xue qi* 女人血氣, "[stagnant] blood and [blocked] qi in females;" and *chan hou xue qi* 產後血氣, [stagnant] blood and [blocked] qi after delivery".

③ PN CD of the qi and blood required as nutrients in the body. *SW* 9: 其充在筋，以生**血氣**, "Its fullness [manifests itself] in the sinews. It serves to generate **blood and qi**". *BCGM* has *yang xue qi* 養血氣, "to nourish blood and qi"; *bu yi xue qi* 補益血氣, "to supplement blood and qi"; *xue qi shuai bei* 血氣衰憊, "exhaustion of blood and qi". Seen as a whole, in the *BCGM* the pathological meaning of *xue qi* 血氣, blood and qi, is referred to more often than the physiological meaning.

Xue re **血熱, blood heat** [30]

PC of diseases associated with heat in blood vessels. *QJYF* 26: 胡瓜，味甘寒有毒，不可多食，動寒熱，多瘧病，積瘀，**血熱**, "*Hu gua* flavor sweet, cold, with poison. Must not be consumed in large quantities. Excites alternating sensations of cold and heat. Increases the severity of malaria, accumulation of stasis [blood], and **blood heat**".

Xue shan **血疝, blood elevation-illness** [2]

PC identical with → *bian yong* 便癰, obstruction-illness in the region of [urine and defecation] relief. *RMSQ* 4: 便癰者，**血疝**也, "Obstruction-illness in the region of [urine and defecation] relief, this is **blood elevation-illness**".

Xue tong **血痛, blood pain** [25]

PC CD of all types of painful conditions caused by stagnant blood that fails to pass on. *ZHF* 4: 治反腰有**血痛**方, "Recipe to cure **blood pain** felt [by a patient] when he turns back his lumbar region".

Xue tuo **血脫, blood loss** [6]

PC identical with → *wang xue* 亡血. *QJYF* 13: **血脫**，色乾燥不澤，飲食不為肌膚, "**Blood loss.** The complexion is that of dryness without glossiness. Ingesting beverages and food does not generate muscles or skin".

Xue wang xing **血妄行, uncontrolled blood flow** [9]

EA PM where, because of uncontrolled counterflow of qi dynamics or excessive presence of evil in the body, the normal movement of blood is disturbed and blood is forced to leave its vessels, manifesting itself as the presence of extravascular blood. *SJZL* 68: 治心肺蘊熱，或恚怒氣逆，使**血妄行**，日久不止, "To cure stored heat in the heart and lung, or qi counterflow stimulated by rage and anger, causing **uncontrolled blood flow** which does not end for a long time".

Xue xia **血下, blood discharge** [13]

IS of bleeding in women through their yin orifice, i.e. vagina. *QJYF* 2: 妊娠**血下**不止，名曰漏胞, "If pregnant women experience an unending **blood discharge**, this is called ,leaking bladder'".

Xue xie **血邪, blood evil** [6] CD of

PCs caused by stagnant blood abiding in the human body. *RHZ* SE *wu ci ji* 烏雌雞：治**血邪**, 破心中宿血及治癰疽, "It cures **blood evil**, breaks blood abiding in the heart, and cures obstruction- and impediment-illnesses".

Xue xu **血虛, blood depletion** [63]

PC of depletion with loss of blood liquid, and hence diminished nourishing function of blood. *SW* 39: 寒氣客於背俞之脈則脈泣，脈泣則**血虛**，**血虛**則痛, "When cold qi settles in the vessels of the back transporters, then the [movement in the] vessels is impeded. When the [movement in the] vessels is impeded, then the **blood is depleted**. When the **blood is depleted**, then pain results".

Xue xu huo kang **血虛火亢, blood depletion with excessive fire** [1]

EA, PM of a → *yin xu huo dong* 陰虛火動, yin depletion with excited fire, resulting from a unilateral insufficiency of yin blood. *BCGM* SE *ren shen* 人參 quotes LYW: **血虛火亢**能食，脈弦而數，涼之則傷胃，溫之則傷肺，不受

補者也, "In the case of **blood depletion with excessive fire**, when [the patient] is able to eat, and when the [movement in the] vessels is string[-like] and frequent, [treatment with] cold substances will harm his stomach; [treatment with] warming substances will harm his lung. This is a situation where supplementation is not accepted".

Xue xuan 血眩, **blood dizziness** [1]

PC of → *xuan yun* 眩運, vertigo experienced by females who suffer from depletion and weakness of qi and blood, and at the same time an intrusion of wind evil. *SWBJQYMJ* Fj: 治產後風虛**血眩**，精神昏昧，荊芥散, "To cure wind [intruding into a state of] depletion with **blood dizziness** and a clouded mind following delivery, [use] the powder with *jing jie*".

Xue yan 血眼, **blood eyes** [6]

PC of newborns with stagnant blood in their eyes as a result of a difficult birth, in serious cases obfuscating the pupil, in light cases causing redness and swelling of the eyes. *HYKY* 4: 議**血眼**：…盛則灌注其睛，不見瞳人；輕則外胞赤腫，上下爛眩, "To define '**blood eyes**': …When [the blood] is abundant, it flows into the eyes and the pupil is no longer visible. In slight cases the eyelids on the outside are red and swollen. Above and below there is festering and vision is blurred".

Xue yi 血翳, **blood shade** [2]

PC of → *nu rou* 胬肉, tumorous flesh-growth, with a red color that is just in a developmental phase. *BCGM* SE *ku hu* 苦瓠 quotes *JYF*: 瘀肉**血翳**皆漸下，不傷睛也, "Excessive flesh and **blood shades** all gradually descend; they do not harm the eyeball".

Xue yong 血壅, **blood obstruction** [4]

① EA PM identical with → *yu xue* 瘀血①, stagnant blood. *NJ* 22: **血壅**而不濡者，為血後病也, "When the **blood is obstructed** [in its movement] and fails to moisten [the body], then the blood was affected by this disease later on".

② PC of rashes and itching accompanied by pain, a condition which, if not cured immediately, will result in suppuration. *CXSYF* quoting *QJF* writes *xue zhu* 血住, blood stoppage. *SYDXF* writes *xue yong* 血臃, blood grossness. *BCGM* has *xue yong* **血壅**, "**blood obstruction**".

Xue yu 血餘, **blood surplus** [9]

① PC of worms growing from the wounds of severed fingers. Rarely seen. *CXSYF* Lj quotes *QJF*: 手十指節斷壞，惟有筋連，無節，肉蟲出，如燈心粗，長數尺。遍身綠毛卷多，名曰**血餘**。治以茯苓、胡黃連煎湯，飲兩盞，愈, "When the ten fingers have been severed so that there are no joints with only sinews connecting the individual parts, and when then worms appear as thick as a lamp wick, and several *chi* long, having curled green hair all over their body, then this is called '**blood surplus**'. One treats this with a decoction with *fu ling* and *hu huang lian*. If one drinks two small cups, this will bring the cure".

② PS of human hair pharmaceutically prepared for use as medication. *LGPZL* SE *yuan qing* 芫蜻：去兩翅足並頭，用**血餘**裹懸於東牆角上一夜，至明取

用, "Discard the two wings, the feet, and the head. Wrap in **blood surplus** and suspend above the edge of the eastern wall for one night. At dawn remove it and use it [for therapeutical purposes]".

Xue yu **血郁, pent-up blood** [1]

PC one of → *liu yu* 六郁, the six types of pent-up [matter in the organism]. Refers to accumulation disease brought forth by stagnant blood. The four limbs have no strength. Patients eat as normal; the movement in the vessels is in the depth. *DXXF* 3: **血郁**者，四肢無力，能食便紅，脈沉, "In the case of **pent-up blood**, the four limbs have no strength. [Patients] can eat [as usual, but] their discharge is red. The [movement in the] vessels is deep inside".

Xue yu **血瘀, blood stagnation** [15]

① AN *xue zhi* 血滯, blood sluggishness; *xue yong* 血壅, blood obstruction. EA PM of a slowed down or locally completely halted blood flow brought forth by such causes as stagnant blood, blocked qi, and cold. This, in turn, may be the cause of further diseases. *ZBYHL* 39: **血瘀**在內，則時時體熱面黄，瘀久不消，則變成積聚癥瘕也, "In the case of internal **blood stagnation**, the body will frequently be hot and the face yellow. If the stagnation lasts over an extended period of time and fails to dissolve, it will generate accumulations and collections, concretion-illness and conglomeration-illness".

② PC identical with → *yu xue* 瘀血③, stagnant blood. *BCSY* SE *hu zhang* 虎杖：主風在骨節間及**血瘀**, "It controls wind present in the bone joints, as well as **blood stagnation**".

Xue yun **血運, blood[-induced brain] movements; vertigo** [71] AN *chan yun* 產運, [brain] movements following delivery.

PC of sudden vertigo brought forth by sudden and violent depletion of qi and blood following parturition. [Patients] pant and vomit. In severe cases this includes a clouded mind. *TPSHF* 80: 產後**血運**，才覺噁心，頭旋，多涕唾，身如在船車上，便速宜服此赤馬通散, "In the case of **blood[-induced brain] movements** following delivery when [the woman] feels nauseous (lit.: has a feeling of a malign center) and the head spins, when she produces much snivel and saliva, and when her body feels as if she were on a boat or carriage, she should quickly ingest this powder with red horse manure".

Xue zao **血燥, blood dryness** [7]

PC of → *zao bing* 燥病, dryness disease, brought forth by a loss and depletion of blood fluid. *YXQY* Lj: 桃仁，氣溫，味甘苦，治大便血結、血秘、**血燥**, "*Tao ren* has warm qi. Its flavor is sweet bitter. It cures stools with blood nodes, blood blockage, and **blood dryness**".

Xue zhang **血脹, blood distension** [7]

PC of a) a feeling of painful distension brought forth by post-delivery internal stagnation of the blood or a failure of the placenta to descend. In extreme cases this is accompanied by dizziness and confusion; the patient passes out. *FRDQLF* 18: 有一親戚婦人，產後胞衣不下，**血脹**，迷悶不記人事, "There was a relative whose placenta did not come down following delivery. She experienced **blood distension**, mental confusion and heart-pressure, and passed out". b) A → *gu zhang* 鼓脹, drum-like distension, accompanied by stagnation of the blood. *TBC* SE *jue chuang* 爵床：甚療**血脹**下氣, "It is very capable of curing **blood distension** and bringing down qi". In the *BCGM*, blood distension mostly refers to meaning a).

Xue zhen tong **血枕痛, pain because of blood-headrest** [1]
PC identical with → *er zhen tong* 兒枕痛, pain because of an unborn infant's blood headrest in its mother's uterus. *BCGM* SE *hu po* 琥珀 quotes *RHZ*: 治產後**血枕痛**, "It cures **pain** following delivery **because of blood headrest**".

Xue zheng **血證, blood condition** [6]
PC identical with → *xue bing* 血病, blood disease. *SHL* 125: 小便自利，其人如狂者，**血證**諦也, "When urine flows spontaneously, and that person behaves as if mad, then this is a sign of a **blood condition**".

Xue zheng **血癥, blood concretion-illness** [4]
PC of → *zheng* 癥, concretion-illness, that forms when stagnant blood collects without dissolving and forms lumps after an extended period of time. *MYBL* SE *zhan si* 占斯：除水，堅積**血癥**，月閉無子, "It eliminates water, hardness accumulations and **blood concretion-illness**, and [cures] blocked menstruation with childlessness".

Xue zhi **血滯, blood sluggishness** [21]
EA identical with → *yue xue* 瘀血①, stagnant blood. *PJBSF* 6: 大抵**血滯**則生瘡，肝為宿血之臟，而決明和肝氣，不損元氣也, "In general, **blood sluggishness** generates sores. The liver is the depot of residual blood. *Jue ming* serves to harmonize liver qi and it does not harm the original qi".

Xue zhi **血痔, blood piles** [13]
PC of → *zhi chuang* 痔瘡, piles sores, associated with a release of clear, red blood in the course of defecation. *ZBYHL* 34: 因便而清血隨出者，**血痔**也, "If fresh blood is released with defecation, this is because of **blood piles**".

Xue zhong **血腫, blood swelling** [3]
PC of → *zhong ji* 腫疾, swelling ailment, brought forth by stagnant blood. *DXXF* 3: 其皮間紅縷赤痕者，此**血腫**也, "When there are red threads and marks in the skin, this is a **blood swelling**".

Xue zhu **血注, blood influx** [1]
PC of sores on the feet brought forth by blood that has flown downward and caused blockages through coagulation. *PJF* 276: 治**血注**脚, "It cures **blood influx** in the legs".

Xun yi mo chuang **循衣摸床, to trace one's garment and stroke one's bedding** [2]
IS of mental derangement making a person unconsciously trace the seems of one's garment, or stroke one's bedding. *SHL* 212: 劇者，發則不識人，**循衣摸床**，惕而不安, "In serious cases, [patients] no longer recognize persons. Their fingers **trace their garment and stroke their bedding**. They are fidgety and find no rest".

- Y -

***Ya* 啞, muteness** [1]

PC a) with an inability to speak as a major sign. This may be a congenital birth defect, or the result of some later illness. *BCGM* refers to "muteness" with the singular character *ya* 啞 once only. *SJZL* 154: 言遲語吃，或**啞**或聵，神氣昏塞，此心形之不備也, "Slow speech, and stuttering, **muteness** and deafness, with clouding and obstruction of the spirit qi, results from an incomplete forming of the physical appearance of the heart". b) Identical with → *ya* 瘂, muteness disease. *BCGM* uses *ya* 啞 in binomes interchangeably with *ya* 瘂, as for example in → *ya bing* 啞病, muteness disease, and → *sheng ya* 聲啞, muteness.

***Ya* 瘂, muteness-illness** [1]

PC following a localized throat disease with difficulty speaking or a very low and deep, rather than mellow and full, voice. *WTMY* 2: 射干湯，主春冬傷寒，秋夏中冷，咳嗽，曲拘不得氣息，喉鳴，**瘂**，失聲，乾嗽無唾，喉中如哽者方, "The decoction with *she gan* is a recipe to control harm caused by cold in spring and winter, being struck by cold in autumn and summer, with cough, a bent body making it impossible to breathe, sounds in the throat, **muteness-illness**, loss of voice, dry cough without saliva, and a feeling in the throat as if one were choking".

***Ya bing* 啞病, muteness disease** [2]

PC identical with → *ya* 瘂, muteness-illness. *PJF* 64: 治**啞病**，以蜩蟟蛻皮，研一錢匕，井花水服, "To cure **muteness disease** grind the amount of a spoon with 1 *qian* of the skin shed by cicadas and ingest with *jing hua shui*".

***Ya bing* 瘂病, disease of muteness-illness** [1]

PC identical with → *ya* 瘂, muteness-illness. *BCGM* Bai bing zhu zhi yao 百病主治藥 quoting the main entry of *chan tui* 蟬蛻：啞病 writes: **瘂病, disease of muteness-illness.**

***Ya chi dong yao* 牙齒動搖, loose teeth** [5]

① IS of unstable roots of the teeth resulting in loose teeth. *SJZL* 120: 風疳之病，其候槽齦虛腫，**牙齒動搖**，侵蝕齒根，腐臭脫落, "The signs of wind-*gan* disease are: depleted and swollen jawbones, **loose teeth**, invasive erosion of the roots of the teeth, resulting in decay with malodorous stench and [teeth] falling out".

② PC with loose teeth as a major sign. *TPSHF* 34: 治**牙齒動搖**，吃食不穩，地骨皮散方, "Recipe for the powder with *di gu pi* to cure **loose teeth**, making eating difficult".

***Ya chi du hei* 牙齒蠹黑, tooth decay with bug blackening** [1]

PC with teeth that have decayed and broken and the remaining stumps assuming a black color. *BCGM* SE *hu tong lei* 胡桐淚 quoting *SJZL* 119: 牙齒歷蠹，齒根黯黑, "The teeth are being eaten away by bugs/worms, and the stumps assume a black color", writes: **牙齒蠹黑, "Tooth decay with bug blackening"**.

Ya chi ji **牙齒疾, tooth ailment** [1]
PC identical with → *chi ji* 齒疾. *BCGM* SE *hu ma* 胡麻 quoting *SXBC*: 有牙齒並脾胃疾人, "Persons with tooth and spleen-stomach ailments", writes: 有**牙齒疾**及脾胃疾人, "Persons with **tooth ailments** and spleen-stomach ailments".

Ya chi teng **牙齒疼, toothache** [1]
PC identical with → *ya tong* 牙痛. *QJYiF* 11: **牙齒疼**，灸兩手中指背第一節前有陷處七壯，下火方愈, "For **toothache**: cauterize seven times the depression in front of the first joint on the back of the middle fingers of both hands".

Ya chi tong **牙齒痛, toothache** [8]
PC identical with → *ya tong* 牙痛. *ZBYHL* 29: **牙齒痛**候…蟲食於牙齒，則齒根有孔，蟲居其間，又傳受余齒，亦皆疼痛, "The signs of **toothache**... Bugs/worms eat the teeth and as a result the roots of the teeth have holes. The bugs/worms reside in these [holes] and spread to the remaining teeth which then all are in pain".

Ya chi xuan ni **牙齒宣䘌, tooth exposure with hidden-worms** [1]
PC identical with → *chi ni* 齒䘌. *BCGM* SE *wu pei zi* 五倍子：止下血，久痢脫肛，**牙齒宣䘌**, "It ends blood discharge, chronic free-flux illness with prolapse of the rectum, as well as **tooth exposure with hidden-worms**".

Ya chu **牙齼, dental discomfort** [1]
PC identical with → *chi chu* 齒齼. *BCGM* SE *fen xi* 粉錫 quotes *WLXGZ*: 食梅**牙齼**，韶粉揩之, "If eating plums results in **dental discomfort**, wipe the [teeth] with powder prepared from *shao fen*".

Ya gan 牙疳, **dental *gan*-illness** [23] AN *chi gan* 齒疳; *ya yin gan chou* 牙齦疳臭, dental and gums *gan*-illness with stench.
PC of → *gan chuang* 疳瘡, *gan*-illness sores, with teeth and the gums festering and emitting a bad stench, the teeth aching and becoming loose, and the appearance of pus and blood. In severe cases teeth and bones turn brittle and rot. *SJZL* 172：治小兒**牙疳**口臭，三靈散方, "Recipe for the 'powder with three magically [effective ingredients]' to cure children's **dental *gan*-illness** with oral stench".

Ya guan bu kai **牙關不開, the jaws do not open** [2]
IS identical with → *ya guan jin ji* 牙關緊急, tightly closed jaws. *SJZL* 14: 如中風涎潮，**牙關不開**者，先用大蒜一瓣，搗爛塗兩牙關外腮上，次用豆淋酒化一丸，揩在牙齦上，即便開口。續用薄荷酒，化服兩丸, "If [a patient] has been struck by wind, if saliva surges and **the jaws do not open**, first pound one garlic section and smear the pulp on the cheeks outside of the jaws. Then take 1 pill dissolved in bean maceration wine and apply this to the gums. [The patient] will immediately open his mouth. Finally he should ingest two pills dissolved in *bo he* wine".

Ya guan jin **牙關緊, tight jaws** [1]
IS identical with → *ya guan jin ji* 牙關緊急, tightly closed jaws. *BYXF* 3: 如**牙關緊**，即撬開灌入, "If the **jaws are tight**, force them open to instill (the medication)".

***Ya guan jin bi* 牙關緊閉, tightly closed jaws** [6]
IS identical with → *ya guan jin ji* 牙關緊急, tightly closed jaws. *BCGM* SE *cong* 葱 quotes *RZTJYF*: 卒心急痛，**牙關緊閉**，欲絕, "Suddenly the heart is tense and painful. The **jaws are tightly closed**. [The patient] is on the verge of dying".

***Ya ji* 牙疾, tooth ailment** [1]
PC identical with → *chi ji* 齒疾. *BCGM* SE *feng xiang zhi* 楓香脂：燒過揩牙，永無**牙疾**, "When roasted and used to brush the teeth, there will never be a **tooth ailment**".

***Ya jin* 牙噤, clenched teeth, lockjaw** [2]
IS identical with → *kou jin* 口噤, clenched jaw. *SJZL* 6: 治急中風，目瞑**牙噤**，不能下藥，用此散，以中指點散子，揩齒三二十次，在大牙左右，其口自開，始得下藥，開關散方, "The recipe for the powder to open the jaws: it cures violent cases of being struck by wind, with the patient's eyes closed and **teeth clenched**, and if he cannot ingest medication, then use this powder. Dip the middle finger into the powder and apply it to the teeth twenty to thirty times, to the left and right of the large teeth. This will cause his mouth to open, and he will be able to ingest medication".

***Ya ni* 牙䘌, hidden-worms teeth** [3]
PC identical with → *chi ni* 齒䘌. *BCGM* SE *wo niu* 蝸牛 quoting *TPSHF*: 齒䘌 writes: **牙䘌**, "**Hidden-worms teeth**".

***Ya shang* 壓傷, injury resulting from pressure** [1]
PC of a → *shang sun* 傷損, injury, received from pressure exerted by a heavy object. *BCGM* SE *da huang* 大黃 quoting *SYJYBZFL*: 木石所壓, "Pressed by wood and stones", writes: 木石**壓傷**, "**Injury resulting from pressure** exerted by a piece of wood and a stone".

***Ya shi* 牙蝕, tooth erosion** [1]
IS of tooth decay resulting from tooth worms. *PJF* 67: 上（銅綠、生白礬、膽礬、麝香）為細末，研勻，上**牙蝕**處, "The above-mentioned substances, *tong lü*, unprocessed *bai fan*, *dan fan*, *she xiang*, are to be finely ground and evenly mixed to be applied to the location of **tooth erosion**".

***Ya si* 壓死, [appearance of] death from being crushed** [4]
PC of → *cu si* 卒死, sudden [appearance of] death, resulting from accidentally being crushed by a heavy object. *SYDXF* 18: 凡墜、**壓死**者, 急安好處, 以手袖掩其口鼻上一食頃, 眼開, 先與熱小便, 若初覺氣能言, 急掰開口以熱小便灌之, "In all cases of [an **appearance of] death** from a fall or **from being crushed**, quickly take [the victim] to a safe place. Then cover the [victim's] mouth and nose with your sleeve as long as it takes to have a meal. When the eyes open, at once pour hot urine [into his mouth]. When he is just regaining consciousness and is capable of speaking, pry his mouth apart with your hands and forcibly instill hot urine into him".

***Ya sou* 呀嗽, creaking cough** [1]
PC identical with → *ga sou* 呷嗽. *TBC* SE *ku hu* 苦瓠：主水腫，石淋，吐**呀嗽**，囊結，疰蠱，痰飲, "It controls water swelling, stone dripping, spit-

ting with **creaking cough**, pouch nodes, attachment-illness with *gu*, and phlegm rheum".

***Ya teng* 牙疼, toothache** [23]

PC identical with → *ya tong* 牙痛. *QJYiF* 11: 治**牙疼**方：蒼耳子（五升）。右一味，以水一斗，煮取五升，熱含之, "Recipe to cure **toothache**: *cang er zi* (5 *sheng*). This single substance is to be boiled in 1 *dou* of water until [only one half, i.e.] 5 *sheng* are left. The hot [liquid] is to be held in the mouth".

***Ya tong* 牙痛, toothache** [116] AN *chi tong* 齒痛; *ya chi tong* 牙齒痛; *ya teng* 牙疼; *chi teng* 齒疼.

PC with pain affecting the teeth and their environment as major sign. *ZBYHL* 29: **牙痛**候…若蟲痛，非針灸可瘥，敷藥蟲死，乃痛止, "The signs of **toothache**…If the pain is caused by bugs/worms, it cannot be cured by needling and cauterization. One applies medication externally to kill the bugs/worms, and the pain ends".

***Ya xuan* 牙宣, tooth exposure** [6]

PC with contracted gums exposing the roots of teeth as a major sign, often accompanied by bleeding gums. *SJZL* 120: 治風蚛牙疼及**牙宣**，七香散方, "The recipe for the 'powder with the seven fragrant substances' cures wind worm-borer teeth with pain, and **tooth exposure**".

***Ya yin gan chou* 牙齦疳臭, *gan*-illness with stench of teeth and gums** [1]

PC identical with → *ya gan* 牙疳, dental *gan*-illness. *BCGM* SE *wu pei zi* 五倍子 quotes *BHJJF*: **牙齦疳臭**：五倍子炒焦一兩，枯礬、銅青各一錢，為末。先以米泔漱淨，摻之, "***Gan*-illness with stench of teeth and gums**: Burned *wu pei zi* 1 *liang*; *ku fan* and *tong qing*, 1 *qian* each. Powderize. First cleanse [the teeth] with the slop from washing rice. Then apply the [powder]".

***Ya yong* 牙癰, dental obstruction-illness** [2]

PC of → *yong* 癰, obstruction-illness, developing from the gums. *QJYF* 13: 喉燥口痛，**牙癰**舌傷, "The throat is dry and the mouth aches, with **dental obstruction-illness** and harm to the tongue".

***Ya zhang* 啞瘴, muteness miasma** [1]

PC of → *zhang nüe* 瘴瘧, miasmatic malaria, accompanied by mental confusion and an inability to speak. *ZNZN* Fj: 惟以其神昏不能言，但噫噫作聲，或全不作聲，謂之**啞瘴**, "If the mind is confused and [the patient] cannot speak, that is, he may utter some sounds or is entirely unable to speak, this is called **muteness miasma**".

***Yan* 黶, black mole; crust; black spot** [p]

① PC a) identical with → *yan zi* 黶子. *MYBL* SE *lu ci shi* 鸕鷀屎：去面黑䵟**黶**志, "It removes facial gloom, and **black moles**, and [other] moles. b) Identical with *dao yan* 倒黶, inverse black mole. *XEWSZWLF* 8: 人齒散，治瘡疹黑**黶**，發搐危困, "Powder prepared from human teeth cures sores, papules, **black moles**, and severe convulsions.

② PM of crust formation on sores, smallpox, or papules. *BCGM* SE *bai mao* 白茅：痘瘡潰爛，難**靨**不乾, "For smallpox sores that fester and do not dry, making **crust formation** difficult".
③ PP of crusts on sores. *BCGM* SE *shui yin fen* 水銀粉 quotes *JSTF*: 下疳陰瘡：輕粉末乾摻之，即結**靨**而愈, "For *gan*-lesions and yin sores in the lower body parts: apply dry *qing fen* powder to them. This will bring the cure by causing the formation of a **crust**.
④ Black spots on any item. *BCGM* SE *ku gua* 苦瓠：凡用苦瓠，須細理瑩淨無**靨**翳者乃佳, "Whenever one uses *ku gua*, only those that have a fine texture, a jade-green color, that are clean, and have no **black spots** or a shade are good".

***Yan an* 眼暗, dim vision** [5]
PC identical with → *mu an* 目暗, unclear vision. *TBC* SE *gan jiang* 乾薑：久服令人**眼暗**, "Ingested over an extended period of time it causes **dim vision**".

***Yan bi* 咽痹, throat blockage** [1]
PC identical with → *hou bi* 喉痹, throat blockage. *SJZL* 93: 手足熱如火，口生瘡舌爛，夜夢驚恐，口中䘌齒牙痛，**咽痹**，服（青蒿丸）五兩, "When [a patient's] hands and feet are hot as fire, his mouth develops sores and the tongue festers, during the night he has terrifying dreams, in his mouth there are hidden-worms teeth with toothache, and in case of **throat blockage**, [it is advisable] to ingest five *liang* [of the pills with *qing hao*]".

***Yan bing* 眼病, eye disease** [1]
PC identical with → *yan ji* 眼疾, ailments of the eyes. *SJZL* 102: 治肝虛眼目昏暗，及一切**眼病**，還睛丸方, "Recipe for the 'pills to return the eyeballs'. It cures liver depletion [resulting in] dim vision, and all **eye diseases**".

***Yan bu li* 咽不利, the throat is not free** [1]
IS identical with → *yan hou bu li* 咽喉不利. *BCGM* Bai bing zhu zhi yao 百病主治藥：痘出不快，便閉，**咽不利**, "Smallpox does not erupt quickly. Defecation is blocked. The **throat is not free**".

***Yan chi* 眼赤, eye redness** [13]
IS, PC identical with → *mu chi* 目赤. *BCJJZ dan shen* 丹參：時人服多**眼赤**，故應性熱, "At that time people who consumed it often developed **eyes redness**. This way they responded to its hot nature".

***Yan fan bu xia* 眼翻不下, eyes turned upward without coming down** [1]
IS identical with → *shang shi* 上視, vision turned upward. *BCGM* SE *deng huo* 燈火 quotes *XEJFMJ*: 眼翻不下者，焠其臍上下, "In case of **eyes turned upward without coming down**, apply hot compresses to above and below the [patient's] navel".

***Yan gan* 眼疳, ocular *gan*-illness** [1]
PC identical with → *gan yan* 疳眼, *gan*-illness eye. *TPSHF* 87: 腦熱目癢，或赤爛生瘡，或生障翳，漸漸遮睛，久而不差，損於眼目，故號**眼疳**也, "The brain is hot and the eyes itch. In some cases they turn red and develop sores. Or they grow an obstructive shade which gradually covers the eyeball. If

this continues for long without being cured it will harm the eyes. Hence this is called '**ocular *gan*-illness**'".

Yan gan **咽乾, desiccated throat** [8]

IS of an uncomfortable feeling of dryness in the throat. *SHL* 263: 少陽之為病，口苦、**咽乾**、目眩也, "When the minor yang [section] has a disease, the mouth has a bitter taste, the **throat is desiccated**, and the eyes are dizzy".

Yan ge bu tong **咽膈不通, gullet occlusion and impassability** [2] AN *yan hou yong se* 咽喉壅塞, gullet congestion.

IS of blocked passage of beverages and food through the esophagus. *LSMC* Mj: 吳茱萸丸，治寒在膈上，噎塞，**咽膈不通**, "Pills with *wu zhu yu* cure cold situated above the diaphragm [resulting in] gullet occlusion with blockage, [that is,] **gullet occlusion and impassability**".

Yan ge yong sai **咽膈壅塞, gullet congestion** [1]

IS identical with → *yan ge bu tong* 咽膈不通, gullet occlusion and impassability. *HJJF* 10: 壯熱狂躁，**咽膈壅塞**，睡臥不安, "Strong heat, crazy jumping. **Gullet congestion**. Inability to sleep calmly".

Yan han **眼寒, cold eyeballs; the eyeballs are cold** [3]

PC of pain in the eyes, tearflow, and night blindness brought forth by wind and cold evil rising to the head and residing there. *SW* 42: 風入系頭，則為目風**眼寒**, "When the wind enters the connection with the head, then this causes eye wind. The **eyeballs are cold**".

Yan hei **眼黑, darkened eyes** [6]

IS identical with → *mu hei* 目黑. *ZBYHL* 4: 有二十三蒸，…九肝蒸，**眼黑**, "There are 32 variants of steaming…The ninth is: liver steaming. [This is the case when] the **eyes are darkened**".

Yan hou **鹽齁, salt roaring** [4] AN *yan xiao* 鹽哮, *xian hou* 咸齁, *xian xiao* 咸鼾.

PC of → *xiao chuan* 哮喘, roaring panting, brought forth by a consumption of excessively salty beverages and food. *BCGM* SE *wu jiu mu* 烏桕木 quotes *ZXF*: **鹽齁**痰喘：桕樹皮去粗搗汁，和飛麵作餅烙熟。早辰與兒吃三四個，待吐下鹽涎乃佳, "**Salt roaring** with phlegm panting: Remove the coarse parts from the *jiu* tree bark and pound to prepare juice. Mix this with loose flour and bake to cakes. Have the child eat three or four in the morning. Once it spits and discharges salty saliva it will be fine".

Yan hou bi se **咽喉閉塞, throat closure** [2]

IS of an inability to drink and eat because of an impassability of the throat resulting from a local swelling, muscle spasm, or an occlusion due to the presence of a foreign object. *QJYF* 7: 若毒氣甚，**咽喉閉塞**不能嚥者，折齒納葱葉口中，以膏灌葱葉中令下, "In case of a severe presence of poison qi, when **throat closure** prevents swallowing, break one tooth out and insert an onion leaf [through the resulting opening] into the mouth. Then instill the [semi-liquid] paste through the leaf. This will make [the throat] move [food] down".

Yan hou bing **咽喉病, diseases of the throat** [1] AN *yan hou zhu bing* 咽喉諸病, all types of diseases of the throat and the tongue.

PC CD of diseases affecting the throat. *BCGM* SE *jin lan shui* 浸藍水：染布水，療**咽喉病**, "The water used for dyeing cloths cures **diseases of the throat**".

Yan hou bu li **咽喉不利, the throat is not free** [6] AN *yan bu li* 咽不利; *yan hou fang ai* 咽喉妨礙, throat obstruction.

IS of a throat disease with pain making swallowing difficult. *ZBYHL* 7: 毒氣上熏，故**咽喉不利**，或痛而生瘡, "Poison qi steams upward with the result that **the throat is not free**. In some cases this is accompanied by pain and the generation of sores".

Yan hou bu tong **咽喉不通, the throat is not passable** [2]

IS of an impossibility to swallow beverages and food. In severe cases breathing is impaired too. *PJF* 204: 木香利膈丸，治寒在膈上，噎塞，**咽喉不通**, " 'Pills with *mu xiang* to open the diaphragm' cure cold above the diaphragm, gullet occlusion with blockage, and when **the throat is not passable**".

Yan hou cu se **咽喉卒塞, sudden throat obstruction** [1]

IS identical with → *yan hou bi se* 咽喉閉塞, throat closure. *BCGM* SE *li* 李 quotes *SYZJ*: **咽喉卒塞**：無藥處，以皂角末吹鼻取嚏, "**Sudden throat obstruction**: When this cannot be dealt with pharmaceutically *in situ*, blow a *zao jiao* powder into the nose to elicit sneezing".

Yan hou fang ai **咽喉妨礙, throat blockage** [1]

IS identical with → *yan hou bu li* 咽喉不利, the throat is not free. *BCGM* SE *chong chu tou xi kang* 舂杵頭細糠 quoting *SJZL* 124: 咽喉如有物噎塞，飲食不下, "The throat has a feeling as if there were a gullet occlusion with a blockage; beverages and food do not descend", writes: **咽喉妨礙**，如有物吞吐不利, "**Throat blockage** as if there were an item that fails to move regardless of whether one intends to swallow it or spit it out".

Yan hou guai zheng **咽喉怪證, strange condition of the throat** [1]

PC with sores growing in the throat, a swelling that does not ache, holes developing after some time that release malodorous qi, and a lack of appetite. *BCGM* SE *gou ju* 枸橘 quotes *QJF*: **咽喉怪證**：咽喉生瘡，層層如疊，不痛，日久有竅出臭氣，廢飲食, "**Strange condition of the throat**: The throat develops sores with several layers as if folded. They do not ache. After an extended period of time they develop a hole to release malodorous qi. [Patients] refrain from drinking and eating".

Yan hou kou chi bing **咽喉口齒病, diseases of the throat, the mouth and the teeth** [1] AN *yan hou kou chi zhu bing* 咽喉口齒諸病.

PC CD of diseases affecting the throat, the oral cavity, and the teeth. *BCGM* SE *huang hua liao* 黃花了 quoting *BCTJ*: 療咽喉口齒, "It cures throat, mouth and teeth", writes: 療**咽喉口齒病**效, "It effectively cures **diseases of the throat, the mouth and the teeth**".

***Yan hou kou chi zhu bing* 咽喉口齒諸病, all types of diseases of the throat, the mouth and the teeth** [1]

PC identical with → *yan hou kou chi bing* 咽喉口齒病, diseases of the throat, the mouth, and the teeth. *BCGM* SE *bo he* 薄荷：利**咽喉口齒諸病**，治瘰癧瘡疥，風瘙癮疹, "It is helpful for **all types of diseases of the throat, the mouth, and the teeth**, and it cures scrofula with pervasion-illness, sores in general and *jie*-illness in particular, wind itching and dormant papules".

***Yan hou kou she zhu bing* 咽喉口舌諸病, all types of diseases of the throat, the mouth and the tongue** [1]

PC CD of diseases affecting the throat, the oral cavity and the tongue. *BCGM* SE *jie geng* 桔梗：甘桔湯，通治**咽喉口舌諸病**, "Decoction with *gan* [cao] and *jie* [*geng*] cures **all types of diseases of the throat, the mouth and the tongue**".

***Yan hou zhong bi* 咽喉腫痹, throat swelling and blockage** [1]

PC identical with → *hou bi* 喉痹, throat blockage. *BCGM* SE *zhu sha gen* 硃砂根：**咽喉腫痹**，磨水或醋嚥之，甚良, "For **throat swelling and blockage**: grind with water or vinegar and swallow. Very good".

***Yan hou zhu bing* 咽喉諸病, all types of throat diseases** [1]

PC identical with → *yan hou bing* 咽喉病, throat disease. *BCGM* SE *liu shui* ·流水：逆流水，主治中風、卒厥、頭風、瘧疾、**咽喉諸病**, "Water flowing contrary to its ordinary direction: it controls by curing wind stroke, sudden recession, head wind, malaria ailment, and **all types of throat diseases**".

***Yan hua* 眼花, blurred vision** [4]

IS of unclear vision, or of a perception of things such as stars or flowers fluttering in front of the eyes. *QJYF* 22: 多四肢沉重、頭痛、心驚、**眼花**, "Often the four limbs feel very heavy. [Patients suffer from] headache, their heart is frightened and their **vision is blurred**".

***Yan hun* 眼昏, dim vision** [7]

IS identical with → *mu hun* 目昏. *QJYF* 6: 凡人少時不自將慎，年至四十，即漸**眼昏**, "When people do not take care of themselves in their youth, when they have reached the age of 40, gradually **dim vision** sets in".

***Yan huo dan du* 烟火丹毒, smoking fire cinnabar poison** [1]

PC of → *dan du* 丹毒, cinnabar poison, starting from the two thighs and the two flanks, and displaying a red color like a fire. *ZLBC* SE *jing tian* 景天 quotes *YSCRF*: 療烟火丹發從背起或兩脅及兩足，赤如火, "It heals smoking fire cinnabar that starts either from the back or from the two flanks and two feet. It is red as fire". *BCGM* SE *jing tian* 景天 in turn quotes this as: 療治**烟火丹毒**，從兩股兩脅起，赤如火, "It cures **smoking fire cinnabar poison** emerging from the two thighs and two flanks, with a redness like fire".

***Yan ji* 眼急, tightness of an eye**[1]

IS identical with → *mu xie* 目斜, slanted eyes a). *TPSHF* 25: 治風，口偏**眼急**，枳殼浸酒方, "To cure wind, with a wry mouth and **tightness of an eye**, [use the] recipe with *zhi ke* steeped in wine".

Yan ji **眼疾, ailments of the eyes** [12] AN *yan bing* 眼病; *yan zhong ji* 眼中疾, ailments in the eyes.

PC identical with → *mu ji* 目疾. *QJYF* 6：此法乃可終生行之，永除**眼疾**, "This [therapeutic] method can be applied throughout one's life. It will rid a person forever of **ailments of the eyes**".

Yan jian **言蹇, impeded language** [1]

IS identical with → *yan yu jian se* 言語蹇澀. *BCGM* Bai bing zhu zhi yao 百病主治藥：風濕痹痛，不遂**言蹇**, "Wind moisture [has led to] blockage and pain. [The limbs] do not follow [one's will] and **language is impeded**".

Yan jin **咽噤, clenched pharynx** [1]

PC of a swollen pharynx making swallowing difficult. *BCGM* SE *qiao* 雀：癰疽瘡癤，**咽噤**齒齲諸症, "[It serves to cure] pathological conditions such as obstruction- and impediment-illnesses, sores and pimples, **clenched pharynx**, and tooth decay".

Yan kou **燕口, swallow's mouth** [3]

PC identical with → *yan kou chuang* 燕口瘡, swallow's mouth sores. *QJYF* 5：治小兒**燕口**，兩吻生瘡方：燒髮灰和豬脂敷之, "Recipe to cure **swallow's mouth** in children, when both lips develop sores: Burn hair to ashes and apply with hog fat".

Yan kou chuang **燕口瘡, swallow's mouth sores** [2] AD *yan kou* 燕口, swallow's mouth.

PC identical with → *wen chuang* 吻瘡, lip sores. *BCSY* SE *bai jia zhu* 百家筯：燒筯頭為灰，傅吻上**燕口瘡**, "Burn the ends of chopsticks to ashes and apply them to **swallow's mouth sores** on the lips".

Yan mei **魘寐, nightmare** [13] AW *meng yan* 夢魘, *hao yan* 好魘, *cu yan* 卒魘, *yan mei* 魘魅, nightmare seduction-specter; *gui yan* 鬼魘, demonic nightmare.

PC of bad dreams with a feeling of being pressed down by demonic beings and finding it difficult to breath. *BJ* SE *she xiang* 麝香：久服除邪，不夢寤**魘寐**, "Ingested over an extended period of time it will eliminate evil, and prevent awaking from **nightmares**".

Yan mei **魘魅, nightmare seduction-specter** [2]

PC identical with → *yan mei* 魘寐, nightmare. *ZBYHL* 23：屈大母指，著四小指內抱之，積習不止，眠時亦不復開，令人不**魘魅**, "Hold the thumb covered by the remaining four fingers. Do this without interruption, even when going to sleep, do not open [the fist]. This prevents a person from being affected by **nightmare seduction-specters**".

Yan mei bao jue **魘寐暴絕, sudden cut-off during nightmare** [1]

PC identical with → *yan si* 魘死, [appearance of] death because of nightmares. *BCGM* SE *fu long gan* 伏龍肝 quoting *QJYF* 25: 鬼魘不悟, "Demonic nightmares and unconsciousness", writes: **魘寐暴絕**, "**Sudden cut-off during nightmare**".

Yan mei si 魘寐死, [appearance of] death from nightmares [1]
PC identical with → *yan si* 魘死. *BCGM* SE *fu long gan* 伏龍肝 quoting *QJYF* 25: 鬼魘不悟, "Demonic nightmares and unconsciousness", writes: 魘寐暴絕, "Sudden cut-off during nightmares". This, in turn, was quoted in *BCGM* Bai bing zhu zhi yao 百病主治藥 as **魘寐死, "[Appearance of] death from nightmares"**.

Yan mo 魘魔, nightmare demon [1]
EA of demons believed to be able to cause → *yan mei* 魘寐, nightmares. *BCGM* SE *xiong huang* 雄黃 quotes *ZWZF*: 辟禳**魘魔**，以雄黃帶頭上, "To turn away **nightmare demons**, carry *xiong huang* on the head".

Yan mu yan hou kou chi zhu bing 眼目咽喉口齒諸病, all types of diseases of the eyes, the throat, the mouth, and the teeth [1]
PC CD of diseases affecting the eyes, the throat, the oral cavity, and the teeth. *BCGM* SE *bo he* 薄荷：頭痛頭風，**眼目咽喉口齒諸病**，小兒驚熱及瘰癧瘡疥，為要藥, "It is an essential medication [for curing] headaches and head wind, **all types of diseases of the eyes, the throat, the mouth, and the teeth**, fright heat in children, scrofula with pervasion-illness, as well as sores and *jie*-illness".

Yan mu zhu bing 眼目諸病, all types of eye diseases [3]
PC identical with → *mu ji* 目疾, ailments of the eyes. *BCGM* SE *xi xin* 細辛：**眼目諸病**，宜用之, "It is to be used for **all types of eye diseases**".

Yan re 眼熱, hot eyes [5]
IS identical with → *mu re* 目熱. *WTMY* 21: 療**眼熱**目赤，生赤脈息肉, "To heal **hot eyes**, and red eyes, and the emergence of tumorous flesh-growths with red vessels".

Yan sheng xi rou 咽生瘜肉, the throat grows tumorous flesh [5] AN *hou zhong sheng rou* 喉中生肉, tumorous flesh-growth in the throat.
PC of → *xi rou* 瘜肉, tumorous flesh-growth, in the throat. *BCGM* SE *yang ti cao* 羊蹄草 quoting *TPSHF* 35: 治懸壅腫及咽喉內有息肉, "It cures uvula swelling and tumorous flesh-growth inside the throat", writes: 懸壅舌腫，**咽生瘜肉**, "Uvula and tongue swelling; **the throat grows tumorous flesh**".

Yan shui bu xia 嚥水不下, drunk water fails to move down [1]
IS identical with → *shui jiang bu xia* 水漿不下, water and broth failing to move down. *WTMY* 23: 升麻湯，療風毒，**嚥水不下**, "Decoction with *sheng ma* cures wind poison and **the failure of drunk water to move down**".

Yan shun 眼瞤, the eyes shiver [1]
IS of eyeballs or eyelids making involuluntery uncontrolled movements. *QJYiF* 16: 頭面風，**眼瞤**，鼻塞，眼暗冷淚方, "Recipe for head and face wind; **shivering eyes**; blocked nose; dim vision with cold tears".

Yan si 魘死, [appearance of] death from nightmares [9] AN *yan mei si* 魘寐死; *yan mei bao si* 魘寐暴絕, sudden cut-off because of nightmare demons.
PC of → *cu si* 卒死, sudden [appearance of] death, resulting from bad dreams while one is asleep. *QJYF* 25: 治**魘死**不自覺者方：慎燈火, 勿令人手動, 牽牛

臨其上即覺, "Recipe to cure **[appearance of] death from nightmares** and unconsciousness: Be careful not to expose [the victim] to a shining light, and let no one touch him. Lead a buffalo to stand above him, and he will regain consciousness".

***Yan sui* 眼睢, squint, strabismus** [2] AN *mu sui* 目睢.
IS identical with → *xie shi* 斜視, squint. *LGPZL* Xu 序：目辟**眼睢**，有五花而自正，五加皮是也。其葉有雄雌，三葉為雄，五葉為雌，須使五葉者，作末酒浸飲之，其目喎者正, " 'When the eyes **squint**, an application of the 'five[-leaves] flower will cause them to return to straight [vision]', is a reference to *wu jia pi*. From its leaves [one can distinguish] male and female variants. [Those with] three leaves are male, [those with] five leaves are female. One must use those with five leaves to prepare a powder and ingest it soaked in wine. Awry eyes will be corrected".

***Yan wo chuang* 燕窩瘡, swallow-nest sores** [2]
PC of → *chuang* 瘡, sores, conditions developing in the nape hollow below the hair line on the back of the head. *BCGM* SE *fei zao jia* 肥皂莢 quotes *ZXF*: 頭耳諸瘡：眉癬、**燕窩瘡**。並用肥皂煅存性一錢，枯礬一分，研勻，香油調，塗之, "All sores affecting the head and ears: eyebrow *xuan*-illness, and **swallow-nest sores**. Use 1 *qian* of *fei zao* (*jia*) prepared with heat maintaining its nature, and one *fen* of *ku fan*. Grind evenly. Mix with *xiang you*, and apply externally".

***Yan xi* 眼瘜, ocular tumor-illness** [1]
PC of a flesh-growth developing in the realm of the eyes. *BCGM* SE *ye ju* 野菊：治癰腫疔毒，瘰癧**眼瘜**, "It cures obstruction-illness with swelling, pin-illness poison, scrofula with pervasion-illness, and **ocular tumor-illness**".

***Yan xiao* 鹽哮, salt roaring** [1]
PC identical with → *yan hou* 鹽齁. *BCGM* SE *zhu ma* 苧麻 quotes *ZXF*: 小兒**鹽哮**：脂麻秸，瓦内燒存性，出火毒，研末，以淡豆腐蘸食之, "**Salt roaring** in children: Bake *zhi ma* straw on a curved tile but maintain its nature. This serves to eliminate its fire poison. Grind to powder. Consume dipped in bland bean curd".

***Yan xie* 眼斜, awry eye** [1]
IS identical with → *mu xie* 目斜 a). *BCGM* SE *zhi* 枳 quoting *BCTJ* SE *zhi shi* 枳實：卒中急風，身直，不得屈伸反覆者, "When one has suddenly been struck by urgent wind, and [as a result] the body is straight, and one is unable to bend and stretch", writes: 中風身直，不得屈伸反覆，及口僻**眼斜**, "When one has been struck by wind, and [as a result] his body is straightened and he is unable to bend and stretch, and the mouth is wry and the **eyes are awry**".

***Yan xuan* 眼眩, visual dizziness** [3]
PC identical with → *mu xuan* 目眩. *MYBL* SE *shu yu* 薯蕷：主頭面游風，風頭**眼眩**, "It controls wind roaming in head and face, and wind head with **visual dizziness**".

Yan ye **咽噎, gullet occlusion** [1]
IS introduced to replace → *yue* 噦, retching. *BCGM* SE *tan huo* 炭火 quoting *QJYiF* 18 卒噦, "Sudden retching", writes: 卒然**咽噎**, "Sudden **gullet occlusion**".

Yan yi **眼翳, eye shade** [5]
PC identical with → *mu yi* 目翳. *WTMY* 21: "深師療**眼翳**方，胡粉注翳上，以療三年翳, "Master Shen's recipe to cure **eye shade**: Drip *hu fen* onto the shade. Shades three years old are cured this way".

Yan yu jian se **言語蹇澀, impeded language** [3] AN *Yan yu jian zhi* 言語蹇滯, Yu jian 語蹇, Yu jian 語謇, Yan jian 言蹇, Yu yan jian se 語言蹇澀, Yu se 語澀.
IS of difficulties in speaking because of an impeded movement of the tongue. Words are projected and cannot be understood easily. *QJYF* 8: 吾嘗中風，**言語蹇澀**，四肢痑曳，處此方日服四服，十日十夜，服之不絕得愈 "When I was struck by wind, my **language was impeded**. The four limbs sagged. I applied this recipe and each day I ingested it four times. I did so for ten days and ten nights and never stopped ingesting. Eventually I was cured".

Yan yu jian zhi **言語蹇滯, impeded language** [1]
IS identical with → *yan yu jian se* 言語蹇澀. *BCGM* SE *wei ling xian* 威靈仙 quoting *HSF*: 此藥治丈夫、婦人中風不語，手足不隨，口眼喎斜…，言語澀滯, "This medication cured males and females struck by wind. They cannot speak, their hands and feet no longer follow their will. The mouth and eyes are slanted … their language is rough and sluggish", writes: 此藥治丈夫婦人中風不語，手足不遂，口眼喎斜，**言語蹇滯**, "This medication cures males and females struck by wind. They cannot speak, their hands and feet do no longer follow their will. The mouth and eyes are slanted. Their **language is impeded**".

Yan yu pi yue **言語僻越, eccentric language** [1]
IS identical with → *pi miu* 僻謬, eccentric and muddled [language]. *MYBL* SE *she tui* 蛇蛻：**言語僻越**，惡瘡，嘔咳, "[It cures] **eccentric language**, malign sores, vomiting and cough".

Yan yun **眼運, visual movements** [1]
IS identical with → *mu yun* 目運. *SJZL* 164: 疼痛寒熱，頭旋**眼運**，精神恍惚, "Pain and alternating sensations of cold and heat. The head spins and [one experiences] **visual movements**. Absent-mindedness. "

Yan zhang **烟瘴, smoky miasma** [1]
EA identical with → *zhang qi* 瘴氣, miasmatic qi ①. *SYJYBZFL* 6 *bai du san* 敗毒散：**烟瘴**之地，或温疫時行，或人多風、多痰、多氣，或處卑濕脚弱，此藥不可缺也, "In regions of **smoky miasma**, during seasonally active warmth epidemics, when people have much wind, phlegm or qi, or if one lives in low-lying moist locations and if his legs are weak, he cannot do without this medication".

Yan zhang **眼障, eye screen** [1]
PC identical with → *mu zhang* 目障. *PJF* 78: 常病**眼障**，全不見物，只用生辰砂一塊，每日眼中擦之, "For diseases as frequent as **eye screen**, when one

cannot see anything, simply take a piece of unprocessed cinnabar and rub it into the eyes day after day".

Yan zhong bi **咽腫痹, throat swelling and blockage** [1]
PC identical with → *hou bi* 喉痹, throat blockage. *BCGM* Bai bing zhu zhi yao 百病主治藥 quoting from the main entry on SE *sheng jiang* 生薑：喉痹毒氣, "Throat blockage poison qi", writes: 生薑汁…**咽腫痹**, "The juice of *sheng jiang* … [serves to cure] **throat swelling and blockage**".

Yan zhong chi mai **眼中赤脈, red vessels in the eye** [1]
PC identical with → *mu zhong chi mai* 目中赤脈. *SJZL* 109: 治**眼中赤脈**，癢痛，時見黑花，杏子膏方, "Recipe for a paste with *xing zi* to cure **red vessels in the eye**, with itching and pain, and occasional vision of dark patterns".

Yan zhong ji **眼中疾, ailments in the eyes** [1]
PC identical with → *yan ji* 眼疾, ailments of the eyes. *YXQY* Lj: 草龍膽，氣寒，味大苦，治兩目赤腫睛脹，瘀肉高起，痛不可忍，以柴胡為主，龍膽為使，治**眼中疾**必用藥也, "*Cao long dan*, its qi is cold; its flavor is very bitter. It serves to cure eyes that are red and swollen, with the eyeball protruding, and excessive flesh rising. The pain is unbearable. With *chai hu* serving as ruler and *long dan* as messenger, for curing **ailments in the eyes**, these are pharmaceutical drugs that must be resorted to".

Yan zi **黶子, black mole** [2]
PC identical with → *hei zhi* 黑痣, on the face. *BCSY* SE *cao hao* 草蒿：燒為灰，紙八九重淋取汁，和石灰去息肉、**黶子**, "Burn to ashes. Place on eight or nine layers of paper and filter water through this. Mix the resulting liquid with *shi hui* to remove tumorous flesh-growths and **black moles**".

Yang **瘍, ulcers** [p]
PC AD of → *chuang yang* 瘡瘍, sores and ulcers. *BJ* SE *shui yin* 水銀：主疥、瘺、痂、**瘍**、白禿, "It controls *jie*-illness, fistulas, crusts, **ulcers**, and white baldness". There are two types of *yang* 瘍, ulcers: *zhong yang* 腫瘍, swollen ulcers, and *kui yang* 潰瘍, festering ulcers.

Yang bi **癢痹, itching with blockage** [1]
IS identical with → *bi yang* 痹癢. *BCGM* SE *wu zhu yu* 吳茱萸 quoting *SLBC* 風瘙癢痛, "Wind, itching, and pain", writes: 風瘺**癢痹**, "Wind, stubborn **itching with blockage**".

Yang dao jue shang **陽道絕傷, harm of yang path severance** [1]
PC identical with → *jue yang* 絕陽, severed yang. *BCGM* SE *lu* 鹿 quoting *SLBC*: 補絕傷, "It supplements severance harm", writes: 補**陽道絕傷**, "It supplements in the case of **harm of yang path severance**".

Yang du **陽毒, yang poison** [30]
① PC a) of → *shang han* 傷寒, harm caused by cold, resulting in a flourishing of only yang qi and a diminution of yin qi, with strong heat and restlessness, a red face with streaks, pain in the throat and bloody sputum as major characteristics. *JGYL* Fj: **陽毒**之為病，面赤斑斑如錦文，咽喉痛，唾膿血, "The disease of **yang poison** is as follows: The face is red and has streaks like a pattern of

brocade. The throat aches. One spits pus and blood". b) Brought forth by being struck by → *xi du* 溪毒, rivulet poison, with ulcers in the body's lower parts that are red as if one had cut the flesh. *ZHF* 7: 當深視下部，若有瘡，正赤如截肉者為**陽毒**, "One should deeply inspect the lower parts [of the body]. If there are ulcers that are purely red as if the flesh had been cut, then this is **yang poison**".
② EA identical with → *du qi* 毒氣, poison qi, with a heat quality. *QJYF* 13: 若臟腑實則為**陽毒**所侵, "The cause of depot and palace repletion is an intrusion of **yang poison**".
③ PQ of pharmaceutical substances with a poisonous nature of massive heat. *TQFLLSF* SE *nao sha* 硇砂：北庭砂所稟陰石之氣，性含**陽毒**之精, "*Bei ting sha* is imbued with the qi of yin stones, and has in its nature the essence of **yang poison**".

Yang du jie xiong **陽毒結胸, bound chest because of yang poison** [1]
PC of → *jie xiong* 結胸, bound [qi in the] chest, brought forth by an exuberant presence of yang poison. *BCGM* SE *qiu jin* 蚯蚓 quotes *SHYY*: **陽毒結胸**，按之極痛，或通而復結，喘促，大躁狂亂, "**Bound chest because of yang poison**: if pressed the pain is extreme. In some cases the [chest] opens and then is bound again. [Patients] pant hectically; they are restless and exhibit madness with confusion".

Yang gui **殃鬼, calamitous demon** [2]
EA identical with → *e gui* 惡鬼, malign demon. *MYBL* SE *sheng ma* 升麻: 主解百毒，殺百精老物**殃鬼**，辟溫疫，瘴氣，邪氣，蠱毒, "It controls the dissolution of all types of poison. It kills all types of ancient spirit beings and **calamitous demons**, and eliminates warmth epidemics, miasmatic qi, evil qi, and *gu* poison".

Yang huang **陽黃, yang jaundice** [2]
PC of a type of → *huang dan* 黃疸, yellow *dan*-illness, characterized by a strong presence of moisture and heat and a weakness of proper qi, as pathological signs, and fever as well as a distinct yellow color of the body, as clinical signs. *SHWZL* Lj: 或服發汗溫中藥太過，加以厚衣蓋覆，仍於陰濕不通風處坐臥，或以火劫之，變為黃病，此乃**陽黃**也，當投寒藥以治之, "It may be that [a patient] has ingested too much medication to make him sweat and warm his center, and that he, in addition, was covered with thick clothes, and was seated or rested lying at a dark, moist place not passed by wind, and if an attempt was made to eliminate [the moisture] by means of fire, and [his illness] then changed to become jaundice, then this is **yang jaundice**. To cure it one must ingest medication of a cold nature".

Yang jue **陽絕, yang cut-off** [3]
PC of a rather serious → *yang xu* 陽虛, yang depletion. *XMLF* 13: 金針丸, 治**陽絕**痞氣, 心腹痛不可忍者, "Golden-Needle Pills cure **yang cut-off** and obstacle-illness qi, with unbearable heartache and abdominal pain".

***Yang mei chuang* 楊梅瘡, red bayberry sores; syphilitic sores** [20] AN *yang mei du chuang* 楊梅毒瘡, red bayberry poison sores.

PC of → *chuang* 瘡, sores, conditions affecting the entire body resulting from an infectious sores poison. *WKLL* 7: **楊梅瘡**：濕勝者，宜先導濕；表實者，宜先解表；裏實者，宜先疏裏, "**Red bayberry sores**: Of those predominantly damp, the moisture needs to be led away first. Of those replete in the outer sphere, the outer sphere needs to be resolved first. Of those replete in the interior, the interior needs to be dredged first".

***Yang mei du chuang* 楊梅毒瘡, red bayberry poison sores** [11]

PC identical with → *yang mei chuang* 楊梅瘡, red bayberry sores. *BCGM* SE *tu fu ling* 土茯苓 quotes *Wang Ji* 汪機：近有好淫之人，多病**楊梅毒瘡**，藥用輕粉，愈而復發, "Nowadays persons who love lewdness often suffer from **red bayberry poison sores**. For a treatment with pharmaceutical drugs one uses *qing fen*. [The disease appears] healed but then breaks out again".

***Yang mei feng* 楊梅風, red bayberry wind** [1]

PC of sinew contraction and aching bones or paralysis brought forth by a consumption of calomel to cure red bayberry sores, i.e. syphilis. *BCGM* Bai bing zhu zhi yao 百病主治藥；土茯苓治楊梅瘡及楊梅風, "*Tu fu ling* cures red bayberry sores and **red bayberry wind**".

***Yang ming bing* 陽明病, yang brilliance disease** [3]

PC in the course of harm caused by cold disease where evil qi has changed to heat and enters the interior causing the yang heat to flourish, with fever, sweating, thirst, vexation and restlessness, a movement in the vessels that is vast, massive, smooth and accelerated, and/or with heat waves in the afternoon, a feeling of distension, fullness and pain in the navel and abdominal region, constipation, a red tongue with a yellow coating, and a deep and accelerated movement in the vessels. *SHL* 182: **陽明病**外證云何？答曰：身熱，汗自出，不惡寒反惡熱也 "A **yang brilliance disease**, what are its external pathological conditions? Answer: The body is hot, and sweats spontaneously. [Patients] have no aversion to cold; on the contrary, they have an aversion to heat".

***Yang ming jing tou tong* 陽明經頭痛, yang brilliance conduit headache** [1]

PC identical with → *yang ming tou tong* 陽明頭痛, yang brilliance headache. *YXZC* 4: 石膏散，治**陽明經頭痛**大效, "Powder with *shi gao* cures **yang brilliance conduit headache**; it is very effective".

***Yang ming tou tong* 陽明頭痛, yang brilliance headache** [3] AN *zheng yang ming tou tong* 正陽明頭痛, proper yang brilliance headache; *shou yang ming tou tong* 手陽明頭痛, hand yang brilliance headache; *yang ming jing tou tong* 陽明經頭痛, yang brilliance conduit headache.

PC of → *tou tong* 頭痛, headache, extending along the course of the yang brilliance conduits resulting from an intrusion of evil qi into the yang brilliance conduits. That is, the pain affects mainly the region of the eyes and the forehead. *SJZL* 24: **陽明頭痛**，不惡寒反惡熱, "In the case of **yang brilliance headache**, [patients] have no aversion to cold; on the contrary, they have an aversion to heat".

Yang qi xia xie **陽氣下陷, defect of yang qi descent** [5] AD *yang xie* 陽陷, yang defect.

PM of an insufficiency of yang qi impairing the physiological dynamics of clear qi rising and turbid qi sinking, which leads to diarrhea, blockage with a feeling of fullness, and dizziness. *BCGM* Bai bing zhu zhi yao 百病主治藥：**陽氣下陷**作泄, "**The defect of yang qi descent** causes diarrhea".

Yang shi bu qi **陽事不起, failure of the yang thing to rise** [6]

PC identical with → *yin wei* 陰痿, dysfunction of the yin [member, i.e. penis]. *PJF* 卷 219: 治臟腑虛冷，元陽正氣虛弱，**陽事不起**, "It cures conditions such as depletion cold affecting the depots and palaces, depletion weakness of original yang and proper qi, and **failure of the yang thing to rise**".

Yang shi bu xing **陽事不行, failure of the yang thing to act** [1]

PC identical with → *yin wei* 陰痿, dysfunction of the yin [member, i.e. penis]. *SYXJ* SE *yang shen* 羊腎：主下焦虛冷，脚膝無力，**陽事不行**, "It controls depletion cold affecting the lower burner, lack of strength in legs and knees, and **failure of the yang thing to act**".

Yang shi bu xing **陽事不興, failure of the yang thing to rise** [1]

PC identical with → *yin wei* 陰痿, dysfunction of the yin [member, i.e. penis]. *PJF* 227: 安腎丸，治男子諸風，五勞七傷，顏色枯朽，手足不遂，語言謇澀，口眼歪斜，筋脈攣急，腰脚疼痛…及**陽事不興**，胃冷精流, "The pills to calm the kidneys cure all types of male wind, the five types of exhaustion and seven types of harm, withered and decayed complexion, when hands and feet do not follow one's wishes, with impaired language, wry mouth and eyes, cramped sinews and vessels, painful lower back and legs … as well as **failure of the yang thing to rise**, and stomach cold with [involuntary] seminal pollution".

Yang shi wei ruo **陽事痿弱, dysfunction of the yang thing** [1]

PC identical with → *yin wei* 陰痿, dysfunction of the yin [member, i.e. penis]. *BCGM* SE *diao* 吊 quotes *BHJJF*: **陽事痿弱**：紫梢花、生龍骨各二錢，麝香少許，為末，蜜丸梧子大。每服二十丸，燒酒下, "For **dysfunction of the yang thing**: *zi shao hua* and unprocessed dragon bones, 2 *qian* each. *She xiang*, a small quantity. Grind to a powder, and prepare pills with honey the size of *wu* seeds. Each dosage comprises 20 pills, to be ingested with brandy".

Yang shui **陽水, yang water** [10]

PC of → *shui zhong* 水腫, water swelling, disease with swelling of the entire body, vexation, constipation and difficult urination. *DXXF* 2: 若遍身腫，煩渴，小便赤澀，大便閉，此屬**陽水**, "When the entire body is swollen, with vexation, difficult and red urination, and constipation, this is **yang water**".

Yang tuo **陽脫, loss of yang [qi]** [1]

PC identical with → *tuo yang* 脫陽. *SJZL* 23: 氣虛**陽脫**，體冷無脈，氣息欲絕，不省人事, "In the case of qi depletion and **loss of yang [qi]**, the body is cold and has no [movement in the] vessels. The breathing of qi is about to be interrupted, and [patients] fail to recognize other people and things".

Yang wei **陽痿, dysfunction of the yang [member]** [4]

PC identical with → *yin wei* 陰痿, dysfunction of one's yin [member, i.e. penis]. *YXRM* 4: **陽痿**不舉，命門脈虛欲脫者，巨勝子丸, "For **dysfunction of one's yang [member]** with its failure to rise and when the [movement in the] vessels of the gate of life is depleted with a tendency toward complete absence, [use] the pills with *ju sheng zi*".

Yang xian **羊癇, sheep epilepsy** [2]

PC of a → *dian xian* 癲癇, peak-illness with epilepsy, which, at the time of its outbreaks, makes the patient's four limbs twitch, and his eyes and tongue protrude. *QJYF* 5: **羊癇**之為病，喜揚目吐舌, "The disease of **sheep epilepsy**: a tendency to raise the eyes and to stick out the tongue".

Yang xie **陽陷, yang defect** [3]

EA PM identical with → *yang qi xia xie* 陽氣下陷, defect of yang qi descent. *BCGM* SE *sheng ma* 升麻：治**陽陷**眩運, 胸脅虛痛, 久泄下痢, "It cures **yang defect** with dizziness, depletion pain in the chest and flanks, as well as long-lasting outflow and discharge with free-flux illness".

Yang xu **陽虛, yang depletion** [29]

PC of depletion with insufficient yang qi, with a decrease of functions, a diminution of reaction, and a lack of yang heat. *LS* 9: 陰盛而**陽虛**，先補其陽，後瀉其陰而和之, "In the case of yin abundance and **yang depletion**, the yang is to be supplemented first, and the yin is to be drained afterwards. This leads to harmonization".

Yang yi **陽易, yang exchange** [1]

PC of a communicable disease acquired by females through sexual intercourse with a male who had just been cured of harm caused by cold. *ZBYHL*8: 男子病新瘥未平復，而婦人與之交接得病者，名**陽易**, "The disease acquired by a woman who had intercourse with a male who had just been cured of the disease without having fully recovered yet, it is called '**yang exchange**'".

Yang zheng **陽證, yang condition** [4]

① PC CD of violent body reactions to heat abundance without qi and blood depletion. *SJZL* 192: 陽證之病, 不可灸也, "Diseases that are **yang conditions** must not be cauterized".

② IS CD of all conditions of body depletion with heat abundance apparant as a high fever and red face, as well as madness with restlessness and constipation. *SHL* 130: 臟結, 無**陽證**, 不往來寒熱, 其人反靜, 舌上苔滑者, 不可攻也, "In the case of a depot bind, with no **yang condition**, and no alternative sensations of cold and heat, if, in contrast, that person is calm and the coating on the tongue is smooth, one must not carry out an attack".

Yao chuang **咬瘡, bite sores** [22] AN *nie chuang* 齧瘡.

PC of → *chuang* 瘡, sores, conditions resulting from bites by any animal or insect. *QJYF* 26: 茴香菜，其子主蛇**咬瘡**久不瘥者，擣敷之, "Fennel: its seeds control snake **bite sores** that have not healed for a long time. Pound and apply them [to the wound]".

***Yao du* 藥毒, pharmaceutical drug poison; drug poisoning** [88]

① EA. The poison in a pharmaceutical substance. *ZHF* 7 has 治卒中諸**藥毒**救解方, "Recipes to cure suddenly being struck by all types of **pharmaceutical drug poison**".

② PC of poisoning brought forth by ingestion of inadequate pharmaceutical substances. *QJYiF* 21: 諸得**藥毒**，以冷水半合，研藥一丸如梧子，服之，二服止, "For all afflictions resulting from **drug poisoning**, grind the medication, one pill of the size of a *wu* seed, with half a *ge* of cold water and ingest it. After two dosages the [poisoning] will be ended". Variants of drug poisoning documented in the *BCGM* include *bai yao du* 百藥毒, poisoning from all types of pharmaceutical drugs; *shi yao du* 石藥毒, poisoning from mineral drugs; *cao shi yao du* 草石藥毒, poisoning from herbal and mineral drugs; *jin shi yao du* 金石藥毒, poisoning from gold and mineral drugs, and *dan shi yao du* 丹石藥毒, poisoning from cinnabor [et al.] mineral drugs.

***Yao du* 咬毒, poisoning resulting from bites** [29] AN *shi du* 螫毒.

PC of poisoning resulting from poison entering the body in the course of a bite or sting by an animal with poisonous glands. *QJYF* 25: 治蜘蛛**咬毒**方, "Recipes to cure **poisoning resulting from the bites** of spiders". Bite poisonings documented in the *BCGM* include *she yao du* 蛇咬毒, snake bite poisoning; *kuang quan yao du* 狂犬咬毒, mad dog bite poisoning; *ying yi yao du* 蠅蟻咬毒, fly and ant bite poisoning; *xie yao du* 蠍咬毒; scorpion bite (sic!) poisoning.

***Yao ji luan* 腰脊攣, lower back and spinal contraction** [1]

IS of bent lumbar region and spine making it difficult to assume an upright position. *RHZ* SE *du zhong* 杜仲：治腎勞，**腰脊攣**, "It cures kidney exhaustion, as well as **lower back and spinal contraction**".

***Yao leng* 腰冷, the lower back is cold** [3]

IS of a feeling of cold in the lower back. *ZBYHL* 5: 其病狀，身重，**腰冷**，腹重如帶五千錢, "The signs of this disease: the body feels heavy; **the lower back is cold**; the abdomen feels heavy as if it carried five thousand strings of cash".

***Yao nüe* 妖瘧, goblin malaria** [1]

PC identical with → *jie nüe* 痎瘧, epidemic malaria. *BCSY* SE *nüe gui* 瘧龜：痎瘧，下俚人呼為**妖瘧**, "Epidemic malaria is called '**goblin malaria**' by vulgar persons".

***Yao rong rong ru zuo shui zhong* 腰溶溶如坐水中, flabby lower back, as if one were sitting in water** [4]

IS of flabbiness and weakness in one's lower back accompanied by a feeling of cold. *NJ* 29: 帶之為病，腹滿，**腰溶溶若坐水中**, "When the belt [vessel] has an illness, the abdomen feels full and [patients] suffer from a **flabby lower back as if they were sitting in water**".

Yao shang 咬傷, harm from a bite [48] AN *nie shang* 齧傷.

PC of a → *shang sun* 傷損, injury, resulting from bites of an animal or a human. *SJZL* 139: 治一切金刃箭鏃傷中，及打撲傷損，貓犬**咬傷**，或至死者，急於傷處摻藥, "To cure all types of injuries from metal [objects, including] blades and arrowheads, as well as injuries from a blow, and **harm from bites** of cats and dogs that may be fatal, attach [this] medication quickly to the location of the injury". *BCGM* lists the following as potential causes of harm from a bite: *zhi quan* 猘犬, rabid dog (AN *zhi gou* 猘狗, *kuang quan* 狂犬, *dian quan* 顛犬, *kuang gou* 狂狗); *wu song* 蜈蚣, centipede; *she xie* 蛇蠍, snakes and scorpions; *she hui* 蛇虺, venomous snake; *zhu chong* 諸蟲, all types of bugs/worms; *bai chong* 百蟲, the hundred/all bugs/worms; *hu quan* 虎犬, tigers and dogs; *ren* 人, human person.

Yao shi 咬螫, bites and stings [2]

EA identical with → *shi ren* 螫人, to sting a person. *BCGM* SE *ren shi* 人屎 quoting *QJYF* 25: 治蛇齧方：人屎厚塗，帛裹即消, "Recipe to cure snake bite: Apply a thick layer of human feces and bandage with silk cloth. This will dissolve it". writes: 毒蛇**咬螫**：人屎厚封之，即消, "If someone was **bitten/stung** by a venomous snake: wrap a thick layer of human feces around it, and it will dissolve".

Yao shi fa 藥石發, outbreak of [stalactite] mineral drug [poisoning] [1]

PC identical with → *ru shi fa* 乳石發, outbreak of stalactite mineral [poisoning]. *BCSY* SE *qian jin teng* 千金藤：**藥石發**, 癲, 雜疹, 悉主之, "It controls **outbreak of [stalactite] mineral drug [poisoning]**, peak-illness, and various types of papules alike".

Yao shi fa dong 藥石發動, outbreak of [stalactite] mineral drug [poisoning] [1]

PC identical with → *ru shi fa* 乳石發, outbreak of stalactite mineral [poisoning]. *KBBC* SE lü dou 綠豆：主丹毒, 煩熱, 風疹, **藥石發動**, 熱氣奔豚, 生研絞汁服, "To master cinnabar poisoning with vexing heat, wind papules, **outbreak of [stalactite] mineral drug [poisoning]**, heat qi with running piglets, grind fresh [*lü dou*], wring to obtain the juice, and ingest".

Yao tou 搖頭, shaking of the head [7]

IS of an uncontrolled swaying and shuddering of the head. *BJ* SE *zao xiu* 蚤休：主驚癇，**搖頭**弄舌, "It controls fright epilepsy, **shaking of the head**, and non-directional movement of the tongue".

Yao ya 咬牙, biting the teeth [2]

IS of involuntary uncontrolled and noisy mutual grinding of the upper and lower teeth. *BCGM* SE *tong cao* 通草 quoting *XEYZZJ* Fj: 視其睡, 口中氣温, 或合面睡, 及上竄切牙, 皆心熱也。導赤散主之, "When the [child] seems to be asleep with warm qi in its mouth, or when it sleeps facing upwards, with its eyes turned upwards, and pressing the teeth upon each other, this is always a case of heat in the heart. The 'powder to draw away redness' will control this", writes: 心熱尿赤：面赤唇乾，**咬牙**口渴。導赤散, "For heat in the heart with red urine, a red face and dry lips, **biting the teeth** and a thirsty mouth, [use] the 'powder to draw away redness'".

***Ye* 噎, gullet occlusion** [23]

① IS of an uncomfortable feeling of painful blockage in the throat, chest, and diaphragm region brought forth by an inability to swallow. This may be caused by bad food, or too hectic swallowing as singular events, or as a major sign of a gullet occlusion disease. *QJYF* 5: 兒**噎**，輒奪其乳，令得息，息已，復乳之, "When children experience **gullet occlusion**, immediately remove them from the breast and let them get some breath. When they have got some breath, continue to breastfeed them".

② PC identical with → *ye bing* 噎病, gullet occlusion disease. *ZHF* 6: 取老牛涎沫如棗核大，置水中，飲之。終身不復患**噎**也, "Take as much as a date pit of an old buffalo's saliva foam, place it in water, and drink this. For your entire life you will never suffer from **gullet occlusion** again".

***Ye bing* 噎病, gullet occlusion disease** [9] AD *ye* 噎; AN *ye ji* 噎疾, gullet occlusion ailment; *ye sai* 噎塞, gullet occlusion.

PC of a → *ye ge* 噎膈, gullet occlusion, where the seat of the disease is in the throat and does not permit beverages or food to pass. *QJYF* 26: 羊肚共飯飲常食，久之成反胃，作**噎病**, "If one regularly consumes sheep stomach together with one's food and beverages, after an extended period this will cause a turned-over stomach and result in **gullet occlusion disease**".

***Ye bu he yan* 夜不合眼, inability to close the eyes at night** [2]

IS identical with → *bu mian* 不眠①, insomnia. *BCGM* SE *deng xin cao* 燈心草 quotes *BHJJF*: **夜不合眼**，難睡。燈草煎湯代茶飲，即得睡, "In case one is **unable to close one's eyes at night** and has difficulties falling asleep, he should boil lampwick rush and drink it instead of tea. This will enable him to sleep".

***Ye bu neng wo* 夜不能臥, inability to lie down to sleep at night** [1]

IS identical with → *bu de wo* 不得臥 b), inability to lie down. *BCGM* SE *can* 蠶 quoting *RZTJYF* 不能睡臥, "Unable to lie down to sleep", writes: **夜不能臥, "Inability to lie down to sleep at night".**

***Ye chou* 腋臭, armpit stench** [4] AN *chou ye* 臭腋， malodorous armpit.

PC of → *hu chou* 胡臭, barbarian stench, as a distinct stench originating from one's armpits. *TBC* SE *chi tong xie* 赤銅屑：以醋和如麥飯，袋盛，先刺腋下脈，去血，封之，攻**腋臭**神效, "Mix with vinegar as if to prepare a wheat dish, and fill this into a bag. First pierce the vessels in the armpit to let blood. Then cover [the wound] with the [bag]. This is wondrously effective in fighting **armpit stench**".

***Ye die* 殗殜, progressing calamity** [6]

PC identical with → *chuan shi* 傳屍, corpse [evil] transmission. *WTMY* 13: 傳屍之疾…以其初得，半臥半起，號為**殗殜**, "The ailment of corpse [evil] transmission...in its initial stages, when one lies as much as he is up, this is called **progressing calamity**".

***Ye ge* 噎膈, gullet occlusion** [64] AN *ge ye* 膈噎.

PC of a blockage preventing food from reaching the stomach, in some cases causing food to be thrown up again. In accordance with notions of different locations of the disease, ancient authors distinguished between → *ye bing* 噎病, gullet occlusion disease, and → *ge bing* 膈病, occlusion disease. *SLBC* SE *dan zhu ru* 淡竹茹：主**噎膈**、鼻衄, "It controls **gullet occlusion**, as well as nosebleed". LSZ: **噎膈**反胃，積塊內癥之病…皆起於七情飲食所致，痰氣鬱結，遂成有形，妨礙道路, "Diseases such as **gullet occlusion**, turned over stomach, accumulation-lumps and internal concretion-illness…are all caused by the seven affects, as well as consumption of beverages and food. Phlegm qi is pent-up and forms nodes, which gradually assume physical shape with the result that they block the way".

***Ye huo dan du* 野火丹毒, wild fire cinnabar poisoning** [2]

PC of → *dan du* 丹毒, cinnabar poisoning, starting from the two feet or from the two flanks on the back. *BCGM* SE *ru xiang* 乳香 quotes *YYXS*: **野火丹毒**：自兩足起。乳香末, 羊脂調塗, "**Wild fire cinnabar poison** emerges from the two feet. Mix *ru xiang* powder and *yang* fat and apply externally".

***Ye ji* 噎疾, gullet occlusion ailment** [11]

PC identical with → *ye bing* 噎病, gullet occlusion disease. *HJJF* 3：撞氣阿魏丸，治五種**噎疾**, " 'Pills with *a wei* to strike the qi' cure five types of **gullet occlusion ailments**".

***Ye ji bing* 野雞病, wild fowl disease** [8] AN *ye ji zhi* 野雞痔, wild fowl piles; *ye ji lou zhi* 野雞瘺痔, wild fowl fistula piles; *ye ji lou chuang* 野雞瘺瘡, wild fowl fistula sore.

PC identical with → *zhi* 痔, piles. *BCSY* SE *rong shou* 狨獸：主五**野雞病**。取其脂傅瘡，亦食其血肉，亦坐其皮，積久**野雞病**皆差也, "It controls five types of **wild fowl disease**. Smear its fat on the lesion, eat its blood and meat, and sit on its skin. This will heal **wild fowl disease** that has lasted for an extended period of time". The term *zhi* 痔, piles, is homophone with the character *zhi* 雉 constituting the second name of the founder of the Han-dynasty Liu Bang's wife Lü Zhi 呂雉. Legend has it that, allegedly to honor the taboo on the term *zhi* 雉, pheasant, as well as its homophones such as *zhi* 痔, piles, in what appears to have beeen a satirical act the emperor's wife was likened to the disease of hemorrhoids in that the latter was designated with the characters for "wild fowl", *ye ji* 野雞, alluding to the "pheasant" (*zhi* 雉) as a fowl living in the wilderness. In later times people may have forgotten these etymological origins and spoke of *ye ji zhi* 野雞痔, wild fowl piles, to clarify the meaning of the term.

***Ye ji lou chuang* 野雞瘺瘡wild fowl fistula sores** [1]

PC identical with → *zhi lou* 痔瘺, piles fistula. *BCSY* SE *tu ba shu* 土撥鼠：主**野雞瘺瘡**, "It controls **wild fowl fistula sores**".

***Ye ji lou zhi* 野雞瘺痔, wild fowl fistula piles** [1]

PC identical with → *zhi lou* 痔瘺, piles fistula. *HYBC* SE *jin xian fan* 金綫礬：主**野雞瘺痔**，惡瘡疥癬等疾, "It controls ailments such as **wild fowl fistula piles**, malign sores, *jie*-illness and *xuan*-illness".

***Ye ji zhi* 野雞痔, wild fowl piles** [2]

PC identical with → *ye ji bing* 野雞病. *BCSY* SE *rong shou* 狨獸：主五**野雞痔**下血, "It controls the five types of **wild fowl piles** with bleeding".

***Ye qi* 噎气, gullet occlusion qi** [3]

① PC identical with → *qi ye* 氣噎① a), qi induced gullet occlusion. *SWBJQYBMJ* Lj: 治產後衝脹，胸中有物狀，是**噎氣**，不降，紫金丹, "For treating surging [qi] and distension following delivery, with a feeling as if there were an object in the chest, this is **gullet occlusion qi** which fails to descend, [use] purple-gold-elixir".

② IS identical with → *qi ye* 氣噎②, qi[-induced] gullet occlusion. *BCGM* Bai bing zhu zhi yao 百病主治藥：雞嗉，**噎氣**不通，燒研，入木香，沉香、丁香、紅棗丸服, "For **gullet occlusion qi** failing to pass on, roast chicken crop and grind it, add *mu xiang*, *chen xiang*, *ding xiang*, and *hong zao*, and ingest as pills".

***Ye re* 夜熱, nocturnal heat** [3]

IS of fever occurring at night and subsiding again at dawn. *DXXF* 2: 大病後陰虛，氣鬱**夜熱**, "In the aftermath of a massive disease, when the yin is depleted, [patients experience] pent-up qi and **nocturnal heat**".

***Ye se* 噎塞, gullet occlusion with blockage** [11]

① PC identical with → *ye bing* 噎病, gullet occlusion disease. *QJYF* 16: 胃腑方設 "**噎塞**第六"，專論各種噎病, "Recipes for the stomach palace are listed in '**Gullet occlusion with blockage** #6'. It focuses on all types of gullet occlusion disease".

② IS of all types of uncomfortable sensations of a blocked passage of qi, water/liquid, and food. *ZBYHL* 20：噎者，**噎塞**不通也, "Gullet occlusion is a **gullet occlusion with blockage**, i.e. no passage".

***Ye shi* 噎食, gullet occluding food** [25]

PC identical with → *ye bing* 噎病, gullet occlusion disease. *PJF* 205: 治**噎食**，用猢猻糞陰乾，燒灰，好酒送下，不過十服立瘥, "To cure **gullet occluding food**, take macaque feces dried in the shade and burned to ashes, and swallow with good wine. After ten intakes at most this will bring a cure".

***Ye si* 暍死, [appearance of] death from sunstroke** [5]

PC of → *cu si* 卒死, sudden [appearance of] death, resulting from an extreme exposure to heat or sunlight. *WTMY* 28: 文仲療夏月**暍死**方。濃煮蓼汁, 灌三升, 不瘥更灌之, "Recipe by Wenzhong to cure **[appearance of] death from sunstroke** in summer. Boil the juice of knotweed down to a viscous liquid, and forcibly instill 3 *sheng* [into the patient]. If this does not cure him, forcibly instill again".

***Ye ti* 夜啼, night crying** [59]

PC of children with incessant crying during the night that calms down only at dawn. *BJ* SE *zha chan* 蚱蟬：主小兒驚癇，**夜啼**, "It controls fright epilepsy in children, as well as their **night crying**".

Ye tong **噎痛, painful gullet occlusion** [1]

IS of a feeling of painful obstruction with pressure in the chest. *BCYY* SE *ha jie* 蛤蚧：喉中氣塞，胸鬲**噎痛**, "For qi blockage in the throat; chest occlusion, and **painful gullet occlusion**".

Ye wo bu an **夜臥不安, lying down at night without finding rest** [1] AW *ye wo bu ning* 夜臥不寧.

IS of shallow sleep at night from which one wakes up easily. *ZBYHL* 34: 轉脈瘺者，因飲酒大醉，**夜臥不安**，驚，欲嘔，轉側失枕之所生也, "The origin of twisted vessels fistula is as follows: [Patients] consumed wine until they were massively intoxicated. They **lied down at night but could not find rest**. They were frightened and experienced an urge to vomit. When they turned [around on their bed] they missed the headrest".

Ye wo bu ning **夜臥不寧, lying down at night without finding rest** [1]

IS identical with → *ye wo bu an* 夜臥不安. *SJZL* 43: 治心氣虛弱驚悸，**夜臥不寧**，沉香散方, "To cure depletion weakness of the heart qi, with fright and palpitation, and when **one lies down at night without finding rest**, [use] the recipe for the powder with *chen xiang*".

Ye wo jing han **夜臥驚汗, fright and sweating during sleep at night** [1]

IS of suddenly waking up in fright from sleep at night and sweating without apparent reason. *BCGM* Bai bing zhu zhi yao 百病主治藥：龍骨止**夜臥驚汗**, "*Long gu* stops **fright and sweating during one's sleep at night**".

Ye wo zi jing **夜臥自驚, spontaneous fright during one's sleep at night** [1]

IS of suddenly waking up in fright from sleep at night without apparent reason. *MYBL* SE *long gu* 龍骨：療心腹煩滿，四肢痿枯，汗出，**夜臥自驚**, "It cures vexation and a feeling of fullness in the heart and abdomen; loss of function of the four extremities; sweating; **spontaneous fright during one's sleep at night**".

Ye yan **噎涎, gullet occlusion with drooling** [1]

IS of a heavy flow of saliva from the mouth. *BCTJ* SE *yi yu* 鮧魚：不可與牛肝合食，令人患風多**噎涎**, "It must not be eaten together with ox liver lest it make a person suffer from much wind and **gullet occlusion with drooling**".

Ye you **腋瘤, armpit tumor** [1]

PC of → *liu ying* 瘤癭, goiter, growing in the armpit. *BCGM* Bai bing zhu zhi yao 百病主治藥 quoting *BHJJF*: 腋下瘤癭, "Tumorous goiter in the armpit", writes: **腋瘤, "Armpit tumor"**.

Yi **疫, epidemic** [23]

PC AD of → *wen yi* 瘟疫, warmth-illness epidemic. *JGYL* Lj: 六畜自死，皆**疫**死，則有毒，不可食之, "When the six types of domestic animals die by themselves, these are always deaths because of an **epidemic.** That is, they are poisonous and cannot be eaten".

Yi **噫, belching** [6]

IS identical with → *yi qi* 噫氣, belching qi. *ZBYHL* 6: 氣自通，得**噫**, "Qi passes spontaneously, and this results in **belching**".

Yi **翳, shade** [p]

① PI of a speckled membrane covering the pupil and impairing vision. *ZBYHL* 48：輕者止生一**翳**，重者乃至兩三**翳**也, "In mild cases only one **shade** grows. In severe cases these may be up to two or three **shades**.

② PC AD of → *mu yi* 目翳, eye shade. *ZHF* 2：若生**翳**者，燒豉二七粒，末，納管鼻中以吹之, "In case a **shade** grows, burn two times seven salted fermented beans, and prepare a powder which is to be blown into the nose through a tube".

Yi bai er shi zhong e feng **一百二十種惡風, one hundred and twenty types of malign wind** [2]

DC: *YXL* refers to *ma hua* 麻花 as: 能治**一百二十種惡風** "It is able to cure **120 types of malign wind**".

Yi bai liu shi zhong e feng **一百六十種惡風, one hundred and sixty types of malicious wind** [2]

DC: *YXL* refers to *gao ben* 藁本 as: 能治**一百六十種惡風**, "It is able to cure **160 types of malign wind**".

Yi bing **疫病, epidemic disease** [3]

PC identical with → *wen yi* 瘟疫, warmth-illness epidemic. *ZBYHL* 26: 因**疫病**死者，肉亦有毒, "[Horses] that have died because of an **epidemic disease**: their meat is poisonous too".

Yi bu xia **衣不下, the placenta fails to descend** [3]

PC identical with → *bao yi bu xia* 胞衣不下. *JXCB* Bao yi bu xia 胞衣不下：歷時既久，或乘冷氣，則血道凝澀而**衣不下**, "After an extended period of time it may be that cold qi will avail itself [of the void]. As a result, the blood will congeal and its path will be rough and **the placenta fails to descend**".

Yi dan **嗌疸, throat *dan*-illness** [1]

PC identical with → *zou ma hou bi* 走馬喉痹, running horse throat blockage. *BCGM* Bai bing zhu zhi yao 百病主治藥：有**嗌疸**，俗名走馬喉痹，殺人最急, "When someone has **throat *dan*-illness**, this is commonly called 'running horse throat blockage'. It kills a person very quickly".

Yi du **疫毒, epidemic poison** [2]

PC of → *yi bing*, 疫病, epidemic disease, with papules, swelling and sores, and sometimes bleeding. *WTMY* 2: 蒲黄湯，療傷寒温病，天行**疫毒**, "Decoction with *pu huang*: to cure harm caused by cold and warmth disease, and heaven-sent **epidemic poison**".

Yi e **噫呃, hiccough** [2]

IS identical with → *e ni* 呃逆①, hiccough with adverse movement of qi. *BCGM* SE *ren shen* 人參 quotes *TPSHF:* 多食則吐，氣引前後，**噫呃**不除, "Eaten in large quantities it causes vomiting, with qi pulling on the front and back. [Patients experience] **hiccough** and are unable to relieve themselves of [what appears to be stuck in their body]".

Yi gan 嗌乾, the throat is desiccated [2]
IS identical with → *yan gan* 咽乾. *SW* 31: 四日太陰受之，太陰脈布胃中絡於嗌，故腹滿而**嗌乾**, "On the fourth day, the major yin [conduits] receive it. The major yin vessels spread into the stomach and enclose the throat. Hence, [patients] have a feeling of abdominal fullness and their **throat is desiccated**".

Yi ji 疫疾, epidemic ailment [11]
PC identical with → *wen yi* 瘟疫, warmth-illness epidemic. *BJ* SE *xu zhang qing* 徐長卿：主鬼物百精，蠱毒**疫疾**，邪惡氣，温瘧, "Controls demonic items and the one hundred spirits; the poison of *gu* and **epidemic ailments**, evil and malign qi, as well as warmth malaria".

Yi ji 異疾, unusual ailment [3]
PC identical with → *guai bing* 怪病, queer disease. *QJYF* 5: 小兒無**異疾**, 惟飲食過度, 不知自止, 哺乳失節, "Children have no **unusual ailments**. It is only that their eating and drinking may exceed limits. They themselves do not know when to stop. Their nursing may be immoderate".

Yi jing 遺精, involuntary emission of seminal fluid [50] AN *xie jing* 泄精, *jing xie* 精泄, *yi xie* 遺泄, *shi jing* 失精, *yi li* 遺瀝.
PC with emissions of seminal fluid independent of sexual intercourse. *HYBC* SE *an xi xiang* 安息香：又主男子**遺精**, "It also controls **involuntary emission of seminal fluid** by males".

Yi ju 異疽, strange impediment-illness [2]
PC of → *ju* 疽, impediment-illness, somewhat similar to a → *yong* 疽, obstruction-illness, with pus like the juice of small beans. They vanish one day and are filled again the next. *BCGM* SE *yun tai* 芸薹 quoting *QJYF*: 疽似癰而小有異, "Impediment-illness reminiscent of obstruction-illnesses but smaller. They are strange", writes: **異疽**似癰, "**Strange impediment-illness** reminiscent of obstruction-illness".

Yi li 疫癧, epidemic pervasion-illness [1]
PC identical with → *wen yi* 瘟疫, warmth-illness epidemic. Probably an erroneous writing of → *yi li* 疫癘. *BCGM* Bai bing zhu zhi yao 百病主治藥, Shang han re bing 傷寒熱病：黑大豆，**疫癧**發腫，炒熟，同甘草煎服, For **epidemic pervasion-illness**: Black beans, thoroughly roasted, should be ingested with a *gan cao* decoction".

Yi li 疫癘, epidemic [12]
PC identical with → *wen yi* 瘟疫, warmth-illness epidemic. *ZHBJF* 2 in the paragraph Zhi zhang qi yi li wen du zhu fang di shi wu 治瘴氣疫癘温毒諸方第十五, "All recipes to cure miasmatic qi, epidemics, and warmth poison, #15", lists a recipe 辟天行**疫癘**, "To ward off heaven-sent **epidemics**".

Yi li 遺瀝, involuntary emission [of seminal fluid] [6]
PC identical with → *yi jing* 遺精. *RHZ* SE *ji li zi* 蒺藜子：止**遺瀝**泄精，溺血, "It stops **involuntary emission** with free flow of seminal fluid, and hematuria".

_Yi li qi_ 疫癘氣, epidemic qi [1]
EA identical with → *yi qi* 疫氣, epidemic qi. *BCGM* SE *ma chi xian* 馬齒莧 quotes *JYF*: 禳解疫氣：六月六日，采馬齒莧晒乾。元旦煮熟，同鹽、醋食之，可解**疫癘氣**, "To ward off epidemic qi: On the sixth day of the sixth month collect *ma chi xian* and dry it. On New Year's Day boil it thoroughly and eat it with salt and vinegar. This can dissolve **epidemic qi**".

Yi lou 蟻瘺, ant fistula [11]
PC of → *lou* 瘺, fistula, with many small swellings that appear strung together mostly around one's neck. In severe cases they cover the entire body. In former times it was believed that this disease results from inadvertently ingesting poisonous semen of ants. Hence for treatment a medication was prepared from animals known to overcome ants. *MYBL* SE *ling li jia* 鯪鯉甲：燒之作灰，以酒或水和方寸匕，療**蟻瘺**, "Burn to ashes and mix with wine or water. One square inch size spoon will heal **ant fistula**".

Yi meng 異夢, wild dreams [1]
IS of wild dreams leaving a person fatigued. *HJJF* 5: 夜多**異夢**，晝少精神, "Those who have many **wild dreams** during the night have little essence spirit during daytime".

Yi miao 翳眇, shade blindness [1]
PC identical with → *mu yi* 目翳, eye shade. *BJ* SE *chang shi* 長石；明目，去**翳眇**, "It clears the eyes and removes **shade blindness**".

_Yi mo_ 翳膜, shade membrane [44] AN *mo yi* 膜翳.
PC identical with → *mu yi* 目翳, eye shade. *WTMY* 2: 若毒氣盛者，眼生**翳膜**, "In the case of abounding poison qi, the eyes will grow a **shade membrane**".

_Yi ni_ 遺溺, loss of urine [17]
IS identical with *yi niao* 遺尿. *SW* 23: 膀胱不利為癃，不約為**遺溺**, "In the urinary bladder, if it does not pass freely, this is a protuberance-illness; if it is unrestrained, this constitutes a **loss of urine.**

_Yi ni_ 噫逆, belching with adverse movement [of qi] [2]
IS identical with → *e ni* 呃逆①, hiccough with adverse movement of qi. *PJF* 138: **噫逆**即咳逆，胃寒所致也, "*Yi ni*, **belching with adverse movement [of qi]**, is identical with *ke ni*, cough with adverse movement [of qi]. It results from cold in the stomach".

Yi niao 遺尿, loss of urine [53] AW *yi niao* 遺溺, *shi niao* 失溺, *xiao bian yi shi* 小便遺失.
IS of uncontrolled and spontaneous loss of urine while awake or asleep or during loss of consciousness. *JGYL* Fj 其人不渴，必**遺尿**，小便數, "Such persons are not thirsty, and they will experience **loss of urine** and frequent urination".

_Yi qi_ 疫氣, epidemic qi [10] AN *yi li qi* 疫癘氣; *li qi* 癘氣; *wen qi* 瘟氣, warmth-illness qi; *wen yi qi* 瘟疫氣, warmth-illness epidemic qi; *wen yi qi* 温疫氣, warmth epidemic qi.
EA bringing forth → *wen yi* 瘟疫, warmth-illness epidemics. *MYBL* SE *ta gan* 獺肝, *rou* 肉：療**疫氣**温病, "It heals warmth disease brought forth by **epidemic**

qi". *QJYF* 9: 屠蘇酒，辟**疫氣**，令人不染温病, "*Tu su* wine wards off **epidemic qi** and prevents a person from being affected by warmth disease".

Yi qi **噫氣, belching qi** [9] AD *yi* 噫, belching.

IS of qi moving upward from the stomach and producing sounds when leaving the throat. *ZBYHL* 21: 令人腹脹氣急，**噫氣**醋臭, "It causes a person to have abdominal distension and experience qi urgency. There is **belching qi** with a vinegar stench".

Yi re **遺熱, left-over heat** [1]

PC identical with → *liu re* 留熱, abiding heat. *SHZG* Mj: 益元散解中暑…汗後**遺熱**、勞復諸疾, "The 'Powder that adds to one's original [qi]', dissolves heatstroke…**left-over heat** after sweating, and all ailments associated with exhaustion relapse".

Yi shi **遺屎, fecal incontinence** [1] AN *da bian bu gu* 大便不固, incontinence of stools.

IS of an inability to control the passage of stools. *QJYF* 28: 病患臥**遺屎**不覺者，死, "Those who unknowingly suffer from **fecal incontinence** while lying down to sleep are bound to die".

Yi shi er bi **一十二痹, the twelve types of blockage** [2]

PC of a large number of → *bi bing* 痹病, blockage diseases. *BCGM* SE *jiu* 酒：菖蒲酒，治三十六風，**一十二痹**, "Wine with *chang pu* cures the 36 types of wind, and the **12 types of blockage**".

Yi si **縊死, [appearance of] death from hanging** [11]

PC of → *cu si* 卒死, sudden [appearance of] death, resulting from an attempt at strangling oneself by committing suicide by hanging. *QJYF* 25: 凡救**縊死**者，極須按定其心，勿截繩，手抱起徐徐解之, "For all attempts to rescue someone who [**appears to have**] **died from hanging**, it is of utmost importance to stabilize the [victim's] heart. One must not cut the rope. Rather one should gently lift [the body] and this way loosen the [strangling]".

Yi suan **噫酸, sour belching** [1] AN *yi tu suan jiang* 噫吐酸漿.

IS of sour liquid from the stomach following belching qi and being moved upward contrary to its normal direction. *ZBYHL* 20: 四肢重，喜臥，喜噦**噫酸**, "The four limbs are heavy. One wishes to lie down/sleep. One tends to retch and experience **sour belching**".

Yi tu suan jiang **噫吐酸漿, belching and spitting of sour liquid** [2]

IS identical with *yi suan* 噫酸, sour belching. *BCGM* SE *tou gou* 頭垢 quoting *PJF* 35: 噫酸漿, "Belching sour liquid", writes: **噫吐酸漿**, "**Belching and spitting sour liquid**".

Yi wen **疫瘟, epidemic warmth-illness** [1]

PC identical with → *wen yi* 瘟疫, warmth epidemic. Not documented in ancient medical literature. Possibly a writing error by LSZ. *BCGM* SE *bing ren yi* 病人衣：天行**疫瘟**。取初病人衣服，於甑上蒸過，則一家不染, "For heaven-sent **epidemic warmth illness**: Take the garments of the first patient and place them on a steamer to have them steam. This will protect the entire household from being affected".

***Yi xie* 遺泄, involuntary emission [of seminal fluid]** [3]
PC identical with → *yi jing* 遺精. *TPSHF* 98: 身力衰殘，夜夢**遺泄**, "The body's strength has declined and is deficient; [he experiences] **involuntary emission [of seminal fluid]** during his nocturnal dreams".

***Yi yin* 溢飲, spillage rheum** [3]
PC of → *yin* 飲②, rheum, disease brought forth by rheum spilling into the four limbs, with an absence of sweating and a feeling of pain and heaviness in the body. *JGYL* Mj: 飲水流行，歸於四肢，當汗出而不汗出，身體疼重，謂之**溢飲**, "When rheum water flows into the four limbs, one should sweat but the sweat does not leave. The body is in pain and feels heavy. This is called '**spillage rheum**'".

***Yi zhang* 疫瘴, epidemic miasma** [1]
PC identical with → *zhang li* 瘴癘, miasmatic epidemic. *KBBC* SE *wu yao* 烏藥：主…天行**疫瘴**, "It controls...heaven-sent **epidemic miasma**".

***Yi zhang* 翳障, shade and screen** [17]
PC identical with → *zhang yi* 障翳, obstructive shade. *BCSY* SE *yuan ci lei* 元慈勒：明目，去**障翳**、風淚、努肉, "It clears the eyes, and removes **shades and screens**, wind tears, and tumorous flesh-growths".

***Yi zhong* 翳腫, shade swelling** [2]
PC identical with → *mu yi* 目翳. *YXL* SE *qing xiang zi* 青葙子：能治肝臟熱毒衝眼，赤障青盲**翳腫**, "It is capable of curing heat poison rushing from the liver depot into the eyes, with resulting red screen, green blindness, and **shade swelling**".

***Yin* 喑, mute; muteness** [7] AW 瘖.
① IS of an inability to produce vocal sounds. *SJZL* 191: 面腫，唇吻不收，**喑**不能言，口噤不開, "The face is swollen. The lips do not hold anything. [Patients] are **mute** and do not speak. The jaws are clenched and do not open".
② PC with muteness as a major sign. *SJZL* 4: 重身而**喑**，十月當復, "A doubled (i.e. pregnant) body with **muteness** will recover after the tenth month".

***Yin* 瘖, muteness-illness** [2]
IS, PC identical with → *yin* 喑, muteness. *SW* 23: 搏陽則為巔疾，搏陰則為**瘖**, "When it strikes at the yang, this causes the ailment of peak[-illness]. When it strikes at the yin, this causes **muteness-illness**".

***Yin* 飲, rheum** [p]
① EA of a clear, thin liquid that is excreted in the course of pathological changes affecting the depots and palaces and that accumulates in the body's cavities and passageways. It may block the passage of qi and blood and thereby become a pathogenic factor. *SYJYBZFL* Mj: 喜怒憂思，致臟氣不行，鬱而生涎，涎結為**飲**，隨氣上厥，伏留陽經，亦使人眩暈嘔吐, "When joy, anger, grief, and pondering block the passage of the qi of the depots, it will be pent-up and gen-

erate saliva. The saliva congeals and forms **rheum**. It follows the qi upwards and abides deep inside the yang conduits. It may also cause dizziness and vomiting". ② PC CD of pathological conditions brought forth by rheum. *ZBYHL* 20: 其為病也，或兩脅脹滿，或心胸煩悶，或眼暗口乾，或嘔逆短氣，諸候非一，故云諸飲, "Its pathology is such that in some cases both flanks experience a feeling of distension and fullness, or the region of heart and chest experiences vexation and pressure, or vision is dim and the mouth is dry, or one vomits with [qi] counterflow and experiences shortness of qi. The signs are many. Hence one speaks of 'all types of **rheum**'". *BCGM* Bai bing zhu zhi yao 百病主治藥: 飲有五：支、留、伏、溢、懸也, "There are five types of **rheum**: propping [rheum], abiding [rheum], deep-lying [rheum], spillage [rheum], and suspended [rheum]".

***Yin bi* 陰痹, yin blockage** [4]

PC of a *bi* 痹① a) blockage disease, brought forth by cold evil that has entered the bones, with aching bones and unbearable pain when touched. *LS* 20: **陰痹**者，按之而不得, "In the case of **yin blockage**: one cannot bear [the pain] if touched".

***Yin bing* 陰病, yin disease** [7]

PC a) identical with → *yin zheng* 陰證. *SW* 5: 陰勝則陽病, 陽勝則**陰病**, "When yin dominates, then this is a yang disease; when yang dominates, then this is a **yin disease**". b) Of external genital parts. *BCGM* Bai bing zhu zhi yao 百病主治藥: **陰病**：陰寒、陰吹、陰腫痛、陰癢、陰蝕、陰脫、產門不合、產門生合、脬損, "**Yin diseases**: Yin cold (cold in the genital region), vaginal flatulence, swelling and pain in the genital region, itching in the genital region, erosion in the genital region, yin prolapse, failure of the birth gate to close, congenital closure of the birth gate, bladder damage".

***Yin bu qi* 陰不起, failure of the yin [member] to rise** [2]

PC identical with → *yin wei* 陰痿, dysfunction of the yin [member, i.e. penis]. *BJ* SE *fu bi* 腐婢：主痎瘧寒熱，邪氣泄痢，**陰不起**, "It controls malaria with alternating sensations of cold and heat, evil qi with free-flux illness, and **failure of the yin [member] to rise**".

***Yin chuang* 陰瘡, yin sores** [53]

PC CD of → *chuang* 瘡, sores, conditions developing in the genital region. *BJ* SE *xia ma* 蝦蟆：主邪氣，破癥堅血，癰腫，**陰瘡**, "It controls evil qi, breaks up concretion-illness and hardness of blood, obstruction-illnesses with swelling, as well as **yin sores**".

***Yin chui* 陰吹, yin flatulence; vaginal flatulence** [5]

PC with air – resembling flatulence – constantly exiting the vagina. *JGYL* Lj: 胃氣下泄，**陰吹**而正喧，此穀氣之實也, "When there is a discharge with outflow of stomach qi, [resulting in] noisy **vaginal flatulence**, this is a sign of a repletion with grain qi".

Yin du **陰毒, yin poison** [80]

① PC a) of → *shang han* 傷寒, harm caused by cold, resulting in a flourishing of only yang qi and a diminution of yin qi, with cold extremities and a greenish facial complexion, pain in the abdomen and affecting the entire body, as well as a deep-lying and fine movement in the vessels. *JGYL* Fj: **陰毒**之為病，面目青，身痛如被杖，咽喉痛, "The disease of **yin poison** is as follows: the face and eyes are greenish. The body aches as if flogged with a stick. The throat aches". b) Brought forth by being struck by → *xi du* 溪毒, rivulet poison, with ulcers in the body's lower parts as if caused by the insect stingers or fish. *ZHF* 7: 若瘡如蠡魚齒者為**陰毒**, "If there are ulcers that appear to result from insect [stingers] or fish teeth, then this is **yin poison**".

② EA identical with → *du qi* 毒氣, poison qi, with a cold quality. *QJYF* 19: **陰毒**內行，臟腑受客邪之氣，則病生矣, "When **yin poison** moves inside and the depots and palaces receive visitor evil qi, a disease is generated".

③ PQ of pharmaceutical substances with a poisonous nature of massive cold". *ZLBC* SE *qian* 鉛 quotes *TQFLLSF*: 錫鉛…服之而多**陰毒**，傷人心胃, "Tin and lead, if one consumes them one ingests much **yin poison**, and this will harm the heart and stomach".

Yin du wei **陰毒痿, yin poison dysfunction** [2]

PC identical with → *yin wei* 陰痿, dysfunction of the yin [member, i.e. penis]. *HYBC* SE *wu shi zi* 無食子：治**陰毒痿**，燒灰用, "To cure **yin poison dysfunction**, burn it to ashes and use them".

Yin fei **喑痱, silence disablement** [1]

PC of → *feng fei* 風痱, wind disablement, together with an inability to speak. *PJF* 225 RE *jin chai shi hu wan* 金釵石斛丸, golden hairpin pills with *shu hu*: 治腎氣內奪，厥逆**喑痱**, "They cure internal loss of kidney qi, recession with counterflow, **silence disablement**".

Yin fu **淫膚, excess skin** [7]

PC of → *xi rou* 瘜肉, tumorous flesh-growths, developing between the white of the eyeball and the eyelid. *BJ* SE *qi cao* 蠐螬：目中**淫膚**，青翳白膜, "**Excess skin** in the eye, greenish shade, white membrane".

Yin gan **陰疳, yin *gan*-illness** [6]

PC identical with → *xia gan* 下疳, lower-region *gan*-illness. *BCGM* SE *deng xin cao* 燈心草：燒灰入輕粉、麝香，治**陰疳**, "Burn to ashes and add *qing fen* and *she xiang*. This will cure **yin *gan*-illness**".

Yin han **陰寒, yin cold; cold in the yin body region** [12]

① EA comprising all types of yin and cold causes of disease. *SJZL* 53: **陰寒**凝結，停滯於胸膈之間, "When **yin cold** has coagulated into nodes, and stays in the section between the chest and diaphragm".

② PC comprising all types of yang depletion and cold abundance. *WTMY* 37: 澀為**陰寒**，弱為陰虛, "When it is rough, this is **yin cold**; when it is weak, this is yin depletion".

③ Cold weather/climate: *SJZL* 73: 若遇**陰寒**，或食冷物則作痛, "If one happens to encounter **yin cold** and consumes cold food, this will cause pain".
④ IS identical with → *yin leng* 陰冷, yin cold. *BJ* SE *song luo* 松蘿：女子**陰寒**腫痛, "[It controls] **cold**, swelling, and pain in the **yin** body region [i.e. private parts] of women".

Yin han **陰汗, yin sweating** [29]
① IS of sweating in the frontal 'yin region', at the scrotum and at the perineum. *WTMY* 13: 夜臥夢泄，**陰汗**痿弱, "Dream ejaculation during night sleep, **yin sweating** and dysfunction with weakness".
② PC with sweating in the yin region as a major sign. *WTMY* 16：一曰**陰汗**，二曰陰衰, "The first is called '**yin sweating**'; the second is called 'yin weakness'".

Yin huang **陰黃, yin jaundice** [5]
PC of a type of → *huang dan* 黃疸, yellow *dan*-illness, characterized by hidden yang and flourishing yin and harmed proper qi as pathological signs, and the absence of fever as well as a dark yellow body complexion as clinical signs. *ZBYHL*12: 但身面色黃，頭痛而不發熱，名為**陰黃**, "When the body and facial complexion are yellow, with headaches and without an effusion of heat, this is called '**yin jaundice**'".

Yin huang **瘾黃, hidden-illness jaundice** [4]
PC identical with → *yin huang* 陰黃. *BCGM* SE *tian gua* 甜瓜 quoting *SLBC* 陰黃黃疸, "Yin jaundice and yellow *dan*-illness", writes: 黃疸**瘾黃**, "Yellow *dan*-illness and **hidden-illness jaundice**".

Yin huo **陰火, yin fire** [35]
① Lightning, also called *tian zhi yin huo* 天之陰火, heaven's yin fire. *BCGM* SE *yin huo yang huo* 陰火陽火：天之**陰火**二：龍火也，雷火也, "Heaven has two **yin fires**, i.e. dragon fire and lightning".
② Fire burning with liquid fuel such as mineral oil. *BCGM* SE *yin huo yang huo* 陰火陽火：地之**陰火**二：石油之火也，水中之火也, "The earth has two **yin fires**, i.e. the fire of mineral oil, and fire in water.
③ PN identical with → *xiang huo* 相火, minister fire. *BCGM* SE *yin huo yang huo* 陰火陽火：人之**陰火**二：命門相火也，三昧之火也, "Man has two **yin fires**, i.e. minister fire in the gate of life, and the three hidden fires.
④ PC identical with → *xu re* 虛熱, depletion heat a). *LSMC* Fj: 時顯熱躁，是下元**陰火**蒸蒸然發也, "When the season is damp, fiercly hot, this may cause a steaming outbreak of **yin fire** from the kidneys".

Yin jing **陰痙, yin spasms** [1]
PC of → *jing bing* 痙病, spasms disease, associated with an inadequacy of yang qi. *BCGM* Bai bing zhu zhi yao 百病主治藥：附子，**陰痙**自汗, "*Fu zi* [cures] **yin spasms** with spontaneous sweating".

Yin ju **陰疽, yin impediment-illness** [6]
PC of → *ju* 疽, impediment-illness, which emerges because a body's yang qi is weak and hence has no strength to ward off evil qi. In general, the affected region is not hot, and the pain is comparatively mild. The color is pale, and the surface is

sunken in. However, the patient's mind is disturbed, and his condition is serious. *BCGM* SE *ya chi* 牙齒 quotes *RZZZF*: **陰疽**不發：頭凹沉黯，不疼無熱，服內補散不起, "Before a **yin impediment-illness** has emerged, its head is sunken in and of a pale color. There is neither pain nor heat. If one ingests a powder for internal supplementation, [the impediment] will not rise".

***Yin leng* 陰冷, yin cold** [14] AN *yin han* 陰寒; *yin zhong han* 陰中寒, cold in the yin [body region].

IS of cold in the sexual organs. *ZBYHL* 4: 陰虛陽弱，血氣不能相榮，故使**陰冷**也, "When the yin is depleted and the yang is weak, the blood and the qi are unable to provide nourishment. This leads to **yin cold**".

***Yin lou* 陰瘺, yin fistula** [1]

PC of → *lou* 瘺, fistula, developing in a female's yin [i. e., genital] region. *RHZ* SE *mu gou yin jing* 牡狗陰莖：犬陰治絕陽及婦人**陰瘺**, "A dog's yin [member; i. e., penis] cures interrupted yang [qi of males] and **yin fistula** in women".

***Yin ni* 陰䘌, hidden-worms in the yin [region]** [3]

PC of → *ni chuang*, 䘌瘡, hidden-worms sores, generated in the genital region. *BCGM* SE *yang* 羊 quotes *BHJJF*: 婦人**陰䘌**：作癢，羊肝納入引蟲, "For **hidden worms in a** woman's **yin [region]**: when they itch, put lamb liver into [the vagina]. It will draw out the worms".

***Yin nüe* 陰瘧, yin malaria** [4]

PC of → *nüe ji* 瘧疾, malaria ailment, associated with a depletion weakness of proper qi. *YXRM* 4: 陽瘧易治，**陰瘧**難愈, "Yang malaria is easy to cure. **Yin malaria** is difficult to heal".

***Yin pi* 飲澼, rheum flush** [5]

PC identical with → *yin pi* 飲癖, rheum aggregation-illness. *BCGM* Bai bing zhu zhi yao 百病主治藥：芫花，胸中痰水，脅下**飲澼**, "*Yuan hua* (cures) phlegm water in the chest, **rheum flush** below the flanks".

***Yin pi* 飲癖, rheum aggregation-illness** [2]

PC of a → *pi* 癖, aggregation-illness, resulting from excessive amounts of fluid that collect below the flanks and are affected by cold. *ZBYHL* 20：**飲癖**者，由飲水過多，在於脅下不散，又遇冷氣相觸而痛, "**Rheum aggregation-illness** results from the failure to dissipate excessive amounts of rheum liquid below the flanks. When they are met by cold qi this results in pain".

***Yin sao* 陰臊, yin stench** [1]

IS of a bad stench emitted from the private parts of males. *BCGM* Bai bing zhu zhi yao 百病主治藥：囊癢，陰汗、**陰臊**、陰疼，皆屬濕熱, "Scrotal itching, yin sweating, **yin stench**, and yin pain, all these [conditions] are associated with moisture and heat".

***Yin shan* 陰疝, yin elevation-illness** [10]

PC of → *shan* 疝, elevation-illness, with massive swelling and pain in the scrotum. *ZHF* 5: 小兒**陰疝**，發時腫痛, "**Yin elevation-illness** in children. Its onset is associated with swelling and pain".

***Yin shen wei ruo* 陰腎萎弱, wilting and weakness of the yin[-member, i.e. penis, and] kidneys [i.e. testicles]** [1]

PC identical with → *yin wei* 陰痿, dysfunction of the yin [member, i.e. penis]. *BCGM* SE *a yue hun zi* 阿月渾子 quoting *HYBC* SE *wu ming mu pi* 無名木皮：主陰腎痿弱，囊下濕癢, "It controls dysfunction and weakness of the yin-kidneys, and wet itching below the scrotum", writes: **陰腎萎弱**，囊下濕癢, "**Wilting and weakness of the yin[-member, i.e. penis, and] kidneys [i.e. testicles]**, and wet itching below the scrotum".

***Yin shen tong* 陰腎痛, yin[-member, i.e. penis, and] kidneys [i.e. testicles] pain** [1]

IS of scrotal pain. *PJF* 249: 治猝**陰腎痛**，以燒牛屎末，和酒敷之, "To cure sudden **yin[-member, i.e. penis, and] kidneys [i.e. testicles] pain**, apply a powder of burned cow dung mixed with wine to the [painful region]".

***Yin shi* 陰蝕, yin erosion** [31] AN *yin shi chuang* 陰蝕瘡, yin erosion sores.

PC of → *yin chuang* 陰瘡, yin sore, forming a festering indentation in the genital region. *BJ* SE *huai mu* 淮木：主久咳上氣，傷中虛羸，女子**陰蝕**，漏下赤白沃, "It controls long-lasting cough with ascending qi, harm to the center with depletion and emaciation, and **yin erosion** of females, as well as leaking discharge with red-white foam".

***Yin shi* 陰虱, yin lice** [3]

PC of a disease caused by lice in the pubic hair with itching in the genital region. *BCGM* SE *yin xing* 銀杏 quotes *LCCF*: **陰虱**作癢：陰毛際肉中生蟲如虱，或紅或白，癢不可忍者, "Itching caused by **yin lice**: worms like lice grow in the flesh at the border of the pubic hair. They may be red or white. The itching is unbearable".

***Yin shi chuang* 陰蝕瘡, yin erosion sores** [3]

PC identical with → *yin shi* 陰蝕, yin erosion. *MYBL* SE *hei shi zhi* 黑石脂：主**陰蝕瘡**, "It controls **yin erosion sores**".

***Yin shui* 陰水, yin water** [4]

PC of → *shui zhong* 水腫, water swelling, disease with swelling of the entire body accompanied by viscous stools, scant but not difficult urination, most often associated with physical depletion and cold. *DXXF* 2: 若遍身腫，不煩渴，大便溏，小便少，不澀赤，此屬**陰水**, "When the entire body is swollen, without vexation, while the stools are viscous and urination is scant but neither difficult nor red, this is **yin water**".

***Yin sou* 飲嗽, rheum cough** [1]

PC of cough resulting from abiding rheum. *WTMY* 9: 深師療五嗽，一曰上氣嗽，二曰**飲嗽**，三曰燥嗽，四曰冷嗽，五曰邪嗽, "Master Shen's cure of the five types of cough - The first is named 'qi cough'; the second is named '**rheum cough**'; the third is named 'dry cough'; the fourth is names 'cold cough'; the fifth is named 'evil [qi] cough'".

Yin ting **陰挺, yin prolapse** [6]

PC identical with → *yin tuo* 陰脫. *QJYF* 30: 照海主**陰挺**，下血，陰中腫或癢，"[To pierce] the *zhao hai* [hole] controls **yin prolapse**, discharge of blood, and swelling as well as itching in [a woman's] private parts".

Yin tong **隱痛, latent pain** [4]

IS of a mild pain seemingly continuing forever, sometimes dormant and sometimes active. *SJZL* 52: 治腎臟風毒，脚弱少力，脚重疼痹，脚腫生瘡，脚下**隱痛**，不能蹈地，脚膝筋攣，不能屈伸，腰膝拘急，風毒流注等疾，石南丸方，"To treat ailments such as the kidney depot affected by wind poison, the legs being weak and lacking strength, legs being heavy and painful, legs being swollen and growing sores, a **latent pain** underneath the legs making it impossible to tread on the ground, legs and knees with sinew contraction making it impossible to bend or stretch them, the lower back and knees cramp and are tense, and wind poison influx, [use] the recipe for pills with *shi nan*".

Yin tong **引痛, pulling pain** [7]

IS of pain at one location pulling on a different location, or radiating into a third location. *ZHF* 4: 胸痹之病，令人心中堅痞忽痛，肌中苦痹。絞急如刺，不得俯仰，其胸前皮皆痛，不得手犯，胸滿短氣，咳嗽**引痛**，煩悶自汗出，或徹引背膂，不即治之，數日害人，"The disease of chest blockage causes a person to have a hard obstacle-illness in the heart accompanied by sudden pain, and suffering from a blockage in the sinews. There is a twisting pain as if pierced, with an inability to bend or lift the body. The skin on the chest is painful all over, and does not allow one's hand to touch it. There is a feeling of fullness in the chest, with a shortness of qi. [Patients] cough with a **pulling pain**. They experience vexation, heart-pressure and spontaneous sweating. In some cases the entire backbone is affected. If this is not cured immediately, after several days it will cause harm to that person".

Yin tong **陰痛, yin pain** [10]

PC with pain in the vaginal region as the major sign. *BJ* SE *sang er* 桑耳：主女子漏下赤白汁，血病，癥瘕積聚，**陰痛**, "It controls, in women, spotting of red and white liquid, blood disease, concretion-illness and conglomeration-illness, accumulations and collections, and **yin pain**". In the *BCGM*, **陰痛**, *yin pain*, is mostly a women's disease.

Yin tui **陰㿗, yin (i.e. scrotal) prominence-illness** [33] AD *tui* 㿗; AN *tui shan* 㿗疝, prominence-illness with elevation-illness.

PC of local swelling and pain affecting a male's private parts. *MYBL* SE *tie jing* 鐵精：療驚悸，定心氣，小兒風癇，**陰㿗**脫肛, "It cures fright with palpation, fixes the heart qi and wind epilepsy in children, as well as **yin prominence-illness** and prolapse of the rectum".

Yin tui **陰癩, yin breakdown-illness** [14] AD 癩.

PC a) AN *tui shan* 癩疝, breakdown-illness with elevation-illness. Identical with → 陰㿗, *yin tui*, yin (i.e. scrotal) prominence-illness. *MYBL* SE *li gu* 狸骨：陰莖，主月水不通，男子**陰癩**, "Its penis controls blocked menstruation, and **yin breakdown disease** of males". b) Identical with → *yin tuo* 陰脫, yin prolapse; prolapse of the uterus. *BCGM* SE *wang gua* 王瓜 quoting *JGYL* Lj: **陰癩**腫亦主之, "It also controls **yin breakdown-illness** with swelling", writes: **婦人陰癩**, "**Yin breakdown-illness** of females".

Yin tuo **陰脫, yin prolapse** [21] AN *yin ting* 陰挺; *zi chang ting chu* 子腸挺出; *chan hou chang chu* 產後腸出, intestinal prolapse following delivery; *chan hou chang tuo* 產後腸脫; *zi gong xia tuo* 子宮下脫; *zi gong tuo xia* 子宮脫下; *chan chang tuo xia* 產腸脫下, prolapse of the birth intestine; *chan chang tuo chu* 產腸脫出; *zi chang tuo xia* 子腸脫下, prolapse of infant's intestine; *zi chang zhui xia* 子腸墜下; *zi chang tuo chu* 子腸脫出; *yin tui* 陰癩,

PC of prolapse of the uterus or the vaginal mucous membrane, in severe cases resulting in a protrusion out of the vagina. *QJYF* 3: 治婦人**陰脫**若脫肛方, "Recipe to cure **yin prolapse** and prolapse of the rectum".

Yin wei **陰痿, yin dysfunction** [71] AN *yang wei* 陽痿, *yin xia wei* 陰下痿, *yin du wei* 陰毒痿, *yang shi bu qi* 陽事不起, *yin bu qi* 陰不起, *yang shi bu xing* 陽事不行, *yang shi bu xing* 陽事不興, *yang shi wei ruo* 陽事痿弱, *jing wei* 莖痿, *yin shen wei ruo* 陰腎萎弱, *yin xiao* 陰消, yin[-member, i.e. penis, and] kidneys [i.e. testicles] dysfunction.

PC of male adults with partial or complete erectile dysfunction, resulting in an inability to have sexual intercourse. *BJ* SE *yang qi shi* 陽起石：腹痛，無子，**陰痿**不起, "Abdominal pain, childlessness, and **dysfunction of the yin[-member]** so that it fails to rise".

Yin xia wei **陰下痿, dysfunction of the yin [i.e. the male member] remaining below** [1]

PC identical with → *yin wei* 陰痿, yin dysfunction. *YXL* SE *bai ji* 白及：主**陰下痿**，治面上皯皰, "It controls **dysfunction of the yin [i.e. male member] remaining below**, and cures facial blisters".

Yin xian **陰癇, yin epilepsy** [2]

PC of → *dian xian* 癲癇, peak-illness with epilepsy, as a yin condition: the disease makes the body feel cold first. The movement in the vessels is deep inside. *ZBYHL* 45: 發時脈沉者，為**陰癇**，內在五臟，外在骨髓，極者難治, "When it breaks out and the [movement in the] vessels is deep inside, this is **yin epilepsy**. Internally it is in the five depots; externally it is in the bones and their marrow. When [the disease] has reached an extreme it is difficult to cure".

Yin xiao **陰消, yin melting** [4]

PC of → *yin wei* 陰痿, wilting of the yin [member, i.e. penis]. *MYBL* SE *shui yin* 水銀：以傅男子陰，**陰消**無氣, "Used to apply to the male's yin [i.e. genital] organ in case of **yin melting** and lack of qi".

Yin xu **陰虛, yin depletion** [49]

PC of depletion with insufficient yin liquid, with essence and blood harmed, and inadequate moisture and nourishment. *LS* 9: **陰虛**而陽盛，先補其陰，後瀉其陽而和之, "In the case of **yin depletion** and yang abundance, harmonization is achieved by supplementing the yin first, and draining the yang afterwards".

Yin xu huo dong **陰虛火動, yin depletion with excited fire** [7] AN *yin xu huo wang* 陰虛火旺.

EA, PM of a depletion of yin essence, yin blood and yin body liquids leaving the yang uncontrolled and allowing depletion fire to flare up. *DXXF* 4: **陰虛火動**耳聾者，亦用四物湯, "[To cure] those suffering from **yin depletion with excited fire** and deafness, one may also use the 'decoction with the four ingredients'".

Yin xu huo wang **陰虛火旺, yin depletion with fire exuberance** [1]

EA, PM identical with → *yin xu huo dong* 陰虛火動, yin depletion with excited fire. *MYZZ* 1: 若勞心好色，內傷真陰，陰血既傷，則陽氣偏勝而變為火矣，是謂**陰虛火旺**勞瘵之症, "If one exhausts the heart and loves sex, thereby harming the true yin, with damage to yin blood, then the yang qi will dominate alone and transform into fire. This is called the pathological condition of **yin depletion with fire exuberance** with exhaustion consumption".

Yin ya **喑啞, muteness** [3] AW 喑瘂, muteness-illness.

PC identical with → *ya* 瘂, muteness-illness. *SLBC* SE *zhi zi* 梔子：主**喑啞**，紫癜風，黃疸, "It controls **muteness**, purple patches wind, and yellow *dan*-illness".

Yin ya **喑瘂, muteness-illness** [1]

PC identical with → *yin ya* 喑啞. *BCGM* Bai bing zhu zhi yao 百病主治藥 quoting from the main entry on *zhi zi* 梔子：主喑啞, "It controls muteness", writes: 去煩悶**喑瘂**, "It removes vexation, heart-pressure, and **muteness-illness**".

Yin yang **陰癢, yin itching** [25]

PC with vaginal itching. *ZHF* 5: 姚療**陰癢**生瘡，嚼胡麻，塗之, "When the Yao cure **yin itching** associated with generation of sores, they chew *hu ma* and smear this on the [affected region].

Yin yang du **陰陽毒, yin and yang poison** [2]

PC CD of → *yin du* 陰毒① a), yin poison, and → *yang du* 陽毒① a), yang poison. *SXBC* SE *jing jie* 荊芥：理筋骨煩疼及**陰陽毒**，傷寒頭痛, "It manages sinews and bones affected by vexing pain as well as **yin and yang poison**, as well as harm caused by cold with headache".

Yin yang yi **陰陽易, yin and yang exchange** [17]

PC of a communicable disease acquired through sexual intercourse by persons who had been cured of harm caused by cold only shortly before. *SHL* 392: "傷寒**陰陽易**之為病，其人身體重、少氣、少腹裏急, "In the case of the disease of harm caused by cold with **yin and yang exchange**, the respective person feels as if his body were heavy. He is short of qi, and there is tension inside his abdomen".

Yin yi **陰易, yin exchange** [6]

PC of a communicable disease acquired by males through sexual intercourse with a female who had just been cured of harm caused by cold. *ZBYHL*8: 婦人得病新瘥未平復，而男子與之交接得病者，名**陰易**, "The disease acquired by a male who had intercourse with a female who had just been cured of the disease without having fully recovered yet is called '**yin exchange**'".

Yin zhen **癮疹, dormant papules** [35] AW *yin zhen* 隱疹. AN *yin zhen feng* 癮疹風, dormant papules wind; *yin zhen feng* 隱疹風.

PC identical with → *feng zhen* 風疹, wind papules. *QJYF* 22 has a paragraph Yin zhen di wu **癮疹**第五, "**Dormant papules**, no. 5: 治**癮疹**百療不瘥者方：景天一升, 一名慎火草, 細搗取汁敷上, 熱炙手摩之, 日三度, 瘥, "A recipe to cure **dormant papules** that does not fail once in a hundred cases: *jing tian*, 1 *sheng*, also called 'the herb that bewares of fire'. Pound well and apply the juice externally by forceful rubbing. Three times daily. This brings the cure".

Yin zhen **隱疹, dormant papules** [7]

PC identical with → *yin zhen* 癮疹. *PJF* 74: 治皮膚瘙癢，**隱疹**赤腫, "To cure skin itching and **dormant papules** with a red swelling".

Yin zhen feng **隱疹風, dormant papules wind** [1]

PC identical with → *yin zhen* 癮疹, dormant papules. *BCTJ* SE *da ji* 大戟：醫家用治**隱疹風**，及風毒脚腫，並煮水熱淋，日再三便愈, "Medical experts use it to cure **dormant papules wind**, as well as wind poison with leg swelling. For both [these ailments] they boil water and pour it hot [on the affected area]. Repeated three times a day, this will bring the cure".

Yin zheng **陰證, yin condition** [9]

PC CD of subdued bodily reactions to an abundance of cold or insufficiency of yang qi. *SJZL* 192: 病有因寒而得, 或**陰證**多寒, "If the cause of the disease is cold, or if this is a **yin condition** with much cold".

Yin zheng shang han **陰證傷寒, yin signs associated with harm caused by cold** [4]

PC identical with → *shang han yin zheng* 傷寒陰證, harm caused by cold with yin signs. *BCYY* SE *tai yin xuan jing shi* 太陰玄精石：**陰證傷寒**，指甲面色青黑，六脈沉細而疾 … 四肢逆冷，咽喉不利，腹疼，亦須佐他藥兼之, "**Yin signs associated with harm caused by cold**: The fingernails and the face are greenish-black; The [movements in the] six vessels are deep inside, fine, and fast … The four limbs have [qi] counterflow and are cold. The throat is blocked. The abdomen aches. This must be assisted by further medication".

Yin zhong han **陰中寒, cold in the yin [body region]** [1]

IS identical with → *yin leng* 陰冷, yin cold. *BJ* SE *gao ben* 藁本：主婦人疝瘕，**陰中寒**，腫痛, "It controls, in females, elevation-illness with conglomeration-illness, **cold in their yin [body region,** i.e. private parts], with swelling, and pain".

Ying **癭, goiter** [p] AN *ying ji* 癭疾, goiter ailment; *ying liu* 癭瘤, goiter tumor; *ying zhui* 癭贅, goiter redundancy; *ying qi* 癭氣, goiter qi; 癭結氣, goiter with bound qi.

PC of a swelling at the front side of the neck to the side of the throat. *SM* 8: **癭**，嬰也，在頸嬰喉也, "*Ying*, **goiter**, is *ying*, to surround. Because at the neck it surrounds the throat".

Ying he **硬核, hard kernel** [2]

PC of → *jie he* 結核, nodular kernel, appearing as a hard swelling. *QJYF* 26: 主癭瘤結氣，散頸下**硬核**痛, "It controls bound qi associated with goiter tumors, and it disperses **hard kernels** with pain below the neck".

Ying ji **瘿疾, goiter ailment** [4]

PC identical with → *ying* 瘿, goiter. *BCTJ* SE *huang yao gen* 黄藥根：療忽生**瘿疾**一二年者, "To cure **goiter ailments** that suddenly developed one or two years ago".

Ying jie qi **瘿結氣, goiter with bound qi** [2]

PC identical with → *ying* 瘿, goiter. *BJ* SE *xia ku cao* 夏枯草：破癥，散**瘿結氣**, "It serves to break up concretion-illness, and to disperse **goiter with bound qi**".

Ying liu **瘿瘤, goiter tumor** [21] AN *liu ying* 瘤瘿 tumorous goiter.

PC identical with → *ying* 瘿, goiter. *BJ* Xu li 序例：癰腫、惡瘡，痔瘺、**瘿瘤**, "Obstruction-illness with swelling, malign sores, piles fistula, and **goiter tumor**".

Ying qi **瘿氣, goiter qi** [20]

PC identical with → *ying* 瘿, goiter. *BJ* SE *bai tou weng* 白頭翁：主温瘧，狂易寒熱，癥瘕積聚，**瘿氣**, "It controls warmth malaria, madness with a change to alternating sensations of cold and heat, as well as concretion-illness and conglomeration-illness, accumulations and collections, as well as **goiter qi**".

Ying sheng chong bing **應聲蟲病, echo-bug disease** [2]

PC of a disease with something in the abdomen issuing sounds echoing human voices. *BCGM* SE *lan* 藍 quotes *QJF*: 腹中有物作聲，隨人語言，名**應聲蟲病**, "There is an item in the abdomen that generates sounds echoing human voices. This is called '**echo-bug disease**'".

Ying teng **硬疼, hardening with pain** [1]

IS identical with → *jian tong* 堅痛. *BCGM* SE *shan yu* 鱔魚 quoting *TPSHF* 71: 婦人乳結硬疼痛, "A nodular hardening with pain in a woman's breast," writes: 婦人乳核**硬疼**, "A pit[-like] **hardening with pain** in a woman's breast".

Ying tong **硬痛, hardening with pain** [4]

IS identical with → *jian tong* 堅痛. *SHL* 149: 若心下滿而**硬痛**者，此為結胸也，大陷胸湯主之, "Whenever there is a feeling of fullness and **hardening with pain** below the heart, this is a case of bound chest. The 'major decoction sinking into the chest' will master this".

Ying zui **瘿贅, goiter redundancy** [4]

PC identical with → *ying* 瘿, goiter. *RHZ* SE *shi hui* 石灰：療冷氣，婦人粉刺，痔瘺疽瘡，**瘿贅**疣子, "It cures cold qi, flour thorns in women, piles fistula and impediment-illness sores, as well as **goiter redundancy** and warts".

Yong **癰, obstruction-illness** [p] AN *yong chuang* 癰瘡, obstruction-illness sores; *yong zhong* 癰腫, obstruction-illness swelling; *yong yang* 癰瘍, obstruction-illness ulcer.

PC CD of acute festering abscesses, with local heat-pain, of a large circumference without reaching deeply, developing from between the skin and subdermal tissue or in bodily cavities. They are often associated with conditions affecting the entire body, and include an aversion to cold and fever. *LS* 81: 熱勝則肉腐，肉腐則為膿。然不能陷，骨髓不為焦枯，五藏不為傷，故命曰**癰**, "When heat dominates the flesh will decay. When the flesh decays it will fester. Still, it will not sink in, and hence the bones and marrow will not be heated to desiccate. The five depots will not be harmed. Hence this is called '**obstruction-illness**' ". LSZ: 深為疽，淺為**癰**。大為**癰**，小為癤, "Those that reach deep inside are impediment-illnesses. Those that are superficial are **obstruction-illnesses**. Large ones are **obstruction-illnesses**. Small ones are pimples".

Yong chuang **癰瘡, obstruction-illness sores** [17] AN *gui yong* 潰癰, festering obstruction-illness; *lan yong* 爛癰.

PC a) identical with → *yong* 癰, obstruction-illness. *BJ* SE *mu dan* 牡丹：安五藏，療**癰瘡**, "It calms the five depots, and cures obstruction-illness sores. b) A differentiating reference to *yong* 癰, abscesses that have begun to fester. This is in contrast to → *yong zhong* 癰腫, obstruction-illness swelling. *ZBYHL* 50: 膿潰之後，其瘡不瘥，故曰**癰瘡**, "When the festering has set in, these sores will not heal. Hence they are called **obstruction-illness sores**".

Yong du **癰毒, obstruction-illness with poison** [11]

PC identical with → *yong* 癰, obstruction-illness. *TPSHF* 71: 治婦人乳腫痛，慮作**癰毒**，宜服此方, "To cure painful swelling of the female breast, and if one assumes that this may develop into an **obstruction-illness with poison**, one should ingest this recipe".

Yong jie **癰癤, obstruction-illness with pimples** [19]

PC CD of → *yong* 癰, obstruction-illnesses, and → *jie* 癤, pimples. *ZBYHL* 32: 五月勿食不成核果及桃、棗，發**癰癤**, "During the fifth month it is not advisable to consume fruit that has not developed a kernel yet, as well as peaches and dates, lest one develop an **obstruction-illness with pimples**".

Yong ju **癰疽, obstruction- and impediment-illnesses** [299]

PC CD of → *yong* 癰, obstruction-illnesses, and → *ju* 疽, impediment-illnesses. *LS* 81: 黃帝曰：夫子言**癰疽**，何以別之？岐伯曰：營衛稽留於經脈之中，則血泣而不行，不行則衛氣從之而不通，壅遏而不得行，故熱。大熱不止，熱勝則肉腐，肉腐則為膿。然不能陷，骨髓不為焦枯，五藏不為傷，故命曰癰。黃帝曰：何謂疽？岐伯曰：熱氣淳盛，下陷肌膚，筋髓枯，內連五藏，血氣竭，當其癰下，筋骨良肉皆無餘，故命曰疽。疽者，上之皮夭以堅，上如牛領之皮。癰者，其皮上薄以澤。此其候也, "Huang Di: 'Now, you, Sir, speak of **obstruction- and impediment-illnesses**. How are they distinguished?' Qi Bo: 'When camp [qi] and guardian [qi] reside in the conduit vessels then the blood stagnates and fails to move. When it fails to move, the guardian qi, as a consequence, is unable to pass. It is stopped-up and cannot move, and this results in heat. In the case of massive heat that fails to end, when the heat dominates the flesh will decay. When the flesh decays it will fester. Still, it will not sink in, and hence the bones and marrow will not be heated to desiccate. The five depots will not be harmed. Hence this is called 'obstruction-illness'. Huang Di: 'What does 'impediment-illness' mean?' Qi Bo: 'When pure heat qi abounds, it sinks into the skin and the muscles. The sinews and the bones desiccate. Internally, this links up with the five depots where the blood and qi are exhausted. Then below the obstruction-illness sinews, the bones and good flesh no longer abound. Hence this is called 'impediment-illness'. The skin above an impediment-illness has died and hardened. It feels above like the skin of a buffalo's neck. The skin above an obstruction-illness is thin and moist. These are their signs".

***Yong ju tou* 癰疽頭, head of obstruction- and impediment-illnesses** [2]
PP CD of → *yong* 癰, obstruction-illnesses, and *ju* 疽, impediment-illnesses. A successful cure requires the removal of such tissue. *TBC e shi* 惡實：吞一枚，出**癰疽頭**, "Swallow one seed. This will bring out the **head of obstruction- and impediment-illnesses**".

***Yong lou* 癰漏, obstruction-illness with leakage** [3]
PC CD of → *yong* 癰, obstruction-illness, and → *lou chuang* 漏瘡, leaking sores. *BCGM* SE *tu fu ling* 土茯苓 quotes a Wang Ji 汪機：近有好淫之人，多病楊梅毒瘡，藥用輕粉，愈而復發，久則肢體拘攣，變為**癰漏**，延綿歲月，竟致廢篤, "Recently people who have indulged in licentiousness have often suffered from red bayberry poison sores. For medication one uses *qing fen*, but once it is cured, [the disease] will break out again. After an extended period of time, the limbs and the body develop cramps and contract, and the [disease] develops into an **obstruction-illness with leakage**. This will last for years before eventually completely maiming [a person]".

***Yong lou* 癰瘺, obstruction-illness with fistula** [3]
PC CD of → *yong* 癰, obstruction-illness, and → *lou* 瘺, fistula. *MYBL* SE *wang bu liu xing* 王不留行：葉似酸漿，子似菘子。而多入**癰瘺**方用之, "The leaves resemble *suan jiang*; the seeds resemble *song* seeds. They are often used in recipes for **obstruction-illnesses with fistula**".

***Yong men* 壅悶, obstruction with heart-pressure** [1]
IS identical with → *yu men* 鬱悶, pent-up [qi] with heart-pressure. *QJYiF* 19: 水煮露蜂房一服五合汁，下乳石熱毒**壅悶**, "Boil honeycomb in water and ingest five *ge* per dosage. This will bring down breast stone, heat poison, and **obstruction with heart-pressure**".

***Yong qi* 壅氣, obstruction qi** [15] AN *yong qi* 擁氣, congesting qi.
① EA identical with → *zhi qi* 滯氣①, sluggish qi. *YXL* SE *mu xiang* 木香：逐諸**壅氣**上衝，煩悶, "It eliminates all **obstruction qi** that rush upward, with vexation and heart-pressure.
② Side effect of pharmaceutical substances, identical with → *zhi qi* 滯氣②, sluggish qi. *SLBC* SE *da dou* 大豆：小兒不得與炒豆食之。若食了，忽食豬肉，必**壅氣**致死, "Children must not eat fried beans. If they eat them and then immediately afterwards eat pork, this will result in **obstruction qi** leading to their death".

***Yong qi* 擁氣, congesting qi** [4]
① EA identical with → *zhi qi* 滯氣①, sluggish qi. *YXL* SE *shao yao* 芍藥：通宣臟腑**擁氣**, "It returns **congesting qi** to a free flow".
② Side effect of pharmaceutical substances, identical with → *zhi qi* 滯氣②, sluggish qi. *SLBC* SE *chun* 蓴：熱食之，亦**擁氣**不下, "If consumed warm, it will [cause] **congesting qi** that fails to descend".

***Yong re* 壅熱, obstruction heat; obstructed heat**[10] AW *re yong* 熱壅; *re yong* 熱擁.

① PC of abundant heat in the interior associated with obstruction of the qi mechanism. *TPSHF* 6: 肺臟**壅熱**，心胸不利, "When the lung is affected by **obstruction heat**, the heart and chest cannot function freely".

② Natural disposition of pharmaceutical substances with a hot nature that are able, if consumed for an extended period of time, to generate congestion disease. *ZLBC* SE *xiao mai* 小麥 quotes *BCSY*: 麵⋯性**擁熱**，小動風氣, "Flour: Its nature is one of **obstructed heat**. It slightly excites wind qi".

***Yong yang* 癰瘍, obstruction-illness ulcer** [3]

PC identical with → *yong* 癰, obstruction-illness. *SW* 12: 其民皆黑色疏理，其病皆為**癰瘍**，其治宜砭石, "Its people all have a black complexion and open [skin] structures. Their diseases are always **obstruction-illnesses ulcers**. For their treatment, pointed stones are suitable".

***Yong zhang* 壅脹, obstruction with distension; to obstruct** [2]

① AN *yong zhang* 擁脹, congestion with distension; *zhang yong*, 脹壅, distension with obstruction; *zhang pi*, 脹痞, distension with an obstacle-illness. IS of a feeling of obstructions with swelling and distension. *TBC* SE *ma fen* 麻蕡：根主產難，衣不出，破血，**壅脹**, "The roots control difficult births, when the placenta fails to descend, bleeding from an injury, and **obstruction with distension**".

② Used as a verb in the sense of "to obstruct". *BCGM* SE *qian niu zi* 牽牛子, LSZ: 予思此乃濕熱之邪在精道，**壅脹**隧路, "I think that this is an intrusion of moisture and heat into the path of essence/semen, where they **obstruct** the internal passageway".

***Yong zhang* 擁脹, congestion with distension** [1]

IS identical with → *yong zhang* 壅脹①, obstruction with distension. *KBBC* SE *ding xiang* 丁香：主温脾胃，止霍亂**擁脹**, "It is capable of warming the spleen and stomach; it stops cholera and **congestion with distension**".

***Yong zhong* 癰腫, obstruction-illness swelling** [242]

PC a) identical with → *yong* 癰, obstruction-illness. *BJ* SE *bai ji* 白棘：主心腹痛，**癰腫**潰膿, "It controls pain in the heart and abdomen, and festering **obstruction-illness swelling**". b) A differentiating reference to obstruction-illnesses that have not begun to fester yet. This is in contrast to → *yong chuang* 癰瘡，obstruction-illness sores. *MYBL* SE *dong xiang qing ce ni kang zhong qing ni* 東向圊廁溺坑中青泥：消**癰腫**，若已有膿即潰, "It dissolves **obstruction-illness swelling**. When pus has formed it will fester".

***You* 疣, wart** [p] AN *you zi* 疣子; *hou zi* 瘊子; *you mu* 疣目, wart eye; *you zhui* 疣贅, wart redundancy.

PC of a pea-size protuberance in the skin. The color is that of normal skin, while the texture of the skin appears rougher than normal. There is no abnormal sensation, such as pain or itching. *QJYF* 23: 苦酒漬鍛石六七日，滴取汁點**疣**上，小作**疣**即落, "Soak *duan shi* in bitter wine for six or seven days. Pour off the liquid and drop on the **wart**. This will make small **warts** fall off very soon".

You chou **憂愁, worrying; depression** [10]

① EA identical with → *you yu* 憂鬱, grief with pent-up [qi]. *NJ* 49: **憂愁**思慮則傷心，形寒飲冷則傷肺, "**Worrying** and pondering harm the heart. A cold body and chilled beverages harm the lung".

② IS of depression brought forth by frequent worrying and much grief. *QJYF* 14: 治心氣不定，五臟不足，甚者**憂愁**，悲傷不樂，忽忽善忘，朝瘥暮劇, "To cure unstable heart qi, and if the [qi of the] five depots is insufficient. In extreme cases with **depression** and sadness and sorrow, and a recurring tendency to be forgetful. In the morning this improves; at night it is serious".

You feng **游風, roaming wind** [19] AN *feng you* 風游, wind roamer.

PC of roaming and sudden pain and itching brought about by → *feng xie* 風邪, wind evil. *ZBYHL* 2: **游風**在於皮膚，逢寒則身體疼痛，遇熱則瘙癢, "If **roaming wind** in the skin encounters cold, the entire body will ache. If it encounters heat, it will itch". Depending on the afflicted body part and actual appearance of symptoms, authors distinguished between → *tou mian you feng* 頭面游風, wind roaming in the head and face, and → *chi bai you feng* 赤白游風, red-white roaming wind. *BCGM* uses *you feng* 游風 in the context of ailments affecting the skin: *you feng feng zhen* 游風風疹, roaming wind with wind macules; *you feng yin zhen* 游風隱疹, roaming wind with hidden macules; *you feng re du* 游風熱毒, roaming wind with heat poison.

You gu **游蠱, roaming *gu*** [4]

PC of a feeling as if an item were stuck in the throat, one that cannot be cleared by either swallowing or vomiting. *BCSY* SE *ran she* 蚺蛇：肉主飛屍，**游蠱**，喉中有物，吞吐不得出者，作膾食之, "The meat controls flying corpse [qi], **roaming *gu*,** with an item stuck in the throat that cannot be made to leave by swallowing or vomiting. Prepare a dish of minced meat and consume it".

You liu **疣瘤, wart tumor** [1]

PC identical with → *liu you* 瘤疣, tumorous wart. *BCGM* SE *zhi zhu* 蜘蛛 quoting *JBF*: **疣瘤**初起：柳樹上花蜘蛛纏之，久則自消, "When a **wart tumor** has just arisen: use [threads produced by] spiders from the blossoms on willow trees to wind around them. After an extended period of time they will dissolve".

You liu **游瘤, roaming tumor** [1]

PC identical with → *dan du* 丹毒, cinnabar poison. *BCTJ* SE *jian dao cao* 剪刀草：塗傅諸惡瘡腫及小兒**游瘤**丹毒, "To be applied externally to all types of malign sores with swelling, as well as **roaming tumors** and cinnabar poison affecting children".

You mu **疣目, wart eye** [24]

PC identical with → *you* 疣, wart. *ZBYHL* 31: 人手足邊忽生如豆，或如結筋，或五個，或十個，相連肌裏，粗強於肉，謂之**疣目**, "When at the side of his hands or feet someone suddenly grows something like a pea, or like a sinew node, sometimes five or even ten together in the flesh, rougher and more unyielding than flesh, then this is called '**wart eye**'".

You qi **游氣, roaming qi** [3]
IS of qi scurrying in the abdomen and making sounds there. *TBC* SE *nü wei* 女萎：霍亂泄痢，腸鳴**游氣**, 上下無常, "In the case of cholera with outflow and free-flux illness, there are sounds in the intestines with **roaming qi** rising and descending irregularly".

You shang huo zhuo **油傷火灼, harm following scorching by oil and fire** [1]
PC identical with → *tang huo shang* 湯火傷, harm caused by boiling water and fire. *BCGM* SE *shi gao* 石膏: quotes *MSF*: **油傷火灼**：痛不可忍。石膏末傅之，良, "For **harm following scorching by oil and fire**: When the pain is unbearable apply *shi gao* powder to it. Excellent".

You wai **右喎, wryness on the right** [5]
IS of → *kou wai* 口喎, wryness of the mouth, manifesting itself as a slanting mouth corner on the right side. *QJYF* 8: 治中風面目相引，口偏僻…又方：酒煮桂取汁，以故布拓病上，正則止，左喎搨右，**右喎**搨左, "Another recipe to cure wind stroke pulling on the face and eyes, with the mouth slanting to one side: Boil *gui* in wine and use the resulting juice to rub on the diseased region. Stop when it has assumed its proper structure again. For wryness on the left, rub on the right. For **wryness on the right**, rub on the left".

You yu **憂鬱, grief with pent-up [qi]** [5]
EA of an irritation of one's sentiments resulting from grief and worrying lasting for an extended period of time. *SYJYBZFL* 12: 石淋, 多因**憂鬱**，氣注下焦，結所食咸氣而成, "Stone dripping is often brought forth by **grief with pent-up [qi]**. When qi flows down into the lower burner it forms nodes with salty qi consumed as food".

You zhi **疣痣, wart and mole** [12]
PC CD of → *you* 疣, wart, and → *zhi* 痣, mole. *PJF* 51: 治**疣痣**黑子，以諸灰雜鍛石熬煎以點之, "To cure **warts, moles**, and black spots, mix all kinds of ashes with *duan shi*, boil this, and then swab them".

You zhong **游腫, roaming swelling** [6]
PC CD of red or white → *dan du* 丹毒, cinnabar poison, activating protrusions, with the swelling not occupying a permanent location. *ZBYHL* 30: **游腫**之候，青、黃、赤、白，無復定色，遊走皮膚之間，肉上微光是也, "The signs of **roaming swelling**: virid, yellow, red – it has no fixed color. It roams in the skin, and there is a mild gloss on the flesh".

You zi **疣子, wart** [4]
PC identical with → *you* 疣, wart. *ZBYHL* 50: 人有附皮肉生, 與肉色無異，如麥豆大，謂之**疣子**，即疣目也, "Someone has a growth of flesh on the skin. The color is not different from that of ordinary flesh. The size ranges from that of a grain to that of a bean. This is called a '**wart**'. It is identical with 'wart eyes'".

You zui **疣贅, wart redundancy** [10]
PC identical with → *you* 疣, wart. *BCJJZ* SE *dong hui* 冬灰：欲銷黑志、**疣贅**，取此三種灰, 和水蒸, 以點之, 即去, "If one wishes to remove a black mole,

or a **wart redundancy**, he should take these three types of ashes and steam them with water. Then use this to swab the [wart redundancy] and it will go away".

Yu **鬱, pent-up [qi]; depression** [p] AN *fu yu* 怫鬱, anger with pent-up [qi].
① AN *yu jie* 鬱結, pent-up [qi] with nodes; *yu e* 鬱遏, pent-up [qi] with containment; *yu yi* 鬱抑, pent-up [qi] with restraint: *yu xu* 鬱蓄, pent-up [qi] with accumulation. EA of pathological qi stagnating and collecting inside the human body. While mostly related to stagnation and collection of qi, *yu* 鬱, accumulation, may also result from stagnation/collection of fire, phlegm, food, moisture, and blood. *SW* 3: 勞汗當風，寒薄為皶，**鬱**乃痤, "If in a state of exhaustion one sweats and encounters wind, and if cold strikes [against the skin], this leads to blotches; in the case of **pent-up [qi]**, this will generate acne".
② AN *you yu* 憂鬱, grief with pent-up [qi]; *you men* 鬱悶, pent-up [qi] with heart-pressure. IS of a feeling of distress and unhappiness. *SHL* 103: 嘔不止、心下急、**鬱鬱**微煩者，為未解也, "In cases in which vomiting does not end, with a [feeling of] tightness below the heart, and **pent-up [qi]** with a slight vexation, it has not been resolved yet".

Yu **傴, hunchback** [2]
IS AD of → *yu lou* 傴僂①. *SW* 52: 刺脊間，中髓為**傴**，"When piercing between [the segments of] the spine, if one hits the marrow, this makes [the patient] become **hunchbacked**".

Yu bing **鬱病, pent-up [qi] disease** [1]
PC of diseases brought forth by pathological qi stagnating and collecting inside the human body. *YXZC* 1: 傷寒大法有四：曰傳經，曰專經，曰即病，曰**鬱病**, "The overall pattern of harm caused by cold is distinguished into four [categories]: transmission through conduits, affecting one particular conduit only, immediate disease, and **pent-up [qi] disease**".

Yu chang qi **育腸氣, birth intestine qi** [4]
PC identical with → *shan qi* 疝氣, elevation-illness qi. *TPSHF* 7: 腎氣虛微，為邪冷之氣所侵，傳注於小腸，則令小腸連陰疼痛，故號**育腸氣**也, "When the qi of the kidneys is depleted, this is because they have been penetrated by evil cold which is then transferred to the small intestine. As a result, the small intestine and, joined to it, the yin [member] are painful. Hence this is called the **birth intestine qi**".

Yu chen **余疹, residual papules** [2]
PC of a slightly painful disease of women following delivery. *YXL* SE *tong jing bi* 銅鏡鼻：主治產後**余疹**刺痛，三十六候，取七枚投醋中，熬過呷之, "To control, following delivery, **residual papules** with a piercing pain, 36 signs, take seven pieces and boil in vinegar. Then sip the [liquid]".

Yu chi **語遲, retarded beginning of speaking; speech retardation** [6]
① PC of children with an inability, at the age of four of five years, to speak. *TPSHF* 89: 治小兒心氣不足，舌本無力，令兒**語遲**，芍藥散方, "To cure children with heart qi insufficiency. The base of their tongue has no strength and

as a result **the beginning of their speaking is retarded**. [Use] the recipe for the powder with *shao yao*".

② IS, often caused by wind stroke, of adults whose language is unclear and whose responses in conversation are retarded. *PJF* 88: 筋急拘攣，**語遲**脈弦，加薏苡仁, "[To cure] tight sinews with cramps and contraction, **speech retardation** and [a movement in the] vessels that is string[-like], add *yi yi ren*".

Yu du **鬱毒, pent-up [heat] poison** [2]

EA of heat poison that stagnates inside the human body and generates accumulations that are difficult to expel. *BCGM* SE *sang zhai hui* 桑柴灰 quotes [Zhu] Zhenheng 震亨：火以暢達, 拔引**鬱毒**，此從治之法也, "To allow the fire to expand freely, one extracts the **pent-up [heat] poison**. This is the therapy pattern of compliance [with the nature of the pathogenic agent]".

Yu e **鬱遏, pent-up [qi] with containment** [9]

EA identical with → *yu* 鬱① pent-up [qi]. *NWSBHL* Fj 寒邪乘之，**鬱遏**陽分，陽不得伸，故發熱也, "When cold evil avails itself [of this depletion, this will result in] **pent-up [qi] with containment** in the yang section. The yang [qi] is barred from extension, and [patients] develop heat as a result".

Yu huo **鬱火, pent-up fire** [12]

PC identical with → *huo yu* 火鬱. *JFFH*: 積温成熱，漸至**鬱火**, "Warmth accumulates and manifests itself as heat. Gradually this will reach [a condition of] **pent-up fire**".

Yu jian **語蹇, impeded language** [2]

IS identical with → *yan yu jian se* 言語蹇澀. *BCGM* SE *lu* 驢 quoting *SYXJ* 言語似澀，一身動搖, "The language seems rough, and the entire body sways", writes: **語蹇**身顫, "**Impeded language** with a trembling body".

Yu jian **語謇, impeded language** [1]

IS identical with → *yan yu jian se* 言語蹇澀. *PJBSF* 1: 竹瀝湯，治中風入脾肝經年，四肢不遂，舌強**語謇**, "Decoction with *zhu li* cures [patients] being struck by wind, with [wind] having entered the spleen and liver for at least a year already, so that the four limbs do not follow their will, the tongue is stiff, and **language is impeded**".

Yu jie **鬱積, pent-up and accumulated** [2]

EA identical with → *yu* 鬱① pent-up [qi]. *DXXF* 3: 吞酸者，濕熱**鬱積**於肝而出, "Acid regurgiation is to say: moisture and heat **pent-up and accumulated** in the liver find their way out".

Yu jie **鬱結, pent-up [qi] with nodes** [19]

EA identical with → *yu* 鬱① pent-up [qi]. *SJZL* 11: 論曰：風瘙瘾胗，其狀有二，皆緣肌中有熱。若涼濕之氣折之，熱結不散，則成白胗。若因風邪所折，風熱相搏，則成赤胗。赤胗得熱則劇，得冷則滅，熱氣**鬱結**於內，故惡熱宜冷, "The discourse states: wind itching and dormant papules have two appearances, with both of them originating from heat in the muscles. If it is affected by cool moisture, the heat will form nodes and cannot dissipate. As a result it forms white papules. If [the heat] is affected by wind evil, wind and heat strike at each other, and this generates red papules. When red papules receive further heat, then they turn serious. If they receive cold, they vanish. When heat **qi is pent-up with nodes** in the interior, [patients] have an aversion to heat and should be treated with cold [medication]".

Yu jing bu wei **玉莖不痿, failure of the jade stalk to return to dysfunction** [1]
IS of male adults with an erection persisting over a long time without returning to a normal condition, associated with an uncomfortable feeling. *BCGM* SE *bu gu zhi* 補骨脂 quotes *QJF*: **玉莖不痿**：精滑無歇，時時如針刺，捏之則脆，此名腎漏, "When the **jade stalk fails to return to dysfunction**: unceasing smooth flow of essence/semen, often accompanied by a feeling as if pierced with a needle. When pinched it feels crisp. This is called 'kidney leakage'".

Yu jing chang ying bu wei **玉莖長硬不痿, long-term hardness of the jade stalk and its failure to return to dysfunction** [1]
IS identical with → *yu jing bu wei* 玉莖不痿, failure of the jade stalk to return to dysfunction. *BCGM* Bai bing zhu zhi yao 百病主治藥：**玉莖長硬不痿**，精出捏之則脆癢如刺針，名腎漏, "**The jade stalk is hard and fails to return to dysfunction for a long time**. When one pinches it while seminal fluid is discharged then it feels crisp and [the patient] experiences an itch as if pierced with a needle. This is called 'kidney leakage'".

Yu jing qiang ying bu wei **玉莖強硬不痿, hardness of the jade stalk and failure to return to dysfunction** [1]
IS identical with → *yu jing bu wei*, failure of the jade stalk to return to dysfunction. *BCGM* SE *jiu* 韭：玉莖強中：**玉莖強硬不痿**，精流不住，時時如針刺，捏之則痛，其病名強中，乃腎滯漏疾也, "Hardness of the jade stalk in the center: When the **jade stalk is hard and fails to return to dysfunction**, with unceasing spontaneous seminal pollution, often accompanied by a feeling as if pierced with a needle. Pinching it generates pain. This disease is called 'hardened center'. This is an ailment of sluggish and leaking kidney [qi]".

Yu kou chuang du **魚口瘡毒, fish mouth sores poison** [2]
PC of festering → *chuang* 瘡, sores, conditions developing in the genital region and in the crevices between the legs and the genital/anal region. *BCGM* SE *fan shi* 礬石 quotes *JJLF*: **魚口瘡毒**：白礬枯研，寒食麵糊調, 傅上，即消, "For **fish mouth sores poison**: Grind dried *bai fan* and mix with a paste made from Cold Dish [Festival] dough. Apply externally and [the sores poison] will disappear".

Yu kou feng **魚口風, fish mouth wind** [1]
PC of the upper lip being swollen and aching, and developing sores. *BCGM* Bai bing zhu zhi yao 百病主治藥：上唇腫痛生瘡，名**魚口風**, "When the upper lip is swollen and aches, this is called '**fish mouth wind**'".

Yu li **餘瀝, residual dribbling** [13]
IS of an inability to completely discharge all urine or ejaculate all semen at once, with a residue dribbling afterwards. *BJ* SE *ku shen* 苦參：主心腹結氣，癥瘕積聚，黃疸，溺有**餘瀝**, "It controls bound qi in the heart and abdomen, concre-

tion-illness and conglomeration-illness, accumulations and collections, yellow *dan*-illness, as well as urinary **residual dribbling**".

Yu lou **傴僂, hunchback** [4] AD *yu* 傴.

① IS of stoop and hunchback making it impossible to assume a straight posture. *ZBYHL* 41: 不欲令見**傴僂**侏儒，醜惡形人, "One does not wish to look at **hunchbacks** and dwarfs, and others with a repulsive physical appearance".

② Appearance of animals with an arched back. *BCYY* SE *lei shu* 鼺鼠：首如馬，身如蝦，背**傴僂**，身有竹節紋，長二三寸。今謂之海馬, "The head is like that of a horse, the body is like that of a shrimp. The spine is **hunchbacked**. The body has lines like the nodes of bamboo. It is two to three *cun* long. Nowadays it is called 'sea horse' ".

Yu mao **鬱冒, pent-up malicious [qi]** [5]

① IS of dizziness affecting the head and eyes, in severe cases with an inability to recognize persons or things. *SW* 74: 暴喑心痛，**鬱冒**不知人, "Suddenly [they] turn mute and their heart aches. They experience **pent-up malicious [qi]**, and do not recognize people".

② PC identical with → *xue jue* 血厥. *PJBSF* 7: 名曰**鬱冒**，亦名血厥，婦人多有之, "It is called **pent-up malicious [qi]**. Another name is 'blood recession'. Women often experience it".

Yu men **鬱悶, pent-up [qi] with heart-pressure** [2]

IS of a feeling of heart vexation and being upset that is difficult to resolve. *WTMY* 28: 凡五月六月，井中及深冢中皆有伏氣，入中令人**鬱悶**，殺人, "Every year during the fifth and sixth months, there is hidden qi in wells and dark graves. If it enters the interior of a person, he will experience **pent-up [qi] with heart-pressure**. It kills a person".

Yu men kuan leng **玉門寬冷, flabby jade gate with cold** [1]

PC with a slack and cold vagina as major signs. *FRDQLF* 8: 治**玉門寬冷**，硫黃末煎湯洗, "To cure a **flabby jade gate with cold**, rinse with the decoction with powderized *liu huang*".

Yu ne **語訥, slowed-down language** [1]

IS of slowed-down speech with an inability to clearly express one's thoughts. *BCGM* Zhu shui you du 諸水有毒：小兒就瓢及瓶飲水，令**語訥**, "When children drink water directly from a ladle or from a jar, this will let their **language slow down**".

Yu qi **鬱氣, pent-up qi** [2]

EA identical with → *qi yu* 氣鬱②. *SWBJQYBMJ* Fj: 宜辛以調上，以咸調下，必折其**鬱氣**，先資其化源, "It is advisable to use acrid [flavor] to regulate above, and to use salty [flavor] to regulate below. It is essential to break open the **pent-up qi**, and to first supply the source of its transformations".

Yu qi chuang **魚臍瘡, fish belly sores** [5] AN *Yu qi ding chuang* 魚臍丁瘡, fish belly pin-sores.

PC of → *chuang* 瘡, sores, conditions resembling the long and narrow shape of a fish belly. They have a white or slightly dark spot in their center, and are red on all four sides. Also, the swelling is painful and liquid seeps from it. *QJYF* 22: 治**魚臍瘡**，頭白腫痛不可忍者方, "Recipe to cure **fish belly sores** with a white top, swelling and unbearable pain".

Yu qi ding chuang **魚臍丁瘡, fish belly pin-sores** [2] AN *yu qi ding chuang* 魚臍疔瘡, fish belly pin-illness sores.

PC identical with → *yu qi chuang* 魚臍瘡, fish belly sores. *ZBYHL* 31: 此瘡頭破之黃水出，四畔浮漿起，狹長似魚臍，故謂之**魚臍丁瘡**, "When the heads of these sores are broken open they will emit yellow water. On all four sides blisters with thick liquid rise. They are long and narrow like a fish belly. Hence one calls them '**fish belly pin-sores**'".

Yu qi ding chuang **魚臍疔瘡, fish belly pin-illness sores** [3]

PC identical with → *yu qi ding chuang* 魚臍丁瘡, fish belly pin-sores. *BCGM* SE *bao yu* 鮑魚 quoting *QJYF* 22: 魚臍丁瘡似新火針瘡, "Fish belly pin-sores look like newly generated fire needle sores", writes: **魚臍疔瘡**似新火針瘡, "**Fish belly pin-illness sores** look like newly generated fire-needle sores".

Yu re **餘熱, residual heat** [4]

PC identical with → *liu re* 留熱, abiding heat. *ZBYHL* 8: 客邪未散，真氣不復，故旦暮猶有**餘熱**如瘧狀, "When visitor evil has not been dispersed, and the true qi has not yet recovered, there will be [outbreaks of] **residual heat** at dawn and dusk, very much like malaria".

Yu re **瘀熱, stagnant heat** [8]

PC resulting from evil heat that has accumulated in the body's interior and stays there for long. *SHL* 236: 此為**瘀熱**在裏，身必發黃, "This is **stagnant heat** in the interior. The body will turn yellow".

Yu se **鬱塞, pent-up [qi] blockage** [1]

EA identical with → *yu* 鬱①, pent-up [qi]. *YXRM* 6: 痰火胸膈**鬱塞**，嘈酸噎氣呑酸，或酒積泄結痛，加黃連、白芍、陳皮各一兩，石膏、甘草各五錢，砂仁、木香各二錢，川芎四錢, "For **pent-up [qi] blockage** in the chest and diaphragm brought forth by phlegm fire, with acid swallowing, burping, and acid regurgitation, as well as for outflow accompanied by twisting pain resulting from an accumulation of wine, add 1 *liang* each of *huang lian*, *bai shao*, and *chen pi*, 5 *qian* each of *shi gao* and *gan cao*, 2 *qian* each of *sha ren* and *mu xiang*, as well as 4 *qian* of *chuan xiong*".

Yu se **語澀, impeded language** [5]

IS identical with → *yan yu jian se* 言語蹇澀. *ZLBC* quotes *XPF*: 又方：治產後中風**語澀**，四肢拘急, "Another recipe: It cures being struck by wind after delivery with **impeded language**, and the four limbs cramping and being tense".

Yu sheng bu chu **語聲不出, loss of voice** [6] AN *yu yin bu chu* 語音不出.

IS identical with → *shi yin* 失音② a). *TPSHF* 35: 荊芥湯，治風熱肺壅，咽喉腫痛，**語聲不出**，或如有物哽, "The decoction with *jing jie* cures wind heat with lung obstruction, throat swelling and pain, **loss of voice**, sometimes with a feeling as if one were choking because of an object [in the throat]".

***Yu shi du* 礜石毒, mispickle mineral poisoning** [1]
EA of the poison of arsenopyrite. *QJYF* 24: **礜石毒**, 用大豆汁、白鵝膏, "For **mispickle mineral poisoning** use *da dou* juice and *bai e* paste".

***Yu shi du fa* 礜石毒發, outbreak of mispickle mineral poisoning** [1]
PC of poisoning resulting from an ingestion of mispickle mineral. *BCGM* SE *yu shi* 礜石：時珍竊謂洪文安之病, 未必是**礜石毒發**, "[I, L]SZ, venture to say, Hong Wen'an's disease was not necessarily an **outbreak of mispickle mineral poisoning**".

***Yu xu* 鬱蓄, pent-up [qi] accumulation** [2]
EA identical with → *yu* 鬱①, pent-up [qi]. *BCGM* SE *tu fu ling* 土茯苓 quotes *BCHB*: 土屬濕，主肌肉，濕熱**鬱蓄**於肌腠，故發為癰腫, "Soil is associated with moisture; it rules muscles and flesh. Now if there is **pent-up** moisture and heat **[qi] accumulation** in the muscles and interstices, this will result in obstruction-illness with swelling".

***Yu xue* 瘀血, stagnant blood** [224]
① AN *ke xue* 客血, visitor blood, *zei xue* 賊血, robber blood. PI of blood flowing for whatever reason into tissue outside of blood vessels and remaining either deep in the body, or in the skin and muscles in the outer regions. *JGYL* Lj: 曾經半產，**瘀血**在少腹不去, "She had had a miscarriage and there was **stagnant blood** in her lower abdomen that failed to leave".
② AN *zhi xue* 滯血, sluggish blood. EA of blood stagnating in the body that may in turn cause further disease because it blocks the passage of qi and blood. *SHL* 237: 本有久**瘀血**，故令喜忘, "[The patient] habitually had **stagnant blood**. This made him tend to be forgetful".
③ AN *xue ju* 血聚, blood collection. PC CD of all conditions caused by stagnant blood. *BJ* SE *an lü* 庵蕳：主五藏**瘀血**，腹中水氣, "It controls **stagnant blood** in the five depots, and water qi (i.e. water) in the abdomen".

***Yu xue qiang xin* 余血搶心, residual blood knocking on the heart** [1]
PC identical with → *chan hou bai xue gong xin* 產後敗血攻心, rotten blood attacking the heart following delivery. *TBC* SE *tu pi mao* 兔皮毛：主產難後衣不出及**余血搶心**, "It controls [conditions where] following delivery the placenta fails to appear, and **residual blood knocks on the heart**".

***Yu yan cuo miu* 語言錯謬, muddled and delirious language** [1]
IS identical with → *pi miu* 僻謬, eccentric and muddled [language]. *MYBL* SE *hu rou* 狐肉：治驚癇，神情恍惚，**語言錯謬**, "It cures fright epilepsy, spirit-affection of absent-mindedness, **muddled and delirious language**".

***Yu yan cuo wang* 語言錯妄, muddled and absurd language** [1]
IS identical with → *pi miu* 僻謬, eccentric and muddled [language]. *HJJF* 5: 治心氣不足，志意不定，神情恍惚，**語言錯妄**, "It cures insufficiency of heart qi, instability of the mind, spirit-affection of absent-mindedness, as well as **muddled and absurd language**".

Yu yan jian se **語言蹇澀, impeded language** [1]
IS identical with → *yan yu jian se* 言語蹇澀. *BCGM* SE *bai hua she* 白花蛇 quotes *BHJJF*: 世傳白花蛇酒，治諸風無新久，手足緩弱，口眼喎斜，**語言蹇澀**, "[The recipe] transmitted through the ages of wine with *bai hua she* cures all types of wind, regardless of whether these are acute or chronic cases, with the hands and feet slack and weak, the mouth and eyes slanted, and **impeded language**".

Yu yan nan chu **語言難出, impeded speech** [2]
IS identical with → *bu yu* 不語①, inability to speak. *BCGM* SE *wei rui* 萎蕤 quoting *SHLZHRS* 9: 鼻息必鼾，語言難, "Breathing through the nose will be snoring; speaking is difficult", writes: 鼻息必鼾，**語言難出**, "Breathing through the nose will be snoring; **speech is impeded**".

Yu yi **鬱抑, pent-up [qi] restraint** [2]
EA identical with → *yu* 鬱①, pent-up [qi]. *YXRM* 4: 凡房勞思恐傷腎，陰虛口中有味，夜熱晝輕者，俱宜四物湯加知、柏、黃芩；甚者，加童便、龜板峻補其陰。有**鬱抑**者，下甲丸, "Whenever after over-indulgence in sex one fears that the kidneys are harmed, with yin depletion and a flavor in the mouth, and with nocturnal heat that is milder during daytime, it is advisable [to use] the decoction with the four items, amended by *zhi* [*mu*], *bai*, and *huang qin*. In severe cases boys' urine and tortoise shell are to be added to quickly supplement the [patient's] yin. In the case of **pent-up [qi] restraint**, ingest pills with [tortoise] shell".

Yu yin bu chu **語音不出, loss of voice** [2]
IS identical with → *yu sheng bu chu* 語聲不出. *HJJF* 2: 三拗湯：治感冒風邪，鼻塞聲重，**語音不出**, "The decoction for the three stubborn [diseases] cures affection by the malicious in the form of wind evil, stuffed nose and heavy voice, and **loss of voice**".

Yu zheng **鬱蒸, pent-up [qi] with steam** [4]
Reference to a rising dense heat qi, either as a vital qi or as a disease qi, either in the natural world or inside the human body. *SW* 67: 其令**鬱蒸**，其變炎爍, "Its commands are **pent-up [qi] with steam**. When it causes changes [it generates] flames and melting".

Yu zhong **瘀腫, stasis swelling** [3]
IS identical with → *qing zhong* 青腫, greenish swelling. *TPSHF* 68: 治毒箭所傷，皮內**瘀腫**疼痛，不可過時，宜服梨母子煎方, "To cure injuries caused by poisonous arrows, with **stasis swelling** of the skin and pain, but not after too long a time, the recipe to ingest boiled *li mu zi* is advisable".

Yuan xue **遠血, distant bleeding** [2]
PC of bleeding where the location of the bleeding in the body is distant from the anus, with defecation first and bleeding afterwards, and the blood assuming a purple, dim coloring. *WTMY* 6: 先便轉後見血，此為**遠血**, "If one defecates first and this changes to bleeding afterwards, then this is '**distant bleeding**'".

Yue **啘, retching** [2] AN *ou yue* 嘔啘; *yue yue* 噦啘; *gan yue* 乾啘, dry retching.
IS identical with → *yue* 噦. *MYBL* SE *niu jiao sai* 牛角鰓：主消渴，止**啘**、泄, "It controls melting with thirst, and ends **retching** and outflow".

Yue **噦, retching** [p] AN *yue ou* 噦嘔, *yue yue* 啘噦; *yue* 啘; *yue qi* 噦氣, retching qi; *yue ni* 噦逆, retching with countermovement [of qi].
IS identical with → *gan ou* 乾嘔, dry vomiting. *SHL* 194：陽明病，不能食，攻其熱必**噦**, "In the case of disease in the yang brilliance [section], if one is unable to eat, attacking the heat will cause **retching**". *BCGM* SE *pi pa ye* 枇杷葉：**噦**者，乾嘔有聲也, "**Retching** is dry vomiting with sounds".

Yue bi **月閉, menstrual blockage** [23]
PC identical with → *jing bi* 經閉. *BJ* SE *bai e* 白堊：主女子寒熱，癥瘕，月閉, "In women it controls alternating sensations of cold and heat, concretion-illness and conglomeration-illness, as well as **menstrual blockage**".

Yue ge **月割, moon eclipse** [2]
PC of → *yue shi* 月蝕, moon eclipse [sores], developing at the ear. *BCSY* SE *gua fu zhuang tou chen tu* 寡婦床頭塵土：主人耳上**月割**瘡，和油塗之，效也, "It controls **moon eclipse** sores at the ears. When applied together with oil it is effective".

Yue hou bu tiao **月候不調, menstrual irregularity** [4]
PC identical with → *yue shui bu tiao* 月水不調. *QJYiF* 7：小五石澤蘭丸，主婦人勞冷虛損，飲食減少，面失光色，腹中冷痛，**月候不調**, "The 'small pills with the five mineral substances and *ze lan*' cure women suffering from exhaustion cold and depletion harm. They drink and eat little. Their facial complexion has lost its glossiness. They feel a cold pain in their abdomen, and they experience **menstrual irregularity**".

Yue hou bu tong **月候不通, menstrual blockage** [1]
PC identical with → *yue shui bu tong* 月水不通. *YXL* SE *shui zhi* 水蛭：主破女子**月候不通**, "It controls breaking up a woman's **menstrual blockage**".

Yue hou bu yun **月候不勻, menstrual irregularity** [6]
PC identical with → *yue shui bu tiao* 月水不調. *RHZ* SE *ma bian cao* 馬鞭草：通月經，治婦人血氣肚脹，**月候不勻**, "It opens the passage of menstruation, and cures females experiencing abdominal distension because of [stagnating] blood and qi, as well as **menstrual irregularity**".

Yue ji **噦疾, retching ailment** [1]
PC with retching as its major illness sign. *BCGM* SE *lu* 鹿 quotes *GJLY*: 小兒**噦疾**：鹿角粉、大豆末等分，相和乳調，塗乳上飲之, "For **retching ailment** in children: Mix equal portions of deer horn powder and soybean powder with milk. Apply to the mother's breast nipples for [the child to consume] while drinking".

Yue jia bing **月家病, menstruant's disease** [1]
PC identical with → *jing bing* 經病, menstrual disease. *BCGM* SE *ma chi xian* 馬齒莧 quotes *HSMF*: 筋骨疼痛：不拘風濕氣、楊梅瘡及女人**月家病**，先用此藥止疼，然後調理, "The sinews and bones ache: Regardless of whether

this involves wind moisture qi, red bayberry (i.e. syphilitic) sores, or a female's **menstruant's disease**, always use this medication to end the pain, and only then begin to take care [of the underlying disease]".

Yue jing bu duan **月經不斷, incessant menstruation** [1]
PC identical with → *yue shui bu zhi* 月水不止. *PJF* 334: 治**月經不斷**，用松茹一斤，淨洗，河水四升半，煮取二升，分二服, "To cure **incessant menstruation**, take one *jin* of *song ru*, cleanse carefully, boil with four and a half *sheng* of river water down to two *sheng*, and ingest in two portions".

Yue jing bu li **月經不利, impeded menstruation** [2]
PC identical with → *jing shui bu li* 經水不利. *ZBYHL* 37: 左手關上脈，足厥陰經也，沉為陰，陰虛者，主**月經不利**，腰腹痛, "The vessel[-movement] above the pass-section of the left hand is that of the foot ceasing yin conduit. [The movement] deep inside is that of yin [qi]. When the yin [qi] is depleted, this is responsible for **impeded menstruation** and pain in the lumbar and abdominal region".

Yue jing bu tiao **月經不調, menstrual irregularity** [7]
PC identical with → *yue shui bu tiao* 月水不調. *QJYF* 4: 杏仁湯，治**月經不調**, "Decoction with *xing ren* cures **menstrual irregularity**".

Yue jing bu tong **月經不通, menstrual blockage** [7]
PC identical with → *yue shui bu tong* 月水不通. *QJYF* 4: 治**月經不通**，心腹絞痛欲死，通血止痛方, "To cure **menstrual blockage**, a twisting pain in the heart and abdomen so severe that one wishes to die, [use] the 'recipe to have blood penetrate and end pain'".

Yue jing bu yun **月經不匀, menstrual irregularity** [1]
PC identical with → *yue shui bu tiao* 月水不調. *RHZ* SE *mao gen* 茅根：根主婦人**月經不匀**, "The root controls a woman's **menstrual irregularity**".

Yue jing bu zhi **月經不止, incessant menstruation** [5]
PC identical with → *yue shui bu zhi* 月水不止. *RHZ* SE *dai zhe* 代赭：止吐血鼻衄，腸風痔瘺，**月經不止**, "It stops vomiting of blood and nosebleeds, intestinal wind with piles and fistulas, as well as **incessant menstruation**".

Yue jing jiu bi **月經久閉, chronic menstrual blockage** [2]
PC of → *jing bi* 經閉, menstrual blockage, which has not been cured for an extended period of time. *PJF* 327: **月經久閉**：肉桂、甘草、黃耆、薑錢棗子、木通、紅花, "For **chronic menstrual blockage**: *rou gui*, *gan cao*, *huang qi*, *jiang qian zao zi*, *mu tong*, *hong hua*".

Yue jing lin bi **月經淋閉, menstrual blockage leading to dripping** [1]
PC of → *lou xia* 漏下, scant uterine bleeding, and → *jing bi* 經閉 menstrual blockage. *BCGM* SE *niu xi* 牛膝 quotes *BCF*: 女人血病：萬病丸，治婦人**月經淋閉**，月信不來, "Blood diseases in women: The 'pills for a myriad diseases' cure a woman's menstrual **blockage leading to dripping**, and complete failure of the monthly period to arrive".

Yue jing ni xing **月經逆行, menstrual counterflow** [2] AN *jing mai ni xing* 經脈逆行; *jing shui ni xing* 經水逆行.

PC of → *jing bing* 經病, menstrual disease, with diminished menstruation and, at the same time, nosebleed, bleeding gums, or even spitting of blood. *BCGM* SE *dang gui* 當歸 quoting *JBF*: **月經逆行**，從口鼻出, "**Menstrual counterflow** leaves [the body] through the mouth and nose".

Yue jing tai guo **月經太過, excessive menstruation** [2]

PC identical with → *jing shui guo duo* 經水過多. *BCSY* Xu 序 (preface): 甘瓜子，止**月經太過**, "Sweet melon seeds stop **excessive menstruation**".

Yue jing yu bi bu lai **月經瘀閉不來, blocked menstruation fails to arrive** [1]

PC identical with → *jing bi* 經閉, menstrual blockage. *BCGM* SE *qi* 漆 quotes *ZNF*: 萬應丸：治女人**月經瘀閉不來**, "The 'pills with myriad responses': they cure a woman's **blocked menstruation that fails to arrive**".

Yue ni **噦逆, retching with adverse movement [of qi]** [15]

① IS identical with → *yue* 噦, retching. *JYJZ* SE *ding xiang* 丁香：治傷寒咳噫不止及**噦逆**不定, "It cures harm caused by cold with unending cough and belching, as well as **retching with adverse movement [of qi]** that cannot be stabilized".

② PC with dry retching without sound. *MYBL* SE *li lu* 藜蘆：療**噦逆**，喉痹不通, "It cures **retching with adverse movement [of qi]**, and a throat that is blocked and impenetrable".

Yue ou **啘嘔, retching** [2]

IS identical with → *yue* 啘, retching. *BCGM* SE *luo le* 羅勒 quoting *JYBC*: 患啘，取汁服半合定, "For suffering from retching, consume one half *ge* of its juice", writes: 患**啘嘔**者，取汁服半合, "Patients suffering from **retching** should consume one half *ge* of its juice".

Yue qi **噦氣, retching qi** [11]

IS identical with → *yue* 噦, retching. *BCSY* SE *xian ren zhang* 仙人杖：主**噦氣**嘔逆, "It controls **retching qi** and vomiting with adverse movement [of qi]".

Yue shi **月蝕, lunar eclipse** [25]

PC of → *chuang* 瘡， sores developing on the ears, nose, face, and to the side of the orifices in the anal and genital region. Various explanations of this disease may be found in pre-modern medical literature. For example, this disease affects children who were conceived when their parents had intercourse during a lunar eclipse. Other reasons given are: drinking during a lunar eclipse, or a child pointing its finger towards the moon. Still others explain the name as reflecting a parallel between the waxing and waning of the moon, and the development of these ulcers, or between the shape of the ulcers below or behind the ears and the shape of a crescent moon. LSZ suggested that these ulcers develop at the time of the new moon. They abound during the full moon, and they weaken when the moon is waning. As these ulcers develop near the ears of children and are difficult to cure, they may eventually result in → *gan* 疳, *gan-illness*. *QJYF* 5: 治小兒**月蝕**瘡，隨月生死方：以胡粉和酥敷之，五日瘥, "Recipe to cure **lunar-eclipse**

sores with surviving and dying in accordance with the [waxing and waning of the] moon: Mix *hu fen* with butter and smear this [on the sores]. They will be cured within five days".

Yue shi **噦食, food retching** [2]

IS of dry retching accompanied by a mouth odor of rotten food. *BCGM* SE *bang* 蚌 quotes *RCF*: 乾嘔**噦食**者，炒粉丸主之, "Dry vomiting and **food retching** is controlled by pills with roasted [clam] powder".

Yue shi gan chuang **月蝕疳瘡, lunar eclipse *gan*-illness sores** [2]

PC of → *yue shi* 月蝕, lunar eclipse, ulcers that persist for a long time without cure and eventually cause a child to gain a yellow complexion and be emaciated. *BCGM* SE *hu* 虎 quotes *SXF*: **月蝕疳瘡**：虎頭骨二兩搗碎，豬脂一斤，熬膏塗之, "**Lunar eclipse *gan*-illness sores**: grind 2 *liang* of tiger bones to pieces, and boil with 1 *jin* of lard to a paste to apply to it externally".

Yue shi shuai shao bu lai **月事衰少不來, the monthly affair is weak and diminished and fails to arrive; minimal or failing menstruation** [2]

IS of an obviously decreased or even entirely absent menstruation. *SW* 40: 病名血枯，此得之年少時，有所大脫血，若醉入房中，氣竭肝傷，故**月事衰少不來**也, "The disease is named blood decay. It is acquired in younger years either [because of] a massive loss of blood or [because] one has entered the [woman's] chambers in a state of drunkenness [with the result that] the qi is exhausted and the liver is harmed. Hence, the **monthly affair is weak and diminished and fails to arrive**".

Yue shui bu ding **月水不定, menstrual irregularity** [2]

PC identical with → *yue shui bu tiao* 月水不調. *YXL* SE *shan zhu yu* 山茱萸：治腦骨痛，止**月水不定**，補腎氣，興陽道, "It cures skull bone pain, ends **menstrual irregularity**, supplements kidney qi, and makes the yang path (i.e. the penis) rise".

Yue shui bu duan **月水不斷, incessant menstruation** [11]

PC identical with → *yue shui bu zhi* 月水不止. *ZBYHL* 37: 婦人**月水不斷**者，由損傷經血，衝脈、任脈虛損故也, "As for **incessant menstruation**, the reason is harm caused to menstrual blood, with both the throughway vessel and the controller vessel being depleted and injured".

Yue shui bu lai **月水不來, menstruation fails to arrive** [2]

PC identical with → *yue shui bu tong* 月水不通. *ZBYHL* 37: 診其腎脈微澀，為不利者，是**月水不來**也, "If diagnosis reveals a slightly rough [movement in the] kidney vessels, with no free passage, then this signals that **menstruation fails to arrive**".

Yue shui bu li **月水不利, menstruation does not flow freely** [3]

PC identical with → *jing shui bu li* 經水不利. *ZBYHL* 37: 婦人**月水不利**者，由勞傷血氣，致令體虛而受風冷, "As for **menstruation that does not flow freely**, the reason is exhaustion that has harmed the blood and qi, causing bodily depletion which then is affected by wind cold".

***Yue shui bu tiao* 月水不調, menstrual irregularity** [10] AN *yue jing bu tiao* 月經不調; *jing hou bu tiao* 經候不調; *jing shui bu tiao* 經水不調; *yue hou bu tiao* 月候不調; *jing mai bu tiao* 經脈不調; *fu ren xue mai bu tiao* 婦人血脈不調; *jing bu tiao* 經不調; *yue hou bu yun* 月候不勻; *yue shui bu yun* 月水不勻; *jing mai bu yun* 經脈不勻; *xue jing bu yun* 血經不勻; *yue jing bu yun* 月經不勻; *yue shui bu ding* 月水不定.

PC CD of irregularities in the periodicity, length and quantity, consistency, and color of menstruation. *ZBYHL* 37: 婦人**月水不調**，由勞傷氣血，致體虛受風冷，風冷之氣客於胞內，傷衝脈、任脈，損手太陽、少陰之經也, "When a woman's **menstruation is irregular**, this may be because exhaustion has harmed her qi and blood to the extent that her body is in a state of depletion and receives wind cold. The qi of the wind cold resides inside her bladder. It harms the throughway vessel and the controller vessel, and it causes injury to the hand major yang and minor yin conduits".

***Yue shui bu tong* 月水不通, menstrual blockage** [7] AN *yue jing bu tong* 月經不通; *jing mai bu tong* 經脈不通; *jing shui bu tong* 經水不通; *tian gui bu tong* 天癸不通; *jing hou bu tong* 經候不通; *jing xue bu tong* 經血不通; *yue hou bu tong* 月候不通; *jing luo bu tong* 經絡不通, impassability of conduits and network [vessels].

PC identical with → *jing bi* 經閉. *MYBL* SE *niu xi* 牛膝：除腦中痛及腰脊痛，婦人**月水不通**, "It eliminates pain in the brain and in the lumbar region and spine, as well as in female **menstrual blockage**".

***Yue shui bu yun* 月水不勻, menstrual irregularity** [1]

PC identical with → *yue shui bu tiao* 月水不調. *QXLF* 63: 調經通治方：治婦人諸疾…**月水不勻**，當歸酒下, "Recipe to regulate menstruation and cure all variants: It cures all types of women's diseases…For **menstrual irregularity**, ingest it with the wine with *dang gui*".

***Yue shui bu zhi* 月水不止, incessant menstruation** [15] AN *jing shui bu zhi* 經水不止; *yue jing bu zhi* 月經不止; *jing xue bu zhi* 經血不止; *jing mai bu zhi* 經脈不止; jing bu zhi 經不止; *yue shui bu duan* 月水不斷; *yue jing bu duan* 月經不斷; *jing shui bu duan* 經水不斷.

PC of a → *jing bing* 經病, menstrual disease, with a duration of bleeding exceding seven days. *TPSHF* 73: 治婦人崩中下五色及下血，或**月水不止**，側柏散方, "To cure women experiencing a collapsing center with discharge in various colors as well as discharge of blood, and also **incessant menstruation**, the recipe for the powder with *ce bai* [is appropriate]".

***Yue shui guo duo* 月水過多, excessive menstruation** [1]

PC identical with → *jing shui guo duo* 經水過多. *HJJF* 9: 膠艾湯，治勞傷血氣，衝任虛損，**月水過多**, "Decoction with [*a*] *jiao* and *ai* cures exhaustion harming the blood and qi, with depletion injury affecting the throughway and controller [vessels, causing] **excessive menstruation**".

***Yue shui zha duo zha shao* 月水乍多乍少, menstruation that is sometimes excessive, other times diminished** [1]

PC of → *yue shui bu tiao* 月水不調, menstrual irregularity, with the quantity of menstrual bleeding sometimes exceeding and sometimes not reaching the average. *ZBYHL* 37: 月水乍多乍少，為不調也, "When **menstruation is sometimes excessive and other times diminished**, then this is irregular".

Yue tan **噦痰, phlegm retching** [1]

Most likely a misspelling of → *yue ji* 噦疾, retching ailment, in *BCGM* Bai bing zhu zhi yao 百病主治藥：鹿角，食後喜嘔，燒研，同人參末，薑湯服。小兒**噦痰**，同大豆末塗乳飲之, "Deer horn: [To treat] a tendency to vomit after having had a meal. Roast and grind, ingest together with *ren shen* powder and a decoction with *jiang*. For children with **phlegm retching**, smear it on the [mother's] breast nipple together with *da dou* powder, and [have the child ingest] it when drinking". In *BCGM* SE *lu* 鹿, quoting *GJLY*, the same recipe is given for the indication "children with retching ailment": 小兒噦疾：鹿角粉、大豆末等分，相和乳調，塗乳上飲之, "For children with retching ailment: mix equal amounts of deer horn powder and *da dou* powder with breast milk, smear on [the mother's] breast nipple and [have the child ingest] it when drinking".

Yue xie **啘泄, retching and outflow** [1]

PC identical with → *ou xie* 嘔泄, vomiting and outflow. *MYBL* SE *niu jiao sai* 牛角鰓：主消渴，止**啘泄**, "It controls melting with thirst and stops **retching and outflow**".

Yue xin bu lai **月信不來, menstrual blockage** [1]

PC identical with → *yue shui bu tong* 月水不通. *PJF* 333: 神仙活命丹，治婦人血氣凝滯，**月信不來**，日漸羸瘦, "The 'spirit-hermit elixir to support life' cures females with congealed blood and sluggish qi, [resulting in] **menstrual blockage**. They gradually lose weight day by day".

Yue xin lai duo **月信來多, excessive menstruation** [1]

PC identical with → *jing shui guo duo* 經水過多. *SLBC* SE *chun* 椿：女子血崩及產後血不止，**月信來多**。可取東引細根一大握，洗之，以水一大升煮，分再服，便斷, "For [treating] a woman's blood collapse and incessant bleeding following delivery, as well as **excessive menstruation**, one may grasp a large handful of its fine roots stretching eastward, cleanse them and boil them with one large *sheng* of water. This is to be ingested divided into several portions, and will end [the bleeding] immediately".

Yue xin se zhi **月信澀滯, impeded menstruation** [1]

PC identical with → *jing shui bu li* 經水不利. *PJF* 233: 治**月信澀滯**，用白蘘荷根細切，煎取二升，空心酒調服, "To cure **impeded menstruation** use the roots of *bai rang he*, chop them finely, and boil the liquid down to two *sheng*. Ingest mixed with wine on an empty stomach".

Yue yue **啘噦, retching** [1]

IS identical with → *yue* 噦, retching. *BCGM* SE *pi pa ye* 枇杷葉quotes *MYBL*: 卒啘不止, "Sudden belching that does not stop". In Bai bing zhu zhi yao 百病主治藥 this is quoted again as: **啘噦**不止, "**Retching** that does not stop".

***Yue yue* 噦啘, retching** [5]

IS identical with → *yue* 噦, retching. *BCGM* Za cao 雜草 quoting *BCSY* SE *yan ru cao* 燕蓐草：亦主噦氣, "It also controls retching qi", writes: 亦止**噦啘**, "It also stops **retching**".

***Yun* 運, movements** [p]

① IS identical with → *tou xuan* 頭旋, spinning head. *BCGM* Bai bing zhu zhi yao 百病主治藥：眩是目黑，**運**是頭旋, "眩 stands for darkness in front of the eyes; 運 stands for a revolving **movement** [perceived] in the head".

② PC identical with → *xue yun* 血運, blood[-induced brain-]movements. *ZBYHL* 43: 亦去血過多，亦有下血極少，皆令**運**, "If blood is removed excessively, and if blood is purged only in very small quantities, all this leads to **movements**".

***Yun dao* 運倒, [brain] movement with falling** [1]

IS identical with → *hun dao* 昏倒, clouding with fall. *BCGM* SE *jing quan shui* 井泉水 quoting *TYJYF*: 中煤炭毒：一時**運倒**，不救殺人。急以清水灌之, "When someone has been struck by coal poison, and for some time has been experiencing **[brain] movement and falls** to the ground, if he is not helped this will kill that person. Quickly forcibly instill clear water into him".

***Yun jue* 運絕, [brain] movement with a cut off [qi flow]** [3]

IS of dizziness and loss of consciousness following a severe form of vertigo. *TPSHF* 80: 產時出血過多，血虛氣極，因此而**運絕**也, "If during delivery she loses too much blood, so that there is an extreme depletion of blood and qi, this will result in **[brain] movement with a cut off [qi flow]**".

***Yun li* 孕痢, pregnancy-related free-flux illness** [5] AN *tai qian li* 胎前痢, free-flux illness preceding delivery; *tai li* 胎痢, embryo-related delivery.

PC of → *li ji* 痢疾, ailment of free-flux illness, affecting women during pregnancy. *BCGM* SE *bai yang* 白楊 quoting *QJYF* 2：白楊皮，治妊娠下痢, "*Bai yang pi* cures pregnancy-related discharge with free-flux illness", writes: 止**孕痢**, "It ends **pregnancy-related free-flux illness**".

***Yun nüe* 孕瘧, pregnancy malaria** [3]

PC of → *nüe ji* 瘧疾, malaria ailment, of pregnant women. *BCGM* Bai bing zhu zhi yao 百病主治藥：生薑汁，露一夜服，**孕瘧**尤效, "*Sheng jiang* juice ingested after having been left exposed for one night is very effective in the treatment of **pregnancy malaria**".

***Yun sou* 孕嗽, pregnancy cough** [1]

PC of coughing during pregnancy. *BCGM* Bai bing zhu zhi yao 百病主治藥：貝母，清肺消痰止咳，沙糖丸食。又治**孕嗽**, "*Bei mu* cools/clears the lung, dissolves phlegm and ends a cough. Ingest the pills with ground sugar. It also cures **pregnancy cough**".

***Yun xuan* 運眩, [brain] movement with dizziness** [1]

IS identical with → *xuan yun* 眩運①, vertigo. *BCGM* SE *xiong qiong* 芎藭 quoting *SWBJQYBMJ* Fj: 頭目眩, "Dizziness affecting head and eyes", writes: 頭目**運眩**, "Head and eyes affected by **[brain] movement with dizziness**".

***Yun yi* 雲翳, cloud shade** [4]

PC of → *mu yi* 目翳, eye shade, which is pale-white and thin. Vision is dimmed as if there were clouds or fog. *PJF* 74: 四物龍膽湯：治目赤暴發，作**雲翳**, "The decoction with four items including *long dan*: It cures sudden affliction with red eyes resulting in a **cloud shade**".

***Yun zhong you yong* 孕中有癰, obstruction-illness during pregnancy** [4]

PC of → *chang yong* 腸癰, intestinal obstruction-illness, developing during pregnancy. *FRLFBY* 15: 治**孕中有癰**。薏苡仁煮汁飲之, "To cure **obstruction-illness developing during a pregnancy** drink the sap obtained from boiling *yi yi ren*".

- Z -

***Za bing* 雜病, miscellaneous diseases** [8]

CD of all internal PC that are not the typical warmth and heat diseases related to the course of the four seasons. *QJYF* 2: （婦人）若是四時節氣為病, 虛實冷熱為患者, 故與丈夫同也。惟懷胎妊而挾病者, 避其毒藥耳。其**雜病**與丈夫同, 則散在諸卷中, 可得而知也, "When [women] have a disease associated with the four seasonal qi, and suffer from depletion or repletion, cold or heat, this is identical with [the diseases affecting males]. Only for those diseases associated with pregnancy they must abstain from poisonous medication. Their **miscellaneous diseases** that are identical with those of males are documented in many chapters and can be learned from there".

***Za chuang* 雜瘡, various sores** [5]

PC CD of all types of nameless → *chuang* 瘡, sores, conditions. *ZHF* 8: 療諸疥癬**雜瘡**，並宜摩之, "To cure all types of *jie*-illness, *xuan*-illnesses, and **various sores**, the [afflicted regions] are to be rubbed with it".

***Zang du* 臟毒, depot poisoning** [32]

PC a) of → *li ji* 痢疾, free-flux illness ailment, resulting from a presence of much heat poison, with pus and even more blood being passed down. *SJZL* 178: 治小兒**臟毒**，久痢下膿血，如聖散方, "Recipes for a powder as if provided by a sage to cure **depot poisoning** in children, with a chronic free-flux illness accompanied by pus and blood. b) Of → *bian xue* 便血, stools with dark, turbid blood. *SJZL* 97: 治**臟毒**，便血不止，龍骨餅子方, "Recipes for cakes with *long gu* to cure **depot poisoning**, [that is,] an unending passage of blood in the stools".

***Zang han* 臟寒, depot cold; depots are cold** [10]

PC brought forth by a depletion of qi in the large intestine leading to a lack of control of incoming cold. *SW* 12: **臟寒**生滿病, "Their **depots are cold** and generate diseases of fullness".

***Zang nüe* 臟瘧, depot malaria** [1]

PC identical with → *wu zang nüe* 五臟瘧, the five types of depot malaria. *BCGM* SE *fu zi* 附子 quoting *JSF* Zhu nüe men 諸瘧門, Section "All types of malaria", Zhu nüe lun zhi 諸瘧論治, "Treatment of all types of malaria:" 七棗湯，治五臟氣虛，陰陽相勝，作為痎瘧, "The 'decoction with seven *zao*' serves to treat qi depletion of the five depots, with yin and yang [qi] dominating alternatingly, resulting in malaria", writes 五臟氣虛，陰陽相勝，發為**臟瘧**, "When the qi in the five depots is depleted, and yin and yang [qi] dominate alternatingly, this effuses as **depot malaria**".

***Zang zao* 臟燥, depot dryness** [3]

PC of women whose spirit is depressed and who feel sad and begin to weep for no apparent reason. *JGYL* Lj: 婦人臟躁，喜悲傷欲哭，象如神靈所作，數欠伸，甘麥大棗湯主之, "When females suffer from depot restlessness, they tend to be harmed by sadness and wish to weep. It seems as if a spirit had caused this. They frequently yawn and stretch their body. The decoction with *gan* [*cao*], [*xiao*] *mai* and *da zao* controls it". *PJBSF* 10: 鄉裏有一婦人數欠伸，無故悲泣不止, 或謂之有祟, 祈禳請禱備至, 終不應。予忽憶《金匱》有一症云：婦人**臟燥**, 悲傷欲哭, 象如神靈所作, 數欠伸者, 甘麥大棗湯。予急令治此藥, 盡劑而愈, "In my home town there was a woman who repeatedly yawned and stretched he body. She was, without reason, overcome by sadness and weeped without end. Someone said she was possessed. Prayers were read and sacrifices were offered, but there was no response. Eventually I suddenly remembered a condition recorded in the *JG*[*YL*] as follows: 'When females suffer from **depot dryness**, when they are harmed by sadness and wish to weep, and if it seems as if a spirit had caused this, with [the patients] frequently yawning and stretching their body, the decoction with gan [cao], [xiao] mai and da zao [is appropriate]'. I hurriedly had this medication prepared for her. After she had taken the entire dosage she was cured". *BCGM* SE *zao* 棗：按許叔微《本事方》云：一婦病**臟燥**，悲泣不止, 祈禱備至。予憶古方治此證用大棗湯, 遂治與服, 盡劑而愈, "In Xu Shuwei's [*PJ*]*BSF* it is said: There was a woman who suffered from **depot dryness**. She was overcome by sadness and weeped without end. Prayers and sacrifices were performed. I remembered an ancient recipe using the decoction with *da zao* to cure this condition. Hence I had it prepared and given to her. After she had ingested the entire dosage she was cured". The *BCGM* mentions this condition three times, always referring to it as *zang zao* 臟燥， depot dryness.

***Zao* 燥, dry; dryness; to dry** [p]

① Condition of matter that contains no moisture or liquid. *SW* 69: 岐伯曰：有喜有怒，有憂有喪，有澤有**燥**，此象之常也, "Qi Bo: They may be joyful or angry, they may be anxious or mournful, they may be humid or **dry**. These are regular [manifestations] of the [heavenly] images".

② EA that may bring about external dryness. One of the six potential climatic excesses. *SW* 5: 風勝則動，熱勝則腫，**燥**勝則乾，寒勝則浮，濕勝則濡瀉, "When wind dominates, there is movement; when heat dominates, there is swelling. When **dryness** dominates, there is aridity; when cold dominates, there is surface [swelling]. When moisture dominates, there is soggy outflow".

③ IS of an uncomfortable feeling or appearance of dryness rather than moisture. *SW* 31: 五日少陰受之，少陰脈貫腎絡於肺，系舌本，故口**燥**舌乾而渴, "On the fifth day, the minor yin [conduits] receive it. The minor yin vessels penetrate the kidneys and enclose the lung. They are attached to the base of the tongue. Hence, the mouth is **dry**, the tongue is desiccated, and one is thirsty".

④ AN *zao bing* 燥病, dryness disease. PC of dryness either brought forth by external conditions or by a lack of body liquids or blood internally. *SW* 71: 其變肅殺雕零，其病**燥**，背瞀胸滿, "The changes [caused by] them include sternness, killing, withering, and falling. The illnesses [caused by] them include **dryness**, back pressure and [a feeling of] fullness in the chest".

⑤ PQ of pharmaceutical substances able to harm human body liquids and bring forth a condition of dryness. *LGPZ* SE *shi gao* 石膏：凡使，勿用方解石，方解石雖白，不透明，其性**燥**, "Whenever it is applied, one must not use *fang jie shi*. *Fang jie shi* is white, but opaque. Its nature is **dry**".

⑥ AN *zao shi* 燥濕, to dry moisture. TA to eliminate moisture evil. *SW* 71: 宜以苦燥之溫之，甚者發之泄之, "Hence this year it is appropriate to use bitter [flavor] to **dry** it, to warm it. In severe cases, effuse it, drain it".
⑦ AN *zao ji* 燥劑, pharmaceutical preparation with a drying effect. Effect of substances or recipes with an ability to dry moisture. *SW* 22: 脾苦濕，急食苦以燥之, "When the spleen suffers from moisture, quickly consume [food with] bitter flavor to **dry** it".

Zao **躁, restlessness** [p]
IS of restlessness with an inability to calm down. *SW* 32: 熱爭則狂言及驚，脅滿痛，手足**躁**，不得安臥, "When the heat is fought [by the proper qi, the patient] talks crazily and is frightened. The flanks are full and painful. The hands and the feet move **restlessly**. [The patient] cannot sleep peacefully".

Zao bing **燥病, dryness disease** [2]
PC identical with *zao* 燥④. *RMSQ* 7: 食之半載，居然生子，其婦**燥病**方愈, "She consumed one half of it and immediately gave birth to a son. The woman was then cured of **dryness disease**". *BCGM* refers to various types of dryness disease: *xia zao* 下燥, dryness below; *shang zao* 上燥, dryness above; *pi zao* 皮燥, skin dryness; *rou zao* 肉燥, flesh dryness; *jin zao* 筋燥, sinew dryness; *gu zao* 骨燥, bone dryness; *fei zao* 肺燥, lung dryness; *gan zao* 肝燥, liver dryness; *shen zao* 腎燥, kidney dryness.

Zao chuan **燥喘, dry panting** [1]
PC of → *chuan zheng* 喘證, panting condition, without phlegm. *BCGM* Li Dongyuan sui zheng yong yao fan li 李東垣隨證用藥凡例：熱喘、**燥喘**，阿膠、五味、麥門冬, "Heat panting, **dry panting**: [for treatment use] *a jiao*, *wu wei* [*zi*], *mai men dong*".

Zao fan **躁煩, restlessness with vexation** [1]
PC should be 㤹 燥，煩, "[heart and lung] dryness with vexation", meaning heart and lung yin depletion with vexation and heart-pressure. *BCGM* quote based on *ZLBC* SE *ou shi jing* 藕實莖：荷葉，止渴，落胞，殺蕈毒，併產後口乾，心肺燥，煩悶，入藥炙用之, "*He ye* stop thirst, make the placenta descend, kill the poison of *xun*, and [cure] dry mouth after delivery, heart and lung dryness, as well as vexation with heart-pressure. Use medicinally after roasting". LSZ abbreviated 心肺燥，煩悶 to 心肺躁煩, changing *zao* 燥, "dry", to *zao* 躁, "restless", thereby severely altering the meaning of this passage.

Zao guo **燥瘑, dry lair-illness** [1]
PC of → *guo chuang* 瘑瘡, lair-illnes sores, that are dry and have no liquid seeping from them. *QJYF* 22: 治**燥瘑**方：用醋和灰塗之, "Recipe to cure **dry lair-illness**: Use vinegar and lime and apply [to the affected region]".

Zao ji **燥劑, pharmaceutical preparation with a drying effect** [6]
TA identical with → *zao* 燥⑦. *RMSQ* 1: 豈獨薑附之儔，方為**燥劑**乎, "How can it be that only in a combination with *jiang* and *fu* [*zi*] it may serve as a **pharmaceutical preparation with a drying effect**?"

Zao jie **燥結, dryness nodes** [16] AN *jie zao* 結燥, binding with dryness; *zao sai* 燥塞, dry and blocked up; *zao se* 燥澀, dryness and roughness; *zao shi* 燥實, dry and solid.

IS of dry and congealed stools that do not pass. *TPSHF* 8: 太陽病以火蒸之，不得汗者，其人必**燥結**, "If patients with a major yang disease are steamed without sweating, they will suffer from **dryness nodes**".

Zao ke **燥渴, dryness and thirst** [11]

IS of an uncomfortable feeling of dryness and thirst. *MYBL* SE *mai men dong* 麥門冬：主身重目黃，心下支滿，虛勞客熱，口乾**燥渴**, "It controls a feeling of bodily heaviness and yellow eyes, propping fullness below the heart, depletion-exhaustion and visitor heat, and a desiccated mouth with **dryness and thirst**".

Zao men **躁悶, restlessness with heart-pressure** [3]

IS identical with → *fan zao* 煩躁, vexation with restlessness. *YHL SE zhi mu* 知母：主治心煩**躁悶**, "It controls heart vexation and **restlessness with heart-pressure**".

Zao re **燥熱, dryness and heat** [13] AW *re zao* 熱燥. CD of → *zao* 燥, dryness, and → *re* 熱, heat.

① Climatic condition of dryness and heat. *SW* 67: 風寒在下，**燥熱**在上, "Wind and cold are below; **dryness and heat** are above".

② EA identified as simultaneous appearance of dryness and heat. *SW* 68: **燥熱**相臨，風火相值, "**Dryness and heat** come down on each other. Wind and fire come into contact".

③ PC brought about by dryness with heat. *SJZL* 10 RE *tian zhu yin zi* 天竺飲子, Indian decoction: 治伏暑、**燥熱**, "It cures latent summerheat, **dryness and heat**".

④ IS of a subjective feeling of dryness and heat. *TPSHF* 17: 治熱病未得汗，**燥熱**，飲水過多, "It cures heat disease without sweating. [Patients feel] **dryness and heat** and drink water excessively".

⑤ Thermoquality of pharmaceutical substances. The nature of pharmaceutical drugs that are able to cure conditions of cold with moisture. *SW* 71: 同寒濕者**燥熱**化, "When they agree in cold and moisture, **dryness and heat** serve to achieve transformations".

Zao sai **燥塞, dry and blocked up** [1]

IS identical with → *zao jie* 燥結, dryness nodes. *BCGM* SE *zao* 棗 qotes *RZZZF*: 大便**燥塞**，大棗一枚去核，入輕粉半錢縛定，煨熟食之，仍以棗湯送下, "When the stools are **dry and blocked up**, take one piece of *da zao* and discard the kernel. Insert one half of a *qian* of *qing fen* into it and close tightly. Cook over a slow fire until done. Then swallow with a decoction with *zao*".

Zao se **燥澀, dryness and roughness; dry and rough** [3]

① IS identical with → *zao jie* 燥結, dryness nodes. *SJZL* 179: 實熱之氣，歸於大腸，故大便**燥澀**而不通也, "The qi of repletion heat turns to the large intestine. Hence the stools are **dry and rough**, and fail to pass".

② SEC identical with → *gan se* 乾澀, desiccated and rough. *SHZG* Lj: 難產或死胎不下，皆由風熱**燥澀**，緊斂結滯而不能舒緩，故產戶不得自然開通也, "In the case of difficult deliveries or if the fetus has died and does not descend, the reason is wind heat has brought about **dryness and roughness**. This makes [the birth canal] be tight with nodular and sluggish [qi] rather than allowing it to relax. Hence the birth gate cannot open by itself".

Zao shi **燥實, dry and solid** [1]
IS identical with → *zao jie* 燥結, dryness nodes. *PJF* 178: 大便**燥實**，小便大利而不甚渴, "The stools are **dry and solid**. The urine flows massively, and [patients] are not very thirsty".

Zao shi **燥屎, dry stools** [2]
SEC of dry stools possibly causing vexation, restlessness, and crazy talking. *SHL* 209: 有**燥屎**也，乃可攻之, "[In this case, the patient] has **dry stools.** This can be attacked".

Zao shi **燥濕, to dry moisture** [38]
TA identical with → *zao* 燥⑥. *SWXJYBS* Liu qi wei bing 六氣為病, Diseases caused by the six qi: 辛熱能發散開通鬱結, 苦能**燥濕**, 寒能勝熱, 使氣宣平而已, "Acrid [flavor] and heat are able to dissipate and to open pent-up [qi] with nodes. Bitter [flavor] is able to **dry moisture.** Cold is able to overcome heat. This way the qi are returned to normal".

Zao sou **燥嗽, dry cough** [3]
PC of → *ke sou* 咳嗽, cough, without phlegm. *WTMY* 9: 五嗽，一曰上氣嗽，二曰飲嗽，三曰**燥嗽**，四曰冷嗽，五曰邪嗽, "The five types of cough: the first is called 'cough with rising qi'. The second is called 'rheum cough'. The third is called ' **dry cough**'. The fourth is called 'cold cough'. The fifth is called 'evil [qi] cough'".

Zao tong **燥痛, dryness and pain** [4]
IS of an uncomfortable feeling of dryness and pain. *ZBYHL* 31: 惡核者，肉裏忽有核，累累如梅李，小如豆粒，皮肉**燥痛**, "In the case of 'malign kernels' there are all suddenly kernels in the flesh. They are strung together like plums. They are as small as beans. The skin and the flesh are marked by **dryness and pain**".

Zao xuan **燥癬, dry *xuan*-illness** [1]
PC identical with → *gan xuan* 乾癬, dry *xuan*-illness. *WTMY* 30: 療**燥癬**方，水銀和胡粉，研令調, 以塗之, "Recipe to cure **dry *xuan*-illness**. Grind *shui yin* and *hu fen* until they have mixed, and apply [to the affected region]".

Zao yang **燥癢, dryness and itching** [4]
IS of an uncomfortable feeling of dryness together with itching. *YXQY* Mj: 筋脈攣急，肌肉頑痹，皮膚**燥癢**, "The sinews and vessels are cramped. The muscles and flesh are numb. The skin is **dry and itches**".

Zao yu **燥鬱, dry and pent-up [qi]** [1]

EA of heat accumulation availing itself of the lung, with harm to the body liquids and qi rising contrary to its proper direction. *PJF* 139: 熱邪乘之，氣則**燥鬱**, "When heat evil avails itself of it, then the qi will be **dry and pent-up**".

Zei feng **賊風, robber wind** [40]

① EA a) of a qi that appears in a season it does not belong to. *SW* 1: 虛邪**賊風**，避之有時, "Depletion evil and robber wind, there are times to avoid them". b) Of a pathogenic wind coming from the South on the day of the winter solstice. *ZBYHL* 1: **賊風**者，謂冬至之日，有疾風從南方來，名曰虛風，此風至能傷害於人，故言**賊風**也, "**Robber wind**, that is to say: on the day of the winter solstice a swift wind comes from the South. It is called 'depletion wind'. This wind can severely harm a person. Hence it is called '**robber wind**'".

② PC caused by **robber wind**. *SJZL* 7: **賊風**：“論曰：邪之中人有四，從所不勝來者，謂之賊邪；與冬至之日，疾風南來，名曰賊風。其義一也。聖人於虛邪賊風，避之有時，以邪從所不勝來，故謂之虛邪。以其竊害中和之氣，故謂之**賊風**。其證痛而不熱”, "The discourse states: There are four types of evil that may harm a person. When it originates from what cannot be overcome, it is called 'robber evil'. When a swift wind arrives from the South on the day of the winter solstice, it is called 'robber wind'. The meaning is the same. The sages protected themselves against depletion evil and robber wind when it was their time. As the evil originates from what cannot be overcome it is called 'depletion evil'. As it steals and harms the qi of central harmony, it is called '**robber wind**'. Its pathological signs are pain without heat". *BCGM* refers to further pathological conditions brought about by robber wind, such as *da ren zei feng* 大人賊風robber wind of an adult, *zei feng wai pi* 賊風喎僻, [facial] wryness caused by robber wind, and *zei feng ma bi* 賊風麻痹, hemp[-like numbness] blockage caused by robber wind.

Zei xue **賊血, robber blood** [4]

PI identical with → *yue xue* 瘀血①, stagnant blood. *MYBL* SE *fei meng* 蜚虻：除**賊血**在胸腹五藏者, 及喉痹結塞, "It removes **robber blood** from the chest, abdomen and the five depots, as well as throat blockage with nodular blockages".

Zeng **黷, speckles** [p]

PC identical with → *gan zeng* 皯黷, dermal dark spots. *BCGM* SE *cu* 醋 quoting *ZHF*: 療面多皯**黷**如雀卵色, "To cure numerous facial dark **speckles** colored like sparrow eggs", writes: 面**黷**雀卵, "Facial **speckles** [resembling] sparrow eggs".

Zeng han **憎寒, to hate cold** [10]

IS identical with → *wu han* 惡寒, aversion to cold. *YBZHL* 42: 冬時嚴寒，人體虛而為寒所傷，即成病為傷寒也。輕者嗇嗇惡寒，噏噏發熱，微咳鼻塞，數日乃止。重者頭痛體疼，**憎寒**壯熱。久不歇，亦傷胎也, "In winter, at a time of severe cold, when the human body in a state of depletion is harmed by cold, the resulting disease is 'harm caused by cold'. In the case of a mild affection, [patients] feel miserable and have an aversion to cold, and shiver and effuse heat. They have a slight cough, and their nose is stuffed. This will end within a few days. In severe cases, they have head and body aches. They **hate cold** and have a strong fever. If this does not end over an extended period of time, it may harm [a pregnant woman's] fetus".

Zha **齇, sediments** [p]AW *zha* 皻, *zha* 皶, *zha* 査

PC identical with → *jiu zha* 酒齇, wine sediments. *BCGM* SE *zi wei* 紫葳 (*hua* 花) quotes *RHZ*: 酒齇热毒风刺风, "[It cures]sedimentsresulting from [a consumption of] wine, heat poison wind, and piercing wind".

Zha **皶, sediments** [p]

PC AD of → *jiu zha* 酒齇, wine sediments. *BCGM* Bai bing zhu zhi yao 百病主治藥：**皶**是血熱，即酒皶, "**Sediments** are [a sign of] blood heat; these are wine sediments".

Zha **皻, sediments** [p]

PC identical with → *jiu zha* 酒齇, wine sediments. *BCGM* SE *hu shi* 槲實：活血，利小便，除面上**皻**赤, "It quickens blood, frees urination, and removes the redness of **sediments** from one's face".

Zha **査, sediments** [p]

PC identical with → *jiu zha* 酒齇, wine sediments. *BCGM* Zang fu xu shi biao ben yong yao shi 脏腑虚实标本用药式 (*wei* 胃)：标病：发热蒸蒸，身前热，身前寒，发狂谵语，咽痹，上齿痛，口眼喎斜，鼻痛鼽衄赤**査**, "Its external diseases: effusion of heat with steaming. The body's front is [at times] hot; the body's front is [at times] cold. [Patients] are mad and their speech is incoherent. They have a throat blockage, and the upper teeth ache. Mouth and eyes are slanted. The nose aches, with runny nose, nosebleed and red **sediments**".

Zha liu **齇瘤, sediment tumor** [3]

PC identical with → *jiu zha* 酒齇, wine sediments. *BCGM* SE *lu feng fang* 露蜂房 quotes *ZHF*: 鼻外**齇瘤**，膿水血出, "A **sediment tumor** growing on the outside of the nose, emitting pus, water and blood".

Zha pao **齇皰, sediment blisters** [14]

PC identical with → *jiu zha* 酒齇, wine sediments. *TPSHF* 40: 治鼻面酒皻皰方。木蘭皮（半斤銼），醋（一斤三年者）。上件藥相和，浸二七日，取焙乾，搗細羅為散。每於食後，以温酒調下一錢, "Recipe to cure the nose and face with wine sediment blisters: *mu lan* skin (one half *jin*, filed), vinegar (one half *jin*, three years old). Mix the pharmaceutical substances listed above and allow to soak for two times seven days. Then roast until dry and pound through a fine sieve to obtain a powder. Ingest one *qian* mixed with warm wine after each meal". *BCGM* SE *mu lan* 木蘭 quotes *GJLY*: 面上**齇皰**：皯黷。用木蘭皮一斤，細切，以三年酢漿漬之百日，晒乾搗末, "[To cure] facial **sediments blisters**: [For] dermal dark spots: use 1 *jin* of *mu lan* skin, finely cut, and soak in three-year-old vinegar for 100 days. Then dry in the sun, and pound to a powder".

Zha pao **皶皰, sediment blisters** [1]

PC identical with → *jiu zha* 酒齇, wine sediments. *BCGM* SE *kou jin tuo* 口津唾：瘡腫、疥癬、**皶皰**，五更未語者，頻塗擦之, "For [treating] sores and swelling, *jie*-illness and *xuan*-illness, and **sediment blisters**, repeatedly apply it and wipe it off again at the fifth watch before [the patient] has begun to speak".

Zha pao **痄皰, sediments blisters** [1]
PC identical with → *jiu zha* 酒齇, wine sediments. *BCGM* SE *xing* 杏（*he ren* 核仁）：去頭面諸風氣**痄皰**, "It serves to remove all types of wind qi and **sediment blisters** from the head and face".

Zha sai **痄腮, mumps** [2] AN *ha ma wen* 蛤蟆瘟, frog warmth-illness.
PC of a communicable disease with painful swelling on both sides of the face below the jaws. *BCGM* SE *chi xiao dou* 赤小豆 quotes *ZSJYF*: 宋仁宗在東宮時，患**痄腮**, "When [Emperor] Renzong of the Song was in the Eastern Palace, he suffered from **mumps**".

Zha zhong **痄腫, mumps swelling** [1]
IS of a swelling of the ears and cheeks in the course of mumps. *BCGM* SE *wo niu* 蝸牛：耳腮**痄腫**及喉下諸腫，用蝸牛同麵研，傅之, "For **mumps swelling** of the ears and cheeks, and all swelling below the throat, grind snails together with flour and attach this [to the affected area]".

Zhai **瘵, consumption; disease** [6]
① PC AD of *lao zhai* 勞瘵, exhaustion consumption. *BCTJ* SE *sheng jiang* 生薑：近世方有主脾胃虛冷，不下食，積久羸弱成**瘵**者, "Among the recipes used in recent times there are those which master depletion cold of the spleen and stomach, with an inability to eat, which, if continuing for an extended period of time, leads to emaciation weakness and generates **consumption**".
② CD of any disease or ailment, with a meaning identical with → *bing* 病, disease, and → *ji* 疾, ailment. *QJYF* preface: 伏羲氏作，因之而畫八卦，立庖廚，滋味既興，痾**瘵**萌起, "When Fu Xi acted he continued the [work of Sui Ren] and drew the eight trigrams. He established cuisines and all the delicious food emerged. [This] gave rise to all types of **disease**".

Zhai chong **瘵蟲, consumption bugs/worms** [1]
EA identical with → *lao chong* 勞蟲, exhaustion bugs/worms. *BCGM* SE *chong bai la* 蟲白蠟：入丸散服，殺**瘵蟲**, "Ingest prepared as pills or powder. It kills **consumption bugs/worms**".

Zhai ji **瘵疾, consumption ailment** [5]
PC identical with → *lao zhai* 勞瘵, exhaustion consumption. *SYJYBZFL* 8: 世醫例以傳屍骨蒸為五勞者，非也。彼乃**瘵疾**，各一門類，不可不知, "Contemporary physicians list it together with → *chuan shi* 傳屍, corpse [evil] transmission, and → *gu cheng* 骨蒸, bone steaming, as one of the → *wu lao* 五勞, five types of exhaustion. This is wrong. These **consumption ailments** constitute a group by themselves. Everybody should be aware of this".

Zhai zhu **瘵疰, consumption attachment-illness** [2]
PC identical with → *lao zhai* 勞瘵, exhaustion consumption. *BCGM* Bai bing zhu zhi yao 百病主治藥：**瘵疰**，有蟲積，屍氣, "**Consumption attachment-illness** includes bug/worm accumulation and corpse qi".

Zhan kuang **譫狂, incoherent speaking and crazy behavior** [2]
IS identical with → *zhan yan* 譫妄, incoherent speaking and movement. *BCGM* SE *da huang* 大黃 quoting *TPSHF*: 熱病狂語, "Heat disease with crazy speaking", writes: 熱病**譫狂**, "Heat disease with **incoherent speaking and crazy behavior**".

Zhan li **戰慄, trembling and shivering** [3]
IS identical with → *zhen han* 振寒, shaking from cold. *SW* 71: 少陰所至為驚惑，惡寒，**戰慄**，譫妄, "Where the minor yin [qi] arrives, there is fright and uncertainty, aversion to cold, **trembling and shivering**, as well as incoherent and absurd speech".

Zhan yan **譫言, incoherent speech** [1]
IS identical with *zhan yu* 譫語. *SW* 31: 腹滿身熱，不欲食，**譫言**, "As a result, the abdomen is full, the body is hot, [the patient] does not wish to eat, and his **speech is incoherent**".

Zhan yan **譫妄, incoherent speaking and absurd movement; delirium** [3]
IS of mental confusion developing in the course of an illness episode, with the patient uttering meaningless statements and engaging in absurd movements. This is often triggered by high fever. *SW* 69: 病反**譫妄**狂越，咳喘息鳴, "Illnesses contrary [to what is normal are:] **incoherent speaking and absurd movement**, jumping in madness, coughing, and panting breath with sounds".

Zhan yü **譫語, incoherent speech** [12]
IS of mental confusion developing in the course of an illness episode, with the patient uttering meaningless statements lacking any coherence. This is often triggered by high fever. *SHL* 29: 胃氣不和**譫語**者，少與調胃承氣湯, "Persons whose stomach qi is unbalanced and who utter **incoherent speech**: give them a small dosage of the 'decoction to regulate the stomach and uphold qi'".

Zhang **瘴, miasma** [24]
①EA identical with → zhang qi 瘴氣①, miasmatic qi. *SJZL* 37: **瘴**者，山川厲毒之氣。"As for **miasma**, this is a violently poisonous qi at the site of mountains and rivers".
② PC identical with → *zhang qi*瘴氣②, miasmatic qi. *SJZL* 37: 又云江山霧氣多**瘴**，凡以其氣鬱蒸而然也。諸家治瘴之法不一, "Also, it is said that the haze of rivers and mountains is full of **miasma**. This is always because of pent-up [qi] steaming. The patterns employed by the experts to cure miasma vary".

Zhang **脹, distension** [719]
① IS of an uncomfortable feeling of being filled to bursting. *SW* 16: 邪氣著藏，令人**脹**, "The evil qi attaches itself to the depots. [This] makes a person [experience] **distension**".
② PC with an uncomfortable feeling of being filled to bursting or with a swelling resulting from abdominal water. *LS* 35: 夫**脹**者，皆在於藏府之外，排藏府而郭胸脅，脹皮膚，故命曰**脹**, "Now, those [qi] that cause **distensions** are situated outside of the depots and palaces. They attack the depots and palaces

and their bulwarks, the chest and ribs, causing the skin to distend. Hence one refers to **distension**".

Zhang **障, screen** [p]
PC AD of → *mu zhang* 目障, eye screen. *YHJW* Fj: 或腫而痛，羞澀多淚；或生**障**，昏暗失明，其症七十有二, "There may be swelling and pain, photophobia, roughness and plenty of tears, or a **screen** may grow that makes vision dim or causes a complete loss of the eyesight. There are 72 such disorders".

Zhang bi **脹閉, distension and closure** [1]
IS of abdominal distension and anuria. *BC* SE *xiao shi* 消石：主五藏積熱，胃**脹閉**，滌去蓄結飲食，推陳致新，除邪氣, "It controls heat accumulation in the five depots, stomach **distension and closure**, cleanses out concretions and nodes of liquid and solid food, pushes out the old and lets the new arrive, eliminates evil qi".

Zhang chuang **杖瘡, cudgel wound** [34]
PC of → *chuang* 瘡, sores, conditions inflicted on the skin or flesh by being struck with a cudgel, including fresh injuries that have not yet become infected, as well as open inflamed sores resulting from injuries some time ago. *QJYF* 25: 治**杖瘡**方：鍛石（七斤），新豬血（一升）。右二味，和丸，熟燒之破，更丸，燒三遍止，為末敷上, "Recipe to cure **cudgel wounds**: *duan shi* (7 *jin*), fresh hog blood (1 *sheng*). These two ingredients are to be formed to pills. Burn them until they break open. Form pills again. Burn three times and then stop. Prepare a powder and apply it to [the wound]".

Zhang ci **脹刺, distension with [a feeling of] being stabbed** [1]
IS identical with → *ci zhang* 刺脹, stabbing distension. *BCGM* SE *tu* 兔 quoting *TBC*: 余血搶心，脹欲死者, "When surplus blood rushes against the heart, this results in distension and one wishes to die", writes: 余血搶心，**脹刺**欲死者, "When surplus blood rushes against the heart, this results in **distension with [a feeling of] being stabbed** and one wishes to die".

Zhang du **瘴毒, miasmatic poison** [4]
EA identical with → *zhang qi* 瘴氣, miasmatic qi① . *QJYF* 12 RE *tai yi shen jing dan* 太乙神精丹：辟**瘴毒**, "Wards off **miasmatic poison**".

Zhang ji **脹急, distension and hectic [movement of qi]** [11]
IS of an uncomfortable feeling of distension with a hectic movement of qi. *ZHF* 4: 夜食便臥，不即消，心腹煩痛，**脹急**, "If at night one goes to sleep immediately after having dined, and if digestion fails to begin immediately, the heart and abdomen will experience irritation and pain, with **distension and hectic [movement of qi]**".

Zhang jian **脹堅, distension with hardness** [1]
IS identical with → *jian zhang* 堅脹, hardness with distension. *BCGM* SE *shi yan* 食鹽 quotes *MSF*: 心腹**脹堅**，痛悶欲死。鹽五合，水一升，煎服, "For **distension with hardness** affecting the heart and abdomen, with pain and heart-pressure so violent that one wishes to die, ingest 5 *ge* of table salt boiled in 1 *sheng* of water".

Zhang li **瘴瀝, miasmatic pervasion-illness** [1]
PC identical with → *zhang li* 瘴癘, miasmatic epidemic; possibly a copying error. *BCGM* SE *jie du zi* 解毒子 quoting a *TBC* quote from *ZLBC*: 主解蠱毒，止煩熱，辟瘴癘，利喉閉及痰毒, "It controls *gu* poison, stops vexing heat, eliminates miasmatic epidemics, and frees throat closure and phlegm poison", writes: 解蠱毒，止煩熱，辟**瘴瀝**，利喉閉及痰毒, "It dissolves *gu* poison, stops vexing heat, eliminates **miasmatic pervasion-illness**, and frees throat closure and phlegm poison".

Zhang li **瘴癘, miasmatic epidemic** [15] AW *zhang li* 瘴瀝, miasmatic pervasion-illness; AN *zhang yi* 瘴疫, miasmatic epidemic; *yi zhang* 疫瘴, epidemic miasma; *wen zhang* 瘟瘴, warmth-illness miasma; *wen zhang* 温瘴, warmth miasma.
PC brought forth by miasmatic qi with a high incidence of violent morbidity. *QJYF* 1: 忽逢**瘴癘**，素不資貯，無以救療，遂拱手待斃，以致夭歿, "If suddenly one is confronted with a **miasmatic epidemic**, and he has nothing in store, there is nothing that could bring help or a cure. All that remains is to expect early death submissively".

Zhang man **脹滿, distension and fullness; distended and full** [162]
① IS a) of an uncomfortable, violent feeling of fullness and heart-pressure. *SW* 45: 陰氣盛於上則下虛，下虛則腹**脹滿**, "When yin qi abounds above, then it is depleted below. When it is depleted below, then the abdomen is **distended and [gives a feeling of] fullness**". In the *BCGM* this type of an uncomfortable feeling of distension and fullness is associated with the regions of the chest, the ribs, the abdomen and limbs and trunk. b) Of a swollen or enlarged abdomen or other body part. *ZBYHL* 19: 積聚成病，蘊結在内，則氣行不宣通。氣搏於腑臟，故心腹**脹滿**。心腹**脹滿**則煩而悶，尤短氣也, "When accumulations and collections bring forth a disease, with internal concretions and nodes, then the passage of qi is blocked, and the qi strikes at the depots and palaces. Hence the heart and abdomen are **distended and full**. Once the heart and abdomen are **distended and full**, vexation and heart-pressure, as well as shortness of qi will follow".
② PC with all types of swelling, distension, and fullness. *QJYF* 8: 附子酒，治大風、冷痰癖、**脹滿**、諸痹方, "Wine with *fu zi*, a recipe to cure massive wind, cold phlegm aggregation-illness, **distension and fullness**, and all types of blockage". *BCGM* Bai bing zhu zhi yao 百病主治藥：**脹滿**，有濕熱，寒濕，氣積，食積，血積, "**Distension and fullness** may be associated with moisture and heat, cold and moisture, qi accumulation, food accumulation, blood accumulation".

Zhang men **脹悶, distension and heart-pressure** [18] AN *fan zhang* 煩脹, irritation and distension.
IS of a feeling of distension associated with vexation and heart-pressure. *TBC* SE *chong wei zi* 茺蔚子：又下子死腹中，主產後血**脹悶**, "It further brings a fetus down that has died in the abdomen, and it controls bleeding with **distension and heart-pressure** following delivery".

Zhang mo **障膜, obstructive membrane** [2]
PC identical with → *mu yi* 目翳, eye shade. *RHZ* SE *bai jiang* 敗醬：治赤眼**障膜**，努肉, "It cures red eyes and **obstructive membrane**, as well as tumorous flesh-growths".

Zhang nüe **瘴瘧, miasmatic malaria** [37] AN → *yue zhang* 瘧瘴, malaria miasma.
PC of the malaria variant of → *zhang qi* 瘴氣, miasmatic qi②. It is more violent than ordinary malaria, and comprises → *re zhang* 熱瘴, heat miasma; → *leng zhang* 冷瘴, cold miasma; → *ya zhang* 啞瘴, muteness miasma; and → *lao zhang* 勞瘴, exhaustion miasma. *WTMY* 1: 又療傷寒近效方，凡胸中惡、痰飲、傷寒、熱病、**瘴瘧**，須吐者方。鹽末（一大匙）。右一味，以生熟湯調下，須臾則吐，吐不快明旦更服，甚良, "Another effective recipe to cure harm caused by cold. A recipe forcing [a patient] to vomit for all cases where [the patient] feels bad in his chest, has phlegm-rheum, was harmed by cold, suffers from heat disease, and **miasmatic malaria**: Salt powder, one large spoon. This substance is to be ingested with fresh hot water. After a short while [the patient] will vomit. If he does not vomit immediately, have him ingest this again the next morning. Very good".

Zhang pi **脹痞, distension with an obstacle-illness** [2]
IS identical with → *zhang yong* 脹壅, distension with obstruction. *BCGM* SE *su sha ren* 縮砂仁：通滯氣，散寒飲**脹痞**, "It penetrates stagnant qi, and disperses cold rheum [causing] **distension with an obstacle-illness**".

Zhang pu shang sun **杖撲傷損, injury from blows with a cane** [1]
PC of → *da pu shang sun* 打撲傷損, injury from a blow, with a cane. *BCGM* SE *san qi* 三七：凡**杖撲傷損**，瘀血淋漓者，隨即嚼爛，罨之即止，青腫者即消散, "For all **injuries from blows with a cane**, with stagnant blood [that has left the vessels] pouring, immediately chew [*san qi*] to a pulp and use this to cover [the afflicted region]. This will end it. In case of greenish-blue swelling, [it is essential to apply] dispersing [medication]".

Zhang qi **瘴氣, miasmatic qi** [29] AD *zhang* 瘴, miasma.
① AN *lan zhang* 嵐瘴, hazy miasma; *shan zhang* 山瘴, mountain miasma; *zhang du* 瘴毒; miasmatic poison; *zhang wu* 瘴霧; miasmatic haze; *yan zhang* 烟瘴; smoky miasma; *zhang yu* 瘴雨, miasmatic rain. EA indicating a steam-like pathogenic qi of moisture and heat characteristic of the mountains and forests of Guangdong and Guangxi. *ZBYHL* 10: 其一日、二日，**瘴氣**在皮膚之間，故病者頭痛惡寒，腰背強重, "During the first or second day the **miasmatic qi** is in the skin. Hence patients suffer from headaches and have an aversion to cold. The lower back and spine are stiff and feel heavy".
② PC CD comprising all diseases supposed to have been brought forth by miasmatic qi. *QJYF* 12 RE *wan bing wan san* 萬病丸散, pills and powders for a myriad diseases: 治風熱**瘴氣**相染滅門, "They cure a merger of wind, heat, and **miasmatic qi** that eradicates entire households".

Zhang teng **脹疼, distension with pain** [1]

IS identical with → *zhang tong* 脹痛. *TPSHF* 27: 治風勞，脾腎虛冷，心腹**脹疼**，骨節煩痛，食少無力，宜服桃仁散方, "To cure wind exhaustion, depletion cold of the spleen and kidneys, **distension with pain** in the heart and abdomen, vexation and pain in the bones and joints, the recipe to ingest the powder with *tao ren* is advisable".

Zhang tong **脹痛, distension with pain** [52] AN *tong zhang* 痛脹, painful distension, *zhang teng* 脹疼, distension with pain.

IS of a painful feeling of → *zhang* 脹, distension. *JGYL* Fj: 九痛丸…兼治卒中惡，腹**脹痛**，口不能言, " 'Pills for the nine types of pain': …also cure sudden strokes by the malign, abdominal **distension with pain**, and inability to speak".

Zhang wu **瘴霧, miasmatic haze** [1]

EA identical with → *zhang qi* 瘴氣, miasmatic qi ①. *YXL* SE *hong dou kou* 紅豆蔻：能治冷氣腹痛，消**瘴霧**氣毒, "It is able to cure cold qi [causing] abdominal pain, and dissolves the poison of **miasmatic haze** qi".

Zhang yi **瘴疫, miasmatic epidemic** [9]

PC identical with → *zhang li* 瘴癘, miasmatic epidemic. *WTMY* 4 RE *chi tang* 豉湯, decoction with salty, fermented beans: 平旦服之，令人不著**瘴疫**, "If consumed in the early morning it keeps a person free from an affection with **miasmatic epidemic**".

Zhang yi **障翳, obstructive shade** [46]

① PC a) CD of → *mu yi* 目翳, eye shade, and → *mu zhang* 目障, eye screen. *ZBYHL* 48: 熱氣蘊積，變生**障翳**, "Massive accumulation of heat qi develops into an **obstructive shade**". b) AN *yi zhang* 翳障, shade screen. Identical with → *mu yi* 目翳, eye shade. *RHZ* SE *shi jue ming* 石決明：明目，殼磨**障翳**, "To clear the eyes, use the hard shell to rub an **obstructive shade**.

② PI of objects impairing vision. *TPSHF* 33: 瞳人中潛生**障翳**，作青白色, "Hidden from outside view an **obstructive shade** develops in the pupil, assuming a greenish white color".

Zhang yong **脹壅, distension with obstruction** [1] AN *zhang pi* 脹痞, distension with an obstacle-illness.

IS identical with → *yong zhang* 壅脹①. *JYBC* SE *e shi* 惡實：根細切如豆，麵拌作飯食之，消**脹壅**, "Cut the root into small pieces the size of beans. Eating a dish prepared of it with flour will eliminate **distension with obstruction**".

Zhang yu **瘴雨, miasmatic rain** [1]

EA identical with → *zhang qi* 瘴氣, miasmatic qi ①. *BCGM* SE *hu* 葫, LSZ: 攜之旅途，則炎風**瘴雨**不能加, "If one takes it along when travelling, one cannot be affected by fiery wind and **miasmatic rain**".

Zhang zhong **脹重, distension and heaviness**[1]

IS of an uncomfortable feeling of an extreme distension. *BCGM* SE *qian niu zi* 牽牛子 LSZ: 治水氣在肺，喘滿腫脹，下焦鬱遏，腰背**脹重**, "It cures the presence of water qi in the lung, panting and a feeling of fullness, swelling and distension. Pent-up and restrained [qi] in the lower burner. The lumbar region and the back feel **distension and heaviness**".

Zhao gu ding **著骨疔, bone-attached pin-illness** [1]

PC of → *ding chuang* 丁瘡, pin sores, which if locally opened by means of a needle will not bleed and also do not let a person feel pain. *PJF* 313: 如針破無血，系是**著骨疔**, "If broken open with a needle it will not bleed. It belongs to the **bone-attached pin-illnesses**".

Zhao shi mu tu **朝食暮吐, eating at dawn, vomiting at dusk** [2]

IS of a vomiting of undigested food in the evening that was consumed in the early morning. *JGYL* Mj: 脾傷則不磨，**朝食暮吐**，暮食朝吐，宿穀不化，名曰胃反, "When the spleen is harmed it cannot rub [the stomach]. **Eating at dawn will result in vomiting at dusk**. Eating at dusk will result in vomiting at dawn. Grains stay without being digested. This is called 'stomach turnover'".

Zhe shang **折傷, fracture** [85] AW *shang zhe* 傷折.

PC of a → *shang sun* 傷損, injury, resulting from an improper bending of an extremity either because of an accident or because of pressure exerted, mostly affecting the bones. *TBC* SE *liang zi mu* 椋子木：主**折傷**，破惡血，養好血，安胎止痛生肉, "It controls **fractures**, breaks through malign blood, nourishes good blood, calms the fetus, ends pain, and generates flesh".

Zhen **疹, disease; papule** [180]

① Identical with *bing* 病, disease. *ZBYHL* 3: 去一切諸勞疾**疹**, "Removes all types of **diseases** associated with exhaustion ailment".

② PC of skin diseases characterised by skin elevations sometimes resembling strings of cash, sometimes hemp seeds or beans. *WTMY* 30: 初發**疹**起，大者如連錢，小者如麻豆, "When it begins, **papules** rise, large ones resembling strings of cash, small ones resembling hemp or beans". *BCGM* refers to various disease names associated with the emergence of papules, such as → *feng zhen* 風疹， wind papules, → *ban zhen* 瘢疹, maculopapular eruption, and → *dan zhen* 丹疹, bolus papules.

Zhen chuang **針瘡, needle wound** [2]

PC of → *chuang* 瘡, sores, conditions resulting from local injuries inflicted by means of needle piercing. *QJYF* 22：魚臍疔瘡，似新火**針瘡**，四邊赤，中央黑， 可針刺之, "Fish belly pin-illness sores appear as fresh fire-**needle wounds**. They are red on all four sides, with a black center. They can be pierced with a needle".

Zhen dou **疹痘, papules and smallpox** [1]

PC identical with → *dou zhen* 痘疹, smallpox with papules. *BCGM* SE *zi cao* 紫草 quotes *JYHF*: 嬰童**疹痘**：三四日，隱隱將出未出，色赤便閉者, "For children with **papules and smallpox**: when on the third and fourth day [papules and smallpox] are still dormant, when they are about to appear, but have not appeared, and when their complexion is red and they suffer from constipation".

Zhen feng **疹風, papules wind** [1]

PC identical with → *feng zhen* 風疹, wind papules. *LGPZL* Xu 序：遍體疹風，冷調生側，附子傍生者曰側子，作末，冷酒服，立差也, "If the entire body is affected by **papules wind**, process lateral [*fu zi* 附子] with cold [wine]. {Those growing to the side of *fu zi* are called *ci zi*, (lit.: lateral [*fu*] *zi*)} Prepare a powder, and ingest with cold wine. Immediately effective".

Zhen han **振寒, to shake from cold** [4] AN *zhan li* 戰慄, shivering; *han chan* 寒顫, trembling from cold.

IS of the body having a fear of cold and shaking involuntarily. *SW* 33: 唾出若涕，惡風而**振寒**, "That which is spit out resembles snivel [from the nose. The patient] has an aversion to wind and **shakes from cold**".

Zhen jing **鎮驚, to press down fright** [8]

TA of using physically heavy pharmaceutical substances, such as metals or minerals, to cure fright wind and fright palpitation. *SJZL* 14: 治心受風邪，**鎮驚**，利頭目，化痰壅，鉛金丸方, "To cure a heart that has received wind evil, **to press down fright**, to disinhibit the head and eyes, to transform phlegm obstruction, [use] the recipe for pills with *qian* (*shuang* 霜) and *jin* (*bo* 箔)".

Zheng **癥, concretion-illness** [p]

PC of abdominal nodes/lumps that are hard and cannot be moved. *ZBYHL* 19: **癥**者，由寒温失節，致腑臟之氣虛弱，而食飲不消，聚結在內，漸染生長。塊段盤牢不移動者，是**癥**也, "**Concretion-illness**: when cold and warmth lose their appropriate measure, and meet depots and palaces in a status of qi depletion and weakness, so that food and beverages are not digested, they collect as nodes internally and gradually grow larger. When these are tightly intertwined bits and pieces that do not move, then this is '**concretion-illness**'".

Zheng chong **怔忡, panic uneasiness** [7]

① IS of extreme → *xin ji* 心悸①, heart palpitation. *TPSHF* 22：風熱上攻，頭旋運悶，喜臥**怔忡**，起即欲倒, "When wind heat rises to attack [above], the head will spin with heart-pressure. [Patients] wish to sleep and experience **panic uneasiness**. When they rise they may fall to the ground".

② PC with panic uneasiness. *BYXF* 1：治**怔忡**不寧，精神昏倦，睡臥不安, "To cure **panic uneasiness** with restlessness, mental disturbance and failure to sleep calmly". LSZ distinguishes among three types of panic uneasiness, those associated with *xue xu* 血虛, blood depletion, those associated with the presence of fire, *you huo* 有火, and those associated with the presence of phlegm, *you tan* 有痰.

Zheng ji **癥積, concretion-illness accumulation** [11]

PC identical with → *zheng* 癥, concretion-illness. *MYBL* SE *shi dan* 石膽：散**癥積**，咳逆上氣，及鼠瘺惡瘡, "It disperses **concretion-illness accumulations**, cough with counterflow and rising qi, as well as mouse fistulae and malign sores".

***Zheng jia* 癥瘕, concretion-illness and conglomeration-illness** [124]
PC CD of → *zheng* 癥, concretion-illness, and → *jia* 瘕, conglomeration-illness. The two terms are often used interchangeably and do not signify two distinctly different conditions. *ZBYHL* 19: **癥瘕**者，皆由寒温不調，飲食不化，與臟氣相搏結所生也, "All cases of **concretion-illness and conglomeration-illness** result from a disharmony of cold and warmth. Beverages and food are not transformed. When they clash with the qi of the depots nodes are formed". *BCGM* Bai bing zhu zhi yao 百病主治藥：癥繫於氣與食，瘕繫於血與蟲, "Concretion-illnesses are associated with qi and food; conglomeration-illnesses are associated with blood and bugs/worms".

***Zheng jian* 癥堅, concretion-illness hardness** [11]
PC identical with → *zheng* 癥, concretion-illness. *BJ* SE *mu dan* 牡丹：除**癥堅**，瘀血留舍腸胃, "It eliminates **concretion-illness hardness**, stagnant blood [that has left the vessels and] abides in the intestines and stomach".

***Zheng jie* 癥結, concretion-illness node** [45]
PC identical with → *zheng* 癥, concretion-illness. *MYBL* SE *hu zhang gen* 虎杖根：主通利月水，破留血**癥結**, "It controls free flow of menstruation, and crushes residual blood [forming] **concretion-illness nodes**".

***Zheng kuai* 癥塊, concretion-illness lump** [24]
PC identical with → *zheng* 癥, concretion-illness. *WTMY* 7: 療心痛**癥塊**硬築，心氣欲絕，當歸湯方, "To cure heartache, **concretion-illness lumps**, and hard structures, when the [movement of] heart qi is about to be cut, [use] the recipe for the decoction with *dang gui*".

***Zheng pi* 癥癖, concretion-illness and aggregation-illness** [19]
PC CD of → *zheng* 癥, concretion-illness, and → *pi* 癖, aggregation-illness. *TBC* SE *mu tian liao* 木天蓼：去風冷**癥癖**，大效, "It removes wind cold, **concretion-illness and aggregation-illness**".

***Zheng shui* 正水, proper water** [4]
PC of → *shui zhong* 水腫, water swelling, disease brought forth by kidney failure due to depletion, and an absence of passage of water. *JGYL* Mj: **正水**其脈沉遲，外證自喘, "In the case of **proper water**: the [movement of the] vessels is deep inside and retarded. External sign: spontaneous panting"

***Zheng tou feng* 正頭風, proper head wind** [1]
PC of → *tou feng* 頭風, head wind, characterized by pain in the front and top of the head. *GJYJ* 16: 偏頭風，川芎湯下。**正頭風**，羌活湯。雷頭風，薄荷湯下, "For hemilateral head wind, ingest it with the decoction with *chuan xiong*. For **proper head wind**, [ingest it with] the decoction with *qiang huo*. For thundering head wind [ingest it with] the decoction with *bo he*".

***Zheng yang ming tou tong* 正陽明頭痛, proper yang brilliance headache** [1]
PC identical with → *yang ming tou tong* 陽明頭痛, yang brilliance headache. *SWBJQYBMJ* Lj: 白芷，治**正陽明頭痛**, "*Bai zhi* cures **proper yang brilliance headache**".

Zheng zhu **癥疰, concretion-illness with attachment-illness** [1]
PC with painful skin as a major sign. *QJYF* 17: 治人皮膚中痛，名**癥疰**方，醋和燕窠土敷之, "Recipe to cure pain in the skin, called '**concretion-illness with attachment-illness**'. Smear [a paste] on it prepared by mixing vinegar and soil obtained from a swallow's nest".

Zhi **痔, piles** [p] AN *zhi bing* 痔病, piles disease; *zhi ji* 痔疾, piles ailment
PC a) identical with → *zhi chuang* 痔瘡, piles sores. *SW* 3: 因而飽食，筋脈横解，腸澼為**痔**, "Subsequent overeating [causes] sinews and vessels to relax. The intestines are flushed, and this leads to **piles**". b) CD of small tumorous flesh-growths in any one of the body orifices. *YXGM* 27: 人於九竅中凡有小肉突出，皆曰**痔**，不特於肛門邊生, "All small flesh-growths in one of the nine orifices are called '**piles**.' Not only those that grow at the side of the anus".

Zhi **痣, mole** [p]
PC of clearly visible colored spots on the skin. They may be even with the skin, or they may rise above the surrounding skin. In general they are considered physiological phenomena. If they become painful, itch, or grow larger, they are considered a PC requiring a treatment. *BCJJZ* SE *mei shi* 梅實：今人多用白梅和藥，以點**痣**, "Today people often use white [pulp of] plums in medications to be swabbed on a **mole**".

Zhi bing **痔病, piles disease** [10]
PC identical with → *zhi* 痔, piles. *ZBYHL* 34: 去心勞、**痔病**, "This will remove heart exhaustion and **piles disease**".

Zhi chong **痔蟲, piles bug** [9]
EA of bugs believed, in former times, to cause → *zhi chuang* 痔瘡, piles sores. *BJ* SE *shi hui* 石灰：殺**痔蟲**，去黑子息肉, "It kills **piles bugs/worms** and removes black dots and tumorous flesh-growths".

Zhi chu **汁出, discharge of liquid** [27]
IS identical with *chu zhi* 出汁. *ZHF* 5: 陰癢**汁出**，嚼生大豆黄，塗之, "In case of itching in the yin (i.e. one's private) parts, with **discharge of liquid**, chew the yellow contents of fresh soy beans, and smear [onto the affected parts]".

Zhi chuang **痔瘡, piles sores** [54]
PC CD of numerous types of anal ailments characterized by protruding swelling, pain and itching, as well as bleeding. *QJYF* 12 RE *lao po wan bing wan* 耆婆萬病丸, "granny's pills for a myriad of diseases": **痔瘡**，塗綿箸上，納孔中，日別易，差止, "For **piles sores** smear on a stick made of silk floss and insert into the [anal] opening. Do not change for a day. Stop when it is cured".

Zhi gou **猘狗, rabid dog** [3]
Identical with → *zhi quan* 猘犬. *BJ* SE *bai tu huo* 白兔藿：主蛇虺、蜂蠆、**猘狗**、菜肉蠱毒，鬼疰, "It controls the poison of snakes, bees, scorpions, **rabid dogs**, vegetables, meat and *gu*, as well as demon attachment-illness".

Zhi he **痔核, piles kernels** [5]
① PC of → *zhi chuang* 痔瘡, piles sores, with a protruding swelling at the anus that may itch and be painful. *BCGM* SE *bie jia* 鱉甲 quoting *BJ*: 陰蝕痔惡肉,

"Erosion in the yin (i.e. genital) region, piles, and malign flesh [growth]", writes: 陰蝕**痔核**惡肉, "Erosion in the yin (i.e. genital) region, **piles kernels**, and malign flesh [growth]".

② PI of protruding piles tissue. *YXZC*5: 秦艽蒼术湯，治**痔核**已破，謂之痔漏, "Decoction with *qin jiao* and *cang zhu* cures **piles kernels** that have broken open. This is called 'piles leakage'".

Zhi ji 痔疾, **piles ailment** [21]

PC identical with → *zhi* 痔, piles. *QJYF* 22: 地黃煎，補虛除熱，散乳石毒，癰癤**痔疾**，悉宜服之方, "*Di huang* decoction supplements depletion and removes heat. It serves to dissipate *ru shi* poison. It should be ingested for all types of obstruction-illnesses with pimples, and **piles ailments**".

Zhi jiang 肢強, **stiff limbs** [2]

IS of stiff limbs with difficulties to move. *TPSHF* 19: 治中風不能語，四**肢強**，宜服天麻散方, "To cure wind stroke with an inability to speak, and when the four **limbs are stiff**, the recipe to ingest the powder with *tian ma* is advisable".

Zhi jing 止驚, **to stop fright** [10] AN *ding jing* 定驚, to stabilize fright; *chu jing* 除驚, to eliminate fright; *pi jing* 辟驚, to break up fright; *jie jing* 截驚, to cut fright.

TA including various means to cure fright wind and fright palpitation. *QJYF* 5: 牛黃，益肝膽除熱，定精神**止驚**, "*Niu huang* adds [qi] to the liver and gallbladder and eliminates heat. It stabilizes the essence spirit and **stops fright**".

Zhi lou 痔漏, **piles with leakage** [71] AW 痔瘺, piles fistula. Mentioned in *QJYF* 22: 青龍五生膏，治癰疽**痔漏**，惡瘡膿血出, "The 'virid dragon paste with five unprocessed ingredients' cures obstruction- and impediment-illnesses, **piles with leakage**, malign sores that fester and release blood".

PC a) of → *zhi chuang* 痔瘡, piles sores, of a rather long duration with repeated, periodical bleeding. *YCZC* 5: 治痔核已破，謂之**痔漏**，大便秘澀，必作大痛, "It serves to cure piles kernels that have already broken open. One calls this '**piles with leakage**'. Defecation is blocked and rough and inevitably causes massive pain". b) Identical with → 痔瘺 a) piles fistula. *QXLF* 51: 初生肛邊，成瘟不破者曰**痔**；破潰而出膿血，黃水浸淫，淋瀝久不止者曰**漏**也, "When they first develop to the side of the anus and form a clustered[-seeds]-illness, but have not broken open yet, they are called '**piles**'. When they have broken open they fester and release pus and blood, and when they are soaked with yellow liquid, which drips for an extended period of time without ending, then it is called '**leakage**'". Also, *BCGM* Bai bing zhu zhi yao 百病主治藥：**痔漏**：初起為痔，久則成漏, "**Piles with leakage**: In the beginning these are piles. After an extended period of time leakage develops".

Zhi lou 痔瘺, **piles fistula; piles and fistula** [72] AN *lou zhi* 瘺痔. Mentioned in *BJ* Xu li 序例：夫大病之主，有…癰腫、惡瘡，**痔瘺**、癭瘤, "Now, the most important massive diseases include … obstruction-illness with swelling, malign sores, **piles fistula**, and goiters with tumors of the neck".

PC a) in the vicinity of the anus with the muscles and flesh being pierced with holes, the sores failing to close and at times releasing pus and blood. *SJZL* 143

: 毒氣浸漬，肌肉穿穴，瘡口不合，時有膿血，故成**痔瘺**, “When soaked with poison qi the muscles and flesh are pierced with holes, the openings of the sores fail to close and at times there is pus and blood. Hence this develops into **piles fistula**”. b) Identical with → *zhi lou* 痔漏 a) piles with leakage. *RHZ* SE *bai lian* 白斂：止驚邪，發背，瘰癧，腸風**痔瘺**, “It ends fright evil, effusion of the back, scrofula with pervasion-illness, intestinal wind and **piles fistula**”. c) CD of → *zhi* 痔, piles, and → *lou* 瘺, fistula. *ZBYHL* 18: 甚者則能成**痔瘺**疥癬，癲癧疽瘍諸瘡, “In severe cases this may generate sores such as **piles, fistula**, *jie*-illness, *xuan*-illness, repudiation-illness, obstruction-illness, impediment-illness, and lair-illness”.

Zhi man **支滿, propping fullness** [11]
IS of an uncomfortable feeling of fullness associated with one of obstruction. *SW* 36: 胃瘧者，令人且病也，善飢而不能食，食而**支滿**腹大, “Stomach malaria: it causes a person to have a *qie*-disease. [Patients] tend to be hungry but cannot eat. When they eat, **propping fullness** results, and the abdomen is enlarged”.

Zhi qi **滯氣, sluggish qi** [52] AN *yong qi* 壅氣, obstruction qi.
① EA of qi that cannot move freely in the body and may cause disease. *QJYF* 12: 五臟**滯氣**，積聚不消，壅閉不通，心腹脹滿. “When the five depots have **sluggish qi**, which accumulates and collects and fails to be dissolved, with blockage and failure of passage, then heart and abdomen will be affected by distension and a feeling of fullness”.
② A side effect of pharmaceutical substances blocking the qi dynamics in the body. *BCYY* SE *li* 栗：小兒不可多食，生者難化，熟即**滯氣**, “Children must not eat too much. [If consumed] raw it is difficult to digest. [If consumed] prepared it causes **sluggish qi**”.

Zhi quan **猘犬, rabid dog** [31]
Identical with → *kuang quan* 狂犬. *ZHF* 7 lists recipes 療**猘犬**咬人方, “To cure people bitten by a **rabid dog**”.

Zhi re **痔熱, piles that are hot** [1]
IS of a feeling of hot → *zhi chuang* 痔瘡, piles sores. *FRDYLF* 8: *kuo yu* 蛞蝓：療**痔熱**腫痛, “It heals **piles that are hot,** swollen, and painful”.

Zhi shi **直視, straight vision** [2]
IS of eyeballs looking straight ahead without being able to freely move around. *QJYF* 3: 大豆紫湯，治產後百病及中風痱痓，或背強口噤，或但煩熱，苦渴，或頭身皆重，或身癢，劇者嘔逆**直視**, “ ’Purple decoction with *da dou*’ cures all types of diseases following delivery, as well as wind stroke and seething heat with spasms; also: stiff back and clenched jaw; also: singular vexing heat with pathological thirst; also: a feeling of heavy pressure in the head and body; also: body itch. In severe cases: vomiting with [qi] moving against its proper direction and **straight vision**”.

***Zhi shi* 痔蝕, piles erosion** [1]
PC of festering → *zhi chuang* 痔瘡, piles sores. *MYBL* SE *qing xiang zi* 青葙子：惡瘡疥虱，**痔蝕**，下部䘌瘡, "Malign sores, *jie*-illness, lice, **piles erosion**, and hidden worms infestation sores in the lower parts".

***Zhi tong* 掣痛, convulsion pain** [10]
IS of pain accompanied by a twitching sensation. *ZHF* 3：身中有**掣痛**，不仁不隨處, "In the body there are locations with **convulsion pain**, numbness, and an inability to follow one's will".

***Zhi tong* 痔痛, painful piles** [4]
PC of pain associated with → *zhi chuang* 痔瘡, piles sores. *SJZL* 141: 治五種**痔痛**，六神丸方, "Recipe for the 'pills with the six wondrous ingredients' to cure the five types of **painful piles**".

***Zhi tong* 支痛, propping [fullness] with pain** [1]
IS of pain in the flanks accompanied by a feeling of propping distension. *SW* 65: 心病先心痛，一日而咳，三日脅**支痛**, "In the case of heart disease, first [the patient experiences] heartache. [After] one day he coughs. [Within the next] three days the flanks [experience] **propping [fullness] with pain**".

***Zhi xue* 滯血, sluggish blood** [15]
EA identical with → *yue xue* 瘀血②，stagnant blood. *SLBC* SE *li yu* 鯉魚：魚鱗，燒烟絕，研，酒下方寸，破產婦**滯血**, "The scales: burn them until the smoke stops. Grind. Ingest one square inch [size spoon] with wine. This breaks through **sluggish blood** in women giving birth".

***Zhi xue* 痔血, piles' bleeding** [5]
PC of bleeding → *zhi chuang* 痔瘡, piles sores. *QJYF* 12: 治吐血、蠱毒、**痔血**，女子腰腹痛，大便後出清血者方, "Recipe to cure blood spitting, *gu* poison, **piles' bleeding**, women's pain in the lower back and abdomen, as well as release of clear blood following defecation".

***Zhi yin* 支飲, propping rheum** [13]
PC of → *yin* 飲②, rheum, disease brought forth by rheum flowing into the lung with panting, cough, alternating sensations of cold and heat, vomiting of foam, and a feeling of cold in the back. *JGYL* Mj: 咳逆倚息，氣短不得臥，其形如腫，謂之**支飲**, "When [patients] cough with [qi] counterflow, and when they need to support themselves to be able to breathe, with shortness of qi and an inability to sleep, and when they have a physical appearance as if swollen, then this is called '**propping rheum**'".

***Zhi zhong* 痔腫, piles' swelling** [3]
PC of swelling associated with → *zhi chuang* 痔瘡, piles sores. *RHZ* SE *zhi qiao* 枳殼：皮膚癢、**痔腫**可炙熨, "It can be applied as hot compresses to cure itching skin and **piles' swelling**".

***Zhong* 腫, swelling; swollen** [ca. 390]
IS of swollen skin or muscles/flesh. *SW* 18: 足脛**腫**曰水, "When the feet and the shins are **swollen**, that is called: 'water'". In the *BCGM*, such swelling may be topical, e.g. *mu zhong* 目腫, swollen eye(s); *she zhong* 舌腫, swollen tongue;

yin zhong 陰腫, swollen private parts, or encompassing the entire body, e.g. *shen zhong* 身腫, swollen body; *ti zhong* 體腫, swollen body; *shen mian ju zhong* 身面俱腫, swollen body and face.

Zhong bi **腫痹, swelling with blockage** [4]

① IS of a blockage of narrow sections of narrow structures such as the throat because of a swelling. *BCGM* SE *zhu sha gen* 硃砂根：咽喉**腫痹**，磨水或醋嚥之，甚良, "For **swelling with blockage** affecting the throat swallow [this substance] ground in water or vinegar. Very good".

② PC of a *bi* 痹① a), blockage disease, with obvious swelling. *ZHF* 8：莽草膏，療諸賊風**腫痹**, "Ointment with *mang cao* cures all types of robber wind and **swelling with blockage**".

Zhong bing **腫病, swelling disease** [4]

PC identical with → *zhong* 腫, swelling. *QJYF* 21: 凡**腫病**須百方內外攻之，不可一概, "For all types of **swelling disease** one must make use of all possible recipes, to be applied for internal and external attack. One cannot employ just one single approach".

Zhong chi **腫赤, swollen and red** [6]

IS identical with → *chi zhong* 赤腫, red and swollen. *ZBYHL* 9: 毒氣從腑臟而出，循於經絡，攻於手足，故手足指皆**腫赤**焮痛也, "Poison qi leaves the palaces and depots. It follows the conduits and network [vessels] and attacks the hands and feet. Hence all fingers and toes are **swollen and red**, and experience a scorching pain".

Zhong da **腫大, swollen and enlarged** [5]

IS identical with → *zhong* 腫, swelling. *JGYL* Mj: 面目**腫大**有熱，名曰風水, "When the face and eyes are **swollen and enlarged**, and hot, this is called 'wind and water'".

Zhong du **腫毒, swelling with poison** [206] AN *du zhong* 毒腫, poison swelling.

PC CD of all types of local swelling that may or may not be purulent, with or without a head, festering or not. *QJYF* 22: 治一切**腫毒**，疼痛不可忍者方, "Recipe to cure all types of **swelling with poison** and unbearable pain".

Zhong du **中毒, poisoning** [54]

PC brought forth by poisonous matter that has entered the body. *JGYL* Lj: 治食生肉**中毒**方, "Recipe to cure **poisoning** after having consumed raw meat".

Zhong e **中惡, struck by the malign** [149] AN *zhong wu* 中忤, struck by the hostile; *cu e* 卒惡, sudden [stroke by the] malign.

PC CD of diseases brought forth by an affection with evil qi or a partial exhaustion of yin or yang qi with sudden loss of consciousness or sudden twisting pain in the heart and abdomen. *MYBL* SE *sheng ma* 升麻: it controls **中惡**腹痛，時氣毒癘，頭痛寒熱, "If one was **struck by the malign**, with abdominal pain, poison epidemics brought forth by seasonal qi, headache with cold and heat spells". Related to → *ke wu* 客忤, a visitor's hostility.

Zhong feng **中風, wind stroke, struck by wind** [277]

① PM of being struck by wind evil. *SW* 42: 飲酒**中風**，則為漏風, "If someone drinks wine and is **struck by wind**, this will cause leakage wind".

② PC a) AN *cu zhong feng* 卒中風, suddenly being struck by wind; *cu zhong* 卒中，sudden stroke; *cu feng* 卒風, sudden wind [stroke]. Sudden loss of consciousness, sometimes accompanied by wry mouth and eyes, unilateral paralysis, and impeded speech. *JGYL* Fj: **中風**歷節病脈證並治, "The disease **struck by wind**, running through the joints: its [associated movements in the] vessels, conditions, and therapy". b) Of external affection brought about by wind evil. *SHL*, 發熱，汗出惡風，脈緩者，名為**中風**, "In the case of an effusion of heat, sweating, an aversion to wind, and a slow [movement in the] vessels, [the condition] is called '**wind stroke**'".

Zhong fu **中腑, palace struck [by wind]** [2]

PC of a mental confusion with an inability to recognize people, brought about by wind stroke. *JGYL*: calls this condition *xie ru yu fu* 邪入於府, "evil has entered the palaces". *SWBJQYBMJ* 2: **中腑**者，面加五色，有表證, "In the case of a **palace struck [by wind**, [one of the respective] five complexions shows in the [patient's] face, as external indicator".

Zhong gu **中蠱, *gu* stroke** [18]

PC identical with → *gu du* 蠱毒②, *gu* poison[ing]. *ZHF* 7: **中蠱**令人心腹切痛，如有物齧，或吐下血, "***Gu* stroke** causes a person to have a cutting pain in the heart and abdomen, as if he were being gnawed by some being. In some cases patients vomit or discharge blood".

Zhong gui **中鬼, demon stroke** [2]

PC of sudden loss of consciousness with blood leaving from mouth and nose. *PJF* 238: 至寶丹，治**中鬼**惡疰，解一切毒, "The "Most Precious Elixir' cures **demon stroke** and attachment-illness by the malign, and dissolves all types of poison".

Zhong han **腫寒, swollen and cold** [1]

IS identical with *han zhong* 寒腫, cold swelling. *BCGM* Zang fu xu shi biao ben yao shi 臟腑虛實標本用藥式：（肾）本病：諸寒厥逆，骨痿腰痛，腰冷如冰，足胻**腫寒**, "The diseases [of the kidneys] themselves: All types of cold with recession and [qi] counterflow, bone dysfunction and lower back pain, the lower back is ice cold, the feet and shins are **swollen and cold**".

Zhong han **中寒, struck by cold; cold stroke; cold center** [14]

PC a) of dizziness and wry mouth brought forth by a strong cold stroke. *SYJYBZFL* 2: 乾薑附子湯，治**中寒**，卒然暈倒…口噤，四肢厥冷, "Decoction with *gan jiang* and *fu zi* cures **cold stroke** with sudden unconsciousness and fall to the ground, ...clenched jaw, and recession cold in the four limbs". b) Identical with → *han zhong* 寒中, cold center. *JGYL* Fj: **中寒**，其人下利，以裏虛也, 欲嚏不能，此人肚中寒, "Patients with a **cold center** experience free-flux illness because of internal depletion. They feel an urge to sneeze but are unable to do so. This is cold in a person's abdomen".

Zhong he **腫核, swelling with kernels** [5] AN *he zhong* 核腫, kernel swelling.
PC of → *jie he* 結核, nodular kernel, developing in the skin with local swelling. *ZBYHL* 31: **腫核**候：凡腫，挾風冷則不消，而結成核也, "The signs of **swelling with kernels**: If it includes wind cold, no type of swelling will dissolve, but eventually develop into a kernel instead".

Zhong ji **腫疾, swelling ailment** [9] AN *zhong bing* 腫病, swelling disease; *zhong qi* 腫氣, qi swelling.
PC of ailments with → *zhong* 腫, swelling, as its main sign. *SJZL* 4: 一切**腫疾**，悉宜鐮割足小指下橫文間。腫在左則割左，在右則割右，血少出則瘥, "In all cases of **swelling ailment**, use a sickle to cut in the horizontal line underneath the small toe. If the swelling is on the left side, cut the left [toe]. If it is on the right side, cut the right [toe]. The cure is achieved when a small amount of blood appears".

Zhong jiang **腫強, swelling and stiffness** [4]
IS of topical swelling accompanied by difficulties moving. *ZBYHL* 30: 舌腫脈脹急，則舌**腫強**, "When the tongue is swollen und the vessels are distended and tight, then this is tongue **swelling and stiffness**".

Zhong jiao re **中焦熱, heat in the central burner** [1]
PC of heat-type diseases affecting the central burner. *QJYF* 20 RE *lan qing wan* 藍青丸, pills with indigo blue: 治**中焦熱**，下痢水穀, "They cure **heat in the central burner**, and discharge of liquid and solid food with free-flux illness".

Zhong jing **中經, to strike a conduit** [1]
PC of an inability to move the hands and feet at will, while at the same time one is mentally fully alert. *JGYL* 5: 邪氣**中經**，則身癢而癮疹, "In the case of evil qi **striking a conduit**, the body itches and has dormant papules".

Zhong ke **腫渴, swelling with thirst** [3]
IS of swelling and distension associated with thirst. *BCBM* Bai bing zhu zhi yao 百病主治藥：大麻仁，脚氣腹痹，浸酒服。**腫渴**，研汁煮小豆食, "*Da ma ren*: consume soaked in wine for leg qi and abdominal blockage. For **swelling with thirst** grind until a juice is produced, and consume it boiled with small beans".

Zhong lan **腫爛, swelling and festering** [5]
IS of topical swelling with festering. *WTMY 29* : 療甲疽瘡**腫爛**生，脚趾甲邊赤肉出，時瘥時發者方, "Recipe to cure impediment-illness sores with **swelling and festering** emerging at the [toe] nails, and red flesh appearing to the side of a toe nail, sometimes healing and then breaking out again".

Zhong lou **腫瘺, fistula swelling** [4]
PC of → *lou* 瘺, fistula, with a rather prominent swelling. *ZJJYJ* 10: 馬刀，**腫瘺**，目痛，肩不舉…支溝主之, "Saber, **fistula swelling**, pain in the eyes, the shoulders cannot be raised, … [A needle pierced into the] *zhi gou* [insertion hole] controls all these".

Zhong man 腫滿, swelling and fullness [69]
IS a) identical with → *fou zhong* 浮腫, surface swelling. *SW* 74: 諸濕**腫滿**，皆屬於脾, "All [diseases with] moisture [causing] **swelling and fullness**, without exception are associated with the spleen". b) Of a topical extraordinary swelling *QJYF* 24: 冷氣漸入陰囊，**腫滿**恐死, "When cold qi gradually enters the scrotum, this results in **swelling and fullness** and fear of imminent death". *BCGM* uses *zhong man* 腫滿 mostly in the sense of a), rarely in the sense of b).

Zhong mu 腫木, swollen and wooden [1]
IS identical with *zhong jiang* 腫強, swollen and stiff. *BCGM* SE *fu long gan* 伏龍肝 quoting *TPSHF* 36: 治重舌，口中涎出，水漿不收...又方：用伏龍肝研如粉，以牛蒡汁調傅之，效, "Another recipe for saliva flowing from the mouth, and when [the patient] refuses to ingest water as well as viscous liquids, mix with *niu ban* juice and apply externally. Effective", writes: 重舌**腫木**，伏龍肝末，牛蒡汁調塗之, "The tongue feels heavy, is **swollen and wooden**. [Take] *fu long gan* powder, mix with *niu bang* juice and apply externally. Effective".

Zhong qi 中氣, central qi; qi stroke [27]
① PN of a qi moved and transformed by the spleen and stomach. *LS* 28: **中氣**不足，溲便為之變，腸為之苦鳴, "If the **central qi** is insufficient, this causes changes in urination, and suffering from intestinal sounds".
② PC of sudden unconsciousness resulting from internal harm caused by one of the seven affections. *ZZYJ* 1: **中氣**，因七情內傷，氣逆為病, "In the case of **qi stroke**, qi moves contrary to its proper direction because of internal harm caused by one of the seven affections, which leads to this disease".

Zhong qi 腫氣, qi swelling [5]
PC identical with → *zhong ji* 腫疾, swelling ailment. *BJ* SE *lu zhi* 麋脂：主癰腫、惡瘡、死肌，寒風濕痹，四肢拘緩不收，風頭**腫氣**，通腠理, "It controls obstruction-illness with swelling, malign sores, dead muscles/flesh, cold, wind, moisture blockage, cramps of the four limbs so that they cannot be pulled in, wind head, and **qi swelling**. It penetrates the interstitial structures".

Zhong re 中熱, struck by heat [2]
PC identical with → *zhong shu* 中暑, struck by summerheat. *JGYLFL* Fj: 太陽**中熱**者，暍是也, "If the major yang [conduit] is **struck by heat,** this is a sunstroke".

Zhong sai 腫塞, swelling with closure [9]
IS of a swollen, distended throat that is obstructed and does not allow free passage. *ZBYHL* 30: 喉裏**腫塞**痹痛，水漿不得入也, "If there is **swelling with closure**, blockage and pain in the throat, neither water nor broth can enter".

Zhong shi 中濕, moisture stroke; struck by moisture; to be moistened [12]
① PC a) identical with *shi bi* 濕痹, moisture blockage. *MJ* 8: 太陽病，關節疼煩，脈沉而緩者，為**中濕**, "If in the case of major yang disease, the joints feel discomforting pain, the [movement in the] vessels is deep inside and retarded, then this is **moisture stroke**". b) Identical with *shui du* 水毒, water poison: *BCGM* SE *suan* 蒜 quoting *ZHF*: 水毒中人：一名中溪，一名中灑，一名水

病, "Water poison strikes humans. Alternative designations are 'struck by a rivulet'; 'struck by sprinkling water'; and 'water disease'", writes: 水毒中人：一名中溪，一名**中濕**，一名水病, "Water poison strikes humans. Alternative designations are 'struck by a rivulet'; '**struck by moisture**'; and 'water disease'".
② Reference to being soaked. *ZLBC* SE *gu yang jiao* 羖羊角 quotes *MYBL*: 勿使**中濕**，濕即有毒, "Do not allow it to **be moistened**. When it is moist it will be poisonous".

***Zhong shi* 腫濕, swelling with moisture** [1]
IS identical with → *shi zhong* 濕腫①. *TPSHF* 82: 斷臍之後，洗浴傷於濕氣，水入臍口，致令**腫濕**，經久不乾也, "If following the cutting of the umbilical cord washing [the newborn child] results in harm caused by moisture qi, water has entered the navel and brings forth **swelling with moisture** which fails to dry for an extended period of time".

***Zhong shu* 中暑, struck by summerheat; heatstroke** [17] AN *zhong ye* 中暍.
PC brought forth by being struck by summerheat during summer, or by ingesting cold when because of burning heat one craves something cooling. *SJZL* 34: 治**中暑**煩躁, 香薷散方, "Recipe for the powder with *xiang ru* to cure **heatstroke** with vexation and restlessness".

***Zhong shui* 中水, struck by water** [11]
① EA of swelling, pain and festering brought forth by water/moisture affecting open sores. *QJYF* 25: 治因瘡腫痛者，皆**中水**及中風寒所作腫, "To cure swelling and pain resulting from sores, these are always swellings resulting from [the sores] having been **struck by water** or wind cold".
② PC identical with → *shui du* 水毒, water poisoning. *BCGM* SE *xi gui chong* 溪鬼蟲 quoting *ZHF* 7: 水毒中人，一名中溪，一名中灑，一名水病, "When water poison enters a person, this is also called 'struck by a rivulet'; 'struck by sprinkling water', and 'water disease'", writes: 溪毒中人，一名**中水**，一名中溪，一名水病, "when rivulet poison strikes a person, this is also called '**struck by water**'; 'struck by a rivulet'; and 'water disease'".
③ Reference to all types of items that have been affected by water. *QJYF* 3: 以不**中水**豬膏一斤，微火上煎, "Take lard that has not been **struck by water** and boil it on a mild fire".

***Zhong teng* 腫疼, swelling and pain** [2]
IS identical with → *zhong tong* 腫痛, swelling and pain. *WTMY* 2: 集驗療毒熱攻手足，**腫疼**欲脫方, "*JiY*[*F*] recipe to cure poison heat attacking the hands and feet, with **swelling and pain** so severe that one wishes to shed [one's limbs]".

***Zhong tong* 重痛, a feeling of heaviness with pain** [8] AN *chen tong* 沉痛.
IS of pain affecting the lumbar region and regions further below accompanied by a sensation of the presence of something heavy descending. *MYBL* SE *bai shi* 柏實：療恍惚，虛損吸吸，歷節腰中**重痛**, "It cures absent-mindedness, depletion harm with panting, pervading joints [wind], and a **feeling of heaviness with pain** in the lower back".

Zhong tong **腫痛, swelling and pain** [387]
IS of a topical swelling associated with a feeling of pain. *SW* 19: 或痹不仁，**腫痛**，當是之時，可湯熨及火灸刺而去之, "In some cases blockage, numbness, **swelling, and pain** [result]. At this time, it can be removed with hot water and poultices, as well as through fire cauterization and piercing".

Zhong wu **中忤, struck by the hostile** [1]
PC identical with → *zhong e* 中惡, struck by the malign. *BCGM* SE *xi jiao* 犀角 quotes *HTF*: **中忤**，中惡鬼氣，其證或暮夜登廁，或出郊外，驀然倒地，厥冷握拳，口鼻出清血, "The signs of being **struck by the hostile**, (i.e.) of being struck by malign demon qi, are such that if one has gone to the latrine during the night or has left the suburbs, one suddenly falls on the ground, with recession cold and clenched fists. Clear blood leaves from the nose and mouth".

Zhong xi **中溪, struck by rivulet** [5]
PC identical with → *shui du* 水毒②, water poisoning. *ZHF* 7: 水毒中人，一名**中溪**，一名中灑，一名水病, "When water poison strikes humans, this may also be called '**struck by rivulet**', 'struck by sprinkling water', 'water disease'".

Zhong xiao **中消, central melting** [2]
PC of → *xiao ke* 消渴, melting with thirst, associated with a diseased central burner. Major signs: patients are constantly hungry and drink and eat much. *SWBJQYBMJ* Xiao ke lun 消渴論：**中消**者胃也，渴而飲食多，小便黄, "In the case of **central melting** the stomach is affected. [Patients] are thirsty, and they drink and eat a lot. The urine is yellow".

Zhong yang **腫癢, swelling and itching** [5]
IS of topical swelling accompanied by itching. *ZBYHL* 36: 經日便**腫癢**，隱胗起，久久亦成瘡, "After a day this turns into **swelling and itching**. Dormant papules rise. Gradually sores will form too".

Zhong yang **腫瘍, swollen ulcer** [4]
PC of → *chuang yang* 瘡瘍, sores and ulcers, that have not opened to fester yet. *SJZL* 133: 周官瘍醫掌**腫瘍**、潰瘍、金瘍、折瘍, "Among the Zhou officials, the physician responsible for sores took care of **swollen ulers**, festering ulcers, ulcers inflicted by metal [weapons], and ulcers resulting from fractures".

Zhong ye **中暍, struck by summerheat; heatstroke** [7]
PC identical with → *zhong shu* 中暑. *JGYL* Lj lists: 療**中暍**方, "Recipes to cure **heatstroke**".

Zhong ying **腫硬, swelling and hardness** [11]
IS of topical swelling which if pressed gives a feeling of hardness. *TPSHF* 25: 治一切風毒筋急，**腫硬**疼痛，摩風膏方, "To cure all types of wind poison causing muscle cramps, **swelling and hardness** with pain, [use the] recipe for the 'ointment that rubs the wind away'".

Zhong zang **中臟, depot struck [by wind]** [1]
PC of a sudden fall into unconsciousness, a heavy tongue, flow of drool, and an impeded speech, brought about by wind stroke. *JGYL* calls this condition *xie ru yu zang* 邪入於藏, "evil has entered into the depots". *SWBJQYBMJ* 2: **中臟**者，

唇吻不收，舌不轉而失音, "In the case of a **depot struck [by wind]**, one cannot pull in the lips, the tongue cannot be turned, and the voice is lost".

Zhong zhang **腫脹, swelling and distension** [34]
IS of a swelling of the body and its four extremities, or of only local swelling, associated with an uncomfortable feeling of distension. *SW* 71: 熱至則身熱，吐下霍亂，癰疽瘡瘍，瞀鬱注下，瞤瘛**腫脹**，嘔鼽衄頭痛，骨節變肉痛，血溢血泄，淋閟之病生矣, "When heat sets in, then the body turns hot. Vomiting, diarrhea, cholera, obstruction-illnesses, impediment-illnesses, sores, ulcers, indistinct vision, pent-up [qi], and outpour below, twitching and spasms, **swelling and distension,** vomiting, stuffy nose, nosebleed, headache, changes of the bones and joints, pain in the flesh, blood overflow, and blood outflow, as well as dripping [resulting from] blockage – such illnesses are produced".

Zhong zhui **腫墜, swelling with sagging** [2]
IS of a topical swelling accompanied by a feeling as if something had dropped. *YXL* SE *mang cao* 莽草：治風痘，疝氣**腫墜**，凝血, "It cures wind impediment-illnesses, elevation-illness qi, **swelling with sagging**, and coagulation of blood".

Zhong zhui **重墜, heavy and sagging** [8]
① PC of a feeling of deep-seated heaviness in the entire body or parts of it, accompanied by a sensation of sagging. *HJJF* 5: 腰痛，或腰間似有物**重墜**，起坐艱辛者，悉能治之, "Cases of lower back pain occasionally with a feeling as if there were some **heavy, sagging** item in the lumbar region, making rising and sitting down very difficult, they can all be cured".
② A characterization of pharmaceutical substances when their mass is very heavy and when they have a tendency to move downwards in the body. *BCGM* SE *jin* 金：豈知血肉之軀，水穀為賴，可能堪此金石**重墜**之物久在腸胃乎, "How does one know that the human body, consisting of blood and flesh and depending on a supply of water and grain, could bear such **heavy and sagging** items as metal and stones in its intestines and stomach?"

Zhou bi **周痹, circling blockage** [14]
PC of a → *bi* 痹① a), blockage disease, roaming up and down with the disease affecting the entire body. *LS* 27: **周痹**者，在於血脈之中，隨脈以上，隨脈以下, "As for '**circling blockage**', it is located in the blood vessels and moves up and down always following the vessels".

Zhu **疰, attachment-illness** [p]
PC AD of → *gui zhu* 鬼疰, demon attachment-illness. *QJYF* 1 RE *da jin ya san* 大金牙散, massive powder with *jin ya*: 帶之辟百邪，治九十九種**疰**, "To carry it on the body drives away all types of evil, and it cures the ninety-nine types of **attachment-illness**". For an alternative interpretation of *zhu* 疰 as "influx-illness", see entry *shi zhu* 尸疰, corpse [qi] attachment-illness.

***Zhu bi* 諸痹, all types of blockage** [8]

PC of all types of blockage disease. *BJ* SE *ge gen* 葛根：主消渴，身大熱，嘔吐，**諸痹**, "It controls melting with thirst, massive body heat, vomiting, and **all types of blockage**".

***Zhu bing* 疰病, attachment-illness disease** [8]

PC identical with → *gui zhu* 鬼疰, demon attachment-illness. *ZLBC* SE *bai jie* 白薇 quotes *BCJJZ*: 陶隱居云：近道處處有，根狀似牛膝而短小爾。方家用，多療驚邪，風狂，**疰病**, "Tao Yinju says: One finds it everywhere adjacent to roads. The root resembles that of *niu xi*, but is shorter and smaller. Prescription controls use it. It often serves to cure fright evil, wind madness, and **attachment-illness disease**".

***Zhu bing* 諸病, all diseases; all types of diseases** [145] AN *zhu ji* 諸疾, all types of ailments; *zhu zheng* 諸證/諸症, all types of [pathological] conditions. CD of all possible sub-classes of

PC, and of all PC in general. Different prefixes refer to the category of diseases referred to in specific, such as *yan mu zhu bing* 眼目諸病, all diseases of the eyes; *tai chan zhu bing* 胎產諸病, all diseases associated with pregnancy and delivery. *LS* 10: 為此**諸病**，盛則瀉之，虛則補之，熱則疾之，寒則留之，陷下則灸之，不盛不虛，以經取之, "For **all** these **diseases** [of qi abundance and depletion], in the case of abundance, drain it; in the case of depletion, supplement it; in the case of heat, make it move fast; in the case of cold, retain it. When it has sunk down, cauterize it; when there is neither an abundance nor a depletion, remove it from the conduits".

***Zhu che zhu chuan* 注車注船, motion sickness** [1]

PC of motion illness, experienced on a car or boat, with heart-pressure and headache, as well as nausea and vomiting. *PJF* 1: 女子小兒多**注車注船**，心悶亂，頭痛，吐, "Women and children often experience **motion sickness**, with heart-pressure and disorganisation, headache, and vomiting".

***Zhu chi* 蛀齒, worm-attachment teeth** [1]

PC identical with → *qu chi* 齲齒, decayed teeth. *HYBC* SE *teng huang* 藤黃：主蚛牙**蛀齒**，點之便落, "It controls worm-borer teeth and **worm-attachment teeth**. Drip them [with it] and they will simply fall off".

***Zhu chong* 諸蟲, all types of bugs/worms** [71]

① EA a) CD of all types of parasites in the human body. *ZBYHL* 18: **諸蟲**依腸胃之間，若腑臟氣實，則不為害，若虛則能侵蝕, "**All types of worms** exist in the intestines and stomach. As long as the depots and palaces are replete with qi they will not cause harm. Once they (i.e. depots and palaces) are depleted they (i.e.bugs/worms) may enter and feed on them". b) CD of all living organisms in the natural world that are able to enter and harm the human body, in severe cases causing intoxication. The spectrum is very broad, ranging from large ones such as snakes to small ones such as toxic microorganisms found in rivulets. *BJ* SE *li lu* 藜蘆：殺**諸蟲**毒，去死肌, "It kills the poison of **all types of bugs/worms**, and removes dead muscles".

② CD of all small living beings that may serve as pharmaceutical substance. *BCJJZ* 1: **諸蟲**，先微炙，亦完煮之，惟螵蛸當中破之, "**All types of bugs/worms** are to be slightly roasted first. Also, they are to be heated in complete form. With the exception of *piao xiao*. These are to be opened [and their inner parts removed first]".

***Zhu chong shang* 諸蟲傷, all types of injury caused by bugs/worms** [4]
PC identical with → *chong shang* 蟲傷, injury caused by bugs/worms. *PJF* 306: **諸蟲傷**，凡諸蟲齒所傷，其類不一, "**All types of injury caused by bugs/worms** [refers to] all types of harm inflicted by the teeth of bugs/worms. There are many types of them".

***Zhu chuang* 諸瘡, all types of sores** [132]
PC CD of all types of → *chuang* 瘡, sores, conditions. *MYBL* SE *zi shen* 紫參：療腸胃大熱，唾血衄血，腸中聚血，癰腫**諸瘡**, "It cures massive heat in the intestines and the stomach, blood spitting and nosebleed, blood collection in the intestines, obstruction-illnesses with swelling, and **all types of sores**".

***Zhu chuang zhong feng* 諸瘡中風, wind stroke via all possible sores** [4] AN *po shang feng zhong* 破傷風腫, wound wind with swelling; *sun chuang zhong feng* 損瘡中風, wind stroke via wounds and sores; *po shang feng shui du* 破傷風水毒, wound wind with water poisoning; *ding chuang zhong feng* 疔瘡中風，wind stroke via pin-illness sores.
PC of swelling and pain brought about by cold, wind, and moisture having entered the human body through an open wound. *WTMY* 29 has a recipe: 備急療**諸瘡中風**寒水露腫痛, "To promptly cure **wind stroke via all possible sores**, with swelling and pain brought about by cold water and dew".

***Zhu du* 疰毒, attachment-illness poison** [2]
EA bringing forth → *gui zhu* 鬼疰, demon attachment-illness, and → *gu du* 蠱毒, *gu* poisoning. *MYBL* SE *guan gu* 鸛骨：主鬼蠱諸**疰毒**，五屍心腹疾, " It controls demon *gu* and all types of **attachment-illness poison**, as well as the five corpse illnesses in heart and abdomen".

***Zhu e* 諸惡, all types of malignity** [2]
PC CD of numerous forms of malign disease. *QJYF* 7: 既覺脈及體內瘥，但當勤服八風散，勿以脚未能行，輕加余治，未必全得要，更生**諸惡**，失此諸治也, "One may have the impression that the movement in the vessels and the situation in the body are all fine. Still one must regularly ingest the 'powder for the eight winds', and one must not carelessly add an additional treatment only bcause the legs cannot walk yet. This is to avoid that after one has done all that was necessary one still generates **all types of malignity** and the treatments initiated turn into a failure".

***Zhu feng* 諸風, all [diseases with] wind** [130]
PC brought about by wind. *SW* 74: **諸風**掉眩，皆屬於肝, "**All [diseases with] wind** [causing] swaying and dizziness, without exception they are associated with the liver". *BCGM* Bai bing zhu zhi yao 百病主治藥, "The Hundred Diseases and The Drugs Capable of Curing Them"; section Zhu feng 諸風, All [dis-

eases with] wind, lists *zhong zang* 中臟, depots struck [by wind]; *zhong fu* 中腑, palaces struck [by wind]; *zhong jing* 中經, conduits struck [by wind]; *zhong qi* 中氣, struck [by wind] qi, *tan jue* 痰厥, phlegm recession; *tong feng* 痛風, pain wind; → *po shang feng*, 破傷風, wound wind; → *ma bi* 麻痹, hemp[-like numbness] blockage. In addition, the *BCGM* refers to many kinds of pathological conditions such as *zhu feng xuan yun* 諸風眩暈, all [diseases with] wind [associated with] dizziness; *zhu feng bu sui* 諸風不遂，all [diseases with] wind [with body parts] failing to respond; *zhu feng tong bi* 諸風痛痹，all [diseases with] wind [associated with] blockage with pain; and *zhu feng sao yang* 諸風瘙癢，all [diseases with] wind [associated with] itching.

Zhu gan **諸疳, all types of *gan*-illness** [13]
PC CD of all types of → *gan* 疳, *gan*-illness. *SJZL* 173: 五疳之外，隨十二經脈血氣所受，變狀不一，故曰**諸疳**, "In addition to the five types of *gan*-illness, there are different types depending on which of the twelve conduit vessels' blood and qi are affected. Hence one speaks of '**all types of *gan*-illness**'".

Zhu gu **疰蠱, attachment-illness with *gu*** [1]
PC CD of → *gui zhu* 鬼疰, demon attachment-illness, and → *gu du* 蠱毒, *gu* poison. *TBC* SE *ku gua* 苦瓠：主水腫，石淋，吐，呀嗽，囊結，**疰蠱**，痰飲, "It controls water swelling, stone dripping, vomiting, creaking cough, pouch nodes, **attachment-illness with *gu***, and phlegm rheum".

Zhu gu **諸蠱, all types of *gu*** [2]
PC CD of all types of → *gu du* 蠱毒, disease resulting from *gu* poison. *BCSY* SE *xi rou* 犀肉：主**諸蠱**，蛇、獸咬毒，功用劣於角, "It controls poison of **all types of *gu***, and bites by snakes and animals. The effects are less strong than those achieved by cupping".

Zhu guan **珠管, pearls in a tube** [8]
PC of → *yan xi* 眼瘜, tumor-illness on the eye, with a crystal clear color reminiscent of pearls in a tube. *ZBYHL* 28, Mu bing zhu hou 目病諸候 lists 目**珠管**候, "Signs of **pearls in a tube** in the eye": 血氣蘊積，衝發於眼，津液變生結聚，狀如**珠管**, "Blood and qi collect massively, and rush against and effuse in the eye. The liquid transforms into nodular collections shaped like **pearls in a tube**". After its first appearance in the *ZBYHL*, the term *zhu guan* 珠管 was quoted in *QJYF*, *WTMY*, *TPSHF*, *SJZL*, and *PJF*, albeit never with an explanatory remark permitting its identification from hindsight. Beginning with the Ming era, no ophthalmological work mentioned it again.

Zhu han **諸汗, all types of sweating** [3]
PC CD of all types of sweating. *JSF* lists a Zhu han men **諸汗門**, "Section: all **types of sweating**". *YXRM* 3: **諸汗**不止者，防术牡蠣湯，外用米粉撲乾, "In **all cases of sweating** that does not end, [ingest] the decoction with *fang* [*feng*], [*bai*] *zhu*, and *mu li*. Externally swab and dry [the sweating body] with ground rice powder".

***Zhu ji* 疰疾, ailment of attachment-illness** [1]

PC identical with → *gui zhu* 鬼疰, demon attachment-illness. *BCJJZ* SE *ling li jia* 鯪鯉甲：方用亦稀，惟療瘡癩及諸**疰疾**爾, "It is rarely used in recipes, as it serves only to cure sores and repudiation-illness, as well as all types of the **ailment of attachment-illness**".

***Zhu ji* 諸疾, all types of ailments** [68]

PC identical with → *zhu bing* 諸病, all types of diseases. *MYBL* SE *tao he ren* 桃核仁：帶下**諸疾**, 破堅閉, 刮取毛用之, "For **all types of ailments** of discharge from below the belt, and to break open hardenings and closures, remove the hair before using it".

***Zhu jing* 諸痙, all types of spasms** [3]

PC CD of various forms of spams disease. *SW* 74: **諸痙**項強，皆屬於濕, "All **types of spasms** and stiff nape are associated with moisture".

***Zhu lai* 諸癩, all types of repudiation-illness** [2]

PC CD of all different appearances of → *lai* 癩, repudiation-illness. *ZBYHL* 2 lists: **諸癩**候, "Signs of **all types of repudiation-illness**". *WTMY* 30 lists: **諸癩**方, "Recipes for **all types of repudiation-illness**".

***Zhu lao* 諸勞, all types of exhaustion** [3]

PC CD of numerous types of depletion detriments. *ZBYHL* 3: 去身一切**諸勞**疾疹, "It removes papules associated with all **types of exhaustion** ailment from the body".

***Zhu li* 諸痢, all types of free-flux illness** [17]

PC CD of all types of → *li ji* 痢疾, ailments of free-flux illness. *ZHF* 2: 天行**諸痢**悉主之, "It controls **all types of free-flux illness** sent by heaven".

***Zhu lin* 諸淋, all types of dripping** [14]

PC CD of all types of → *lin bing* 淋病, dripping disease. *ZBYHL* 14: **諸淋**者，由腎虛膀胱熱故也, "**All types of dripping** are caused by kidney depletion and urinary bladder heat".

***Zhu lou* 諸漏, all types of leakage** [2]

PC of all types of → *lou chuang* 漏瘡, leaking sores. *QJYF* 22: 治癰疽膿血內漏，**諸漏**敗壞，男發背、女乳房及五痔，蝟皮散方, "Recipe for the powder with hedgehog skin to treat obstruction- and impediment-illnesses with internal leakage of pus and blood, **all types of leakage** from destroyed and rotten [sores], effusion of the back in males, [sores affecting] female breasts, and the five types of piles".

***Zhu lou* 諸瘻, all types of fistula** [15]

PC CD of all types of → *lou* 瘻, fistula. *MYBL* SE *di yu* 地榆：止膿血，**諸瘻**，惡瘡，熱瘡, "It ends [release of] pus and blood, **all types of fistula,** malign sores, and heat sores".

***Zhu nüe* 諸瘧, all types of malaria** [21]

PC CD of all types of → *nüe ji* 瘧疾, malaria ailments. *ZHF* 3 lists 治寒熱**諸瘧**方第十六, "Recipes to cure **all types of malaria** with alternating sensations of cold and heat, No. 16".

***Zhu qi* 疰氣, attachment-illness qi** [12]

① PC identical with → *gui zhu* 鬼疰, demon attachment-illness. *MYBL* SE *bai jie* 白芥：子，主射工及**疰氣**, "The seeds control the archer [bug's poison] and **attachment-illness qi**".

② EA of a turbid qi issued by demonic beings or encountered on burial grounds and in mountain forests that is capable of bringing forth demon attachment-illness. *QJYF* 1: 江南度世丸，治萬病癥結積聚，伏屍長病，寒熱**疰氣**流行皮中, "The 'pills from South of the Yangzi transcending ages' cure a myriad of diseases of concretion-illness nodes, accumulations and collections, as well as chronic hidden corpse [qi] disease, alternating sensations of cold and heat, and **attachment-illness qi** flowing in the skin".

***Zhu qi* 注氣, influx qi** [3]

PC identical with → *gui zhu* 鬼疰, demon attachment-illness. *SYXJ* SE *tao he ren* 桃核人：主傳屍鬼氣，咳嗽痃癖，**注氣**, "It controls corpse [evil] transmission of demon qi, cough, string-illness with aggregation-illness, and **influx qi**".

***Zhu qi* 諸氣, all types of qi [disease]; all qi; all types of qi [quality]** [44]

① PC CD of all types of → *qi bing* 氣病, qi disease. *SW* 74: **諸氣**膹鬱，皆屬於肺, "**All** [diseases with] pent-up **qi** [resulting in heart-]pressure, are without exception associated with the lung". In the *BCGM* the vast majority of 諸氣 is with this meaning.

② CD of all types of physiological qi. *SW* 10: 諸血者皆屬於心，**諸氣**者皆屬於肺，此四肢八溪之朝夕也, "All blood is tied to the heart. **All qi** is tied to the lung. This is the morning and the evening of the four limbs and the eight ravines".

③ CD of all types of qualities of pharmaceutical substances. *YXQY* Lj: 凡同氣之物必有諸味，同味之物必有**諸氣**, "Among all items with identical qi [quality] one will find all types of flavors. [Among all] items with identical flavors one will find **all types of qi [quality]**".

***Zhu qin shou shang* 諸禽獸傷, all types of harm caused by birds and four-legged animals** [1]

PC possibly based on a misreading of an original textual passage by LSZ. The original text refers to injuries received by birds and animals, not to harm caused by birds and animals to humans. *BCGM* SE *tian cai* 菾菜 quoting *BCSY*: 搗絞汁服之，主冷熱痢，又止血生肌，人及禽獸有傷折，傅之立愈, "Pound and wring out the liquid to be ingested. This controls cold-heat free-flux illness. Also, it ends bleeding and generates muscles. Furthermore, if externally applied it will immediately cure all types of harm received by humans, fowl and four-legged animals", writes: 搗汁服，主冷熱痢，又止血生肌，及**諸禽獸傷**，傅之立愈, "The liquid obtained through pounding is to be ingested to control cold-heat free-flux illness. Also, it ends bleeding and generates muscles. Furthermore, if externally applied it will immediately cure **all types of harm caused by birds and four-legged animals**".

Zhu re **諸熱, all types of heat** [38]

PC CD of many types of disease that are all brought about by → *re* 熱, heat. *LS* 1: 刺**諸熱**者，如以手探湯, "To prick **all types of heat** one proceeds [as fast as if] testing hot water with a finger". *BCGM* has *tian xing zhu re* 天行諸熱, all types of heaven-sent heat; *chan hou zhu re* 產後諸熱, all types of heat following delivery; *xiao er zhu re* 小兒諸熱, all types of heat affecting children. Also, there is mention of *zhu re bing* 諸熱病, all types of heat disease; *zhu re lao* 諸熱癆, all types of heat with exhaustion; *zhu re du* 諸熱毒, all types of heat poison.

Zhu shi **諸濕, all types of moisture** [5]

PC CD comprising all types of → *shi bing* 濕病, moisture disease. *SW* 74: **諸濕**腫滿，皆屬於脾, "**All types of moisture** [causing] swelling and fullness are without exception associated with the spleen".

Zhu shou shang **諸獸傷, all types of harm caused four-legged animals** [2]

PC CD of bodily injuries received from animals attacking by biting, kicking, or scratching. *BCGM* Bai bing zhu zhi yao 百病主治藥：**諸獸傷**：虎、狼、熊、羆、豬、貓、犬、猘、驢、馬、鼠咬，人咬, "**All types of harm caused by four-legged animals**: tiger, wolf, bear, brown bear, pig, cat, dog, rabid dog, donkey, horse, as well as rat bites, and human bites".

Zhu tong **疰痛, attachment-illness pain** [3]

PC of sudden extremely violent pain brought forth by attachment-illness. *QJYiF* 19:（鹿）角主貓鬼中惡，心腹**疰痛**, "(Deer) horn controls malign stroke by a cat demon, with **attachment-illness pain** in the heart and abdomen".

Zhu tong **注痛, influx pain** [6]

IS of pain erratically changing its location. *SJZL* 52: 腰胯**注痛**，脚膝無力, "The lower back and hips have **influx pain**. The legs and knees lack strength".

Zhu wu **疰忤, attachment- illness and [presence of] the hostile** [26]

PC of sudden piercing pain in the heart and abdomen, sometimes accompanied by nausea and trepidation. It comes and goes for a while, and cannot be cured over an extended period of time. *QJYF* 17: 大附著散，治五屍**疰忤**與前狀同者方, " 'Large adhesion powder' cures the five types of corpse [qi causing] **attachment-illness and [presence of] the hostile**, with an appearance similar to that mentioned above".

Zhu wu **注忤, influx of the hostile** [3]

PC identical with → *zhu wu* 疰忤, attachment-illness and [presence of] the hostile. *BCSY* SE *gui chi* 鬼齒：主中惡**注忤**，心腹痛, "It controls stroke by the malign and **influx of the hostile**, with pain in heart and abdomen".

Zhu xia **注下, outpour discharge** [8]

① IS of an extremely urgent outpouring of watery diarrhea. *ZBYHL* 25: 蟲上食五臟，熱盛煩毒，**注下**不禁, "Bugs/worms rise to gnaw on the five depots. Heat abounds, with vexing poison. Unending **outpour discharge**".

② PC identical with → *shui xie* 水泄, watery outflow. *SW* 69: 民病瘧、少氣咳喘、血溢、血泄、**注下**, "People suffer from malaria, being short of qi, coughing and panting. There is blood overflow, blood outflow, and **outpour discharge**".

Zhu xia **注夏, summer influx** [1]

PC of headache and weakness of the legs, with failing appetite and a feverish body, during summer when it is moist and hot, with children particularly affected. *DXXF* 1: **注夏**屬陰虛，元氣不足，夏初春末，頭疼脚軟，食少體熱者, "**Summer influx** is an example of yin depletion. The original qi is insufficient. In early summer, at the end of spring one experiences headaches and weakness of the legs. [Patients] eat less and their body is hot".

Zhu xian **諸癇, all types of epilepsy** [11]

PC of all types of → *xian* 癇, epilepsy, regardless of their varying etiologies or appearances. *BJ* SE *fang ji* 防己：主風寒，温瘧，熱氣，**諸癇**, "It controls wind cold, warmth malaria, heat qi, and **all types of epilepsy**".

Zhu xian **豬癇, hog epilepsy** [2]

PC of a → *dian xian* 癲癇, peak-illness with epilepsy, which, at the time of its outbreaks, makes the patient's four limbs twitch, accompanied by a tendency to spit foam. *QJYF* 5: **豬癇**之為病，喜吐沫, "The disease of **hog epilepsy**: [patients] tend to spit foam".

Zhu xie **注泄, outpour outflow** [1]

PC identical with → *shui xie* 水泄, watery diarrhea. *SJZL* 74: 腹脹下利，有如注水之狀，謂之**注泄**，世名水瀉, "An abdominal swelling with a free-flux illness resembling an outpouring of water, this is called '**outpour outflow**'. A common designation is 'watery diarrhea'".

Zhu xin tong **疰心痛, attachment-illness heartache** [1]

PC identical with → *gui zhu xin tong* 鬼疰心痛, demon attachment-illness heartache. *BCGM* Bai bing zhu zhi yao 百病主治藥 quoting the main text: 鬼疰心痛, demon attachment-illness heartache", writes: **疰心痛**, "**Attachment-illness heartache**".

Zhu xu **諸虛, all types of depletion** [28]

PC CD of all types of → *xu zheng* 虛證, depletion condition. *QJYF* 13: 當歸湯，治心腹絞痛，**諸虛**，冷氣滿痛方, "Decoction with *dang gui*, a recipe to cure twisting pain in the heart and abdomen, **all types of depletion**, cold qi, and a feeling of fullness with pain".

Zhu xue **諸血, all types of blood; all types of bleeding** [41]

① PS CD of blood liquid of all types of animals. *BCSY* SE *zhu xue* **諸血**：**諸血**，味甘，平。主補人身血不足, "**All types of blood**: the flavor is sweet, [qi] is balanced. They control supplementing insufficiency of blood in a person's body".

② PC CD mainly of all types of bleeding conditions, sometimes also of extravascular stagnant blood conditions. *SJZL* 15: "產後**諸血**，漏下赤白, "**All types of bleeding** after delivery, (i.e.) a leaking of red-white [liquid]".

***Zhu yang tou tong* 諸陽頭痛, all types of yang headache** [1]
PC CD of → *tai yang tou tong* 太陽頭痛, major yang headache; *yang ming tou tong* 陽明頭痛; yang brilliance headache, and *shao yang tou tong* 少陽頭痛, minor yang headache. *YXQY* Lj SE *xi xin* 細辛：止**諸陽頭痛**，諸風通用之, "It ends **all types of yang headache**, and can be used [for treating] all types of wind".

***Zhu yu* 諸鬱, all types of pent-up [qi]** [9]
PC CD of all types of accumulation disease. *DXXF* 3: 蒼朮、撫芎，總解**諸鬱**，隨證加入諸藥, "*Cang zhu* and *fu xiong* are able to resolve **all types of pent-up [qi]**. They are to be added to all types of medication on the basis of the signs [exhibited by a patient]".

***Zhu zheng* 諸證, all types of pathological conditions** [35]
① PC identical with → *zhu bing* 諸病, all types of diseases. *QJYF* 5: **諸證**各根據脈形為治, "**All types of pathological conditions** are to be treated in accordance with the physical appearance of the [movement in the] vessels".
② CD of all sub-groups of IS, or of all IS in general. *BCYY* SE *zhu ye* 竹葉：是夜**諸證**皆定, "That night **all pathological conditions** were stabilized".

***Zhu zheng* 諸症, all types of pathological conditions** [5]
PC, IS CD identical with → *zhu zheng* 諸證. *BCGM* SE *sha cao xiang fu zi* 莎草香附子 quoting *JSF*: 婦人氣盛於血, 變生諸證, "When in a woman qi is more abundant than blood, this will give rise to all types of pathological conditions", writes: 婦人氣盛血衰, 變生**諸症**, "When in a woman qi abounds while the blood is weak, this will give rise to **all types of pathological conditions**".

***Zhu zhi* 諸痔, all types of piles** [3]
PC CD of numerous types of → *zhi chuang* 痔瘡, piles sores. *ZBYHL* 34: 有一方而治之者，名為**諸痔**，非為諸病共成一痔, "As there is one identical recipe to cure them, one speaks of '**all types of piles**'. It is not so that all types of diseases bring forth one identical type of piles".

***Zhu zhong* 諸腫, all types of swelling** [11]
PC underlying all types of → *zhong* 腫, swelling. *ZBYHL* 31: 其候非一，故謂之**諸腫**, "It has more than one sign. Hence one speaks of '**all types of swelling**'". In the *BCGM*, *zhu zhong* 諸腫 includes edematose swelling and swelling associated with sores/ulcers. *BCGM* Bai bing zhu zhi yao 百病主治藥：**諸腫**，有風腫、熱腫、水腫、濕腫、氣腫、虛腫、積腫、血腫, "**All types of swelling** includes wind swelling; heat swelling; water/edematose swelling; moisture swelling; qi swelling; depletion swelling; accumulation swelling; blood swelling".

***Zhu zhu* 諸疰, all types of attachment-illness** [2]
PC CD of all types of → *zhu bing* 疰病, attachment-illness disease. *MYBL* SE *jin ya* 金牙：主鬼疰，毒蠱，**諸疰**, "It controls **all types of attachment-illness**, such as demon attachment-illness, and poisonous *gu*".

***Zhua ku* 爪枯, nail dryness** [3]
IS of one's nails drying and becoming thin and soft, and losing their luster. *SW* 10: 多食辛，則筋急而**爪枯**, "If one consumes large quantities of acrid [food], then the sinews become tense and the **nails dry**".

Zhua shang **爪傷, injury from claws** [3]

PC of a → *shang sun* 傷損, injury, of skin and flesh resulting from being scratched by the claws of an animal. *BCGM* SE *su* 粟 quoting *ZHF* 7: 熊虎爪牙所傷, "Injured by the claws and teeth of bears and tigers", writes: 熊虎**爪傷**, "**Injury from the claws** of bear and tiger".

Zhua shang **抓傷, injury from scratching claws** [6]

PC of a → *shang sun* 傷損, injury, of skin and flesh resulting from being scratched by the claws or nails of an animal or human. *BCGM* SE *fen xi* 粉錫 quotes *BHJJF*: **抓傷**面皮：香油調鉛粉搽之，一夕愈, "**Injury** of facial skin **from scratching claws**: Mix *xiang you* with *qian fen* and apply externally. It will heal overnight".

Zhuan bao **轉胞, contorted bladder** [11]

PC identical with → *zhuan pao* 轉脬. *JGYL* Lj: 問曰：婦人病飲食如故，煩熱不得臥，而反倚息者，何也？師曰：此名**轉胞**，不得溺也，以胞系了戾，故致此病。但利小便則愈，宜腎氣丸主之, "Question: When a woman suffers, although she has drunk and eaten as usual, from vexing heat and cannot lie down to sleep, and on the contrary, she must prop herself up to breathe, why is this so? Master: This is called '**contorted bladder**'. [Patients] are unable to pass urine. This disease results from a twisted bladder connection. However, once the passage of urine is freed they are cured. The 'pills for kidney qi' are suitable for controlling this".

Zhuan jin **轉筋, contorted sinews** [121]

IS of a contraction of sinews and vessels in the extremities and the body with a feeling of pain as if something were twisted. *SW* 77: 身體解散，四肢**轉筋**, "The [patient's] body will disintegrate; the **sinews** in his four limbs will become **contorted**".

Zhuan pao **轉脬, contorted bladder** [16] AN *zhuan bao* 轉胞.

PC of a distended, tight and painful urinary bladder because of a blockage of the 'bladder connection' (*bao xi* 胞系, i.e. the urethra) and resulting inhibition of the flow of urine. *YXRM* 4: 脬系轉戾，臍下並急而痛，小便不通，名曰**轉脬**, "[A condition where] the bladder connection is contorted-twisted, with both tightness and pain felt below the navel, as well as urinary stoppage, this is called '**contorted bladder**'".

Zhuan shi **轉食, regurgitation of food** [3]

IS identical with → *tu shi* 吐食, vomiting of food. *PJF* 173: 翻胃**轉食**，面黃瘦乏, "When the stomach is upset and in the case of **regurgitation of food**, the face becomes yellow and [patients experience] emaciation and weariness".

Zhuang re **壯熱, strong heat** [69]

IS of a fever with a strong heat force. *JGYL* Lj: 救卒死而**壯熱**者方, "Recipe to rescue those with a sudden [appearance of] death and **strong heat**".

Zhui shang **墜傷, damage from a fall** [2]

PC identical with → *zhui sun* 墜損. *WTMY* 29：療男子虛勞，**墜傷**內損，吐血不止，欲死，面目黑如漆者，悉主之方, "To cure depletion exhaustion in males, **damage from a fall** and internal injuries, unending blood spitting with a desire to die, and face and eyes turning black like lacquer, this recipe controls all of this".

Zhui sun **墜損, injury from a fall** [6] AN *sun zhui* 損墜; *duo shang* 墮傷, damage from a fall; *zhui shang* 墜傷.

PC of → *shang sun* 傷損, injury, resulting from a fall from somewhere high. *WTMY* 29: 近效療墜損方，生地黃一斤，分為三份。右每服取一份, "The *JXF's* recipe to cure **injuries from a fall**: divide 1 *jin* of fresh *di huang* into three portions. Of these take one portion for each ingestion".

Zhui tai **墜胎, to cause an abortion; spontaneous abortion** [3]

① identical with → *duo tai* 墮胎①, to cause an abortion. *MYBL* SE *she xiang* 麝香：婦人產難，**墜胎**, "[To cure] women who experience difficult births, and to **cause an abortion**".

② PC identical with → *duo tai* 墮胎②, spontaneous abortion. *RHZ* SE *pu huang* 蒲黃：婦人帶下，月候不勻，血氣心腹痛，妊孕人下血**墜胎**，血運血癥，兒枕急痛, "[It cures] women's [diseases of] discharge from below the belt and menstrual irregularities, as well as heart and abdominal pain resulting from blood and qi [stagnation]. In pregnant women [it cures] discharge of blood and **spontaneous abortion**, blood[-induced brain] movements and blood concretion-illness, as well as [formation of] an infant's headrest (i.e. a lump of coagulated blood in the uterus resembling an infant's headrest) with tightness and pain".

Zhui tong **錐痛, stabbing pain** [2]

IS identical with → *ci tong* 刺痛, piercing pain. *SYDXF* 10: 手足甲忽然長倒生肉刺，如**錐痛**不可忍。吃葵菜，自愈, "Toenails and fingernails suddenly grow and pierce into the flesh. One feels an unbearable **pain as if stabbed** by an awl. Eat *kui cai* and this will heal as a result".

Zhuo bing **濁病, turbidity disease** [1]

PC of turbid urine. *BCGM* SE *qian shi* 芡實 quotes *ZXF*: 分清丸：治**濁病**, "The 'pills to separate and clear': they cure **turbidity disease**".

Zhuo chuang **灼瘡, sores resulting from scorching** [2]

PC identical with → *huo chuang* 火瘡, fire sores. *BCSY* SE *jing jing* 荊莖：其洗**灼瘡**及熱焱瘡，有效, "Effective if used to rinse **sores resulting from scorching** and sores resulting from heat and flames".

Zhuo lan **灼爛, festering because of scorching** [1]

PC identical with → *huo chuang* 火瘡, fire sores. *MYBL* SE *jing jing* 荊莖：療**灼爛**, "Heals **festering because of scorching**".

Zhuo li **濁瀝, turbid trickle** [2]

PC of turbid urine accompanied by difficult urination. *BCGM* Bai bing zhu zhi yao 百病主治藥：蒼术，脾濕下流，**濁瀝**, "*Cang zhu*, [it cures] spleen moisture with downard outflow, and **turbid trickle**".

***Zhuo lin* 濁淋, turbid dripping** [2] AN *lin zhuo* 淋濁, dripping turbidity.

PC of frequent and painful urination. The appearance of the urine is turbid; in extreme cases it seems to be mixed with pus and blood. *ZZYJ* 2: 清心連子飲，**濁淋**, "The 'drink with *lian zi* that clears the heart', [it cures] **turbid dripping**".

***Zhuo yi* 濁遺, turbid emission** [1]

PC CD of → *bai zhuo* 白濁, white turbidity, and → *yi jing* 遺精, seminal emission. *BCGM* SE *fu ling* 茯苓：**濁遺**帶下：威喜丸, "For **turbid emission** and [discharge from] below the belt: [use] the 'powerful happiness pills'".

***Zi bai dian ban* 紫白癜斑, purple and white patches and macules** [2]

PC identical with → *zi bai dian feng* 紫白癜風, purple and white patches wind. *BCGM* SE *bei mu* 貝母 quotes *DSTJYF*: **紫白癜斑**：貝母、南星等分為末, 生薑帶汁擦之, "For **purple and white patches and macules**: equal amounts of *bei mu* and *nan xing* are to be ground to powder. Mix with *sheng jiang* juice and rub on [the diseased region]".

***Zi bai dian feng* 紫白癜風, purple and white patches wind** [3] AN *chi bai dian feng* 赤白癜風, red and white patches wind; *dian feng* 癜風, patches wind; *zi bai dian ban* 紫白癜斑, purple and white patches and macules.

PC of a joint occurrence of → *zi dian feng* 紫癜風, purple patches wind, and → *bai dian feng* 白癜風, white patches wind. *FKJYMF* 19: 當歸散，治皮風，**紫白癜風**, "The powder with *dang gui* cures skin wind, and **purple and white patches wind**".

***Zi chang bu shou* 子腸不收, failure of the infant's intestine to recede** [2]

PC identical with → *yin tuo* 陰脫, yin prolapse. *BCGM* SE xie **蠍** quoting *WSBJ* 18: 治婦人子腸下不收…全蠍（不以多少）。右為末, 口噙水, 鼻內嗃之, 立效, "To treat women whose infant's intestine has come down and fails to recede: …Take several complete scorpions and grind to powder. Have [the woman] hold water in her mouth and inhale [the powder] through her nose. Immediately effective", writes: **子腸不收**，全蠍炒，研末。口噙水，鼻中嗃之，立效, "For **failure of the infant's intestine to recede**: roast complete scorpions and grind them to powder. Have [the woman] hold water in her mouth and inhale [the powder] through her nose. Immediately effective".

***Zi chang ting chu* 子腸挺出, prolapse of the infant's intestine** [1]

PC identical with → *yin tuo* 陰脫, yin prolapse. *BCGM* SE *bi ma* 蓖麻：女人胎衣不下，**子腸挺出**, "[It cures] women whose placenta fails to be discharged, and those with **prolapse of the infant's intestine**".

***Zi chang tuo chu* 子腸脫出, prolapse of the infant's intestine** [2]

PC identical with → *yin tuo* 陰脫, yin prolapse. *PJF* 360: **子腸脫出**，吳茱萸三升，酒五升，煎取二升，分溫三服, "For **prolapse of the infant's intestine**: *wu zhu yu*, 3 *sheng*; wine, 5 *sheng*. Boil down to 2 *sheng*. Ingest divided into three portions".

Zi chang tuo xia **子腸脫下, prolapse of the infant's intestine** [1]
PC identical with → *yin tuo* 陰脫, yin prolapse. *BCGM* Bai bing zhu zhi yao 百病主治藥, Yin tuo 陰脫：狐陰莖，並主產後**子腸脫下**, "Fox penis, it also controls, following delivery, **prolapse of the infant's intestine**".

Zi chang xian chu **子腸先出, prior appearance of the infant's intestine** [1]
IS of → *pan chang chan* 盤腸產, birth with a twisted intestine. *FRDQLF* 17: 趙都運恭人，每臨產則**子腸先出**，然後產子。產子之後，其腸不收，甚以為苦，名曰盤腸產, "Whenever the wife of the official Zhao Duyun approached the moment of delivery, **the infant's intestine appeared first**, and only then did she give birth to a child. After the child was born, its intestine failed to recede. This caused her extreme suffering. It is called 'birth with a twisted intestine'".

Zi chang xian xia **子腸先下, prior descent of the infant's intestine** [1]
IS of → *pan chang chan* 盤腸產, birth with a twisted intestine. *BCGM* Bai bing zhu zhi yao 百病主治藥, Chan nan 產難, Difficult births: 生產，**子腸先下**，產後不收, "During birth **the child's intestine descends first**, and fails to retreat after the birth is complete".

Zi chang zhui xia **子腸墜下, prolapse of the infant's intestine** [1]
PC identical with → *yin tuo* 陰脫, yin prolapse. *BCGM* SE *wu pei zi* 五倍子：收脫肛、**子腸墜下**, "[It serves] to draw in a prolapsed rectum and a **prolapsed infant's intestine**".

Zi dian **紫癜, purple patches** [1]
PC identical with *zi dian feng* 紫癜風, purple patches wind. *BCGM* SE *qie zi* 茄子：治癜風，用茄蒂蘸硫、附末摻之，取其散血也。白癜用白茄蒂，**紫癜**用紫茄蒂，亦各從其類耳, "To cure patches wind dip the footstalks of eggplants into sulphur and *fu* [*zi*] powder and apply externally. This will remove the dissipated blood. For white patches use white eggplant footstalks; for **purple patches** use purple eggplant footstalks. This, too, is to act in accordance with their categories of likeness".

Zi dian feng **紫癜風, purple patches wind** [3] AD *zi dian* **紫癜**, purple patches.
PC of purple skin macules or dots without pain or itching. *SJZL* 18: **紫癜風**之狀，皮膚生紫點，搔之皮起而不癢痛是也, "The appearance of **purple patches wind**: the skin develops purple dots. If scratched the skin rises but does not itch or ache".

Zi fan **子煩, child[-induced] vexation** [7]
PC of vexation with heart-pressure experienced by women during pregnancy. *ZBYHL* 42: 妊娠而煩，故謂之**子煩**也, "It is called '**child[-induced] vexation**' because this type of vexation occurs during pregnancy".

Zi gong bu shou **子宮不收, failure of the infant's palace to recede** [2]
PC identical with → *yin tuo* 陰脫, yin prolapse. A prolapse of the uterus or vaginal mucous membrane, in severe cases resulting in a protrusion out of the vagina that fails to recede into its original position. *SYDXF* 15: 磁石散，治**子宮不收**，名瘣疾, "Powder with *ci shi* cures an **infant's palace** that fails to recede. This is called 'demonic ailment'".

***Zi gong tuo xia* 子宫脱下, prolapse of the infant's palace** [1]
PC identical with → *yin tuo* 陰脱, yin prolapse. *BCGM* SE *bi ma* 蓖麻 quotes *ZXF*: 子宫脱下：蓖麻子仁、枯礬等分，為末，安紙上托入, "For **prolapse of the infant's palace**: grind equal amounts of *bi ma zi* seeds and *ku fan* to powder. Put this on a piece of paper and use it to push [the uterus back] into [the vagina]".

***Zi gong xia tuo* 子宫下脱, prolapse of the infant's palace** [1]
PC identical with → *yin tuo* 陰脱, yin prolapse. *BCGM* SE *zhu* 竹 (*dan zhu gen* 淡竹根)：同葉煎湯，洗婦人子宫下脱, "Together with a decoction of the leaves [it may be used] to rinse a woman's **prolapsed infant's palace**".

***Zi han* 自汗, spontaneous sweating** [90]
① IS of a sudden profuse sweating while one is awake without having overexerted oneself with any activity, or being affected by hot weather or wearing overly warm clothing. Also, pontaneous sweating as an illness sign does not include sweating associated with fever, with the intake of medication, or sweating associated with extreme pain. *SHL* 6: 風温為病，脈陰陽俱浮，自汗出，身重, "When wind and warmth cause a disease, the [movements in both the] yin and yang vessels will be at the surface. There is **spontaneous sweating** and the body feels heavy".
② PC with spontaneous sweating while one is awake without having overexerted oneself with any activity, or being affected by hot weather, or wearing overly warm clothing. *ZBYHL* 8: 夫諸陽在表，陽氣虛則自汗, "Now, all yang [qi] is in the [body'] external sections. In the case of yang qi depletion **spontaneous sweating** results".

***Zi li* 自利, spontaneous free flow** [6]
IS identical with → *xie xie* 泄瀉 ①, outflow. *SHL* 273: 太陰之為病，腹滿而吐，食不下，自利益甚，時腹自痛, "When the major yin [conduit] is affected by disease, the abdomen has a feeling of fullness, and one cannot eat. This goes along with extreme **spontaneous free flow**. At times the abdomen develops spontaneous pain".

***Zi lin* 子淋, infant's dripping** [3]
PC of a → *lin bing* 淋病, dripping disease, affecting women during pregnancy. *ZBYHL* 42: 妊娠之人，胞繫於腎，腎患虛熱成淋，故謂子淋也, "In pregnant persons the uterus bladder is tied to the kidneys. When the kidneys suffer from depletion heat, this generates dripping. Hence it is called **infant's dripping**".

***Zi mao* 子冒, infant's assault** [3]
PC identical with → *zi xian* 子癇, infant's epilepsy. *WTMY* 33：妊娠忽悶，眼不識人，須臾醒，醒復發，亦仍不醒者，名為痓病，亦號子癇病，亦號子冒, "When during pregnancy [a woman] suddenly experiences heart-pressure and fails to recognize other persons with her eyes, regains her consciousness after a while, and develops the same ailment after she has regained her consciousness, or, in some cases, does not regain consciousness at all, this is called 'cramp

disease'. It is also called 'child[-bearing] epilepsy disease', and also '**infant's assault'**".

Zi qi **子氣, infant's qi** [2]

PC identical with → *ren shen shui zhong* 妊娠水腫, edematose swelling during pregnancy. *FRDQLF* 15: 妊娠自三月成胎之後，兩足自脚面漸腫腿膝以來，行步艱辛，以至喘悶，飲食不美，似水氣狀。至於脚指間有黃水出者，謂之**子氣**，直至分娩方消, "After three months of pregnancy the fetus has formed. The [pregnant woman's] two feet gradually develop a swelling spreading from the surface of the legs to the thighs and knees. Walking is difficult. Eventually [the pregnant woman] develops panting and heart-pressure. She finds no pleasure in drinking or eating. The appearance is like that of water qi. Eventually yellow water is excreted from between the toes. One calls this **infant's qi**. This will end only after delivery".

Zi ru yu ji **字乳余疾, ailments in the aftermath of delivery** [4]

PC identical with → *chan hou yu ji* 產後余疾. *MYBL* SE *sang jing shi* 桑莖實：主**字乳余疾**，輕身益氣, "It controls **ailments in the aftermath of delivery**, relieves the body of its weight, and increases qi".

Zi shang chong xin **子上衝心, an infant rises and clashes with the heart** [1] AN *tai qi shang chong* 胎氣上沖, fetal qi rises and clashes [with the heart]; *tai shang chong xin* 胎上衝心, a fetus rises and clashes with the heart; *tai shang qiang xin* 胎上搶心, a fetus rises and knocks at the heart; *tai dong shang bi* 胎動上逼, fetal movement pressing upward; *tai dong shang ge* 胎動上膈, fetal movement rising towards the diaphragm; *tai dong po xin* 胎動迫心, fetal movement pressing against the heart.

PC of pregnant women experiencing chest and abdominal distension and a feeling of fullness, with hectic panting in serious cases, and vexation, restlessness and a failur to calm down. *SLBC* SE *pu tao* 葡萄：妊孕人，**子上衝心**，飲之即下，其胎安, "When a pregnant woman experiences that her **infant rises and clashes with the heart**, drinking this will bring it down, and the fetus will be pacified".

Zi si fu zhong **子死腹中, an infant's death in the abdomen** [21] AN *tai si fu zhong* 胎死腹中, a fetus' death in the abdomen; *si tai bu xia* 死胎不下, a dead fetus fails to descend; *ren shen tai si* 妊娠胎死, fetal death during pregnancy; *si tai zai fu* 死胎在腹, a dead fetus in the abdomen; *tai si bu xia* 胎死不下, a fetus has died and fails to descend.

PC of a fetus' death, during pregnancy or in the course of delivery, in the uterus and its failure to be born spontaneously for an extended period of time. *QJYF* 2: 治產難，或半生，或胎不下，或**子死腹中**, "To cure difficult birth, or a miscarriage, or failure of the fetus to descend, or **an infant's death in the abdomen**".

Zi xian **子癇, infant's epilepsy** [6]

PC of spasms disease affecting women during pregnancy. *ZBYHL* 42: 妊娠而發者，悶冒不識人，須臾醒，醒復發，亦是風傷太陽之經作痓也，亦名**子癇**, "When it breaks out during pregnancy, [patients] experience heart-pressure and do not recognize others. After a short while they regain consciousness. Once they have regained consciousness another outbreak follows. This is a spasms [disease] brought forth by wind harming the major yang conduit. Another name is **infant's epilepsy**".

***Zi yi* 自縊, hanging oneself** [3]
PC identical with → *zi yi si* 自縊死, [appearance of] death from suicide by hanging. *ZBYHL* 23: 以繩物系頸, 自懸掛致死, 呼為**自縊**, "To take a rope, tie it around the neck, and hang oneself to cause death, this is called '**hanging oneself**'".

***Zi yi si* 自縊死, [appearance of] death from hanging oneself** [2] AD *zi yi* 自縊, hanging oneself; 卒縊垂死, suicide by hanging.
PC of → *cu si* 卒死, sudden [appearance of] death, resulting from an attempt at committing suicide by hanging. *ZHF* 1: 以葱刺耳…亦治自縊死, "Pierce the ear with a scallion. … This also cures **[appearance of] death from hanging oneself**".

***Zi zang feng* 子臟風, infant's depot wind** [4]
PC of wind evil residing in the uterus, with swelling and pain in the external genital region. *BCGM* SE *fang feng* 防風：得葱白能行周身，得澤瀉、藁本療風，得當歸、芍藥、陽起石、禹餘糧療婦人**子臟風**, "With *cong bai* it is able to pass through the entire body; with *ze xie* and *hao ben* it heals wind; with *dang gui*, *shao yao*, *yang qi shi*, and *yu yu liang* it heals women with **infant's depot wind**".

***Zong chi* 縱弛, relaxed; to slacken** [1]
IS identical with → *huan* 緩①. *PJF* 154: 鬱怒傷肝，則諸筋**縱弛**, "When pent-up [qi] and anger harm the liver then all sinews will **slacken**".

***Zong huan* 縱緩, relaxed; to slacken**[4]
IS identical with → *huan* 緩①. *LS* 8: 有熱則筋弛**縱緩**，不勝收，故僻, "If heat is present, then the sinews will **slacken**, and cannot be used to contract [the limbs]. This results in wryness".

***Zou* 皺, wrinkles** [p]
IS CD of all wrinkles appearing with the desiccation of exposed skin. *SLBC* SE *mi* 麋：（茸）於漿水中研為泥，塗面，令不**皺**，光華可愛, "[Young antlers] ground in starch liquid to a pulp, if smeared on the face will prevent the development of **wrinkles** and help to preserve a shiny, lovable appearance".

***Zou jing huang* 走精黃, running-essence yellow** [2]
PC of → *huang dan*, yellow *dan*-illness, with face and eyes all yellow, dizziness and sleepiness, the four limbs in pain, the tongue purple and its surface with fissures. *SJZL* 61: 病患惛惛饒睡，四肢疼痛，面目俱黃，舌上紫色，甚則舌面坼裂，及加黑色，此是**走精黃**, "When one suffers from dizziness and sleepiness, the four limbs being in pain, face and eyes being all yellow, and a purple color on the tongue, and in severe cases the tongue surface developing fissures and an additional black color, this is **running-essence yellow**".

***Zou ma gan* 走馬疳, running horse *gan*-illness** [6]
PC identical with → *zou ma ya gan* 走馬牙疳, running horse dental *gan*-illness. *TPSHF* 34: 治**走馬疳**，蝕落牙齒，齦腫有膿水，宜用藥綿方, "To cure **running horse *gan*-illness**, with teeth eroding and falling out, and gums swell-

ing and losing pus and water, it is advisable to use a recipe for a medicinal cotton [to apply to the gums]".

Zou ma hou bi **走馬喉痹, running horse throat blockage** [6] AN *yi dan* 嗌疸, throat *dan*-illness.

PC identical with → *ji hou bi* 急喉痹, acute throat blockage. *SJZL* 122: 治咽喉腫痛及**走馬喉痹**，硼砂丸方, "The recipe for pills with *peng sha* cures a swollen and aching throat, as well as **running horse throat blockage**".

Zou ma ji gan **走馬急疳, running horse acute *gan*-illness** [1]

PC identical with → *zou ma ya gan* 走馬牙疳, running horse dental *gan*-illness. *BCGM* Bai bing zhu zhi yao 百病主治藥 quoting *QYXJ*: 走馬牙疳, "Running horse dental *gan*-illness", writes: **走馬急疳, "Running horse acute *gan*-illness"**.

Zou ma ya gan **走馬牙疳, running horse dental *gan*-illness** [19] AD *zou ma gan* 走馬疳, running horse *gan*-illness; AN *zou ma ji gan* 走馬急疳, running horse acute *gan*-illness.

PC of → *ya gan* 牙疳, dental *gan*-illness, that develops abruptly and turns into a serious condition, with festering decay beginning at the teeth and gums and eventually causing the teeth to erode and fall out. It passes through four stages: → *peng sha* 崩砂, collapsing sand; → *kui cao* 潰槽, bursting trough; → *xuan lu* 宣露, exposure; → *fu gen* 腐根, rotten root. *XEWSZWLF* 20: 治小兒**走馬牙疳**, "To cure **running horse dental *gan*-illness** in children".

Zou pi qu chuang **走皮趨瘡, sores running through the skin** [1] AN *bei yang chuang* 悲羊瘡, sorrow sheep sores.

PC of → *chuang* 瘡, sores, conditions with moisture covering cheeks and the entire top of the head and possibly reaching to the two ears. They itch and produce liquid, with irregular periods of activity and dormancy. *BCGM* SE *zi wei* 紫葳 quoting *RZZZF*: **走皮趨瘡**：滿頰滿頂，浸淫濕爛，延及兩耳，癢而出水，發歇不定, "**Sores running through the skin** cover cheeks and the entire top of the head with soaking moisture and festering extending to the two ears. They itch and produce liquid, with irregular periods of activity and dormancy".

Zou tong **走痛, running pain** [8]

IS of a pain affecting the extremities and body that appears to move from one location to another without apparent regularity. *TPSHF* 25: 治一切風及肢節**走痛**不可忍者，神效麝香丸方, "Wondrously effective recipe for pills with *she xiang* to cure all types of wind and unbearable **running pain** affecting extremities and joints".

Zou zhu **走注, running influx** [22] AN *zou zhou* 走疰, running attachment-illness.

PC of pain moving in the limbs and body so that the exact location of the pain cannot be determined. *ZBYHL* 24: 邪氣隨血而行，或淫奕皮膚，去來擊痛，遊走無有常所，故名為**走注**, "Evil qi moves with the blood, in some cases affecting the skin. A pain as if from a hit comes and goes. It roams around without a place to stay. Hence this is called '**running influx**'".

Zou zhu **走疰, running attachment-illness** [1]

PC identical with → *zou zhu* 走注, running influx. *PJF* 89 RE *shen li yuan* 神力圓, bolusses with divine power: 治手足失力…**走疰**作痛及癱緩等疾, "They cure hands and feet that have lost their strength, … as well as ailments such as **running attachment-illness** causing pain, paralysis and slackening".

Zu ding **足釘, foot pin** [1]

PC of a swelling rising on both foot soles. On top of it it develops sores like a black bean. It is hard like a metal pin. *BCGM* SE *fu zi* 附子 quotes *QJF*: **足釘**怪疾：兩足心凸腫，上生黑豆瘡，硬如釘，脛骨生碎孔，髓流出，身發寒顫，惟思飲酒, "The strange illness of **foot pin**: On the soles of both feet a swelling emerges. On top of it there grow sores like a black bean. They are as hard as a nail. The shinbones turn brittle and develop holes from which marrow is released. The body shivers from cold. [Patients] have but one desire: to drink wine".

Zu du **鏃毒, arrowhead poison** [2]

EA identical with → *jian du* 箭毒, arrow poison. *BCGM* SE *bei zi* 貝子 quotes *QJiF* 藥箭**鏃毒**：貝齒燒研，水服三錢，日三服, "For [harm caused by] **arrowhead poison** on a medicated arrow: roast cowrie shells and grind to powder. Ingest 3 *qian* with water. Three times a day".

Zu jian **足趼, callous feet** [2], AN *jiao jian* 脚趼, callous legs.

PC brought forth by excessive friction with the skin of the feet being injured, hardened, developing blisters, and giving a feeling when walking as ifstepped on a foreign body, accompanied by pain. *BCGM* SE *ban xia* 半夏 quoting *BHJJF*: 遠行**足趼**，方同上, "For **callous feet** after a long walk, the recipe is identical with thenamed above".

Zui liu **贅瘤, redundancy tumor** [2]

PC identical with → *liu* 瘤, tumor. *BCSY* SE *zhi dang* 蛭蟷：主一切疔腫，附骨疽蝕等瘡，宿肉**贅瘤**, "It controls all types of sores, such as pin-illness with swelling, as well as impediment-illnesses attached to the bones, and abiding flesh **redundancy tumors**".

Zui sou **晬嗽, brittle days cough** [2]

PC of cough in children within the first 100 days of their life. *BCGM* SE *bei mu* 貝母 quoting *HYXS* 百日內嬰孩，咳嗽有痰, "When the cough of children within the [first] 100 days of their life includes phlegm", writes: 小兒**晬嗽**，百日內咳嗽，痰壅, "**Brittle days cough** of children: This is cough within the first 100 days with phlegm obstruction".

Zuo ban chuang **坐板瘡, sores from sitting on the plank** [4]

PC of → *chuang* 瘡, sores, conditions developing on the buttocks and legs where one has been in contact with a wooden seat or chair. *BCGM* Bai bing zhu zhi yao 百病主治藥：胡麻生嚼，塗**坐板瘡**, "Chew fresh *hu ma* and smear the pulp on **sores from sitting on the plank**".

Zuo chuang **酢瘡, acid sores** [2] AN *cu chuang* 醋瘡, vinegar sores.

PC of → *chuang* 瘡, sores, conditions with a small and hard tip. *BCSY* SE *xian ren cao* 仙人草：主小兒**酢瘡**，煮湯浴，亦搗傅之, "It controls **acid sores** among children. Boil to prepare a decoction to be used for bathing.may also pound it to a pulp and apply externally".

***Zuo ma yong* 坐馬癰, horse-riding obstruction-illness** [1]
PC of → *yong* 癰, obstruction-illness, developing at the tips of the coccyx. It also develops where pressure is exerted when horse-riding. *BCGM* SE *fang che xian* 紡車弦：坐馬癰，燒灰傅之, "For **horse-riding obstruction-illness**: burn to ashes and apply externally".

***Zuo wai* 左喎, wryness on the left** [5]
IS of → *kou wai* 口喎, wryness, manifesting itself as slanting mouth corners on one's left side. *QJYF* 8: *QJYF* 8: 治中風面目相引，口偏僻…又方：酒煮桂取汁，以故布拓病上，正則止，**左喎**搨右，右喎搨左, "Another recipe to cure wind stroke pulling on the face and eyes, with the mouth slanting toside: Boil *gui* in wine and use the resulting liquid to rub on the diseased region. Stop when it has assumed its proper structure again. For **wryness on the left**, rub on the right. For wryness on the right, rub on the left".

***Zuo wo bu an* 坐臥不安, sitting and lying without finding rest** [3] AN *zuo wo bu de* 坐臥不得; *zuo xi bu de* 坐息不得, sitting without finding rest.
IS of patients who, because of vexation or rapid qi flow, feel uncomfortable in whatever position they assume with their body. *TPSHF* 6: 肺萎，咳唾如稠膠，日夜計升以上，**坐臥不安**，脅肋疼痛, "Lung wilting: cough and spittle are thick like glue, and by day and night the quantity exceeds*sheng*. [Patients] when **sitting or lying find no rest**. The flanks ache".

***Zuo wo bu de* 坐臥不得, inability to sit or lie down** [2]
IS identical with → *zuo wo bu an* 坐臥不安, sitting and lying without finding rest. *WTMY* 36: 療小兒上氣急滿，**坐臥不得**方, "Recipe to cure children with rapid qi rise and a feeling of fullness, as well as an **inability to sit or lie down**".

***Zuo xi bu de* 坐息不得, inability to sit and rest** [1]
IS identical with → *zuo wo bu an* 坐臥不安, sitting and lying without finding rest. *YXL* SE *ma dou ling* 馬兜鈴：主肺氣上急，**坐息不得**, "It controls rapid rise of lung qi, with an **inability to sit and rest**".

***Zuo zhang* 作脹, to distend** [7]
IS identical with → *zhang* 脹, distension. An uncomfortable feeling of being filled to bursting in the abdominal region. *SYDXF* 6: 感應丸，治積食停滯，脾胃**作脹**, "The 'pills that elicit a reaction' cure food accumulation and stagnation. The spleen and stomach **distend**".

***Zuo zhong* 作腫, to develop a swelling** [6]
IS identical with → *zhong* 腫, to swell; swelling. *QJYiF* 22: 治石發熱，熱結生腫堅起。始**作腫**，宜下之, "To cure an effusion of heat resulting from [the consumption of this] mineral, with heat nodes generating swelling with hardness. When the **swelling** is about **to develop**, it is advisable to purge it with a discharge".

3. Appendix 1

Book Titles Referred to and Quoted in the Dictionary Entries

BaSF:	*Bao shi xiao er fang* 鮑氏小兒方	Pediatric book. Early Ming era, or before. Lost.
BBSJ:	*Bing bu shou ji* 兵部手集	Recipe book. Tang era, early 9th century.
BCBS:	*Ben cao bie shuo* 本草別說	Materia medica book. Full title: *Chong kuang bu zhu shen nong ben cao jing bing tu jing* 重廣補注神農本草經并圖經. Song era, 1092.
BCF:	*Ji sheng ba cui fang* 濟生拔粹方	Recipe book. Yuan era, 1315.
BCGM:	*Ben cao gang mu* 本草綱目	Materia medica book. Ming era, 1593.
BCHB:	*Ben cao hui bian* 本草會編	Materia medica book. Ming era, ca. 1522~1539.
BCJJZ:	*Ben cao jing ji zhu* 本草經集注	Materia medica book.Liang era/North-South division. 500.
BCMQ:	*Ben cao meng quan* 本草蒙筌	Materia medica book. Ming era, 1565.
BCSY:	*Ben cao shi yi* 本草拾遺	Materia medica book. Tang era, 739.
BCTJ:	*Ben cao tu jing* 本草圖經	Materia medica book. Song era, 1061.
BCYY:	*Ben cao yan yi* 本草衍義	Materia medica book. Song era, 1116.
BCYYBY:	*Ben cao yan yi bu yi* 本草衍義補遺	Materia medica book. Yuan era, 1358 or earlier.
BHJJF:	*Bin hu ji jian fang* 瀕湖集簡方	Recipe book. Latter period of 16th century.
BJ:	*Shen nong ben cao jing* 神農本草經	Materia medica book. Presumably Han era.

BQSYZJYLJ:	*Bian Que shen ying zhen jiu yü long jing* 扁鵲神應針灸玉龍經	Acupuncture book. Yuan era, ca. 1295.
BYF:	*Bai yi fang* 百一方	General reference to books including the Tang era *Zhou hou bai yi fang* 肘後百一方, and the Song era *Bai yi xian fang* 百一選方.
BYTY:	*Bao ying ti yao* 保嬰撮要	Pediatric book. Ming era, 15th-16th century.
BYXF:	*Shi zhai bai yi xuan fang* 是齋百一選方	Recipe book. Southern Song era, 1196.
CJ:	*Cha jing* 茶經	Book on tea. Tang era, ca. 756~760.
CSXZ:	*Chi shui xuan zhu* 赤水玄珠	Medical case histories. Ming era.Not found in *BCGM*. 1573.
CXSYF:	*Chuan xin shi yong fang* 傳信適用方	Recipe book. Southern Song era, 1180.
CYLHSF	崔元 亮海上方	Recipe book. Tang era, early 9th century.
DMF:	*Dou men fang* 斗門方	Recipe book. Northern Song era or earlier.
DNBS:	*Duo neng bi shi* 多能鄙事	Book on agriculture. Ming era.
DRF:	*Du ren fang* 杜壬方	Recipe book. Northern Song era, first half of 11th century.
DSTJYF:	*De sheng tang jing yan fang* 德生堂經驗方	Recipe book. Yuan era.
DTQL:	*Dong tian qing lu* 洞天清錄	Miscellaneous contents. Song era, between 1237 and 1252.
DXF:	*Dan xiang fang* 單驤方	Recipe book. Northern Song era.
DXSJ:	*Dan xi shou jing* 丹溪手鏡	Book on clinical medicine. Early Ming era.
DXXF:	*Dan xi xin fa* 丹溪心法	Book on clinical medicine. Ming era, 1481.
DXZFXY:	*Dan xi zhi fa xin yao* 丹溪治法心要	Book on clinical medicine. Ming era, 1543.

DXZY:	*Dan xi zuan yao* 丹溪纂要	Book on clinical medicine. Ming era, 15th century.
FKBW:	*Nü ke bai wen* 女科百問	Gynecological book. Song era, 1279.
FKCY:	*Fu ke cuo yao* 女科撮要	Gynecological book. Ming era, 16th century.
FKJYMF:	*Feng ke ji yan ming fang* 風科集驗名方	Recipe book. Yuan era, ca. 1300.
FRDQLF:	*Fu ren da quan liang fang* 婦人大全良方	Gynecological book. Southern Song era, 1237.
FRLFBY:	*Fu ren liang fang bu yi jiao zhu* 婦人良方補遺校注	Gynecological book. Ming era, 15th century.
FYHXF:	*Fan ye he xiang fang* 范曄合香方	Miscellaneous contents. Southern Dynasties Song, 5th century.
GJF:	*Kai yuan guang ji fang* 開元廣濟方	Recipe book. Tang era, 723.
GJLY:	*Gu jin lu yan* 古今錄驗	Recipe book. Tang era, ca. 7th century.
GJYJ:	*Gu jin yi jian* 古今醫鑒	Book on clinical medicine. Ming era, 1576.
GSJYF:	*Gong shi jing yan fang* 龔氏經驗方	Recipe book. Ming era.
GZQF:	*Guai zheng qi fang* 怪證奇方	Book on internal medicine. Ming era, 1544.
GZYL:	*Ge zhi yu lun* 格致餘論	Book on medical theory. Yuan era, 1347.
HFJ:	*Hong fei ji lun* 鴻飛集論	Ophthalmological book. Ming era, 1556.
HJJF:	*Tai ping hui min he ji ju fang* 太平惠民和劑局方	Recipe book. Northern Song, 1107~1110.
HNHLJ:	*Huai nan hong lie jie* 淮南鴻烈解; Huai nan zi	Miscellaneous contents. Western Han era, 179~122 BCE.
HRXT:	*Huo ren xin tong* 活人心統	Book on internal medicine. Ming era, 1539.

HSF:	*Hai shi fang* 梅師方	Recipe books of identical title by different authors. Song era and later.
HSJYF	*Hai shang ji yan fang* 海上集驗方	Recipe Book. Tang era.
HSMF:	*Hai shang ming fang* 海上名方	Recipe book. Song era, 1165~1173.
HSYT:	*Han shi yi tong* 韓氏醫通	Book on clinical medicine. Ming era, 1522.
HXKY:	*Huo xin kou yi* 活幼口議	Pediatric book. Yuan era.
HYBC:	*Hai yao ben cao* 海藥本草	Materia medica book. Tang era to Five Dynasties era, 10th century.
HYKY	*Huo you kouyi* 活幼口议	Pediatric book. Yuan era.
HYQS:	*Huo you quan shu* 活幼全書	Pediatric Book. Ming era, 1495.
HYXS:	*Huo you xin shu* 活幼心書	Pediatric book. Yuan era, 1294.
JBF:	*Jian bian dan fang* 簡便單方	Recipe book. Ming era, 1522~1566.
JDTF:	*Ji de tang jing yan fang* 積德堂經驗方	Recipe book. Ming era.
JFBJF:	*Ji feng bei ji fang* 雞峰備急方	Recipe book. Southern Song era, 1133.
JFPJF:	*Ji feng pu ji fang* 雞峰普濟方	Recipe book. Song era.
JgXF:	*Jing xiao fang* 經效方	Recipe book. Northern Song era, or earlier.
JGYL:	*Jin gui yao lue* 金匱要略	Book on harm caused by cold. Han era, ca. 3rd century.
JiuJF:	*Jiu ji fang* 救急方; *Ji jiu liang fang* 急救良方	Recipe book. Northern Song era, or earlier. Ming era.

JiXF:	*Ji xiao fang* 集效方	Recipe book of identical title by three different authors, two of Northern Song era,of Ming-era. Full titles: *Yan shi xiao er fang lun* 閻氏小兒方論, 1119; *San feng zhang zhen ren shen su wan ying fang* 三豐張真人神速萬應方.
JiYF:	*Ji yan fang* 集驗方	Recipe book. Northern Zhou era, 6th century.
JJF:	*Ji ji fang* 濟急方	Recipe book. Full title: *Ji ji xian fang* 濟急仙方. Yuan era.
JJLF:	*Jiu ji liang fang* 救急良方	Recipe book. Ming, 1550.
JSF:	*Ji sheng fang* 濟生方	Book on clinical medicine. Southern Song era, 1253.
JSL:	*Ji shen lu* 稽神錄	Daoist book. Five Dynasties to Early Song era, 955.
JSTF:	*Ji shan tang jing yan fang* 積善堂經驗方	Recipe book. Ming, ca. 16th century.
JWYS:	*Jie wei yuan sou* 解圍元藪	Book on leprosy. Ming era, 1550.
JXCB:	*Jing xiao chan bao* 經效產寶	Gynecological book. Tang era, 847~859.
JXF:	*Jin xiao fang* 近效方	Recipe book. Tang era, 713-741.
JYBC:	*Jia you bu zhu Shen nong ben cao* 嘉祐補註神農本草	Materia medica book. Song era, 1060.
JYBJF:	*Ji yan bei ju fang* 集驗背疽方	Book on external medicine. Southern Song era, 1196.
JYF:	*Jing yan fang* 經驗方	Recipe book of identical titles by different authors of various eras.
JYHF:	*Jing yan hou fang* 經驗後方	Recipe book. Northern Song era, or earlier.
JYJC:	*Huang you jian yao ji chong* 皇祐簡要濟眾方	Recipe book. Northern Song era, 1051.
JYZF:	*Ji yao zhu fang* 集要諸方	Recipe book possibly with full title Yi lin ji yao 醫林集要 of Ming era.

KBBC:	*Kai bao xin xiang ding ben cao* 開寶新詳定本草 *Kai bao chong ding ben cao* 開寶重定本草	Materia medica book. Song era, ca. 973, and 974.
LBLY:	*Ling biao lu yi* 嶺表錄異	Book on geographical sceneries. Tang, 10th century.
LCCF:	*Liu chang chun fang* 劉長春方	Recipe Book. Full title: Mi chuan jing yan fang 秘傳經驗方. Ming era.
LGPZL:	*Lei gong pao zhi lun* 雷公炮炙論	Materia medica book. Song era.
LH:	*Lun heng* 論衡	Philosophy book. Eastern Han, 1st century CE.
LNWSF:	*Ling nan wei sheng fang* 嶺南衛生方	Recipe Book. Song era, 1264.
LS:	*Ling shu* 靈樞	Book on medical theory. 2nd centry BCE to 2nd century CE.
LSh:	*Lei shuo* 類說	Miscellaneous contents. Southern Song era, 1136.
LSJYF:	*Lin shi jing yan fang* 藺氏經驗方	Recipe Book. Ming era, or earlier.
LSMC:	*Lan shi mi cang* 蘭室秘藏	Book on clinical medicine. Jin/Yuan era, ca. 1251.
LSZ:	Li Shizhen 李時珍	Physician, author and team leader of *Ben cao gang mu* compilation. Ming era, 1518~1593.
LTY:	Le Tianyi 羅天益	Physician and author. Yuan era, 13th century.
LXJ:	*Lu xin jing* 顱囟經	Pediatric book. First quoted in → *ZBYHL* of 610.
LYW:	Li Yanwen 李言聞	Physician, author and father of → LSZ. Ming era, 15th-16th century.
MJ:	*Mai jing* 脈經	Book on pulse diagnosis. Wei era to Jin era, 3rd century.
MSF:	*Mei shi fang* 梅師方	Recipe Book. Sui or Tang era.
MTKH	Mao ting ke hua 茆亭客話	Anthology of novels. Northern Song era.

MXBT:	*Meng xi bi tan* 夢溪筆談	Miscellaneous contents. Northern Song, 11th century.
MYBL:	*Ming yi bie lu* 名醫別錄	Materia medica book. Wei era to Jin era, ca. 3rd century.
MYZZ:	*Ming yi za zhu* 明醫雜著	Book on clinical medicine. Ming era, 1502.
NJ:	*Nan jing* 難經	Book on medical theory. Later Han era, 1st – 3rd century.
NKTY:	*Nü ke ti yao* 女科撮要	Gynecological book. Ming era, 16th century.
NWSBHL:	*Nei wai shang bian huo lun* 內外傷辨惑論	Book on internal medicine. Jin/Yuan era, 1232.
PJBSF:	*Lei zheng pu ji ben shi fang* 類證普濟本事方	Book on clinical medicine. Southern Song era, 12th century.
PJF:	*Pu ji fang* 普濟方	Recipe book. Ming era, 1406.
PWL:	*Pi wei lun* 脾胃論	Book on internal medicine. Jin/Yuan era, ca. 1249.
QJF:	*Zhi qi ji fang* 治奇疾方	Recipe book. Southern Song era.
QJYF:	*Qian jin bei ji fang* 千金備急方	Comprehensive medical book. Tang era, 652.
QJYiF:	*Qian jin yi fang* 千金翼方	Comprehensive medical book. Tang era, 682.
QJZJ:	*Qi ju za ji* 起居雜忌	Miscellaneous contents. Age/author unknown.
QKMY:	*Qian kun sheng yi mi yun* 乾坤生意秘韞	Recipe Book. Ming era, ca. 15th century.
QXLF:	*Qi xiao liang fang* 奇效良方	Recipe Book. Ming era, ca. 1449.
QYXJ:	*Quan you xin jian* 全幼心鑒	Pediatric book. Ming era, 1468. Also quoted as → *Huo you xin shu* 活幼心書.
RCF:	*Ren cun tang jing yan fang* 仁存堂經驗方	Recipe Book. Yuan era.

RHZ:	*Ri hua zi zhu jia ben cao* 日華子諸家本草	Materia medica book. Song era, 968~975.
RMSQ:	*Ru men shi qin* 儒門事親	Comprehensive medical book. Jin era, ca. 13th century.
RYBC:	*Ri yong ben cao* 日用本草	Materia medica book. Yuan era, 1329.
RYJY:	*Ru yi jing yao* 儒醫精要	Book on medical theory. Ming era, 1528.
RZTJYF:	*Rui zhu tang jing yan fang* 瑞竹堂經驗方	Recipe Book. Yuan era, 1326.
RZZZF:	*Ren zhai zhi zhi fang* 仁齋直指方	Book on clinical medicine. Southern Song era, 1264.
SBC:	*Shu chong kuang ying gong ben cao* 蜀重廣英公本草	Materia medica book.Five Dynasties, Later Shu era, 938~964.
SHBZG:	*Shang han bai zheng ge* 傷寒百證歌	Book on harm caused by cold. Song era, 1132.
SHL:	*Shang han lun* 傷寒論	Book on harm caused by cold. Eastern Han era, ca. 3rd century.
SHLS	*Shang han liu shu* 傷寒六書	Encyclopedic book on harm caused by cold. Ming era, 1436~1449.
SHLY:	*Shang han lei yao* 傷寒類要	Book on harm caused by cold. Northern Song era, ca. 11th century.
SHLZHRS:	*Shang han lei zheng huo ren shu* 傷寒類證活人書	Book on harm caused by cold. Northern Song era, 1108.
SHMLL:	*Shang han ming li lun* 傷寒明理論	Book on harm caused by cold. Jin era, ca. 1142.
SHWZL:	*Shang han wei zhi lun* 傷寒微旨論	Book on harm caused by cold. Northern Song era, 1086.
SHZBL:	*Shang han zong bing lun* 傷寒總病論	Book on harm caused by cold. Northern Song era, before 1100.
SHZG:	*Shang han zhi ge* 傷寒直格	Book on harm caused by cold. Jin era.
SHZZZS:	*Shang han zheng zhi zhun sheng* 傷寒證治準繩	Book on harm caused by cold. Ming era, 1602.

SJSY:	*Shan ju si yao* 山居四要	Book on daily health regimen. Yuan era, 1360.
SJZL:	*Sheng ji zong lu* 聖濟總錄	Recipe Book. Northern Song era, ca. 1111~1117.
SLBC:	*Shi liao ben cao* 食療本草	Book on pharmaceutically used victuals. Tang era, ca. 713~739.
SLGJ:	*Shi lin guang ji* 事林廣記	Miscellaneous contents. Song era.
SLQL:	*Shi liu qiu lu* 使琉球錄	Historiography. Ming era, second half 16th century.
SM:	*Shi ming* 釋名	Etymological book. Eastern Han era, ca. 200 CE.
SQF:	*Shi quan bo jiu fang* 十全博救方	Recipe Book. Northern Song era.
SS:	Shen shi 深師	Medical books/recipe books named after physician and author of this name. Southern dynasties, Song/Qi era.
SSB:	*Sheng sheng bian* 生生編	Recipe Book. Ming era.
SSJXF:	*San feng Sun zhen ren shen su wan ying fang* 三豐張真人神速萬應方	Recipe Book. Ming ca. 15th/16th century.
SSLF:	*Su Shen liang fang* 蘇沈良方	Recipe Book. Southern Song era, 11th century.
SSSM:	*Shang shu*. Shuo ming 尚書 說命	One of the Confucian classical texts. Contents of pre-Han era, and later.
SW:	*Su wen* 素問	Book on medical theory and treatment. Han era, 2nd century BCE to 2nd century CE, with additions until Tang era.
SWBC:	*Shi wu ben cao* 食物本草	Book on pharmaceutically used victuals. Ming era, 16th century.
SWBJQYBMJ:	*Su wen bing ji qi yi bao ming ji* 素問病機氣宜保命集	Book on medical theory. Jin era, 1186.
SWXJYBS:	*Su wen xuan ji yuan bing shi* 素問玄機原病式	Book on medical theory. Jin era, 1186.

SXBC:	*Shi xing ben cao* 食性本草	Book on pharmaceutically used victuals. Southern Tang, ca. 937~957.
SYCZYS:	*San yuan can zan yan shou shu* 三元參贊延壽書	Book on daily health regimen. Yuan era, 1291.
SYDXF:	*Shi yi de xiao fang* 世醫得效方	Recipe book. Yuan era, 1337.
SYJYBZFL:	*San yin ji yi bing zheng fang lun* 三因極一病證方論	Book on disease etiology. Southern Song era, 1174.
SYSF:	*Shou yu shen fang* 壽域神方	Recipe book. Ming era, ca. 1403~1424.
SYSS:	*Shi yao shen shu* 十藥神書	Book on depletion conditions and blood spitting of unclear origin. Ca. Yuan/early Ming era.
SYXJ:	*Shi yi xin jing* 食醫心鏡	Book on pharmaceutically used victuals. Tang era, late 9th century.
SYZJ:	*Shu yuan za ji* 菽園雜記	Mscellaneous contents. Ming era, ca. 1488-1505.
SZRF:	*Shao zhen ren fang* 邵真人方	Recipe Book. Full title: *Mi chuan jing yan fang* 秘傳經驗方. Ming era, ca. 1459.
SZRSJ:	*Sun zhen ren shi ji* 孫真人食忌	Book on pharmaceutically used victuals. Unclear origin.
SZYS:	*Shen zhai yi shu* 慎齋遺書	Book on clinical medicine. Ming era, 1573.
SZZF:	*Shi zai zhi fang* 史載之方	Recipe Book. Northern Song era, 1085.
TBC:	*Xin xiu ben cao* 新修本草	Materia medica book. Tang era, 659.
TBYF:	*Shi yi tong bian yao fa* 世醫通變要法.	Book on clinical medicine. Ming era, 1539.
TPSHF:	*Tai ping sheng hui fang* 太平聖惠方	Recipe Book. Song era, 978-992.
TQFLLSF:	*Tai qing fu lian ling sha fa* 太清服煉靈砂法	Daoist book. Song era, or earlier.
TXL:	*Wai ke tong xuan lun* 外科通玄論	Book on external medicine. Ming era.

TYBC:	*Tang ye ben cao* 湯液本草	Materia medica book. Yuan era, ca. 1298.
TYJYF:	*Tang Yao jing yan fang* 唐瑤經驗方	Recipe Book. Ming era, or earlier.
TYWF:	*Tan ye weng fang* 談野翁方	Recipe Book. Ming era, ca. 15th century.
WKJY:	*Wai ke jing yi* 外科精義	Book on external medicine.Yuan era, 1335.
WKJYao:	*Wai ke jing yao* 外科精要	Book on external medicine.Southern Song era, 1263.
WKJYF:	*Wai ke ji yan fang* 外科集驗方	Book on external medicine.Ming era, 1498.
WKLL:	*Wai ke li li* 外科理例	Book on external medicine.Ming era, 1531.
WKZZ:	*Wai ke zheng zong zhi* 外科正宗	Book on external medicine.Ming era, 1617.
WRXXEF:	*Wang Ri xin xiao er fang* 王日新小兒方	Pediatric book. Ming era.
WSBJ:	*Wei sheng bao jian* 衛生寶鑒	Comprehensive medical book. Yuan era, 1281.
WSYJF:	*Wei sheng yi jian fang* 衛生易簡方	Recipe book. Ming era, 1423.
WSZX	*Wei sheng za xing* 衛生雜興	Recipe book. Ming era.
WTMY:	*Wai tai mi yao* 外台秘要	Recipe book. Tang era, 752.
XCWKJYF:	*Xian chuan wai ke ji yan fang* 仙傳外科集驗方	Recipe book for external medicine. Yuan era, ca. 13th century.
XEDZFL:	*Xiao er dou zhen fang lun* 小兒痘疹方論	Pediatric book. Song era, ca. 13th century.
XEJFMJ:	*Xiao er jing feng mi jue* 小兒驚風秘訣	Pediatric book. Ming era.
XEWSZWLF:	*Xiao er wei sheng zong wei lun fang* 小兒衛生總微論方	Pediatric book. Southern Song era.

XEYZZJ:	*Xiao er yao zheng zhi jue* 小兒藥證直訣	Pediatric book. Northern Song to Yuan era, 1119.
WLXGZ:	*Wu lei xiang gan zhi* 物類相感志	Miscellaneous contents. Song era.
XJ:	*Xian jing* 仙經	Daoist text. Unclear origin.
XMLF:	*Xuan ming lun fang* 宣明論方	Full title: *Huang di su wen xuan ming lun fang* 黃帝素問宣明論方. Recipe book. Jin era, 1172.
XPF:	*Xiao pin fang* 小品方	Recipe book. Jin era.
XQF:	*Xuan qi fang* 選奇方	Recipe book. Song era, ca. 13th century.
XQYJ:	*Xi qiao ye ji* 西樵野記	Miscellaneous contents. Ming era, ca. 1522-1566.
XSLSXDMF:	*Xian shou li shang xu duan mi fang* 仙授理傷續斷秘方	Book on external medicine. Unclear origin. Possibly Song era to Ming era.
XSTCF:	*Xu shi tai chan fang* 徐氏胎產方	Gynecological book. Ming era, ca. 14th/early 15th century.
XTS:	*Xin Tan shu* 新唐書	Historiography. Song era, 1044-1060.
XZF:	*Xiu zhen fang* 袖珍方	Recipe book. Ming era, 1390-1415.
YD:	*Lei gong yao dui* 雷公藥對	Materia medica book. Unclear origin.
YDXL:	*Yu deng xu lu* 餘冬敘錄; 餘冬序錄.	Miscellaneous contents. Ming era, 1528.
YEMB:	*Yang e man bi* 養痾漫筆	Miscellaneous contents. Southern Song era, ca. 1265-1274.
YFZY:	*Yi fang zhai yao* 醫方摘要	Recipe book. Ming era, 1572.
YHCF:	*Yao He chong fang* 姚和眾方	General reference to Yao Hechong’ s recipe books. Tang era.
YHJW:	*Yin hai jing wei* 銀海精微	Ophthalmological book. Ming era, 14th/15th century.
YJQW:	*Yuan ji qi wei* 原機啟微	Ophthalmological book. Ming era, 1370.

YJSJYF	*Yu Jiang shi jing yan fang* 禹講師經驗方	Recipe book of unknown origin.
YJWY:	*Yü ji wei yi* 玉機微義	Comprehensive book on clinical medicine. Ming era, 1368.
YJZ:	*Yi jian zhi* 夷堅志	Miscellaneous contents. Southern Song era, after 1198.
YKFH:	*You ke fa hui* 幼科發揮	Pediatric book. Ming era, 1579.
YKLC:	*You ke lei cui* 幼科類萃	Pediatric book. Ming era, 1536.
YLFQS	*Yang lao feng qin shu* 養老奉親書	Book on daily health regimen. Northern Song era to Yuan era, 1307.
YLJY:	*Yi lin ji yao* 醫林集要	Comprehensive medical book. Ming era, 1482.
YLQF:	*Yong lei qian fang* 永類鈐方	Recipe book. Yuan era, 1316-1331.
YS:	*Yi shuo* 醫說	Miscellaneous contents. Southern Song era, 1189-1224.
YSCRF:	*Yang shi chan ru ji yan fang* 楊氏產乳集驗方	Gynecological book. Tang era.
YSJCF:	*Yang shi jia cang fang* 楊氏家藏方	Recipe book. Southern Song era, 1178.
YSLYF:	*Ye shi lu yan fang* 葉氏錄驗方	Recipe book. Song era, 1186.
YSZL:	*Tai ding yang sheng zhu lun* 泰定養生主論.	Book on daily health regimen. Yuan era, 1338.
YSZY:	*Yin shan zheng yao* 飲膳正要	Book on pharmaceutically used victuals. Yuan era, 1330.
YTBW:	*Ying tong bai wen* 嬰童百問	Pediatric book. Ming era, ca. 15th century.
YXFM:	*Yi xue fa ming* 醫學發明	Book on clinical medicine. Jin/Yuan era, ca. 1251.
YXGM:	*Yi xue gang mu* 醫學綱目	Comprehensive book on clinical medicine. Ming era, late 14th century.
YXJC:	*Yi xue ji cheng* 醫學集成	Comprehensive book on clinical medicine. Ming era, 1515.

YXL:	*Yao xing lun* 藥性論	Materia medica book. Unclear origin; possibly before Song era.
YXQY:	*Yi xue qi yuan* 醫學啟源	Comprehensive medical book. Unclear origin.
YXRM:	*Yi xue ru men* 醫學入門	Comprehensive medical book. Ming era, 1575.
YXZC:	*Yi xue zheng chuan* 醫學正傳	Comprehensive book on clinical medicine. Ming era, 1515.
YYXF:	*Yong yao xin fa* 用藥心法	Materia medica book. Yuan era, ca. early 13th century.
YYXS:	*You you xin shu* 幼幼新書	Pediatric book. Song era, 1150.
YYZZ:	*You yang za zu* 酉陽雜組	Miscellaneous contents. Tang era, ca. 860.
YZ:	*Yao zhun* 藥准	Recipe book. Northern Song, ca. late 11th century.
ZBF:	*Zhi bao fang* 至寶方	Full title: *Chong tong yan ling zhi bao fang* 眾童延齡至寶方. Pediatric book. Tang era.
ZBYHL:	*Zhu bing yuan hou lun* 諸病源候論	Book on disease etiology. Sui era, 610.
ZBZZZS:	*Za bing zheng zhi zun sheng* 雜病證治準繩	Book on internal medicine. Ming era, 1602.
ZHBYF:	*Zhou hou bai yi fang* 肘後百一方	Recipe book. Southern Qi era, 500.
ZHF:	*Zhou hou bei ji fang* 肘後備急方	Recipe Book. Jin era, ca. 4th century.
ZJJYJ:	*Zhen jiu jia yi jing* 針灸甲乙經	Acupuncture book. Wei/Jin era, ca. 260.
ZJSHL:	*Zhu jie shang han lun* 註解傷寒論	Book on harm caused by cold. Jin era, ca. early 12th century.
ZJZSJ:	*Zhen jiu zi sheng jing* 針灸資生經	Acupuncture book. Southern Song era, ca. 1180~1195.
ZLBC:	*Zheng lei ben cao* 證類本草	Materia medica book. Northern Song era, late 12th century.
ZMML:	*Zi mu mi lu* 子母秘錄	Gynecological and pediatric book. Tang era.

ZNF:	*Zhi nan fang* 指南方	Recipe book. Northern Song era, ca. 11th century.
ZNZN:	*Zhang nüe zhi nan* 瘴瘧指南	Book on internal medicine. Ming era, 1609.
ZQZSHL:	*Zhang Qing zi Shang han lun* 張卿子傷寒論	Book on harm caused by cold. Late Ming era.
ZSF:	*Zhang shi fang* 張氏方	Recipe book. Possibly early Ming era.
ZSJYF:	*Zhu shi ji yan yi fang* 朱氏集驗醫方	Full title: *Lei bian Zhu shi ji yan yi fang* 類編朱氏集驗醫方. Recipe book. Southern Song era, 1265.
ZSYT:	*Zhang shi yi tong* 張氏醫通	Comprehensive book on clinical medicine. Qing era, 1695.
ZWZF:	*Zhang Wen zhong fang* 張文仲方	Recipe book. Tang era, 7th/8th century.
WSZX:	*Wei sheng za xing* 衛生雜興	Recipe book. Ming era.
ZXF:	*Zhai xuan fang* 摘玄方	Recipe book. Identical title of different books. Ming era.
ZYGLF:	*Zhen yuan guang li fang* 貞元廣利方	Full title: *Zhen yuan ji yao guang li fang* 貞元集要廣利方. Recipe Book. Tang era, 796.
ZYMZ:	*Zheng yin mai zhi* 症因脈治	Comprehensive book on clinical medicine. Ming era.
ZZJ:	*Zhong zang jing* 中藏經	Book on medical theory. Unclear origin.
ZZN:	*Zhen zhu nang* 珍珠囊	Full title: *Jie gu zhen zhu nang* 潔古珍珠囊; *Dong yuan zhen zhu nang* 東垣珍珠囊. Materia medica book. Song era, 13th century.
ZZNYXF:	*Zhen zhu nang yao xing fu* 珍珠囊補遺藥性賦	Full title: *Zhen zhu nang bu yi yao xing fu* 珍珠囊補遺藥性賦. Materia medica book. Early Ming era.
ZZYJ:	*Zheng zhi yao jue* 證治要訣	Comprehensive book on clinical medicine. Ming era, ca. 14th century.

4. Appendix 2

Pharmaceutical Substances Referred to in the Dictionary Entries.

Note: 1. The earlier a text mentioning pharmaceutical substances was compiled, the less certain one can be that today's botanical identification of a substance applies. 2. The botanical species given in the following list may not include all species covered by a Chinese plant name. Here only the most common identifications are provided as a first hint at the nature of a pharmaceutical substance referred to in a quote. 3. Substances of animal origin are given with their vernacular meaning. 4. Minerals are listed with their English names rather than chemical formulas wherever possible.

A bo le	阿勃勒	Cassia fistula L.
A jiao	阿膠	Ass hide glue
A wei	阿魏	Ferula assa foetida L.
A yue hun zi	阿月渾子	Pistacia vera L.
Ai	艾	Artemisia argyi Lèvl. et Vant.
Ai ye	艾葉	Leaves of → *Ai*
An lü	庵藺	Artemisia keiskeana Miq.
An shi liu	安石榴	Punica granatum L.
An xi xiang	安息香	Styrax benzoin Dryand.
Ba dou	巴豆	Croton tiglium L.
Ba ji tian	巴戟天	Morinda officinalis How.
Ba jiao	芭蕉	→ *Gan jiao* 甘蕉.
Ba qia	菝葜	Smilax Chinensis L.
Bai	柏	Platycladus orientalis (L.) Franco
Bai bi	敗筆	Decayed writing pen
Bai bu	百部	Stemona sessilifolia (Miq.) Franch. et Sav.
Bai bu gen	百部根	Roots of → *Bai bu*
Bai cao shuang	百草霜	Soot
Bai e	白堊	Chalk. Kaolin (bolus alba)
Bai e	白鵝	White goose
Bai e fen	白堊粉	→ *Bai e* 白堊
Bai fan	白礬	Alum
Bai fu zi	白附子	Aconitum coreanum (Levl.) Rapaics
Bai hao	白蒿	Artemisia sieversiana Ehrhart ex Willd.

Bai he	百合	Lilium brownii F.E. Brown ex Miellez var. viridulum Baker
Bai hu	白虎	→ *Shi hui* 石灰
Bai hua she	白花蛇	Embroidered pit viper
Bai ji	白棘	1. Zizyphus jujuba Mill. var. spinosa (Bunge) Hu ex H. F. Chow 2. Paliurus ramoissimus Poir.
Bai jia zhu	百家筯	Household chopsticks
Bai jiang	敗醬	Patrinia scabiosaefolia Fisch. ex Trev.
Bai jiang can	白僵蠶	Silkworm
Bai jiao	白膠	White glue prepared from deer antlers
Bai jie	白芥	Sinapis alba L.
Bai jing qiu yin	白頸蚯蚓	Earthworm with a hundred necks
Bai ju	白苣	Lactuca sativa L. var. romana Hort.
Bai la	白蠟	White wax
Bai lian	白蘞	Ampelopsis japonica (Thunb.) Makino
Bai ma jing	白馬莖	White horse penis
Bai ma yan	白馬眼	White horse eye
Bai mang bo	敗芒箔	Decayed bamboo tray
Bai mao	白茅	Imperata cylindrica (L.) Beauv. var. major (Nees) C. E. Hubb.
Bai piao	敗瓢	Broken gourd ladel
Bai pu xi	敗蒲席	Decayed rush mat
Bai qian	白前	Cynanchum stauntonii (Deone.) Schltr. ex Lèvl.
Bai qiu yin	白蚯蚓	White earthworm
Bai rang he	白蘘荷	Zingiber mioga Rose
Bai shao	白芍	→ *Shao yao* 芍藥
Bai shi	柏實	Fruit of → *Bai* 柏
Bai shi ying	白石英	Milky Quartz; crystalline silica
Bai shi zhi	白石脂	Kaolin (bolus alba)
Bai shi zi	白師子	"White lion". An apotropaic item: a white stone carved to resemble a lion
Bai tian gong	敗天公	Decayed bamboo hat
Bai tou weng	白頭翁	Pulsatilla chinensis (Bge.) Regel

Bai tu huo	白兔藿	Cynanchum caudatum Maxim.
Bai wei	白薇	Cynanchum atratum Bunge
Bai xian	白鮮	Dictamnus angustifolius G. Don ex Sweet.
Bai xian pi	白鮮皮	Skin of → *Bai xian* 白鮮
Bai xiong ji rou	白雄雞肉	Meat of a white rooster
Bai yang	白楊	Populus davidiana Dode
Bai yang pi	白楊皮	Skin of → *Bai yang* 白楊
Bai ye	柏葉	Leaves of → *Bai* 柏
Bai ying	白英	Solanum lyratum Thunb.
Bai you ma	白油麻	Light colored seeds of → *Hu ma* 胡麻
Bai zhi	白芷	Angelica dahurica (Fisch. ex Hoffm.) Benth. et Hook f. ex Franch. et Sav. cv. Hanbaizhi
Bai zhu	白朮	Atractylodes macrocephala Koidz.
Ban bian lian	半邊蓮	Lobelia chinensis Lour.
Ban bian shan	半邊山	Alternative name of *shui ku mai* 水苦蕒Veronica undulata Wall.
Ban mao	斑貓	Mylabris
Ban mao	斑蝥	→ *Ban mao* 斑貓
Ban tian he	半天河	Midday river; water that accumulates in the openings of the posts of bamboo fences and in tree holes
Ban xia	半夏	Pinellia ternata (Thunb.) Breit.
Bang	蚌	Clam
Bao	鴇	Bustard
Bao yu	鮑魚	Abalone
Bei mu	貝母	Fritillaria unibracteata Hsiao et K.C. Hsia
Bei ting sha	北庭砂	Sal Ammoniac
Bei zi	貝子	Arabic cowrie shell
Bi ba	蓽茇	Piper longum L.
Bi ba	蓽撥	→ *Bi ba* 蓽茇
Bi jie	萆薢	Dioscorea hypoglaucae Palib
Bi ma	蓖麻	Ricinus communis
Bi ma zi	蓖麻子	Seeds of → *Bi ma* 蓖麻
Bian qing	扁青	Azurite

Bian xu	萹蓄	Polygonum aviculare L.
Biao	鰾	→ *Biao jiao* 鰾膠
Biao jiao	鰾膠	Swimming bladder; fish glue
Bie	鱉	Soft-shelled turtle
Bie jia	鱉甲	Turtle shell
Bing lang	檳榔	Areca catechu L.
Bing ren yi	病人衣	A sick person' s garments
Bo he	薄荷	Mentha canadensis L.
Bo lao	伯勞	Shrike
Bo luo hui	博落回	Macleya cordata (Willd.) R. Br.
Bo mu	檗木	Phellodendron amurense Ruppr.
Bo pi	檗皮	Identical with *Huang bo* 黄檗, bark of Phellodendron amurense Ruppr.
Bo shang liu huang	舶上硫黄	White sulphur
Bu gu zhi	補骨脂	Psoralea corylifolia L.
Cai ju ji shi	蔡苴機屎	Excrement of elks with two heads
Can	蠶	Silkworm
Can tui	蠶退	Silkworm sloth
Cang er	蒼耳	→ *Cang er zi* 蒼耳子
Cang er zi	蒼耳子	Xanthium sibiricum Patr. Ex Widder
Cang zhu	蒼朮	Atractylodes lancea (Thunb.) DC.
Cao dou kou	草豆蔻	→ *Dou kou* 豆蔻
Cao hao	草蒿	Artemisia annua L.
Cao jue ming	草決明	→ *Qing xiang* 青葙
Cao long dan	草龍膽	Gentiana scabra Bge.
Cao wu	草烏	Aconitum kusnezoffii Reichb
Cao zhi zhu	草蜘蛛	Grass spider
Ce bai	側柏	→ *Bai* 柏
Ce zi	側子	Aconitum carmichaeli Debx.
Cha	茶	Tea
Chai hu	茈胡	→ *Chai hu* 柴胡
Chai hu	柴胡	Bupleurum chinense D.C.
Chan chu	蟾蜍	Toad

Chan fu ren mai shang cao	產死婦人冢上草	Herbs growing on the tomb of a woman who had died during delivery
Chan hua	蟬花	Cordyceps cicadae Shing
Chan su	蟾酥	Dried venom of toads; toad cake
Chan tuo	蟬蜕	Cicada slough
Chang pu	菖蒲	Acorus gramineus Ait. (M. Br.)
Chang shan	常山	1. Dichroa febrifuga Lour. 2. Root of Orixa japonica Th.
Chang shan shu qi	常山蜀漆	Root of → *Chang shan* 常山, Dichroa febrifuga Lour.
Che qian	車前	Plantago asiatica L.
Che qian zi	車前子	Seeds of → *Che qian* 車前
Chen lin mi	陳廩米	Oryza sativa L.
Chen pi	陳皮	Dried tangerine or orange peels
Chen sha	辰砂	Cinnabar
Chen xiang	沉香	Aquilaria agallocha (Lour.) Roxb.
Cheng zi pi	橙子皮	Orange peels
Chi fu ling	赤茯苓	→ *Fu ling* 茯苓
Chi he	赤赫	Unidentifible, obsolete substance
Chi jian	赤箭	Gastrodia elata B.
Chi shao yao	赤芍藥	Root of → *Shao yao* 芍藥. *Paeonia veitchii* Lynch.
Chi shi zhi	赤石脂	Red halloysite
Chi tong xie	赤銅屑	Red copper crumbs
Chi tou	鴟頭	Owl head
Chi xian	赤莧	Amaranthus tricolor, L.
Chi xiao dou	赤小豆	Vigna umbellata (Thunb.) Ohwi et Ohashi
Chi zhi	赤芝	→ *Zhi* 芝
Chong bai la	蟲白臘	Insect wax. Wax excreted by Ericerus pela on the twigs of Fraxinus chinensis or Ligustrum lucidum
Chong chu tou xi kang	舂杵頭細糠	Hulls pounded finely with the pestlehead: Ricebran
Chong tai yan	重台根	Paris polyphylla Smith var. yunnanensis (Franch.) Hand.
Chong wei	茺蔚	*Leonurus japonicus* Houtt.

Chong wei zi	茺蔚子	Seeds of → *Chong wei* 茺蔚
Chu	楮	Broussonetia papyrifera (L.) Vent.
Chu ji	樗雞	Red cicada
Chu sheng qi dai	初生臍帶	Umbilical cord of a first child
Chuan bao yu sheng	穿鮑魚繩	A rope pierced through an abalone
Chuan di tai	船底苔	Moss growing on the hulls of boats. Algae
Chuan jiao	川椒	→ *Shu jiao* 蜀椒
Chuan shan jia	穿山甲	Pangolin
Chuan xiong	川芎	→ *Xiong qiong* 芎藭
Chun	椿	→ *Chun chu* 椿樗
Chun	蓴	Brasenia schreberi J. F. Gmel.
Chun chu	椿樗	Ailanthus altissima (Mill.) Swingle
Ci gu	慈姑	Sagittaria trifolia L. var. sinensis (Sims.) Makino
Ci huang	雌黃	Orpiment
Ci mu	慈母	Unidentifiable type of trees
Cong	蔥	Allium fistulosum L.
Cong bai	蔥白	→ *Cong* 蔥
Cong zhi	蔥汁	Juice of → *Cong* 蔥
Cu	醋	Vinegar from millets, rice, wheat, or barley
Cu jiang cao	酢漿草	Oxalis corniculata L.
Cu lin zi	醋林子	Embelia subcoriacea C. B. Clarke
Da dou	大豆	Glycine max (L.) Merr.
Da dou chi	大豆豉	Bean relish, fermented soybeans
Da dou huang	大豆黃	The fermentation pellicle which forms on the top of bean powder
Da dou huang juan	大豆黃卷	Dried bean sprouts of → *Da dou* 大豆
Da hong xia zha	大紅蝦鮓	A fermented preparation: Minced red shrimps mixed with rice porridge and salt and allowed to ferment.
Da huang	大黃	Rheum palmatum L.
Da huang feng	大黃蜂	Hornet
Da ji	大戟	Euphorbia pekinensis Rupr.

Da ma	大麻	Cannabis sativa L.
Da ma ren	大麻人	Seeds of → *Da ma* 大麻
Da ma ren	大麻仁	Seeds of → *Da ma* 大麻
Da mai	大麥	Hordeum vulgare L.
Da qing	大青	1.Clerodendrum cyrtophyllum Turcz. 2. Isatis tinctoria L.. Indigo plant.
Da suan	大蒜	→ *Hu* 葫
Da yan	大鹽	Crude salt
Da zao	大棗	Ziziphus jujuba Mill. var. inermis (Bunge) Rehd.
Dai mao	瑇瑁	Hawksbill turtle
Dai zhe	代赭	→ *Dai zhe shi* 代赭石
Dai zhe shi	代赭石	Red Haematite, Bloodstone
Dan fan	膽礬	→ *Shi dan* 石膽
Dan sha	丹砂	Cinnabar, vermilion
Dan shen	丹參	Salvia miltiorrhiza Bunge
Dan xiong ji	丹雄雞	Red rooster
Dan zhu bing gen	淡竹並根	Bamboo with roots
Dan zhu gen	淡竹根	Phylostachys nigra var. henonis, (Mitford) Stapf ex Rendle
Dan zhu ru	淡竹茹	Bamboo shavings
Dang gui	當歸	Angelica sinensis (Oliv.) Diels
Dao	稻	Oryza sativa L. var. glutinosa Matsum.
Deng gua	冬瓜	Benincasa hispida (Thunb.) Cogn.
Deng hui	冬灰	"Winter ash". Ashes from grass and firewood accumulated in a stove during winter
Deng huo	燈火	Lamp wick fire
Deng xin cao	燈心草	Juncus effusus L.
Deng zhan you	燈盞油	Lantern cup oil
Di bu rong	地不容	Stephania delavayi Diels
Di dan	地膽	Beetle
Di fu	地膚	Kochia scoparia (L.) Schrad.
Di fu zi	地膚子	Fruit of → *Di fu* 地膚
Di gu pi	地骨皮	Lycium chinense Mill

Di huang	地黃	Rehmannia glutinosa (Gaertn.) Libosch. ex Fisch et Mey.
Di yu	地榆	Sanguisorba officinalis L.
Diao	吊	Fabulous creature with a snake' s head and an alligator' s body. Its fat is called *diao zhi* 吊脂
Diao teng	釣藤	Uncaria rhynchophylla (Miq.) Miq. ex Havil.
Ding xiang	丁香	Syzygium aromaticum (L.) Merr. et Perry
Dong bi tu	東壁土	Soil from a wall facing East
Dong hai fu ren	東海夫人	Mussels
Dong kui zi	冬葵子	Malva verticillata L.
Dong xiang qing ce ni kang zhong qing ni	東向圊廁溺坑中青泥	Greenish mud from a urinary pit in a latrine facing east
Dou chi	豆豉	→ *Da dou chi* 大豆豉
Dou kou	豆蔻	Alpinia katsumadai Hayata
Du fu yu	杜父魚	Sculpin
Du guan cao	都管草	Angelica kiusiana Maxim.
Du huo	獨活	Angelica pubescens Maxim. f. biserrata Shan et Yuan
Du ruo	杜若	Pollia japonica Hornst.
Du zhong	杜仲	Eucommia ulmoides Oliv.
Duan shi	鍛石	→ *Shi hui* 石灰
E shi	惡實	Arctium lappa L.
Fa pi	髮髲	Human hair removed from one' s head by cutting
Fan	礬	→ *Bai fan* 白礬
Fan shi	礬石	→ *Bai fan* 白礬
Fang che xian	紡車弦	Spinning wheel string
Fang feng	防風	Saposhnikovia divaricata (Turcz.).
Fang ji	防己	Aristolochia heterophylla Hemsl.
Fang jie shi	方解石	Calcite, chalk, calcspar
Fang kui	防葵	Peucedanum japonicum Thunb.
Fei fan	飛礬	→ *Bai fan* 白礬
Fei lian	蜚蠊	Cockroach
Fei lian	飛廉	Carduus crispus L.

Fei meng	蜚虻	Gadfly
Fei shi	榧實	Torreya grandis Fort. ex Lindl..
Fei zao jia	肥皂莢	Gymnocladus chinensis Baill.
Fen xi	粉錫	White lead, ceruse
Feng	蚌	Clam
Feng mi	蜂蜜	Honey
Feng xiang zhi	楓香脂	Liquidambar formosana Hance
Fu bi	腐婢	Flower of → *Chi xiao dou* 赤小豆
Fu ling	茯苓	Poria cocas (Schw.) Wolf
Fu long gan	伏龍肝	Oven earth
Fu pen zi	覆盆子	Rubus chingii Hu
Fu qi mo	釜臍墨	The black residue on a pan base after burning grass
Fu rong	芙蓉	→ *Lian hua* 蓮花
Fu she	蝮蛇	Pallas pit viper
Fu shen	茯神	Poria cocos (Schw.) Wolf
Fu shi	浮石	Pumice stone, porous lava
Fu xiong	撫芎	Ligusticum sinense Oliv.
Fu zi	附子	Aconitum carmichaeli Debx.
Gan	柑	Citrus chachiensis Hort.
Gan cao	甘草	Glycyrrhiza uralensis Fisch
Gan di huang	乾地黄	Dried → *Di huang*
Gan guo	甘鍋	Crucible used for melting metal utensils
Gan jiang	乾薑	Zingiber officinale Rosc.
Gan jiao	甘蕉	Musa sapientum L.
Gan ju hua	甘菊花	Flower of → *Ju* 菊
Gan lan	橄欖	Canarium album (Lour.) Raeusch.
Gan lan	甘藍	Brassica oleracea L. var. capitata L.
Gan lan he	橄欖核	Fruit of → *Gan lan* 橄欖
Gan pi	甘皮	Possibly *gan pi* 柑皮, peel of Citrus chachiensis Hort.
Gan qi	乾漆	Resin of → *Qi* 漆
Gan song xiang	甘松香	Nardostachys chinensis Batal.
Gan sui	甘遂	*Euphorbia kansui* T. N. Liou ex T. P. Wang

Gan zhe	甘蔗	Saccharum sinensis Roxb.
Gang tie	鋼鐵	Steel
Gang zi	剛子	→ *Ba dou* 巴豆
Gao ben	藁本	Ligusticum sinense Oliv.
Gao liang jiang	高良姜	Alpinia conchigera Griff.
Ge	葛	→ *Ge gen* 葛根
Ge fen	蛤粉	Clam shell powder
Ge gen	葛根	Pueraria lobata (Willd.) Ohwi
Ge li	蛤蜊	Clam
Ge shang ting chang	葛上亭長	Epicauta hirticornis Haag-Rutenberg
Gen dang zi	莨菪子	Hyoscyamus niger L.
Gen huang	根黃	Unidentifiable
Gong nu xian	弓弩弦	Crossbow string
Gou	狗	Dog
Gou bao	狗寶	A dog' s gallbladder/kidney stone
Gou ji	狗脊	Cimbotium barometz (L.) J. Smith
Gou ju	枸橘	Poncirus trifoliata (L.) Raf.
Gou qi	枸杞	Lycium barbarum L.
Gou she cao	狗舌草	Senecio kirilowii Turcz.
Gou shu	構樹	Broussonetia papyrifera (L.) L' Her ex Vent
Gou teng	鉤藤	→ *Diao teng* 釣滕
Gou wen	鉤吻	Gelsemium elegans (Gardn.et Champ.) Benth.
Gu jin hui	故錦灰	Ashed old brocade
Gu sui bu	骨碎補	Drynaria fortunei (Kunze) J. Smith
Gu wen qian	古文錢	Old copper coins
Gu yang	羖羊	Ram
Gu yang jiao	羖羊角	A ram's horn
Gu zi	菰子	→ *Tu jun* 土菌
Gua di	瓜蒂	Melon fruit base
Gua fu zhuang tou chen tu	寡婦床頭塵土	Dust from the head of a widow's bed
Gua lou	栝蔞	→ *Gua lou* 栝樓

Gua lou gen	栝樓根	Root of → *Gua lou*
Gua lou shi	栝蔞實	Fruit of → *Gua lou*
Gua lou	栝樓	Trichosanthes kirilowii Maxim.
Guan fen	官粉	→ *Fen xi* 粉錫
Guan gu	鸛骨	Bones of a crane
Guan gui	官桂	Quilled bark of → *Gui*
Guan jun	雚菌	White fungi growing in marsh lands
Guan zhong	貫眾	Dryopteris crassirhizoma Nakai
Gui	桂	Cinnamomum cassia Presl.
Gui chi	鬼齒	"Demons' teeth". Rotten bamboo roots
Gui fan	鬼扇	Belamcanda chinensis (L.) DC.
Gui gai	鬼蓋	Coprinus atramentarius (Bull. ex Fr.) Fr.
Gui jia	龜甲	Tortoise shell
Gui jiu	鬼臼	Dysosma versipellis (Hance) M. Cheng ex Ying
Gui xin	桂心	→ *Gui* 桂
Gui zhi	桂枝	Twigs of → *Gui* 桂
Ha jie	蛤蚧	Gecko
Hai ge	海蛤	Clam
Hai hong dou	海紅豆	Adenanthera pavonina L. var. microsperma (Teijsm. et Binnend.) Nielsen
Hai jin sha	海金沙	Lygodium japonicum (Thunb.) Sw.
Hai tong pi	海桐皮	Erythrina variegata L. var. orientalis (L.) Merr.
Hai zao	海藻	Sargassum fusiforme (Harv.) Setch.
Han fang ji	漢防己	→ *Fang ji* 防己
Han hao chong	寒號蟲	Flying squirrel
Han shui shi	寒水石	→ *Ning shui shi* 凝水石
He	荷	→ *Lian'ou* 蓮藕
He li lei	訶黎勒	Terminalia chebula Retz.
He ming cao	合明草	Aeschynomene indica L.
He shou wu	何首烏	Polygonum multiflorum Thunb.
He ye	荷葉	Leaf of → *Lian'ou* 蓮藕
He zi	訶子	→ *He li lei* 訶黎勒
He zi rou	訶子肉	Flesh of → *He li lei* 訶黎勒

Hei dou	黑豆	Glycine max (L.) Merr.
Hei shi zhi	黑石脂	Black halloysite
Hong dou kou	紅豆蔻	*Alpinia galanga* (L.) Willd.
Hong hua	紅花	→ *Hong lan hua* 紅藍花
Hong lan hua	紅藍花	Carthamus tinctorius L.
Hong zao	紅棗	Ziziphus jujuba Mill.
Hou pu	厚朴	Magnolia officinalis Rehd. et Wils.
Hu	狐	Fox
Hu	葫	Allium sativum L.
Hu	虎	Tiger
Hu	鵠	Swan
Hu cong	胡蔥	Allium cepa L.
Hu dou	胡豆	→ *Sha yuan ji li* 沙苑 芰藜
Hu fen	胡粉	→ *Fen xi* 粉錫
Hu gu	虎骨	Tiger bones
Hu gua	胡瓜	Cucumis sativus L.
Hu huang lian	胡黃連	Picrorhiza scrofulariiflora Pennell.
Hu jiao	胡椒	Piper nigrum L.
Hu lu	葫蘆	Lagenaria siceraria (Molina) Standl.
Hu ma	胡麻	Sesamum indicum L.
Hu ma you	胡麻油	Oil from the uncooked seeds of → *Hu ma* 胡麻
Hu po	琥珀	Amber
Hu rou	狐肉	Fox meat
Hu shi	槲實	Fruit of Quercus dentata Thunb.
Hu shu pi	槲樹皮	Bark of Quercus dentata Thunb.
Hu sui	胡荽	Coriandrum sativum L.
Hu tao	胡桃	Juglans regia L.
Hu tong lei	胡桐淚	Resin of Populus euphratica Oliv.
Hu yan ke nei tu	胡燕窠內土	Soil from the nest of a golden-rumped swallow
Hu yan ke tu	胡燕窠土	Soil from the nest of a golden-rumped swallow
Hu yin jing	狐陰莖	Fox penis
Hu zhang	虎掌	Arisaema thunbergii Bl.

Hu zhang	虎杖	Polygonum cuspidatum Sieb. et Zucc.
Hu zhang gen	虎杖根	Root of → *Hu zhang* 虎杖
Hua jiao	花椒	→ *Qin jiao* 秦椒
Hua ru shi	花乳石	Dolomite
Hua rui shi	花蕊石	Ophicalcite
Hua shi	滑石	Soapstone, talcum
Huai	槐	Sophora japonica L.
Huai jiao	槐膠	Glue prepared from → *Huai* 槐
Huai mu	淮木	Timber found as relics from ancient city dwellings
Huai shi	槐實	Fruit of → *Huai* 槐
Huai xiang zi	蘹香子	Foeniculum vulgare Mill.
Huan kun zhi	浣褌汁	Liquid resulting from washing trousers
Huang bo	黃柏	Phellodendron Chinense Schneid.
Huang bo	黃檗	→ *Huang bai* 黃柏
Huang da dou	黃大豆	Yellow soybean → *Da dou* 大豆
Huang dan	黃丹	→ *Qian dan* 鉛丹
Huang fan	黃礬	Yellow-colored alum
Huang han she	黃頷蛇	Beauty rat snake
Huang hua liao	黃花了	Unidentifiable
Huang huan	黃環	Wisteria chinensis, DC
Huang jin xie	黃金屑	Yellow gold crumbs
Huang jü pi	黃橘皮	Yellow peel of ripe → *Jü* 橘
Huang kui zi	黃葵子	Seeds of Abelmoschus moschatus (L.) Medik
Huang lian	黃連	Coptis chinensis Franch.
Huang ming jiao	黃明膠	Glue prepared from the hide of deer or oxen
Huang qi	黃芪	→ *Huang qi* 黃耆
Huang qi	黃耆	Astragalus membranaceus Bunge var. mongolicus (Bunge) P. K. Hsiao
Huang qin	黃芩	Scutellaria baicalensis Georgi, Sc. amoena C.H. Wright
Huang shi zhi	黃石脂	Yellow clay
Huang tu	黃土	Loess

Huang yao gen	黃藥根	Dioscorea bulbifera L.
Huang yao zi	黃藥子	Clematis terniflora DC
Hui hua	槐花	Sophora japonica L.
Hui xiang	茴香	Foeniculum vulgare Mill.
Huo	藿	Bean leaves
Huo shi	活師	Tadpole
Huo xiang	藿香	Agastache rugosa (Fisch. et Mey.) O. Kuntze
Ji	雞	Chicken
Ji	薺	Capsella bursa-pastoris (L.) Medic.
Ji	稷	Panicum miliaceum L.
Ji mi	稷米	→ *Ji* 稷
Ji bi zhi li huang pi	雞胜胵里黃皮	The yellow skin inside a bird's stomach
Ji chang cao	雞腸草	Trigonotis peduncularis (Trev.) Benth.ex Baker et Moore
Ji ji	及己	Hepatica nobilis Schreb. var. asiatica (Nakai) Hara
Ji li	蒺藜	Tribulus terrestris R.
Ji li zi	蒺藜子	Seeds of → *Ji li* 蒺藜
Ji mi	稷米	Panicum miliaceum L.
Ji mi	穄米	→ *Ji mi* 稷米
Ji ni	薺苨	Adenophora trachelioides Maxim.
Ji ti bi sheng	屐屜鼻繩	String used to tie a wooden sandal to the ankles
Ji tou shi	雞頭實	Seeds of Euryale ferox Salisb.
Ji xue cao	積雪草	Centella asiatica (L.) Urban
Ji yu	鯽魚	Bream
Ji zi	雞子	Chicken egg
Jia jian	甲煎	Made from operculum of the sea-snail mixed with lignum Aloes, musk and various medicinal flowers
Jia su	假蘇	Schizonepeta multifida (L.) Briq.
Jia ya	家鴨	White duck
Jia yu	嘉魚	Fish of unclear identification
Jia zhu rou	豭豬肉	Meat of a male piglet
Jian dao cao	剪刀草	Sagittaria trifolia L.

Jian dao gu	剪刀股	Ixeris debilis A. Gray
Jiang	姜	→ *Sheng jiang* 生薑
Jiang huang	薑黃	Curcuma longa L.
Jiang qian	姜錢	"Ginger coin". A round slice of ginger the size of a copper coin.
Jiang shi	姜石	"Ginger stone"; gravel.
Jiang shui	漿水	Vinegar produced by fermentation of millet-like grains
Jiang zhen xiang	降真香	Acronychia pedunculata (L.) Miq.
Jiao long	蛟龍	The flood dragon
Jiao yu pi	鮫魚皮	Shark skin
Jie du zi	解毒子	Stephania epigaea H.S. Lo.
Jie geng	桔梗	Platycodon grandiflorus (Jacq.) A. DC.
Jin	金	Native gold
Jin cao	藎草	Arthraxon hispidus (Thunb.) Makino
Jin hua	金花	Lonicera japonica Thunb.
Jin lan shui	浸藍水	Water that was used to prepare indigo
Jin shu	槿樹	Althaea frutex Hort. ex Mill.
Jin xian fan	金線礬	Fibroferrite
Jin xing shi	金星石	Biotite; golden or brown Mica
Jin ya	金牙	Iron pyrites
Jing	粳	Oryza sativa L.
Jing hua shui	井花水	Splendid well water; collected between the 3rd and fifth hour at the day of Li qiu 立秋 (Aug 7)
Jing jie	荊芥	Schizonepeta tenuifolia Briq.
Jing jing	荊莖	Stem of Vitex negundo L. Var. cannabifolia (Sieb. Et Zucc.) Hand.- Mazz.
Jing li	荊瀝	Sap from the stems of Vitex negundo L. Var. cannabifolia (Sieb. Et Zucc.) Hand.- Mazz
Jing mi	粳米	→ *Jing* 粳
Jing quan shi	井泉石	Stones from wells and springs
Jing quan shui	井泉水	Water from wells and springs
Jing san leng	京三棱	Sparganium stoloniferum (Graebn.) Buch.-Ham. ex Juz.

Jing tian	景天	Hylotelephium erythrostictum (Miq.) H. Ohba
Jing zhong tai ji ping	井中苔及萍	Moss and duckweed growing in a well
Jiu	酒	Wine
Jiu	韭	Allium tuberosum Rottl. ex Spreng.
Ju	櫸	Zelkova schneideriana Hand.-Mazz.
Ju	橘	Citrus reticulata Blanco
Ju	菊	Dendranthema morifolium (Ramat) Tzvel.
Ju hua	菊花	Flower of → *Ju* 菊
Ju jiang	蒟醬	Piper betle, L.
Ju pi	橘皮	Peel of *Ju* 橘
Ju sheng zi	巨勝子	→ *Hu ma* 胡麻
Ju you	橘柚	Tangelo
Juan	絹	Silk
Juan bai	卷柏	Selaginella involvens Spr.
Jue chuang	爵床	Rostellularis procumbens (L.) Nees.
Jue ming	決明	Cassia tora L.
Jue ming zi	決明子	Seeds of → *Jue ming* 決明
Jun da	莙薘	Beta vulgaris L.
Ke	珂	Inferior type of jade
Kong gong nie	孔公糵	Middle part of the stalactite which posesses a hole in the centre.
Kong qing	空青	Malachite, large hollow variety
Kou jin tuo	口津唾	Saliva
Ku ao	苦芺	Cirsium lineare Thunb.
Ku cai	苦菜	Sonchus oleraceus L.
Ku fan	枯礬	Burnt alum
Ku hu	苦瓠	Lagenaria siceraria (Molina) Standl. var. microcarpa (Naud.) Hara
Ku ju	苦苣	1. *Ixeris chinensis* (Thunb.) Nakai subsp. *versicolor* (Fisch. ex Link) Kitam. 2. → *Ku cai* 苦菜
Ku shen	苦參	Sophora flavescens Ait.
Ku zao	苦棗	Eleutharrhena macrocarpa (Diels) Forman
Ku zhu ru	苦竹茹	Bitter bamboo shavings

Ku zhu sun	苦竹筍	Bitter bamboo shoots
Kuai	鱠	Chinese herring
Kuan dong hua	款冬花	Tussilago farfara L.
Kui	葵	Malva verticillata L.
Kui cai	葵菜	→ *Kui* 葵
Kui gen	葵根	Roots of → *Kui* 葵
Kun bu	昆布	Laminaria japonica Aresch.
Kun dang	褌襠	Crotch of trousers
Kuo yu	蛞蝓	Slug
La xue	臘雪	"Snow of the *la* 臘-period"; winter snow collected in the twelfth month of the lunar year.
Lai fu	萊菔	Raphanus sativus L.
Lai lan	萊藍	Herbal drug of unclear identity
Lan	藍	1. (*Liao lan* 蓼藍) Polygonum tinctorium Lour. 2. (*Song lan* 菘籃) Isatis indigofera L. 3. (*Ma lan* 馬藍) Baphicacanthus cusia (Nees) Bremek 4. (*Mu lan* 木藍) Indigofera tinctoria L.
Lan dian	藍澱	Indigo, "Blue sediment"
Lan shi	藍實	Fruit of → *Lan* 藍
Lang dang	莨菪	Hyoscyamus niger F.W.Schmidt
Lang dang zi	莨菪子	Seeds of → *Lang dang* 莨菪
Lang du	狼毒	1. Stellaria chamaejasme L. 2. Euphorbia fischeriana Steud. 3. Aconitum lycoctonum L.
Lao ya suan	老鴉蒜	→ *Shi suan* 石蒜
Lei shu	鸓鼠	Flying squirrel
Lei wan	雷丸	Fungus Omphalia lapidescens Schroet.
Li	李	Prunus salicina Lindl.
Li	栗	Castanea molissima L.
Li chang	鱧腸	Eclipta prostrata L.
Li he ren	李核仁	Kernel of → *Li* 李
Li lu	藜蘆	Veratrum nigrum L.
Li mu zi	梨母子	Citrus limon

Li shi	理石	Variety of gypsum, alabaster
Li shi	蠡實	Iris lactea Pall. var. chinensis (Fisch.) Koidz.
Li shu gen	李樹根	Root of the → *Li* 李 tree
Li yu	鯉魚	Carp
Li yü	鱧魚	Snakehead
Li yü dan	鯉魚膽	Carp gallbladder
Li zhi he	荔枝核	Litchi stones
Lian fang	蓮房	Seedpod of → *Lian ou* 蓮藕.
Lian hua	蓮花	Flower of → *Lian ou* 蓮藕.
Lian ou	蓮藕	Nelumbo nucifera Gaertn.
Lian qiao	連翹	Forsythia suspensa (Thunb.) Vahl.
Lian shi	楝實	Fruit of Melia azedarach L.
Lian zi xin	蓮子心	Dried young cotyledon and radicle of ripe seeds of Nelumbo nucifera Gaertn.
Liang zi mu	椋子木	Cornus macrophylla Wallich.
Liao	蓼	Polygonum hydropiper L.
Liao qiao	蓼蕎	Allium macrostemon Bge.
Liao zi	蓼子	Polygonum criopolitanum Hance
Lin shi	淋石	Bladder stones excreted with the urine
Ling huo	零藿	1. Agastache rugosa (Fisch. et Mey.) O. Kuntze 2. Pogostemon cablin (Blanco) Benth.
Ling li	鯪鯉	Pangolin
Ling li jia	鯪鯉甲	Pangolin shell
Ling ling xiang	零陵香	Ocimum basilicum L.
Ling xiao hua	凌霄花	Campsis grandiflora (Thunb.) K. Schum.
Ling yang	羚羊	Antilope
Ling yang	麢羊	Fabled *ling*
Ling yang jiao	羚羊角	Antilope horn
Liu	柳	Salix babylonica L.
Liu chu mao ti jia	六畜毛蹄甲	Hair and hoof nails of the six domestic animals
Liu hua	柳華	Cotton down of the seeds, including the catkins, of → *Liu* 柳
Liu huang	硫黄	Sulphur

Liu shui	流水	Running water from rivers and creeks
Long chi	龍齒	Dragon teeth, fossil bones and teeth of extinct reptiles and mammals, furnishing Ca and P
Long dan	龍膽	Gentiana scabra Bunge
Long dan cao	龍膽草	→ *Long dan* 龍膽
Long gu	龍骨	→ *Long chi* 龍齒
Long nao	龍腦	→ *Long nao xiang* 龍腦香
Long nao xiang	龍腦香	Dipterocarpus tubinatus Gaertn. f.
Long tai	龍胎	Possibly petrified fossils
Long zhu	龍珠	Tubocapsicum anomalum (Franch. et Sav.) Makino
Lou gu	螻蛄	Mole cricket
Lou lan zi	漏籃子	Aconitum carmichaeli Debx.
Lou lu	漏蘆	Rhaponticum uni-florum (L.) DC
Lu	蘆	Phragmites communis Trin.
Lu	鹿	Deer
Lü cao	葎草	Humulus scandens (Lour.) Merr.
Lu ci	鸕鷀	Cormorant
Lu ci shi	鸕鷀屎	Cormorant urine
Lü dou	綠豆	Vigna radiata (L.) R. Wilczak
Lu er	鹿茸	Pilose deer horn
Lü fan	綠礬	Green Vitriol, Ferrous sulphate
Lu gan shi	爐甘石	Zincspar, zinc carbonate
Lu jian	鹵鹼	Alkali
Lu jiao	鹿角	Deer horn
Lu mao	驢毛	Donkey fur
Lü qing	綠青	Malachite, fine granular variety; basic copper carbonate
Lu ru	驢乳	Donkey milk
Lü ru	藺茹	Euphorbia ebracteolata Hayata.
Lü ru	閭茹	→ *Lü ru* 藺茹
Lu zhi	麋脂	Elk fat
Lu zhong chong	蘆中蟲	Insects collected from common reed

Luan hua	欒華	Koelreuteria paniculata Laxm.
Luo bo	蘿卜	Raphanus sativus L.
Luo fen	螺粉	Powder prepared from spiral shells
Luo kui	落葵	Basella alba L.
Luo le	羅勒	Ocimum basilicum L.
Luo shi	絡石	Trachelospermum jasminoides (Lindl.) Lem.
Luo si	螺螄	Spiral shell, snail
Luo su	落蘇	Solanum melongena L.
Luo xin fu	落新婦	Astilbe chinensis (Maxim.) Franch.et Sav.
Ma	馬	Horse
Ma bian cao	馬鞭草	Verbena officinalis L.
Ma bing lang	馬檳榔	Capparis masaikai Lévl.
Ma bo	馬勃	Calvatia lilacina (Mont. et Berk.) Lloyd
Ma bo	麻勃	→ *Da ma* 大麻
Ma chi xian	馬齒莧	Portulaca oleracea L.
Ma dao	馬刀	Razor clam
Ma dou	麻豆	→ *Yun shi* 雲實
Ma dou ling	馬兜鈴	Aristolochia contorta Bunge
Ma fen	麻蕡	1. Flower of → *Da ma* 大麻. 2. Capsule with seeds of → *Da ma* 大麻
Ma hua	麻花	Flower of → *Da ma* 大麻
Ma huang	麻黃	Ephedra sinica Stapf.
Ma lan	馬蘭	Kalimeris indica (L.) Sch.-Bip.
Ma lin	馬藺	Iris pallasii Fisch. var. chinensis Fisch.
Ma lu	馬陸	Millipede
Ma pi bo	馬窠勃	Calvatia lilacina (Mont. et Berk.) Lloyd
Ma ren	麻仁	Seeds of *Da ma* 大麻
Ma xian hao	馬先蒿	Pedicularis resupinata L.
Ma xie	麻鞋	Hemp sandals
Ma ya xiao	馬牙硝	→ *Mang xiao* 芒硝.
Ma ya xiao	馬牙消	→ *Mang xiao* 芒硝.
Ma you	麻油	Oil of sesamum indicum L.
Ma zao	馬藻	Potamogeton crispus L.
Ma zi	麻子	Seeds of *Da ma* 大麻

Mai men dong	麥門冬	Ophiopogon japonicus (L.f.) Ker-Gawl.
Man jing shi	蔓荊實	Fruit of Vitex trifolia L.var. simplicifolia Cham
Man jing zi	蔓菁子	→ *Man jing shi* 蔓荊實
Man li yu	鰻鱺魚	Eel
Man li yü zhi	鰻鱺魚脂	Fat of → *Man li yu* 鰻鱺魚
Mang cao	莽草	Illiceum lanceolatum A. C. Smith
Mang xiao	芒消	Mirabilite. Glauber's salt
Mao	貓	Cat
Mao gen	茅根	Root of Imperata cylindrica Beauv. var. major (Nees) C. E. Hubb.
Mao xiang hua	茅香花	Inflorescence of Hierochloe odorata (L.) Beauv.
Mei	梅	Armeniaca mume Sieb. [Prunus mume Sieb. et Zucc.]
Mei shi	梅實	Fruit of → *Mei* 梅
Meng shi	礞石	Micacous earth
Mi	蜜	Honey
Mi feng	蜜蜂	Honey bee
Mi hou tao	獼猴桃	Actinidia chinensis Planch.
Mi jiao	麋角	Elk horn
Mi la	蜜蠟	Bee wax
Mi meng hua	蜜蒙花	Buddleia officinalis Maxim.
Mi rou	麋肉	Elk meet
Mi tuo seng	蜜陀僧	Lithargyrum
Mi wu	蘼蕪	Young leaves of → *Xiong qiong* 芎藭
Mi zhi	麋脂	Elk fat
Ming	茗	Camellia sinensis L.
Ming fan	明礬	Alum
Mo li	茉莉	Jasminum sambac (L.) Ait.
Mo yao	沒藥	Commiphora Myrrha Engl.
Mu bie zi	木鱉子	Momordica cochinchinensis (Lour.) Spreng.
Mu dan	牡丹	Paeonia suffruticosa Andr.
Mu dan pi	牡丹皮	Bark of the root of → *Mu dan* 牡丹
Mu fu rong	木芙蓉	Hibiscus mutabilis L.

Mu gou yin jing	牡狗陰莖	Dog's penis
Mu gua	木瓜	Chaenomeles speciosa (Sweet) Nakai
Mu gua he	木瓜核	Kernels of → *Mu gua* 木瓜
Mu gui	牡桂	→ *Gui* 桂
Mu he	木核	Fruit pit of unclear identity
Mu jin	木槿	Hibiscus syriacus L.
Mu lan	木蘭	Magnolia amoena Cheng; M. sieboldii K. Koch.
Mu li	牡蠣	Oyster
Mu lian	木蓮	Ficus pumila L.
Mu meng	木虻	Awl-fly
Mu tian liao	木天蓼	Actinidia polygama (Sieb. et Zucc.) Maxim.
Mu tong	木通	→ *Tong cao* 通草
Mu xiang	木香	Aucklandia lappa Decne
Mu zei	木賊	Hippochaete hiemale (L.) Borher
Na qi xi	那耆悉	Tree of unclear identity growing in the south-west of China
Nan xing	南星	→ *Tian nan xing* 天南星
Nao sha	硇砂	Sal ammoniac, Ammonium chloride
Ni bai yin	溺白垽	Sediments of human urine
Nie mi	糵米	Malted grains from rice, millets, barley, beans
Ning shui shi	凝水石	Calcareous Spar; Gypsum
Niu	牛	Ox; cow
Niu bang bo tuo	牛蒡餺飥	Cooked wheaten food prepared from Arctium lappa, L.
Niu gan	牛肝	Ox liver
Niu huang	牛黃	Bovine bezoar
Niu jiao	牛角	Ox horn
Niu jiao sai	牛角鰓	The bone in an ox horn
Niu shi	牛虱	Ox louse
Niu xi	牛膝	Achyranthes bidentata Bl.
Nü wei	女萎	Clematis apiifolia DC.
Nüe gui	瘧龜	Turtle and shellfish
Ou shi	藕實	Seeds of → *Lian ou* 蓮藕.

Ou shi jing	藕實莖	Seeds and stalk of → *Lian ou* 蓮藕.
Peng e zhu	蓬莪术	Curcuma aeruginosa Roxb.
Peng sha	蓬砂	Borax, Sodiumborat
Pi li zhen	霹靂針	Meteorites, minerals containing iron
Pi pa	枇杷	Eriobotrya japonica (Thunb.) Lindl.
Pi pa ye	枇杷葉	Leaves of → *Pi pa* 枇杷
Pi shuang	砒霜	Arsenic
Po xiao	朴硝	→ *Po xiao* 朴消
Po xiao	朴消	Crude Glauber's Salt, Mirabilite; Sodium sulphate
Pu huang	蒲黄	Pollen of Typha orientalis Presl.
Pu sa shi	菩薩石	Quartz
Pu sun	蒲筍	Shoots of Typha orientalis Presl.
Pu tao	葡萄	Vitis vinifera L.
Qi	漆	Toxicodendrum vernicifluum (Stokes) F. A. Barkl.
Qi cao	蠐螬	Dung beetle
Qi cao kou ye	蠐螬口液	Spittle of the dung beetle
Qi lin jie	騏麟竭	Daemonorops draco Bl.
Qian	鉛	Lead
Qian cao	茜草	Rubia cordifolia L.
Qian dan	鉛丹	Minium; red oxide of lead, lead tetroxide Pb_3O_4.
Qian fen	鉛粉	Ceruse, lead carbonate
Qian gen	茜根	Root of Rubia cordifolia L.
Qian guang shi	鉛光石	Unidentifiable mineral
Qian hu	前胡	Peucedanum praeruptorum Dunn.
Qian jin teng	千金藤	Stephania japonica (Thunb.) Miers
Qian niu zi	牽牛子	Pharbitis nil (L.) Choisy
Qian shi	芡實	Euryale ferox Salisb. ex DC..
Qian shuang	鉛霜	Lead acetate
Qian sui lei	千歲蘽	Vitis flexuosa Thunb.
Qiang huo	羌活	Notopterygium incisum Ting ex H. T. Chang
Qiang lang	蜣螂	Dung beetle

Qiao	雀	Sparrow
Qiao mai	蕎麥	Fagopyrum esculentum Moench.
Qiao nao xiong	雀腦芎	→ *Xiong qiong* 芎藭
Qiao weng	雀瓮	Cocoon of the slug-caterpillar
Qie	茄	→ *Qie zi* 茄子
Qie gen	茄根	Root of → *Qie zi* 茄子
Qie zi	茄子	Solanum melogena L.
Qin bai pi	秦白皮	Dried bark of Fraxinus rhynchophylla Hance
Qin gui	秦龜	Turtles found in the mountains of Qin
Qin hua	芹花	Celery flowers
Qin jiao	秦椒	Zanthoxylum amatum DC.
Qin jiao	秦艽	Gentiana macrophylla Pall.
Qin pi	秦皮	Fraxinus rhynchophylla Hance
Qing dai	青黛	Indigo prepared from → *Lan* 藍, different Indigo-plants, with lime
Qing fan	青礬	→ *Lü fan* 綠礬
Qing fen	輕粉	→ *Shui yin fen* 水銀粉
Qing hao	青蒿	Artemisia carvifolia Buch.-Ham.ex Roxb.
Qing jing gan shi xin fan	青精乾石䭀飯	Rice/ Oryza sativa L; Gramineae. "dried black rice", rice boiled with the shoots of Vaccinium bracteatum Thunb., Ericaceae, to dye it black.
Qing lang gan	青琅玕	1. Obtained from the sea: Coral 2. Obtained from the mountains: Malachite
Qing mu xiang	青木香	→ *Mu xiang* 木香
Qing xiang	青葙	Celosia argentea L.
Qing xiang zi	青葙子	Seeds of → *Qing xiang* 青葙
Qing yan	青鹽	→ *Rong yan* 戎鹽
Qing yang gan	青羊肝	A black sheep's liver
Qing yu	青魚	Black carp
Qing zhu ru	青竹茹	Green shavings of Bambusa tuldoides Munro
Qiu	楸	Catalpa bungei C.A. Mey.
Qiu jin	蚯蚓	Earthworm
Qiu shi	秋石	Processed sediments obtained from human urine

Qu	麴	Yeast
Qu	曲	→ *Qu* 麴
Qu mai	瞿麥	Dianthus superbus S.
Qu yu	鴝鵒	Myna
Qu yu rou	鴝鵒肉	Myna flesh
Que luan	雀卵	Sparrow eggs
Que shi	雀屎	Sparrow droppings
Que weng	雀瓮	Cocoon of the slug caterpillar
Ran she	蚺蛇	Boa constrictor
Ran she dan	蚺蛇膽	Gallbladder of boa constrictor
Rang he	蘘荷	Zingiber mioga (Thunb.) Rosc.
Rao hua	蕘花	Wikstroemia canescens (Wall.) Meissn.
Re tang	熱湯	Hot, boiled water
Ren dong	忍冬	Lonicera japonica Thunb.
Ren kui	人傀	Human monstrosities
Ren niao	人溺	Human urine
Ren niao	人尿	Human urine
Ren ru	人乳	Human milk
Ren ru zhi	人乳汁	→ *Ren ru* 人乳
Ren shen	人參	Panax ginseng C. A. Meyer
Ren shi	人屎	Human feces
Ren shi	人虱	Lice gathered from humans
Ren xue	人血	Human blood
Ren zhong bai	人中白	White sediments collecting on the bottom of a urine receptacle
Ren zi	荏子	→ *Su zi* 蘇子
Rong shou	狨獸	Marmoset, Hapale Jacchus
Rong yan	戎鹽	Crystal salt. “Salt from the Rong”: crystallized salt brought from Gansu and Beizhili in the West of China.
Rou cong rong	肉蓯蓉	Saline cistanche
Rou dou kou	肉豆蔻	Myristica fragrans Houtt.; Nutmeg..
Rou gui	肉桂	→ *Gui* 桂
Ru gan zi	乳柑子	Mandarin orange
Ru shi	乳石	Stalactites

Ru xiang	乳香	→ *Xun lu xiang* 薰陸香.
Ru zhi	乳汁	Human milk
Rui he	蕤核	Prinsepia uniflora Batal.
Rui xiang	瑞香	Daphne acutiloba Rehd.
San leng	三棱	Scirpus flaviatilis (Torr.) A.Gray
San qi	三七	Panax notoginseng (Burk.) F.H. Chen ex C. Chow
Sang	桑	Morus alba L.
Sang bai pi	桑白皮	→ *Sang gen bai pi* 桑根白皮
Sang chai hui	桑柴灰	Ashes from mulberry fire wood
Sang chai huo	桑柴火	Fire from mulberry wood
Sang du chong	桑蠹蟲	Mulberry tree grub
Sang er	桑耳	Fungi growing on mulberry trees (Auricularia auricula (L. ex Hook.) Underw.
Sang gen bai pi	桑根白皮	Mulberry tree root bark
Sang ji sheng	桑寄生	Mistletoe
Sang jing shi	桑莖實	Mulberry stem and fruit
Sang piao xiao	桑螵蛸	Egg capsule of mantis
Sang shang ji sheng	桑上寄生	"Mulberry epiphyte", Taxillus chinensis (DC) Danser
Sha ren	砂仁	Fruts of Amomum villosum Lour.
Sha tang	沙糖	Saccharum sinensis Roxb.
Shan zha	山查	Fruit of Crataegus pinnatifida Bunge
Shan zha he	山楂核	Seeds of Crataegus pinnitifida Bunge
Shan dou gen	山豆根	Sophora tonkinensis Gagnep.
Shan hu	珊瑚	Coral
Shan jiang	山姜	Alpinia japonica (Thunb.)
Shan xing	山杏	Prunus armeniaca var. ansu Maxim.
Shan yao	山藥	→ *Shu yu* 薯蕷
Shan yu	鱔魚	Eel
Shan zhi zi	山梔子	Gardenia fruit
Shan zhu yu	山茱萸	Cornus officinalis Sieb. et Zucc.
Shang lu	商陸	Phytolacca acinosa Roxb.
Shao fen	韶粉	→ *Qian fen* 鉛粉

Shao jiu	燒酒	Brandy
Shao shang sha	杓上砂	Sand scooped up with a ladle
Shao yao	芍藥	Paeonia lactiflora Pall.
She	麝	Musk dear
She chuang zi	蛇床子	Fruit of Cnidium monnieri (L.) Cuss
She gan	射干	Belamcanda chinensis (L.) DC.
She rui cao	蛇芮草	Alternative writing of *she wang cao* 蛇罔草, i.e. *chi di li* 赤地利, Fagopyrum dibotrys (D.Don) Hara
She tui	蛇蜕	Snake slough
She xian	蛇銜	Potentilla Kleiniana Wight et Arnott
She xiang	麝香	Musk
Shen qu	神曲	Medicated leaven
Shen zhen huo	神針火	"Fire of the spirit-needle": ancient method of moxibustion which employs a needle from peachwood taken at the fifth day of the fifth month.
Sheng di huang	生地黃	Unprocessed → *Di huang* 地黃
Sheng fan	生礬	Alum
Sheng jiang	生薑	Zingiber officinale Rosc.
Sheng ma	升麻	Cimicifuga foetida L.
Sheng qi	生漆	Fresh lacquer
Sheng xiao	生消	→ *Xiao shi* 消石
Shi	柿	Persimmon
Shi	豕	Pig
Shi cao	蒒草	Carex kobomugi Ohwi.
Shi chang sheng	石長生	Adiantum monochlamys Eaton
Shi ci mu	石刺木	Thorny epiphyte of trees of unclear identity
Shi dan	石膽	Chalcanthite, copper sulphate
Shi di	柿蒂	Calices of the fruit of → *Shi* 柿
Shi gao	石膏	Gypsum fibrosum, calcium sulphate
Shi hu	石斛	Dendrobium nobile Lindl.
Shi hu sui	石胡荽	Centipeda minima (L.) A. Br. et Ascher.
Shi hui	石灰	Limestone, calcium carbonate
Shi jue ming	石決明	Mussel of the family Haliotidae

Shi liu	石榴	Punica granatum L.
Shi liu chi	石硫赤	Sulphur, amorphous red; allotropic form
Shi liu huang	石硫黃	Sulphur, natural yellow sulphur
Shi long chu	石龍蒭	Juncus setchuensis L.
Shi long rui	石龍芮	Ranunculus sceleratus L.
Shi long zi	石龍子	Lizards
Shi mi	石蜜	Saccharum sinensis Roxb.
Shi nan	石南	Photinia serrulata Lindl.
Shi she	石蛇	"Stone snakes"; Ammonite.
Shi shi	豕屎	Pig dung
Shi suan	石蒜	Lycoris radiata (L'Herit.)
Shi ting zhi	石亭脂	Red sulphur
Shi xian	石莧	Lippia nodifera Rich.
Shi yan	石燕	"Stone swallows", fossil shells
Shi yan	食鹽	Cooking salt
Shi yan zi	石燕子	Petrified fossil of Cyrtospirifer sinensis Gr.
Shi yin chen	石茵陳	→ *Yin chen hao* 茵陳蒿
Shi yu	鰣魚	Reeves shad
Shou di huang	熟地黃	Processed → *Di huang* 地黃
Shou gong	守宮	Gecko, house lizard
Shu	秫	Setaria italica (L.) Beauv.
Shu	鼠	Mouse; rat
Shu bi	梳篦	Comb
Shu dan	鼠膽	Gallbladder of a rat
Shu er	鼠耳	Ear of a rat
Shu fu	鼠婦	Pill bug
Shu jiao	蜀椒	Zanthoxylum bungeanum Maxim.
Shu mang	鼠莽	→ *Mang cao* 莽草
Shu qi	蜀漆	Dichroa febrifuga Lour.
Shu yang quan	蜀羊泉	Sagina japonica (Sw.) Ohwi
Shu yu	署預 薯蕷	Dioscorea opposita Thunb.
Shu yu niao	鸀鳿鳥	Unidentifiable water fowl
Shu zhan zi	鼠粘子	Ripe fruit of Arctium lappa L.
Shui jing	水精	Rock-crystal, transparent quartz

Shui lang dang	水莨菪	→ *Lang dang* 莨菪
Shui mu	水母	Jellyfish
Shui ping	水萍	Spirodela polyrhiza (L.) Schleid.
Shui qin	水靳	Oenanthe javanica (Bl.) DC.
Shui she	水蛇	Water snake
Shui su	水蘇	Stachys japonica Miq.
Shui ta	水獺	→ *Ta* 獺
Shui xian	水仙	Narcissus tacetta L. var. chinensis Roem.
Shui yin	水銀	Quicksilver, mercury
Shui yin fen	水銀粉	Calomel, mercurous chloride
Shui ying	水英	Plant of unclear identity, possibly a type of knotweed
Shui zhi	水蛭	Leech
Si chun	絲蓴	→ *Chun* 蓴
Si gua	絲瓜	Luffa cylindrica (L.) Roem.
Si ren chen ji xi	死人枕及席	Headrest and mat of a dead person
Sigua	絲瓜	Luffa cylindrica (L.) Roem.
Song	菘	Brassica campestris L.
Song jie	松節	Joints of pine twigs
Song luo	松蘿	Usnea longissima Ach.
Song pi	松皮	Pine bark
Song ru	松茹	Erroneous designation for *chuan ru* 船茹, slices of skinned bamboo stem used to stop up holes in a boat.
Song xiang	松香	Colophony; pine resin
Song ye	松葉	Pine needles
Song zhi	松脂	→ *Song xiang* 松香
Su	粟	Setaria italica (L.) Beauv.
Su	蘇	→ *Zi su* 紫蘇
Su fang mu	蘇方木	Cesalpinia sappan L.
Su he xiang	蘇合香	Liquidambar orientalis Mill.
Su mi	粟米	Millet
Su sha ren	縮砂仁	Amomum villosum Lour.
Su zi	蘇子	Seeds of → *Zi su* 紫蘇

Suan	蒜	Allium sativum L.
Suan jiang	酸漿	→ *Cu jiang cao* 酢漿草
Suan tou cao	酸頭草	→ *Shi suan* 石蒜
Suan zao	酸棗	Zizyphus jujuba Mill. var. spinosa (Bunge) Hu ex H. F. Chow
Suan zao ren	酸棗仁	Stones of → *Suan zao* 酸棗
Suo cao gen	莎草根	Root of Cyperus rotundus L.
Suo cao xing fu zi	莎草香附子	Rhizoma of Cyperus rotundus L.
Suo sha	縮砂	Amomum villosum Lour.
Ta	獺	Otter
Ta gan	獺肝	Otter liver
Tai yin xuan jing shi	太陰玄精石	Selenite
Tan huo	炭火	Charcoal fire
Tang yi	唐夷	A beast of prey mentioned in ancient literature
Tao	桃	Amygdalus persica L.
Tao fu	桃符	A charm made from peachwood → *Tao* 桃; hung in front of the entrance door to scare away demons and ghosts
Tao he ren	桃核人; 桃核仁	Seeds of → *Tao* 桃.
Tao hua	桃花	Blossom of → *Tao* 桃
Tao hua shi	桃花石	Marmor (white and red), calcium carbonate
Tao ren	桃仁	→ *Tao he ren* 桃核仁
Tao xiao	桃梟	Fruit of → *Tao* 桃, hanging on the tree all winter and gathered in early spring.
Teng huang	藤黃	Garcinia morella Desv. (M.J.)
Ti hu	醍醐	Finest cream
Tian cai	菾菜	Beta vulgaris L. var. cicla L.
Tian e	天鵝	Swan
Tian gua	甜瓜	Cucumis melo L.
Tian hua fen	天花粉	→ *Gua lou* 栝樓
Tian liao zi	天蓼子	Seeds of Actinidia polygama (Sieb. Et Zucc.) Miq

Tian luo	田螺	→ *Si gua* 絲瓜
Tian ma	天麻	Gastrodia elata BL.
Tian men dong	天門冬	Asparagus cochinchinensis (Lour.) Mer.
Tian ming jing	天名精	Carpesium abrotanoides L.
Tian nan xing	天南星	Arisaema heterophyllum BI.
Tian shu shi	天鼠屎	Bat's droppings
Tian xian teng	天仙藤	Aristolochia debilis Sieb. et Zucc.
Tian xiong	天雄	Aconitum carmichaeli Debx.
Tian zhong luo	田中螺	Farmland snails, river snails
Tie ding	鐵釘	Iron nails
Tie jing	鐵精	Black oxide of iron, ferrous oxide
Tie ruo	鐵爇	Residue produced by heating bamboo or peach stones on an ax blade
Tie xiu	鐵鏽	Rust, ferrous oxide
Tien ting li	甜葶藶	Lepidium latifolium L.
Ting li	葶藶	Lepidium apetalum Willd.
Tong	桐	Paulownia fortunei (Seem.) Hemsl.
Tong cao	通草	Akebia quinata (Thunb.) Decne
Tong jing bi	銅鏡鼻	"Copper mirror's nose". Grip to hold an ancient mirror produced from tin, copper and gold.
Tong lü	銅綠	→ *Tong qing* 銅青
Tong qing	銅青	Verdigris, zingar, basic copper acetate
Tong tuo mu	通脫木	Tetrapanax papyriferus (Hook.) K. Koch
Tong xie	銅屑	Copper crumbs
Tou gou	頭垢	Filth scraped from one's head/hair
Tu	兔	Hare
Tu ba shu	土撥鼠	Marmot
Tu dang gui	土當歸	Aralia cordata Thunb.
Tu fu ling	土茯苓	Smilax glabra Roxb.
Tu gua	土瓜	→ *Wang gua* 王瓜
Tu hong shan	土紅山	Local species of → *Chang shan* 常山
Tu pi mao	兔皮毛	A hare's skin and hair
Tu tou gu	兔頭骨	A hare's skull bone
Tu zi	菟絲子	Cuscuta chinensis Lam.

Tuan	猯	Chinese badger
Tujun	土菌	Sarcodon fuligineo-albus (Fr.) Quél.
Tun	豚	Suckling pig
Tuo	鼉	Chinese alligator
Tuo zhi	駝脂	Camel fat
Wa	蛙	Frog
Wa na qi	膃肭臍	Penis and testes of an ursine seal
Wa song	瓦松	Orostachys fimbriatus (Turcz.) Berg. and O. japonicas (Maxim.) Berg.
Wa zeng	瓦甑	Clay steamer
Wan dou	豌豆	1. Pisum sativum L. 2. Cicer arietinum L.
Wan jiao	蔓椒	Zanthoxylum nitidum (Roxb.) DC.
Wang bu liu xing	王不留行	Vaccaria segetalis (Neck.) Garcke
Wang gua	王瓜	1. Trichosanthes cucumeroides (Ser.) Maxim. 2. in *BCGM*:Thladiantha dubia Bunge
Wang sun	王孫	Paris bashanensis Wang et Tang
Wei	蝟	Hedgehog
Wei ling xian	威靈仙	Clematis chinensis Osbeck.
Wei mao	衛矛	→ *Wei mao* 衛茅
Wei mao	衛茅	Euonimus alatus (Thunb.) Sieb.
Wei rou	蝟肉	Meat of → *Wei* 蝟
Wei rui	萎蕤	Polygonatum odoratum (Mill.) Druce
Wei xian	薇銜	Senecio nikaensis Miq..
Wen mu niao	蚊母鳥	Nightjar
Wo luo	蝸螺	Snail
Wo niu	蝸牛	Snail
Wu	鶩	Duck
Wu ci ji	烏雌雞	Black hen
Wu fan	烏飯	→ *Qing jing gan shi xin fan* 青精乾石䭀飯
Wu gou xue	烏狗血	A black dog's blood
Wu gu wa	烏古瓦	Ancient, blackened roof tiles
Wu gua long	五爪龍	→ *Wu lian mei* 烏蘞莓
Wu hui	烏喙	→ *Wu tou* 烏頭

Wu jia	五加	Acanthopanax gracilistylus W.W. Smith
Wu jia pi	五加皮	Bark of → *Wu jia* 五加
Wu jing	蕪菁	Brassica rapa L.
Wu jiu mu	烏桕木	Sapium sebiferum (L.) Roxb.
Wu lan	吳藍	Indigo plant from Wu
Wu lan si can	烏爛死蠶	Black and rotting dead silkworm
Wu lian mei	烏蘞梅	Cayratia japonica (Thunb.) Gagnep.
Wu ling zhi	五靈脂	Droppings of the flying squirrel
Wu mei	烏梅	"Black plums", → *Mei* 梅 gathered half ripe and smoked.
Wu ming mu pi	無名木皮	Tree bark of → *A yue hun zi* 阿月渾子
Wu ming yi	無名異	Pyrolusite, manganese dioxide
Wu pei zi	五倍子	Galla Chinensis
Wu song	蜈蚣	Centipede
Wu tong	梧桐	Firmiana platanifolia (L.f.) Marsili
Wu tou	烏頭	Tuber of Aconitum carmichaelii Debeaux
Wu wei zi	五味子	Schisandra chinensis Turcz. Baill.
Wu xin cao	無心草	1. Li Shizhen suspects it to be identical with *Wei xian* 薇銜. Senecio palmatus Pall. 2. Gnaphalium luteoalbum L. subsp. affine
Wu xiong ji	烏雄雞	Black rooster
Wu yao	烏藥	Lindera aggregata (Sims.) Kosterm.
Wu ye teng	五葉藤	Ipomoea cairica (L.) Sweet
Wu yi	蕪荑	Seeds of Ulmus macrocarpa Hance
Wu you	屋游	Weissia controversa Hedw.
Wu yu	烏芋	Eleocharis dulcis (Burm. f.) Trin. ex Henschel
Wu zei yu	烏賊魚	Cuttlefish
Wu zei yu gu	烏賊魚骨	Sepia bone
Wu zhu yu	吳茱萸	Evodia rutaecarpa (Juss.) Benth.
Wu zi	梧子	Firmiana platanifolia (L.f.) Marsili
Xi er	枲耳	Xanthium sibiricum Patrin ex Widder
Xi gui	蠵龜	Loggerhead turtle
Xi gui chong	溪鬼蟲	A rivulet's demon bug
Xi jiao	犀角	Rhinoceros horn
Xi lin zhi	錫吝脂	Stibnite (antimony ore), natural alloy of silver

Xi rou	犀肉	Rhinoceros meat
Xi xin	細辛	Asarum heteropoides Fr. Schmidt var. manshuricum (Maxim.) Kitag.
Xi'er	枲耳	Xanthium sibiricum Patrin ex Widder
Xia ku cao	夏枯草	Prunella vulgaris L.
Xia ma	蝦蟆	Frog
Xian ren cao	仙人草	1.Clematis paniculata Th. 2.Mesona chinensis Benth.
Xian ren zhang	仙人杖	Decayed shoots of Phyllostachys nigra (Lodd. ex Lindl.) Munro var. henonis (Mitf.) Stapf ex Rendle
Xian shi	莧實	Seeds of → *Xian* 莧, Amaranthus mangostanus L.
Xiang bai zhi	香白芷	Root of Angelica dahurica (Fisch. ex Hoffm.) Benth. et Hook
Xiang fu	香附	Cyperus rotundus L.
Xiang lu hui	香爐灰	Ashes in an incense burner
Xiang ru	香薷	Elsholtzia ciliata (Thunb.) Hyland.
Xiang you	香油	Sesame oil
Xiao dou	小豆	Vigna angularis [Willd.] Ohwi & H. Ohashi
Xiao mai	小麥	Triticum aestivum L.
Xiao mai qu	小麥曲	Wheat starter
Xiao shi	消石	→ *Xiao shi* 硝石
Xiao shi	硝石	"Flux Stone", Potassium Nitrate
Xie	薤	Allium macrostemon Bunge
Xie	蠍	Scorpion
Xie bai	薤白	Bulb of → *Xie* 薤
Xin yi	辛夷	Fallen leafs of Magnolia liliflora Desr.
Xing	杏	Armeniaca vulgaris Lam.
Xing he ren	杏核人; 杏核仁	Seeds of → *Xing* 杏
Xing ren	杏仁	Seeds of → *Xing* 杏
Xing shi	杏實	Fruit of → *Xing* 杏
Xing zhi	杏枝	Twigs of → *Xing* 杏
Xing zi	杏子	Seeds of → *Xing* 杏
Xiong	熊	Bear

Xiong huang	雄黃	Realgar (red). arsenic disulphide
Xiong qiao shi	雄雀屎	Droppings of a male sparrow
Xiong qiong	芎藭	Ligusticum chuanxiong Hort.
Xiong zhi	熊脂	Bear fat
Xu chang qing	徐長卿	Cynanchum paniculatum (Bunge) Kitag.
Xu duan	續斷	Dipsacus asperoides C.Y.Cheng er T.M. Ai.
Xu sui zi	續隨子	Euphorbia lathyris L.
Xuan cao	萱草	Hemerocallis citrina Baroni
Xuan cao gen	萱草根	Root of Hemerocallis L.
Xuan fu hua	旋覆花	Inula japonica Thunb.
Xuan gou gen	懸鉤根	Root of Rubus corchorifolius L.
Xuan hua	旋花	Calystegia sepium (L.) R. Br.
Xuan ming fen	玄明粉	Sodium sulfate powder
Xuan shen	玄參	Scrofularia ningpoensis Hemsl.
Xue jie	血竭	→ *Qi lin jie* 騏麟竭
Xun	蕈	unspecified fungus
Xun cao	熏草	Ocimum basilicum L.
Xun lu xiang	薰陸香	Mastic.
Xun lu xiang ru xiang	熏陸香乳香	→ *Xun lu xiang* 薰陸香
Ya chi	牙齒	Teeth
Ya zi	牙子	Agrimonia pilosa Ledeb.
Yan fang	雁肪	Wild geese fat
Yan hu suo	延胡索	Corydalis yanhusuo W. T. Wang
Yan jiao	煙膠	Black residue in a kitchen range or kiln that deposits by burning firewood.
Yan ru cao	燕蓐草	Herbs growing in a swallow's nest
Yan shu	鼴鼠	Mole
Yang	羊	Sheep
Yang lu mu	楊櫨木	Weigela japonica Thunb. var. sinica (Rehd.) Bailey
Yang qi shi	陽起石	Tremolite-Asbestos, silicate of lime and magnesia
Yang rou	羊肉	The meat of sheep
Yang shen	羊腎	Sheep kidney

Yang shi	羊屎	Sheep dung
Yang ti	羊蹄	Rumex japonicus Houtt.
Yang ti cao	羊蹄草	→ *Yang ti* 羊蹄
Yao zi	藥子	Aesculus chinense Bge.
Ye ju	野菊	Dendranthema indicum (L.) des Moul.
Ye tuo	野駝	Wild camel; Bactrian camel
Ye tuo zhi	野駝脂	Fat from the Bactrian camel
Ye zhu	野豬	Wild boar
Ye zhu dan zhong huan	野豬膽中黃	Yellow stuff collected from a wild boar's gall-bladder
Yi dai	衣帶	Girdle
Yi mu cao	益母草	Leonurus japonicus Houtt.
Yi tang	飴糖	Oryza sativa L.
Yi weng	蠮螉	Solitary wasp
Yi xue zhong chu tu	蟻穴中出土	Soil collected from an ant's cave
Yi yi	薏苡	Coix lacryma-jovi L. var. ma-yuen (Romanet) Stapf
Yi yi ren	薏苡人	Identical with → *Yi yi ren* 薏苡仁
Yi yi ren	薏苡仁	Seeds of → *Yi yi* 薏苡
Yi yu	衣魚	Silverfish
Yi yu	鮧魚	Sheat fish; Chinese welsh
Yi zhi zi	益智子	Alpinia oxyphylla Miq.
Yin chen	茵陳	→ *Yin chen hao* 茵陳蒿
Yin chen hao	茵陳蒿	Artemisia scopariia Waldst. et Kit.
Yin di liu quan	陰地流泉	Water flowing from a well at a shadowy location
Yin hua	銀花	Lonicera Caprifolium Mill.
Yin huo yang huo	陰火陽火	Yin fire and yang fire
Yin xing	銀杏	Ginkgo biloba L.
Yin yang huo	淫羊藿	Epimedium brevicornum Maxim.
Yin yu	茵芋	Skimmia reevesiana Fort.
Yin zhu	銀硃	Vermilion, mercuric sulphide
Ying shi bai	鷹屎白	White elements from a hawk's/eagle's droppings

Ying shi bai	鷹糞白	→ *Ying shi bai* 鷹屎白
Ying su ke	罌粟殼	Opium poppy capsule
Ying yu	蘡薁	Vitis adstricta Hance
Ying zi tong	罌子桐	Vermicia fordii (Hemsl.) Airy-Shaw
Yu	榆	Ulmus pumila L.
Yu	玉	Nephrite, Jade
Yu bai pi	榆白皮	White elm bark
Yü bao du	玉胞肚	→ *Mu dan* 牡丹
Yu jin	鬱金	Curcuma longa L.
Yu li ren	郁李仁	Seeds of Prunus humilis Bunge
Yu pi	榆皮	Elm bark
Yu quan	玉泉	Aqueous liquid assumed to result from molten jade
Yu shi	礜石	Arsenopyrit
Yu xie	玉屑	→ *Yu* 玉
Yu yu liang	禹餘糧	→ *Shi cao* 蒒草
Yuan ci lei	元慈勒	A tree resin imported from Persia, reminiscent of Borneo Camphor
Yuan hua	芫花	Daphne Genkwa Sieb. et Zucc.
Yuan jing	芫菁	Beetle
Yuan qing	芫蜻	Blister fly
Yuan qing	芫青	→ *Yuan qing* 芫蜻
Yuan zhi	遠志	Polygala tenuifolia Willd.
Yue wang yu suan	越王余筭	Coral-type animal
Yun mu	雲母	Mica, Muscovite
Yun shi	雲實	Cesalpinia decapetala (Roth) Alston
Yun tai	芸薹	Brassica campestris L.
Zao	棗	Zizyphus jujuba Mill.
Zao fan	棗礬	→ *Lü fan* 綠礬
Zao jia	皂莢	Gleditsia sinensis Lam.
Zao jiao	皂角	Identical with → *Zao jia* 皂莢
Zao ren	棗仁	Seeds of → *Zao* 棗
Zao rou	棗肉	Fruit flesh of → *Zao* 棗

Zao xiu	蚤休	Paris polyphylla Smith var. chinensis (Franch.) Hara
Zaojia	皂莢	Gleditsia sinensis Lam.
Ze lan	澤蘭	Lycopus Iucidus Turcz. var. hirtus Regel
Ze lan zi	澤蘭子	Seeds of → *Ze lan* 1 澤蘭
Ze xie	澤瀉	Alisma orientale (Sam.) Juz.
Zeng dai hui	甑帶灰	Ashes obtained through burning cattail ribbons used to seal jars or cauldrons
Zha chan	蚱蟬	Cicada
Zha er cao	札耳草	Plant of unclear identity
Zhan	占斯	Taxillus nigrans (Hance) Danser
Zhan	氈	Felt
Zhang cai	樟材	Camphor tree timber
Zhang liu	樟柳	→ *Shang lu* 商陸
Zhang lu	章陸	Phytolacca acinosa Roxb.
Zhe gu	鷓鴣	Chinese francolin, partridge
Zhen sha	針砂	Needle filings
Zhen shao mu	震燒木	Tree or timber struck by lightning
Zhen zhu	真珠	Genuine pearl
Zhi	枳	Citrus aurantium L.
Zhi	雉	Phesant
Zhi dang	蛭蟷	→ *Zhi zhu* 蜘蛛
Zhi ke	枳殼	→ *Zhi shi* 枳實
Zhi li	陟厘	Spirogyra nitida (Dillw.) Link
Zhi ma	脂麻	→ *Hu ma* 胡麻
Zhi mu	知母	Anemarrhena asphodeloides Bunge
Zhi shi	枳實	Fruit of Citrus aurantium L.
Zhi zhu	蜘蛛	Spider
Zhi zi	卮子	→ *Zhi zi* 梔子
Zhi zi	梔子	Gardenia jasminoides Ellis
Zhong ru	鍾乳	Stalactite
Zhu	术	Atractylodes macrocephala Koidz.
Zhu	豬	Pig
Zhu	竹	Bamboo
Zhu	豕	Pig

Zhu dan	豕膽	Hog gall
Zhu du chong	竹蠹蟲	Bamboo grub
Zhu gen	苧根	Root of → *Zhu ma* 苧麻
Zhu li	竹瀝	Sap processed from Phyllostachys nigra (Lodd. ex Lindl.) Munro var. henonis (Mitf.) Stapf ex Rendle
Zhu ma	苧麻	Boehmeria nivea L.
Zhu rou	豬肉	Pork
Zhu ru	竹茹	Shiraia bambusicola P.Henn.
Zhu sha	硃砂	→ *Dan sha* 丹砂
Zhu sha gen	硃砂根	Ardisia crenata Sims.
Zhu sun	竹筍	Shoots of Phyllostachys nigra (Lodd. ex Lindl.) Munro var. henonis (Mitf.) Stapf ex Rendle
Zhu ti	鮧鮧	Air bladders of various types of fish
Zhu tie qi	諸鐵器	Various iron utensils
Zhu tong qi	諸銅器	Copper ware
Zhu xin xue	豬心血	Blood from the heart of a pig
Zhu xue	諸血	All types of blood
Zhu ye	竹葉	Bamboo leafs
Zhu yi	豬胰	Hog pancreas
Zhu yu	茱萸	→ *Shu yu* 藷蕷
Zi	梓	Catalpa ovata G. Don.
Zi bai pi	梓白皮	White bark of Chinese catalpa
Zi bei	紫貝	Purple cowries
Zi bei cao	紫背草	Senecio nudicaulis Buch.-Ham. Ex D. Don.
Zi cao	紫草	Arnebia euchroma (Royle) Johnst.
Zi ge	紫葛	Ampelopsis delavayana (Franch.) Planch.
Zi jin	紫金	Schisandra sphenanthera Rehd. et Wils.
Zi jing	紫荊	Cercis chinensis Bunge
Zi lan hui	紫藍灰	Ashes obtained from burning an herbal substance of unknown identity
Zi ran tong	自然銅	Copper pyrites, copper iron sulphides
Zi shao hua	紫梢花	Freshwater sponge
Zi shen	紫參	Polygonum bistorta L.

Zi shi	磁石	Magnetite
Zi shi ying	紫石英	1. Amethyst, purple quarz 2. Fluorspar, calcium fluorid
Zi su	紫蘇	Perilla frutescens (L.) Britt. var.arguta (Benth.) Hand.-Mazz.
Zi teng	紫藤	Wisteria sinensis Sweet.
Zi wan	紫菀	Aster tataricus L. f. Purple aster.
Zi wei	紫葳	Campsis grandiflora (Thunb.) Loisel ex K. Schum.
Zuo ye he cao	昨葉何草	Orostachys fimbriatus (Turcz.) Breger